The
Book of Health

The
Book of Health

A MEDICAL ENCYCLOPEDIA FOR EVERYONE

THIRD EDITION

Compiled and Edited by

Randolph Lee Clark, B.S., M.D., M.Sc., D.Sc. (Hon.)

President, The University of Texas System Cancer Center; Professor
of Surgery, M. D. Anderson Hospital and Tumor Institute of The
University of Texas System Cancer Center; Fellow of the American
College of Surgeons; Member of the President's Cancer Panel

and

Russell W. Cumley, B.A., M.A., Ph.D.

Editor and Head, Department of Publications, and Professor of
Medical Journalism, M. D. Anderson Hospital and Tumor Institute
of The University of Texas System Cancer Center; Professor of
Medical Journalism, Division of Continuing Education of The University of Texas Health Science Center at Houston.

 Van Nostrand Reinhold Company
NEW YORK CINCINNATI TORONTO LONDON MELBOURNE

Van Nostrand Reinhold Company Regional Offices:
New York   Cincinnati   Chicago   Millbrae   Dallas

Van Nostrand Reinhold Company International Offices:
London   Toronto   Melbourne

Library of Congress Catalog Card Number: 72-12256
ISBN: 0-442-01606-9

Manufactured in the United States of America

Published by Van Nostrand Reinhold Company
450 West 33rd Street, New York, N.Y. 10001

Published simultaneously in Canada by Van Nostrand Reinhold Ltd.

15   14   13   12   11   10   9   8   7   6   5   4   3   2

Library of Congress Cataloging in Publication Data
Clark, Randolph Lee, 1906-   ed.
  The book of health.

  1. Medicine, Popular.   I. Cumley, Russell Walters,
1910-   joint ed.   II. Title.
RC81.C59   1973   616   72-12256
ISBN 0-442-01606-9

FOREWORD TO THE THIRD EDITION

The human body is one of the most complex and perfect of all machines. It is the primary concern of each of us. A knowledge of its normal development and abnormal manifestations will enable the patient to recognize the need for medical advice and, by a general understanding of his problem, equip him to co-operate intelligently with his physician in the treatment recommended. There are many things about the body and about the various diseases that the doctor does not have time to explain—things the patient should know in order to hold up his end of the medical partnership between physician and patient. It is hoped that these necessary explanations, which the physician often has to omit, may be found here.

In these pages there is unfolded the story of the body's development, the changes it undergoes from birth until death, and the diseases which may attack it. Interwoven, is the story of the great contributions to medical knowledge from the dawn of antiquity to the present day. Historically, we believe the book to be unique in that many of today's physicians and scientists destined for future renown have edited the accounts of their contributions to medicine. Further, the care in its preparation and the expertness of knowledge of those who assisted, make *The Book of Health,* an acceptable source of information for the student of physiology and hygiene, and for those preparing themselves for the study of medicine, nursing, dentistry, and technology.

In this edition of *The Book of Health,* additional information has been added to every chapter—from new knowledge about how life begins (with the development of the science of fetology) to almost a situation of life after death (with the advent of heart transplantation). Many of these new facts are outgrowths of the "Space Age" of the 'sixties. During that decade and the early years of the 'seventies, the concentration on using every bit of new knowledge and improved technological procedures has advanced diagnostic abilities, patient care methods, and research techniques. The improved methods of education of physician, scientist, and layman, and the increase in the number of dedicated people in the allied health sciences fields, has aided in bettering the welfare of man.

Because of the newer technological means of probing the innermost workings of the cell, man now has additional knowledge of antibodies and antigens, of amino acids and enzymes. Great advances have occurred in diagnosis: there are earlier diagnoses of various types of cardiovascular diseases and sickle cell anemia, of endocrine and genetic disorders. The scourge of cancer is steadily being weakened by improved means of early diagnosis and research into chemotherapy and immunotherapy for many cancers of the different anatomic sites. There is a vast expansion in the hope of actually conquering cancer by the judicious implementation of the National Cancer Act which has been legislated in the United States and which, as it is implemented, will begin an era of international cooperation by physicians and scientists who are involved with cancer.

It is hoped that this edition of *The Book of Health,* as the previous two editions, will allow the layman to be better informed regarding his own body and will assist him in better communicating with his physician. The joint knowledge and efforts of layman, physician, and other health workers will continue to contribute to the improved welfare of man.

R.L.C.
R.W.C.

v

EDITORIAL BOARD

DECEASED EDITORIAL BOARD MEMBERS

Directing Medical Editor:	Randolph Lee Clark, M.D.
Executive Editor:	Russell W. Cumley, Ph.D.
Writers:	S. S. Arnim, D.D.S.; Jorge Awapara, Ph.D.; Dorothy M. Beane, B.A.; Ernest Beerstecher, Jr., Ph.D.; Suzanne Beerstecher, M.A.; Elwood Briles, Ph.D.; Ruth Briles; Sidney O. Brown, Ph.D.; John James Bunting, M.D.; Ora Blanche Burright, M.S.; Dorothy Cato, M.D.; Sally Connelly, B.A.; Barbara Cox, B.S.; Mary Ann Crossley, B.A.; Chris Cusick, R.N.; Jan Devereaux, M.A.; Carol Lee Dimopoulos, B.S.; Leon Dmochowski, M.D., Ph.D.; Lucille Fenton; Susan Birkel Freitag, B.A.; Lucile Grebene; Margaret R. Harrington, B.S.; Evelyn Bubendorf Heinze, B.S.; Joseph C. Ireland, Ph.D.; Judith James, B.A.; Chauncey D. Leake, Ph.D.; Mary Lucille Magee, M.D.; Eleanor Macdonald, A.B.; Charles J. Maisel, B.S.; Manley Mandel, Ph.D.; James Leslie McCary, Ph.D.; Lois Hill Pearson, B.A.; L. O. Pearson, B.S.; Anita Reiner, M.A.; Joan Joyce Sellers, B.J.; Russell Smith, D.D.S.; S. E. Stapleton, M.D.; Sylvia Stapleton; Hubertus Strughold, M.D.; L. W. Sundquist, M.D.; J. B. Trunnell, M.D.; Mary Walker, R.N.; M. R. Wheeler, Ph.D.; Wendelyn White, M.A.; Marian G. Williams; Patricia Wolf, B.S.; E. Staten Wynn, Ph.D.
Copy Chief:	Joan E. McCay, M.A.
Art Director:	Joseph F. Schwarting, B.F.A.
Artists:	Reese Brandt, Joseph F. Doeve, Gero Von Le Fort, Grace Hewitt, Clinton Howard, Joseph F. Schwarting, William Shields, Eugene Trentham
Photographers:	James Dean, W. S. Eastman, Donald Kelly, R. A. Kolvoord, Walter J. Pagel, B. S. Sallee, F. W. Schmidt, G. W. Webb
Assistants:	Carol Flynn, Belinda Hartenberger, Marilyn Haxton, Pamela Hester, Susan Huey, Elizabeth Klomp, Diane Shoquist, and Bonnie Somyak
Index:	Walter J. Pagel, B.A.
Copy Chief, Former Editions:	Barbara Atwell Browning
Production Director, Former Editions:	Gladys Schneider Spaeter, R.N., B.A.
Research Librarian, Former Editions:	Mary C. Smith, B.A.

CONTENTS

LIST OF COLOR PLATES

1 LIFE BEGINS

HOW IT BEGINS

All life comes from existing life. The structural basis of life is the cell; from it new life develops by division and growth.

In the 17th century, an English scientist, Robert Hooke, observed that living tissue was composed of a multitude of "small chambers" which he called *cells*. The human body is made up of many kinds of cells which differ greatly in shape and function, yet all these cells have several basic features in common.

The living substance which comprises the major part of a cell is called *protoplasm*. It is an extremely complex, watery-appearing fluid in which tiny droplets of nutrients and waste products are suspended. Protoplasm has been called "the basis of life." The characteristics which distinguish living matter from dead matter—the capacity to grow, to reproduce, and to adapt to altered environment—originate within the protoplasm of the cell. The most liquid part of the protoplasm is called the *cytoplasm*, and the firm outer covering is called the *plasma membrane*. The plasma membrane permits substances, such as waste products, to leave the cell and allows nutrients and oxygen to enter it. It also serves as a barrier to the entrance of extraneous substances. The less liquid, more jellylike part of the cell, usually located near the center, is the *nucleus*, the center of cellular activity.

The cells of the human body are of two general types—*somatic* cells and *germ* cells; each contains the important and essential nucleus. The somatic cells are "body cells." They make up the various tissues and organs of the body such as the skin, brain, and muscles. The germ cells are the reproductive or sex cells of the body. They arise from cells set aside early in the development of a new individual.

Human germ cells were first seen in the latter part of the seventeenth century by scientists working with the crude microscopes of those days. But the significance of the germ cells was not understood until the middle of the nineteenth century. It was then that the true nature of the cell was recognized, and it was from this recognition that *embryology*, the science dealing with the origin and development of the individual, had its beginning.

The body of the new individual arises from the union of two germ cells—one germ cell, the *sperm*, coming from the male parent, and the other germ cell, the egg or *ovum*, coming from the female parent. The two cells fuse to form a single large cell from which the myriad somatic and germ cells arise. Through this union of the sperm and the egg, hereditary characteristics of both parents are brought together in their offspring.

The chromosomes and genes

The factors determining heredity are located on small rodlike bodies found in the nucleus of the germ cell. These bodies take up certain stains or dyes more readily than other parts of the cell and have been given a name derived from the two Greek words *chroma* (color) and *soma* (body)—hence, the name *chromosome* or "color body." Along each chromosome lie numerous structures called *genes*. The genes are so small that they cannot be seen even with the micro-

1

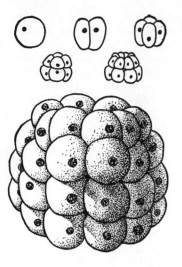

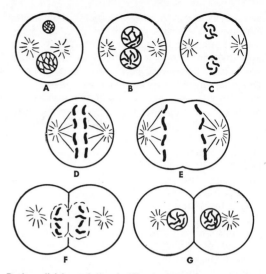

The fertilized ovum commences to divide in a stepwise manner, each division being numbered, and the number of cells after each division being twice the number that existed previously. In this way, the complex human body is able to originate from the single, original, fertilized ovum.

During division of the fertilized ovum, the sperm becomes a nucleus (A) and the nuclei break up into chromosomes (B) which move toward poles (C) and pair off (D) as the cell begins to divide (E). The chromosomes again become nuclei (F) and the two cells separate (G) to continue the process.

scope, but what they lack in size they make up in effect. They are the basic units of inheritance which a child receives from his parents and transmits to his offspring.

The number of chromosomes in the cells of the various species of animals varies, but the normal number for a given species is constant. The normal somatic and *immature* germ cells of man contain 23 pairs or a total of 46 chromosomes. The *mature* sperm or egg contains only one member of each of the 23 chromosome pairs. Thus, the total chromosome number for the species is kept constant. When the sperm unites with the egg, each contributes a set of 23 chromosomes, restoring the full complement of 46 chromosomes to the fertilized egg. Following this union, the fertilized egg begins a series of cell divisions which are the first external signs of development.

Cell division

Fertilization is followed by a brief period of restricted cell division. During this period, the protoplasm converts the nutrients of the egg into new protoplasm, and important changes take place in the chromosomes. At this stage of development the chromosomes do not appear as small rodlike structures, but as long, thin threads. The tiny genes along these threads possess the remarkable power of making exact duplicates of themselves from the material surrounding them. When this process of duplication is complete, a new chromosome thread lies beside each old chromosome; that is, each of the original 46

chromosomes of the fertilized egg has an exact duplicate lying parallel to it. The cell is now ready to divide. Because of forces within the cell, and because of the nature of certain of the genes along the chromosome, the two chromosome threads of each of the duplicated 46 chromosomes move apart. The result is that a representative of each of the original 46 chromosomes of the fertilized egg moves to one or the other end of the cell. Meanwhile, the outer membrane of the cell and the cytoplasm divide. When the process is complete, two cells exist where before there was only one. This process is repeated by each cell until the millions of somatic cells of the body are formed.

This type of division is sufficient for the somatic cells; but if the germ cells could divide only in this manner, they would contain 46 chromosomes and the fertilized egg 92 chromosomes. Thus, the number of chromosomes in each subsequent generation would be doubled. Nature escapes this doubling by a special type of division, which reduces the chromosome number of the germ cells. This type of cell division, *reduction division*, differs from ordinary cell division in that *whole chromosomes and not chromosome threads* are separated. The 46 chromosomes of the reproductive cells come together, forming 23 pairs; one member of each pair is contributed by the mother and the other member by the father. The members of a pair of chromosomes carry genes affecting the same traits but these genes are not necessarily alike. (For example, one chromosome may carry genes for blue eyes and light hair and its partner carry genes for dark eyes and dark hair.) Each whole chromosome consists of two duplicate threads which remain bound together throughout reduction division; however, while the chromosomes are paired, there may be an exchange of genes (*crossing over*) between the threads of one chromosome and the threads of its chromosome partner. In this manner a part of the genes from the paternal and maternal grandparents may be brought together in a single chromosome. After crossing over occurs, the chromosomes separate, and the cell divides in such a manner as to include only one chromosome from each pair in the resulting two cells. Reduction division is followed by simple equational division in which the two duplicate threads of each of the 23 chromosomes are separated and are included in two cells of 23 chromosomes each. The exchange of genes by crossing over and the chance distribution of chromosomes from the mother and father are important sources of variation in each new generation. Reduction in chromosome number and exchange of genes are the principal features of the *maturation* or "ripening" of the germ cells and take place in the sex glands—the ovaries of the female and the testes of the male.

HEREDITY

Do you want a boy or a girl? This is one of the questions a pregrant woman often asks of herself. Sex, however, cannot be determined by the mother and cannot be changed during pregnancy. Sex is determined at the moment of fertilization and depends upon the type of sperm that penetrates the egg. It has been pointed out that the fusion of the ovum and sperm brings together the hereditary contributions of both parents; they are the link between parents and their offspring.

All ova are alike as regards their sex-producing potentialities, but the spermatozoa are of two kinds. Each mature germ cell possesses 23 chromosomes. In the egg, one of these is the X chromosome. The sperm also has a total of 23 chromosomes, one of which is an X or a Y. The X and Y are called sex-determining or sex chromosomes, and the 22 remaining chromosomes are called *autosomes*. If the egg is penetrated by a Y-bearing sperm, a boy develops; if an X-bearing sperm penetrates the egg, a girl develops. Since equal numbers of X- and Y-bearing spermatozoa are formed during the cell divisions leading up to the maturation of the spermatozoa, the two sexes should be produced in equal numbers. Actually, the ratio is about 106 boys to every 100 girls among whites in the United States, and between 102 and 103 boys to every 100 girls among negroes.

It is not the action of the X and Y chromo-somes alone which determines sex. Sex is determined by the genes which these chromosomes and which the autosomes carry. The X chromosome appears to carry genes for femaleness, and the autosomes and Y chromosome carry genes for maleness. Early in embryonic development, sex is not defined. However, as development progresses in an embryo of XX constitution, the genes for femaleness exert their effect and female characteristics develop. The embryo of XY constitution possesses the femaleness genes of the X in only a single dose; this is not sufficient to outweigh the effect of the maleness genes in the autosomes and Y chromosome; consequently, a boy develops.

Some sexual anomalies have been traced to improper distribution of sex chromosomes. In Klinefelter's syndrome, apparent males fail to form spermatozoa, and exhibit eunuchoid traits. They have the usual 44 autosomes plus two X chromosomes and one Y chromosome. In Turner's syndrome, the individual is of female appearance, but the gonads are practically absent, consisting only of streaks of connective tissue. Such individuals have 44 autosomes, only one X and no Y chromosome: a total of 45 chromosomes.

Developmental anomalies can be attributed not only to the sex chromosomes, however. Mongolism, or mongolian idiocy, results from the presence of an extra autosome. Thus, there are 45 autosomes plus XX or XY, making a total of 47 chromosomes.

How genes act

In recent times, our understanding of many aspects of living processes has been provided by research in molecular biology. One of the most dramatic events in this explosion of biological knowledge was the unraveling of the structure of the principal chemical component of the nucleus. *Deoxyribonucleic acid*, or *DNA*, had been known for a century to be a chemical particularly characteristic of the nucleus of all cells. At the beginning of the second half of this century, it was well established that the DNA was the target of the mutation-causing radiations and was the chemical entity involved in inheritance.

The unraveling of the structures of DNA became an exciting problem, solved by James D. Watson, Francis Crick, and Maurice Wilkins. DNA is an exceedingly long molecule made up of four principal bases (*adenine, guanine, cytosine, and thymine*), each of which is connected through a sugar, *deoxyribose*, to a phosphate which connects to the next sugar. The important element in the structure of DNA is that the molecule is made of two chains organized in a regular maneuver, so that an adenine on one chain always faces a thymidine on the other, and guanine and cytosine are similarly paired. The duplication of genetic information is easy to understand in light of this structure. The action of the genes was further elucidated so that the copying of a genetic message into a complementary molecule of ribonucleic acid (RNA) was readily shown. These molecules act as the actual informational sequence for the production of proteins.

While many of the details of this flow of information from the gene to a protein have been established through researches using microbes, the exact details of all the regulatory controls resulting in the balanced activities of a cell and of the differential development of cells (all with the same DNA and genetic potential) into complex tissues, organs, and organisms still remain largely unknown. Further knowledge of these processes may be expected to be of aid in the management of hereditary diseases such as *diabetes mellitus* and in the control of congenital malformations of the fetus such as are occasioned by the effects of drugs and diseases on the pregnant woman.

How genes behave

Usually there is not a simple, direct connection between a given gene and a given trait or characteristic. Many genes act together in the development of a certain structure; and a single gene, acting with many other genes, often influences the development of more than one character. Genes were recognized as discrete units by the Austrian monk, Gregor Mendel, in 1866. Up to that time, heredity had been considered a blending of bloods, or the result of a solution in which the heredities of parents, grandparents, and great-grandparents were dissolved. Even though Mendel's important discoveries regarding the nature of inheritance were made in 1866, their significance was not realized until nearly a half century later. It was in 1900 that the science of heredity had its real beginning.

Working with garden peas, Mendel found that genes exist in pairs, the two members of which are not necessarily alike. When seeds were formed, he found that the members of each pair of genes separated independently of the other pairs. Later, when the chromosomes were found to be the carriers of the genes, it became evident that this *independent assortment* of genes was in reality a chance sorting.

It is now known that genes are located along almost the entire length of each chromosome, and that each gene occupies a definite place or *locus*. The arrangement of genes for any given member of a chromosome pair is ordinarily identical. The genes occupying a given locus on each chromosome of a pair are partners, or *alleles*. Occasionally one member of a pair of

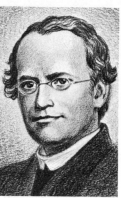

MENDEL, Gregor Johann (1822-1884) Austrian botanist. Often called the father of genetics, he discovered a principle of inheritance known as the *Mendelian Law*. Although he worked almost entirely with leguminous plants, the principles that he established are applicable to the study of animals, and are the basis of our understanding of human inheritance. He was an unknown monk during his lifetime, and his work was discovered after his death.

alleles becomes changed or fails to reproduce itself exactly. This change is called a *mutation*. Mutations are basic sources of hereditary variability.

A drawing of the various chromosomes showing the location of the genes along the chromosomes and the distance between the genes is called a *chromosome map*. Mapping of the chromosomes in man is incomplete because of the great complexity of human inheritance, the lack of information regarding many human traits, the great number of genes involved, and the impossibility of performing large numbers of definitive experiments. One authority has estimated that each cell of the body contains between 5000 and 120,000 pairs of genes.

Single factor inheritance

In his work with peas, Mendel found that one member of a pair of alleles frequently exerted an influence which to a large extent dominated over the effect of the other allele. Such an allele is called a *dominant* allele and the opposing allele is called a *recessive* allele.

The first case of dominant Mendelian inheritance demonstrated in man was short-fingeredness or *brachydactyly*. The allele for this defect is dominant. If a capital letter is used to represent the dominant gene for brachydactyly (B) and a lower case letter is used to represent the recessive allele (b), the inherited constitution, or *genotype*, of an individual may be represented in symbols. Thus, the genotype of a person who received a dominant gene for brachydactyly from each of his parents would be represented as BB. Such an individual would be *homozygous* for the alleles for brachydactyly. A person inheriting both recessive alleles (bb) would also be *homozygous*, but would not have short fingers. To distinguish between these two types of homozygosity, the first person may be referred to as homozygous-dominant and the second as homozygous-recessive. Opposed to the homozygous condition (*homo* meaning like), is the *heterozygous* condition (*hetero* meaning different). Consequently, an individual who received the recessive allele (b) from one parent and the dominant allele (B) from the other parent is heterozygous (Bb) for the trait. Since the gene for brachydactyly is dominant, a heterozygous individual would have the defect just as would a homozygous-dominant individual. As regards brachydactyly, these two people would appear to be very much alike or of the same *phenotype*. (Phenotype comes from the Greek word *phainein,* meaning *to show*.) However, it seems that in man a dominant *defect* is usually more extreme when homozygous; consequently, homozygous brachydactyly would doubtless be more pronounced than would heterozygous.

The difference in genotype and phenotype is important, for it is not the genes which a man *appears* to posses that he passes on to his children, but the genes he *actually* possesses. For example, a man homozygous for brachydactyly will pass the character to all of his children regardless of whether his wife is homozygous for the dominant gene, heterozygous, or homozygous for the recessive gene. However, a man heterozygous for the brachydactyly allele (Bb) could very well expect approximately half of his children to have fingers of normal length if his wife has normal fingers. If his wife is also heterozygous for the dominant allele, his children will have one chance in four of having fingers of normal length. Only if his wife is homozygous for the dominant gene for brachydactyly must all of his children have the trait.

Another trait or disease that is caused by a dominant allele is *Huntington's chorea.* This is a nervous disorder which usually appears late in life. It is said that of the 1000 or more people in America affected with Huntington's chorea, all descended from three men, probably brothers, who came to America in about the year 1630. The descendants of this trio scattered over the New England states, and many were involved in early witchcraft trials, because the odd symptoms of the disease aroused the suspicions of superstitious persons.

Many family-specific traits may be controlled by dominant genes, as was the protruding lower lip and underslung jaw of the Austrian royal family, the Hapsburgs. This dominant phenotype can be traced back to the fourteenth century.

Other human traits may be caused by recessive alleles. It has been pointed out that the effect of a recessive allele is largely masked by a dominant allele. Hence, in order for the recessive allele to be well expressed as phenotype, it must be present in a homozygous condition. An example of recessive inheritance is the most common form of complete albinism. Albino individuals lack the dark pigment granules which are normally deposited in the skin, hair, and in the iris of the eye. Children from the marriage of two albinos will be albino. Children from the marriage of an albino to a heterozygous nonalbino (Rr) would have one chance in two of being without the defect, since they would have equal chances of receiving either allele from their heterozygous parent. (In the symbol, Rr, the small r is used to designate the albino allele, and R the allele for normal pigmentation.) Expressed differently, half of the children from such a marriage would be expected to be albinos; all would carry an albino allele from their albino parent. All children from the marriage of an albino to a homozygous nonalbino (RR) should have normal pigmentation; however, all would be heterozygous (Rr), since they would receive one allele for normal pigmentation from their nonalbino parent and an allele for albinism from their albino parent. In order for nonalbino parents to have children with recessive albinism, both must be heterozygous (Rr) for the recessive albino gene. One-fourth of their children would be expected to be albinos, and three-fourths should have normal pigmentation. However, half of their children would be heterozygous for the recessive allele and could transmit it to their children in turn.

Eye color is caused by the reflection of light from granules of pigment deposited in the connective tissue of the iris. In the case of blue eyes, the pigment is deposited only in the rear of the iris. Gray eyes may be caused by pigmented connective tissue in the front of the iris or by scattered pigment in front of the iris, in addition to that deposited in the back of the iris. Green eyes result when diffuse yellow or brown pigment is deposited in the front of the iris. If pigment in front of the iris is concentrated, brown eyes will result. Differences in eye color are not always sharp and are not inherited in a direct, simple fashion. So little is known about the inheritance of gray and green eye colors that their transmission cannot be predicted with any certainty. Brown-eyed parents can expect most of their children to have brown eyes, since the genes for brown eyes are usually dominant to the genes for other eye colors, especially blue. If both parents have blue eyes, their children may have blue eyes. Occasionally gray, green, or brown eyes are found among children having one brown-eyed and one blue-eyed parent; the same eye colors may even be found among children whose parents are both blue-eyed. Some of the difficulty in predicting eye color arises from the fact that genes for a particular color may not be completely expressed. Thus, a person may be genotypically brown-eyed but appear blue-eyed because of other modifying factors which restrict pigmentation in the front of the iris.

It has been suggested that both light hair and light eye colors have arisen as mutations from the dark hair and eye colors originally present in human populations, and that the mutations have occurred often, in such a way that the genes for a given eye or hair color are not alike. Various shades of hair color from blond to black are caused by varying amounts of *melanin,* a dark pigment which is deposited in the central core of each strand of hair. The color of the hair is dependent upon the amount of pigment deposited; light hair has less pigment. Genes for dark hair appear, in large measure, to mask the effect of genes for lighter hair color. Dark-haired parents usually have dark-haired children, but may have fair-haired children if their genotype contains masked genes for light hair. Genes for red hair, when homozygous, usually show their effect unless in combination with genes for very dark hair. The ranges in hair color from red-blond to auburn may be due to combinations of homozygous genes for red hair with genes for blond and brown hair. People with light blond hair are usually regarded as homozygous for the genes for light hair. Gray hair appears to be caused by changes that usually come with age or disease. Less pigment is deposited in the core of the hair, less oil is secreted, and the structure of the hair changes. Premature grayness seems to "run in families" and thus may be controlled to some extent by heredity.

Sex-linked inheritance

The characters discuseed so far are controlled by genes located on the autosomes. Inheritance from genes located on the sex chromosomes is called *sex-linked inheritance.* The X chromosome is longer than the Y, and carries some genes which are not represented on the Y. The smaller Y chromosome also carries a few genes that are not represented on the X. The genes on the X having "partners," or alleles, on the Y are inherited somewhat as if they were on the autosomes.

Red-green color blindness is caused by a recessive gene which is to be found only on the X chromosome and is sex-linked in inheritance.

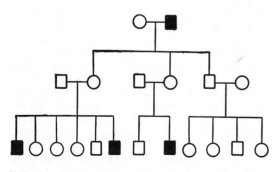

Pedigree of a family with red-green color blindness. Circles are women and squares men, who are mostly affected by it. Darkened figures are those afflicted with this sex-linked disorder.

The defect is not passed from father to son, but from mother to son. The reason for this is simply that a son does not receive an X chromosome from his father but a Y. If his mother has only one recessive allele from red-green color blindness, she will not have the defect; but since she is heterozygous for the allele, she is often spoken of as a "carrier." Women have two X chromosomes, and the dominant normal allele on one X masks the effect of the recessive allele on the other. Since a man has only one X, there can be no normal allele to mask the action of the gene for color blindness if it is present. All of the daughters of a color-blind man would be carriers of the defect. They would have the defect only if their mother were a carrier, or color-blind. Since the gene for this defect is relatively rare in the total population, such marriages seldom occur. Therefore, the number of women who are red-green color-blind is much lower than the number of men so affected. (For further discussion of color blindness, see Chapter 17, "The Eye: *Color blindness.*")

Hemophilia, a "bleeding" disease in which the blood does not clot properly, provides a good example of sex-linked inheritance. Part of the interest of this disease lies in its presence in many royal families of Europe. From the descendants of Queen Victoria of England, the recessive allele for hemophilia was transmitted to the royal families of Russia, Spain, and Germany. The disease is inherited in the same manner as red-green color blindness. Men having the disease often do not live to reproductive age; therefore, the disease is usually transmitted by mothers who are carriers. As with red-green color blindness, it is theoretically possible for a woman to be homozygous for the allele for hemophilia and have the disease; actually this seldom, if ever, happens. Occasionally women who have only one allele for hemophilia are partial bleeders; and in such cases, the recessive allele for hemophilia appears not to be completely dominated by the normal allele. (For further discussion of hemophilia, see Chapter 6, "Blood and Blood-Forming Organs.")

Other characteristics appear more often in one sex than in the other, and are not sex-linked but are *sex-influenced.* The genes for these traits are located on the autosomes and are present in both sexes. Their effectiveness seems to be partially controlled by hormones. Pattern baldness occurs more frequently in men than in women. The allele for this type of baldness seems to be dominant in men so that only one allele is necessary to produce baldness. If a woman receives two alleles for baldness, she may be bald. (For further discussion see Chapter 8, "The Skin: *Baldness.*")

Inheritance which is caused by independently-acting genes is called *multiple-factor* inheritance. Characteristics which are controlled by multiple-

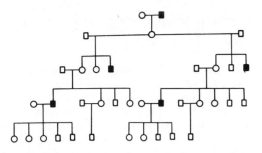

Pedigree of a family in which hemophilia is inherited. Squares indicate men, circles women. The darkened figures indicate those afflicted.

factor inheritance are usually those which cannot be separated into readily recognizable classes. Height, body weight, mentality, and many other traits which show a continuous gradation from one level to another may be controlled by multiple-factor inheritance. Part of the variation in these characteristics is caused by the modifying effect of environment, both internal and external. A person may have those genes which ordinarily would produce tall stature; but if his mother's health is poor during pregnancy, or if he is not adequately nourished during childhood, his genes for tallness may never exert their full effect. This is also true for other similarly inherited traits.

Studies of identical twins have contributed information as to the importance of environment and heredity to the development of *characters* showing a continuous gradation. ·It was found that while identical twins reared apart might be quite different as regards mental and emotional traits, they were much more alike in these traits than people taken at random. Physical traits, such as body length, seem to be influenced to a lesser extent by environmental factors.

Genetic counseling

The scientific study of genetics has revealed in recent years that many common disorders, some serious and some of little consequence to the health of the afflicted individual, have a genetic basis; in other words, these diseases are passed from parent to child, through the generations. As has been explained, some family members may only carry the trait and not actually be affected by it; however, their children may develop the characteristic.

In most cases, the characteristics passed from one generation to another are simply familial characteristics. In some cases, however, the propagated trait may be a serious disease. An astounding number of serious disorders have a genetic etiology. These include Down's syndrome (mongolism), mental retardation, errors in metabolism, some blood disorders (hemophilia is probably the best known of these), and

even certain forms of cancer. As more research is done, many more disorders will undoubtedly be shown to have a genetic basis.

Enough study has now been devoted to genetically related diseases to determine the frequency with which a particular disorder will develop in the children of parents with certain characteristics. Knowing the probability of their having a child affected with a serious disease, these parents may elect to take that chance, or they may decide to forego having their own children and to adopt children instead.

The experts who are able to give parents this information about the likelihood of bearing children with an inherited disorder are called genetic counselors. Most often, the person who gives genetic information or advice is a physician, by virtue of the fact that genetic disorders are medical problems. However, genetic counselors may also be guidance counselors, family counselors, and public health nurses. Many medical centers have genetic counseling services from which a family may seek advice.

Genetic counseling may be administered at any time, but most experts agree "the sooner, the better." If both husband and wife are carriers of a certain disorder, the chances are vastly increased that their children will have it also, and this may not be desirable. Ideally, such a couple should be informed of this before they begin to have children. Unfortunately, however, many couples bear one or more afflicted children before they are informed of the genetic nature of their children's condition. Genetic counseling in such cases could have saved the frustration of bringing into the world children who are often economic and emotional burdens to their families.

Most authorities agree that more and more families are going to need genetic counseling in the future. This is because improved medical and supportive health techniques have now made it possible to keep alive individuals with serious genetic diseases, whereas formerly these people died very early and did not survive long enough to reproduce.

Inheritance of skin color

Pigmentation of the skin is controlled by multiple-factor inheritance. Since variations of skin color within a race are not always readily identified and may be partly environmental, knowledge of skin color inheritance has had to come mainly from study of negro-white marriages. When a negro without white ancestry marries a white without negro ancestry, their children are typically intermediate in color, or *mulattoes*. Children from the marriage of a typical mulatto to another typical mulatto may vary in skin color from the black of the negro grandparent to the light color of the white grandparent. It has been estimated that the color differences in negroes and whites are controlled by from two to four pairs of alleles. It is possible for a white-skinned person of negro-white ancestry to have all the genes of the white genotype. Children from such a person married to a white or similar near-white should all be white. Children from the marriage between two near-whites are seldom much darker than their parents, and some would have light skin color. If a near-white marries a white, their children are usually no darker than their near-white parent; there is no well-established evidence that a very dark or black child could be born to them.

Races

The main races are the Caucasoid (white), Mongoloid (yellow), and Negroid (black). Most of the characteristics that distinguish these and other races appear to be controlled by multiple-factor inheritance which, as pointed out, depends upon the action of several genes. The variation in distinguishing characteristics from race to race is more likely to be caused by a difference in the frequency of certain genes than by the complete presence or absence of these genes. While there are observable differences between races, the variations within a race are, in most respects, as great as or greater than those between races.

Races probably arose mainly from geographical isolation of peoples, so that they married only their own kind. These groups were usually large enough that no great numbers of genes became homozygous, and, therefore, there was much genetic variability. The great movement of people from place to place in modern times has broken down most racial barriers until today many groups which are thought of as races are bound together more by cultural, religious, and historical ties than by apparent or real physical similarity.

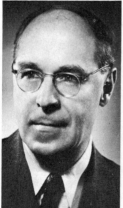

MULLER, Hermann Joseph (1890-1967) American geneticist. He is world famous for his researches upon the changes that may occur in genes (mutations), and was the first man to be able to induce such changes artificially by the means of X-rays. His work on the genetics of lower forms of life provided a theoretical basis for many of our present ideas regarding the nature of genes. In 1946, Muller was awarded the highly coveted Nobel prize for his research in the field of genetics.

REPRODUCTIVE ORGANS AND HORMONES

A hormone is a glandular secretion which is released directly into the blood stream. In this way, the secretions of special glands are carried all over the body and can have an effect on other glands and organs in widely separated parts of the body. The action of the reproductive hormones first takes on importance at *puberty,* the time of sexual maturity. At this time, mature development of the sex glands (*gonads*) is initiated through stimulation by a secretion of the *pituitary* gland. In recent years, scientists have been studying the chemistry of pituitary hormones, and these studies are important with regard to the question of control of growth. A major achievement in these studies has been the determination of sequence of amino acids for ovine and bovine luteinizing hormone. This is the first determination of the complete amino acid sequence of this particular pituitary hormone from any species. Since the luteinizing hormone controls ovulation in the female, it is also of great interest to those concerned with population control. The pituitary gland is located at the base of the brain, and one substance in its anterior part is called the *gonadotrophic* (gonad-influencing) hormone. This hormone stimulates the gonads to secrete their hormones; these, in turn, stimulate the growth of the reproductive organs and influence the gradual appearance of the *secondary sex characteristics*—such as the well-rounded bust and hips of a woman and the deeper voice and beard of a man.

The primary hormone of the female gonads (*ovaries*) is *estrogen*. It acts with the gonadotrophic hormone to stimulate the growth of the egg within the ovaries. Estrogen also controls the development of the accessory organs of reproduction, and brings about the onset of menstruation.

The ovaries are located close to the back and side in the lower part of the abdominal cavity. The egg develops in the wall of one of these ovaries. As it ripens, the cells about it multiply and surround it to form a sac (*follicle*). The egg then remains in this follicle until maturation is complete.

Many such follicles are formed within each ovary, and it is within these follicles that the eggs or ova can be found in all stages of development. When an egg is mature, it is expelled from the ovary; this is *ovulation*. Ovulation alternates between the two ovaries. Normally, ovulation occurs about 14 days prior to the beginning of menstruation. Most women ovulate every 28 or 29 days, from puberty until the menopause.

After the egg is discharged from the ovary, it passes into the fringe-like end of the Fallopian tube, which leads to the womb (*uterus*). It is

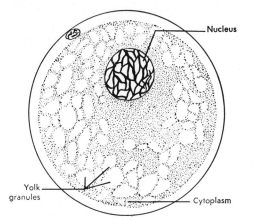

This greatly enlarged illustration of a single human ovum shows the nucleus which controls the cell's manifold activities, the large amount of cytoplasm wherein most of the physiological processes take place, and some of the nutritional yolk granules which are suspended within the cytoplasm.

within the Fallopian tube that fertilization of the egg, by the sperm from the male, usually occurs. This tube is so small that the slightest obstruction can prevent the egg from reaching the womb. Such obstruction is a common cause of childlessness, or sterility. A sterile woman may have a doctor check her tubes to see if obstruction is the cause of her sterility. This is done by blowing a gas through the tubes. If the gas passes through, it is assumed that the egg can pass through and reach the womb. Sometimes the spermatozoa are capable of moving up a tube which is only partially blocked, but the larger fertilized egg cannot move past the obstruction and into the uterus. In such rare instances, if the egg is fertilized and still is unable to move into the uterus, *tubular* or *ectopic pregnancy* occurs.

Following ovulation, the follicle which discharged the egg acts as a new gland, the *corpus luteum*. It increases in size and secretes the hor-

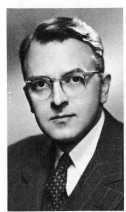

ALLEN, Willard Myron (1904-) American physician. Working with Dr. G. W. Corner he discovered the hormone progesterone in 1929. The secretion of this hormone by the corpus luteum prepares the lining of the uterus to receive an ovum when one becomes fertilized. Progesterone is one of several hormones that control the female sex cycle and consequently it plays a most important role in the processes of reproduction. *Edwyn Portrait.*

mone *progesterone*. This hormone acts with estrogen to produce changes in the lining of the uterus which, presumably, make it more receptive to the fertilized egg. If fertilization does not take place, the corpus luteum ceases to function just before the next menstrual period. This is followed by a sloughing off of the extra tissue built up in the uterus and by the accompanying bleeding which constitutes menstruation. If fertilization occurs, the corpus luteum generally continues to produce progesterone, which acts to prevent further ovulation or menstruation.

Normally, the egg remains in the Fallopian tube for about 24 hours after ovulation. If fertilization has not occurred, it passes through the uterus and is discharged during menstruation. If fertilization occurs, the egg attaches itself to the wall of the uterus and continues its development.

The uterus is shaped like a pear, the neck *(cervix)* of which projects into the *vagina*. The tube-like vagina leads from the cervix to the outside of the body. The vagina serves as an outlet for menstrual fluid and is the "birth canal." During the sex act, the male organ of copulation *(the penis)* enters the vagina and ejects spermatozoa. The vagina is lubricated by a fluid which is manufactured in the glands of the cervix. Normally, this secretion is not excessive or bloodstained. If excessive or stained secretions occur, a physician should be consulted.

The spermatozoa are developed within the male gonads, or testes, which correspond to the ovaries of the female. The two testes lie outside the abdominal cavity and are suspended between the thighs in a pouch of skin called the *scrotum*. Long, coiled seed-bearing tubes *(seminiferous tubules)* are contained in the inside of the testes. Located between these tubes are groups of cells which secrete *androgen*, the hormone of masculinity and the male counterpart of estrogen. (For a more detailed discussion of various hormones, see Chapter 10, "The Endocrine System," and Chapter 15, "The Reproductive System.")

The mature spermatozoa were called "semen animals," by the Dutch scientist van Leeuwenhoek when he first observed them in 1677. And indeed, they do look and behave like small, delicate animals. There is a head, which contains the important nuclear material, a short neck, and a "body," or connecting piece between the neck and the tail. The lashing motions of its thread-like tail make it possible for the sperm to move.

The transformation of simple germ cells to mature spermatozoa takes place in the seminiferous tubules. When the transformation is complete, the spermatozoa receive nourishment from the cytoplasm of "nurse cells" which lie along the walls of the seminiferous tubules. From these tubules, the spermatozoa move to another

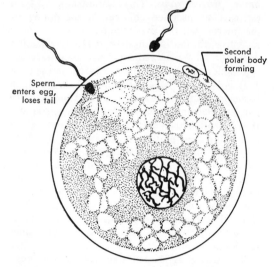

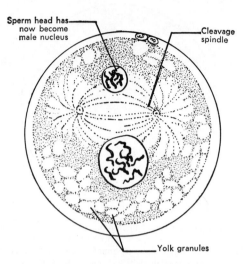

Sperm entering an ovum. Polar bodies are small cells which, when cast off, carry with them the extra set of chromosomes that result from reduction division. Only one sperm enters the ovum.

Fertilized egg cell showing spindle-shaped structures at its poles. Before cell division, chromosomes rearrange and become attached to spokes of the spindles, as is illustrated on page 2.

coiled tube, the *epididymis,* where they are stored.

The fluid, *semen,* in which millions of spermatozoa are suspended is ejected by the male at the climax of sexual union. This fluid is made up of the secretion of several accessory sex glands, the most important of which is the *prostate* gland. The prostate surrounds the *ejaculatory duct* through which the spermatozoa pass into the *urethra.* The urethra, which also serves for the passage of urine, is the tube running through the penis.

Usually, the penis is a relatively soft organ, but in order for it to place the spermatozoa into the vagina, it normally hardens. This hardening of the penis is called *erection.* The many blood vessels which supply the penis become swollen by an increase in blood supply and cause the penis to become firm.

Fertilization

At the climax of copulation, muscular contraction forces the semen through the urethra of the penis and into the vagina. The spermatozoa then proceed into the uterus and on to the Fallopian tube, where fertilization takes place.

Unlike the ovaries, which produce only one egg each month, the testes produce spermatozoa continually. Literally millions of spermatozoa are ejaculated at one time, yet only one enters the egg. Spermatozoa or egg may remain alive in the uterine tube, prior to fertilization, for a day or more, sometimes for as long as seven days. They must then enter into the process of fertilization or die.

Fertilization is complete only after one of the spermatozoa penetrates the egg, and the nuclear material of the egg and the sperm unite to form a new nucleus. This union of sperm and ovum restores to the nucleus the full number of chromosomes, half of which come from the sperm and the other half from the ovum. Following the fusion of the two nuclei, a rapid series of cell divisions begin from which a baby develops.

THE UNBORN

At the moment the sperm cell of the human male meets the ovum of the female and the union results in a fertilized ovum *(zygote),* a new life has begun. But before being born into the world, the new organism will have acquired an age which may vary from a premature 26 weeks to a postmature 46 weeks.

Medical science has not yet devised a method of computing the exact age of a child at birth, because the precise date of ovulation of the mother is not established. Although most authorities agree that ovulation occurs about 14 days prior to the beginning of menstruation, it is recognized that such an estimate is hardly more than an average, and that mature eggs *(ova)* may be liberated either sooner or later. Therefore, it is not known how long the new life inhabits the womb before birth, except in rare cases in which the exact occasion of a fruitful coitus is surely known. But regardless of the length of time spent in the womb by the unborn life, it goes through six preparatory stages before becoming a full-term infant.

Six stages of development

First of these stages is fertilization within one of the *Fallopian tubes,* which extend from each side of the top of the womb *(uterus).* It is believed that fertilization takes place within the first 24 hours following sexual intercourse. Almost immediately after fertilization of the ovum, the second stage begins. This stage is concerned with the process of cell division. The single-celled zygote becomes a multicelled *embryo.* The term *embryo* covers the several stages of early development from conception to the ninth or tenth week of life. The early embryo is barely visible without the aid of a microscope; it is considerably smaller than the periods which end the sentences upon this page. The initial series of cell divisions occur as the fertilized egg passes down the Fallopian tube.

Although cell division is still going on in the third stage, when the embryo reaches the womb, the cell cluster has not increased appreciably in size. Up to this time the embryo is free in the uterus. By the end of the tenth day of development, the fertilized ovum begins to burrow its way into the wall of the uterus. This process is known as *implantation,* the fourth stage. It takes about two weeks for the embryo to begin to obtain food from the maternal blood vessels; during this time the developing embryo is probably nourished by the uterine substances it absorbs.

During the fifth stage, the growing new life attains an age of eight to ten weeks, has definitive vital organs, as well as partial ability to balance itself within its fluid environment. When these organs are formed, the future individual is called a *fetus.*

In the sixth stage of prenatal development, the fetus is prepared for and experiences birth, at which time it becomes a *viable infant,* capable of existing as a separate entity in the outer world.

The first weeks of life

During the fourth stage of development, which coincides with the first two or three weeks after conception, the new life is still not much taller than the capital letters upon this page. It can barely be seen and gives little evidence of its presence in the womb. By the third week after conception the embryo indicates its position in the womb by a small elevation. In the weeks since fertilization of the ovum, the weight of the resulting embryo has increased about 10,000 times, its length about 15 times.

Within the first weeks of growth, the outer layers of embryonic cells are undergoing development and providing nourishment; at this time, too, changes are taking place in the thick disc of inner cells (the *blastodisc*) which gives rise to the embryo proper. The uppermost layer of cells of this disc separates from the remainder to form a cavity known as the *amniotic cavity* and the upper layer thus becomes the *amnion.* The cavity remains filled with fluid throughout the prenatal period so that the developing child leads an aquatic existence during the entire period of prenatal life. The amnion is one of the important membranes covering the developing fetus. In this central cell mass, the outer layer of cells on the underside split off to form what is known as the *yolk sac.* The lowermost cells of the blastodisc becomes the *endoderm.* The embryonic structure now appears to be a flattened disc between two hollow sacs *(vesicles).* The upper of these vesicles is the amnion, and the lower is the yolk sac. The relationship of these structures is shown on the accompanying diagram.

The cells of the embryonic disc segregate to give rise to three main layers of cells which form the definitive organs of the body. The outermost of these cell layers is the *ectoderm,* the middle is the *mesoderm,* and the innermost is the *endoderm.* The middle germ layer, as it is called, rapidly sends out migrant cells which line the entire sac. These mesoderm cells which migrate to the outside of the hollow sphere unite with the external layer to form the *chorion,* a part of which later becomes the *placenta* or the organ by which the fetus obtains food from the mother's blood. Another layer of mesoderm spreads out in a sheetlike fashion to surround the yolk sac. A relatively large amount of mesoderm adheres to the outer membranes to form the body stalk which later will become the *umbilical* cord through which the fetus will receive its nourishment.

Between the second and eighth weeks after conception the three germinal layers differentiate,

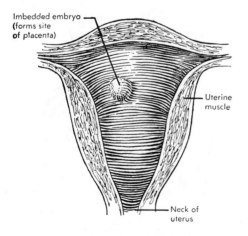

Imbedded embryo
(forms site
of placenta)

Uterine muscle

Neck of uterus

On about the tenth day of its growth, the human embryo becomes embedded in the soft uterine wall. Another two weeks are required before it will derive nourishment through the new placenta which will develop at the site of the attachment.

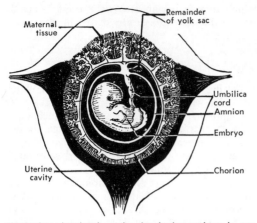

Illustration showing how the developing embryo is protected within the uterus by the chorion and the amnion. Here the growing child is completely surrounded by amniotic fluid, and derives its entire nutrition from maternal blood through its umbilical cord which is connected to the placenta.

divide, and combine with each other to lay down the basic body structures, from which the more complicated organism grows. All of the infant body is derived from combinations of the three germinal layers of the embryonic disc. From the mesoderm come supporting structures—muscles, bones, and connective tissues—as well as kidneys, blood and blood vessels, the lymphatic system, and the organs of generation. From the ectoderm are derived the skin and its glands, the hair, the nails, the lens of the eye, the internal and external ear, the mouth and teeth, the mammary glands, the nervous system, and the lower part of the rectum. From the endoderm evolve the respiratory tract, except for the nose; the digestive tract and its glandular outgrowths, including the liver, the pancreas, and the gall bladder; the bladder, and portions of the reproductive organs.

The primitive streak

During the early part of the third week, the embryonic disc changes shape, so that from the upper surface it appears as an elongated, egg-shaped structure. The cells in the central portion of this disc thicken and form a slight ridge which is known as the *primitive streak*. At one end of this streak, a small knob appears which marks the beginning of the head; in front of this knob the head process forms. The mesoderm is thought by many authorities to give rise to a solid, compact, elongated mass of tissue, the *notochord*. This structure grows forward as well as backward to form the beginning of the backbone. The notochordal tissue continues well into the head region, and on each side of it are formed the bones of the base of the skull.

The primitive streak with its head process divides the embryonic disc into right and left halves. This primitive streak is the first evidence of polarity—cells growing at opposite poles in opposite directions. In the postnatal human animal this polarity of development is clearly evident. An example is the manner in which muscles and tissues grow in opposite directions away from the axis of the spinal cord.

A groove soon courses along the primitive streak, deepens, and presently forms a connecting canal between the amniotic and yolk sac. This is the *neurenteric canal*, forerunner of the *neural* canal. The neural canal is the forerunner of the entire nervous system, including the brain and the spinal cord.

Having organized the area in which will lie the future head of the embryo, the primitive knot shifts, enlarges into an "end bud," and from this bud the lower half of the body arises.

During the third week of prenatal life the embryo is still a tiny organism the size of a large English pea, and the embryonic disc is about the size of the head of a pin. The body now begins to assume a cylindrical form instead of its previously flattened shape. This change is produced by the edges of the embryonic disc growing downward and enclosing the underlying structures. Concomitantly the underlying endoderm rolls itself into a tube which is to form the digestive system, or as it is properly called, the "gut." The mesoderm gathers itself into a number of small segmentally-arranged bundles called *somites*, which later give rise to the deeper layers

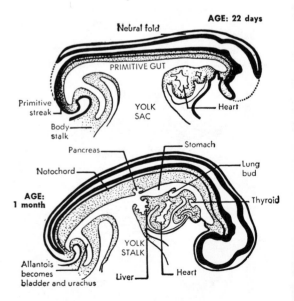

By the end of the third week the embryo has commenced to fold over and assumes a more cylindrical form instead of its previously flat one. During this early period traces of most of the important body structures can first be observed.

of the skin and to the muscles and bones. These somites are formed in rapid succession, so that sometimes they are used as an index to the age of the embryo.

Differentiation of the primitive organ systems

Near the end of the third week the embryo has formed the beginnings of most of the important organ systems. The anterior or front end of the neural tube closes and the primitive brain starts forming. On either side of the brain, early in the fourth week, is to be found the first sign of the eyes. These are called the *optic vesicles;* they grow out from the brain and appear as bulges on either side of the early head. Back of or posterior to the future eyes are the *auditory vesicles,* which represent the beginning of the ears.

Toward the end of the fourth week of prenatal life, the original three divisions of the brain called the forebrain, midbrain, and hindbrain now become five divisions. By a symmetrical growth the brain makes a series of bends which cause the head region to curve downward with respect to the remainder of the body. The cranial nerves which later innervate the face begin their formation during this fourth week.

The spinal cord, which is formed from the neural tube, becomes thickened on the underside to develop the primitive nerve cells. Previously, when the margins of the neural tube had formed, there were left behind small clusters of cells. These clusters of cells, by uniting with the upper and lower sides of the neural tube, form the spinal nerves. These nerves grow outward from the spinal cord to innervate the organs of the body as they are being formed.

The heart is formed by the union of two blood vessels underneath the head. The united tube thus formed grows rapidly in length and bends around itself to form the letter "S." Thus by bending back upon itself the *ventricle,* or main pumping organ of the heart, is formed. Rapidly it changes into an incomplete, four-chambered structure. The heart begins to beat during the third week and continues beating throughout the life of the individual.

The lungs develop from endodermal tissue by forming a bud, which later branches into two lung buds. Each lung bud forms two *bronchi,* from which later are formed the *bronchioles* and finally the *air sacs.*

The primitive gut gives rise to some of the glands such as the thyroid, pancreas, thymus, and parathyroid. From the gut, a pouch grows downward and invades the circulatory system to form the liver. The hind part of the digestive system produces a pouch known as the *allantois* which remains relatively undeveloped in human beings during most of embryonic life. The urinary bladder may be considered a remainder of part of the allantois. The limbs first appear during the fourth week as tiny buds from the midside region and from the hind region of the

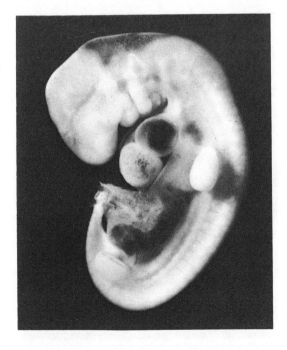

Photograph of a 29-day human embryo, magnified 9 times. *Courtesy Carnegie Institution, Washington.*

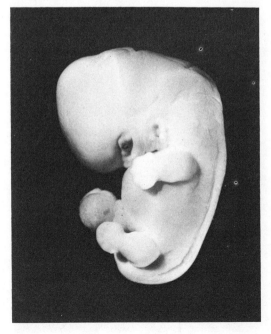

Photograph of a 37-day human embryo, magnified 4 times. *Courtesy Carnegie Institution, Washington.*

embryo. They later develop into the arms and legs of the fetus.

Early fetal development

After the first eight weeks the embryo has become a fetus; that is, it now roughly resembles the ultimate adult human being. Prior to this time it would have been impossible to determine by observation whether the embryo was that of a human being, pig, goat, dog, or monkey.

During the third month, there is a rapid growth of the fetus so that by the end of the third month the weight has increased eight- to tenfold. The facial features have shown a marked change; the eyes have migrated inward so that they are no longer on the sides of the head. A bulging high forehead, a small slitlike ear, widely separated nostrils, and a large slitlike mouth characterize the earlier part of the third month's development. The upper limbs show sufficient development so that one may readily discern the fingers, wrist, and the forearm. The lower limbs are relatively smaller and less developed. The liver begins to function during this period. The intestine becomes a coiled structure. At the beginning of the third month the internal organs of reproduction have become sufficiently developed to enable one to distinguish between the sexes. The external genitalia, however, are still in the asexual stage, so that externally both sexes appear the same. Some of the bones are beginning to calcify.

The umbilical cord

Living a parasitic life, the unborn depends for its nourishment, oxygen supply, and the removal of its waste products, upon the mother's blood supply. From the original multicelled embryo, accessory arrangements have developed apace with the growth of the fetus. These, in conjunction with maternal contributions, provide mechanisms to give the embryo nourishment from the mother. From the larger sac which was contained within the covering membrane and surrounded by ectoderm cells, a two-way cord (*umbilical cord*) develops. This is the connecting structure between the embryo and the placenta. It is attached to the middle of the fetal abdomen.

The placenta

The original covering membrane (*chorion*), in co-operation with certain accommodating cells of the womb, evolves the *placenta*, which is commonly known as "the afterbirth."

Through the placenta, the bloods of mother and fetus circulate independently, and in entirely separate channels. Maternal blood empties into pockets (*sinuses*) in the placenta, from which food materials are absorbed through the thin walls, to pass into the fetal circulatory system. By a reverse process, waste material is picked up by the maternal blood. In addition to providing oxygen and taking up gaseous and fluid wastes from the fetus, the placenta acts as a

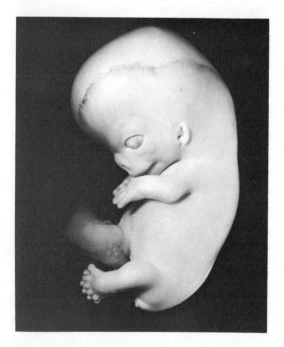

Photograph of a 42-day human embryo, magnified 3.5 times. *Courtesy Carnegie Institution, Washington.*

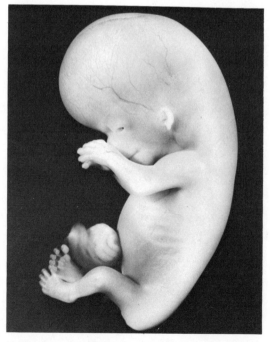

Photograph of a 56-day human embryo, magnified 2 times. *Courtesy Carnegie Institution, Washington.*

digestive area for adjusting foodstuffs in the maternal blood stream to meet the absorption capabilities of the fetus.

The supportive role of the placenta is essential to fetal health and well-being. Besides keeping the fetus alive, the placenta has the additional function of preparing the uterus and birth canal for the delivery. Several hormones are manufactured by the placenta; these are for use sometimes by the mother and sometimes by the fetus. Should the placenta falter in any of its supportive endeavors, the fetus is in trouble.

If the protective functions of the placenta are impaired, noxious products of the fetal metabolism enter and cause disturbances in the maternal blood. The severe and continued vomiting sometimes experienced in pregnancy may be associated with the incomplete functioning of the placenta. In most cases, the placenta prevents infections from reaching the fetus, although sometimes it fails to protect against such diseases as syphilis, smallpox, and German measles. After the birth of the baby, the placenta is expelled from the uterus.

The protected fetus

When the placenta and the umbilical cord have been formed—during the first eight weeks of unborn life—the fetus rests within a closed membrane *(amniotic sac)* which fills the inside of the womb. This fluid-filled sac absorbs shock, equalizes pressure, prevents the fetus from adhering to its protective enclosure, and provides nourishment.

After the first eight weeks, the primitive but fast-developing muscular and nervous system of the fetus allows it spontaneous movement. Within the amniotic sac, the tenant has room to rearrange its posture. During the seventh week the middle vestibule of the ear becomes functionally alive. This development allows the embryo to balance itself. The semicircular canals of the middle ear are structures providing for maintenance of static equilibrium throughout life. At birth of the baby, they are of adult size.

From the fourth month to birth

During the fourth month, there is considerable development of the abdomen so that the head is less out of proportion to the remainder of the body. Hair begins to appear on the head. During this time, the mother becomes aware of movements of the arms and legs.

During the fifth month the lower abdomen and legs become proportionately larger. The legs and arms show vigorous, active movements during this month. A thin silky hair, which disappears during the succeeding weeks, is deposited over the surface of the body. During the sixth month, the fetus increases in size and the organs

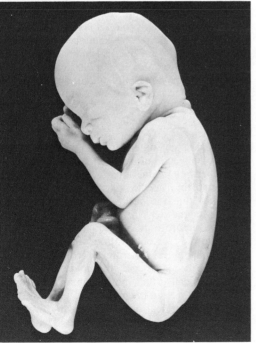

Photograph of a 4-month human fetus, reduced to about one-half its actual size. Note disproportionate head size. *Photography by F. W. Schmidt.*

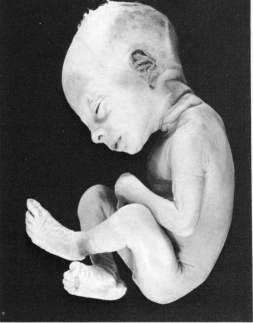

This 6-month human fetus is between one-half and one-third its actual size. Body is now more proportionate to head. *Photography by F. W. Schmidt.*

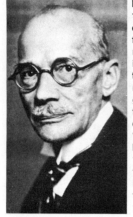

HIS, Wilhelm (Senior), (1831-1904) German anatomist and embroyologist. He was the first person to study the human embryo as a whole and is generally considered to be the founder of modern human embryology. His monograph on the embryology of the chick is regarded as a classic; his greatest work, 'Anatomie menschlicher Embryonen', was published in 1885. He invented a microtome, an instrument for making thin sections of tissues for microscopical examination.

in complexity. The embryo is lean, with little fat immediately beneath the skin. The skin is protected by a thick, oily secretion of the external glands. Eyelashes and eyebrows are present, and the eyelids have become separate.

The seventh, eighth, ninth, and tenth lunar months are characterized by the maturation of the fetus. There is a layer of fat deposited beneath the skin during the last two months of unborn life. This fat protects and nourishes the infant during its early existence in the external world. During these last months before birth, the organs carry on their functions in much the same manner as they will in the external world. The fetus swallows amniotic fluid which passes through the walls of the stomach and the intestine. The kidneys likewise may function slowly and discharge their contents into the amniotic fluid. Rhythmical movements occur in the intestine and the stomach, but their contents are not emptied into the amniotic fluid. During this period the mother's body is active in the elimination of waste material from the fetal body.

In the ninth lunar month, redness which heretofore has been considerable in the fetal skin, now fades. The body becomes rounded; the nails project. Weight is from five and one-half to six

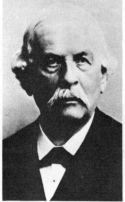

KOELLIKER, Rudolph Albert von (1817-1905) Swiss histologist, anatomist and zoologist. He was the first to recognize that the spermatozoa originate as cells in the testis. Koelliker also described the function of the spermatozoa in the process of fertilization and is especially remembered for his pioneer work in embryology. He is well known for his isolation of the cells of smooth muscle, and for his studies on the structure of certain types of nerve cells.

pounds. The fetal infant is complete except for the finishing touches which are accomplished in the tenth and last lunar month before birth.

As the fetal body produces glandular secretions and excretions in preparation for changes to be encountered through birth, the body becomes firm, sturdy, and round. By the time the baby is ready to be born, its many body functions—heartbeat, blood pressure, temperature regulation and, as it is being born, its breathing—have been correlated.

Study of the Fetus

Within the past several years, there has been a tremendous upswing in the knowledge about the fetus. Problems which had confounded obstetricians for centuries were being ironed out, and it was becoming possible to treat the new life as a patient on his own, and not just as part of the mother. The medical discipline dealing with treatment of the fetus is known as *fetology.*

The technique which has yielded the most information about the tiny fetus is known as *amniocentesis,* extraction and analysis of some of the amniotic fluid from the sac surrounding the baby. Study of this fetal fluid yields clues to many obstetrical problems, for example, the complications that arise in the unborn children of mothers who are Rh-negative, diabetic, or hypertensive. A fairly exact estimate of fetal age can be determined from study of this fluid, and the sex of the baby can be determined. This test indicating the sex of the fetus is not recommended simply on the basis of curiosity of the parent, however. Amniocentesis is done only when there are medical indications of possible malfunction, for it is a surgical procedure which must be done only under the most carefully controlled conditions. In addition, a chromosome study can be done when there is the possibility of a genetic abnormality such as mongolism.

There are several other diagnostic techniques which also yield information for the fetologist. The fiberoptic camera is a miniature camera connected to a needle which is inserted into the uterus. Within the needle are fibers that refract light into the lens. Although this instrument yields a picture only one square inch in size, it does allow direct observation of the fetus.

Another useful instrument which is widely used in Europe is the illuminated endoscope. Sometimes called the amnioscope, this instrument is inserted through the cervix and placed directly against the cervical membrane at any time from the thirtieth week of pregnancy on. The color of the amniotic fluid is indicative of whether the fetus is in distress and/or ready for delivery.

Another diagnostic technique which has been adapted for fetal study is the use of ultrasonic echo sounding in the measurement of the size of the head of the fetus. A pulsed beam of ultrasound passing through the fetal head is partially reflected by the skull margins and by the variable density within the brain. A given echo indicates the size of the fetal head. This can be an accurate aid in the determination of fetal size and weight. In addition, serial determinations can indicate the rate of fetal growth.

Enemies of the unborn

For many years, *rubella*, or *German measles* as it is sometimes called, has been known to be capable of causing birth defects, especially deafness and mental retardation, in children whose mothers had the infection during the first three months of pregnancy. This usually mild disease now appears to be on the way out, however, for laboratory researchers have devised a vaccine which is receiving widespread use and which should prevent infection in those vaccinated with it.

Preventing infection of the fetus is the principal objective of rubella control. This can best be achieved by eliminating the transmission of virus among kindergarten and early school-age children, who are the major source of infection for susceptible pregnant women.

The rubella virus vaccine is prepared in cell cultures of avian or mammalian tissues and is administered as a single subcutaneous injection. Approximately 95 percent of those who are vaccinated develop antibodies. Long-term protection is likely, but its exact duration has yet to be established. Almost no side-effects are associated with the refined vaccine now in use.

Live rubella virus vaccine should be given to boys and girls between the age of one year and puberty. Vaccine should not be administered to infants less than one year old because of possible interference from rubella antibodies from the mother which are still present in the child.

Pregnant women should not be given the vaccine because of the possibility of infecting the fetus. Women of child-bearing age should be considered for vaccination only when the possibility of pregnancy in the following two months is nil. A medically acceptable method for the prevention of pregnancy should be followed during the two-month period following vaccination.

In addition to the rubella virus, it is now known that other virus infections in the mother may lead to infection in the baby. Depending on the type and severity of the infection, abortion or stillbirth may result, normal development of some of the organs may be prevented (for example, the deafness which often occurs in children of rubella-infected mothers), or the baby may be so infected that its first days or weeks of independent life are an uphill struggle against disease.

Apparently, viruses may infect the fetus at any time from the first few days after conception until immediately before delivery. The incidence of virus infections in fetuses is not known, but it is expected that such infections may account for some otherwise unexplained disorders of the fetus and newborn child.

In the early 1960s, one of the most horrifying examples of how damaging influences from the outside can reach the fetus via the maternal blood stream was brought to light. In December 1962, a tranquilizing and sleep-inducing drug *thalidomide* was taken off the open market, and all samples were recalled.

This drug, which had been believed to be safe enough even to be given to babies, was causing a rare malformation in infants of mothers who took the drug during the sixth to eighth week of pregnancy, the period during which the limbs are forming. The most common malformation was *phocomelia* or *"seal limbs,"* in which the arms and legs were often absent and there were seallike "flippers" in their place. Phocomelia was also often accompanied by internal abnormalities, even some affecting the heart. About one third to one half of the babies were stillborn or died within a few days of birth. (The drug is also believed to cause a generalized permanent neuritis, invariably painful and sometimes disabling, in some adults who took the drug.)

After much laboratory work, it was determined how thalidomide works. The thalidomide molecule contains both a form of glutamic acid and a form of phthalic acid. Glutamic acid is a common substance, whose derivatives are used as flavor additives for meat and beer. Phthalic acid is an uncommon drug component moderately irritating to the skin. In thalidomide, the structural combination of glutamic and phthalic acids is most unusual and is capable of causing such deformities as phocomelia in infants.

In the countries (primarily West Germany and Great Britain) in which the thalidomide crisis was most overwhelming, treatment and rehabilitation centers have been set up to train the victims to manage for themselves. The patients are fitted with prostheses early and are given the care and encouragement needed to teach them to become self-sufficient. Interestingly, the thalidomide children seem to have above average intelligence, a factor which helps to overcome the other handicaps.

Another threat to fetal life, an incompatibility between the Rh blood factor in mother and child, has recently been studied intensively, and methods have been devised to control this condition and even to prevent it. (For a more detailed discussion of the Rh factor and medical aspects of treating it, refer to Chapter 6, "Blood and Blood-Forming Organs.")

The most remarkable method of treatment, however, is for those fetuses who show evidence of the disease *erythroblastosis fetalis* in an advanced or dangerous stage. These fetuses are given transfusions of Rh-negative cells before they are born, via the technique of *intrauterine transfusion*.

To accomplish intrauterine transfusion, the mother is prepared as if for a laparotomy. Using fluoroscopy to locate the fetus precisely, a needle is inserted through the mother's adbomen, through the amniotic sac, and into the peritoneal cavity of the fetus. Although the procedure must be done under the most exact medical and surgical conditions, it is successful 80 percent of the time. Usually, several transfusions are necessary, from the twenty-eighth to the thirty-fourth week of the pregnancy, and the baby is generally delivered slightly earlier than usual.

Some fetologists prefer to administer the transfusion in a somewhat different manner. The mother is anesthetized and a hysterotomy is performed (the uterus is opened). The fetus is then manipulated so that its lower limbs and lower abdomen are brought through the site of the incision and out into the doctor's hands. The transfusion is then administered either directly into the baby's peritoneal cavity or into a femoral vein or artery. Injection into the peritoneal cavity seems to be the less hazardous of the two methods and is just as effective. For some as yet unexplained reason, fetuses and newborn infants are able to absorb the red blood cells injected into the peritoneal cavity into their lymphatic systems and from there into the main blood stream of the body.

PREGNANCY

The period of pregnancy is initiated by the union of the sperm and egg. At the moment of fertilization of the egg *(conception)* a new life begins; and if implantation of this fertilized egg occurs, it continues to grow as a parasite within the uterus of the mother. The period of pregnancy is also referred to as the period of *gestation,* and its duration from conception to full-term birth varies between 265 and 285 days.

Conception initiates changes in a woman's body which vary from month to month. The doctor, by observing these changes, is able to diagnose pregnancy and guard the development of the unborn child. The early symptoms of pregnancy are the first outward expression of these changes; they are not definitive signs, because conditions other than pregnancy may produce them.

The first symptom of pregnancy usually is a missed menstrual period. Unless more than ten days have passed, however, since the period was supposed to have begun, the delay should not be regarded as a symptom; a strong fear of pregnancy is thought to be a common cause for delay of the menstrual period. Change in climate, some abdominal tumors, and certain diseases, such as anemia or tuberculosis, may suppress menstruation.

Nausea is often another early presumptive sign of pregnancy; it may occur first about two weeks past the date of the first missed menstrual period and normally does not last beyond the first six weeks of pregnancy. Nausea is also called "morning sickness"; however, it also occurs frequently in the late afternoon. No one completely understands what causes it. Only one-third of all pregnant women suffer from both nausea and vomiting; one-third experience feelings of nausea some time during the day but not to the point of actually vomiting; the remaining one-third do not experience the discomfort at all. Other bodily disorders, such as indigestion, may be responsible for nausea, hence this symptom alone should not be regarded as a definite sign of pregnancy. However, any case of severe or prolonged nausea should be called to the physician's attention.

Changes in the breasts may be significant symptoms, particularly in women who are pregnant for the first time. About the fourth week of gestation most women experience a feeling of fullness similar to premenstrual symptoms, but more intense. Such feelings are often accompanied by a tingling sensation, and enlargement of the breasts. The nipples enlarge, and the pigmented areas (the *areolae*) surrounding them become darker, wider, and are often puffy.

Frequent urination is another early indication of pregnancy. As the uterus enlarges, it stretches the base of the bladder and produces a sensation of a full bladder. The pressure on the bladder diminishes somewhat when the uterus expands beyond the pelvic region and into the abdomen. This occurs at about the tenth or twelfth week of pregnancy, and the frequent desire to urinate is then relieved. When the head of the infant drops farther into the pelvic regions, near the end of gestation, the woman is once more troubled by frequency of urination.

If a woman has experienced any of the presumptive symptoms just discussed, it is advisable for her to consult with her regular physician or with an obstetrician, a doctor who specializes in the care and treatment of women during pregnancy. The doctor will question her about any of the symptoms she may have observed. Since none is an infallible sign of pregnancy, he will probably make a complete examination.

The examination may begin with the breasts in order to check any changes the patient may have noticed. The abdomen will also be examined, because as early as the twelfth week there is usually a slight swelling of the abdomen just

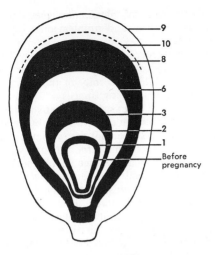

This illustration indicates the relative size of the uterus at successive months during a normal pregnancy. The original pear shape of the human uterus is completely lost in the later months of pregnancy as it fills out to accommodate the tremendously increased size of the developing fetus.

below the navel. This is caused by the enlarging uterus, and the doctor may be able to feel this swelling before it has been observed by the patient. Ordinarily, the vulva and the lining of the vagina are pinkish in color; about the sixth week of pregnancy they may acquire a typically bluish hue. At this time the secretion of the glands in the genital tract may be greater than is usual. The condition of the uterus can be examined by the doctor's gloved fingers. About the sixth week of pregnancy the uterus loses its normal pear shape, and the cervix, or lower portion of the uterus, becomes quite soft. The examination of the condition of the uterus is important, and if the patient relaxes, she will find that the examination requires little time, and is normally performed without pain.

There are now several reliable, immunologically based laboratory tests which can diagnosis pregnancy in a matter of minutes. These tests require an early morning specimen of urine, of which part is put on a slide and read under a microscope and part is used for a tube test in which a "ring" can be noted in the treated urine in the tube. The tests are almost 100 percent effective in diagnosing uncomplicated pregnancies, are very high in diagnosing abnormal pregnant conditions (tubular pregnancy or the presence of disease in the placenta), and can even indicate when a spontaneous abortion has been incomplete.

These immunological pregnancy tests have now largely replaced the formerly popular "rabbit" and "frog" tests, which were accurate in 95 to 98 percent of cases. Both of those tests

made use of hormone (*gonadotrophin*) which appears in the urine shortly after implantation occurs. The early presence of this hormone in the urine of a pregnant woman appears to be caused by the activity of the surface layer of the cells covering the embryo. In the first of these tests, a small quantity of the woman's concentrated urine is injected into the ear vein of a nonpregnant, female rabbit (some laboratories use mice). If the woman is pregnant, the injected urine should contain gonadotrophic hormones which produce changes in the ovaries of the injected animal within 48 to 72 hours. The second test makes use of a female South African frog. Within 18 hours after the injection of urine from a pregnant woman, the frog will lay a great many eggs. These tests are moderately expensive, but extremely useful in special cases.

Between the fourth and fifth months of pregnancy, fetal development is far enough advanced so that a positive diagnosis can be made from clinical signs. The sound of the fetal heart beat, heard by an experienced physician, is the most positive sign of pregnancy. Near the end of the fifth month, he should be able to feel the fetus move within the uterus. The term used to denote the time when these movements are first recognized is *quickening*. It is an old word based on the superstition that life rushed suddenly or quickly into the unborn child. Women often refer to it as "feeling life."

X-ray diagnosis of pregnancy is rarely possible until after the 14th week, because until about that time the skeleton of the fetus is not far enough advanced to show in the x-ray pictures. X-ray diagnosis is seldom necessary, however, because other types of conclusive evidence are available.

Hygiene of pregnancy

Once it is established that a woman is pregnant, she should be examined by her physician at periodic intervals specified by him. Besides giving

ZONDEK, Bernhard (1891-1966) Israeli gynecologist and endocrinologist. In 1928 with Selmar Aschheim, he designed one of the first reliable laboratory tests for pregnancy, and in that same year they isolated prolan-A and prolan-B, the gonadotrophic hormones of the anterior pituitary gland which control the reproductive endoctrine activities of the ovary. His distinguished contributions did much to clarify our present day understanding of the female sexual cycle.

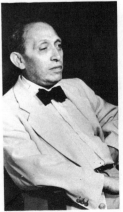

the expectant mother a complete physical examination, the doctor will inquire into her medical history. He will ask about childhood diseases, surgery, and serious accidents she may have had; he will want to know the history of any previous pregnancies. If there are any special family traits or hereditary diseases in the family, he should be told about them. Many of the questions may seem irrelevant to her, but they are all essential to a complete and competent medical safeguard during pregnancy. Therefore, the woman should answer them truthfully and completely.

The taking and recording of the blood pressure is an important part of each office visit during pregnancy. A rise in blood pressure is often the earliest symptom of *toxemia*, a disease which is caused by a kidney disturbance. Analysis of the urine will demonstrate the presence or absence of albumen which also may be an indication of toxemia.

A sample of blood is taken during one of the early visits to the doctor. The blood is usually typed as to a blood group and Rh factor. (For discussion of blood groups and the Rh factor, see Chapter 6, "Blood and Blood-Forming Organs: *Blood types*.") A part of the blood will be used to determine the presence or absence of syphilis. It is important that no pregnant woman have syphilis, for the causative organism of this disease is one of the few that can pass through the placental barrier to the unborn child. Once the disease establishes itself in the baby, abortion or stillbirth may follow. If syphilis is diagnosed early in pregnancy, treatment can be started which may curb the disease and allow the baby to develop normally.

A test will be made on the cells of the blood, because anemia often is associated with pregnancy. The red coloring matter of the blood (*hemoglobin*), contains a large quantity of iron. As the requirements of the unborn baby for iron are largest during the last two or three months of pregnancy, the test for hemoglobin may be repeated during that interval. If the blood is low in hemoglobin, the physician suggests a special diet, rich in iron and supplemented by iron in tablet form.

The diet ordered by the physician will add to the well-being of the expectant mother and the developing child. The body of the unborn baby must be built from substances which are available in the mother's blood; demands for increased nourishment are also made by the enlarging uterus. This does not mean that a pregnant woman must consume large quantities of food; it does mean that the diet should be well-balanced, and should include all of the essential minerals and vitamins. Iron, calcium, and phosphorous are not required in large amounts by the unborn child until the last two or three months of pregnancy, but in order to insure a sufficient supply the diet should be high in these elements throughout pregnancy. The doctor may have to modify the diet if conditions arise which warrant changes.

Laxative foods, cereals, fruits, leafy vegetables, and water aid in the elimination of waste from the body. Regular elimination is important during pregnancy, but laxative drugs should be avoided if possible. Highly seasoned, rich foods should not be eaten. Fatty foods aggravate nausea, or cause it; protein foods, however, are needed for the normal development of the infant. Less salt should be used, since there is a definite relationship between the amount of water retained in the tissues of the body and the amount of salt consumed. If the storage of water becomes excessive during pregnancy, it is probable that the physician will suggest a salt-free diet. This does not mean that the amount of water consumed should be curtailed, for drinking sufficient water during pregnancy seems to help to prevent disturbances of the kidneys. Only when unusual conditions arise will the doctor suggest that the amount of water be cut down. The physician's advice as to alcohol and coffee consumption will vary with the condition and habits of individual patients.

The doctor will help the patient watch her weight during pregnancy; this is not to control the size of the baby, but to keep the mother herself from gaining too much weight. Weight easily gained during pregnancy may be difficult to lose later. If the doctor's advice as to diet is strictly adhered to, a woman need not worry about weighing more after pregnancy than she did before.

A pregnant woman should continue to lead a normal, active life unless her doctor directs otherwise. Plenty of rest is important, but so are recreation and moderate exercise. Violent or unusual activities should be avoided, and any type of activity should be stopped before the expectant mother becomes tired. A woman who is employed may wish to keep working during pregnancy. She should consult her doctor about this;

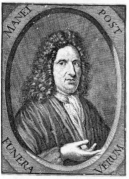

DEVENTER, Hendrik van (1651-1724) Dutch obstetrician. He is very famous for his many notable medical observations on the membranes of the placenta and on the normal human pelvis. He is often called the father of modern midwifery, because of his many contributions to the knowledge of female physiology during pregnancy. Van Deventer was also one of the first persons to devote serious attention to the physiology as well as to the mechanism of labor.

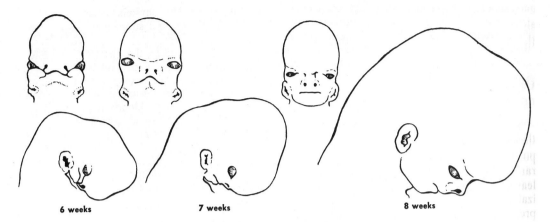

6 weeks   **7 weeks**   **8 weeks**

Illustration showing the size and typical appearance of the head of a human embryo as it develops during the first two months of life within the body of the mother. The profiles show the comparative sizes of the head at given ages. It is later during the third month of its growth that the eyes grow closer together and the embryo commences to assume a more nearly human appearance. These pronounced changes in its size and appearance mark the start of the *fetus* stage of development and the end of the *embryo* stage which has preceded it.

his advice will be given on the basis of the type of work required of her and her general condition during pregnancy.

Although there is still some controversy regarding the actual disadvantages of the practice, it is known that women who smoke heavily during pregnancy (ten or more cigarettes per day) bear babies who are smaller than average at birth. Some studies have even indicated that more spontaneous abortions, stillbirths, or deaths soon after birth occur in infants of women who are heavy smokers. Also, it is thought that these women are more apt to give birth prematurely. On the other side of the argument, however, some researchers believe that some of the usual disorders of pregnancy, most particularly, the "toxemia of pregnancy," occurs less frequently among smoking than among non-smoking mothers. Obviously, much more research needs to be done in this area. It may be that smoking is associated with some underlying disturbance, such as emotional strain, which would cause the differences between smokers and nonsmokers.

The sweat and oil (*sebaceous*) glands of the skin become more active during pregnancy. Daily baths not only help these glands carry out their function of elimination more effectively, but are relaxing and refreshing. The doctor's advice as to shower or tub baths should be followed; generally shower or sponge baths should replace tub baths during the last six weeks before the baby is born.

Special attention should be given the breast and nipples. Daily care helps to prepare the nipples for nursing, and the doctor usually gives specific instructions about such care. Between the fourth and sixth months of pregnancy a sticky, silvery-white fluid may begin to exude from the nipples. This is the precursor of milk and is called *colostrum*. During the last month of pregnancy, the colostrum may flow freely. In such cases, it is advisable for the woman to wear absorbent pads in the brassiere to protect the clothing. To prevent irritation, the expectant mother should wash the breasts and nipples often with warm water and mild soap; a soft cloth should be used and the breasts should be thoroughly dried. Application of sterile oil may also be recommended.

A moderate vaginal discharge (*leucorrhea*), especially during the last two months of pregnancy, is to be expected. If it becomes profuse or causes irritation or itching, the doctor should be notified. Douches should not be taken during pregnancy without consulting the physician first.

Doctors usually advise against sexual intercourse during the first three months of pregnancy, because of the possibility of abortion; and during the last two months or six weeks of pregnancy because of the possibility of infection of the birth canal. Between these periods intercourse in moderation is harmless.

Clothing should be attractive as well as comfortable during pregnancy, since a woman's feeling of well-being is greatly affected by her appearance. If a woman is accustomed to wearing high heels, her doctor may not object to her wearing them during pregnancy. Low heels, however, are usually recommended since equilibrium is likely to be uncertain and high heels may aggravate backache, a common discomfort in pregnancy. Many women wear a well-fitting maternity corset after the first four months; such a garment supports the uterus without binding and may help to prevent backaches. Brassieres which support the breasts without binding them are recommended. Tight clothing, particularly garters, should be avoided, as they may provoke the development of *varicose veins*. Varicose veins are a common ailment in pregnancies, particularly after the first confinement. They are caused by the enlarging uterus, which may obstruct the flow of blood from the lower part of the body, especially the legs.

Calculation of approximate date of confinement

The woman and her physician should calculate the expected date of confinement. This makes it possible to make hospital reservations and to arrange for the care of mother and child after they leave the hospital. Since the exact time of fertilization is difficult to determine, the period of pregnancy usually is estimated by counting 280 days from the first day of the last regular menstrual period; this is not the exact length of gestation, since it usually includes an interval of approximately 15 days between the first day of the last menstruation and ovulation, and fertilization. The date of confinement may also be approximated by counting *back* 90 days from the first day to the last menstruation and adding seven days to that date. For example, if the first day of the last menstruation was November 20, count back 90 days to August 22, and add to that seven days. Thus, August 29 of the following year would be the expected day of confinement. This should not be considered the exact date on which the baby will be born, for fullterm births may occur two weeks following or one week preceding that day.

As pregnancy progresses, the physician will want to see the pregnant woman more often, perhaps once a week during the last month. The date of confinement cannot be determined exactly; the position of the uterus during the last weeks will help the doctor decide when the baby is most likely to be born.

The role of hormones in pregnancy

Following conception, menstruation and ovulation normally cease for the period of pregnancy. The *corpus luteum* secretes a hormone, *progesterone* which acts with the hormone of the ovaries, *estrogen*, to produce changes in the uterus which prepare that organ for the implantation of the developing embryo. Cessation of ovulation is caused in part by the high level of estrogen maintained in the system during pregnancy; this estrogen inhibits the secretion of the follicle-stimulating hormone of the *pituitary gland*.

Growth changes which occur in the uterus following conception are brought about by the interaction of estrogen and progesterone. Estrogen acts as a growth-promoting substance in the

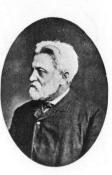

CREDE, Karl Siegmund Franz (1819-1892) German gynecologist. He is famous for his introduction of the use of one percent silver nitrate in the eyes of the newborn to prevent gonococcal infection of the eyes, which usually causes blindness. Credé is also known for his invention of an incubator for premature infants, and *Credés* method for stimulating contractions of the uterus. These advances have contributed greatly to the low mortality in childbirth.

uterus by increasing the blood supply to that organ and causing some increase in cell number. Progesterone brings about an increase in cell number in all of the tissues of the uterus, particularly in the smooth muscles.

Estrogen plays an important role in the growth and development of the breast at puberty and again during pregnancy. It acts with progesterone to bring about the further development of the glands of the breast which secrete milk (the *mammary glands*). The actual onset of milk production (*lactation*), however, is caused by one of the hormones of the pituitary gland. The secretion of this last-mentioned hormone appears to be inhibited during pregnancy by the large amounts of estrogen present; therefore, the flow of milk does not occur until after delivery.

In the pregnant woman, the placenta is a source of estrogen, augmenting that created by the ovaries. Also, the placenta secretes large amounts of progesterone and estriol, another steroid hormone. The fetus and placenta act as an integrated unit as far as production and metabolism of steroid hormones are concerned. This is mainly because of the differential enzyme systems of the two organs, which complement each other and which change as pregnancy advances.

The reason why large amounts of steroids are present in the fetus is not clear, but it is assumed that these are necessary for the intrauterine growth and development of the fetus and in preparation for extrauterine life.

As more information is accumulated about the production and metabolism of steroids in the fetus and placenta and their excretion in the maternal blood or urine, measurement of these substances will give information about fetal growth and development.

Relaxin is another ovarian hormone; it is responsible for the relaxation or motility of the joints in that part of the mother's skeleton (the *pelvis*) through which the fetus must pass at delivery. Late in pregnancy, this increased motility

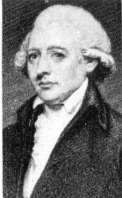

CRUIKSHANK, William Cumberland (1745-1800) English surgeon, studied the passage of the ovum through the Fallopian tube and the uterus. Although an epileptic, he became one of the outstanding anatomists and physicians of his time. Also famous for his many important contributions to the understanding of the function of blood and the lymphatic system. His anatomical teachings had a profound effect upon the training of many physicians of his time.

of the joints of the pelvis may be such as to interfere with walking.

In an effort to avoid confusion, only a brief account of the roles of some of the hormones affecting pregnancy has been given. Indeed, their complete roles are not known, and scientists are currently studying the varied and far-reaching effects of these hormones. (For further discussion of hormones, see Chapter 10, "The Endocrine System," and Chapter 15, "The Reproductive System.")

After delivery and the consequent loss of the placenta as a source of hormones, the estrogen and progesterone levels in the body are sharply reduced and the cycles of menstruation and ovulation are again established.

The capacity to reproduce

The capacity to reproduce depends upon general body health and proper function of the glands and organs of reproduction. Any woman of childbearing age who wants children but does not become pregnant should consult a doctor. Often the cause of sterility is simple and can be corrected under the doctor's guidance; at other times the cause is obscure, or it may be some malfunction of the organs or glands which cannot be readily diagnosed or corrected. It should be pointed out that it is not always the woman who is sterile; in about one third of all cases of sterility, the cause lies with the husband instead of the wife. (For further discussion of sterility, see Chapter 15, "The Reproductive System.")

Disorders of pregnancy

It is best that a woman visit a physician before she becomes pregnant, to see if she is physically fit to bear children. Certain diseases such as diabetes mellitus usually can be kept in control, but the added burden of pregnancy often causes serious complications. Women with active tuberculosis probably should not have children; if they

become pregnant, they need special care from the very beginning. In some cases, heart disease makes pregnancy precarious. For women with these disorders, early diagnosis of pregnancy may be invaluable.

The majority of the complications of pregnancy can be avoided or quickly corrected if the expectant mother knows something of the symptoms of the more common disorders and reports them promptly to her doctor. Vaginal bleeding or "spotting," may be the first signs that an *abortion* or *miscarriage* is about to take place. These terms refer to the birth of a fetus before it has developed sufficiently to live. It has been variously estimated that one out of every five to 20 pregnancies ends in miscarriage, and most of these occur between the second and third months.

Many mothers worry needlessly about "marking" their babies before birth by some fright, shock, or desire they may experience. An understanding of the most simple facts of heredity should prove the foolishness of such superstitions.

During pregnancy, a woman may feel well, but notice some swelling of the hands and feet—particularly in the morning. This and any dimness of vision should be reported to the doctor as they may be early symptoms of toxemia. Chills, fever, and pain between the hips and ribs may be indicative of *pyelitis*, an inflammation of the lower part (*pelvis*) of the kidney. Neither of these conditions should cause serious trouble if it receives early attention.

Multiple pregnancy

Multiple pregnancy means that more than one child is developing in the uterus at the same time. If there is any indication of this condition, the physician will make an x-ray picture of the abdomen. Twins are the most common multiple pregnancy, and occur once in every 88 births. Twins are of two types, *fraternal* and *identical*. Seventy percent of all twins are fraternal twins; they are the result of the fertilization of two separate ova by two separate spermatozoa. *Identical* twins develop from a single fertilized egg; just what causes an egg to divide in such a manner as to produce two individuals is not understood. A tendency toward twinning appears to "run" in some families.

Other types of multiple pregnancies are triplets, quadruplets, and quintuplets. Triplets may be expected once in every 7744 births; other types of multiple pregnancies occur even less frequently. Once it is established that multiple pregnancy exists, the calculated date of confinement should be moved back 14 days, for such pregnancies usually are terminated about two weeks earlier than single births.

Although multiple births have always been considered to be simply phenomena of nature, recent evidence has proved that some drugs can

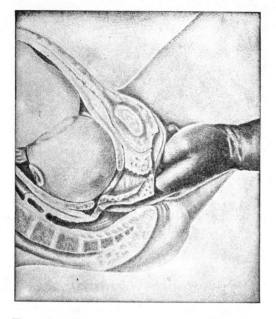

The various stages of labor may be frequently checked by the physician. This is done by inserting his finger into the mother's rectum and feeling the cervix through adjoining tissues.

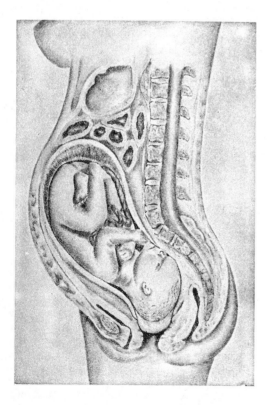

At the very beginning of birth and the height of uterine contraction, the uterus exerts pressure on the amnion, which in turn forces the birth canal to open and permits the fetus' head to drop down.

influence the number of children conceived at one time. Extracts of gonadotropin, the hormone secreted by the pituitary gland which controls ovulation, were given to barren women in an attempt to enable them to conceive. Surprisingly, many women conceived not only one, but several fetuses, some as many as six. In many cases, the fetuses have survived and appear to be healthy children. However, in some instances, the physical demands required in the nurturing of more than one fetus have been overwhelming, and one or more of the infants in a multiple birth group were still-born or died shortly after birth.

Although it is now recognized that the potential for enabling previously infertile women to bear children is available, much study is still required. For optimum use in the future, it will be necessary to regulate use of the medication so that better control of multiple conception is achieved.

As pregnancy begins its last 30-day "round" the physician will explain the signs of approaching labor. The mother-to-be will be on the lookout for rhythmic contractions of the uterus or the sudden gush of water from the vagina; these may mark the onset of labor—the climax of pregnancy.

BIRTH OF A BABY

The advent of a new child in the home is an exciting event and full of promise. It is also time for the closest co-operation with the family physician, in order to insure a healthy beginning for the new arrival.

Well before the expected date of birth, the future mother should pack a bag as if for a weekend trip, and have it handy for immediate departure to the hospital. In it she should put a minimum of two nightgowns, a bathrobe, a pair of slippers, several handkerchiefs, a toothbrush, toothpaste, comb, and brush. The telephone numbers of her doctor, his assistant, and the hospital previously selected should be written down in a definite, easy-to-locate place.

There are two major signs, the appearance of either of which indicates that labor is beginning; however, both may be absent. There may be a passage of a small amount of water, other than urine. This is caused by rupture of the water-filled *amnion* (the sac in which the baby lies during pregnancy—also called the "bag of waters"). Sometimes the initial sign of approaching birth is a bloodstained discharge of mucus from the vagina (called the "show").

However, it is the occurrence of *labor pains* which usually sends the woman to the hospital. The pains are caused by rhythmic contractions of the womb (*uterus*) and feel like abdominal cramps. If a hand is placed over the abdomen during a contraction, the womb will feel very hard; then it relaxes when the cramp subsides. This is the chief method of differentiating true labor pains from false pains. If the baby is actually on its way, the first few labor pains will be slight, at intervals of 15 to 30 minutes. Gradually, they become more intense, longer, and occur more frequently. False pains do not increase in this way. In fact, if there is *any doubt* as to whether pains are true labor pains or false pains, then they are probably false pains.

From the frequency of the pains, the woman can usually tell when the doctor should be called and when she should be taken to the hospital. The usual duration of labor in women who have never borne children is 12 to 18 hours. The second and all other children can usually be delivered in 6 to 10 hours. Therefore, any panic or 80-mile-per-hour trips to the hospital are uncalled for, because there is almost always plenty of time if the pains are recognized soon enough.

Natural labor is triggered by the release of the hormone *oxytocin* from the pituitary gland in the brain. This hormone stimulates the uterus to begin its contractions. At times, it may be desirable to either bring about (induce) labor by artificial means or to delay its natural onset. A variety of medications is available for these needs. To induce labor, the most effective and widely used method is the slow intravenous administration of oxytocin. Usually a synthetic, manufactured oxytocin is used for this purpose. When properly managed, there is little danger involved in this practice. At times, it is necessary only to stimulate the uterus to begin contractions, and the oxytocin may then be discontinued as the uterus takes over on its own.

It is more difficult to delay labor than to induce it, but this may be necessary, as when a baby might be born too prematurely. Alcohol may be used for this purpose, as it apparently inhibits the natural release of oxytocin by the pituitary gland. Muscular relaxants also may be helpful, and tranquilizers are sometimes useful, since fear and other strong emotions are known to increase uterine activity.

The progress of labor

Childbirth is brought about by muscular contractions of the womb. These contractions cause the child to pass down through a canal, shaped somewhat like the "L" in a stovepipe, to the vulva, and from the vulva to the outside world. The process can be divided into three stages. First, the womb contractions cause dilation and relaxation of the neck of the birth canal (the *cervix*). Second, the child is pushed out of the womb, through the vagina, and to the outside, and lastly, the *placenta* (the organ which furnished the child with nourishment during preg-

nancy—often called the "afterbirth") is expelled from the womb after the child is born.

With the onset of the first pains, labor begins. As the uterus contracts, it compresses the fluid sac surrounding the baby. The sac in turn exerts hydraulic pressure against the neck of the cervix, causing it to open gradually.

When the cervix is opened sufficiently to allow the baby to be born, the sac, if not already broken, may rupture, and the second stage begins.

The second stage

With the first child, the second stage lasts an average of about one hour, but mothers with previous children may go through this stage in a much shorter period of time. Seldom does this stage last over two hours. In 96 percent of births, the top of the child's head is the first part of its body to present itself at the opening of the vagina. This is often the most difficult and painful part of childbirth. Indeed, the birth of a child is essentially the birth of the head. As the result of the uterine contractions with its accompanying pains, the head will gradually emerge farther. To understand what is happening to the baby, a comparison may be made with the method an adult would use to get through a hole in a fence. First, he would duck his head, and then put it through. Then, he would turn his body around to get his shoulders out. After lifting his head to look about, he then would turn back around and pull the rest of his body through. The baby performs in the same manner. Meanwhile, the bones in its head overlap slightly to make the head a little smaller.

Either just before or just after the head begins to emerge, the physician may make an incision in the wall of the vulva (an *episiotomy*). This gives the head more room, and prevents any jagged tears in the vulva, which are more difficult to heal and repair.

Throughout the second stage of birth, the mother may assist the uterus in expelling the baby by "bearing down" with each contraction. That is, she strains the muscles in her diaphragm, back, and abdomen every time the womb contracts. Because this voluntary aid of the mother is necessary for most births, the physician probably will not put the mother to sleep. However, various gases (nitrous oxide, cyclopropane, and others) may be administered to lessen the intensity of the pains. Many obstetricians have employed nerve blocks for this purpose. When this method is used, only the sensory nerves and not the motor nerves are blocked.

Natural childbirth

The technique of giving birth to children without benefit of anesthesia is becoming widespread throughout the world. There are two different schools of *natural childbirth*, as it is commonly called. The English school, which was begun by Dr. Grantly Dick-Read almost 50 years ago, is usually referred to as *childbirth without fear*. The *psychoprophylaxis* method, which is based on Russian practices, was perfected by French Dr. Fernand Lamaze, who stressed that it be called *childbirth without pain*. The method which is used most in the United States is the psychoprophylaxis method of Lamaze.

Dr. Dick-Read's theory was that pain in childbirth is increased by many psychological factors including mental tiredness, ignorance of labor, and the often inconsiderate attitude of doctors and assisting personnel during labor. Fear, based on lack of understanding and preparedness, is one of the main causes of pain. To overcome the fear, Dr. Dick-Read advocated prenatal training in muscular relaxation, so that during childbirth the woman might divorce her attention from the activity of the uterus and thereby disregard the pain.

Psychoprophylaxis carries Dr. Dick-Read's principles a step further. Since early in the century, Russian obstetricians had been using Pavlov's principles of conditioned reflexes to train women to react in certain ways during childbirth. Drawing upon both the English and Russian knowledge, Lamaze undertook a complete program of educating women about the principles of pregnancy and childbirth, instructing them in the changes that will occur in the body during delivery and how to react to and work with these changes. He stressed that women must actively participate in labor and childbirth.

Followers of the Lamaze method teach the importance of the "verbal analgesic." Pavlov's dog learned to salivate at the ringing of a bell because he had heard a bell ring each time he was fed—in other words, each time he began to salivate. Likewise, women who use the psychoprophylactic method train themselves to respond to the spoken word. This may then be used during labor by the obstetrician or his attendant to help the woman continue to react as desired at each step in the process of labor and delivery. In addition, the husband is present during labor and delivery, helping his wife relax, giving her moral support, and helping keep her participation exact by using the verbal reminders. He has trained with her and been educated in the method with her during the pregnancy. His presence during birth is invaluable to the mother.

There are several advantages in having a baby without anesthetic. When the mother is awake, she is able to cooperate with the obstetrician and respond to his commands. The baby is not anesthetized, and starts life on his own on a more alert basis. Furthermore, possibly 12 to 15 percent of women who usually would be considered candidates for caesarian section may be able to deliver their babies via the more usual vaginal route if they are schooled in the techniques of natural childbirth.

As the Lamaze practitioners point out, childbirth without pain is not childbirth without effort. However, many women who have experienced the satisfaction and joy of seeing and participating in the birth of their babies believe that there is no better way of bringing a new life into the world.

The use of forceps

If the combination of womb contractions and "bearing down" are not sufficient to deliver the child's head, it may be necessary to use forceps. These are special clamps which are applied to the baby's head and manipulated by the doctor to guide the head and add some traction. The device was invented by a family of seventeenth century obstetricians, the Chamberlens. For many years, the Chamberlens kept the tools a secret, and passed them along from father to son through successive generations. Finally, one member of the line, Hugh Chamberlen, sold the secret to the College of Physicians at Amsterdam, in order to relieve pressing family debts. Thus, the world was denied the benefit of forceps for a hundred years because of the selfishness of one family.

Another instrument now in use in the delivery of babies is one which was originated by a British surgeon in 1706 and rediscovered by a Swedish obstetrician in the 1950s. Believed to be more gentle than forceps, the *vacuum extractor* (like a small suction cup) consists of a metal cup with a rubber hose leading to a pump that pumps air out instead of in. The metal cup is applied to the baby's head at the opening of the birth canal. Pressure is reduced by half and a quantity of scalp is drawn into the cup, forming a "chignon" on the top of the baby's head. Usually, gentle pulling is exerted with the extractor at the same time that uterine contractions are forcing the baby forward; traction is relaxed when the uterus relaxes. At times, however, steady traction is maintained.

There seem to be no aftereffects on the child delivered with this instrument, except for the "chignon" which slowly returns to normal and is usually completely gone by the end of seven days. Likewise, the effect on the mother is usually negligible. The vacuum extractor is less painful than forceps and the instrument is not inserted into the vagina, thus lessening the risk of infection.

Use of the extractor is indicated when the first or second stage of labor has become prolonged or when there is fetal distress and it is desirable to deliver the baby quickly.

Also being tested as an adjunct to labor and delivery is a decompressor unit which completely surrounds the mother from the armpits down. The instrument reduces the exterior pressure on the abdominal wall, allowing the uterus to accomplish its contractions more successfully and with greater results than when it was "fighting" the abdominal muscles. Discomfort is reduced and the duration of labor is shortened, allowing mothers to come to the final stages of birth in a more relaxed and vigorous state. This device is presently being used largely in Great Britain and South Africa.

After the head is brought completely outside, with or without mechanical assistance, there is a short pause in the contractions. Then, they resume and the shoulders, trunk, and lower extremities are delivered. This takes only a short time in comparison with the birth of the head. Usually, at this stage of the delivery, there is a pause of a few minutes, before the placenta is expelled.

BIRTH OF A BABY

Photography . . . Robert A. Kolvoord.

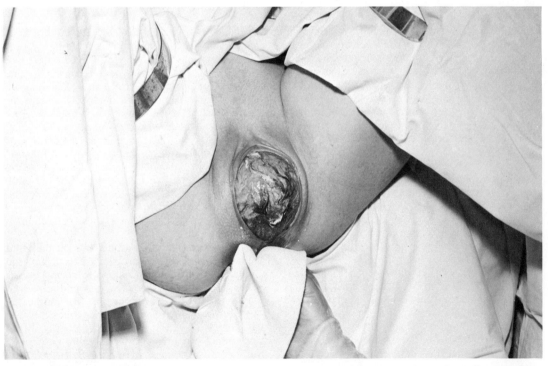

The photograph above illustrates what is technically known as the second stage of the birth of the child. The baby has passed through the fully dilated birth canal (uterine cervix) and is now in the vagina. The top part of the child's head is just beginning to appear. This stage of birth is generally the most painful part of delivery, and it usually necessitates the administration of some type of anesthetic, either in the form of a gas or a nerve block. The "bearing down" of the mother combined with the contraction of the uterus, however, causes the head of the child to emerge gradually in a manner that normally prevents injury to mother or child.

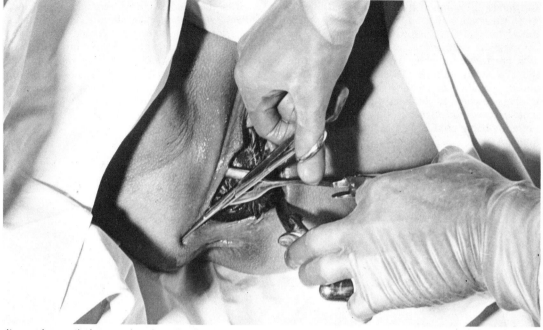

It may frequently happen that the vulva is not sufficiently large to permit the passage of the child without some tearing of the tissues of the mother. In order to prevent such a tear that might be difficult to repair, the attending obstetrician may make a medial or lateral incision of the vulva to enlarge the opening. The operation is usually performed, if necessary, just as the head begins to emerge, and provides an added safety factor for maternal health. It is called an episiotomy, and the clean incision that is made is readily repaired after the delivery of the child is completed and heals in a short time, leaving no unpleasant aftereffects.

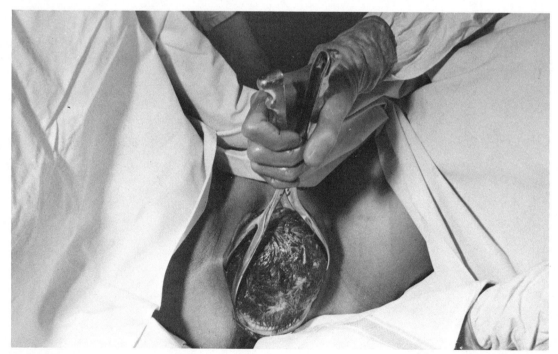

In many cases the natural forces of the mother's bearing down and the contractions of her uterus are not sufficient to expel the head of the child in an expeditious manner, and the attending obstetrician may see fit to use forceps to assist in the process. This procedure has resulted in the saving of many lives. Only a gentle wrist action is necessary in the use of the forceps, and no force that might injure the child is employed in the procedure. Any fear that might exist concerning the use of the forceps is unfounded since the measure is beneficial to both the mother and child, and is a standard procedure that has been employed safely for a great many years.

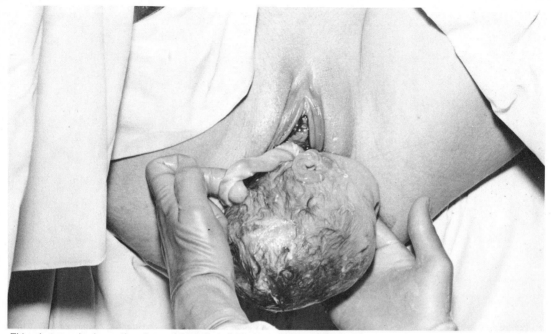

This photograph shows the stage of birth just following delivery of the head of the child. In this picture, a portion of the umbilical cord may be seen in the obstetrician's finger. It may be noted by a comparison with the preceding picture that the baby has now turned around (rotated). This is but one in a series of such turns that the child makes during the process of delivery. These rotations are performed in such a manner as to facilitate the passage of the various parts of the body through the birth canal and out from the vulva with a minimum of strain on child and mother. At this point, the most difficult stage of birth is usually past.

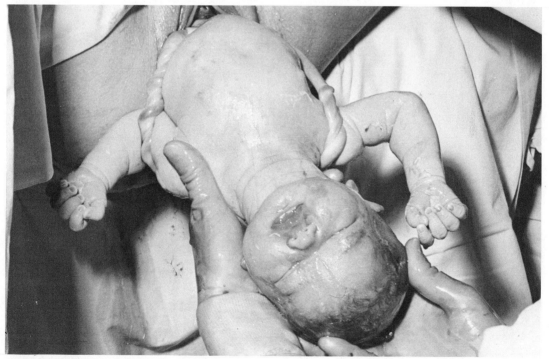

A short period of time elapses after the birth of the head of the child before the contractions commence again. When this happens, the trunk, legs and arms of the child are delivered. Once the baby is completely out of the mother's body, the second stage of the birth process is ended. Within the following half hour, the placenta or afterbirth will also be delivered; but this will involve no such complex process as the birth of the child itself. The doctor may give gentle assistance to the delivery of the placenta and will examine it carefully to ascertain that no part remains in the womb to bring about possibly severe complications later.

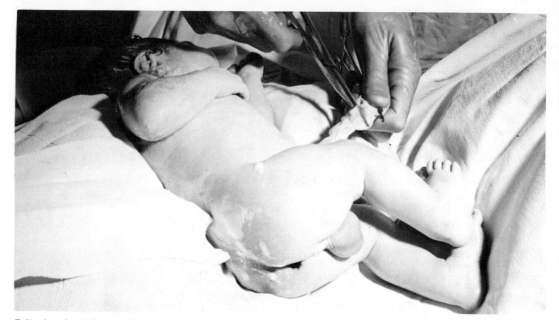

Following the delivery of the baby, the attention of the obstetrician is turned from the mother to the needs of the new individual. If respiration has not already started, this may be stimulated by stroking the child's back or by a gentle slap on the buttocks. The baby must then be carefully cleaned off after the physician has completed tying and cutting the umbilical cord, which is no longer necessary to sustain the infant's life. A drop of silver nitrate solution is placed in the eyes, identification is assured by taking a footprint, and delivery of the child is complete. The physician must now attend to seeing that the entire placenta is expelled.

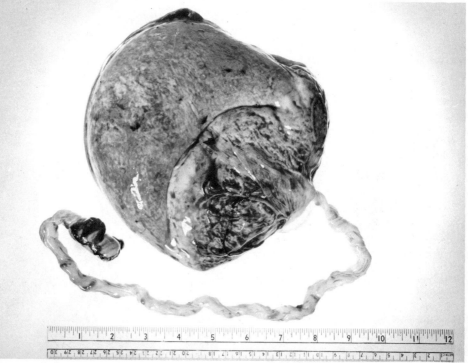

The photograph above shows the placenta and the attached portion of the umbilical cord, following its delivery. The placenta has served the fetus as a means of respiration, nutrition, and excretion during its prenatal period. Blood from the fetus passes through the cord to the placenta, where it comes in close proximity, but does not mix, with the maternal blood. The necessary materials then for the child's nourishment, as well as its waste products, pass between the two blood streams. Careful examination of the placenta by the physician assures that no small part of it remains behind, as it could be a source of hemorrhage to the mother.

Immediate care of mother and infant

The physician now has two patients, mother and child. If the child has not cried yet, the doctor will either stroke its back or give it a few gentle taps on the buttocks. A lusty cry should result, which starts the child breathing. Next, the doctor clamps and cuts the *umbilical cord*, which joined the child to the placenta during pregnancy and was the avenue through which nourishment entered the infant's body. The remaining short stump of the cord will dry up in a few days and will separate spontaneously at the navel.

After the cord has been cut, the physician turns the baby over to a nurse or an assistant. Any mucus present is removed from the nose and throat of the infant with a rubber-tipped syringe. A drop of silver nitrate solution (one percent strength), or an equally effective agent, is put in each of the child's eyes to prevent blindness that may result from gonococcal infection. A footprint and a bead bracelet or necklace bearing the family name are the usual means by which the baby is identified.

The physician has turned his attention to the mother after handing the baby to his assistant. Within about three to eight minutes after the baby is born, the placenta is expelled, usually by manual pressure. The doctor carefully examines the placenta in order to make absolutely certain that every section of it has been expelled. Even a small amount of placental tissue left in the womb can cause hemorrhage.

When the complete placenta has emerged and has been examined, the physician then repairs any torn areas about the vulva, including the episiotomy. These lacerations seldom give the woman future difficulty, and the scars are small or nonexistent.

The mother now is returned to her hospital room. Her womb will continue to contract intermittently for some hours, but there is little pain.

Unusual births or complications

What has gone before has been a description of a normal birth. This is what happens in the great majority of cases. However, even though they occur rarely, there are many types of abnormal births. The most frequent are those connected with presentation of parts of the body other than the head. There may be *breech* delivery, in which the buttocks are first to come out. Likewise, there can be *face presentation, shoulder presentation*, and so on. Often, the physician will have reason to predict these unusual deliveries several weeks before the baby arrives. In such cases, he may be able to change the position of the baby before birth by manipulation from the outside of the womb. If, however, these conditions go unsuspected or the danger of

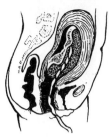

Immediately after the baby has been born, it is handed to the nurse by the doctor. Attention must now be given by the doctor to the proper expulsion of the placenta, or 'afterbirth.' It is usually expelled with the aid of some gentle manual pressure on the part of the attending physician, within about three to eight minutes after completion of the process of birth of the child itself.

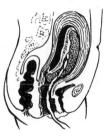

In the process of its expulsion, the placenta must come away from the wall of the uterus to which it has been attached, and follow the same path to the outside of the body that the baby has taken before it. The delicate tissues connecting the placenta to the true wall of the uterus have been prepared for the separation by the various hormonal changes that occur at this time.

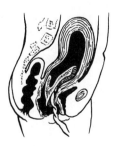

The separated placenta with its attached portion of the umbilical cord is expelled through the birth canal largely by contraction of the uterus and gentle manipulation by the physician. Premature or incomplete separation may cause severe hemorrhaging from the previous point of attachment on the uterus and consequently may bring danger to the life of the new mother.

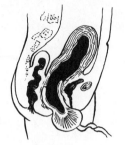

When the placenta has finally been expelled from the body, the physician will examine it thoroughly to determine whether any part of it may still remain attached to the uterus. Even a small piece left behind can bring about severe hemorrhaging in the uterus. This can be especially severe, particularly if the uterus has lost its contractile powers, during the birth process.

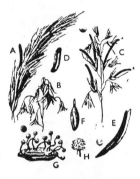

Drawing of the *ergot* mold (*Claviceps purpurea*) growing on rye at early (A) and late (B) stages, and on oats (C). The bundles of mold appear as dark spurs on the rye (D) and oats (E). The granules eventually germinate, those from rye (F) finally appearing as in (G), and forming small beaded stalks (H). Ergot is the source of an important drug that has long been used in obstetrics to stimulate contractions and to stop bleeding after birth of the child.

switching the child's position is too great, the labor will be prolonged.

Another factor that influences labor is the shape and size of the mother's pelvis. If pelvic space is not ample for delivery, the doctor may resort to a cesarean section—as he also may have to do in cases of abnormal positioning of the baby, for abnormal bleeding, or for women with tumors. In some cases, he allows a period of "trial labor" to determine whether the head can go through the canal. When it is proved that normal delivery is impossible, he undertakes the surgical procedure.

A *cesarean section* is the removal of the child from the womb by surgical incision through the abdomen. A woman can undergo as many cesarean sections as necessary in bearing her children. With present-day techniques, there is no truth to the old wives' tale that three is the upper limit for this surgical type of delivery. Furthermore, a

woman may deliver a baby vaginally after having had cesarean sections for previous births. Cesarean section is not known to have been performed on a live woman until 1500. In that year, a Swiss pig breeder's wife underwent labor and was unable to deliver the child. Her husband had often performed the operation on his pigs; thus, he felt justified in doing the same with his wife. He was successful in saving wife and child, and many a mother and child since his time owe him a debt of gratitude.

Another person whose memory should be respected by modern women is Dr. Ignaz Semmelweis. A hundred years ago, childbed fever (*puerperal sepsis*) killed thousands of women annually. It seemed that only those mothers who bore their children in hospitals succumbed to the disease. Indeed, women of that day often pleaded to be allowed to give birth in the gutters rather than in the hospitals. In 1846, Semmelweis, a young Viennese physician, suggested that childbed fever was carried by the doctors themselves. He observed that the physician often went directly from autopsies—where their fingers had dabbled in pus—to attend women in labor *without washing their hands*. An order was given his students, insisting they wash their hands in chlorine water before assisting at a birth. In two years, deaths from childbed fever at his hospital dropped from 459 annually to 45.

Instead of offering their thanks, the medical profession of the time was outraged at Semmelweis' suggestion that they infected their own patients. His doctrine was highly ridiculed for many years; possibly as a result of this ridicule, Semmelweis went insane. His ideas, however, were eventually accepted. Today, childbed fever is rarely a problem—thanks to the efforts of this scientific martyr and newer methods of combating infection.

THE NEW MOTHER

A hospital is the most advantageous place in which a baby can be born. With a staff of trained nurses, technicians, interns, and physicians, the hospital is equipped to attend quickly to the several emergencies which may arise during and shortly following childbirth. Further, a short hospital stay can give the mother a great deal of rest she may not get at home.

The six weeks following the birth of the baby are sometimes called the "lying-in" period. It is a period of convalescence; the doctor calls it the *puerperium*. Four to ten days of this time are usually spent in the hospital; the physician is the best judge as to when the new mother can safely go home.

During recent years, doctors have begun to advocate early rising following delivery. There

CESAREAN SECTION

Photography . . . F. W. Schmidt.

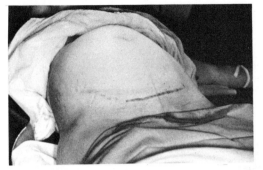

This photograph of the first step in a cesarean section shows the point at which the incision will be made. This incision may also be made higher.

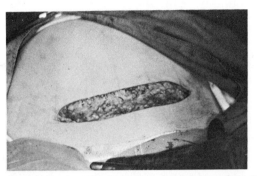

The incision is made just long enough to permit easy delivery of the child. This photograph shows an early stage, at which the incision has been made.

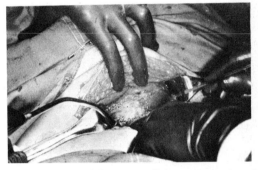

In order to expose the uterus, it is necessary to cut through layers of fatty abdominal tissue and underlying tissues of the peritoneal membrane.

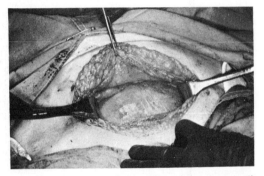

The incised tissues are held aside and the strong walls of the uterus are finally exposed. An incision in it makes the baby available for delivery.

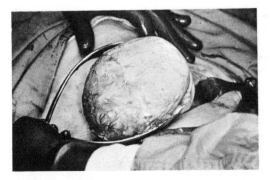

Using either his hands or a pair of forceps, the physician brings the baby's head into position for easy withdrawal from within the uterus.

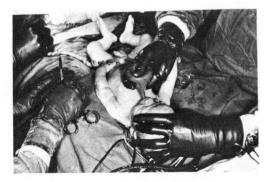

After the baby is delivered, mucus is removed and he is treated like any other newborn. The incision in the mother's abdomen is then repaired.

are many advantages to this. Circulation is better, thus reducing the chances of phlebitis (milkleg); bowel and bladder function are more normal; weakness is prevented; and drainage of the vagina and uterus is improved. There is no evidence that early rising is detrimental to the mother's health.

Changes take place in the body of the pregnant woman to accommodate the fetus and to prepare for its delivery; when the period of pregnancy is over, other changes are to be expected. The uterus, which increases 30 times in bulk during pregnancy, reduces to normal size again; the total blood volume, the heart output per beat, the basal metabolic rate, and many other body activities return to their pre-pregnancy state. During pregnancy the glands of the breasts are prepared for the production of milk. The function of the breasts after birth is discussed in detail later in this section.

Care of the new mother is merely a continuation of the care given her during the period of pregnancy and after the baby is delivered. The mother's genitals are thoroughly cleaned, and any tears or incisions made during the delivery are repaired. If there has been excessive bleeding or shock, the doctor may order a transfusion of whole blood or of *plasma*. Plasma is the liquid portion of the blood only, the cells having been removed.

Changes in the uterus

The major change in the body of the new mother is the decrease in the size of the abdomen brought about by the birth of the baby. There is still a bulge in the region of the navel, but this too, will decrease in size within a few weeks.

Shortly after the birth of the baby, the uterus becomes tightly contracted. This clamps together the spaces in the wall of the uterus to which the placenta was connected and reduces the flow of blood. At this time, the uterus is about the size of a grapefruit and weighs about two pounds; it shrinks until, by the end of six weeks, it is about the size of a lemon and weighs only from one to two ounces. This returning of the uterus to normal size is referred to as *involution*. During the first few days after birth of the baby, the uterus continues to contract and to expel clots of blood; these contractions may cause menstrual-like cramps called *afterpains*. These may be more severe following each pregnancy, and in women who nurse their babies. The stimulation of the breast by nursing causes renewed contraction of the uterus and hastens its involution.

In the course of involution, the cells of the smooth muscles of the uterus lose fluid and shrink; a part of this fluid is absorbed into the circulatory system and a part mingles with the vaginal discharge. This discharge is called *lochia.*

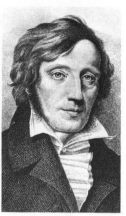

BAER, Karl Ernst von (1792-1876) Estonian embryologist and anthropologist. Famous for his discovery in 1827 of the mammalian ovum. He is generally regarded as the father of modern embryology and as one of the founders of the modern science of descriptive anatomy. With Heinrich Christian von Pander he first described the presently accepted idea of germ-cell growth. His studies formed the basis for the later work of many other investigators in this field.

It is made up principally of the disintegrating lining of the uterus. During the first four or five days after labor, this discharge is profuse and contains blood. Gradually it diminishes in quantity, contains less and less blood, and becomes brownish in color; finally it is scant in amount and pale yellow. Lochia generally disappears about the 15th day after delivery. It is likely to increase when the new mother first resumes her normal activities. If the discharge becomes profuse and red after two or three weeks, it may indicate trouble and should be reported to the doctor.

The lochia is absorbed by sterile sanitary pads or the so-called "sanitary" napkins. The genital organs require the same careful attention given a wound following surgery. The sterile sanitary pads are changed frequently, and for the first few days the vulva is cleansed several times a day with warm sterile water or mild antiseptic solution.

Changes in the breast

The production of milk (*lactation*) is an entirely new function for the body. Usually, it begins three to five days after the birth of the baby. When lactation starts, the blood supply to the breasts is increased, causing congestion in the blood vessels of the breast region. The breasts feel heavier, hot, and tender; associated with this, there may be painful swelling in each armpit. Occasionally there may be a slight fever. This condition usually lasts 24 to 48 hours; if there is much pain, the doctor will order the application of a binder and may prescribe aspirin or other drugs to relieve the discomfort.

If the breast milk becomes hard and caked, it may cause an inflammation of the breast known as *mastitis*. The temperature goes up suddenly and there is an area of extreme tenderness in the affected breast. If this occurs, the doctor will want to know at once, so that he can initiate proper treatment and observe the breast to make sure that abscesses do not form. If the mother is nursing her baby, it may be weaned from the breast and placed on a formula. Usually temperature and tenderness disappear in about two days.

Nursing the baby

Not all mothers can nurse their babies. Occasionally, the breasts do not produce milk, or do so only for a short while. If the new mother is in poor physical condition, or has some disease such as tuberculosis, her doctor will order her not to nurse her baby. Care is taken to prepare a formula well-suited to the infant's needs.

The doctor usually urges the new mother to nurse her baby, if she can do so. This is because the milk of the breast provides the new baby with the quality of food it needs; it may contain substances which protect the baby from disease; it is readily available when needed; it has no chance to spoil; and it is economical.

If the new mother decides to nurse her baby, the child will be brought to her for the first feeding within about 24 hours after delivery. At this time, there is no milk in the breast, but the first secretion of the breast (*colostrum*) satisfies the infant's hunger and has a needed laxative effect. At the first feeding, a nurse will probably instruct the new mother in proper hygienic precautions to be observed during the nursing period. The hands should be thoroughly washed with warm soapy water, rinsed, and dried. The breasts should be washed with warm sterile water before and after each nursing. Between feedings, the nipples should be covered by a soft, clean cloth or gauze held in place by a nursing brassiere, which also supports the breasts. The nursing breast should be treated gently, supported, and not injured. During the first few days, the baby should be allowed to nurse only five or ten minutes at a time.

The quantity of milk produced by a mother varies. During the first few days of lactation, about three ounces of milk is produced at each feeding. By the end of the first week, this amount may be increased to four ounces; by the end of the second week five ounces or more may be produced. The glands which secrete milk are partially controlled by the nervous system; if the mother is worried or upset, less milk is produced. Plenty of rest, a nutritious diet and adequate fluids are important for good milk production.

The quality of milk is dependent upon the food the mother eats. This means plenty of milk and protein foods, for the production of high quality milk. Excessive drinking of alcoholic liquors and smoking should be avoided.

Women who nurse their babies do not begin to menstruate as early as those who do not nurse their babies. Menstruation may be absent for the entire nursing period; however, it usually begins again within eight or nine months after delivery,

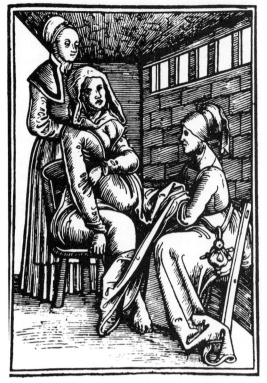

Woodcut (16th century) of midwife at a delivery. The patient is seated upon an obstetrical chair between two attendants. *Bettmann Archive.*

even though the mother is still nursing her baby. A woman who does not nurse her baby can expect menstruation to start between six and ten weeks after delivery. If a woman nurses her child for a time and then weans it, menstruation usually follows in about four to six weeks. Even if menstruation is absent during the period a mother nurses her child, *ovulation* (the ripening and discharging of eggs from the ovaries) may still occur, and accordingly, it is possible but not probable that she may become pregnant again.

Hygiene during the puerperium

Most women can begin to eat regular meals within 24 hours after delivery. A well-balanced diet is just as important during this period of convalescence as it was during pregnancy. Plenty of fluids are necessary, because fluids are lost from the body in unusual amounts during this time. Nursing mothers should have the equivalent of about four quarts of fluid a day, at least one quart of which should be milk.

Occasionally, women have trouble urinating during the first day or two after the birth of the baby. If elimination is long delayed, the doctor or a nurse will insert a fine rubber tube, a *catheter,* into the bladder to remove the urine.

This process may have to be repeated for several days until normal bladder function returns. It may be a nuisance, but is not painful or serious.

An effort should be made to prevent constipation and hard stools, after the delivery. As the bowels are usually sluggish at this time, the doctor may prescribe a mild laxative or warm, saline enemas every night for a brief period.

To assist the abdominal muscles in tightening, and to help the uterus in assuming its normal position, the doctor usually recommends certain exercises. These are selected according to the needs and condition of the individual patient.

Most physicians ask that the new mother come to the office for a final examination when the baby is six weeks old. The doctor checks the condition of the vagina, cervix, and uterus which should have returned to normal size and position by this time. Any tears or lacerations resulting from childbirth should have healed. If such is not the case, the doctor will start proper treatment. He also will examine the abdomen and the breasts, and will check the mothers' blood to determine whether she is anemic.

Many doctors advise that their patients postpone sexual intercourse for two full months after delivery, and certainly until after the six weeks' check has been made. The interval that may be allowed between pregnancies depends largely upon the individual's particular health and circumstances. The mother should discuss this with her physician.

2 THE CHILD

THE PREMATURE

Most authorities regard as premature any infant weighing 2500 grams (5½ lbs) or less at birth. This includes infants with a low birth weight who may be full-term and those who are underterm, but heavier than normal.

Barring deformities and inappropriate care, the premature infant's chance of survival increases with each added week spent in the womb. The stage of development and usually the size and weight of the premature infant are dependent upon the number of weeks between conception and birth. Infants born within 36 to 37 weeks after conception are fairly well-developed and have only slightly reduced chances for survival. Premature infants born within 32 to 36 weeks from conception retain fine fetal hair (*lanugo*) on their cheeks, shoulders, and backs. Their skin is loose, with little fat beneath it; at this stage of development, the infant may weigh from three and one-half to four pounds. Hunger can be registered with a cry, but the baby is weak. Careful supervision and care are necessary if it is to live.

The baby who begins existence outside the womb within 28 weeks after conception starts life with a handicap; such an individual lacks approximately twelve weeks of development. When born within 28 to 32 weeks of conception, the infant requires constant medical supervision. Such a fetal infant weighs about two pounds. Arms, legs, and hands are underdeveloped. The neck is long, and the head does not seem firmly attached. The skin is wrinkled and furrowed; the tissues beneath appear flabby. The infant never seems wholly asleep nor wholly awake. Although limited movements are made when it is disturbed, activities are poorly sustained. An infant at this stage of development cannot maintain a constant body temperature and cannot nurse.

Care of the premature infant

In the premature infant, the transition from *fetus* to infant must take place outside the womb. If the child is to live, the environment of the womb must be closely imitated. In the womb, the fetus is kept warm by the mother's body heat, and it is surrounded by a cushioning and protective fluid. Nutrients and oxygen are supplied from the blood stream of the mother by an organ which attaches the fetus to the mother (the *placenta*); the placenta also serves as a barrier to some infections which might attack the fetus. Consequently, the premature infant requires warmth, humidity, easily-digested food, and an environment free from infectious agents.

The skin and mucous membranes of some premature infants are blue at birth, and many such babies are too weak to breathe efficiently. Some hospitals have equipment for the care of such infants; this includes beds or incubators with automatically controlled temperatures and humidity. The nursery is isolated, and precautions are taken to prevent infection. The child is handled no more than is necessary, and is seldom removed from the incubator. Most premature infants require breast milk, which may be furnished by the hospital if the mother is unable to nurse the child. The chance of survival of a premature infant is enhanced when it is born in a hospital, or is taken there soon after birth.

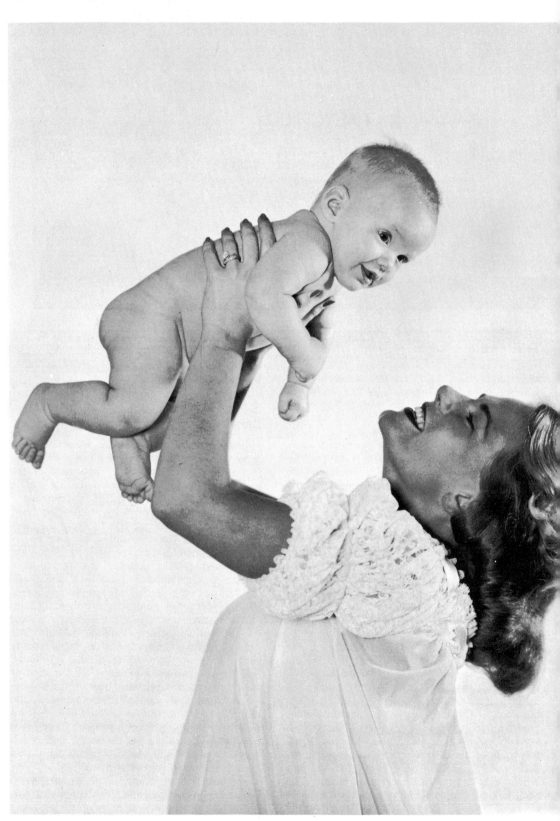

Mother and Child . . . *Photograph by Underwood & Underwood.*

THE NURSERY

Photography . . . Bob Sallee, Houston, Texas

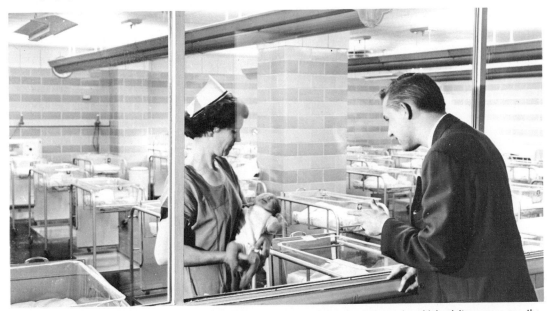

A modern hospital nursery. Note sanitary conditions that prevail and the manner in which visitors may see the new baby without coming in contact with him. Some hospitals require their nurses to wear masks in the nursery; others however, permit the nurses to attend the babies unmasked. Picture Series: *Courtesy of Hermann Hospital, Houston.*

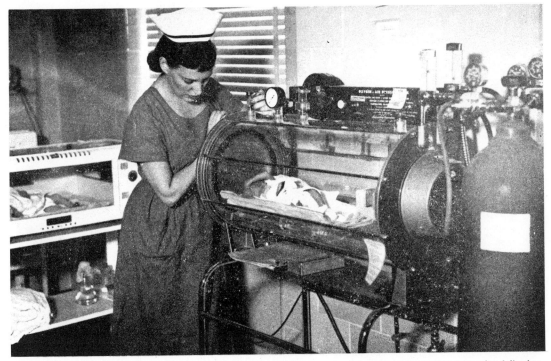

The modern hospital nursery contains special equipment needed for any of the emergencies that may arise following birth of the infant. Here are shown two of the more up-to-date types of incubators which are required for providing prematurely born infants with an ideal environment until they have developed to the extent that a baby crib suffice.

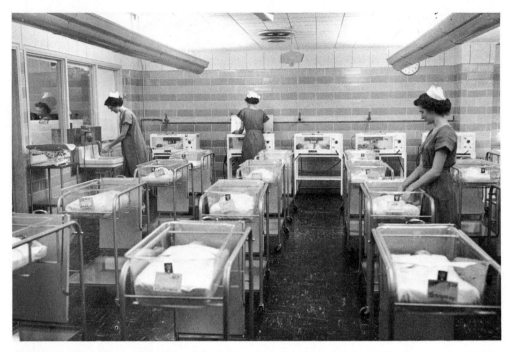

The infant is brought to the nursery immediately following delivery, and spends the first few days of his life in a sanitary environment which protects against respiratory infections and many other contaminations. Proper feeding of the child is insured by personnel who are especially trained for this type of nursing. Incubators are against wall in background.

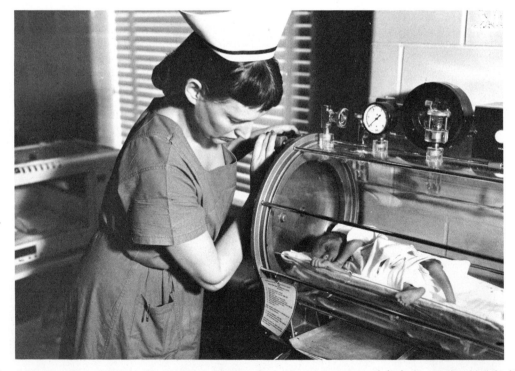

The premature infant shown in this special incubator, often referred to as an *air-lock,* is greatly aided in his earliest days following birth by the artificial environment that can be provided for him within it. Proper temperatures, humidities, and pressures can all be maintained in this air-tight type of incubator. The baby shown here is just a few hours old.

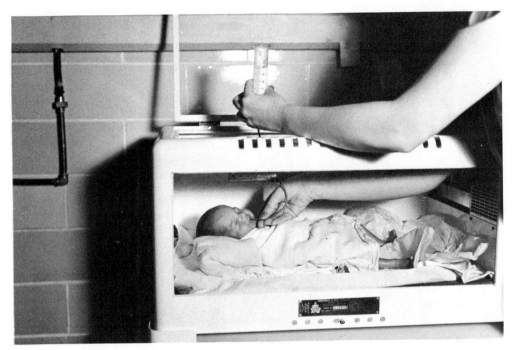

Incubators such as the one shown in this photograph can maintain the body temperature of the prematurely born infant within a normal range, and thus reduce the dangers of a premature birth. The feeding of such infants requires special techniques, as do many of the details of their care. Premature babies remain in incubator until they attain a specified weight.

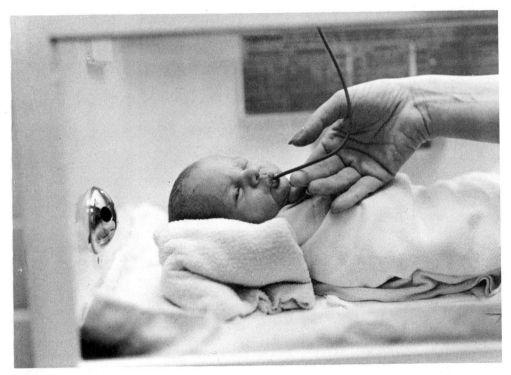

The process of feeding the premature infant through a stomach tube, known as *gavage,* may be necessary for some days. Many advances in the care of such babies have now made the hazard of early birth relatively minor, compared to what it was only a very few years ago. Specialized training and equipment are the key to this progress.

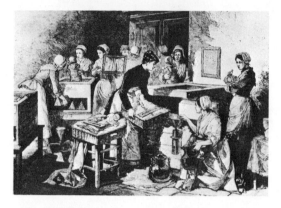

Picture of incubators for infants devised by Dr. Achard of Paris in 1884. Jars of hot water in the bottom provided warmth. *Bettman Archive.*

Feeding the premature infant

Late premature infants—those born 34 to 37 weeks from conception—can swallow, and may be fed from a nursing bottle supplied with a special nipple having a small bulb. Such infants may also be fed by means of a medicine dropper with a piece of rubber tubing attached; the tube is placed in the infant's mouth, and the milk is expressed slowly through the tube. Premature babies who cannot swallow often are fed through a rubber tube *(catheter)* attached to the barrel of a glass syringe. This method of feeding requires training and skill, for the tube is passed directly into the stomach.

Growth of the premature infant

Premature infants who are free from physical defects usually respond to the care given them during the first few months of life. After the period of initial development, they usually are able to consume artificial milk preparations, and show a resistance to disease similar to that of a full-term infant. The poorly developed body of the premature infant gradually assumes the appearance of a full-term infant. The neck shortens and the abdomen and chest fill out. The head shows increased growth, and the face becomes fatter. By the time the premature child is two or three years old, he begins to "catch up" in growth and development with children who were full-term at birth; by the time he is four to six years old, his development often equals that of other children in his age group.

THE FIRST YEAR OF LIFE

The body of the newborn infant is quite different from that of an adult or child. The head makes up as much as one fourth of the total body length. The face of the newborn child is small compared to the high forehead and large rear area of the head. On the top of the infant's head just back of the forehead is a "soft spot" *(fontanel)*. It is a space in the skull where the bones have not fused. It is covered under the outer skin by a tough membrane, and disappears within the first two years. The lower jawbone of the infant (the *mandible*) is not so well developed as the upper (the *maxilla*), causing the infant to have a receding chin. The face of the newborn appears wider than it really is, because of deposits of fat (the *sucking cushions*) in his cheeks. The neck is short, the shoulders narrow. The abdomen is normally protuberant because the muscles of the abdomen are weak and the internal organs are large. The arms and legs are small in proportion to the rest of the body, and the legs appear bowed. The quality and color of the hair are not necessarily related to the texture and color of hair the child will have later in life.

As soon as the child is born, he or she is weighed, cleansed, and tested for a metabolic imbalance known as PKU (phenylketonuria). PKU must be detected in the hours following birth and corrected by diet to prevent mental retardation. The condition is inherited, but also can occur spontaneously.

The stump of the *umbilical cord* usually sloughs off on the sixth to the tenth day. It must be given the same care as a wound, kept clean and dry, and covered lightly with a sterile dressing.

The eyes of the newborn infant cannot focus; and he has little true vision. Eye control develops slowly; it is nearly three months after birth before the child can focus distinctly. Most infants are deaf at birth, because of a mucus-like material which fills the cavity of the *middle ear*. As this fluid drains into the throat, hearing improves. Taste and smell are fairly well developed at birth. The skin of the newborn child is sensitive to heat and cold; the baby will react promptly when touched, but his sense of pain is not acute.

The bones of a newborn baby are soft and flexible; he is therefore less prone to bone fractures and dislocations than adults.

It is better not to leave a baby on his stomach for the first few weeks of life. He should be provided with a firm mattress; pillows and constricting clothing should be avoided.

The young infant makes many random, uncoordinated movements with his arms and legs when awake. He can also cough, sneeze, swallow,

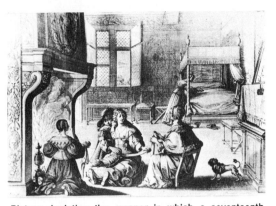

Picture depicting the manner in which a seventeenth century mother swaddled a baby by binding it with a long strip of cloth. *Bettmann Archive.*

and suck. Sucking motions are present at birth and become associated with feeding. Sucking alone is satisfying, and the infant learns the muscular and nervous coordination necessary to place his fist in his mouth for this form of satisfaction.

How the child grows

The first two years of life may be regarded as infancy. Physical and mental growth proceed rapidly during the first half of this period. All infants pass through similar stages of growth, but there is variation in the time a given stage is reached. During this first year, the infant should be checked at frequent intervals by a physician.

When stretched out, the average newborn American baby is 20 inches long. By the end of the third month, the length increases by about 20 percent; and by 50 percent by the first birthday. Most American babies weigh from six to nine pounds at birth. During the first three months of life, the gain is about an ounce a day; by the end of the fifth month, the weight has usually doubled, and the child has increased threefold in weight by the first birthday.

The infant's head appears large for his body at birth, yet it grows rapidly during the first year of life. Although the baby is "top-heavy," he can usually balance his head by the end of the 16th week of life. The trunk, arms, and legs grow and fill out noticeably during the first two years of life; however, the legs and arms will not be proportionate in size to the remainder of the body until the child reaches adolescence. By the time the child starts to walk, the legs frequently will have straightened.

The soft bones of the infant become firm by the deposition of calcium and other salts *(ossification)*. Retarded skeletal development may be indicative of poor health or faulty nutrition.

Dental development

The age of the child at the time of tooth eruption and the sequence with which the teeth erupt are partially controlled by heredity, and partially influenced by nutrition and the growth of the skull. The *primary* deciduous teeth are called "baby" or "milk" teeth; they are smaller and not so hard as the permanent teeth. The baby usually "cuts" his first teeth between six and eight months after birth. These teeth are generally the lower two in front; these two teeth and the two upper front teeth are called the *central incisors,* and on either side of them are the *lateral incisors.* The upper incisors usually erupt between the eighth and twelfth months; the lower lateral incisors appear between the seventh and tenth months. The *cuspids,* or "canine" teeth, usually erupt at the age of 16 to 20 months. The first four *molars* appear from the tenth to the 16th month. The second four molars may erupt as late as the 20th to the 30th months.

Teething may be associated with irritability, mild fever, and disturbed sleep. While the child is teething, he may want to chew constantly on objects and to put his hands in his mouth. A clean, hard object, such as a "teething ring," that withstands chewing and sterilizing, helps him in cutting his teeth.

How the child learns

Learning begins early in life. Through the development of his senses—smell, taste, touch, sight, and hearing—the infant is able to explore his environment, and learning begins. Even the newborn infant responds to light, sound, and pressure. Through muscular activity, he responds to what he sees, feels, or tastes. This ability to control and direct muscles begins with the eye muscles and extends gradually until there is some control of the hands and feet by the end of the first year of life.

From birth the baby cries when hungry. Early in life he comes to associate his mother's presence with the care of his needs and with comfort. When he is able to remember this association, he may stop crying when she approaches, even before she has fed or comforted him.

At four weeks of age, he briefly follows a moving object with his eyes, but his tightly curled hands cannot reach out. He listens, cries, and grunts. By 16 weeks he holds his head erect and can see his hands. His eyes follow a rattle a little farther. He is no longer "two-fisted" but still lacks control over the arm muscles. He puts together sight and sound, and "notices" when he sees or hears his food being prepared.

At 28 weeks, muscle control includes the trunk and hands. The baby can sit up and grasp a rattle or other object, but he is not able to let go of it voluntarily. He sucks and bangs things and passes them from hand to hand. He crows, squeals, and recognizes tones of voices. He is interested in himself and his private enterprises.

The baby who is 40 weeks old stands up by holding on, and enjoys the household world. His hands are controlled enough to poke and pluck. Better use of the face and tongue muscles permits him to take in food more easily. He imitates facial expressions and gestures and has one or two "words" in his vocabulary. He is a little more independent, can hold his bottle and feed himself, likes people, and waves "bye-bye." Social responsiveness and better motor control allow him to play "pat-a-cake." A little more maturity has made him aware of strangers and strangeness.

Most one-year-old children can crawl rapidly, are almost ready to stand alone, and can walk with support. The child of this age can release voluntarily the things he has picked up, and he can put a block in a pan. He repeats words and suits actions to them; for example, he gives up objects when commanded. He squeals to get attention and has added one or two words to his gibberish. He enjoys being the center of attention and repeats the acts that amuse his audience. He can show fear, anger, affection, sympathy, and jealousy. He is beginning to influence and adjust to emotions of others. He cooperates a little in being dressed and fed.

Crying

Crying begins at birth. Through crying, air is brought into the infant's lungs, and breathing begins. The "birth-cry" may be uttered during the process of birth or shortly thereafter. The first gasp of air must be strong enough to expand the lungs sufficiently for them to function.

Crying is the baby's way of expressing discomfort and hunger. As the baby grows older, his cry of hunger should become less frequent, because his stomach can hold more food at each feeding. By the time he is four to six months old, his mind is active enough so that his attention can be diverted for a time from his hunger. The infant often cries in the evening because of colic (indigestion and gas).

If the child finds he can get what he wants by crying, he may develop the crying habit and frequently will continue to cry for things when he is old enough to ask for them. It is well to try to curb the crying early by ignoring it when nothing is wrong.

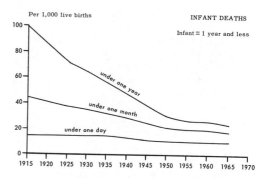

This drawing depicts the decrease in deaths between the years 1915 and 1966 occurring in infants under one year of age. Better control of infections is largely responsible for this decline.

Feeding

The newborn infant is usually offered water within twelve hours after birth. Breast feedings usually are not started until 24 hours after birth. In most cases, the first breast feedings are eight hours apart, and the feeding periods not longer than five minutes; alternate breasts are offered at each feeding. The baby does not get milk at these first feedings; *colostrum,* the precursor of milk, is the first secretion of the breast. During these early feedings, the infant learns to nurse; he is born with a sucking reflex, but he must learn to swallow.

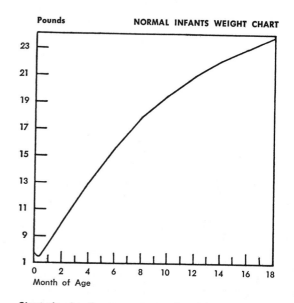

Chart showing the average rate of gain in weight of a normal healthy infant for the first eighteen months. Variations of several pounds are normal.

The infant should be taught to be awake and active during the feeding period and should learn to suck until satisfied. Breast-fed infants generally empty a breast in ten to 15 minutes; small infants may require 15 to 20 minutes. Artificially-fed babies should empty their bottles in similar lengths of time.

The infant should be "burped" after each feeding; sometimes it is necessary to burp the infant during the feeding period also. To burp the baby, he should be held erect over the adult's shoulder and patted gently on the back; this gives the contents of the stomach a chance to settle toward the bottom and the air swallowed with the milk a chance to rise to the top and be expelled. When the infant has been fed and burped, he should be placed in his bed; if he is placed on his right side, the contents of the stomach can empty more readily, thus lessening the possibility of "spitting up" (regurgitation).

Most full-term, healthy infants require nourishment about once in four hours; small infants may require feedings every three hours. The time of feeding should be scheduled to correspond to the infant's periods of hunger. The rhythm of these periods is determined by the time required for the infant's stomach to become empty. A rigid clock schedule seldom corresponds to the infant's natural digestive rhythm; therefore, the mother may find it best to feed the infant a little early at one feeding, if he is awake and demanding food, and a little later at the next, if he is asleep at the scheduled feeding time. Crying between feedings does not always mean that the infant is hungry, because infants seldom require food more often than once in three hours. As the baby grows, his stomach can hold more food at each feeding. During the first month of life, most infants require six or seven feedings a day. The feedings usually begin at six a.m.; they are three hours apart during the day and four hours apart during the night (6-9-12-3-6-10-2). If the baby does not awaken for a feeding, he should be awakened within half an hour of the proper time, except for the two a.m. feeding. This feeding is usually the first the baby can do without. As the infant begins to awaken later and later for the two a.m. feeding, it is advisable to withhold the ten p.m. feeding about an hour. In this way, the infant gradually learns to sleep until four or five a.m., and generally both the ten p.m. and the two a.m. feedings can be eliminated by the time the baby is six months old.

Nursing stimulates the production of milk in the mother's breast. If the infant does not empty the breast at each feeding period, milk production may decline. During the first few weeks of the baby's life, it may be necessary for the mother to empty her breast artificially. Usually, it is advisable to alternate the breasts in feeding the infant. The increased nursing and emptying of the breast often stimulates the production of more milk. If too much milk is produced, it may be advisable to offer both breasts at each feeding, but to have the infant only partially empty each one. If the mother does not produce an adequate supply of milk, supplementary bottle feedings are required.

Occasionally, an infant develops jaundice from mother's milk. In such a case, the physician changes the child over to cow's milk. Unusual allergies to milk are sometimes also seen, but are very rare.

Bottle-fed infants are supplied nourishment from prescribed formulas. Cow's milk is usually used in formulas. If formulas are adjusted to the infant's individual need, the artificially-fed infant should thrive about as well as the breast-fed infant.

Nipples and nursing bottles should always be clean, and the holes in rubber nipples should not be too large. The mother should wash her hands before each feeding; and if her baby is breast-fed, she should wash her nipples with a soft cloth or cotton which has been dipped in sterile water before and after each feeding.

Vitamin C is usually added to the infant's diet by the time he is two weeks old; it may be given as ascorbic acid dissolved in water, or in the form of orange juice. Vitamins A and D in the form of concentrated oil are added to the diet between the second and third weeks of life. Precooked cereals and egg yolk are usually the first solid foods; they are offered the baby between the third and fourth months. Strained fruits and vegetables are added shortly thereafter. Meat and fish are usually a part of the diet as the baby approaches his first birthday.

The physician usually suggests that weaning be started when the baby is eight or nine months old. Breast feedings are gradually replaced by bottle or cup feedings; some babies transfer easily from breast to cup, and some need bottle feedings for a few weeks before they will start drinking from a cup.

Sleeping

The newborn infant sleeps 18 to 20 hours a day. The periods of sleep last from two to three hours, and usually are interrupted by hunger. As his stomach grows and he consumes more food, his periods of hunger are farther apart, and he can sleep longer at a time. When he is six months old, he sleeps less—16 to 18 hours a day—and should be able to do without feeding during the night. By the time he is a year old, the baby sleeps about twelve hours at night and has two naps a day, one in the morning and one in the afternoon. After the second year, the child no longer requires the morning nap.

CIRCUMCISION

Photography . . . F. W. Schmidt.

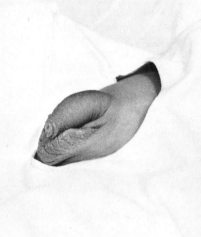

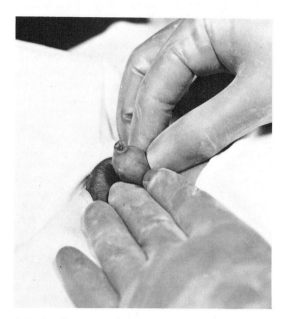

1 Circumcision may be performed immediately after birth, and in several ways. The technique depicted here is in wide use. Above, the area surrounding the penis has been sterilized and draped with a special circumcision towel.

2 In the first step of the operation, the prepuce or foreskin must be retracted from the head of the penis. This must be done carefully to prevent tearing of delicate prepuce and glans tissues; it may be done with moist gauze.

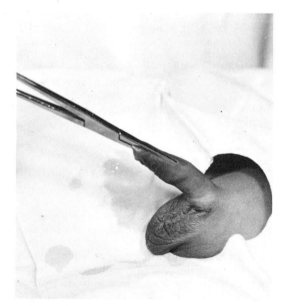

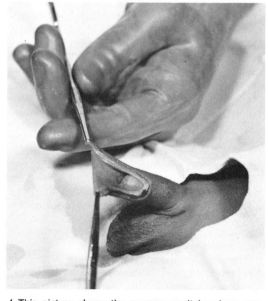

3 The prepuce is folded over the head of the penis. A grooved directing instrument is inserted between the foreskin and head of the penis. The prepuce is then cut by a scissors which is slid alongside the directing instrument.

4 This picture shows the prepuce as it has been cut. Two small hemostats are clamped onto the edge of the prepuce near the incision, and the prepuce is stretched out. At this point it may be necessary to separate any adhesions.

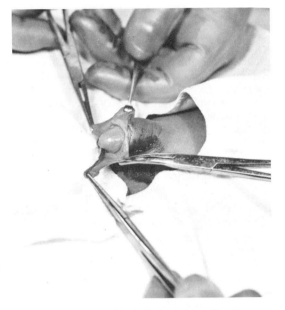

5 The extended foreskin is incised down the side opposite the first incision, producing the appearance shown here. The folds of the foreskin are cut away, leaving enough mucosa to suture the foreskin to the surrounding skin.

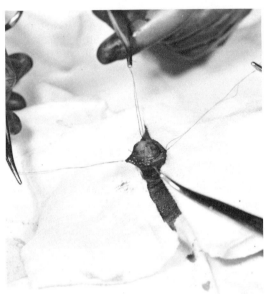

6 The foreskin has now been removed and the initial sutures put in place. The outer skin must be tied to underlying remnant of mucosa so that no damage occurs in head of penis. Remaining foreskin disappears during healing.

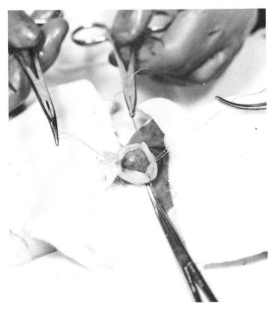

7 When the circumcision has been completed, a sterile dressing is applied to the area to prevent infection and irritation. Dressing usually consists of a piece of vaseline gauze. The gauze may be tied to sutures to keep it in position.

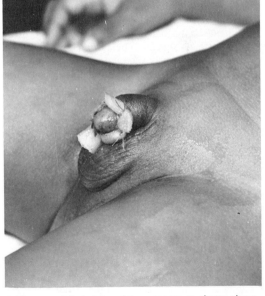

8 The completed circumcision appears as shown above. The wound will rapidly form a dry scab, which after a few days will drop off, leaving a clean scar. Careful attention to the wound is necessary, but complications are very rare.

The newborn child usually sleeps well in a basket with sides high enough to prevent drafts. His clothing should be soft and absorbent; long loose clothing becomes twisted as the infant squirms. As the baby grows, he should be provided with a bed of his own. A firm, long-staple cotton or hair mattress is appropriate for young children. If a sleeping bag is not used, flannelette or heavy cotton knit pajamas with feet attached should be worn in cold weather.

Bathing

Frequent bathing in infancy is desirable. The bath should be given in a warm room, between 70° and 75° Fahrenheit, and at about the same time each day.

During the first part of the bath, it is best to leave the diaper on the baby; and all of the body except the part being washed is kept covered with a flannel square or a large, soft bath towel. The baby's face should be washed first. A special small cloth should be used; soap should not be used. The corners of the eyes and the outer channels of the ears may be washed with separate cotton swabs which have been dipped in boiled water. Hardened crusts of mucus in the nose may be gently removed with cotton swabs moistened with boiled water; a separate swab should be used for each nostril, and for each eye and ear. The mother should not attempt to clean the mouth. The mouth may be gently squeezed open by pressing the jaws with the thumb and fingers; this allows the mother to inspect the gums and tongue for signs of irritation or disease. Usually the infant's head does not need to be washed more often than three or four times a week. The remainder of the infant's body is merely sponged off, not submerged; this procedure is carried out until the navel is completely healed. When healing of the navel is complete, the baby may be placed in a tub containing about two inches of water and at a temperature between 99° and 105° Fahrenheit, or just comfortably warm when tested with the mother's elbow. During this part of the bath, the baby should be securely held and his head supported. His trunk, arms, and legs are lathered with a mild soap, then thoroughly rinsed. The baby is then lifted gently from the tub and wrapped in a large, absorbent towel and patted dry. The neck and body creases should be inspected for accumulations of fuzz or powder. Excessive use of talcum powder causes irritation. Powder should be used sparingly on the baby, and care should be taken that it is not inhaled. Genitals should be cleaned with moist, sterile cotton. In cleaning the genitals of girl babies, the cleansing motions should always be toward the *anus*. It is necessary to push back gently the foreskin of uncircumcised boy babies to clean the penis thoroughly; it should always be pulled back into its original position.

Clothing the baby

The infant's clothing should be simple, soft, and absorbent. Diapers, cotton shirts, and night-gowns are essential. Shirts and gowns that slip on over the feet or that wrap around the baby and tie are preferred. Cotton is the preferred material for these garments, because it is absorbent and easy to launder. Bootees, stockings, sweaters, a coat and cap or a zipper bag with attached hood may be necessary in cold weather. The number of diapers and shirts needed is dependent to a large extent on laundry facilities available.

Illness in infancy

Infants are especially susceptible to respiratory infections and disturbances of the digestive tract. During seasons when respiratory infections are prevalent, they should be kept at home and away from people as much as possible. The food should be free from contamination and feeding equipment should be carefully sterilized.

Weak, undernourished babies often develop a fungus infection of the mouth known as *thrush* which produces white patches; the disease is caused by an organism normally present in the mouth, but it does not ordinarily produce disease in healthy or older children.

Infants are born with a certain amount of immunity to "children's diseases" such as mumps and measles; however, specific immunizations against certain diseases should be started within the first year of life. If certain diseases are prevalent in the area in which he lives, the infant's doctor will usually start immunizations during the first six months. Immunizations against smallpox, diphtheria, tetanus, and whooping cough are usually made by the time the baby is a year old. In some areas, vaccinations against

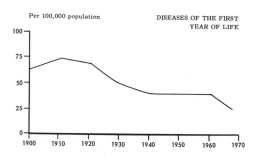

This chart depicts the decline in death rates for diseases peculiar to the first year of life. There are now 25-30 deaths per year per 100,000 persons.

typhoid or certain tropical diseases may be necessary before the child is two years old.

Fever

Fever should never be ignored, because it is a symptom of some disturbance in the body. A rectal thermometer is the best way of taking the temperature of an infant. The bulb of the thermometer should be greased before it is inserted into the rectum. The thermometer need not be inserted beyond half an inch, and should be left in the rectum for two minutes; the person taking the temperature should hold the thermometer and the infant's feet during this interval. Rectal temperatures are normally about a degree higher than temperatures taken by mouth. The thermometer should be cleansed thoroughly with soap and *cold* water before it is put away.

Convulsions

Sudden high fever in infants and small children can cause convulsions (called febrile convulsions) Such episodes, while frightening to the unprepared parent, do not usually have any serious aftereffects.

After calling the doctor, steps to take are outlined in Chapter 23, "Physical Injuries and First Aid." Simply, while the convulsion is going on, the mouth and tongue should be protected from being bitten by placing a small folded washcloth along the teeth. When the rigidity and shaking subside, keep the child lying down, but tilt his head back and pull up the jaw to free the tongue from blocking the throat and breathing passages. Blueness of face is caused by lack of breath. Breathing into the child's mouth will not help unless the tongue is free.

Convulsions not caused by high fever are more serious. They may be triggered by poisoning, head injury, nutritional deficiencies, disease, or inherited tendency. Convulsive-like attacks

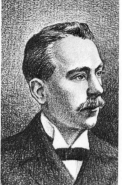

BORDET, Jules Jean Vincent (1870-1961) Belgian bacteriologist and pathologist. Well known for his work in immunity which won him the Nobel prize for physiology and medicine in 1919. His studies in serology and serotherapy have had important results. The bacillus causing whooping cough and the vaccine for its prevention both were developed by Bordet, who also is credited with helping to develop a test reaction for gonorrhea.

are sometimes brought on by emotionally disturbed children who deliberately hold their breath to gain attention.

Since some forms of tranquilizers may also produce convulsions in infants, give the child nothing until the doctor prescribes something.

Colds

The common cold is the most frequent form of illness in childhood. The symptoms of colds in infancy are fever, restlessness, irritability, and loss of appetite. The initial symptoms of more serious diseases, such as measles or poliomyelitis, are similar to symptoms of the common cold; therefore, a physician should examine a baby who has a cold and fever.

Croup

Croup is a term usually applied to a sudden spasm of the opening between the vocal cords *(glottis)*. It often follows a respiratory infection such as a cold. A baby with croup has a barking cough and noisy breathing. Croup causes a suffocating feeling which frightens the baby.

Since croup is a general term that can cover several specific causes treatment should not be given without first checking with the doctor.

Colic

Colic is a discomfort in the abdominal region, the onset of which is very sudden. A baby with colic cries hard, draws his arms and legs to his body, and clenches his fists. A hot water bottle placed on the abdomen, or a warm enema may provide temporary relief from colic. To prevent colic, the baby should not be allowed to suckle too fast. Burping after each feeding also helps prevent colic; it is especially necessary during the first six months of life. Pain similar to colic may have many more serious causes; therefore, discomfort that seems to be caused by colic should be reported to the doctor.

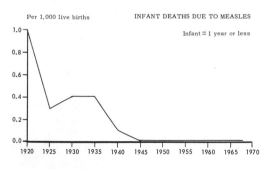

The death rate in infants under one year of age due to measles in the United States has dropped to zero, but the disease still presents a threat.

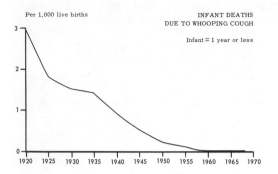

Per 1,000 live births

INFANT DEATHS
DUE TO WHOOPING COUGH

Infant = 1 year or less

Deaths in children less than one year of age resulting from whooping cough have declined during the past forty years, and are now exceedingly rare.

Vomiting

Vomiting is a common occurrence during infancy. When it occurs shortly after a feeding, it may be caused simply by the child's overeating or the mothers' failure to burp him. Vomiting is often an initial symptom of an infectious disease, and it may be caused by nervous and emotional disturbances. Sensitiveness to certain foods and intestinal obstruction may cause vomiting in some infants.

Diarrhea and constipation

Frequent, green-colored, watery stools with varying amounts of mucus may indicate *diarrhea*. An infant with diarrhea should be isolated from other children, for it may be caused by an infectious disease. However, loose stools are not always an indication of infection; they may be caused by overfeeding or an improper formula. In mild cases of diarrhea, the doctor may recommend withholding food for a 24-hour period and giving only weak tea. Severe cases of diarrhea may be caused by the presence of disease-producing organisms in the intestine. In such cases, diarrhea usually is accompanied by fever and requires longer treatment.

Abnormally infrequent stools may indicate constipation; however, as long as the stools are soft and smooth, the infant probably is not constipated. Hard stools, loss of appetite, and abdominal pain may also be symptoms of constipation. Hard, bloody stools and prolonged constipation should be called to the doctor's attention. Chronic constipation may be the result of a faulty diet; the physician may adjust the baby's formula so that it contains more sugar, because sugar has a laxative effect. Fruit juices and cereals reduce the tendency toward constipation. The mother should encourage the baby to empty the bowels shortly after a meal.

The muscles of the intestines then are most active.

Rashes

The skin of babies is subject to rashes. *Diaper rash* may be caused by the chafing effect of soiled diapers. It may also be caused by the presence of bacteria which come from the intestines and become established in the skin of the buttocks. These bacteria act on the baby's urine and produce ammonia, which irritates the skin. When this condition occurs, diapers must be washed with care and given a final rinsing in a saturated solution of boric acid. The irritated area of the skin should be kept as dry as possible and dusted with borated talcum powder.

Prickly heat also attacks babies. It usually affects the face, neck, and chest. This disorder occurs more often in warm climates, but even in cool weather it may affect a child who is over-dressed; flannel pajamas are frequent offenders. If it persists, a physician should be consulted. Indeed, a doctor should be consulted about any rashes, for many are similar in their early manifestations, and must be diagnosed before proper treatment can be given. Exzema, a painful itching rash, which may be related to an allergy, requires a physician's care. Some of the preparations used for other kinds of rashes may irritate exzema.

Infant deaths

Sudden death of an infant, who may have had the best of care, is always a sorrow and a puzzle. Physicians believe that these sudden unexplained deaths (or crib deaths) may be caused by heart attacks. Viral attacks may be another cause.

Although crib deaths are rare, infant mortality in the United States is not. During the first 12 months of life, 23.8 of every 1000 U.S.

PARK, William Hallock (1863-1939) American physician and bacteriologist. Active in the introduction of diphtheria antitoxin, and one of the great contributors to the development of bacteriological diagnosis and serum treatment which eventually conquered the disease. He was one of the first to study the relation of infected milk to infant diseases and led to the movement for bacteriological control of municipal milk supplies.

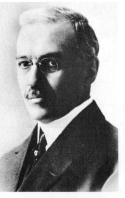

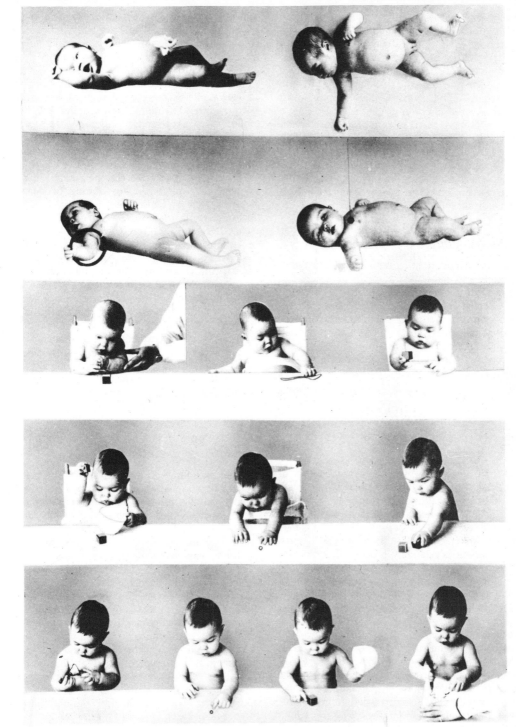

These pictures illustrate stages in the mental growth of the baby. Pictures were taken at intervals during the baby's first year of life, and are arranged chronologically in the usual reading order. The following figures and legends indicate age of the baby in weeks, and his activities. 1) Holds head to side, 6) stares at wall, 8) holds ring without inspecting it, 12) follows object, 16) looks fixedly at block, 20) contacts spoon, 24) grasps block on sight, 28) bangs block, 32) rakes pellet, 36) goes after second block, 40) pokes bell, 44) picks pellet between finger and thumb, 48) recovers block under cup, 52) puts crayon to paper. *Photographs and caption adapted from (a) Arnold Gesell: How a Baby Grows, Harper & Bros., N. Y., (b) Gesell and Ilg: Infant and Child in the Culture of Today, Harper and Bros., N. Y., (c) Gesell and Amatruda: Developmental Diagnosis: Normal and Abnormal Child Development. Copyright 1944 and 1947 by Arnold Gesell.*

babies die. The U.S. is in twelfth place behind other nations in preventing infant deaths. The Department of Health, Education, and Welfare state the causes of infants' dying are respiratory malfunction, low birth weight, premature birth, and malformations. Poor maternal health, malnutrition and lack of sanitation and health services are the underlying causes.

Ten years ago, the first case of a heart attack in a child under 12 years of age was reported. Today it is known that cardiovascular malformations occur in six of every 1000 births. Physicians report that such malformations account for 50 percent of infant deaths from congenital defects during the first year of life.

Hyaline membrane disease

The most common cause of death in both premature and full-term infants in the hours following birth is respiratory difficulty. About half such affected infants are found to have an excess of pink fluid clinging to the membranes of the bronchial tubes. This condition is now called hyaline membrane disease. Although still a mystery, doctors believe it is produced by a lack of oxygen supply to the fetus in the period before birth.

THE YOUNG CHILD

The rapid growth which is characteristic of infancy slows down after the child is two years old. Between the ages of two and six, he grows relatively more in height than in weight. He appears tall and thin in comparison. Growth in general is slow between the sixth and tenth years; gain in weight is relatively greater than increase in height. Weight is influenced more by nutrition than is height. A child may increase in height during a serious illness, yet lose in weight.

Each child has an inherited pattern of skeletal development. Irregularities in bone development may be caused by ill health, abnormal glandular function, or malnutrition. In the embryo, bones begin development as connective tissue, which gradually changes to *cartilage,* which forms the model for the hard bones of the adult. Deposition of certain salts, chiefly calcium phosphate, causes the bones to harden *(ossification)*. Ossification begins in spots called *ossification centers.* The rate of ossification is an index of growth, because the maturation of the skeleton is correlated with the development of the remainder of the body.

No new muscles are acquired after birth, but those that are present increase in weight about 40 times by maturity. The period of greatest muscular growth usually takes place between the ages of five and six years. Since muscle growth is dependent upon liberal amounts of proteins, foodstuffs rich in this material should be generously included in the diet during childhood.

The organs of digestion are not completely mature until the child reaches sexual maturity *(puberty).* The young child requires a diet consisting largely of mildly seasoned, easily digested foods. The capacity of children's stomachs is small, and periods of hunger are more frequent than in adults. Light, in-between-meal snacks are definitely of benefit.

In early childhood, the heartbeat becomes slower and stronger than in infancy. Between the ages of four and ten, there is a lag in the development of the heart. This is most marked when the child is about seven. A similar lag occurs in adolescence. The lungs continue to develop until at least middle childhood. The rate of breathing becomes deeper and more regular in early childhood than it was in infancy. The other organs of the body enlarge in size according to their function. Examination by a physician should be made at least twice a year to determine whether the child is growing in a normal and healthy fashion. With most children, it is intellectual and personality development rather than physical growth that is the difficulty or the delight of the parents.

Chronological mental and emotional growth and development

Mental and emotional growth follows patterns also. These are often misunderstood because too many adults are unaware that children must learn most of the concepts which older people take for granted. Parents reasonably do not expect a one-year-old child to dress himself or a three-year-old to be able to read. However, they do not realize that the child must learn even such elementary physical concepts as time and space. Even less do they understand that ethical concepts, such as obedience, truthfulness, responsibility, and consideration for others, must be learned. Often behavior which worries or irritates the parents can be understood in terms of the child's development; knowing this gives the clues and cues to dealing with such phases during the formative years.

At 18 months: In the sixth months following the first birthday the child gains about two to three pounds in weight and two to three inches in height. The number of teeth usually doubles. His food intake may be less than at one year. He can eat with a little assistance. Much messing and smearing over should not upset the mother. He has learned to walk and to control his hands enough to build a tower with three blocks, or turn the pages of a book, several at a time.

Voluntary control over *sphincter mucles* is just beginning, and toilet training may start. The baby becomes interested in this function and may grunt, cry, or express facially his desire to have a bowel movement. If the mother watches the child, she may soon determine when the bowels are apt to move and can put him on the "potty-chair" at the expected time. Children of this age should not be kept on the seat more than ten minutes. They should never be scolded or shamed for accidents or failures to perform, and parents must maintain a casual, friendly attitude. By the time the baby is one and one-half years old, he usually stays dry for about two hours, and bladder training can begin. Before the bladder can retain urine that long, it is useless to try. Often at the beginning of training, a child will tell his mother *after* he urinates. This is not done to tease her, but because he is learning that he should tell her, although he still lacks control. Girls usually achieve bladder control earlier than boys, and so are easier to toilet-train, and have fewer relapses.

A vocabulary of about ten words is normal at this age, but it will be another six months before words are put together to form sentences. The child is beginning to understand a little of the difference between "you" and "me." He is upset by sudden changes and may react to them by lying down, screaming, or struggling. This defiance is not agressive, but rather an attempt to master the anxiety of the new and unfamiliar. He hits the air rather than the intruder. When he is more socially mature, he may slap the person. He is best handled by gradual and gentle changes. Scolding and verbal persuasion mean little because words mean little to him.

The two-year-old: In the past six months, the child usually has gained two pounds and four teeth. Better balance and more flexible knees and ankles enable him to run. He can go up and down the stairs alone, "marking time" on each step, can kick a ball, but cannot make short turns or sudden stops. He likes rough and tumble play and expresses emotions by jumping, screeching, and "dancing." Now he can string beads, hold a glass with one hand, and build a tower a foot or so high. The memory is longer; he looks for missing toys and recalls events of the day before. He is beginning to note the difference between black and white.

The two-year-old is apt to be bursting with words and may have a vocabulary containing as many as 1000 words, but the average American child of two years has a vocabulary of about 200 words. Names of things and people predominate. The child understands better if one calls his name, instead of addressing him with the pronoun "you." Two-year-old children like stories about themselves. Temper tantrums tend to make their appearance at this stage, and are best handled by adroit distraction before they begin. If the child does have a tantrum, parents must guard against showing emotional upset, also. It is much better to ignore the child during this performance.

The three-year-old: A child at this age has not learned to be unselfish, because the family life has revolved around the baby. Three-year-old children help some with dressing—finding armholes and pulling off stockings. They get tangled up trying to put things on, but do not want help. They mimic their elders, including emotions—such as "guilt" over relapses of bladder control, but they do not really feel it. Although they like vigorous motions, they are becoming interested in finer ones, such as drawing. They can match simple forms and make sentences with three words. They have strong desires to please adults, but are capable of strong but brief outbursts of temper, rolling on the floor, and screaming. Fears of specific things may develop at about this time. They like the company of other children although they usually do not play *with* them in an organized fashion. Three-year-olds are aggressive in play, will yank things away from playmates, and bat them over the head, with no remorse. Parents should not get too excited about this. Putting them with older children who will stand up for their own rights may help. At this stage they begin to learn to share things with others, but may often refuse to do so. These apparently opposite displays of behavior may puzzle parents. They are, however, part of the developmental process.

The four-year-old: Muscle control is growing at four years of age. This child can skip and jump but cannot hop. He can lace his shoes and undress himself. He goes to the toilet by himself with little or no help. Parents should begin to wonder and investigate if he is still having toilet accidents.

The four-year-old talks all the time. Long and involved conversations are his way of making social contacts and strengthening his use of words. His thinking shows more generalizations, abstractions, and awareness of different kinds of things. His mind put together facts, and he asks many questions. He cannot tell the difference between truth and fiction. Past and future mean little to this "bossy," more independent child.

The five-year-old: This year closes early childhood. The sense of balance has improved. More complicated motions, such as combing the hair and brushing the teeth, are done well. He handles a crayon with greater ease; but a downward, oblique stroke is the hardest for him, so that he cannot copy a diamond-shaped figure readily.

The five-year-old's sense of time is growing; this is evidenced by his ability to carry play over from one day to the next. However, he lives mostly in the here and now. There is more relation between idea and execution. Unlike the four-year-old, he has his idea before he draws it. He has trouble discriminating the fanciful from the real, and he likes being taught. The five-year-old is more practical, accurate, and relevant. His attention span is longer. Questions continue but are more pointed; they are for information rather than socialization or practice in speaking. He knows about 2000 words.

He knows his right hand from his left but may not recognize right from left in others. His power of reasoning is limited. Nightmares occur in many children of this age. One cause is anxiety about possible separation from the parents.

The five-year-old is relatively independent. Many children of this age show some competence in caring for younger children. He has pride in possession, in accomplishments, and in going to school, and is sometimes polite and tactful. He has confidence in others and is a social conformist. He enjoys dressing up in masquerade. He may be deceptive, but he also has an elementary sense of shame. Although usually stable and self-confident, the child may have fears which seem unreasonable.

The six-year-old: This is an age of change, both physical and mental. Most of the sinuses are well-developed, and the tonsils may be large. The six-year-old child is usually exposed to more diseases than he was at five, and is apt to have ear, nose, and throat infections. The skin and mucous membranes seem more sensitive. Some six-year-olds seem to tire easily and complain of legs and arms aching, and may shriek with minor hurts. The milk teeth are shedding, and the first permanent molars appear.

New feelings and thoughts are appearing also, and mothers may wonder "what's gotten into him?" In almost the same breath, the six-year-old tells his mother he loves her and hates her. He slams, attacks, and runs in and out. This is not badness or perversity; it is merely that he has not learned to control these new feelings. Furthermore, his world suddenly enlarges and changes when he starts to school. He is faced with strangers whose demands and values are different from those at home. He dawdles, tries too hard, quarrels, and accuses others. He is now challenged by the new world opened to him by school. He learns through either creative or motor activity, or both. He loves to win and may use any means to do so.

Genital inspection, comparison, and exhibition are not uncommon at this time. He asks about babies, but is not especially interested in the father's role. Play now turns into more clearly defined male and female activity.

The appetite is good, but parents should not insist that the child eat all that is asked for. Table manners may vanish. Children of this age may eat with their hands, swing their legs, and talk with full mouths. Lapses in bowel control at this age may occur because the child is not yet accustomed to the school toilet. Getting the child home from school promptly or having his toilet at noon at home may prevent this. The six-year-old may strongly demand the clothes that are popular with his group, but does not take care of his clothes.

Tension finds many outlets: wriggling, scratching, nail-biting, screaming, temper tantrums, etc. The six-year-old is "sassy" and ready to fight. While this attitude is distasteful to parents, it is a sign that the child is trying to act on his own. He usually says "no" to any personal request; but if given time and tactful opportunity, he will usually comply.

The seven-year-old: The seven-year-old is not so active as the six-year-old, but is more vocal. Some children of this age complain of muscular pains, especially of knee pains, and they tire easily. But they do not dawdle so much as formerly.

The seven-year-old child has become more thoughtful. He is more aware of other people and relationships with them. This makes him a

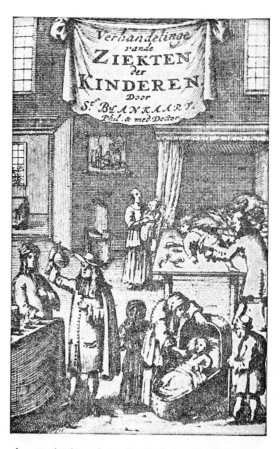

A reproduction of the frontispiece of a seventeenth century book by Stephan Blankaart, *The First Treatise on Diseases of Children. Bettman Archive.*

worrier, and somewhat fearful. Cautious in approaching new problems, he is more apt to withdraw from stressful situations than before. He becomes angry with himself and cries from disappointment, or when he feels that people do not like him. He tries to control his tears and sometimes succeeds.

The seven-year-old is more aware of himself and his body; he becomes modest. He is sensitive about his deviations from what others expect of him. He withdraws if laughed at or criticized, is busy with his own activities, and at times is inattentive and unhearing. He frets about getting places on time; he is interested in magic, but is also beginning to question many things. He is skeptical about Santa Claus, and may ask "why should I?" in response to instructions. He still has sexual curiosity though he may say or do little about it. He is interested in birth and prenatal development. Boy-girl pairs are common in school, and many of them plan to marry and move in with mother.

The seven-year-old wants a place in the family and is ready to take some light household responsibilities, such as emptying wastebaskets or making up his bed. Like the five-year-olds, they may assume a big brother or sister role to a younger child. Girls are frequently closer to the father and may be jealous of his attention toward the mother. The reverse is true of boys.

While he has a wonderful time with playmates, the seven-year-old is less intense than the six-year-old and can enjoy playing alone. Discrimination against the opposite sex is beginning. He can learn to swim, and bats better than he catches. He is adept at meeting strangers. He makes social contacts by physical means, perhaps by throwing a ball at a visitor.

In school he finds reading easier than spelling. He loves to color. He may be forgetful, and often others must reason with him. He can compromise but may be stubborn once his mind is made up. He wants and tries to be good, and is developing firmer ethical standards. He is gaining a concept of religion and may have some confusion with the idea of death.

The eight-year-old: This is an expansive, dramatic age, but one that is demanding of the mother's attention.

In physical fields, the eight-year-old is courageous and venturesome. Motions are faster and smoother. The ravenous appetite may need supervision. Some of these children can cut their own meat, but many do not do this for another year or two. Table habits are characterized by bolting of food and belching. Although he goes to bed later, he sleeps well. The eight-year-old is apt to try many things in a "know-it-all" way, but his interest is short. He needs encouragement and help in order to stick to a job. He is dramatic about most things, including himself. At about this age, boys become interested in their fathers' activities and want to do things with them. Girls turn their interest to their mothers. The child of this age feels his superiority and is less the big brother or sister with younger children than he was earlier. A bulletin board of daily chores helps him to accept responsibilities and keeps the parents from "yelling" at him. "Bosom" friendships are formed, and play is peaceful for longer periods of time. This play often dramatizes events or movies; but the girls, like their mothers, are prone to sit and "talk about things." Table games—checkers, dominoes, etc.—are important, but the child delights in magic and the absurd.

The eight-year-old is usually interested in school and may tell his mother more about it than he did in the earlier grades. Less interested in the teacher than formerly, he is more interested in his group. He likes variety and shifts more easily from subject to subject. He wants to know all about everything. He collects things and loves catalogues. His venturesome and curious attitude toward the world includes further questioning about sexual matters. Girls are especially apt to ask about sexual matters and are beginning to be inquisitive about menstruation. Their questions should be answered in a matter-of-fact, simple, intelligent way. When there is more open display of sexual interest, the parents must show understanding and care in handling the situation, rather than shaming and punishing them. Their play needs fairly close supervision.

The eight-year-old has begun to perceive that adults are not infallible. Cause-and-effect are more apparent to him; therefore, he likes to argue, and alibis are common. Time concepts are better established. He is interested in past events, but lacks chronological judgement. Space concept is also better established. He roams farther, and becomes interested in geography. By now he can tell the right hand from the left hand on another person—another special concept. Children of eight are often quite "money-mad," a trait parents can use as a motivation for other things as well as for teaching a child money values.

Children are now aware of the opposing forces of good and evil and want to be good. They need help in determining "good" and "bad," as they may regard them as absolutes. The sense of ownership is better established, and they are less apt to take something that belongs to another child. Because of the interest in money, they may take the household change. Parents are often upset by this, regarding it as much more serious than the seven-year-old's pilfering of pencils and erasers. If the child is given an allowance or is permitted to earn money, he has an opportunity to learn both property and money value. The eight-year-old child is becoming more truthful, at times even to his own detriment. His mother usually is the one to whom he confesses. If she is friendly, tolerant, and tactful, he will continue to feel free to tell her of misdeeds and failures. The eight-year-old has a continued religious interest. He has learned that everyone, including himself, will die. He begins to get a sense of himself as a person. The world and its forces are better understood.

The nine-year-old: The nine-year-old is neither quite a child nor an adolescent. For the most part, he does not depend on the parents or the group for motivation, but on himself. He thinks things over and plans for future action. He can work on several things for several hours at a stretch. An excellent pupil, he is willing to tackle nearly anything reasonable for his age and tries to perfect his skill by doing the same thing over and over. He has some power of self-appraisal. He measures not only his own behavior, but that of parents and other members of the family, and wants them to act "properly." He is better organized within himself and is more dependable, obedient, and easier to get along with. He may flare up with impatience, but not for long.

Eating is better controlled—the voracious appetite has tamed down, or the poor appetite is better. He is open and positive about food likes and dislikes. He can cut his meat and mind his table manners in company. Baths and bedtime are accepted without particular emotion. He still has to be reminded to brush his teeth. As at earlier ages, he has not learned to be neat about hanging up clothes.

COMMUNICABLE DISEASES OF CHILDHOOD

The series of pictures on this and the following pages portray some of the more characteristic symptoms of the common childhood diseases. All pictures are from Medichrome slides, by courtesy of Clay-Adams, New York. Sources of these are as follow: The picture of ringworm is from the collection prepared in cooperation with Dr. Rhoda W. Benham, Department of Dermatology, College of Physicians and Surgeons, Columbia University, New York. The picture of rheumatic fever was made in cooperation with Drs. Nathan Pensky and Natalie D. Goldberg, New York. Close-up of the arm in chicken pox is by Dr. Adolph Weinzirl of Portland, Oregon. The remaining slides were prepared by Dr. Franklin H. Top, Director, Division of Communicable Diseases and Epidemiology, Herman Kiefer Hospital and Detroit Department of Public Health.

He is not as squirming as before, but lets out tension in scuffling or in the finer motions, picking at fingers or fiddling. He slouches awkwardly and gets into unusual positions.

Nine-year-old children are loyal to friends and family, and are prone to admire members of their own sex. However, the two sexes are mutually disdainful of each other. In spite of this, they tease each other about getting married, and may be interested in kissing games in a playful and impersonal way. Hero worship is beginning at this age.

Only a little stimulus is needed to keep a nine-year-old in the right direction. Meeting a rude person may be all he needs to make him change spontaneously. The old fears have diminished; but more concrete worries, such as school grades, take their place. Having himself under better control, he does not need to be as boastful or aggressive. He still wants to please and likes praise, but he is not dependent on it. Some nine-year-old children are not well-organized and are wrapped up in their own activities. They may resent interference. Planning with these children ahead of time, or leaving written orders, helps get around this.

The nine-year-old is serious and businesslike. He is interested in learning and often collects an amazing array of facts about things that appeal to him. This intellectual trait makes his appraisal of himself and others more accurate.

He likes school, and may talk about it at home. Individual skills show up at this age. Because the nine-year-old is rather emotional and self-critical, it is important to make sure he can handle his work. Failure discourages him more than a younger child, and there is considerable classroom competition. Many ethical concepts develop. The child now has a better developed sense of fair play; he may be appealed to on this basis. He accepts blame justly assessed. His conscience is beginning to grow and often troubles him, despite his excuses and alibis. He is easily disciplined, and often threatened denial of a favorite pastime is enough to bring him into line.

The ten-year-old: At ten years of age, the child gives a fairly accurate picture of the sort of adult he will be, with regard not only to talents, but also to personality traits.

He is more relaxed with himself and his skills. He no longer has to practice the same thing time after time, but goes easily from one activity to another. His nervous system is controlled and integrated well enough so that he can talk at the same time he is working with his hands.

A child of ten years has a mind which is open to reason. Because of this, he is receptive to ideas and prejudices, either good or bad. Parents too often are unaware of his elementary ideas of such social problems as crime and racial

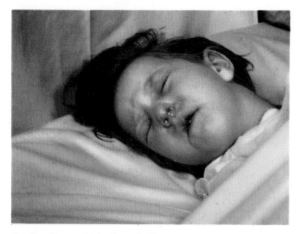

Scarlet fever, 10th day of illness

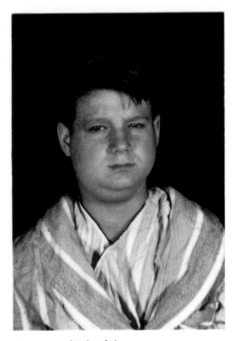

Mumps multiglandular

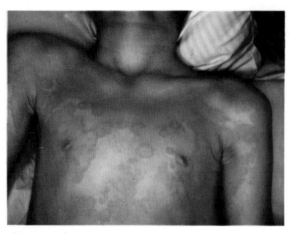

Rheumatic fever

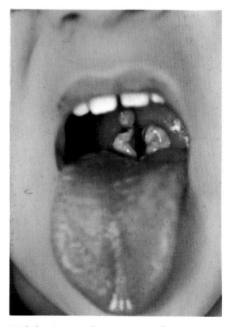

Diphtheria, membrane in mouth,
4th day of illness

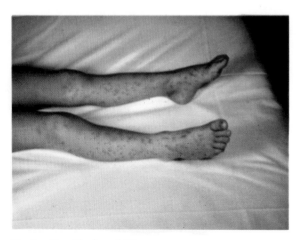

Meningitis, 4th day of illness

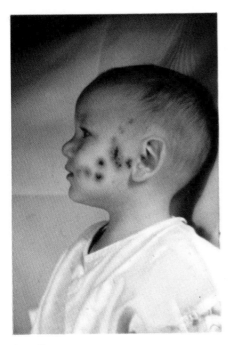

Impetigo

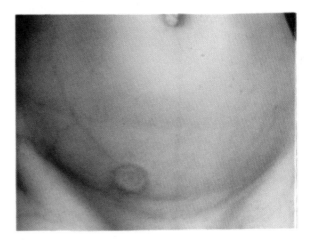

Ringworm

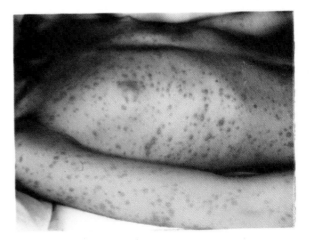

Chickenpox

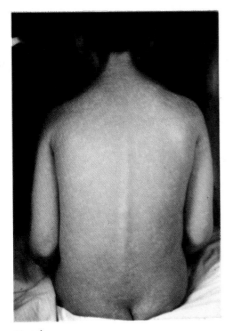

Measles

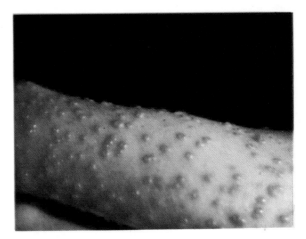

Chickenpox

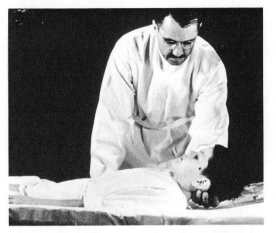

One of the characteristic symptoms of poliomyelitis is the stiff neck which is portrayed in the above photograph.

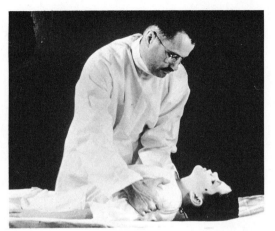

In poliomyelitis the paralysis of the neck muscles makes it impossible for the patient to hold his head erect.

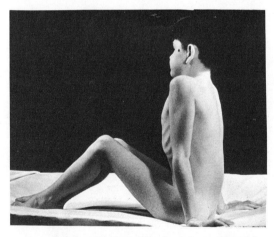

A characteristic stiffening of the back is another of the characteristic symptoms in some cases of poliomyelitis.

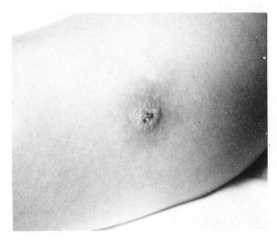

Site of a smallpox vaccination shows the appearance of an old scar with reaction exhibited by a new innoculation.

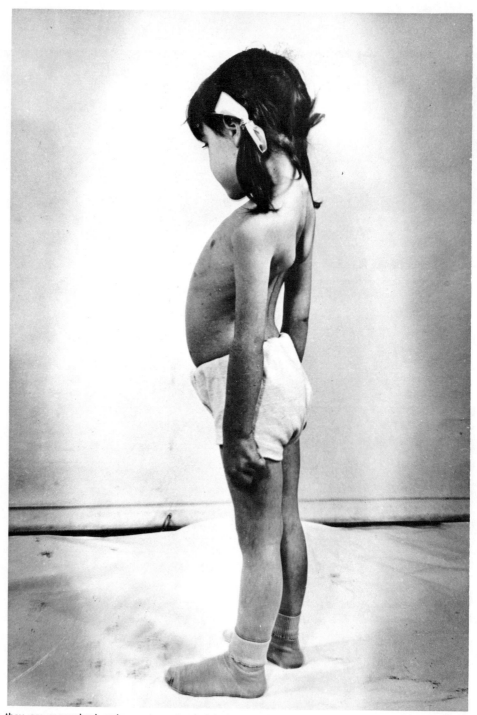

When they are recognized early, many postural defects seen in children can be remedied by proper corrective exercises and physiotherapy. Postural defects similar to that exhibited in the child pictured here can be caused either by poor posture habits or by more serious disorders such as poliomyelitis. Various mechanical devices aid in their correction.

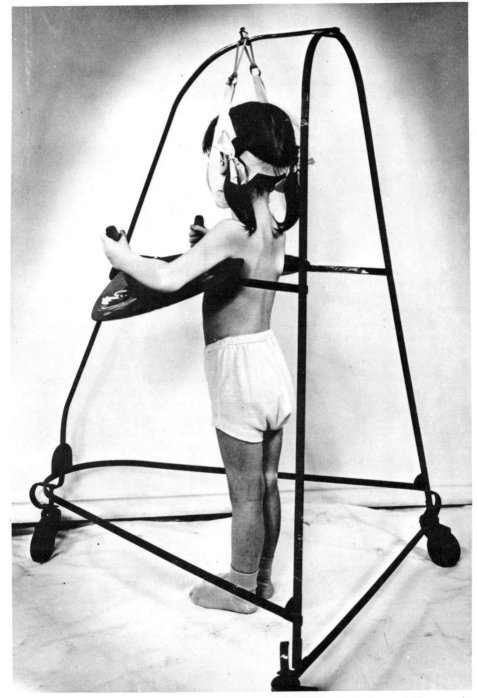

The 'walker' is a commonly employed corrective mechanism. Further details concerning corrective exercises and physiotherapy may be found in Chapter 9, "Skeleton and Muscles." *These Photographs by Courtesy of Inez Porter, Photography Department, St. Luke's Hospital, Chicago, and Medical Radiography and Photography, Copyright 1952.*

minorities. This is the time to plant liberalizing ideas.

Ten is a great age for gangs and secrets and for communication in notes or codes. These are not shared with members of the opposite sex. The boys wrestle and scuffle with each other as a sign of comradeship, while the girls write notes and gossip with one another.

The psychological differences in the sexes are apparent now. The girls show signs of approaching adolescence in their concern over their clothes, appearance, etc. Their interest in family life shows not only in their play but also in their awareness of emotional relationships and financial worries within the family.

Thus, by ten the child has acquired a clearer idea of himself, the world, and others in it. If he feels his world a friendly one, his adjustment is likely to reflect this. If he feels the world is hostile, he tends to react accordingly. Although the turbulent teens await him, they "do not transform the child, but they continue him."

Discipline

Parents should assume the role of a leader who deals with the child in a firm, friendly manner, considering his feelings. This does not mean that the child should rule the household, because he must learn that parents have rights which must be respected. If provided with firm and friendly control, he will have less anxiety. He will not always respond to this control, and punishment may be necessary at times. If the form of punishment used breaks the heart or spirit, it is wrong. Before age three, "take the consequen-

ces" type of punishment is of no help, because the baby is too young to understand. It is of little use before age *six*. Making a child feel guilty or ashamed has no place in his rearing. Parents should say what they have to say in clear, firm, unmistakable terms. They should not nag and harangue him for misdeeds. Threats to a child only carry a dare. If it is to be done, as taking skates away from him when he goes into the street, it is only fair to warn of this penalty beforehand. Parents should not make threats unless they are prepared to carry them out; they should be consistent in their demands and allowances. Children are thrown into confusion when their parents are inconsistent and vacillating in their disciplinary measures. When the parents punish the child for infraction of rules and then permit the rules to be violated, the child quite naturally loses his standard of conduct. In general, the child responds better to love than to punishment; better to respect than to threats; and better to relaxed and natural parents than to stern, overconscientious ones.

BEHAVIOR PROBLEMS

Behavior problems are not necessarily activities that are troublesome to the parents or other authorities. They are persistent patterns of reaction that interfere in relationships with other people or the satisfaction of needs. They are not emotional illnesses in themselves, but a sign that something physical or emotional is wrong in the child's life. What the problems are depends on the age and development of the child. They probably change and grow as the child matures, if the underlying causes of the problems are not corrected, or if he does not learn healthy ways of dealing with them.

A child's difficulty in getting along well in the world may arise from several sources. It may come from a physical condition that partially or totally handicaps him. The situation in which he lives or unpredictable events may trouble him. Or there may be specific emotional factors involved.

Emotional factors

Every child, regardless of his physical condition or his external environment, grows up in some sort of emotional atmosphere to which he must adjust. The parents set the emotional tone of the home; and if there are behavior problems, one place to look for the cause is in the parent-child relationship. If the child is acting in a way that is unacceptable to the parents, they should examine themselves to see if

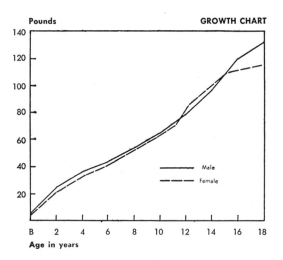

Chart showing average growth rate of boys and girls up to 18 years of age. *From Measurement of Man by Harris, Jackson, Paterson, and Scammon, Copyright 1930, The University of Minnesota Press.*

the fault lies with them. By becoming parents, men and women do not lose their own emotional conflicts, nor do these conflicts necessarily become less. Indeed, having children may create new conflicts or stir up old ones. In turn, the parents' troubles often stem from their own unhappy childhood. It has been shown that children of "good" fathers and mothers tend to grow up to be "good" fathers and mothers themselves. Marital problems of the parents often lead to unhealthy attitudes toward the children. If one parent displays more affection toward the child than toward the mate, the mate is apt to become jealous of the child without being aware of it. If the parents cannot make enough money to support the family properly, another child is often regarded as an additional burden.

Some studies indicate that the attitude and behavior of the mother are stronger influences on the formation of the child's personality than those of the father. This does not mean that the father cannot have an equally important part in rearing the child—if he will accept it. The child certainly should have happy relations with both parents.

Of greatest importance is the degree to which the parents accept or reject the child. A parent who is unable to demonstrate affection and approval because of his own emotional difficulties may appear as hostile and unloving to the child as a person who actually dislikes him. Parents reject their children for many reasons. Matrimonial unhappiness is one; a constantly quarreling couple about to separate or divorce will find less pleasure in the child than a well-adjusted couple. In some instances, pregnancies may be planned and looked forward to as a means of stopping certain behavior in the mate. Thus, a child conceived to liven the husband's failing ambition or to stop the wife's flirtations may be resented and rejected if the baby's arrival does not have the desired affect on the mate. The parents may be unstable, neurotic people who are incapable of good relationships with anyone. The arrival of a baby places responsibility on such parents, and thereby may deprive one or the other parent of the privilege of being a "child." Rejection may be so open that the child is given away to foster parents.

Parents may delude themselves into thinking that nagging, scolding, and punishment are for the child's correction. Subtler forms of rejection are no less damaging and perhaps harder for the child to combat. The sign of rejection may be little more than a derisive shrug of the shoulders or a hard and unsympathetic expression. It may be a cold, unemotional attitude of the parent who frowns on fondling and cuddling the child so that he "won't be spoiled." Or perhaps praise is not granted lest the child become too impudent. At other times rejection causes the parents to feel guilty, so that they try to compensate for their own discomfort by lavishing the child with constant false affection. Their constant apprehension—that the child might get sick and die, that he will get into trouble, that he might not be able to do things—betrays the underlying hostile feelings. Constant insistence that the child be perfect in every way shows the hostile refusal to accept him as he is and the attempt to make him over.

The child's response to rejection depends largely on the form it takes. "The neglected child retaliates with delinquency or other forms of hostile aggressiveness; the spoiled child gets back by dominating the spoilers; the coerced child of perfectionistic parents often comes to look for reasons of parental disapproval within himself and faces life with perpetually guilty insecurity."

The child who is truly accepted is usually a well-adjusted, cooperative, friendly, and cheerful person. He takes care of his own and others' property, and he is less confused and rebellious. He evaluates himself realistically and faces the future with more confidence.

Dominance-submission

The degree to which the parent dominates or submits to the child is an important factor in the parent-child relationship. It depends more on the personality of the individual parent than on the marital adjustment. The mother is more apt to go to extremes than the father, because the care of the children is primarily the mother's duty. Her need to dominate or submit is easily satisfied in the home. The father's need is usually satisfied in his work outside the home. A dominating parent may be as accepting or rejecting as a submissive one. The dominating parent closely supervises or restricts the child's choices and activities. Such a mother is especially prone to be ambitious for her child socially and intellectually. He is beaten, cajoled, or persuaded into a life not of his own choosing, depending on the feelings the parent has for him. Submissive parents are ruled by the child. These parents may be merely lax, careless, and easygoing, or simply not interested enough to put reasonable curtails on the child's behavior. Sometimes the parents seem to need to indulge the child and to get actual enjoyment from submitting to his whims and tyranny. The parents do this while complaining loudly and protesting ineffectually.

Children of dominating parents are better socialized than are the children of submissive parents. They show their more acceptable behavior by being courteous and obedient, and have good attitudes in school. But, they have traits that cause trouble for them too. They may be more sensitive, self-conscious, submissive, shy, and seclusive, and find difficulty in self-expression. Children of submissive parents may be irresponsible and disobedient, lacking in sustained interest and attention. On the positive side, these children are forward and can express themselves effectively and are more dominating and independent themselves.

Other attitudes

Other children in the home, or grandparents there, also subject the child to their own attitudes. But again, the parents set the tone. If they are genuinely loving, they will see that each child gets affection and approval in tokens acceptable to him. Differences arising among the children will be settled justly but with the minimum intrusion. All the children will be protected from unreasonable demands or unhealthy attitudes of others.

A grandparent, according to his feeling about the child, may have an effect on the child equal to that of the parent. Another problem arises when grandparents or other adults live with the family: the problem of authority. The adults may use the child to force certain concessions and ways of behaving from one another. The child himself may try to play one of them against another for his own needs. In either case, the child is apt to be confused by conflicting commands and resentful of too many bosses.

When the child goes to school, his emotional world has new and strange additions to it. If he has found home and the people in it loving and accepting, he will assume that the rest of the world and its occupants are the same. Although this assumption cannot be uniformly true, his behavior is less apt to provoke hostility from his new world. If the persons in his home have been hostile and rejecting, he will feel as though all the world is the same way, and act according to this belief. Warm, accepting teachers can help change his behavior patterns. A child, rejected the first six years of his life, cannot change his pattern of behavior overnight when he finds an understanding teacher. Indeed, he will go out of his way to test this acceptance until he can be sure that the teacher's warm feelings remain regardless of what he does. If the teacher fails to meet these tests, she becomes a replica of the parents, and the child has no haven anywhere. If she passes the tests, she may be able to heal a part of the damage already done.

Environment

Money and luxuries neither prevent nor cause behavior problems. The location of the home is important as it gives the child an idea of what the world in general is like. For example,

if he sees the neighbors frequently quarreling or brawling, he perhaps assumes that the whole world is hostile and aggressive. It makes a difference if his family is accepted or rejected by the neighbors. If the family has to move often, the child finds it hard to get a sense of belonging to any group. He feels lonely and may stay to himself rather than risk another loss. With the feeling of "what's the use" he may resort to daydreaming and excessive masturbation, since he may feel that these activities are more reliable sources of pleasure than friends whom he may soon have to leave. Extreme crowding at home may destroy the child's sense of individuality. In an effort to "hold on to himself," he may become irritable and boastful to cover up his strain.

Physical causes

Behavior problems may arise as the child unsuccessfully attempts to adjust to some physical difficulty. The condition may make it hard for the child to compete with or keep up with other children of his own age. It may cause his fellows or his parents to reject him. If these things happen, the child will become anxious, feel unworthy, and react by becoming more aggressive or by withdrawing.

A child with a physical handicap is aware that he is different from other children. If the parents have handled him lovingly and intelligently, this probably will have no serious effect on his personality. If they have failed, he may feel ashamed and inferior and unable to face other difficulties. He may withdraw into a world of his own. He may demand the center of attention by picking arguments, fighting, lying, or stealing.

Mental retardation

Mentally retarded children show poor judgment, see little relation between cause and effect, and are easily led. The parents, unaware of the child's diminished intellectual powers, try to train him as they would a normal child. When he is slow in sitting up crawling, walking, etc., they have the first inkling that something is the matter and redouble their efforts with him, trying desperately to prove their suspicions wrong. Although the child responds with his best effort, nevertheless he fails often and begins to feel that he is worthless and disappointing to his parents and that they do not like him. When at last the parents must admit their child's difficulty, they begin to feel not only pity and sympathy, but also resentment, irritation, guilt, and hopeless apprehension. To protect themselves from their hostile feelings, they may become overprotective to the child and not allow him to do even what he is able, holding him back from trying new activities. They may feel ashamed of him or be openly irritable and rejecting. Any of these reactions lessens the child's security, places additional burdens on him, and decreases the use of the capacities he does have. This critical attitude may be mirrored by brothers, sisters, other children, and adults who are not members of the family. The retarded child, his resentment now thoroughly aroused by this constant barrage of hostility, may become destructive and aggressive. If he cannot respond by fighting back, he may try to escape by running away from home, playing hooky from school, and avoiding other children his own age. He may be teased and annoyed until he loses all control and commits a violent act in retaliation. He may be led into delinquency by anyone who seems to be good to him, repaying this person with obedience. He is often the scapegoat for more intelligent friends. If he does not become delinquent, he finds it hard to get a job, harder to hold one, and may be forced into a life of petty thievery, vagrancy, and begging.

Brain injury

The behavior difficulties of the child whose brain is injured by disease or accident are somewhat different from those of the mentally retarded, though retardation may also be a factor. This child shows normal mental and personality development until the particular illness or injury. After the injury, the child is extremely active, finding it impossible to be still even when threatened and punished, and is distractable and impulsive. He is given to explosive outbursts of anger and aggressiveness and destroys things at home and in school. He may respond well to certain medication, but occasionally some of these children have to be put in special institutions.

Undetected partial blindness or deafness may create serious difficulties for the child. Children are curious and conscious of their abilities in relation to other children. A first-grade child, unable to hear or see clearly, cannot recognize the sounds and letters he must learn in order to read. He thus misses a basic vocabulary which he cannot make up for in higher grades. The confusion of the printed page becomes greater, and the child becomes more tense and anxious. If he is regarded as stupid by the teachers or fellow students, the emotional factors become greater. Feeling disliked and disapproved of, he may react by hating school and by being truant from it, or he may resort to crying and temper tantrums to quell his inner fears.

Dyslexia

A child who has difficulty learning to read and write may not be brain damaged or mentally retarded. Unfortunately, many children with the condition known as minimal brain dysfunction or dyslexia exist as "shadow children" and are never properly helped.

Dyslexic children are of normal or above normal intelligence. Because of lack of certain neurological connections in the brain, visual signs and symbols do not make much sense to them. They are "mirror readers" of words and numbers and often secretly compensate for their inability to learn to read by memorizing things read to them.

Some dyslexic children are overactive, or hyperkinetic. Some may have emotional problems compounded by frustration and lack of understanding from parents and teachers. They may be physically clumsy. Left-handedness is sometimes a sign of reversed muscular dominance, but not a symptom of dyslexia by itself.

Minimal brain dysfunction is inherited and is passed on to boys four times as often as to girls. When adequately helped, all can achieve satisfactory intellectual progress. Phonetic approaches to reading work better for those with a slight degree of dyslexia.

Eye exercises do not aid such children to overcome dyslexia. The American Association of Ophthalmologists warns against such fraudulent treatment.

Some drugs are administered to overactive children to calm them and energize their minds. Such drugs will not aid those children who are not dyslexic.

Diagnosis and treatment of dyslexic children is made by neurologists. There are special clinics for neurological disorders in every large city or university center. Pediatricians are knowledgeable sources of information and for referral.

How behavior problems are expressed

Behavior problems in general are the child's reaction to, and attempt to solve, his problems. He will do this with whatever means he has. Certain functions such as eating, sleeping, toilet habits, or sexual acts may serve as the outlet. Refusal to eat may be rebellion at nagging, oversolicitous parents or an attempt to get attention from indifferent ones. One child may wet the bed because he is encouraged to remain infantile, while another may wet to spite a harsh mother. Impaired intellectual functions such as speech and learning may point up the problem. A child may be slow in talking because he is mentally retarded, partially deaf, or because "smothering has retarded growth and prolonged the stage of pouting and crying." Poor school work and even failing grades do not necessarily mean mental retardation. This happens in children of superior intelligence when insecurity, frustration, and anxiety make them incapable of learning. Temporary slumps may come if there is anxiety about dissension in the home, illness or death in the family, or jealousy of another brother or sister enjoying the mother alone at home.

It is seen that the same symptoms may come from many different causes. Therefore, each behavior problem must be dealt with individually if it is to be solved successfully.

What can be done

Intelligent parents who are sympathetic and sensitive to the child's needs can handle most behavior problems themselves. They are not shocked, angered, or panicked by undesirable attitudes or behavior of their child. Instead, they look for the cause. Any child in a new situation, such as starting to school or the arrival of a new baby in the family, will probably become tense and anxious and show some type of behavior difficulty. The parents' role here is to help in the solution rather than act as a judge and jury. Realities, such as school or a new sister, must be accepted. If the parents support the child's self-confidence and self-esteem, these become constructive experiences rather than the groundwork of future difficulties. Sometimes the problems are small—whose game is to be played, for instance —and the wise parent does not interfere. Sometimes the problem is too big for solution and may have to be removed altogether—an older, hateful bully may have to be forbidden to play with younger children. Parents can see their own insecurities mirrored in the child and should control these as much as possible when dealing with him or with others in his presence. Parents who have good understanding of themselves can see some of their habits or attitudes which have a bad effect, and many can change these without seeking outside help.

Sometimes troublesome behavior persists after the parents have conscientiously tried to understand and correct the cause, or the trouble may be thought of as physical illness. In either case, they may take the child to a physician. He may find some physical condition that explains the difficulty and prescribe the proper remedy. For example, a hearing aid for a partially deaf child may be the answer. If there is something physically wrong, the child ought to be told in general, reassuring terms what it is, what can be done, and how the remedy will make him more comfortable. Children adjust better to chronic handicaps that are more easily recognized. Thus, a crippled child is apt to be less rebellious than a diabetic child who does not realize that he is sick and yet must tolerate injections and strict diets.

If the symptom has an emotional rather than a physical basis, the physician may treat the child himself or refer the family to a psychiatrist or child-guidance clinic. In some cases, he may see readily the harmful influence to which the child is reacting. Some parents may be able to alter the influence on their own initiative, once it is recognized and understood. In other cases, it is necessary for both the parents and the child to have special treatment. It does little good to help a child rid himself of unhealthy reactions to parental rejection, overprotection, or domination if the parents do not rid themselves of these unhealthy attitudes. "They are neither villains nor fools," but their behavior as parents is determined by their own emotional conflicts. If they sincerely want to help their child, they will not be angry or offended when psychiatric help is suggested. Rather, they will welcome it as another method of understanding themselves and the child. They must have expert advice to be ready for the altered behavior of the child, since this may vary considerably from their preconceived ideas of the way he should behave. A shy, quiet, withdrawn child in the process of gaining self-confidence may have a period of overactive aggression before he "settles down" into a more mature pattern. In some cases, other special forms of treatment may be needed, such as speech correction or remedial reading. They may be used alone or with psychotherapy.

Behavior problems are more easily prevented than cured. When the baby is born, good parents give him a sense of security by fondling and cuddling him. They meet his needs as promptly and completely as possible. Thus, they do not insist that he wait four hours to get his milk when he awakes hungry in three hours. Solid foods are introduced gently, and no issue is made if the baby refuses them at first. The baby can be prepared for weaning, his first major privation, by allowing him to drink small amounts of liquid from a spoon and then a cup while he is being "cuddled." Toilet training is a function that should start when the child himself is ready for it, rather than when the time is set arbitrarily according to the calendar. Parents need have no fear of spoiling the child by openly showing love and approval in terms a child can understand. Genuine love is what the child must have. Material luxuries, showy "sacrifices," or strict adherence to the "rules" of child rearing are no substitutes. Acceptance means respect for their child as an individual, not merely as their baby. It does not mean full condonation of everything he does. The child must be accepted for what he *is* rather than what he *does*. If this is firmly fixed in his mind, he can take correction without feeling rejected. Parents should be consistent in their attitudes toward him. Friendliness interrupted by hostility is very anxiety-provoking. Even consistent hostility is easier for the child to adjust to, because he can at least hate without guilt. The demands made on the child should also be consistent. A child should be able to predict what he can do today by what he was allowed to do yesterday. Only by consistent attitudes does the child know how he stands with other people.

Parents must not only fill the child's physical and emotional needs, but prepare him realistically for the world in which he lives. His repeated failure of reasonable conformity to the group will lead to his rejection by many other people later on. Thus, the question of parental authority complicates the picture—to accept the child without reservation and yet to insist on certain patterns of behavior seems impossible and paradoxical. If parents can anticipate problems before they arise, much can be done to ease the child into them unobtrusively by previous preparation of the child for new experiences. Many impasses can be avoided by offering the child positive action rather than only forbidding action. When correction is necessary, the parents should be sure the child understands that criticism is applied to the act rather than to himself. Most of the time, the fully accepted child will conform to family patterns because of friendly relations between him and his parents. The parents should not expect the child to conform more closely to these standards than they themselves.

Children grow up to be normal, healthy individuals, survive many errors on the part of the parents, and suffer through many whippings and scoldings, if they feel a real sense of love and interest in them as worthwhile persons.

THE TEEN-AGER

Growth during the first ten years of life proceeds at a fairly uniform rate. The child's desires usually keep pace with his ability to meet his needs. However, during the adolescent or teen-age period, there is disharmony between physiological development, growth, and emotional maturation. The teen-ager becomes a blend of maturity and immaturity in body, mind, and emotion. A little knowledge and understanding on the part of mature people can usually aid in bringing the teen-ager through this trying period.

Puberty

Puberty, which refers to the sexual maturation of the individual, is only part of adolescence. Puberty and adolescence begin in the girl at eleven to 15 years of age; boys lag about a year behind. The average age for puberty in girls in the United States is around 13.5 years and in boys 14.5 years. Adolescence in most American youths terminates at about 19 years of age. Adolescence extends from puberty to the attainment of adulthood. The first half of adolescence is characterized more by physical growth and change; the latter half brings more intellectual and emotional changes.

Adolescent growth varies widely between individuals; failure to realize this may cause unnecessary anxiety to both parents and child. Growth rate is influenced by the state of health and nutrition. Not only is there variability in the growth of different individuals, but growth within the single individual is not harmonious. Certain parts of the body grow while others lag behind. The child may grow tall without putting on weight, or he may show more sexual maturity than maturity of the digestive organs. This organ imbalance leads to organ instability. Thus, laziness and awkwardness result. In the average boy, the period of greatest height increase is from about 12 to 14.5 years, although they continue to grow until about the age of 18. They gain most of their weight between the ages of 13 and 16. Girls grow tallest from about 10.5 to 14 years; maximum weight development is from about ages 11.5 to 14.5. As much as 6 inches in height and 25 pounds in weight may be gained within a single year.

Parents and children may show concern about growth and maturation (timing and degree of development of secondary sexual characteristics) during the adolescent years. The evaluation of growth data is difficult at all ages, but is particularly so during puberty. Individual variability in growth patterns is the rule, and the variation may be extreme, especially during the pubertal spurt phase. Since the slow maturer and a rapid maturer of the same age may appear four or five years apart in age, the published curves and graphs for "normal" growth must be examined with care. Genetic influences may be strong and may explain the difference.

Puberty in the boy is marked by growth of the sexual organs and the beginning of their functions. Boys are usually more aware of maturity than are girls. "Wet dreams" (*nocturnal emissions*) may occur at night and are often the source of embarrassment and fright for the boy. He may be plagued by *erections* at inopportune moments. Secondary sexual changes may add to his discomfort. His voice deepens; his shoulders broaden; his muscles harden; his legs lengthen; his hands and feet grow disproportionately large. Appearance of the beard and necessity for shaving are subject to many comments. The adolescent boy is almost certain to masturbate; this may be to a greater or lesser extent, according to the degree he is driven by increasing physical and emotional tension.

Adolescent girls have somewhat different difficulties. Arrival of the first menstrual period may be a shocking and frightening event to the girl who has not been prepared; or if she was improperly prepared, she may find this a revolting experience. Menstrual irregularity and pain are common the first year or so, usually without significance; but unless the girl and the parents both understand this, there may be some anxiety. During her periods, the adolescent girl may be irritable, and she is almost always anxious about stains on her clothes. The broadening of hips, development of breasts, and appearance of pubic hair usually parallel the beginning of menstruation, but are subject to wide variation. The girl who has been improperly taught by her family may find her new femininity embarrassing and unacceptable. Both boy and girl teen-agers are self-conscious about acne and other skin eruptions characteristic of the adolescent period. Unlike her brother, a girl is quite upset by the appearance of heavy hair on the face and arms. Driven by many of the same tensions as the adolescent boy, she too may masturbate.

Regardless of how the teen-ager, boy or girl, accepts sexual development—either with great pride and interest or with embarrassment and secretiveness—both are preoccupied with their bodies and unable to take their growth for granted.

Obesity is often a problem in this period and may be a factor in delayed puberty. Whether the condition is the result of poor eating habits, of emotional instability, or of endocrine dysfunction, it merits careful investigation.

In delayed onset of puberty, sound physical and mental hygiene solves most of the problems of an endocrine nature. This conservative approach utilizes the inherent forces of the body which allow the transition to be made normally. The child whose adolescent period is delayed should be under the care and observation of a physician, so that when the indications for therapy are clear, he may begin as early as is deemed necessary.

Emotional factors in adolescence

To ignore the emotional factors in adolescence is really to ignore the most crucial and important aspect of the adolescent years. The physical changes could be handled relatively easily by these young people if that were all they had to deal with; but many other problems come about as a result of, and in addition to, these bodily changes. No longer a child, the teen-ager has many childish wishes and habits. Not an adult, he has many adult emotions and adult problems. He longs for the pleasures of childhood, yet rebels against the restrictions imposed on children. He longs for the pleasures of adulthood and rebels against the responsibilities. The family's attitude often is as inconstant as the teen-ager's. They alternately dominate him as though he were an irresponsible child, and yet, demand adult attitudes from him. This easily results in feelings of estrangement, confusion, and isolation in the teen-ager. Since he is unable to understand his peculiar position in the family, he

often loses his former intimate contact with his parents. He masks his insecurity with cockiness or rationalizes his isolation with arrogance.

Normally, adolescence should be a period in which the main emotional ties with the parents begin to give way to wider interests and relationships. Usually this is accomplished with a good deal of rebellion against all forms of authority, particularly parental authority. The teen-ager may begin to think his parents do not know what is going on in the modern world. The more strenuous the parents are in efforts to keep their children from becoming emotionally mature, the more apt the rebellion is to be pronounced and painful. One mark of emotional maturity is the ability to say "no," to decide things for oneself despite the opinion of others, and to go ahead in the face of opposition. However, when the child begins to exhibit this type of behavior, many parents feel their authority threatened. They begin to wonder what happened to their formerly obedient child and why he has suddenly become so difficult. He may show his new status by merely discarding his former good manners, or by the excessive use of slang to bewilder his elders. He may be careless in his dress and hygiene in order to show his revolt. A phase quite marked in adolescence, the wish to reform the whole social and economic system, is based not only on revolt against the established forms, but also on a certain amount of idealism.

The teen-ager has less fear of showing his aggression than does the young child. Normally, the aggression finds its outlets in hard-fought games and sports, in arguing, or perhaps in reckless driving. Every generation has its psychological equivalent of the "hot rod." Parents should not be too shocked if they learn of petty pilfer-

(text continued on p. 69)

DEVELOPMENT OF THE FEMALE BREAST

Photography . . . F. W. Schmidt.

The following series of photographs of front and side views of girls at different ages from eight to fourteen years illustrate the normal changes that occur in the development of the breasts during puberty. The exact age at which any particular phase of development occurs depends largely upon the individual child, the racial stock from which she originates, and still other factors, so that any particular stage may appear a year or two earlier or later. There is also considerable variation in the rate of development and in anatomical appearance, so that no absolute set of standards may be established, but rather broad normal ranges of breast growth, size, and shape.

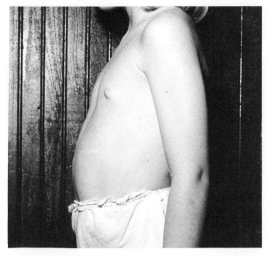

8 years of age

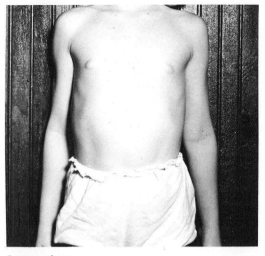

8 years of age

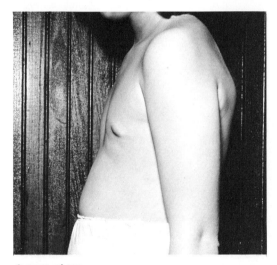

9 years of age

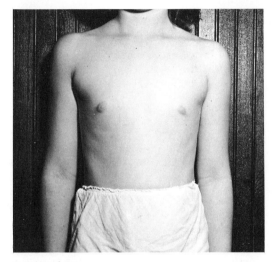

9 years of age

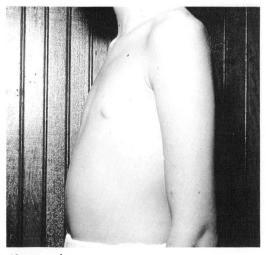

10 years of age

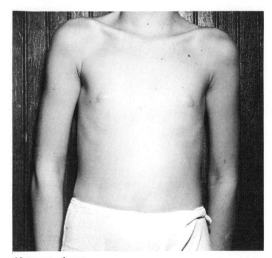

10 years of age

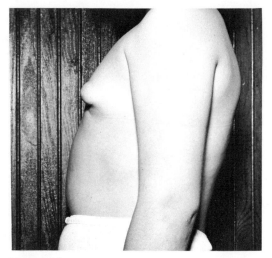

11 years of age

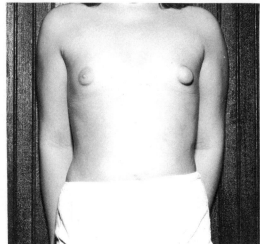

11 years of age

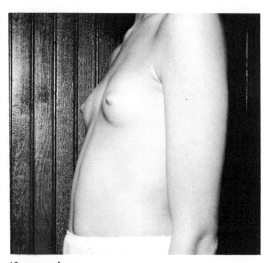

12 years of age

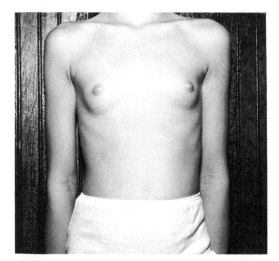

12 years of age

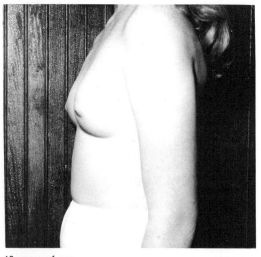

13 years of age

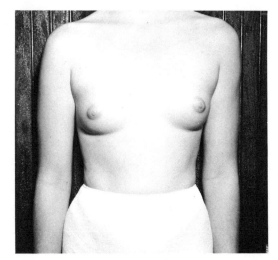

13 years of age

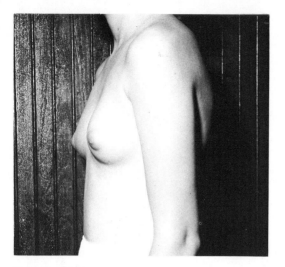

14 years of age   14 years of age

ing or lying during this period. These more serious asocial forms of aggression and rebellion should be handled kindly, but justly punished. Both overharsh punishment and overprotection for this behavior invite later trouble.

Group identification

Apparently paradoxical with this rebellion against authority is the conformity to the group so paramount in the teen-ager's thinking. Adolescents may set up their own moral standards and values and exert the pressure of those standards on other teen-agers. Psychiatrists call this "adolescent peer-culture." Boys and girls desiring the approval of their friends must follow the fashion of their set in matters of morals, dress, speech, etc. This encourages social participation, group loyalty, and individual achievement and responsibility. It also brings about certain problems. At times, particularly in the smaller groups, cliques may dominate either the school or the church, electing their own candidates to school offices and setting the social pace to the exclusion of those teen-agers not accepted. Those excluded from the social life of the reigning set attempt to make life for themselves with other unaccepted adolescents. This rejected group may react with defiant behavior, rowdyism, truancy, etc., which isolate them even more from their other schoolmates. The individual who cannot make the grade with either group may be either delinquent, or bookish and withdrawn, depending on his inner needs. School may then seem to be a prison from which he tries to escape, and the school authorities may be rather heavy-handed with him. Some parents of unaccepted children alternately punish the children and accuse the school authorities of favoritism. Often the leaders of the ac-

cepted set are leaders by virtue of their families' wealth and prestige, and deviant groups are excluded on a financial basis. The teachers of the school may fall in with the leaders in the social groups, because they represent "the best families." This makes the unaccepted teen-agers even more bitter and frustrated.

The emotional life of adolescence is full of paradoxes. Utterly self-centered, the teen-ager is nevertheless capable of much self-sacrificing devotion. He turns from the gang to complete solitude. Idealism of the loftiest sort is present side by side with the most selfish materialism. Sensitive himself, he can be cruelly inconsiderate of others. Sensual indulgence may alternate with asceticism.

But why is he like this? With oncoming sexual maturity, the teen-ager finds many new and disturbing changes in himself and his relation to the world. He tries various ways of dealing with his changing body and emotions in order to regain the stability and security he once had. Sexuality as a part of the personality must be accepted, as must other adult roles. Because of the prohibitions imposed on him during childhood, the adolescent has a mistrust of many "body instincts," especially those which are primarily sexual. He may refuse any sort of pleasure normal for his age. The renunciation may be only mild, such as giving up nice clothes or parties. Occasionally one sees this carried to extremes so that the teen-ager is denying himself any physical comforts. Then there may be a sudden break through this defense, followed by indulgence in all that he formerly prohibited. Increased intellectual activity, delving into problems of the abstract and unfamiliar, often occurs. The sweep of problems that the teen-agers discuss and try to solve may be immense.

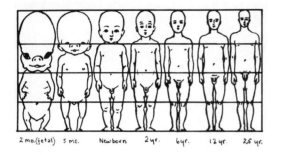

2 mo.(fetal) 5 mo.   Newborn   2 yr.   6 yr.   12 yr.   25 yr.

This drawing illustrates the relative size of the head and trunk in persons of various ages. *From Growth by Robbins, Brody, Hogan, Jackson, and Greene, Copyright 1928, The Yale University Press.*

In an effort to break away from parental ties, the teen-ager forms many new and experimental relationships. "Hero-worship" is a common type of emotional attachment at his age. Usually an older person is the object—a teacher, an adult friend, or a movie actor or singer. There does not have to be even an acquaintance between the teen-ager and his adored one. This sort of attachment is, of course, a substitute for the abandoned parent.

Romantic attachments begin also. The boy-girl relationship may come on gradually or suddenly. The affair blazes high, burns brightly, then goes out as suddenly as it began; the love is transferred to someone else, and the pattern is repeated. The reason for this is that the loved one has failed to live up to the ideal the lover has of him; quarrels ensue, and the disillusioned one starts a search for the ideal lover again. Unwise associations are to be expected, but parents should not use their authority to stop them. This may drive the friendship underground and lessen the parents' already tenuous influence over the teen-ager. The wise parent refrains from critical or comical comments on his youngster's current "crush." Instead, he is encouraging and quietly thankful that this normal transition has occurred. Moreover, the teen-ager is learning how to appraise the opposite sex and to select more wisely in the future.

When interest in one particular boy or girl develops to the exclusion of all others, teen-agers begin to "go steady." They have little interest in group activities but prefer to enjoy movies, dances, or long rides with the loved one. Probably, they will indulge in a certain amount of "necking" or "petting." These activities are practiced almost universally. They provide an outlet for some of the sex drive that is so strong at that time; they are not abnormal nor a sign of depravity. Movies and their glamorous love scenes, little chaperonage, broken home life—all these contribute to the teen-ager's preoccupation with "petting." Fear of not being popular, infatuation,

curiosity, feeling of obligation to their dates, lack of courage, and the idea that petting is expected of them are other reasons they indulge. But, whatever the immediate cause, the basic reason for their sexual overtures is the simple fact that they are arriving at sexual maturity and are subjected to the basic sexual drives without which the race would doubtless perish.

The end of adolescence

Physical maturity is reached when the body has its final height and has assumed adult proportions. The secondary sexual characteristics are fully developed, and the sexual functions have been established. While physical maturity is easy to assess, emotional maturity is much more difficult. People who become angry at trivial things, who depend on older members of the same or opposite sex for their happiness, who are easily hurt, or who run away from reality, are not emotionally mature adults. To accept reality is difficult and is the characteristic of maturity. To know one's limitations, to be able to work with them contentedly, and to suit one's life to one's capacities, is to be emotionally mature. To search for thrills, to refuse to compromise, is adolescent.

Social immaturity is characterized by blind loyalty to one's friends or blind prejudice against other people. Emancipation from the parental ties does not mean calloused indifference to the parents, because that is also adolescent in nature. A true adult loves his parents, takes their desires into consideration, but makes his own decisions and lives his own life. The teen-ager may feel insecure in various social relationships. While an adult may feel this way in the beginning of a relationship, he adjusts quickly to ordinary and recurrent social situations. An adolescent conforms rather rigidly to his own small group of friends. Of course, this same thing is seen in adults.

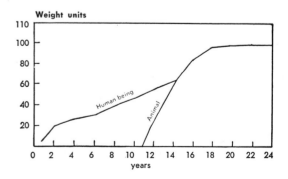

Weight units

The early growth of the child is much more gradual than that of most other animals. This chart illustrates the slow growth rate of a human being compared to the relatively fast rate of other animals.

Parents who are rigid and authoritarian are bound to be disturbed by rebellion in their children. Those parents who are emotionally immature will feel threatened at the realization that their children are growing up and that they themselves are no longer "young." Even good parents are apt to be confused and occasionally hurt if they forget their own adolescence and their sense of humor.

But how are these unpredictable young people to be dealt with? A certain amount of responsibility should be expected of the teen-ager in the home. The duties of homework, passing his courses in school, helping keep the yard, and washing windows now and then are not too much to ask. Girls should help with housework and learn the art of homemaking as they grow up. An allowance, not too small, yet not too exorbitant, with bonuses for extra work has worked out well for some parents. These near-adults should not be forced to beg and tease like children for money and privileges; this only encourages other childish attitudes. Unwise use of money and privilege is to be expected. These may be valuable lessons if the parents can point out the errors in a warm, friendly way without preaching a sermon. The teen-ager should solve problems of his own making, make his own apologies, and accept his own responsibilities with as little help or interference as possible. The teen-ager needs, along with romance, social activities, and hobbies to provide sublimation of his emotions and energies. A part-time job, with remuneration, is valuable experience. Work that will take too much of the time from studies, however, will defeat its purpose.

Parents should be alert for danger signals pointing to the teen-ager's failure to handle his problems. An ascetic mode of existence maintained too long or too rigorously must be investigated. Parents are often foolishly thankful that their child is a quiet, aloof intellectual who does not bother them with hoards of hungry friends and silly crushes. They should realize that such withdrawal is an unhealthful substitute for human relationships. Teen-agers who are preoccupied almost exclusively with abstract subjects such as mathematics, physics, religion, and philosophy are more likely to be mental patients than mental giants. Indifference to the current fads of the group indicates a feeling of estrangement and isolation. Too slavish conformity to the group may also indicate insecurity in the feeling of belonging.

The ideal parents allow the child to grow up without passing on to him their own maladjustments. They are willing to modify the routines of the home and its appearance to a reasonable degree. They offer security in time of stress. They are willing to try to provide guiding models of attitude and behavior. They are also willing to be stimulating and interesting companions.

The turbulence of adolescence is greatly calmed by parents who are willing to become friends and to be sought out as other friends. If the old relationship assumes this new form, the parents take pride in an adolescent who will become a mature, stable adult.

CHILDHOOD DISEASES

Chicken pox

Chicken pox (*varicella*) is an acute, contagious disease marked by eruptions of the skin. It is generally regarded as a disease of childhood, but adults may also contract it. Children of all ages may be affected, although newborn infants are thought to possess some degree of temporary immunity. The *incubation period* (time from exposure to onset of the disease) is usually 11 to 19 days.

Manner of transmission: Chicken pox is caused by a virus and is usually transmitted directly from person to person and occasionally by indirect contact through the air or by contact with objects used by an infected person. An infected person may transmit chicken pox about two days before the rash appears and up to 14 days afterward. The period of infectiousness averages about 14 days. One attack of chicken pox ordinarily produces permanent immunity to the disease. Relapses and second attacks are rare.

Symptoms: A slight rise in temperature, loss of appetite, headache, and backache are sometimes the initial symptoms of chicken pox, but often a rash or skin eruptions appear first. The initial skin eruptions are reddened spots (*macules*) about the size of a pinhead; they characteristically appear first in patches on the trunk, although occasionally a typical lesion or sore is seen on one of the hands or feet, or on the face, before eruptions appear on the trunk. Within a few hours after the appearance of the macules, they enlarge and a small blister (*vesicle*) filled with a clear fluid forms in the center of each spot. The fluid turns yellow after about 24 hours, and a crust or scab forms within 36 hours. The crust peels off in from five to 20 days, the time depending on the depth to which the skin has been penetrated. All of the eruptions do not appear at once, but in series or crops; the length and the severity of the disease is dependent in part upon the number of series of eruptions that are produced. By the third or fourth day after the onset of chicken pox, eruptions may be seen in all stages of development. Ordinarily, the patches of eruptions are most prevalent on the back and chest and decrease in number toward the hands and feet. In severe cases, almost all of the body may be covered, including the palms of the hands, soles of the feet, and lining of the mouth and vagina. Usually, the temperature does not exceed 102°, but in severe cases it may rise to 104° or 105° and remain elevated for four or five days.

Contrary to previous beliefs, the crusts of the sores are not infectious.

What to do: Chicken pox is usually a mild disease requiring little special treatment. Even in cases which appear to be mild, however, a physician should make the diagnosis, as well as look for indications of complications. In its early stages, chicken pox is easily confused with more serious diseases, such as smallpox. The doctor usually advises that the patient be kept in bed as long as new patches or eruptions appear and as long as there is any elevation of temperature. Since chicken pox is contagious, the patient should be isolated from members of the family who have not had the disease, especially very young or weak children, and he should be kept from school and all other public places until all crusts have fallen off. He should be isolated for his own protection, also; his resistance to other infections is lowered while he is infected with chicken pox.

Itching of the eruptions may be alleviated by oral antihistaminics or by applications of calamine lotion or other lotions which the physician may recommend. The patient, his bed, and clothing should be kept scrupulously clean. Tub baths should be discontinued for a week to ten days after the beginning of the disease and replaced by sponge baths. Care should be taken during the application of soothing lotions and sponge baths not to rub the scabs off the lesions.

Complications: A common complication of chicken pox is deep ulceration of the lesions. This may occur when the patient has been undernourished, or may result from scratching the eruptions. The fingernails of the chicken pox patient should be kept short and his hands washed at least three times a day with soap and warm water.

Cotton mittens or gloves can be given to the child so he will not open the healing crusts with scratching. Parents of infected children should be prepared to give them diversionary entertainment to keep them quiet and still.

Of the secondary infections which infrequently follow chicken pox, *erysipelas, suppurative adenitis,* and *impetigo* are the most common. Erysipelas is an acute infection characterized by a spreading inflammation of the skin and the tissues beneath it. The causative agent is a bacterium of the Streptococcus group. In suppurative adenitis, pus forms in or near the glands of the neck, causing local swelling. Impetigo is an acute, contagious, inflammatory skin disease which may alter the appearance of the chicken pox lesions, causing them to become arranged in undulations or to resemble flakes of bran,

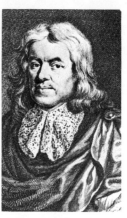

SYDENHAM, Thomas (1624-1689) English physician. Nicknamed the 'English Hippocrates' because of his simple approach to diagnosis and remedy, and generally regarded as the 17th century's greatest clinician. The first to differentiate between measles and scarlet fever, he also introduced the cooling method of treating smallpox. His writings include Latin treatises on epidemics, gout, smallpox, venereal diseases, pathology, and therapeutics.

when crusting begins. When eruptions occur in the mucous membrane inside the eyelids (*conjunctiva*), a severe inflammation known as conjunctivitis may result. *Optic neuritis* and post-varicella encephalitis are rare complications. Chicken pox in the first four months of pregnancy may cause malformations and severe or fatal chicken pox in the fetus. Appropriate measures should be considered. Pneumonia and otitis media (inflammation of the middle ear) are also possible complications of chicken pox.

Measles

Measles is a contagious disease marked by high fever, inflammatory infections of the mucous membrane, and a red, blotchy rash. Although more than 95 percent of all cases of measles occur in persons under 15 years of age, advancing age does not lessen susceptibility. Epidemics of measles usually occur every two or three years. Deaths due to measles are few. Seventy-five percent of the deaths which occur are among children under five years of age. Measles is almost unknown under six months of age (congenital measles may be fatal), and is rare under one year.

There are several forms of measles. The milder kind is called rubeola, also known as the "red" measles. The "German" measles or "black" measles is more properly known as rubella.

Rubella

When rubella infects a young child, the symptoms usually run their course without complications. However, rubella is a serious threat to unborn babies especially in the first three months of development inside the womb. Infants born to mothers who had measles in the first trimester of pregnancy may be born malformed, blind, or deaf. Sometimes deafness develops several years after birth and becomes a serious problem in learning.

For this reason, an effective rubella vaccine was developed. The vaccine, which should be given to a child at nine to 12 months of age, may produce a slight fever and short illness. Women who do not know if they have had the disease can go to a doctor to have a simple blood test to determine whether they are immune. All women should do this several months in advance of planning a pregnancy since the vaccine cannot safely be given to pregnant women.

With mass immunization by active vaccine, epidemics of measles will probably disappear. Population pools of unvaccinated children now result in epidemics every six to nine years, whenever a new "crop" grows up to go to school.

Manner of transmission: The causative agent of measles is a virus which attacks the upper respiratory tract and probably invades the blood stream. It is transmitted chiefly through the air by droplets expelled during talking, coughing, or sneezing, and rarely through articles freshly soiled by the discharges of an infected person. The communicable period of a child with measles is generally from four days before to five days after he has contracted it. The virus which produces measles may be present two or three days before a rash appears and for several days after it disappears. The virus dies quickly in the open air.

A school child who has been exposed to measles may be permitted to go to school for as long as he has no symptoms of the disease. Since measles usually develops eight to ten days after exposure, the child should be examined every morning from the eighth to the fourteenth day following exposure. The rash usually appears 96 hours after the appearance of the first symptoms. If the mother or school nurse observes any symptoms of what appears to be a cold, or if the child has fever, the doctor should make an examination. The child should be kept at home in bed until it is determined whether he has measles.

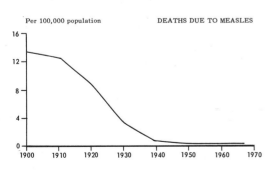

Per 100,000 population   DEATHS DUE TO MEASLES

While in 1900 over one person in 10,000 died of measles each year, this rate has now dropped so that there is less than one death per 100,000.

Symptoms: The onset of measles typically occurs in two stages. The first stage closely resembles a cold, and is marked by a running nose, sneezing, a fluctuating fever, head and back pains, and chills. Appendicitis-like abdominal pain may precede the rash by four or five days. The second stage begins two or three days later and is marked by the appearance on the mucous lining of the mouth, and possibly on the eyelids, of spots peculiar to measles. These spots (*Koplik's spots*) are bluish white and are surrounded by slightly raised, reddened areas. The eyes become inflamed and are sensitive to light. On the third or fourth day, the patient may be troubled with an incessant and violent cough, upper respiratory congestion, and dryness of the mouth and throat; the temperature is usually between 103° and 104° Fahrenheit. Following the onset of fever, a rash appears behind the ears and on the forehead, face, and neck. Later, the entire body is covered with a blotchy, red rash. After the eruption is widespread, the fever usually ceases. Within three or four days, the eruptions fade and dry, leaving the skin mottled.

Complications: Measles is not a trivial disease. Secondary infections of considerable seriousness frequently occur. Involvement of the eyes, ears, and lungs is not uncommon. *Pneumonia* is a complication which should be guarded against. *Encephalitis,* sleeping sickness, is a rare complication.

What to do: When it is known that a child has been exposed to measles, or when there is an epidemic in the neighborhood, consultation with a physician is advisable. Serum treatments which modify the severity of the disease are now available and may be administered by the physician. When the symptoms of the measles appear, the child should be put to bed and isolated from all members of the family who have not had the disease. Isolation is important for the patient's own protection; secondary infections may be brought in by visitors. A doctor should be called.

The clothing and hands of the person attending the patient should be kept clean. The patient should be kept in bed for the duration of the disease. The sickroom should be well-ventilated, but free from drafts, warm (about 70° Fahrenheit) and humid, to help any respiratory difficulties. No drugs or laxatives should be given which are not prescribed by the physician. As a result of prolonged fever, the patient may be dehydrated; fluids should be given freely. Food should be kept light as long as fever is present. Upon the physician's advice, oral antihistaminics and soothing lotions may be used to relieve the itching of the skin. A child who has measles should be kept in bed until his temperature has been normal for at least three days. In some cases, the eyes may become sensitive to light. Keep the room dark and clean the eyes with water to clear away any secretions.

The child should be watched for two weeks or more for secondary infections. Tuberculosis may be activated. Sudden changes in the child's condition, such as pain in the chest, worsening cough, ear pain, or unusual sleepiness should be reported immediately to the physician.

Scarlet fever

Scarlet fever (*scarlatina*) attacks the mucous membranes of the nose and throat. It is usually caused by *Streptococcus scarlatinae*, a member of a group of bacteria which occurs in chains. Scarlet fever organisms invade the blood and may produce poisonous products (*toxins*). These toxins cause dilatation of the blood vessels of the skin, which, in turn, brings on a rash, and later leads to the destruction of the outer layer of skin cells. However, the scarlet fever germ may produce inflammation of tonsils, sinuses, and mastoids, without producing a skin rash.

The disease-producing organisms enter the body through the nose and throat, or through a wound in the skin. They live in the secretions of the nose and throat, in pus from an infection, as in the ear, or in abscesses which penetrate the skin. Quarantine for scarlet fever is usually not practiced any more because of the large number of people without symptoms who are "carrying" the organism.

Half of the cases of scarlet fever occur among children between the ages of three and eight, and 90 percent among persons under 15 years of age. Babies under six months of age seldom have the disease. It is uncommon among adults, because many of them had the disease during childhood. One attack of scarlet fever usually produces immunity. Second attacks *with rash* are rare. Immunization has been tried, but the results were not too satisfactory, so attempts to attain permanent immunity by injected materials have largely been abandoned. Antiserum which combats the effects of the toxin in the blood also has been produced commercially. However, there are many people who react to the foreign serum in their blood stream, making this mode of treatment rather hazardous. In the past few decades, the disease has become milder and various drugs have aided in removing some of its more serious effects.

Symptoms: In a typical case of scarlet fever, chills, fever, and sore throat occur within a few days after exposure. The tongue has a white coating, the tonsils may be swollen, and the throat is very red. The patient usually experiences headache, nausea, and vomiting, but may not appear seriously ill until the rash is evident. There may be minute red spots on the palate before similar eruptions occur on other parts of the body—the neck, chest, groin, or back. The affected skin has a uniformly red flush and feels

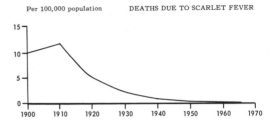

Per 100,000 population   DEATHS DUE TO SCARLET FEVER

As in the case of most other infectious diseases, the number of deaths caused by scarlet fever has now declined appreciably in the United States.

hot, dry, and roughened; occasionally, there may be itching. If the face is attacked, the rash leaves an unaffected pale circle around the mouth and nose. In dark-skinned persons, the rash may not be apparent except on the palms of the hands and the soles of the feet.

Fever may persist until the rash fades, which takes place in from two to seven days after its first appearance. When fever ceases, the throat symptoms begin to clear and the tongue loses its white coating. If the taste buds are swollen, clearing of the tongue reveals a violently red "strawberry tongue," which is one of the typical signs of scarlet fever. Although the rash may recede and reappear, it usually is followed by the appearance of scales resembling bran on the neck and chest. A week or two later, large patches of dead skin may scale from the fingers, toes, and buttocks, and there may be some loss of hair. Inflammation in the neck area may persist for two or three weeks.

What to do: Competent medical care, with sulfonamide and antibiotic therapy, and bed rest are indicated as soon as the first symptoms appear. In mild cases, bed rest should continue for at least two weeks, and longer in severe cases, according to the physician's advice.

The doctor may recommend an ice bag for the head to relieve discomfort occasioned by fever; mild gargles may be used to remove mucous congestion in the throat; and aspirin may be prescribed to control the fever. Any swelling of the neck, pains in the ears, redness or scantiness of the urine, fever fluctuations, or pains in the joints should be reported promptly to the doctor.

Strict isolation of the patient is necessary. Only persons attending the patient should go near him as long as discharges from nose and throat persist.

Complications: Except for its infrequent severe and fatal forms, scarlet fever is less dreaded for the disease itself than for its aftereffects, which may include enlargement of the lymph nodes of the neck, permanent deafness, diseased kidneys, convulsions, or damage to the liver, spleen, heart, and spinal cord. With adequate medical attention, however, most scarlet fever patients recover without serious organic aftereffects. Some children who have had other serious infections such as rheumatic fever may be given continuous antibiotic treatment.

Mumps

Mumps (*epidemic parotitis*) is a contagious disease characterized by swelling of the salivary glands located below the ear and below the angle of the jaw (*parotid, submaxillary,* and *sublingual glands*). The parotid glands, which are located just below and in front of the ears, are the ones principally affected. Mumps is primarily a disease of children and young adults; in rare instances it occurs late in life. It usually occurs in children between the ages of five and 15; children between the ages of seven and nine seem particularly susceptible. Infants appear to be entirely immune for the first eight or ten months of life, and those under two years of age are only slightly susceptible.

Although a mumps vaccine has been developed, it is generally given to older children or adults, rather than infants. This is because mumps can have serious complications in adults but children escape without aftereffects. Since the vaccine is not permanent, it is desirable for young children to have the disease, thus acquiring permanent immunity naturally. With rare exceptions, one attack involving the salivary glands on both sides of the face provides permanent protection against recurrence. A skin test can detect with 75 percent reliability those who have had mumps in the past.

Manner of transmission: Mumps is caused by invasion of the salivary glands by a virus. It is transmitted almost entirely through direct contact with an infected person, although 40 percent of exposed people may not have apparent infection but can infect others. The virus is present in the saliva and in the secretions of the nose. It may be present in secretions for up to seven days before symptoms develop and for nine days after swelling subsides. The incubation period of mumps (the time from exposure to the appearance of first symptoms) is usually 13 to 21 days.

Symptoms: The most characteristic feature of mumps is swelling about the ears and jaws; it is often the first recognizable symptom of the disease. A sudden rise in temperature (between 104° and 105° Fahrenheit) with or without vomiting and headache may also be a first symptom. The swelling of mumps is firm, and typically obliterates the angle of the jawbone, giving the face a pale, shiny, and bloated appearance. Enlargement may extend along the neck; the degree of swelling varies with the severity of the attack. Characteristically, swelling appears first on one side and then the other. The interval between enlargement of the opposite

sides may be up to twelve days or so; in some cases, the second side never swells. The swelling in each side generally lasts from a week to ten days; usually the swelling reaches its peak on the third day and gradually subsides thereafter.

The early stages of the disease are marked by high fever (104° to 105°), headache, pain in the back, reddened taste buds, and loss of appetite; there may be an excess of saliva, or the mouth and throat may be abnormally dry. The initial high temperature gradually subsides, but the patient usually has a mild fever as long as there is any swelling.

What to do: Among children, mumps is generally considered harmless when detected early and if the patient is given prompt treatment. A physician should be consulted immediately when the first signs appear; some other diseases are marked by swelling of the various glands of the neck, and each requires different management. Except in severe and complicated cases of mumps, relatively little medical attention is required. Bed rest is necessary as long as the glands are swollen and the temperature elevated.

In some cases, swelling is painful and may be relieved by applications of moist heat or ice packs, whichever provides more relief to the patient. Most victims of mumps complain of pain when opening the mouth, in chewing, or in swallowing cold fluids. Acid foods and drinks may increase the pain and should be avoided, as should highly seasoned foods and foods requiring chewing. A soft diet with plenty of fluids should be provided as long as there is swelling or elevated temperature. Fever and swelling seldom persist longer than a week to ten days; the patient should be kept in bed until free of both for at least two days. The child should remain isolated and quiet for a week following the disappearance of all symptoms of the disease. Mumps during the first four months of pregnancy may cause fetal malformations, and appropriate measures should be considered.

Complications: Involvement of the sex glands (*testes* or *ovaries*) is a common complication of mumps. When the testes are involved, the infection is known as *orchitis.* This condition occurs once in every four to five cases of mumps among male patients between the ages of 15 and 25; very young boys are seldom affected. Orchitis may precede the swelling of the salivary glands, but usually does not develop until seven to ten days after symptoms of mumps are observed. Orchitis typically begins with a high fever followed by intensely painful swelling of one or both testes; pain radiates to the lower abdomen, the groin, and the thigh, and then subsides within a few days. Permanent shrinkage of the involved gland may follow; when both testes are involved, sterility may result. Among females, a similar infection may involve the breasts (*mammitis*) or the ovaries (*ovaritis*). Such cases are less common and are more difficult to detect than orchitis.

Pancreatitis, an inflammation of the pancreas gland, may precede, occur with, or, as is usual, follow a typical case of mumps. Intense abdominal pain and persistent vomiting are characteristic of pancreatitis.

Mumps may involve the central nervous system and cause an inflammation *(meningoencephalitis);* this complication is seldom dangerous and recovery is rapid.

Whooping cough

Whooping cough *(pertussis)* is an acute, contagious disease caused by the bacterium, *Hemophilus pertussis.* Inflammation occurs in or near the windpipe and induces violent and strangling attacks of coughing which terminate in a loud, harsh, vibrating "whoop" on inspiration.

Whooping cough is one of the most distressing and fatal of childhood diseases. It is readily communicable from material coughed or sneezed through the air, or from contact with contaminated materials. Coughing may project infectious material to a distance of six feet or more, although the infection is most communicable during the catarrhal stage before coughing begins. The disease is contagious from the first appearance of symptoms to about the sixth week. The cough may last much longer, usually from secondary organisms or from habit. An attack which lasts from four to six weeks confers prolonged, but not necessarily permanent, immunity.

The greatest incidence is among children from six months to eight years of age. Comparatively few severe cases occur among persons older than twelve years. The diseases occurs at all seasons and among all races. Although most persons recover, there are a few who die, especially those under one year of age. Mortality is higher among females.

The first symptoms may occur from five to twelve days after exposure, with ten days as an average incubation time. A typical case of whooping cough begins with an ordinary "cold," and a dry, hacking cough, which gradually increases in severity. After a few days, the cough becomes violent, and occurs in bouts separated by an hour or more. An attack usually consists of ten or twelve explosive coughs, each followed by a characteristic intake of breath and a "whoop." The face may become bloated, the tongue projected, the eyes rolled up, the pulse rapid, and the body wet with perspiration. Tenacious mucus is expelled from the throat, and vomiting is frequent. The seizures may occur half a dozen times a day, or approximately once an hour; generally, they are more annoying at night. The disease may persist either with

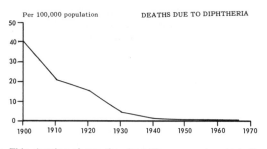

This drawing shows the dramatic manner in which the death rate per 100,000 population due to diphtheria has dropped since 1900 to its present value.

or without whooping or vomiting; violent sneezing or hiccuping may be present instead of the cough. Severe cases may exhaust the child, and infants may require artificial respiration. The spasmodic stage usually lasts about a month, but may persist for two or three months, declining and returning with every cold, especially in winter. Elevation of temperature is not expected in whooping cough, and if present, indicates a complication.

What to do: The child who has been exposed to whooping cough should be watched carefully for symptoms for at least ten days. On the appearance of the first symptom, the physician should be consulted. He may consider it desirable to administer antibiotics or immune serum.

The patient with whooping cough should be isolated from all other children, and so long as there is fever, he should be kept in bed in a well-ventilated room. Elevating the head with pillows may add to the patient's comfort. A rubberized covering on the pillows will protect them from the infectious matter coughed up by the child. All equipment used by the child should be sterilized. Every infant beyond the age of two months should be immunized by at least three injections at monthly intervals of one cubic centimeter of a mixture of pertussis and poliomyelitis vaccines and diphtheria and tetanus toxoids (DPTP). A doctor's care is vital for the child with whooping cough because of possible complications, among them hemorrhaging, middle ear infections, pneumonia, or convulsions.

Diphtheria

Diphtheria is an acute, contagious, and infectious disease caused by the diptheria bacillus *(Corynebacterium diphtheriae),* and characterized by the formation of a tough false membrane on mucous surfaces, principally of the throat. Usually, diphtheria attacks the upper respiratory passages, and may infect the tonsils, the soft palate, the pendulant tip behind the palate *(uvula),* the nasal passages, and sometimes the *vagina* and *conjunctiva*. Diphtheria bacilli produce a soluble poison *(toxin)* which gains access to the internal organs—heart, liver, kidneys, intestines—and causes inflammation of these organs and of the central nervous system. The disease occurs most frequently among children between the ages of one and ten years. Communication of the disease is from sneezing and coughing of a convalescent or other carrier, or less frequently, from contaminated articles. Diphtheria is increasing because of the slack enforcement of toxoid immunization; the 1970 epidemic in San Antonio, Texas points to the necessity of being sure each child is immunized routinely.

Diphtheria may develop within two to seven days after the person has been exposed to the disease. Symptoms include a sore throat, fever, drowsiness, headache, and vomiting. Yellow or gray patches may appear on one or both tonsils. These patches are difficult to remove, and the tissue beneath may bleed when they are removed. The false membrane of diphtheria may begin in the nasal passages, or the larynx may be the first area affected. In untreated cases, the patches spread rapidly; death may follow within six to ten days after onset of the disease, from paralysis caused by the toxin, or from obstruction of the larynx. Not only is the disease itself dangerous, but its damaging aftereffects are serious. Convalescence is long and troubled, because of damage to the heart, kidneys, and nervous system.

If symptoms of diphtheria exist, a doctor should be called at once. When proper treatment is administered during the first 24 hours of the disease, recovery is almost certain. The patient should be isolated in bed in a well-ventilated room. Medical care under supervision of a doctor is necessary. Antitoxin and antimicrobial drugs are usually given by the physician. All those who had intimate contact with the child are quarantined until their nose and throat cultures are negative.

Diphtheria immunity: The "Schick test" is a method of testing for diphtheria immunity. In performing the test, toxin from diphtheria organisms is injected into the arm. If a person is susceptible, an area of redness develops around the point of injection within a few days.

Susceptible persons may be protected against diphtheria by injections of *toxoid,* a material derived from diphtheria toxin by treating the toxin with a chemical *(formalin)* and then aging the mixture. This greatly weakens the toxin, so that it causes only a mild reaction when injected. Toxoid is capable of inducing the formation of protective substances *(antibodies)* in the blood. In communities where toxoid has been administered to almost all children, the disease has been practically eliminated. The age of four months is considered the most favorable time

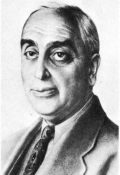

SCHICK, Bela (1877-1967) Austrian pediatrician. Developed the Schick test for natural immunity from diphtheria, a procedure employing superficial inoculation of the individual with diphtheria toxin; a negative reaction indicates immunity. Schick was honored by British and American universities. He was one of the founders of the Academy of Pediatrics and co-authored a book "Child Care Today."

for immunization. Every infant beyond the age of two months should be immunized by at least three injections at monthly intervals of one cubic centimeter of a mixture of diphtheria and tetanus toxoids and pertussis and poliomyelitis vaccines (DPTP).

Tonsils and adenoids

The *tonsils* are the circular band of spongy, lymphoid tissues in the throat, which guard the entrances to the digestive and respiratory tracts. Situated on top of each side of the hind part of the tongue are the *lingual tonsils*. Above them, on either side of the entrance to the throat, are two prominent lymphoid masses, the *palatine tonsils*. These are usually referred to as "the tonsils." On the upper, rear wall of the funnel-shaped cavity (the *pharynx*), leading from the nasal and mouth cavities, is the *pharyngeal tonsil*, commonly called "the adenoids." A thin capsule of connective tissue encloses each tonsil. The lingual and pharyngeal tonsils are embedded in the mucous membrane; the palatine tonsils are partially embedded.

Healthy tonsils perform a valuable protective function for the body. They are a part of the *lymphatic system*. This system, which is spread throughout the body, is an elaborate aggregation of tissue containing a substance, *lymph,* which is made up of plasma and colorless blood corpuscles *(leucocytes)*. Leucocytes also are called "white blood corpuscles," and also are present in the blood stream. The leucocytes of the body engulf invading bacteria and degenerated tissue cells. Structures similar to the tonsils are scattered throughout the body; they are known as *lymph nodes;* in these nodes the lymph is filtered and the leucocytes increase in number.

Enlarged tonsils and adenoids: Enlarged tonsils and adenoids frequently indicate recurring attacks of infection which may be so mild as to pass unnoticed. Because they act as a filter, the lymph nodes in the neck enlarge noticeably during an attack of tonsilitis.

What to do: The young child affected with

tonsillitis should be isolated from other children of the family and put to bed. Prompt diagnosis and treatment by a physician are essential. Ice packs or warm fomentations may be recommended to relieve pain about the throat and neck. Early administration of drugs, particularly the antibiotics, does much to reduce the serious complications and aftereffects of tonsillar infection. Some of these complications are deafness, kidney disease, and rheumatic fever and other heart diseases. The danger of delirium, convulsions and damage to the heart is lessened if fever can be held in check. The doctor often recommends sponge baths or lukewarm enemas and prescribes suitable drugs to combat the fever. The patient should be kept in bed until the inflammation subsides and until the temperature has been normal for 48 hours.

Removal of diseased and enlarged tonsils and adenoids which obstruct the nasal passages and throat often is beneficial and improves the general health of the child. If attacks of tonsillitis are recurrent, such surgery may be necessary.

3 THE BODY

HOW IT FUNCTIONS AS A MACHINE

In ancient times, superstition and medical practice were so hopelessly intermingled that there was virtually no real understanding of how the body functions. Hippocrates, a Greek physician who lived over 400 years before Christ, made the first clear distinctions between medical truth and fancy and therefore has been called the "Father of Medicine." Galen, a Greek physician who lived about 100 A.D., was the first man to study the roles played by the various parts of the human machine. He was so influential in his time, in fact, that his writings were regarded as authoritative for over thirteen hundred years after he died. It was not until the sixteenth century that the Flemish physician, Vesalius, clearly described for the first time the parts of the human body, and Paracelsus, a Swiss, laid the foundations of modern pharmaceutical chemistry. The fact that the blood *flowed* through the body was not recognized for still another hundred years. Despite the fact that these and other men devoted their lives to combating ignorance, the modern physician still finds this one of his greatest problems. A clear insight into the structure and function of the human body is of great importance to everyone. It is necessary for the maintenance of good health and assists a sick patient in cooperating with his doctor. An enlightened person makes a good patient.

The human body has often been called the most nearly perfect of any machine. Much of the mystery surrounding the functions of the body arises through a lack of understanding of the simple manner in which the various parts of the human machine operate. It is true that many of the details of body function are yet to be discovered, but anyone who has some idea of how an automobile or a steam engine works can also gain a good understanding of how the body operates. The basic principles are identical, but the body is more complex than even the best machines that man has invented. Not only can it replace many of its parts as they become worn, but it can also make other machines like itself, and human beings have consciousness, which machines lack.

The fuel for the human machine consists of the food that is consumed. The body burns this fuel at a *low temperature* (98.6° Fahrenheit), so low in fact, it might not seem that the food burns in the usual sense at all. But the combustion of the food is very real, and a pound of fat, when burned by the body, gives off as much heat as it would if the fat were burned in a flame. When fuel is burned in the body oxygen is required just as it is for any other flame. Certain parts of the body have been adapted to distribute oxygen and food to the various areas where they are utilized. Part of the heat that is formed is lost from the surface of the body, just as heat is lost from a steam or gasoline engine, but some of it can be made to do useful work. The movements of the body which are caused by the contraction of muscles require such energy. When death occurs, the supply of fuel and oxygen is cut off and the entire machine stops. And, since the parts of the human machine rapidly deteriorate when deprived of nourishment, the machine cannot be started again. The durability of the human body can well be realized when one considers that the heart is a pump which works continuously day and night throughout a lifetime.

How the body is built from smaller parts

It is easy to see that the fundamental difference between an automobile and the man who drives it is that the driver possesses *life*. Not all of the body is actually living, however, since some of it is made up of material that once had life, but has subsequently lost it. The hair, the outermost layer of the skin, the enamel of the teeth, and the ends of the fingernails are not living, just as the shell of an oyster is only an inanimate mineral deposit laid down by the oyster, but nevertheless part of it. The urine is not living, nor is the fluid material *(plasma)* of the blood, and yet these materials serve important body functions that cannot be dispensed with.

Protoplasm is the term used to designate the basic living material of the body. Chemists can analyze protoplasm and show that it contains many different substances, and it has been found to be highly organized. The protoplasm of the average human body contains about 65 percent oxygen, 18 percent carbon, 10 percent hydrogen, and 3 percent nitrogen. These elements are combined in a great variety of ways to make the tens of thousands of substances of which the body is composed. The other four percent of the body's composition is made up of most of the other chemical elements, such as calcium, phosphorous, sodium, potassium, sulfur, chlorine, magnesium, and iron. Iron is presesnt in the body to the extent of only 0.01 percent, but it is, nevertheless, important. Other substances, such as cobalt and iodine, are present in the body in amounts far less than this, but are still critical for body activities.

Protoplasm is the simplest substance that possesses the ability to reproduce itself, to absorb nutriment, and to use this for the production of energy. In appearance, it is a semi-gelatinous, grayish to colorless fluid. Most of the vital life processes occur within the protoplasm of the body, and it is therefore within this material that most drugs have their ultimate effect.

Cells

The human body is made up of billions of microscopic packages of protoplasm called *cells*. The size of these cells varies greatly, but most of them are so small that a million of them would not be much larger than the head of an ordinary pin. Each little cell may be thought of as having a life of its own; after a human being dies, it may require hours, even days, before all the cells of his body are dead.

All animals and plants are made up of cells.

Some lower forms of life, such as bacteria, may be nothing more than a single cell, while larger plants and animals are built up by gluing together many of these cells into a larger mass. The human body itself begins as a single cell. This cell divides to form two cells, and these divide in turn to form four, and so on, until the complete body, consisting of billions of cells, results. As the human embryo forms, like cells organize the body according to the genetic "blueprint" each cell carries within itself.

The chief activity of all cells is to transform energy. How it does this, at a low temperature and in a watery environment, is a constant source of amazement to engineers. Coal, for instance, requires a 900° centigrade temperature for combustion. Cells gather energy from the breakdown of food at a molecular level. They use the energy to grow, to eliminate waste material, to reproduce by splitting in two *(mitosis)*, to move about the body, and in their special tasks. In addition to energy transformation, cells have properties that contribute to the welfare of the body as a whole. From the single-celled, fertilized egg comes specialized cells that make up the complex body. Cells specialize more and more as the body grows. In the adult, the cells have differentiated to a point where certain kinds of cells no longer reproduce. Reproduction is left to the eggs and spermatozoa. The specialized cells perform the work of muscles, arteries, lungs, and kidneys. To do this, they work together.

All cells contain a *nucleus* that is a center for reproduction and carries the genetic code. It contains deoxyribonucleic acid (DNA) which produces ribonucleic acid (RNA). The RNA organizes the essential amino acids into the proteins necessary for life. The nucleus is made up of protoplasm called *nucleoplasm.*

Outside the nucleus, the rest of the cell is composed of large, complex molecules and membrane. It contains protoplasm called *cytoplasm.* Within this network are *lysosomes,* pockets of digestive enzymes that break up big molecules of fat and protein. The food is passed on to the *mitochondria* for further digestion. *Ribosomes* are parts of the cell used for storing RNA.

Although the cells of the human body may all resemble each other in some respects, their appearance may vary greatly if they come from parts of the body that perform vastly different jobs. Some nerve cells which transmit messages from one part of the body to another may have specialized projections which are as much as a yard long. They are so fine and threadlike, however, that they are invisible to the unaided eye. Some of the white blood cells behave like independent little animals, frequently leaving the blood and traveling throughout the other areas of the body.

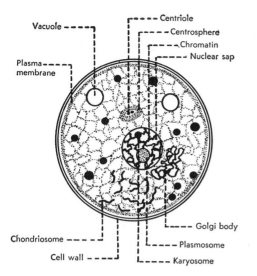

Vacuole
Plasma membrane
Centriole
Centrosphere
Chromatin
Nuclear sap
Golgi body
Plasmosome
Karyosome
Chondriosome
Cell wall

Enlarged drawing of a typical cell, showing its more important internal structures. *Chondriosomes (mitochondria)* are particles in which certain chemical activities seem to be concentrated. The *vacuoles* are special storage regions, while *Golgi bodies* are usually believed to have some secretory function. The *centrosphere*, containing *centrioles*, functions in normal cell division. Nuclear materials, composed of *chromatin*, are suspended in the nuclear sap. The *karyosome* and *plasmosome* are associated with the activity of the chromosomes.

These traveling cells remove bacteria and small particles of waste material. They have no particular shape, and readily change in appearance. Many cells of the respiratory passages have small hairlike bristles projecting from them with which the cells push dust and mucous material toward the outside of the body, thereby preventing the lungs from filling with waste. The cells of the brain are most delicate and require much more exact living conditions than many of the others. Brain cells are the only cells in the body which do not reproduce. If a brain cell dies, therefore, it cannot be replaced. Muscle cells are elastic, and can shrink or stretch like a rubber band. Many of the cells which line the stomach and intestines manufacture large amounts of special chemicals necessary for the digestion of food.

Tissues

When a large number of cells with the same special function work together, they are called a *tissue*. A body tissue, then, is made up of billions of cells which look more or less alike and all of which contribute the same general type of special service to the body. Five different types of tissue may be distinguished in the human body.

The cells which make up the surface of the body and the linings of the various internal tubes and cavities constitute the *epithelial* tissue. They protect the various surfaces of the human body. Some of the epithelial tissue in the skin produces perspiration which aids in the control of body temperature. Others of these tissues in the stomach and intestines produce certain chemicals which aid in the digestion of food. Thus, the epithelial tissues themselves may be specialized in a variety of ways.

The bones and cartilage are referred to as *connective* or *supporting* tissue because their chief function is structural. The connective tissue is the chief source of *collagen*, the principal, fibrous protein in the body. *Muscle* tissue makes possible the various movements of the human being. *Nerve* tissue consists of cells which transmit messages from one part of the body to another. The blood and lymph are also generally regarded as tissues, because they contain cells which are specialized to perform a number of important duties. For example, the red blood cells carry oxygen to the other tissues and the white blood cells destroy disease-producing organisms. The tissue that is formed when a cancer occurs in the body is distinguished by the fact that its cells lose their ability to perform any particular function except proliferation.

Organs

Although the body is made up of many different tissues all having special functions, these tissues are arranged in an intricate and orderly fashion which enables them to cooperate with each other. When several kinds of tissue are grouped together, they are called an *organ*.

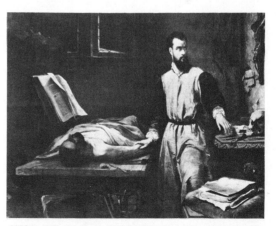

VESALIUS, Andreas (1514-1564) Flemish anatomist. He wrote an outstanding classic on the subject of anatomy entitled *De Humani Corporis Fabrica*. This remarkable book with its many magnificent wood engravings is still in print and further, it is still studied by anatomists. *Bettmann Archive.*

MAJOR FORMS OF TISSUE

Photography . . . F. W. Schmidt.

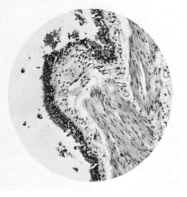

Respiratory Epithelium

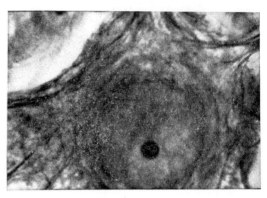

Nerve Cell Body

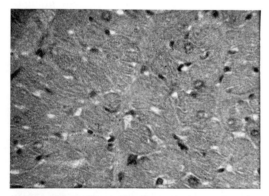

Cardiac Muscle Fibers Cut Transversely

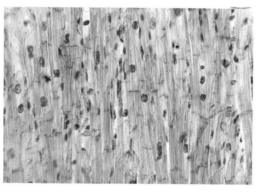

Cardiac Muscle Fibers Cut Longitudinally

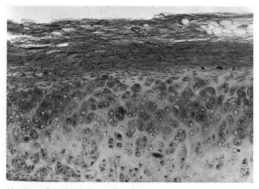

Hyaline Cartilage from Trachea

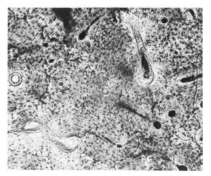

Macerated Bone Cut Transversely

When a number of organs work together as a unit in the human body, they are referred to as a *system*. The circulatory system, the nervous system, and the digestive system are examples of such groupings of organs. The liver may be taken as an example of an organ which is composed of many different kinds of tissues. Some of the liver tissues are responsible for safely ridding the body of waste materials, while others are involved in making blood cells. The liver also contains tissues involved with the storage of iron, and with many of the important parts of the body chemistry. It contains muscle tissue, connective tissue, and epithelial tissue. Among the other important organs might be mentioned the eyes, the ears, the endocrine glands, the heart, the lungs, the kidneys, the stomach, and the spleen. When all of the organs and special tissues are joined in their proper order, the result is the highly complex human being.

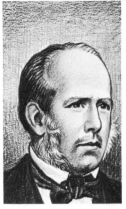

SHARPEY, William (1802-1880) English physiologist and anatomist. Generally acknowledged as having established the science of physiology in England. Sharpey is also credited with the important discovery of the ciliary action in some members of the Protozoa. In addition, he assisted Quain in the task of writing the well-known and still-used volume, *Elements of Anatomy*. Sharpey is famous for his work as an educator during the 38 years that he taught.

Tissue growth

Man has two of many important organs. While there is only one heart, one liver, and one spleen, there are two eyes, ears, lungs, kidneys, reproductive glands, arms, and legs. Normally we use both members of the pair, but should accident or disease befall one of them, the other is able to take over the task for both and perform it with a considerable degree of success. The human body can replace small amounts of some of the tissues when they are destroyed. The process of wound healing involves a replacement. Tissue also forms around plastic implants such as are used to repair arteries and replace heart valves. Through use of nonreactive materials and special meshes, the body will accept and hold in place these sewn-in implants. This kind of regeneration is different from the replacement of tissues which occurs as cells normally wear out and are succeeded by new ones.

In the course of a normal lifetime, the ability of the cells of the tissues to replace themselves as they become worn out continues without interruption. A red blood cell normally survives in the blood stream for about three or four months before it becomes worn out or is destroyed and must be replaced. Over a period of many years, however, the restorative ability of the body generally falls behind: part of the aging process.

Occasionally, a small area of the body may lose control over its normally systematic and careful replacement of cells, and start making new cells at an uncontrolled and rapid rate. Usually, such an occurrence subsides after a short time and no harm is done, but if this process continues, the result is called a cancer. Such a growth in the epithelial tissue is called a carcinoma, while a cancer in other types of tissue may be called a sarcoma.

The fuel that feeds the flame of life— nutrition

Food actually serves two important purposes: it supplies building materials for growth and repair, and it provides the energy that is necessary for all life processes. The summation of all the changes that the food undergoes in the body is referred to as *metabolism*. The rate at which the body burns fuel for energy is called the *metabolic rate*. Life by its very nature involves changes of many kinds, changes in location when a person moves about, and movements of the heart and other internal organs, even when the individual remains very still. All these movements of the body require energy, just as the movement of a steam locomotive requires energy from the burning of coal or oil. In addition to the visible changes in the body, many of the complex and invisible chemical processes that go on within the cells also require energy. The body heat is in itself an indication that such energy is constantly being formed by the body from the combustion of food materials. During exercise we become warm because of the greater amount of heat liberated from the energy required for the vigorous movements of the body. Fireflies are so organized that they convert some of their energy into light, and electric eels convert some of their energy into dangerously powerful electrical currents. All forms of life require energy, however, to drive the basic machinery of their bodies. Part of the food that is eaten may be stored as fat to serve as a reserve fuel supply when the food is not so plentiful. Some persons appear to carry much greater reserve supplies of fuel than are likely to be necessary. When people starve, the body can survive for long periods of time on fuel reserves, sometimes for as long as two months. The ultimate result is that the vital processes terminate when the energy-giving fuel supplies are exhausted.

When coal is burned in a machine to produce energy, it combines with oxygen from the air and gives off another gas, carbon dioxide, as a waste material. Similarly, when the food is burned in the body to produce energy, it combines with oxygen from the air, and carbon dioxide is given off from the lungs as a waste material. A given amount of food produces the same amount of carbon dioxide whether burned in the body or in a flame, and in both cases the amount of heat given off is the same. Amounts of heat are generally stated in Calories (with a capital C), a Calorie being the amount of heat required to raise the temperature of one kilogram of water one degree centigrade. The burning of some foods produces more Calories than others. Thus, a pound of fat, when completely burned, will yield over 4200 Calories, while a pound of sugar, starch, or lean meat will yield less than half of this amount.

The energy requirements of the average grown person demand that each day's food be capable of giving about 3000 Calories, although this figure varies, depending upon the amount of energy necessary for various occupations. This amount of heat would be sufficient to warm ten gallons of water to the boiling point.

The body of a seamstress may require five or ten extra Calories per hour. If the human body is to perform hard physical labor, such as sawing wood or gardening, it may need as much as 300 or 400 extra Calories per hour. A student involved in study requires very little extra energy, and it has been pointed out that one hour of intense mental effort requires no more extra Calories than could be found in one-half of a salted peanut. For reasons other than this, however, mental effort may be as exhausting as effort of a physical kind.

The actual process of energy production from food is not unique to any one part of the body,

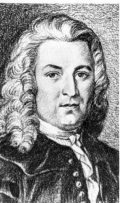

HALLER, Albrecht von (1708-1777) Swiss physiologist. Wrote an outstanding treatise on physiology, *Elementa Physiologiae Corporis Humani.* Although the volume is generally regarded as an important historical work, containing as it did an organization of the physiological knowledge of the eighteenth century, it also set forth Haller's important theory of irritability, involving the contraction of muscles as the result of stimulation applied to the nerves.

but occurs in every single one of the billions of body cells. Every living body cell has the ability to burn food in the presence of oxygen and to produce energy by this process. The energy given off as body heat is simply the summation of the heat produced by all of the cells. The energy needed for a muscle to contract is produced by the muscle cells, and the energy for a heartbeat is produced jointly by the muscle cells of the heart. Each cell thus makes not only enough energy for the continuation of its own life, but some additional energy to serve the purposes of the particular tissue group of which that cell is a member.

The burning of the body fuel occurs within the protoplasm of the individual cells. When fuel is burned outside the body, as in a machine, the process occurs rapidly, and so much heat is given off in so short a period of time, that part of the energy is converted to light energy and a flame appears. If the human body were to use a week's supply of Calories in only a minute or so, it too might ignite and burn with a bright flame. The cellular material of the body contains a complex system of chemical substances which are able to slow down the burning of the food to the point where only a very little heat is liberated at any one time.

Some of the energy released when the food is burned in the body can be stored in special forms ready for use in sudden emergencies and hence does not immediately leave the body as heat. Such special storage forms of energy occur most frequently in muscles and other tissues in which long periods of little activity are followed by sudden exertion. Many of the intricate details of how the body uses its energy are still only partially understood.

In addition to being a supply of energy, the food also serves as a source of building materials for the construction of new tissues during growth, and for the replacement of tissues which

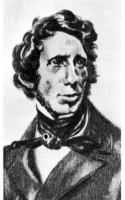

WÖHLER, Friedrich (1800-1882) German chemist. Started the modern study of the chemistry of metabolism by discovering that benzoic acid, taken orally, becomes hippuric acid which is excreted in the urine. He also made extensive studies in biological chemistry, including the synthesis of urea. This latter work alone created a revolution in the thinking of organic chemists of the day. In 1827-28, he isolated the metals aluminum and beryllium.

are being continually broken down during the course of the body's activities. While fats, sugars, and starches are for the most part important in the diet as energy sources, food materials called proteins are of basic importance as raw materials for tissue construction. Indeed, most animal tissues are largely composed of proteins, and lean meat is one of the best nutritional sources of this valuable material. Protein, when taken into the body, is broken down into smaller building blocks of which it is composed *(amino acids)*, and these are transported to all of the tissues. Each of the body cells is able to re-arrange the amino acid units into the particular kind of protein necessary in that cell. The processes by which the cells are able to rebuild or to reproduce themselves are obviously complex, but they generally occur whenever the need arises and the necessary building materials are present. During the growth of children, when there is wound healing, or in certain diseases in which the tissues are broken down, a diet containing large amounts of protein is therefore of particularly great importance.

Many other materials are necessary in the diet, for several different reasons. While water often is not thought of as a food because it does not supply energy, it is still indispensable for life, since it accounts for about 70 percent of the body weight. Minerals are required in the diet as structural materials for teeth and bone. They also enter into the structure of other tissues, such as the red pigment of the blood cells. Traces of rare metals are also needed by the tissues. Copper and manganese, for instance, are needed in minute amounts for enzyme systems. Metals are provided through plants we eat that have absorbed the metals from the soil, and from the water we drink. Vitamins are necessary in the diet largely because they, too, enter in a special manner into the body chemistry, helping to control the processes in which energy and body materials are produced. In some instances, the vitamins enter into the struc-

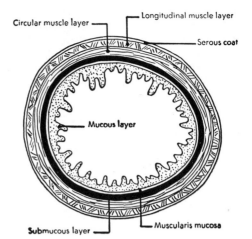

Circular muscle layer — Longitudinal muscle layer — Serous coat — Mucous layer — Submucous layer — Muscularis mucosa

This schematic illustration of a cross-section of the intestine shows the efficient manner in which the various layers of the intestinal wall fit together in such a way as to permit the several kinds of movement of which the intestine is capable. The circular and longitudinal muscle layers, by working together, are able to cause circular constrictions to pass along the length of the intestine *(peristalsis)*. These rhythmic constrictions force the food along in a fashion that promotes its ready absorption by the intestinal mucosa after it has been digested.

ture of body tissues, as in the case of vitamin A, which makes up a part of the light-sensitive portions of the eye. When one of the many essential raw materials needed by the human body is missing from the diet, the life process slows down and eventually comes to a stop, since the human machine, like any other machine, can operate efficiently only when all its vital parts are in good working order.

How food is transported to the cells

Since the food which a person eats must be divided among the billions of cells of the body, it necessarily must be broken down to very small pieces. To accomplish this, the human body has a thorough digestive system which not only grinds the food mechanically, but even breaks it up chemically into exceedingly small particles. The circulatory system is then responsible for the distribution of the food among the individual body cells.

Digestion is aided by the way food is prepared. Cutting food finely and cooking it may accomplish some of the same steps toward digestion that the body would have to perform. For this reason, proper and adequate food preparation is important for babies as well as for older people whose natural digestive processes cannot take care of all the food they eat.

The body begins its work of digestion as soon

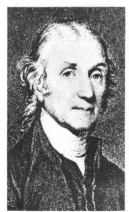

PRIESTLEY, Joseph (1733-1804) English clergyman and chemist. He published the first account of the isolation of gaseous oxygen, and gave it the name, 'dephlogisticated air'. Priestley studied the production of oxygen by green plants under the influence of sunlight. He is also credited with the discovery of a number of gases, including carbon monoxide, sulphur dioxide, pure hydrochloric acid gas, and several of the oxides of nitrogen.

as food enters the mouth. The mouth is the front end of a long tube *(alimentary canal)* which extends throughout the trunk of the body. Foods entering this tube are worked into proper form as they pass along it, and the unusable part of what we eat is finally excreted from the other end, or anus. Man may, in one sense, be considered as hollow, since the material in the digestive tract is not truly in the body tissues. Large numbers of bacteria live in certain parts of this digestive tube without disturbing the body in any way because they are "outside" the body tissues.

The teeth are important parts of the beginning of this digestive tube. Normally, they are arranged so that they can grind the food into very small pieces. At the same time, this grinding serves the purpose of mixing the food thoroughly with the saliva of the mouth. The saliva begins at once to digest the food by means of an *enzyme* in it *(ptyalin)* which breaks down into much smaller pieces the relatively large starch particles, such as are found in bread and potatoes. The saliva that is swallowed with the food continues to act on the starch even after the food reaches the stomach. The saliva also serves another purpose, that of moistening the food to make it easier to swallow.

When food is swallowed, it takes about twelve seconds for it to reach the stomach. Water and other fluids, however, may reach the stomach in as little time as one second, and may pass rapidly through it. Once in the stomach, the food is subjected to the action of the digestive juice which is formed by the stomach lining *(gastric juice)*. The gastric juice contains hydrochloric acid and a number of other more complex substances *(enzymes)* which start changing the food into simpler chemical materials. Most important of these enzymes is *pepsin*, which stimulates the breakdown of proteins into amino acids. The digestive juice oozes from the cells lining the stomach, while at the same time the stomach muscles contract and stretch, causing its shape to change constantly. This churning of the food may break up larger pieces of food, but its most important function is the proper mixing of the food with the digestive juices. Milk is a liquid which would pass immediately through the stomach were it not that the gastric juice contains an enzyme *(rennin)* which stimulates its coagulation or solidification; consequently, the milk also may be digested in the stomach. Rennin prepared from the stomachs of farm animals is used to coagulate milk as the first step in making cheese.

It might be said that the stomach is engaged only at the beginning of the important part of digestion, even though it succeeds in breaking the food down into small pieces. When the food passes into the first twelve inches of the intestines (the *duodenum*), it is further broken down by duodenal digestive juices into exceedingly small, submicroscopic particles. The digestive secretions of the intestine are quite alkaline, as contrasted with highly acidic juices of the stomach. If the food were not thoroughly chewed, the inside of the larger pieces of food could not be reached by the digestive juices of the stomach or intestines. Such pieces of food are not digested, and are lost in the feces.

The digestive juices of the intestine come only partially from the cells lining the intestine. Much of the work is done by fluids or digestive juices made in other organs of the body, and carried to the intestine by special tubes or ducts. The bile duct, for example, brings bile from the liver,

Some Important Digestive Enzymes and What They Do

Enzyme	Where Found	Work Performed
Ptyalin	Saliva	Commences starch digestion
Pepsin	Gastric juice	Commences protein digestion
Rennin	Gastric juice	Curdles milk
Trypsin	Pancreatic juice	Digests proteins
Chymo-trypsin	Pancreatic juice	Digests proteins
Steapsin	Pancreatic juice	Digests fats
Amylop-sin	Pancreatic juice	Converts starch to maltose
Lactase	Pancreatic juice	Digests lactose (milk sugar)
Amylases	Intestinal juice	Digest carbohydrates
Proteases	Intestinal juice	Digest proteins
Lipases	Intestinal juice	Digest fats

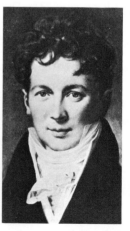

MAGENDIE, François (1783-1855) French physiologist. He is famous for having made important studies of the function of the heart and parts of the brain, the specific action of drugs on various parts of the body, and the chemistry of the blood and lymph. He also investigated many details of the flow of blood in the veins, and the mechanics of swallowing and vomiting. He is generally credited with having given the earliest description of cerebrospinal fluid.

which aids in the digestion of fatty materials. The pancreas is another organ which manufactures digestive juices, and these are sent to the intestine by means of the pancreatic duct. The pancreatic juice is probably the most important of all the digestive juices because it completes the digestive process. It contains starch-digesting enzymes (*amylases*), fat-digesting enzymes (*lipases*), and protein-digesting enzymes (*proteases*).

So it is that the body produces digestive chemicals in the mouth, the stomach, the intestines, and in various organs connected with the intestines. The minute particles (*molecules*) which result from the digestive process are sufficiently small that the individual cells throughout the whole body can use them for fuel and building material.

Not all the food which is eaten can be digested, however, and the indigestible part which remains continues to be moved along the length of the intestine. As this mass travels, large amounts of water which have been drunk or have come from the digestive juices are absorbed from it, and it assumes a firmer consistency. This material might perhaps be regarded as the scrap material that is thrown out by any factory. Most factories make use of some of the scrap material, however, and the human "factory" is no exception. The lower part of the intestine is filled with countless billions of bacteria. These bacteria, far from being harmful, are extremely valuable helpers in the work of the body. As they grow and reproduce, using the body's waste for food, they manufacture considerable amounts of vitamins. These vitamins are cast off by the bacteria and are absorbed into the body in pure form. Newborn babies are apt to acquire a serious vitamin K deficiency during the first few days of life because it takes several days for the bacteria to become established in their intestines. The intestinal bacteria work with the body in a state of mutual cooperation, and the body would not be normal without them. (For a more detailed discussion of digestion, see Chapter 13, "The Digestive System: *What It Is and Does.*")

Circulation

Distribution of digested food to the many cells of the body is done by the blood and the circulatory system. The blood is a liquid, but it contains many kinds of cells suspended in it. It does not flow freely through the body, but is confined within a complex system of tubes (*circulatory system*). It is kept constantly flowing by the heart, a hollow muscular organ which alternately contracts and relaxes. When the heart relaxes, blood flows into it from the tubes (*veins*), and when it contracts, the blood is

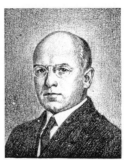

CARREL, Alexis (1873-1944) French surgeon. Introduced a technique for keeping tissues alive in laboratory flasks after removal from the body. He was able to show that arteries can be stored and then transplanted later on. Carrel was probably the first man to transplant a kidney from one animal to another. He developed an important surgical method for sewing blood vessels together. In 1912, he was awarded the Nobel prize.

squeezed out into other tubes (*arteries*) leading away from it. These main arteries, which may be an inch in diameter, have many branches, and the branches in turn have even smaller branches. These smallest branches, too small to be seen without a microscope, are called capillaries, and they form a fine network or mesh throughout the body. If one were to trace out a capillary, he would find that these tiny tubes, rather than branching further, tend to coalesce or join with other capillaries, in the way that small streams may join to make a river. These larger tubes are then called veins, and they lead back to the heart.

As the blood passes through the capillaries, a portion of it leaks out through their walls and into the surrounding tissues. This fluid, called *lymph*, lacks red cells, and is the liquid which directly bathes most of the tissue cells. The lymph is collected into small vessels or tubules which connect with still larger ones in much the same manner as in the circulatory system. The lymph finally flows through the lymphatic system back into the venous circulation largely by way of the *thoracic duct*. Along the course of the lymphatic system are occasional nodes which may filter out debris and prevent the discharge into the blood stream of foreign particles that may have been collected from the tissues. The lymph is important because it aids in distributing food and other materials among the cells, and in preventing the spread of infection.

Since the blood flows by or near all of the cells of the body, it offers a means of distributing food to the cells. The walls of the intestine are surrounded by an extra dense mesh of capillaries. Most of the digested food from the intestine passes into special cells lining it, and these cells in turn pass the food through their walls, through the walls of the capillaries and then into the blood. Much of the fat, however, is first picked up by the lymph and transported by it to the blood. The digested food particles dissolve in the blood and are carried along with it to the veins and finally to the heart cavity. This passage of food from the cavity (*lumen*) of the intestine into the blood is called *absorption*, and can take place only when the food is properly digested. The heart forces the food-bearing blood through the arteries and into the capillaries. The cells of the body can then remove the nourishment from the blood flowing in nearby capillaries. (For a more detailed discussion of circulation see Chapter 7, "The Heart and Circulation: *What It Is and Does*;" and Chapter 6, "Blood and Blood-Forming Organs: *What They Are and Do*.")

HOW CHILDREN GROW

The following sequence of pictures, taken in the laboratory of Dr. Nancy Bayley at the University of California's Institute of Child Welfare, portrays the normal process of body development from childhood through adolescence. The youngest of the children shown are four years of age, while the oldest are 18 years old. The boy and girl in each set are the same age, so that some idea may be obtained of the growth differences that occur. As a girl approaches maturity, her growth tends to slow down, while a

normal boy usually grows steadily until his full height has been attained, and thus becomes larger than a girl of the same age. Periods of slow growth may be followed by spells of accelerated growth, however, and youngsters who shoot up rapidly may not continue their pace during adolescence. Usually the girl's increase in height ceases at around 13 years of age, while the main growth of a boy continues until he is about 17 years old. During development the boy's shoulders tend to become broader than his hips, while the girl's hips tend to become proportionately wider than her shoulders. However, the range of normal variation in growth is broad.

Prediction of height of the adult from his size as a child is difficult, and can only be performed successfully with the aid of x-ray studies of his bone structure. If the child is still growing, a cap of soft, growing bone will appear in the x-ray picture, at the end of each finger joint. If the cap has hardened and become part of the mature bone of the joint, no further growth will occur. The factors which control development of the skeleton are not completely known, but include both hereditary and hormonal influences. The carefully controlled investigations of workers such as Dr. Bayley on children throughout their period of development have made it possible to predict with some accuracy the course of a child's growth, and thus guard against preventable growth defects.

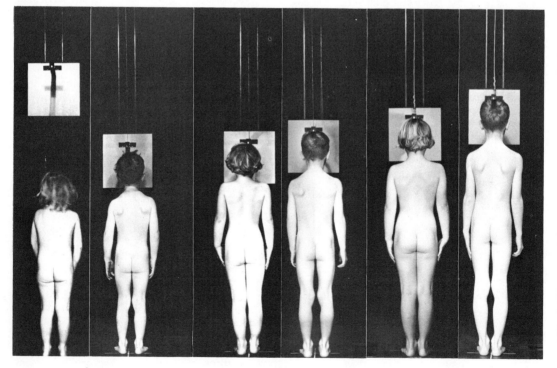

4 years   6 years   8 years

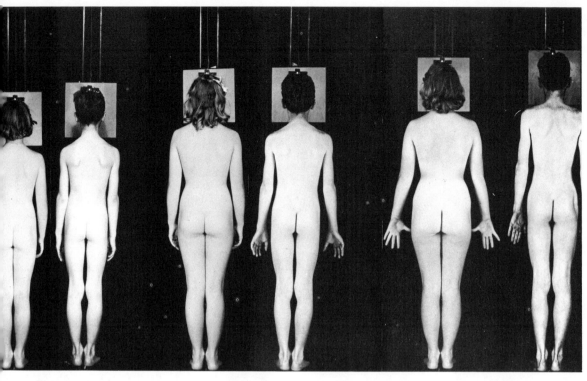

10 years   12 years   14 years

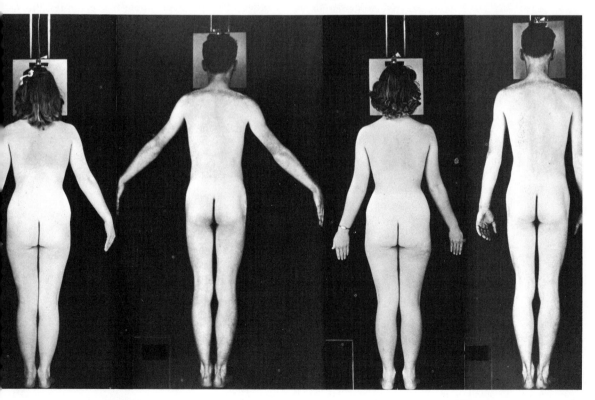

16 years   18 years

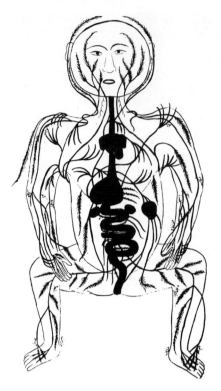

This drawing taken from an ancient Persian manuscript was meant to depict the distribution of the major veins in the human body. Until about three hundred years ago, much of the knowledge of human physiology and anatomy was based purely on superstition and conjecture. Nevertheless, some old drawings such as that above show a truly remarkable degree of accuracy. *Bettmann Archive.*

Respiration

The cells of the body, having received fuel for energy, must also obtain a supply of oxygen, for like an ordinary flame, the combustion inside the cells cannot take place without this element. The oxygen, like nourishment, is carried by the blood, but in a much different manner than that in which food is carried.

An aeration or ventilation system is needed to load the blood with oxygen, and the lungs serve this purpose. The windpipe (*trachea*) serves as an intake and exhaust pipe for the lungs, and also contains the voice box. The lungs may be thought of as balloons or sacks which fill with air when the chest and diaphragm are expanded, and expel air when they are compressed. Unlike balloons, however, the lungs are not simply hollow spaces, but instead contain a maze of small passageways and compartments (*alveoli*) into which the air rushes. Because they are broken up into such small compartments, the lungs have a tremendous surface area. This

is important because only oxygen touching the inside surface of the lungs can pass into the blood, whereas oxygen in the center of a mass of air cannot. The actual area of the lining material of the lungs is about 65 square yards or 30 times as great as the total area of the entire outside surface of the body. The lining of the lungs of young children is pink. In normal adults, however, who have lived for many years in the vicinity of large industrial cities where there is considerable smoke, the lungs will be blackened by carbon which has been inhaled.

The blood has a large number of cells suspended in it. Most of the cells are red and give the blood its typical color. This red color is caused by pigment (*hemoglobin*) which has the ability to pick up oxygen from the air and transport it to the cells, where it is released. One of the main arteries leading from the heart, the pulmonary artery, forces the blood into the capillaries in the walls of the lungs. The air which is drawn into the lungs when a person inhales contains about 20 percent oxygen. This oxygen diffuses through the cells lining the lungs and into the capillaries in much the same way that air will eventually diffuse out of an inflated balloon. Oxygen, unlike the food supplied from digestion, will not dissolve appreciably in the liquid part of the blood, and so it must be grasped by the hemoglobin inside the red blood cells. When the hemoglobin contains large amounts of oxygen, it becomes a bright red. The oxygenated blood passes quickly from the lungs into veins leading to the heart, and the heart pumps this bright red, oxygen-bearing blood out to the cells of the body along with the dissolved food. As the red cells pass through the tiny capillaries of the body tissues, the body cells take the oxygen from the hemoglobin and use it to burn the food which they get at the same time. When the hemoglobin loses its oxygen to the body cells, it becomes a darker shade of red, and so venous blood returning to

WARBURG, Otto (1883-1970) German physiological chemist. He developed a highly sensitive instrument for measuring oxygen and carbon dioxide metabolism in small amounts of tissues and cells. The device is used extensively in metabolic studies throughout the world today, and is generally known as *Warburg's manometer.* In 1931, he won the Nobel prize in medicine for his brilliant experimental work on the function and structure of certain enzymes.

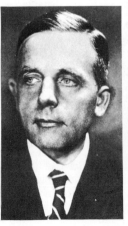

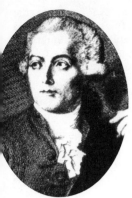

LAVOSIER, Antoine (1743-1794) French chemist. Noted for his statement of the important theory of the indestructibility of matter. Most of Lavoisier's work in the field of chemistry was concerned with coordinating and evaluating the previous work of others. He was responsible for devising a new and highly improved system of nomenclature for the chemicals known at that time, including the term "oxygen," and invented the gasometer, a machine employed in measuring gases.

the heart appears darker than arterial blood. In a real sense, therefore, the blood may be pictured as a highly efficient and intricate fuel supply system for the human machine. Its versatility as a transportation system is great, and it carries much cargo other than fuel and oxygen, as will be demonstrated below.

How waste materials are carried from the cells

The normal activities of the cells of the body invariably result in the formation of large amounts of waste materials. These waste materials may arise from the burning of fuel, as ashes remain after the burning of wood, or they may be left over from building activities, just as carpenter's shavings are left after a house is built. They are the leftover portions of fuel which the human machine cannot use, and consequently they must be eliminated.

There are several organs which are specially developed to remove these waste materials. Most important among these are the lungs, the kidneys, and the skin.

The lungs

The lungs have been described as the organs by which oxygen is obtained. When food is burned with oxygen, another gas is formed, *carbon dioxide*, most of which is of no further use to the body. The carbon dioxide coming from the cells passes into the blood just as the oxygen passed out of it. The red cells do not carry it away, however, since it dissolves easily in the liquid part of the blood much the same as the carbon dioxide dissolves in the liquid part of carbonated beverages. Blood passing among the cells of the body dissolves the carbon dioxide and carries it to the heart which then pumps it

to the lungs. At the same time that the red cells are picking up oxygen in the lungs, the plasma is giving up carbon dioxide. This gas mixes with the air in the lungs and is expelled. The respiratory rate is controlled by a small area in part of the brain, without conscious effort on the part of the individual. This portion of the brain is controlled in turn by the amount of carbon dioxide dissolved in the blood, so that this gas does serve an important function in the body. It is excess carbon dioxide therefore rather than lack of oxygen that causes us to breathe faster. The carbon dioxide dissolved in the blood is also important in preventing the body from becoming overly acid or alkaline.

Exhaled air contains more carbon dioxide than does inhaled air, and it also contains more water. This can be demonstrated by breathing on a piece of glass or on a metallic object. The water of the breath condenses on the cool object, and it can be expected that the amount of water lost in this way over a period of time would be considerable. This water comes from the lining of the lungs, and it must be replaced by the blood. Hence, it might be said that the lungs are a means of getting rid of excessive amounts of water. The evaporation of water from the lungs also has a slight cooling effect which aids the body in maintaining an even temperature. Fur-bearing animals which have no sweat glands in their skin must rely on this process almost entirely for their temperature control. The panting of a dog in warm weather enables the dog to speed up this important cooling process.

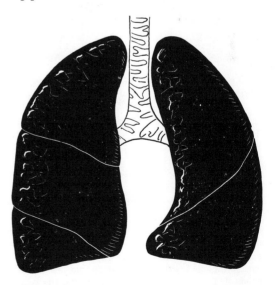

These are the lungs. The lungs are the ventilating system and comprise one part of the cooling system of the human body. Pumping over one thousand times each hour, their capacity is such that they are able to move over 3000 gallons of fresh air into the body in a single day.

The lungs also aid in ridding the body of other volatile substances dissolved in the blood. Any liquid dissolved in the blood which evaporates easily, such as the alcohol which remains there after the drinking of intoxicating beverages, or acetone which may occur in the blood of persons with diabetes, leaves the blood as a vapor in much the same way as carbon dioxide, and can consequently be smelled on the breath. The lungs and windpipe therefore serve as the exhaust pipe of the human machine. (For further discussion of respiration, see Chapter 5, "The Respiratory System: *What It Is and Does.*")

The kidneys

By far the greatest part of the job of ridding the body of waste materials is performed by the kidneys. These two organs, one located on each side of the lower back, contain a complex system of blood capillaries. As blood passes through them, some of the water and most of the undesirable chemicals are removed from it. The resulting water solution of wastes flows through a system of tubes in the kidneys and on out into the urinary *bladder*. This process of "filtering" the blood goes on continuously in the kidneys, and the blood that leaves them goes back to the heart in a purified form.

The kidneys, when functioning properly, are able to excrete most of the waste materials of

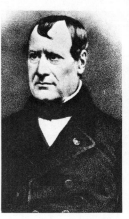

FLOURENS, M. J. P. (1794-1867) French physiologist and anatomist. Universally famous for having made important discoveries concerning the relationships of brain centers to various body activities. By removing the cerebellum of pigeons, he showed that this center controlled coordination and balance. In a similar manner he showed that removal of the cerebrum caused a loss of mental activity, and that removal of the cortex caused blindness.

the body. They also cause the loss of a great deal of the body's water. The material dissolved in the urine consists of *urea*, salt, and much smaller amounts of a variety of other substances. Nitrogen, which enters the body in the form of protein, leaves it as urea.

Ordinarily, the kidneys also excrete considerable amounts of substances from the blood which are not really waste materials. It is normal for small amounts of vitamins, sugar, and amino acids (protein building blocks) to be excreted in this manner so that they must be continually replaced in the body by the diet. Occasionally even a few red cells or some protein from the plasma will be lost in the urine. (For further discussion of kidney function, see Chapter 14, "The Urinary System: *What It Is and Does,* and *The Kidney.*")

The Skin

Certain types of cells in the skin also work toward relieving the body of waste materials, although their role is much less impressive than that of the kidneys. The sweat glands of the skin, in carrying out their major function of controlling the temperature of the body, excrete sweat or perspiration. Sweat is largely water, but it contains also small amounts of chemicals taken from the blood. Some of these may be purely waste materials, although as in the kidneys, other material such as vitamins may be lost. When profuse sweating occurs, the loss of certain minerals from the blood, particularly salt, may become very important, and the body must find some means of getting new supplies of these things. In a temperate climate, about one-fifth of the water consumed is lost by evaporation from the skin; about three-fifths is lost in the urine. The balance of the water passes out of the body in the expired air and the feces.

The sweat glands, along with the lungs, are the principal means of maintaining a constant

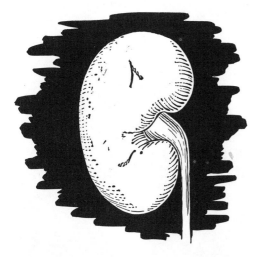

This is a kidney. The two kidneys of the human body contain over ten square yards of active filtering surface which they utilize continuously to purify the incoming blood. They are the single most important system that the body has for ridding itself of its waste materials. Over a quart of blood is purified by the two kidneys every minute, during which period about one teaspoonful of urine is usually formed. This urine is then transported via the ureters to the bladder, where it is stored until it can be conveniently excreted by way of the urethra.

body temperature. As perspiration evaporates into the air, the skin is cooled. As the blood flows through the tiny capillaries near the surface of the skin, it too is cooled and flows back into the interior of the body and cools it. When the body is exposed to cooler temperatures, however, most of the surface capillaries are constricted so that less blood flows through them and the blood on the surface of the body will *not* be cooled. When it is particularly cold, the body warms up by some other means. In this case, we *shiver* as the muscles rub rapidly back and forth, thereby creating heat by the muscular work performed and a resultant increase in the metabolic rate. (For further discussion see Chapter 8, "The Skin: *What It Is and Does*.")

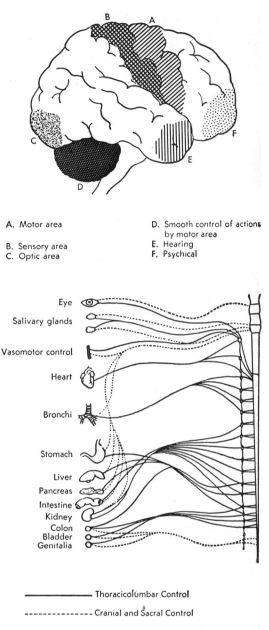

A. Motor area

B. Sensory area

C. Optic area

D. Smooth control of actions by motor area

E. Hearing

F. Psychical

Eye

Salivary glands

Vasomotor control

Heart

Bronchi

Stomach

Liver

Pancreas

Intestine

Kidney

Colon

Bladder

Genitalia

———————— Thoracicolumbar Control

-------------- Cranial and Sacral Control

Keeping the parts of the human machine in harmony

The many different activities going on in the human machine require coordination of the work of the various tissues and organs, if the body is to work smoothly and healthfully. Coordination is also involved when the body reacts to changing conditions around it. The senses of taste, sight, hearing, feeling, and smelling are useful only when there are some means of reacting to their stimulations. All of the body activities are under strict regulation by a system composed of the brain, the spinal cord, and the nerves which spread throughout the body. This system is aided by a group of chemical regulators or *hormones* circulating in the blood, which help to control the tissues and individual cells.

The nervous system

Nerve cells are found throughout the body. In the brain and spinal cord, they are massed together in tremendous numbers, while elsewhere they are far more sparse. Some are quite small, but the cells which connect the brain and spinal cord to the other parts of the body sometimes may be a yard long. The nerves have the function of transmitting messages from one part of the human machine to another. This is done by complicated chemical and electrical changes. The brain may be pictured as the central switchboard of a complex telephone or telegraph system, through which messages must pass in order to reach their proper destination.

Sometimes we can exert control over the activities of the nerves, as when we think, or when we use the various senses. When the brain directs an arm to move, this is frequently at the will of the individual and he is at least remotely aware of it. The group of nerves that have activities which are under our conscious control are referred to as the *voluntary* system. Most of the

Diagram showing some of the different areas of the human brain and spinal cord which control the various functions and parts of the anatomy. The brain may be considered to be the central electronic control station for the human machine, and the spinal column is the major pathway over which messages to and from it travel to the different areas of the body. Motor areas of the brain are necessary for the voluntary movements of the body, while the sensory areas are essential to the proper reception of messages picked up by the sense organs. The presence of disease processes or injuries in these areas may cause corresponding difficulties in movement or sensation. A disorder of the spinal column may not only block out the nerves leaving the spine at that point, but if it is severe enough, may also prevent nerve impulses from passing that location to and from points beyond it.

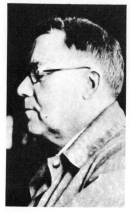

CANNON, Walter (1871-1945) American physiologist. He is credited with being the first person to suggest the relationship which exists between the various emotions and the endocrine glands. His classical experiments with athletes under tension and with angered cats started an important new trend in the study of physiology by showing that anxiety, fear, anger, and other strong emotions influence the functioning of the endocrine system in a pronounced manner.

nerve cells belonging to the voluntary nervous system are located in the brain and spinal cord, but there are other nerve cells that can be willfully used which connect these with the skin, the eyes, the ears, the nose, the muscles and, in fact, all of the parts of the body.

The outer layer of the brain (cerebral cortex) is the part of the brain which in man is different from that of other animals. It is highly developed in human beings, and gives us, among other advantages, the power to reason.

There is another important group of nerve cells in the body called the autonomic nervous system, over which the individual has much less control. Some of the cells of this system are located in the brain, but many of them are also found in the spinal cord and in smaller collections of nerve cells (ganglia) which are located in parts of the body other than the head. The autonomic nervous system is invaluable to the body, because it coordinates all the internal activities of the human body. Digestion, respiration, perspiration, excretion, and other activities which must go on constantly, even though the individual may be sleeping or unconscious, are all under its control.

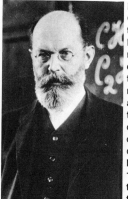

FISCHER, Emil (1852-1919) German chemist. First man to have synthesized a number of highly complex, naturally occurring organic compounds. Included among these were dextrose, mannose, fructose, caffeine, uric acid, purines, and polypeptides. He was recognized as one of the most outstanding organic chemists of the last century, and he received the Nobel prize for chemistry in 1902. He also introduced the barbiturates as sedatives.

Although basically the individual may have no voluntary control over the automatic nerves and the activities which they coordinate, this system still may be influenced by conscious thoughts. While one is not able to cause the heart to beat faster at will, the beat may become faster when one's emotions are aroused. Most influences of this type are quite desirable, for when one suffers fear and wishes to run, the muscles will need more fuel and oxygen and the increased heart rate will supply them.

Frequently, the voluntary and the involuntary systems can work together effectively in the absence of strong emotion. The involuntary system, for example, coordinates most of the digestive processes, but it remains for the voluntary system to supply the food and to release the undigested remains. In the case of breathing and of blinking the eyes, action is controlled most frequently by the involuntary system, but can also be modified somewhat by the voluntary system.

Repetition of frequently occurring signals to and from the brain is avoided by certain shortcuts or reflexes. When a reflex is established, the "thinking" is done outside of the brain in one of the ganglia or small groups of nerve cells along the spinal column. The body automatically moves away from a source of pain, and the eyes automatically squint at the sudden appearance of bright light by the use of such reflexes. A complete "wiring diagram" of all the nerve connections in the human body would be far more complicated than one for any manmade machine, but in many ways it would appear similar. (For further discussion see Chapter 11, "The Brain and Nervous System: *What It Is and Does.*")

The endocrine glands

The endocrine glands assist the brain and nervous system in coordinating the different parts of the body. These glands manufacture certain chemicals (hormones) which influence the activities of one or more body structures. Part of the adrenal glands, for example, sends out large amounts of the hormone adrenalin. This chemical substance is carried along by the blood stream throughout the entire body. When this hormone reaches those parts of the body which are sensitive to it, the work of the chemical begins. The adrenal glands are particularly active under conditions of stress, either from outside the body or from upsets within. Adrenalin is needed under such conditions because it prepares the human machine for an emergency. It causes the heart to beat faster, increases the rate of breathing, and sends greater supplies of fuel to the tissues. The outer portion of the adrenal glands, unlike the inner part which manufactures adrenalin, produces a number of hormones that regulate many other aspects of the body chemistry, and particularly the amounts of mineral salts in the various tissues. Thus, the adrenal glands, although located just above the kidneys, are able to affect the entire body.

Another important endocrine gland which assists the nervous system is the *pituitary* gland, at the base of the brain. This gland manufactures several different hormones, each of which has a different effect upon the tissues of the body. Hormones from the pituitary act as growth-stimulators of children, assist in the process of sexual maturing, and help to maintain many other functions of the body which are of importance throughout life. The pituitary gland is particularly important because it assists the brain in coordinating the activity of other endocrine glands, and for this reason has been called the "master gland." Disorders of the pituitary gland may, therefore, be of particularly grave significance.

The *thyroid* is another important endocrine gland, and is located in the neck. It produces a hormone *(thyroxin)* which regulates the general speed of most of the chemical reactions in the cells of the body. If the thyroid gland is too active, the individual may be highly nervous, one who moves and talks at a rapid rate. An underactive thyroid by contrast causes the individual to be of a much slower nature. Still other glands, the sex glands or *gonads,* help to control many of the characteristics of masculinity or femininity, prepare the female body for childbearing, and influence many of the details of the body chemistry. The *parathyroid* glands in the neck help to control the proper levels of calcium in the body. A portion of the pancreas, the islets of Langerhans, manufactures the hormone *insulin* which is important in regulating the amount of sugar in the blood. Part of the digestive process is stimulated by hormones secreted from small glands in the walls of the intestinal tract. The *thymus* gland, which lies just above the heart, and the *pineal* gland, which is located at the base of the brain are thought to be associated with the process of growth and development.

The endocrine glands, which are partially under the control of the nervous system, work with the latter to keep the various parts of the body in the best possible harmony. The endocrines are, however, somewhat less important than the nervous system, in that, if they do not function properly, the hormone products frequently can be derived from the corresponding glands of lower animals. No such substitute can be found for the human brain. When a defect occurs in its system of nerve connections, serious consequences arise which often cannot be easily remedied. The strange behavior of individuals

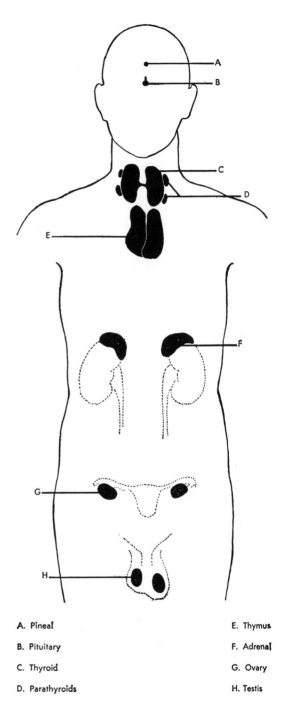

A. Pineal

B. Pituitary

C. Thyroid

D. Parathyroids

E. Thymus

F. Adrenal

G. Ovary

H. Testis

Distribution of the major endocrine glands. The endocrine glands have no direct connecting ducts like other secretory glands, but they preside in a rather mysterious fashion over some of the human body's most important functions, including physical growth, sex, nutrition, and many involuntary activities. If the glands do not function properly, the individual may develop into an idiot, a giant, a runt, a bearded lady, or even a "carnival fat man."

with mental disease sometimes requires long and careful treatment to reestablish the proper interrelationships and functions of the brain cells. Some persons who have no such trouble can, however, by their mental outlook cause a derangement of other parts of the body. The indigestion caused by eating while in a bad mood is one form of such an upset. (For further discussion of the endocrine glands see Chapter 10, "The Endocrine System.")

How the body duplicates itself

Throughout life, the cells of the body continue to reproduce themselves either for the purpose of growth or in order to replace cells which have been destroyed. Many cells, such as those lining the gut, may be replaced nearly every day; others are replaced more slowly. When, however, the cells of the body duplicate themselves in such a way as to produce a completely new human individual, the process is of a different nature. Reproduction is one of the characteristics of living things, and is essential for the maintenance of every species, since all living individuals inevitably die.

In order for a new individual to develop from the body, special types of cells must be manu-

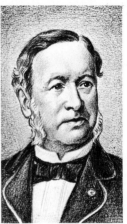

SCHWANN, Theodor (1810-1882) German anatomist. He was the founder of the biological theories of fermentation and putrefaction. Although better known for his thorough investigations of the nature of yeast cells, his studies of the action of the bile in the processes of digestion and absorption were also highly important. He recognized the ovum as a complete cell, and is credited with the discovery of pepsin and with proposing three major anatomical laws.

factured. These are called sex cells, *sperm* when produced by the male body, and eggs *(ova)* when manufactured by the female body. They are produced in parts of the sex organs, which are present in the body from birth, but are not as a rule able to function in reproduction until the individual has reached puberty.

The changes which occur in the body at puberty depend to a considerable extent upon the endocrine glands, particularly the pituitary gland and the glands of the reproductive organs *(gonads)*. Since all the endocrines work to some degree in bringing about puberty, the individual shows widespread changes in appearance, in body function, and in personality. (For further discussion see Chapter 2, "The Child: *The Teen-Ager.*")

The mature female body usually produces one egg about every 28 days. The male body, however, produces millions of sperm, and the production is usually continuous. In each case, the individual reproductive cells contain thousands of submicroscopic particles each of which has the power to transmit some body characteristics of the parent. It is these particles or *genes* which are responsible for the resemblance of a child to his parents.

When a sperm and an egg unite, they lose their separate cellular forms and become a new single cell which is the beginning of the new individual. During this process the genes from the two parents are brought together in the new cell so that the resulting person will take part of his characteristics from each parent. Genes from the parents also give essential deoxyribonucleic acid (DNA) and ribonucleic acid (RNA) to each new cell. It is DNA and RNA that contain the blueprint of the body. The newly formed cell or fertilized egg begins to grow, and becomes implanted within the womb of the mother. First it divides into two cells and then these two cells divide, as do the resulting cells. This process of growth and division is contin-

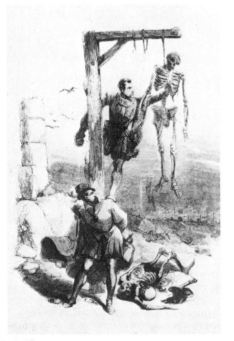

Andreas Vesalius, the great Flemish anatomist of the Renaissance, contributed more to his field than did any other man of his period. He acquired most of his information from human bodies stolen from gallows and dissected in secret. *Bettmann Archive.*

ued until hundreds, thousands, and finally billions of cells have been formed. When the new unborn individual is still only a few weeks old, it begins to take the shape of a human body. As it continues to grow, all of the organs and tissues of the adult are formed.

Development of the new individual within the body of the mother requires approximately nine months. During this period within the mother, the child grows at a more rapid rate than ever again in its life. Under the influence of the endocrine glands, the body of the mother meanwhile changes to meet the special needs of the child. The process of childbirth in itself is one that is brought on by changes in the amounts of the various hormones in the mother's blood. The infant is born at the time in its development when it no longer requires the amount of protection afforded by the mother's body. However, the human machine has by no means completed the duplication of itself at childbirth. It is only after puberty that the body may be regarded as fully developed. (For further discussion of reproduction, see Chapter 1, "Life Begins," Chapter 10, "The Endocrine System;" and Chapter 15, "The Reproductive System.")

How the body is able to move

One of the main reasons why the human body requires fuel is for the production of the necessary energy for motion. Many of the movements of the body are obvious and commonplace, but a number of others are seldom considered. The heart is in constant motion throughout life, as are the lungs and the digestive tract. All of these movements are caused by the contraction and relaxation of muscle cells which are banded together to form *muscles*. A number of structures are necessary, however, for the muscles to be effective. Without the skeleton, for instance, the

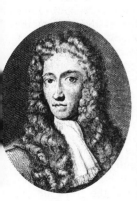

BOYLE, Robert (1627-1691) English physicist. Proposed and proved what is now known as *Boyle's law:* that at any given temperature, the gas volume varies in inverse proportion to the amount of pressure exerted upon it. Experimenting with an air pump and jars containing mice, he was able to make major contributions to the knowledge of the nature of respiratory processes. His many important discoveries were instrumental in earning him the title, Father of Modern Chemistry.

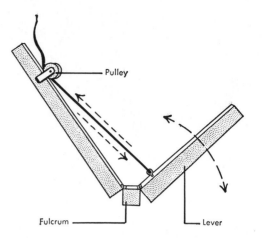

Pulley, fulcrum, and lever. This diagram illustrates the principle employed by the body for the movement of the arms and legs. When a muscle contracts, it produces the same effect as a pull would produce on the end of a rope. The joints serve as fulcrums to which the moving parts are attached.

body would be a relatively formless blob of flesh with little power to travel about. Much of the skeleton acts as a series of levers on which the muscles may pull to produce motions of a useful kind.

There are generally considered to be 206 bones in the human skeleton. In addition, there are several small bonelike structures in the ears, and very small accumulations of bone may grow at places along the larger bones where there is irritation. Some of the bones, such as the 22 that go to make up the skull, serve principally as a protective casing for more delicate organs. The brain, the inner ears, the eyes, and the pituitary gland are protected by the skull. Bones which have red bone marrow may also be considered as protective since the marrow is the site where many of the blood cells are manufactured. The 24 rib bones serve as a protective cage for the heart and lungs in addition to acting as levers. The spine consists largely of 24 bones *(vertebrae)* which protect the spinal cord of the nervous system, act as hinges upon which the ribs may swing, and also as levers for various muscles.

All of the bones are made up of cells which are surrounded by considerable amounts of mineral material. These cells are arranged in layers around the central marrow part of the bone and are connected with each other by small canals. A layer of cells (the *periosteum*) also surrounds the outer surface of the bone as a membrane. Cartilage or gristle is bonelike material which lacks any appreciable amount of mineral deposit and so can bend slightly even though it is quite rigid. The cellular structure of the bone permits

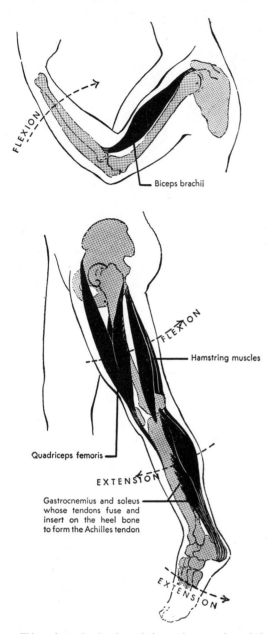

Biceps brachii

FLEXION

FLEXION

Hamstring muscles

Quadriceps femoris

EXTENSION

Gastrocnemius and soleus
whose tendons fuse and
insert on the heel bone
to form the Achilles tendon

EXTENSION

This schematic drawing of the major muscles of the leg and forearm shows how they are able to work upon the bones of the skeleton to cause the latter to perform as levers. A contraction or shortening of the *biceps brachii* muscle causes the long bones of the forearm to flex toward the body upon a pivot at the elbow. A contraction of the *quadriceps femoris* muscle pulls the entire leg forward upon a pivot at the hip joint. The *gastrocnemius* and *soleus* muscles are endowed with a dual function, flexing the leg and extending the foot forward in walking. Muscles such as these, which act upon bones in such a manner as to produce a leverage effect, generally have much longer fibers than muscles which bring about the movements in the softer tissues, such as the heart, the tongue, the blood vessels, and the various organs of the intestinal tract.

even the solid framework of the human machine to renew itself constantly as it becomes worn.

Muscles consist of groups of long muscle cells assembled in such a way that when they contract there will be a shortening of the muscle as a whole. The muscle fibers which are under voluntary control, such as those that cause the body to move about, are quite large and long and appear to be striped or *striated*. The involuntary muscles, such as those in the stomach and intestine, contain somewhat smaller cells and are sometimes referred to as smooth or *unstriated* muscles. The muscle cells of the heart constitute still a third type somewhat intermediate in appearance between the other two. The skeletal muscles are connected to the bones by fibrous bands called *tendons*. A pulled muscle or a sprain usually results from injury at the point of attachment of tendons.

Each muscle has a number of nerves which transmit the impulse that causes the muscle to contract. Close cooperation between the nervous and muscular systems therefore is essential for the proper motion to take place in the human body.

The action of the involuntary muscles is largely independent of the skeletal system, and depends upon the particular manner in which the muscles are organized. Thus, some of the intestinal muscles tend to circle the intestine and by contracting cause the size of this tube to become smaller. This constriction progresses down the gastrointestinal tract in "ripples" (*peristalsis*) forcing the contents of the intestine to move slowly downwards. The heart muscles form four chambers. When the muscles of one of these chambers contract, the chamber becomes smaller and the blood is forced out. These chambers are equipped with small one-way valves so that when the muscle again relaxes, blood flows into the enlarging chamber from another direction.

Breathing is caused by the work of two sets of muscles which function together in increasing the size of the chest cavity. One set of these muscles in the chest draws the ribs upward and outward, while the muscles of the floor of the chest cavity, the *diaphragm*, pull downward. These movements tend to create a vacuum between the lungs and the ribs into which the lungs expand, at the same time sucking in air. When the muscles relax, the cavity in the chest decreases, the lungs collapse, and air is forced out. The lungs have no muscles of their own, and breathing is entirely dependent upon the rhythmic movements of the diaphragm and chest muscles. When these become paralyzed, breathing is only possible in an artificial respirator or iron lung which takes over the work of the chest muscles. The normal process of breathing requires no conscious effort, because the muscles function in a rhythmic fashion under the control of the involuntary nervous system.

The automatic and continuing movements of the body are scarcely less remarkable than those motions that can be made voluntarily. The voluntary muscles have the ability to propel the human machine forward at a speed of over twelve miles per hour and to lift weights of several hundreds of pounds. This is possible largely because of the excellent system of levers and joints that are provided by the skeleton. The bending and straightening of any of the limbs at the joints is caused by the contraction and relaxation of opposing pairs of muscles. Each of such skeletal muscles is connected at its ends to the two bones that are to change position with respect to each other. Training of the muscles and nerves which are responsible for such movements may cause their activities to become almost automatic in some cases. The fingers of a skilled pianist provide a striking example of such *neuromuscular* training in which many of movements are entirely automatic and not singly commanded.

One of the most sensitive systems of nerve and muscle coordination is that which keeps the human body upright. From a system of *semicircular canals* adjoining the inner ear, nervous impulses are sent out which cause the skeleton to shift position in order to maintain its balance. This delicate balance is only achieved through practice, since infants do not possess it. Manmade machines are able to maintain an even stance by the use of a gyroscope, but such machines are unable to restore a balance when it is once lost. The "gyroscope" in the human machine is, moreover, a self-lubricating one that will normally operate throughout a lifetime. (For further discussion see Chapter 9, "The Skeleton and Muscles: *What They Are and Do.*")

How the body reacts to the world around it

Many of the activities of the human being are caused by events that occur in the world around it. The body is able to see, hear, taste, and smell things. It is able to feel pain or changes of temperature or a contact with some other object. These abilities are essential to survival. They are possible only because of complex specializations of the nervous system *(receptors)* which are able to detect these various influences. These special abilities are not, however, limited to human beings. Indeed, man-made devices are able to detect light, sound, and touch but are not able to interpret properly that which is detected. The human brain is the crucial part of the system which integrates the sensations and interprets them into usable information. Many lower animals have a similar system, but their brains cannot reason out a complex series of deductions from what they perceive.

The simplest of the sensations are those that are produced in the skin. A great many nerves end on the surface of the body, and the area in the immediate vicinity of such a nerve ending becomes a detector of injury to the skin. Such naked nerve endings are the receptors of painful sensations and when stimulated send a signal to the brain that we interpret as pain. They may also send a signal to the muscles controlling a portion of the body to withdraw the area from the source of pain. Such a signal may not pass through the brain but may be short-circuited through a reflex arc. Thus, when the hand

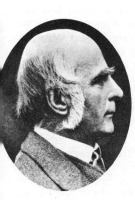

GALTON, Francis (1822-1911) English anthropologist and geneticist. Believed to be the founder of the science of eugenics. Galton made studies of the thought processes of people of different intelligence levels, and originated numerous techniques for mental testing. Galton also suggested that genius is inherited. His detailed studies of patterns in human fingerprints established fingerprinting as the most important means of criminal identification now employed in general police practice.

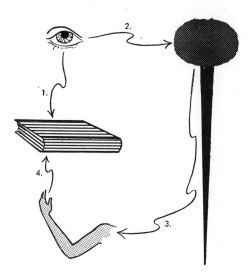

Diagram showing how an idea is transformed by the body into an appropriate action. 1. The eye sees the book; 2. a stimulus is sent from the eye to the brain; 3. the brain sends an impulse down the spinal cord to the muscles of the arm; 4. the muscles are energized to move the arm toward the book.

touches a hot stove or is pricked by a pin, it is jerked away without conscious deliberation.

A great many of the nerve endings in the body's surface serve the purpose of detecting a touch or cold or warmth. In each of these three cases, there are separate nerve endings for the particular sensation. The nerve endings in each case also contain specialized structures or sense organs which make the nerve effective. When the body is touched in a certain area, for instance, the specialized touch-sensitive nerve endings are stimulated, and they send a message to the brain to inform us that a particular portion of the body is touched. If we then wish to move away from the object that touches us, the brain sends a message to the proper muscles to withdraw that part of the body. Some areas of the body are much more sensitive to touch than others. The nose, for example, is 15 times more sensitive than the back of the forearm. Nerve endings which detect cold and warmth are much less numerous in the skin than those which detect touch or pain.

Many of the nerve endings in the body are able to detect strong vibrations or loud sounds, but the human possesses a set of highly specialized organs to make the reception of sound more sensitive and accurate. The human ears are exceedingly complex devices that possess a delicate discriminating ability. The outer ear consists of a funnel to help collect the sound, and a tube which directs the sound against a tightly stretched membrane, the *eardrum*. On the inner side of this membrane (the *middle ear)* are a series of levers that magnify and transmit the vibrations to the *inner ear*. Fluids in a complex set of canals in the inner ear then vibrate against a highly sensitive series of nerve endings which are able to send messages to the brain. The brain then interprets the various sounds. The human ear is not so sensitive as some microphones, but it is able to pick up much more delicate "shadings" of sound.

The senses of taste and smell similarly depend on specialized sets of nerve endings and frequently they are more sensitive than any manmade device in their ability as detectors. They are important aids in sensing various dangers that may threaten the body and in stimulating the digestive system.

The eye is one of the most delicate devices of the human body. It works much like a camera, yet it is more complex and sophisticated than any man-made machine. It contains a transparent front window behind which is a *lens* that focuses the light entering the eye. The opening into the interior of the eye, the *pupil*, is controlled by a muscle, the colored *iris,* which relaxes or contracts to control the amount of light that enters. The interior of the eye is filled with a transparent fluid. The light-sensitive portion of the back of the eye (the *retina*), consists of many highly specialized nerve endings. The image of anything that we see is focused on this bed of nerve endings, which when stimulated by the light, transmits a message through the optic nerve to the brain. Some of the nerves of the eye are specially sensitive to particular colors, and others work best in dim light. The eye therefore is a more adaptable camera than is likely to be built by man.

When the body has been made aware of the activities going on around it, frequently it is necessary for it to make some adjustment. The neuromuscular and skeletal systems perform the motions of the body which assist greatly in this regard. Communication between individuals is possible because of the voice box or *larynx*. In the larynx are the *vocal cords,* which are really folds in the lining of the larynx rather than true cords. These may be stretched to become taut and produce high sounds when air is forced through the voice box on its way to or from the lungs. When the vocal cords are relaxed, they vibrate much more slowly and produce lower sounds. The *spoken* words are those sounds as modified by the lips, the nasal passages, and the tongue. By associating a great variety of different sounds with meanings, man has been able to communicate with his fellows in a much more effective manner than any of the lower animals.

All of the processes of sensory perception, voluntary movement, and vocal communication rely on the brain for their coordination. The brain is the most complex part of the human being. In it are stored not only the abilities to direct the body's many functions, but also the historical records of the life of the human, the memory. The brain is divided into a number of parts which are responsible for various tasks, but the outer layers of the large hemispheres that occupy most of the skull are the portions that make the human being so effective. In this *cerebral cortex* occur the mental processes which distinguish man from the lower animals. When portions of the cortex are lost or destroyed, corresponding losses occur in memory or ability. The brain is therefore in every sense the major control panel of the human. (For further discussion, see Chapter 11, The Brain and Nervous System.)

The conflict of the body with the world around it

Because the earth is a highly competitive place in which many different organisms are fighting for survival, a great number of things can happen to the human body to cause its breakdown. To combat these, the body has a highly organized series of defenses against disease or injury.

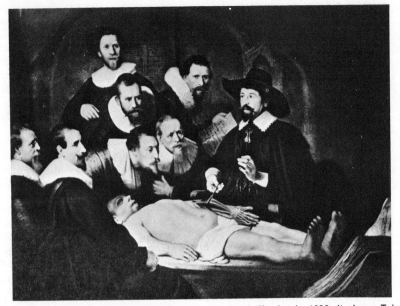

The Anatomy Lesson, by Rembrandt. The original picture was painted life-size in 1632. It shows Tulp, the Dutch physician and anatomist, lecturing on parts of the body. At the time, Rembrandt was 25 years old. *Mauritshuis.*

The skin constitutes a strong barrier against invasion of the body by microorganisms. It also prevents water and other materials from indiscriminately entering or leaving the body. Each of the openings into the interior of the human has special safeguards against invasion of the body by bacteria. The eyes have lids which cover and protect them, and the tears have certain germicidal properties. The lips provide a barrier to invasion of the mouth. The openings of the ears come to a blunt end at the eardrum. The nose, throat, and lungs possess special cells which tend to eject or break down invading material. All these are important to guard the body not only against disease, but against pollutants in the air and soil.

Despite all of these safeguards, disease-producing organisms occasionally do get into the tissues. These might be bacteria, fungi, or molds; protozoa or viruses such as those that cause measles, mumps, and smallpox; or viruses that can pass through the finest filter, causing influenza, poliomyelitis, rabies, and the common cold. The body still has, however, a number of weapons with which to fight such invaders. Frequently, the microorganisms are attacked and devoured by certain of the white blood cells. These cells travel out of the circulatory system and through the tissues. They are of the greatest importance in combating disease, and when the body becomes infected with some microorganism, unusually large numbers of them appear in the blood and tissues. They are present in large numbers in the lymphatic system which drains the tissues, and make this system, with its gourd-like lymph nodes, particularly important in the body's resistance to disease.

The body has a protective system called *immunity*. Immunity is actually a reaction. When a foreign invader such as a virus attacks, the body produces specific chemical substances to combat the particular offender. The invader is an *antigen*—the defenders are *antibodies*. Antibodies are produced by the lymphatic system and remain in the bloodstream a long time to prevent recurrence of the disease.

Natural immunity is enjoyed by some people from birth. Active immunity is produced by having the disease and conquering it, thus building up a standing army of antibodies. It is also produced by inoculation of a very mild form of the disease to deliberately produce antibodies. Passive immunity is obtained by inoculation of serum from an animal that has had a disease and has produced antibodies to it. Thus, the serum contains the antibodies necessary to fight off infection. Finally, if the infection is localized, the body may simply wall off the area by forming around it dense fibrous tissue. Such a defense is commonly employed by the body in combating tuberculosis.

The body is able to survive injury and unpleasant surroundings by means of various mechanisms. Thus, it can exist in extremes of

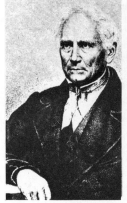

PURKINJE, Johannes (1787-1896) Czech physiologist. Made an extensive study of the structure and function of the human eye. He originated the technique of viewing the retinal blood vessels by the images that may be seen with special light conditions (Purkinje's images). He also is noted for his important descriptions of the microscopic anatomy of muscle fibers, brain cells, and sweat glands, and for his studies on the processes of ovulation and digestion.

heat and cold and maintain its temperature by means of perspiration, breathing, and shivering. Its ability to form blood clots gives it protection against undue fluid loss from wounds. The involuntary nervous system working with the hormone, adrenalin, prepares the parts of the body for extreme physical exertion, such as is necessary in combat. The normal processes of tissue repair prevent the human machine from rapidly wearing out. It is hard to picture a machine that is so well prepared for survival. A reasonable amount of care of the body is necessary, however. A lack of proper care is among the most common causes of the breakdown of the body.

The efficiency of the body

The human body cannot work around the clock. It must have a regular opportunity to catch up on its repair activities, and to dispose of wastes that have accumulated during the day faster than they could be discarded. During sleep the entire body slows down. The liver stores starches needed for the next day. The kidneys clean the blood. The rate of metabolism is at its lowest, being just sufficient to keep the vital parts of the body in operation. The blood pressure drops; the pulse rate is slower; and breathing is irregular and slowed down. The body is less sensitive to stimulation by pain, light, or sound. Even its temperature drops by one degree. Researchers have discovered that man goes to sleep when his muscles become tired and must relax. The natural sleeping time is from six to nine hours in every 24. Even lying down and closing the eyes helps the body.

Does the brain need sleep? Since it does not have muscles, it does not tire in the same way the body does. It keeps on working even though the muscles of the eyelids are so tired they must close. But there is evidence that the brain needs sleep for another reason. Dreaming is an essential activity of the brain during sleep. People

volunteering for a sleep experiment were awakened whenever sensors measuring their brainwaves detected dreaming. They exhibited strange behavior after a few days until they were allowed to dream without interruption. Dreaming may be as essential to the brain as rest is to the muscles and organs.

Just how much work is actually obtained for the fuel that has been fed the body? When gasoline is burned in an engine, only about one-eighth of the energy released can be captured to drive the motor, and the remainder is lost in the form of the heat that is given off. Such an engine is said to have an efficiency of 12.5 percent because it wastes 87.5 percent of the fuel through the loss of heat. Some diesel engines have a 32 percent efficiency because they can put some of this heat to useful purposes. If we were to calculate the energy used and the work produced by a person performing strenuous work, we would find that the efficiency of the human machine is about 20 percent. Much of the fuel burned by the body is converted to heat to maintain the body temperature and is lost by the body to the surroundings without doing any real work. Since the human body cannot work regularly the full 24 hours of a day, its efficiency is in reality even lower, perhaps about ten to twelve percent. Nevertheless, the human body is built to last a great many years.

During the course of a day, the human body performs a huge amount of work. The passage of fluids across the various tissue membranes alone requires effort. Over a pint of water is forced through the skin each day. In warm climates and when the body is subject to extreme exertion, over two quarts of water may be lost in this manner. The kidneys perform a much greater amount of work than this, filtering over 150 quarts of fluids a day. If their total filtering surface were spread out, it would occupy about ten square yards. The heart beats over a hun-

DESCARTES, René (1596-1650) French anatomist and philosopher. Famous for having written the first book on physiology, De l'Homme, which was published after his death. Although the book was in many ways more of a philosophical than technical one, it eventually became the background for a great deal of research on human physiology. His studies on the human eye and other related optical systems led to the establishment of the important principle of optical refraction.

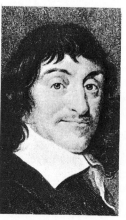

dred thousand times a day, and during this time over 1,500 gallons of blood are pumped through it. The blood may travel through the circulatory system at speeds as high as one mile per hour and exert a pressure of two pounds per square inch or more. A single red blood cell may make over two complete circuits of the body in a single minute. Over ten million red cells are destroyed every second in this hectic race, and these must be replaced at an equally rapid rate.

The nerves must carry millions of messages every day, and the eyelids blink thousands of times to cleanse and lubricate the eye. All of these things, when added together, mean a tremendous amount of work. A day in the life of the human body is certainly a full one.

4 DISEASE-PRODUCING ORGANISMS

VIRUSES

Of the many lower forms of life, only relatively few are capable of producing disease, and many, indeed, are beneficial to the higher animals. The very smallest of the disease-producing organisms, invisible by the microscope, are called *viruses*. By about the year 2500 B.C., the Chinese had identified smallpox and knew that this disease was transmissible. They could not know, however, that it was caused by a virus. The ancient Greeks knew that rabies was transmitted by the bite of dogs, without knowing that it was also caused by a virus. The Hebrews compared the bite of a rabid dog to that of a venomous snake. Venom in Latin means "virus." In the year 50 A.D., Celsus, a Roman physician, wrote, "Rabies is caused by a virus." However, this remarkable statement should be read as meaning that he was aware of rabies being caused by a virus which was "something which could produce a disease." The concept of infectious diseases was metaphysical until the time of Pasteur and Koch. Through their work, the agents of infectious diseases were identified as microbes. Pasteur was able to prove that rabies was a specific infectious disease caused by an agent which he considered to be a small microbe because he was unable to see it. Koch discovered the tubercle bacillus. About the end of the nineteenth century, a Russian scientist Iwanowsky discovered that the juice of tobacco plants with symptoms of mosaic disease remained infectious after filtration through filters retaining microbes. He concluded that the infectious agent was a small microbe. Soon afterwards, a Dutchman, Beijerinck, confirmed the filterability of tobacco mosaic virus, but arrived at the conclusion that tobacco mosaic disease was caused not by a small microbe but a *fluid infectious principle*. This recognition of a difference between the infectious agent of tobacco mosaic disease and microbes or bacteria makes Beijerinck the first scientist to recognize viruses as a new class of disease-producing agents. Almost at the same time, two German scientists, Loeffler and Frosch, discovered the virus responsible for foot-and-mouth disease of cattle. At the beginning of the twentieth century, Reed, an American physician, and his colleagues discovered the viral cause of a human disease: yellow fever.

By 1910, the following diseases had been found to be of viral origin: rabies, poliomyelitis, yellow fever, smallpox and cowpox, dengue fever (or breakbone fever), and sand fly (*Phlebotomus*) fever. Although rabies and smallpox only then came to be recognized as viral diseases, protective measures against smallpox had been known since the time of Jenner, an eighteenth century English country practitioner. Preventative measures against rabies had been known since the time of Pasteur (mid-1800s). During 1910–1920, other diseases were found to be caused by viruses: herpes simplex (fever blisters), herpes zoster (shingles), varicella (chicken pox), measles (rubeola), inclusion conjunctivitis, and warts (verruca). During the 1930s, a considerable number of other diseases were found to be of viral origin: influenza, mumps, German measles (rubella), certain types of meningitis (lymphocytic choriomeningitis), and certain types of brain inflammation caused by arthropods (mosquitoes, ticks, and mites). During the 1940s, certain diseases of the liver (infectious hepatitis, serum hepatitis) and Colorado tick fever were found to be caused by viruses. In 1948, Coxsackie (name of a town in New York state) viruses responsible for a number of diseases were discovered in the stools of children. Shortly afterwards so-called "adenoviruses" were discovered as the cause of a number of respiratory diseases and febrile catarrhs. Recently, a new group of viruses has been discovered and described as ECHO viruses. These viruses were at first considered orphan viruses or viruses in search of disease, because they were discovered before they could be associated with any known disease in man. They are now known to cause meningitis with or without a rash, fever with or without a rash, and diarrhea in infants and in children. Thus, during the past few years many scores of hitherto unknown viruses have been discovered in the intestinal and respiratory tracts and, to a lesser extent, in the blood of man.

Viruses affect not only animals and man, but almost every type of living organism, including insects, fish, and frogs, as well as flowering plants and some of their pests such as red spiders, or spider mites, and also bacteria.

Definition of viruses

Viruses are ultramicroscopic entities which differ greatly in their biochemical organization from all microorganisms, such as bacteria and other one-celled plants and animals. For instance, they are pure nucleoproteins, i.e., they possess a core composed of only one of the nucleic acids, ribonucleic acid (RNA) or deoxyribonucleic acid (DNA), but never both. This nucleic acid core is coated with a sheath of protein. In the laboratory, this protein coat can be removed with phenol and the bare nucleic acid will produce the same symptoms of disease in test animals and tissue cultures as the whole virus.

In 1970, Dr. Howard M. Temin made the discovery that RNA tumor viruses contain enzymes in virions which allow synthesis of DNA from an RNA template. Dr. Sol Speigelman confirmed Temin's finding which supports the hypothesis that information can be transferred from RNA to DNA; this had previously been thought impossible.

Viruses differ also from bacteria in that they have no enzyme system of their own and so are obliged to the host cell for the use of its biochemical machinery (obligate parasitism). The viral nucleic acid soon gains genetic control of the host cell and alters its chemical organization to produce the type of protein and nucleic acid required for replication of the virus. Although symptoms may not appear immediately, these host cells remain as latent foci of infection ready to become active when physiological or psychological factors so alter the cellular environment that natural host resistance is lowered. Fever blisters and shingles are examples of this process.

Viruses differ also from bacteria in that they do not respond to chemotherapeutic agents such as antibiotics and sulfonamide drugs. Although these drugs destroy many infectious microorganisms, they in no way alter the course of viral diseases.

During the past twenty years, a large number of viruses have been discovered. This progress in the discovery of new viruses has been brought about by the application of new or improved scientific methods, such as the use of newborn animals, the employment of tissue culture (susceptible cells grown in test tubes in special nutrient fluids) for the isolation of viruses, and the use of the electron microscope for the study of the submicroscopic structure of virus-infected cells. There have been great triumphs of chemotherapy, i.e., the cure of bacterial infections with chemicals, such as the sulfonamide drugs and antibiotics, and substances produced by living organisms, such as penicillin or streptomycin. This control of diseases caused by bacteria has undoubtedly been a contributing factor to the upsurge in the discovery of new viruses as causative agents of a number of diseases. It is of interest that many types of cancer in animals of various species have recently been found to be caused by viruses, but there is no reproducible proof as yet that any type of cancer in man is caused by or associated with a virus infection.

Properties of viruses

One of the most important properties which led to the discovery of viruses is their ability to pass through filters retaining cells and bacteria. The ultramicroscopic size of viruses and filterability through filters which hold back bacteria indicate that viruses are made up of individual units or particles of a considerable size range. Some bacteria may be even smaller than the largest virus, so that filterability is now no longer considered as a special property of viruses. They may vary in size from 300 millimicrons (pox) to 16 millimicrons (tobacco plant necrosis virus). To understand the size of viruses, one has to realize that one millimicron is 1/1000 of a micron and the micron is approximately 1/25,000 of an inch. The smallpox virus is 230 × 300 millimicrons in size and is considered a large-sized virus. Mumps virus measures 170 millimicrons, rabies virus 150 millimicrons, measles virus 140 millimicrons, and influenza virus 100 millimicrons. These are the medium-sized viruses. Among the small-sized viruses, poliomyelitis virus and Coxsackie virus

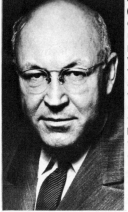

STANLEY, Wendell Meredith (1904-1971), American biochemist. He was the first man to obtain a virus in pure form when in 1935 he was able to isolate the virus that is the causative agent of mosaic disease in tobacco plants. Stanley also determined the chemical nature of viruses, and thus laid the fundamental groundwork for the many subsequent studies in this important field. He shared the Nobel prize with J. H. Northrop and J. B. Sumner in 1946.

measure 28 millimicrons. The shape of most viruses is spherical, although there are some notable exceptions, as some plant viruses may be rodlike or hexagonal in shape with short or long tails. The shape and structure of viruses came to be recognized properly through the use of the electron microscope, which utilizes a beam of electrons as a source of light. Electrons have a much smaller wave length than light rays and permit, therefore, observation of objects much smaller than those seen with the light microscope. Objects as small as 0.5 millimicron may be seen in their natural surroundings, i.e., infected human or animal cells cut into slices 1/1,000,000 of an inch thick. This is a great advance in our knowledge of the physical properties of viruses. It permits the study of viruses during the various stages of their development within cells and, thus, a study of their relationship to various cell components. Electron microscope studies of viruses within cells, combined with the study of cells stained by various fluorescent dyes, may in the future produce a rational basis for our understanding of how to treat patients with viral diseases.

Electron microscope studies of viruses in slices of infected tissues have shown their internal structure. There exists an essential similarity in the structure of bacterial, plant, insect, mammal, bird, and human viruses. They are composed of an internal dense center which is the nucleic acid and which is surrounded by one or more protein membranes. Recently, chemical studies have shown that the nucleic acid is the carrier of viral infectivity. These studies, combined with electron microscope studies, have localized the nucleic acid in the dense center of the virus particle.

Most viruses are destroyed by heating at 60°C., although there are some viruses which are resistant to this temperature (serum hepatitis virus). They withstand freeze-drying and high doses of irradiation and are resistant to treatment with antibiotics and chemotherapeutic agents.

Much higher concentrations of chlorine are required to kill viruses than to kill bacteria. Bactericidal agents such as Lysol and Roccal kill only some of the viruses. Organic iodine, formalin, and dilute hydrochloric acid destroy resistant viruses such as poliomyelitis virus.

In present-day studies of viruses, tissue culture, which is based on cultivation of animal or human cells in a strictly controlled nutritional environment in test tubes or flasks, has been most helpful in isolation of viruses and in the diagnosis for their presence. Under certain conditions, viruses grown on monolayers of cells form characteristic plaques of centers of cell destruction. The size and appearance of these centers are helpful in ascertaining the presence of different types of viruses in the examined tissues. Tissue culture is used nowadays for the preparation of vaccines such as the poliomyelitis vaccine of Salk.

Viruses can also be grown in embryonated chicken eggs in which different viruses produce characteristic lesions or immune antibodies. These again are used as the basis for isolation and diagnosis of viruses. There are vaccines based on the growth of viruses in embryonated chicken eggs—for example, influenza vaccine.

By various changes of the environment in which viruses multiply, certain types of virus progeny during their multiplication can be selected and isolated by various techniques. Such types, or so-called "mutants," have the same antigenic or immunizing properties as the parent virus without its infectivity. In this way, live virus vaccines are produced.

Virus-host relationship

Many viruses, during their multiplication within cells, produce abnormal structures called inclusion bodies. The staining properties and localization of such structures within cells are of considerable diagnostic help in such diseases as rabies or, for example, in differentiating mild cases of smallpox from severe cases of chicken pox.

Viruses, on entry into the cells of a susceptible host, may produce different types of infection. Clinical or apparent infections occur when the host develops symptoms characteristic of the particular virus disease. For example, the virus of measles almost always produces an apparent or clinical infection with a long-lasting immunity. Other viruses may also produce inapparent or subclinical infections—for example, influenza virus. Some viruses may cause either clinical (apparent) or subclinical (inapparent) infections and then persist as latent infection for a considerable length of time (infectious

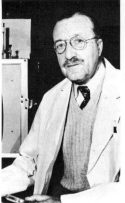

hepatitis) or for a lifetime (herpes simplex or fever blister virus). In the latter case, the virus may become periodically activated and a latent infection becomes apparent.

The question of whether the viruses produce a true poison or toxin has been the subject of intensive research. It is now believed by many investigators that the viruses do produce toxins, but that the toxic substance cannot be separated from the virus particle. The reason for this belief is that if large quantities of some purified viruses are injected into a laboratory animal, an effect is produced so rapidly that one may conclude that an active toxin is present. The role that these toxins play in disease production is not clearly defined.

Immunity to viral diseases

Immunity is the power of living organisms to resist and overcome infections. The human body has several different ways of preventing and combating infection from viral agents. Immunity to many viral diseases may be produced in the individual by his having the disease and recovering from it. In a number of viral diseases, infection almost invariably produces lifelong immunity. Viruses of smallpox, specific types of poliomyelitis, measles, mumps, and yellow fever induce lasting immunity. Persons who have suffered from an attack of these diseases have in their circulating blood substances (antibodies) which will neutralize or give specific reactions with the viruses. Frequently, viruses can be recovered from such immune hosts. It is not understood how the viruses manage to survive in the immune hosts. The persistence of viral agents does not explain the permanent immunity in some viral diseases.

In other viral diseases, such as influenza, common cold, Coxsackie infections, and poliomyelitis, there exists an apparent absence of durable immunity. This is due to the clinical manifestations of these diseases being caused by a group of related but immunologically different viral agents. Thus, infections with influenza Type A virus will not confer immunity against influenza Type C virus, or infection with Type I poliovirus will not elicit immunity to Type III poliovirus. The respiratory infections caused by adenoviruses or various diseases produced by Coxsackie viruses may occur frequently in the same individual because of the many immunologically different types of these viruses, although immunity to one particular type may persist.

Active immunity, which develops in people following mild or subclinical infections with viruses, is the same as in persons who developed severe illness. In many viral diseases, such as smallpox, measles, rabies, and chicken pox, infection produces symptoms typical of the diseases. In other viral infections, only a small number of infected people may develop a typical illness. Only comparatively few persons infected with poliomyelitis virus develop paralytic symptoms, while the majority develop a brief, often poorly defined illness. Such people have active immunity similar to that of persons who have recovered from a severe disease.

Passive immunity may be produced in normal persons by the injection of serum or certain chemically extracted fractions of serum from actively immunized persons or animals. This type of immunity is employed for conferring a rapid although temporary immunity to certain viral diseases—for example, measles and infectious hepatitis.

Immunity may be produced artificially by injecting a virus that has been weakened, so that the person has only a light case of the disease; upon recovery he remains immune for varying lengths of time. The injection of the weakened virus is known as *vaccination*.

The virus may be weakened by infecting another animal species, such as a calf or a rabbit. After these animals have acquired the disease, the organism may be reisolated and the process repeated. After several repetitions of this procedure, the virus may be so weakened that it no longer produces a severe disease, and yet it will produce immunity. The vaccine for smallpox is produced from infecting a calf, while that of yellow fever or influenza is produced from the infection of developing chick embryos. By drying the spinal cord of rabbits that have rabies, a vaccine may be produced which is effective in preventing the disease from developing in individuals who have been bitten by a rabid animal.

Aside from the vaccines that are produced with weakened virus and injected in small amounts, others are made from large amounts of "killed" or inactivated virus. When a large amount of this vaccine is injected, it stimulates the body to produce neutralizing substances in

TABLE OF REPRESENTATIVE VIRUS DISEASES

Common/ Technical Name of Disease	Body Regions Involved	Mode of Transmission/ Incubation Period	Main Symptoms of Disease	Control
Smallpox *Variola*	General (skin)	Direct contact (droplets); indirect by infected articles 12 days	Onset sudden or gradual. High fever, headache, backache, skin eruption starting as elevated spots which turn into vesicles which in turn become pussy and form crust. After crusts fall off, pink scars appear and leave well-known pock marks.	Vaccination with calf lymph or membranes of infected chick embryos. Primary vaccination of babies 4-6 mos. old; revaccination before entering school and again at 16 or later. Revaccination every two years or more often.
Measles *Rubeola*	General (skin)	Direct contact (droplets) 10-14 days	Fever, symptoms of cold, conjunctivitis, spots in the mouth, generalized rash over the whole body which disappears within 5-10 days without leaving any aftereffects. Disease less severe in children over 5 years.	During epidemic, children under 5 years should be kept at home. Passive immunity in exposed persons by inoculation of normal adult human sera. Inactivated virus grown in tissue culture now used for vaccination.
German Measles *Rubella*	General (skin)	Direct contact (droplets) 14-21 days	Symptoms of cold, enlargement of lymph nodes at the back of the neck, skin rash lasting only 2-3 days.	Mild disease. No control required. Deliberate exposure of girls before childbearing age recommended. Dangerous disease during first three months of pregnancy. If exposure occurs, serum from convalescent patients recommended but not very effective.
Chickenpox *Varicella*	General (skin)	Contact (droplets) 12-16 days	Fever, symptoms of cold, rash on the trunk, then limbs and face. Successive rashes may appear, so that spots, vesicles, and crusts appear at the same time. Spots in the mouth and throat. Mild but highly infectious disease.	None is available. Ultraviolet light reduces epidemics, but does not prevent spread of the disease.
Devil's grip, epidemic muscle pain or myalgia *Pleurodynia* (*Coxsackie virus disease*)	General (muscle)	Contact, flies, cockroaches 2-9 days	One of the diseases produced by the newly discovered Coxsackie viruses. Sudden onset, fever, pain in the neck or side of the chest or abdomen. May last 2-14 days or longer.	None is available.
Breakbone fever *Dengue fever*	General	Mosquitoes 4-8 days	Fever, headache, pains in the joints, back, muscles, and eyeballs. Skin rash for a few days. Prolonged (several weeks) convalescence.	Antimosquito measures. Vaccine available but not tried on a large scale.
Sandfly fever *Phlebotomus*	General	Sandfly, a small midge 3-6 days	Itching skin spots for 5 days, headache, fever, stiffness of neck and back, abdominal pain, conjunctivitis. Complete recovery.	Insect repellents, insecticides.
Exanthem subitum *Roseola infantum*	General (skin)	Probably contact 10-14 days	Exclusively infants 6 months to 3 years old. Sudden onset of fever, rash like in measles follows disappearance of fever. Complete recovery.	None.
Mountain tick fever *Colorado tick fever*	General (skin)	Ticks 4-6 days	Sudden onset, fever, headache, backache, vomiting. After 2 days without symptoms, reappearance of fever and other symptoms for 2-4 days.	Suitable clothing in tick-infested regions. Live vaccine from chick embryos infected with the virus.
Hydrophobia *Rabies*	Brain and nerves	Bite of a rabid animal 2-16 weeks or longer	Headache, nausea, vomiting, fever, swallowing produces muscle spasm in the throat, fear of water, convulsions, paralysis, death.	As soon as possible, washing of the wound with soap or detergent. Immune serum (passive immunization) on the day of bite, followed by vaccination with virus killed by phenol or ultraviolet light in 14 daily injections.

Common/ Technical Name of Disease	Body Regions Involved	Mode of Trans-mission/ Incubation Period	Main Symptoms of Disease	Control
Infantile paralysis *Poliomyelitis, Heine-Medin disease*	Spinal cord and brain	Contact, house flies, fleas, food, water 7-14 days, may be shorter or longer up to 4 weeks	Mild disease (abortive) most common form with fever, headache, nausea, vomiting, sore throat, full recovery in a few days. Nonparalytic disease has symptoms of the abortive illness with stiffness of the neck and back; full recovery. Paralytic disease follows symptoms already mentioned with muscle paralysis or with paralysis of respiratory or blood vessel centers in the brain.	Attenuated live virus (Sabin), used as a vaccine and taken by mouth, has superceded the earlier Salk vaccine and is now widely used.
Brain inflammation ("sleeping sickness") *Encephalitis (or meningoencephalitis); equine, St. Louis, Japanese, Russian encephalitis*	Brain and spinal cord	Arthropods (mosquitoes, ticks, mites) 4-21 days	Sudden fever, headache, vomiting, generalized pains, drowsiness, stupor, stiffness of the neck, twitching, convulsions, mental confusion. Aftereffects: blindness, deafness, mental defects, paralysis, epilepsy.	No specific vaccination as yet available. Antiarthropod measures.
Meningitis *Aseptic meningitis (Coxsackie virus-produced disease). Encephalomyocarditis*	Involvement of meningi. These viruses may produce heart muscle inflammation with blisters (herpangina)	Contact, feces, fleas 3-9 days	Variable symptoms according to the type of Coxsackie virus. Dangerous only in newborn infants with heart or brain inflammation.	No specific measures.
Meningitis *Aseptic meningitis produced by ECHO viruses*	Involvement of meningi with occasional mild paralysis	Contact, feces Short, probably a few days	Summer epidemics of fever and rash, especially among young children, diarrhea in infants, summer epidemics with or without rash. Recovery is complete.	No effective control measures available at present.
Common cold *Acute rhinitis, acute coryza*	Respiratory tract	Contact 2-5 days	Headache, cough, nasal discharge, mild fever. Average person suffers from at least two attacks a year.	No effective control measures available at present.
Flu *Influenza*	Respiratory tract	Contact (droplets) 1-2 days	Fever, muscular pain, chills. May be complicated by pneumonia which also may be caused by bacteria invading lungs.	Vaccines made of live weakened virus more effective if several strains of virus are included or made of virus responsible for epidemic.
Viral pneumonia *Primary atypical pneumonia*	Respiratory tract	Droplets 7-14 days	Headache, cough, fever, involvement of lungs.	No specific control.
Acute respiratory disease *Adenovirus diseases*	Respiratory tract	Contact a few days	Fever, inflamed throat, cough, conjunctivitis, running nose, inflammation of larynx, pneumonia.	Vaccine made of three different types of virus killed with formalin. Limited use, mostly among military personnel.

TABLE OF REPRESENTATIVE VIRUS DISEASES (Continued)

Common/ Technical Name of Disease	Body Regions Involved	Mode of Transmission/ Incubation Period	Main Symptoms of Disease	Control
Fever blisters *Herpes simplex or febrilis*	Skin or mucous membranes	Contact, saliva, stools, contaminated articles	Repeated localized vesicles on the skin or between skin and mucous membrane. Eczema. Vesicular eruption in the mouth of small children.	No specific control or treatment.
Shingles *Herpes zoster*	Skin and sensory nerves	Contact, droplets 7-14 days	Fever, severe pain in the skin or mucous membrane. Vesicles on the skin along the route of the nerve on the trunk, head, or neck.	None available.
Molluscum contagiosum	Skin	Direct or indirect contact 14-50 days	Small, pink, wartlike tumors on the face, arms, back. May occur as epidemic more frequently in children than adults. Several months before recovery takes place.	No specific treatment. X-rays may help sometimes.
Warts *Verruca*	Skin	Direct or indirect contact 1-8 months	Wart-shaped bodies on the skin. Disappear spontaneously.	No specific measures or treatment available.
Mumps *Epidemic parotitis*	Salivary glands, reproductive organs, occasionally central nervous system	Direct contact, droplets, contaminated articles 12-21 days	Swelling of the salivary glands on one or both sides. Mild disease in children, more severe in adults, may involve testes or ovaries.	No specific successful control, although vaccine available.
Epidemic jaundice and homologous serum jaundice *Infectious hepatitis and serum hepatitis*	Liver	Direct contact, food, water, injection of human infected blood 10-40 days; 45-160 days	Fever, vomiting, weakness, jaundice. Infectious hepatitis more severe in adults than in children.	Sanitation procedures. Use of normal adult serum during incubation period of infectious hepatitis gives protective action.
Mononucleosis, glandular fever, kissing disease	Lymph nodes, spleen	Probably contact	Fever, malaise, enlarged lymph nodes, spleen, monocytes and lymphocytes.	No specific measures.

the blood *(antibodies)* which persist for a prolonged period of time. Vaccines for sleeping sickness of horses and human beings *(equine encephalomyelitis)* and for influenza have been produced by this method. The viruses are inactivated by the use of ultraviolet light or by formaldehyde.

In some cases, it has been shown that an active virus injected into the skin will not produce a disease, but stimulates the body to form neutralizing substances. Had the same virus been taken into the body by way of the nasal membranes, it would have produced the disease. Thus, the entrance of a virus into the body by a route different from that to which it is habituated may stimulate the formation of immunity.

The body normally produces antibodies which will neutralize the viruses or their products. One may extract from the blood of an animal certain proteins which contain the majority of the antibodies. By various technical processes, relatively pure substances may be obtained. Upon injection, these substances will act in the same manner as the antibodies produced naturally in the human body. Partial immunity to measles may be obtained by injection of the immune fraction from the blood of individuals who have recently had the disease and recovered. Some viral diseases may be prevented by injection of an active virus along with the antibody substances. This method is used by veterinarians in immunizing against hog cholera.

Methods of transmission of viral diseases

Viruses may be present in various parts of the organism, including the blood and secretions of the body. They also may exist for varying periods outside the body, depending on the environment. World-wide epidemics of viral diseases are caused by viruses which have man as their only natural reservoir. In such cases, the spread occurs by direct contact with the infected persons or with their contaminated environment. Transmission may occur through droplets, sneezing and coughing, excreta, or contaminated articles (fomites).

Many viral diseases are transmitted to man by mosquitoes, mites, ticks, fleas, and sand flies (so-called "arthropods"). Few diseases are transmitted from man to man by these means. Most of these diseases are transmitted by arthropods from wild animals (even snakes) and birds, which are the principal hosts. In this case, man is an accidental host. In some viral diseases, arthropods may act as permanent hosts with accidental transmission to man. In arthropods, viruses will persist throughout their natural life span without ill effect, while in vertebrates and man most viruses produce a violent reaction, mostly of short duration, during which the host either succumbs, or survives and develops immunity and may become a carrier for the virus. Some virus diseases may also be spread by contaminated food—for example, poliovirus and infectious hepatitis. Rabies is transmitted through the bite or wound produced by an infected animal. Relatively few viral diseases are waterborne; however, the spread of *infectious hepatitis,* a disease of the liver, has been traced to water. Milk has also been considered as a transmitting agent for infectious hepatitis.

Prevention and treatment of viral diseases

International quarantine regulations are still in force against yellow fever, smallpox, and epidemic typhus. Temporary limitation of freedom of the exposed or affected persons, disinfestation or decontamination, and vaccination of susceptible persons are part of the sanitary practices. Quarantine has been abandoned or modified for patients or contacts with mumps, measles, German measles, chicken pox, and poliomyelitis because of the lack of good results in controlling spread of these diseases.

For active immunization against smallpox and yellow fever, there are vaccines available which are safe and efficient. These vaccines contain safe, live, attenuated viruses. There are also vaccines which consist of noninfectious (killed) virus and are used against poliomyelitis, influenza, and epidemic typhus. They have to be administered repeatedly at various intervals of time to keep up immunity. For example, Salk vaccine against poliomyelitis has to be administered to all persons under forty in three doses, the first two at monthly intervals, followed after six months by a third dose and a "booster" shot every year. Vaccine composed of live but attenuated (deprived of virulence) strains of poliovirus is now available in pills or liquid form. It has been employed extensively in all developed countries and the disease is now a rarity. Painstaking tests are now being carried out to ascertain the absence of other viruses in such vaccines produced from tissue cultures of monkey kidney cells infected with the different strains of poliovirus.

There is no doubt that the next few years will see the development of new and improved vaccines against adenoviruses which produce respiratory diseases, and against measles and influenza, to mention only some viral diseases.

Passive immunization with immune serum against measles and infectious hepatitis must be carried out before exposure or before the onset of clinical disease to prove effective.

There is as yet no specific treatment for viral diseases, but there is little doubt that it will become available in due course because of the present intensive efforts to find proper therapeutic measures.

Classification of virus-produced diseases

The viruses which affect human beings may be divided into certain categories, relating to the portion of the body they attack. Those which have an affinity for the skin are called *dermatropic* viruses; those which primarily affect the lungs are called *pneumotropic* viruses. Some cause disease of the nervous tissue, hence are said to be *neurotropic*. Others may damage the body as a whole, and are termed *generalized* viral diseases. The above classification will be used in this chapter.

Dermatropic viral diseases

The principal dermatropic viruses are those producing smallpox, measles, German measles, chickenpox, shingles, and warts. These diseases seem to be transmitted chiefly by droplet infection from the upper respiratory tract and by direct contact. Prior to the nineteenth century, smallpox was regarded as the most dreaded of diseases. It occurred in epidemics which left behind bodily disfigured or depleted populations. About 95 out of every 100 persons had the disease at some time during their lives. Vaccination, first developed by Jenner in 1798, has been the chief method of combating the disease. At the present time, only a few sporadic cases occur in the United States. (For a more complete discussion of this disease, consult Chapter 8, "The Skin: *Smallpox.*")

Measles is perhaps the most contagious of all human diseases. Most people have it during childhood. Measles is a dermatropic viral disease characterized by a typical skin rash. German measles (Rubella) is a viral disease so mild that quite often it is undetected. However, if a woman contracts the disease in the first or second trimester of pregnancy, her child may be stillborn or afflicted with multiple birth defects which may include congenital heart disease, deafness, cataracts, orthopedic problems, and mental retardation. A new vaccine for this disease is now available and a drive is underway to vaccinate children of school age throughout the country. However, the vaccine contains live viruses and so cannot be given to pregnant women. Since approximately 85 percent of women in the United States have natural immunity to rubella, a blood test should be made before giving a woman the vaccine.

Herpes simplex is a dermatropic viral disease which will attack various parts of the body to produce a large number of different symptoms. Perhaps the most common manifestation of this disease is "cold sores" or "fever blisters," which often occur about the mouth. *Herpes zoster* or shingles is a disease which is characterized by the distribution of large blister-like sores along the course of a nerve. (For a more complete discussion of this subject, see Chapter 8, "The Skin: *Dermatitis.*")

Molluscum contagiosum, a disease which causes round, wartlike structures on the skin, is caused by a virus. Warts of children and sometimes of adults owe their existence to a dermatropic virus.

Neurotropic viral diseases

Of the neurotropic group, the poliomyelitis virus is perhaps the best known. The method of transmission is unknown, but the virus may be isolated from houseflies and the solid waste material *(feces)* and sputum of infected individuals. It is also known to exist in the intestines of infected individuals.

Rabies is another of the neurotropic viral diseases. An effective vaccine was first devised by Louis Pasteur, which prevents the development of the disease; once rabies develops, however, it terminates fatally. Other neurotropic viral diseases are the "sleeping sickness" types of diseases *(encephalitis)*, which are believed to be transmitted from large animals to man, by the mosquito. In addition, the recently discovered Coxsackie and ECHO viruses may attack the nervous system. (Poliomyelitis, rabies, and other neurotropic diseases are discussed more fully in Chapter 11, "The Brain and Nervous System.")

Pneumotropic viral diseases

The pneumotropic viruses are those which have a particular affinity for the lungs and bronchial system. The virus of influenza is of this type. Influenza is ordinarily a rather mild disease characterized by fever, headache, and pains in the back and leg muscles. These symptoms persist for about a week and are followed by recovery. Should the influenza viral infection be accompanied by a bacterial infection, as was thought to be the case during the world-wide epidemic *(pandemic)* of 1918, then it may be a much more serious, pneumonia-like disease.

The virus that is thought to be the cause of the common cold is the pneumotropic type. This virus may initiate the cold, while other microorganisms may be responsible for the variety of symptoms which accompany the disease. Much research is in progress on this, the commonest of all human diseases. *Primary atypical pneumonia* or "virus pneumonia" is considered a viral infection; however, the specific causative organism has not been definitely identified. As in the case of the other pneumotropic viral diseases, there are a multitude of bacteria which may be found associated with this disease. The pneumotropic viral diseases are spread by droplet infection which enters the body by way of the upper respiratory tract. (Pneumonia and influenza are discussed further in Chapter 5, "The Respiratory System.")

Mumps is also a viral disease. The virus enters the body through the upper respiratory system and affects primarily the salivary glands. This infection may spread to other parts of the body, especially the testes and ovaries. Other respiratory viral diseases include diseases produced by the newly discovered adenoviruses.

Generalized viral diseases

The generalized viral diseases include yellow fever, pleurodynia (epidemic myalgia or devil's grip), dengue, sandfly fever, and Colorado tick fever.

The story of the discovery, in 1900, of the method of transmission of yellow fever, a virus disease, by a mosquito, *Aedes aegypti,* is a dramatic chapter in medical history. Doctor Walter Reed and his associates were able to show that the virus that causes the disease can be transmitted only by the bite of a female mosquito which has previously become infected through feeding on the blood of a person during the first few days of his attack. The mosquito is able to transmit the disease for ten to twelve days thereafter. Prior to this discovery, yellow fever was one of the most deadly diseases in the tropics and along the southern seacoast of the United States. There have been few cases of yellow fever in the United States since that time (the last epidemic in the United States occurred in New Orleans in 1905), but it remains a threat, since there is a reservoir of this disease in the monkey population of South America. Vaccination seems effective in preventing this disease. (Yellow fever is discussed further in Chapter 24, "Tropical Diseases.")

Dengue, or breakbone fever, is a painful viral disease of comparatively short duration transmitted by the same mosquito *(Aedes aegypti)* that transmits yellow fever. Sandfly fever is a similar disease spread by small biting flies.

In addition to the viral diseases that readily fall into the above classification, there are still others that relate to specific body parts. Thus, a virus causes jaundice, a liver disorder; another causes warts; still another causes encephalitis, in which the brain and spinal cord are involved.

Viruses and cancer

The last ten years have witnessed an amazing progress in the studies on viruses as causative agents of infectious diseases. During the same time a considerable number of viruses have been found to be the cause of various types of cancer in animals of the most diverse species.

Benign warts, papilloma, and *molluscum contagiosum* of man each have a well-established viral etiology so that these relatively benign tumors are known to be the result of virus affecting man. Many of the adenoviruses of man are capable of producing experimental cancers when injected into newborn animals. The papovavirus of monkeys does not cause any natural tumor in its normal host, but will produce tumors in hamsters. This virus will infect many animal cells (including human) in tissue cultures and cause a change in the cells which is termed *cell transformation.* There is a great parallel between the growth of transformed cells and the growth of cancer cells in the test tubes as well as in the living host. The field of research of the role of viruses as cause of cancers in man is relatively new, but experimentation is progressing rapidly. One interesting, though speculative, by-product of these researches into the genetic interactions between viruses and their hosts is the possibility of "genetic engineering." It may eventually become possible to restore genetic functions which are lacking or defective in an animal or human by attaching the gene in question to the appropriate segment of viral DNA and then introducing it into the cells lacking the function.

At the present time evidence is accumulating that viruses may play a part in at least certain types of human cancer, for example, leukemia. Virus particles have been observed by means of the electron microscope in thin slices of human leukemic lymph nodes surgically removed from patients with various types of leukemia. Similar virus particles have also been found in cells of leukemic lymph nodes grown in test tubes and examined in the electron microscope. Cell-free extracts of such lymph nodes have been reported to induce leukemia in animals. Much additional evidence must be accumulated before the virus particles can be accepted as the causative agents of human leukemia. Nevertheless, a beginning in the study of viral origin of human cancer has been made. There is every hope that application of the methods of study which gave such excellent results in the case of animal cancers, such as tissue culture, use of newborn animals, electron microscopy, and biochemical methods, will help in our future understanding of at least some types of cancer in human beings and lead to its successful prevention and treatment.

The rickettsial diseases

There is a group of submicroscopic organisms which in structure at one time appeared to be midway between the larger viruses and the smaller bacteria. These are known as the *rickettsiae.*

It is clear that these minute organisms are true bacteria, possessing typical bacterial cell walls and membranes, both types of nucleic acid (DNA and RNA) and the biochemical machinery for protein synthesis and enzymatic activities. Like the viruses, probably all of these tiny organisms require living cells for growth. The rickettsiae require an intermediate host, which is usually a bloodsucking insect, in order for the organism to be transmitted from individual to individual. While many of the organisms pass into the bloodstream by the bite of the insect, the organism may be deposited on the skin in the excrement of the insect.

The distribution of these diseases depends on the distribution of the insect carrier. Thus, typhus, which is carried by the human body louse, is world-wide in distribution. In the louse, the rickettsial bodies multiply in the intestinal lining and escape through the intestine by the excrement. The organism then enters the blood by an abrasion produced when the person scratches. A big outbreak occurred in the Korean campaign among the Chinese soldiers. There is also another variety of typhus, *murine* (rat) typhus, which is a disease of both rats and man. It is transmitted from rat to rat, and rat to man, by means of the rat flea. A typhus vaccine produced from organisms grown on chick embryo cultures is effective in preventing these diseases. The spread of typhus, following World War II, was curtailed by the use of DDT as a delousing agent.

Rocky Mountain spotted fever, another

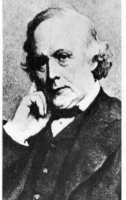

LISTER, Joseph (1827-1912) English surgeon. Lister is universally famous for his introduction of the practice of sterile techniques in surgery. The painstaking care that he employed in order to keep a surgical operation free of infectious microorganisms was at first very unpopular with his medical colleagues, but it rapidly proved its tremendous value in preventing the many complications caused by various types of surgical infections. *Bettmann Archive.*

rickettsial disease, is transmitted by the bite of the wood or dog tick. The rickettsiae are found in all organs of the tick including the egg cells, whereby a new generation of ticks is infected. The use of a vaccine furnishes some immunity to persons continuously exposed.

Some relatively unknown or rare diseases may suddenly become serious threats. This was the case in World War II, when many American soldiers fighting in the South Pacific became victims of *scrub typhus* or tsutsu-gamushi fever. This serious disease is transmitted by the bite of a small mite or "chigger." The use of chemical repellents for the insect is about the only method devised for combating this disease. Bullis Fever, a similar disease believed to be conveyed to man by the tick *Amblyomma americanum,* was first encountered at Camp Bullis, Texas, during 1942 and 1943. Another rickettsial disease called *Q fever* is prevalent among slaughter house workers who probably inhale dried excrement from infected ticks that are carried on the hides of the slaughtered animals.

The chlamydia

The agents of the disease, *psittacosis (ornithosis), lymphogranuloma venereum,* and *trachoma* are another group of minute bacteria which until recently had been considered to be large viruses; but it is now known that they contain both types of nucleic acid, their own enzyme system, and biochemical machinery for making protein. Like the rickettsia, they are obligate intracellular parasites. Most of these organisms live in a well-balanced state of latent infection in their normal hosts. For example, the agent of psittacosis causes, for the most part, a subclinical infection in birds. When spread to man (through handling or by inhalation of infected dried bird feces), human beings may develop the same sort of subclinical in-

fection. More commonly, the disease appears as a sudden atypical pneumonia about seven to ten days after exposure. Clinically, the disease may resemble either bronchial pneumonia, influenza, or typhoid fever. Mortality is generally high in untreated cases; the tetracycline antibiotics have been effective in treatment of the disease.

Lymphogranuloma venereum is a venereal disease caused by an agent in this group. Latent or subclinical infections also appear to be common with this infection. The initial site of infection is usually marked by a small papule which bursts to leave a small ulcer or chancre. The agent rapidly spreads through the lymphatic system and causes infection and enlargement of the nearest lymph node. Chronic inflammation of these glands may persist for years. Treatment with sulfonamide drugs and tetracyclines has given good results.

Two diseases of the eye, *trachoma* and *inclusion conjunctivitis,* are caused by members of the chlamydia group. Both diseases may lead to blindness through the scarring of the tissues involved in the diseases. Trachoma is spread by fingers and fomites (any substance other than foods that may harbor the organism) and it is estimated that about one-half billion people in the world are infected, with perhaps 20 million blinded in tropical and subtropical lands. The disease can be treated with sulfonamides and ophthalmic tetracycline. Modern hygienic practices could reduce the spread. Inclusion conjunctivitis is basically an infection of the adult genital tract and is a typical venereal disease. As in gonorrhea, the eye of the newborn is infected during passage through the birth canal. Some swimming pool infections of the eye may occur, but adequate chlorination easily controls this vector of infection.

The mycoplasmas

A group of bacteria are permanently devoid of rigid cell walls, and consequently are rather formless. The first organism of this type had been shown to be the causative agent of contagious bovine pleuropneumonia. As additional organisms of this type were isolated from human beings and domestic animals, they were termed pleuropneumonia-like organisms, (abbreviated PPLO). These bacteria are minute and due to their plasticity of form can pass through filters which retain most ordinary bacteria. They can be cultivated on cell-free media although most of the parasitic forms require the presence of serum or ascitic fluid for growth. Many bacteria can be grown under conditions where the rigid cell wall cannot be formed and thus these L-forms resemble mycoplasmas superficially. The mycoplasmas breed true to type, while the L-forms of bacteria can regain their structure. The relation of the mycoplasmas to bacterial L-forms is not known. In human beings, both forms can be found in many tissues and exudates with no apparent pathological condition. Two diseases of man are unequivocally proven to be caused by *mycoplasmas. Mycoplasma hominis* type 1 produces an acute respiratory disease marked by sore throat and tonsil involvement. Approximately 50 percent of normal adults give evidence of having acquired antibodies to this agent. *M. pneumoniae* is one of the many agents which can cause primary atypical pneumonia. In man, this syndrome can be almost inapparent to a severe upper respiratory disease. The mycoplasmal diseases are refractory to treatment with antibiotics which interfere with cell wall synthesis (such as penicillin or bacitracin) and the sulfonamides are likewise generally ineffective. Tetracycline antibiotics are effective.

BACTERIA

The *bacteria* are one-celled microscopic organisms which do not have a well-defined nucleus. These organisms divide by a process known as *fission;* they grow longer in one direction, and then pinch into two separate individuals. The bacteria may appear under the microscope as small rodlike bodies, tiny spheres, or corkscrewlike cells. They may adhere to each other or live separately. They are measured by the micron, approximately 1/25,000 of an inch, and vary in size.

Because bacteria are small in size, man did not realize for centuries that they existed. It was not until the seventeenth century that a Dutch lens grinder, Antonj van Leeuwenhoek, first observed these organisms in a drop of stagnant water. Their significance remained unknown until the latter half of the nineteenth century when the French chemist, Louis Pasteur, began research on the cause of fermentation. Before this time, men thought that organic material— that is, substances of plant or animal origin— would spontaneously decompose in the presence of air. Pasteur demonstrated that fluids such as meat, broth, milk, and wine subjected to prolonged boiling would not decompose until some unboiled material was admitted. This suggested the presence of unseen organisms— bacteria—and their role in the decomposition or fermentation of food. The application of his discovery led to the preservation of food and the *"pasteurization"* process for the purification of milk. Lord Lister, the great English surgeon, was the first to apply the discoveries of Pasteur to medicine and to develop antiseptic techniques in surgery, which he reported in 1867.

Most of the thousands of types of bacteria are not harmful to human beings; indeed, many are so essential that our lives depend on them. Were it not for the bacteria, animal waste matter and the bodies of dead plants and animals would accumulate in such abundance that living beings would perish for lack of space in which to exist. In addition to the destruction of waste matter, the enrichment of the soil depends on microorganisms; certain bacteria take *nitrogen* from the atmosphere and combine it into a form that green plants can use for growth and development. Bacteria likewise are essential to the production of foods such as buttermilk and cheese, and in the preparation of linen, the tanning of leather, curing of tobacco, and many chemical manufacturing processes. Unfortunately, among the bacteria there are some that attack the living bodies of man and animals and produce disease; these are known as *pathogens*.

Types of bacteria

On the basis of their shapes, bacteria may be grouped into three main divisions. The first of these are rod-shaped and are called *bacilli* (singular: *bacillus*). The bacilli often have small, whiplike structures known at *flagella*, with which they are able to move about. Some bacilli have oval, egg-shaped, or spherical bodies in their cells, known as *spores*. Under adverse conditions, dehydration, and in the presence of disinfectants, the bacteria may die, but the spores may be able to live on. The spores germinate when the conditions become favorable, and form new bacterial cells. Some are so resistant that they can withstand boiling and freezing temperatures and prolonged desiccation.

A second-type of bacteria is the *cocci* (singular: *coccus*) which are spherical or ovoid in shape. The individual bacterial cells of this group may occur singly (*Micrococcus*), in chains (*Streptococcus*), in pairs (*Diplococcus*), in irregular bunches (*Staphylococcus*), and in the form of cubical packets (*Sarcina*). The coccus does not form spores and usually is *nonmotile* —that is, it does not move about.

A third group of bacteria are the curved or bent rods. Of these, the genus *Vibrio* is composed of bacteria that are comma-shaped; and the genus *Spirillum* consists of those that are twisted and spiral in form. All members of this group are motile, but none forms spores; however, some of these bacteria form a gelatinous capsule or covering by which they are probably protected from adverse environmental conditions. Still another group of spiral-shaped bacteria are known as the *spirochetes*, one of which is the cause of syphilis.

Bacteria also may be classified on the basis of their requirements of free atmospheric oxygen.

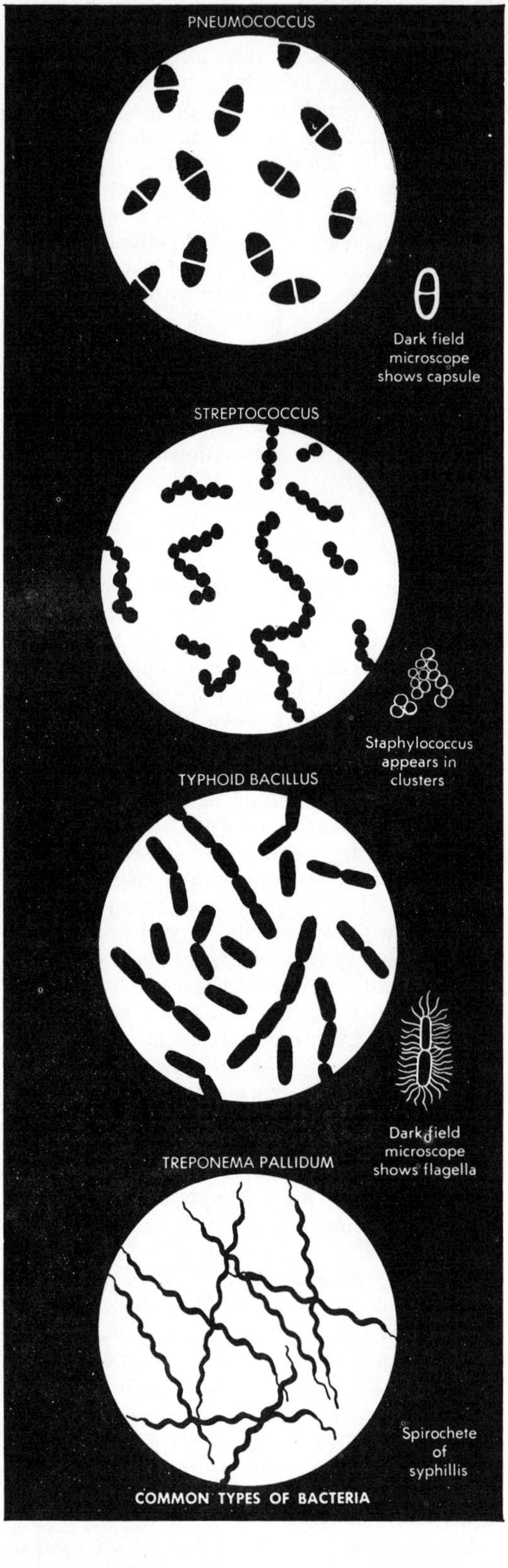
PNEUMOCOCCUS
Dark field microscope shows capsule
STREPTOCOCCUS
Staphylococcus appears in clusters
TYPHOID BACILLUS
Dark field microscope shows flagella
TREPONEMA PALLIDUM
Spirochete of syphillis
COMMON TYPES OF BACTERIA

Those which require atmospheric oxygen are called *aerobic* (air-living); those which cannot live in the presence of atmospheric oxygen are called *anaerobic*; those which do well with oxygen but can get along without it are termed *facultative* anaerobes.

Bacteria are dependent upon the proper temperature for life and reproduction; and the various species of bacteria may differ widely in their temperature requirements. Most of the disease-producing (*pathogenic*) bacteria thrive best at body temperatures; others may live and multiply in much cooler temperatures; while still others live in hot springs. Freezing, as a rule, does not destroy bacteria, but prevents their reproduction. High temperature, conversely, quickly kills many bacteria. For instance, most disease-producing organisms in milk may be killed by raising the temperature to 143° Fahrenheit and maintaining it for 30 minutes. This process is called *pasteurization*, and is used widely for milk and other foods. Most nonsporeforming, disease-producing microorganisms, including the bacteria, are destroyed by boiling water. In the spore stage, some bacteria must be heated to 240° Fahrenheit for a considerable period of time, in order that the spores be destroyed. These high temperatures are best obtained by steam under pressure. For this reason, a pressure cooker must be used to assure that home-canned foods do not spoil.

Destruction of bacteria

Bacteria may be killed by the action of chemicals called *disinfectants*. A substance which prevents infection or inhibits growth of microorganisms is called *antiseptic*. Some of the most potent disinfectants are phenol or carbolic acid and related compounds. Free chlorine gas is an excellent disinfectant, as are hypochlorites, solutions of which are marketed under various trade names. Drinking water is often treated with chlorine gas to render it safe for drinking purposes. Tincture of iodine used on some cuts and other wounds has good disinfecting power. Bichloride of mercury and other mercury-containing compounds, mercurochrome, merthiolate, and phenylmercurinitrate are often used as disinfectants and antiseptics. Alcohol in a 50 to 70 percent solution, as found in common rubbing alcohol, is a dependable disinfectant. Highly advertised mouth washes and gargles have low antiseptic properties and should not be relied upon to prevent colds, sore throat, or tooth decay. All effective antiseptics are poisonous to living tissue, to some extent, and should not be administered promiscuously to infected areas.

In recent years, much emphasis has been placed on *bacteriostatic* agents. These substances prevent or slow down the rate of bacterial

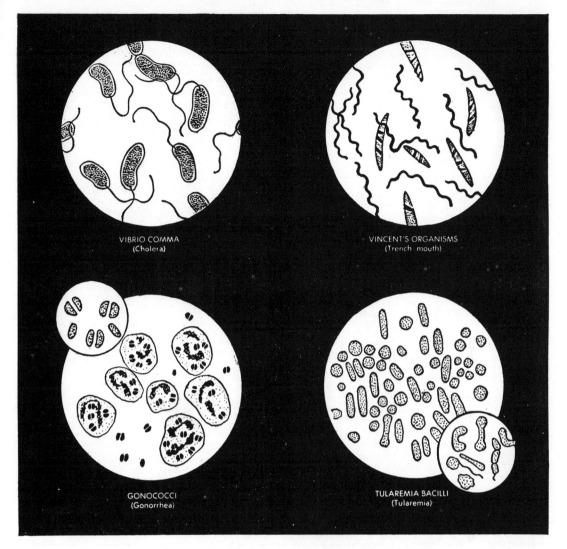

VIBRIO COMMA
(Cholera)

VINCENT'S ORGANISMS
(Trench mouth)

GONOCOCCI
(Gonorrhea)

TULAREMIA BACILLI
(Tularemia)

COMMON TYPES OF BACTERIA

growth and reproduction, so that the natural protective mechanisms of the body can overcome the infection. These chemicals include the sulfonamide group such as sulfathiazole, sulfadiazine, sulfanilamide, sulfasuxidine, and sulfaguanidine. These drugs are valuable in the treatment of patients with certain diseases; however, if taken indiscriminately, they can produce serious symptoms or death.

The use of *antibiotics* is even a newer development in medical science. These are substances produced by other living organisms which inhibit the growth of bacteria or destroy them. One of the most important of these agents is penicillin, which was discovered by Alexander Fleming (1881–1955) in 1928. Sir Alexander Fleming shared the 1945 Nobel prize in Medicine and Physiology for this discovery which revolutionized therapy for infectious microorganisms. This substance was isolated from a green mold that is often found growing in nature. While in general, this substance is not toxic to living tissue, it is quite active against many species of bacteria.

Streptomycin also has been isolated from a soil microorganism. Streptomycin inhibits the growth of some microorganisms which are not affected by either penicillin or the sulfonamides. Numerous other antibiotic agents have been isolated from fungi, other bacteria, or even from green plants. Some of these are chloromycetin, aureomycin, polymixin, neomycin, and Terramycin. There are few known bacterial diseases, the effects of which cannot be mitigated if the proper antibiotic is used early in the course of the disease. Tetanus and botulism are exceptions. These diseases are the manifestations of extremely potent toxins produced by the bacteria, rather than symptoms caused by infections

TABLE OF REPRESENTATIVE BACTERIAL DISEASES

Common Name of Disease	Technical Name of Disease	Organism Responsible	Body Regions Involved	Mode of Transmission	Incubation Period	Symptoms
Septic sore throat	Streptococcus sore throat or tonsillitis	Streptococcus (several species)	Throat and nasal membranes	Droplet and direct contact	3 to 5 days	Sore throat often accompanied by fever and a cough.
Scarlet fever	Scarlatina	Streptococcus (*Streptococcus scarlatinae*)	Throat, tonsils, and often other tissues	Carrier, direct contact, droplet and food	3 to 5 days	Sore throat, headache, fever, swollen tongue, pink or red rash, rapid pulse, and "strawberry tongue."
Pneumonia	Pneumococcal pneumonia	Diplococcus (*Diplococcus pneumoniae*)	Respiratory tract, including the lungs	Droplet	Variable	Chills, pain in the chest, rusty sputum, rapid breathing, abdominal pain, jaundice.
Spinal meningitis	Epidemic meningitis	Diplococcus (*Neisseria intracellularis*)	Respiratory tract, nervous system, and sometimes blood	Carrier, droplet	1 to 5 days	Severe headache, violent vomiting, high fever, delirium, and rigid neck and back. Rash may be present.
Clap	Gonorrhea	Diplococcus (*Neisseria gonorrhoeae*)	Reproductive organs	Sexual intercourse	2 to 8 days	Redness, swelling, penile or urethral discharge, and frequent and burning urination.
Typhoid and paratyphoid fevers	Enteric fever	Short rod (*Salmonella typhosa*) (*Salmonella paratyphi*)	Intestine	Flies, food, feces, water, and carriers	10 to 14 days	Fever, nausea, vomiting, severe abdominal pain, chills, and diarrhea.
Bacillary dysentery	Shigellosis	Short rod (*Shigella dysenteriae*)	Intestine	Flies, food, feces, water, and carriers	1 to 4 days	Fever, nausea, vomiting, severe abdominal pain, blood in the stools, and diarrhea.
Whooping cough	Pertussis	Small short rod (*Hemophilus pertussis*)	Respiratory tract	Droplets projected during cough	7 to 14 days	Coldlike symptoms. Series of coughs followed by a whoop.
Bubonic plague	Pestis	Short rod (*Pasteurella pestis*)	Blood, spleen, liver, and lymph nodes	Rat flea spreads disease from rat to man	2 to 10 days	Sudden onset, high fever, vomiting, hot dry skin, thirst, black spots on skin, lymph nodes in groin swollen.
Rabbit fever	Tularemia	Short rod (*Pasteurella tularensis*)	Lymph nodes, spleen, liver, kidneys, and lungs	Contact with animals that have the disease	1 to 10 days	Sudden onset, chills, fever, nausea, and vomiting. Prostration. Local sore and enlarged regional lymph nodes.
Undulant fever	Brucellosis	Short rod (*Brucella abortus*)	General infection throughout the body	Milk and direct contact with animals	5 days to 3 weeks	Periods of fever alternating with periods of normal temperature, recurrent attacks, loss of weight, backache, weakness and insomnia.
Lockjaw	Tetanus	Sporeforming rod (*Clostridium tetani*)	Nervous system	Organism in soil; enters through wound	2 to 40 days	Spasms of muscles and convulsions. Lockjaw.
Gas gangrene	Gas gangrene	Sporeforming rod (*Clostridium perfringens*)	Wounded areas	Organism in soil; enters through wound	Variable	Gassy swelling of the wounds, foul odor.
Botulinus	Botulism	Sporeforming rod (*Clostridium botulinum*)	Nervous system	Organism produces poison in food	18 to 66 hours	Severe gastrointestinal upset, vomiting and diarrhea, fatigue, disturbance of vision, paralysis.
Tuberculosis or consumption	Phthisis or tuberculosis	Irregular rod (*Mycobacterium tuberculosis*)	Lungs, bones, and other organs	Direct contact, droplet infection, food and milk	Variable	Symptoms vary with the organ affected, cough, fever in the evening, fatigue, loss of weight, x-ray pictures show infection in the lungs.
Syphilis	Lues	Spiral-shaped organism (*Treponema pallidum*)	Blood and nervous system	Direct contact, chiefly sexual intercourse	10 to 90 days	A hard, painless sore or chancre on the genitalia, variable types of skin eruptions, and serious tissue destruction in any part of the body.
Diphtheria	Diphtheria	Irregular rod (*Corynebacterium diphtheriae*)	Respiratory tract	Carrier, direct contact, droplet and food	1 to 7 days	Sore throat, fever, vomiting, prostration, formation of a gray membranous deposit in the throat, difficult breathing.

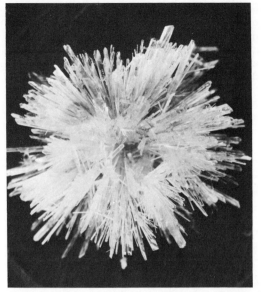

Photomicrograph of crystals of penicillin magnified about 300 times. This material appears as a fine white powder. *Copyright Cutter Laboratories.*

of the microorganisms themselves. If used without medical supervision, antibiotics may lead to severe rashes, swellings, and other more serious symptoms. As bacteria have developed penicillin resistance, through mutation and selection, the development of a wide range of synthetic penicillins has provided more than adequate replacements for the natural substance. These drugs constitute the most effective weapons in the treatment of most diseases of bacterial origin when properly administered. Despite the relatively low toxicities of the penicillins, a small proportion of the human population demonstrates severe reactions (allergic and anaphylactic), so various precautions must be observed.

Transmission of bacterial diseases

Bacterial diseases may be transmitted in a number of ways. The common respiratory diseases, such as sore throat, pneumonia, and whooping cough are distributed by small droplets of sputum and nasal secretions. These are propelled into the air for a considerable distance when an infected person sneezes or coughs. The droplets may carry many living bacteria which would be sources of infection should they come in contact with the mucous membranes of a susceptible person.

Other diseases are transmitted by direct contact of individual to individual. The respiratory diseases may be transmitted by this method also. Sexual intercourse is the method by which venereal diseases such as syphilis and gonorrhea are usually spread. Further, since many bacteria live until they are dried, diseases may be transmitted through indirect contact with persons through objects that they have handled.

Some diseases are transmitted by water, milk, and foods which have become contaminated by persons who have the disease or who carry the organisms that cause the disease (carriers). Typhoid and typhoid-like fevers, cholera, and certain diarrheas, all of which are intestinal diseases, may be transmitted in this manner. Insects are also carriers of bacterial diseases. Many intestinal infections are transmitted by the housefly.

Disease-producing bacteria usually cannot penetrate the unbroken skin; hence they must enter by means of wounds, abrasions, or scratches, or by the natural openings of the body. The diseases which accompany wounds of the skin include blood poisoning, gas gangrene, and tetanus. The organisms causing anthrax and glanders in human beings often enter through wounds.

The practice of sanitation and the prevention of infection rest upon a knowledge of how a disease is transmitted and upon the ability of the individual person to avoid the source of infection. Governmental agencies also assist in prevention through the enforcement of sanitary laws and codes, and by the construction of properly designed water and sewerage systems. The control of insects likewise is chiefly a municipal problem and conducted by trained technicians. Much of the responsibility for detecting the beginnings of epidemics of disease rests with local health units. (The control of disease through sanitary procedures is further discussed in Chapter 25, "Environmental Health and Sanitation.")

Resistance to disease

The most important means of resisting infection is to prevent the entrance of microorganisms into the body. The skin is the principal barrier,

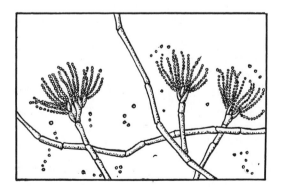

The above drawing of the mold, *Penicillium notatum,* shows characteristic fruiting organs of the genus. Penicillin is obtained from this fungus.

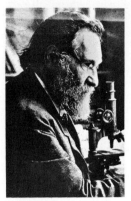

METCHNIKOFF, Elie (1845-1916) Russian biologist who spent much of his life in France. He is universally famous for the important theory that he developed concerning the mode of ingestion of living bacteria by certain of the white blood cells. He also studied methods of syphilis prevention. Metchnikoff's many notable investigations into the mechanisms of immunity to various infectious diseases earned him the Nobel prize with Paul Ehrlich, in 1908.

since few bacteria can enter through the unbroken skin. The secretions of the skin and the mucous membranes of the throat also may retard bacterial invasion. The digestive juices of the stomach and intestine destroy most of the bacteria which are swallowed with food.

Once bacteria have gained entrance into the tissues of the body, a number of important defensive measures are mobilized to resist the invaders. The blood is the carrier of many substances which combat disease. The *white blood cells* take bacteria into their protoplasm, and thereby digest or destroy them. The liquid part of the blood (*plasma*) contains substances which cause the bacteria to clump or adhere to each other, thereby enabling the blood cells to dispose of them more efficiently. Once an infection is established in the body, numerous white blood cells migrate to the area and form a living wall which helps prevent the spread of the infection. They make up a large part of the pus that is so frequently seen in infection. Many bacteria produce poisonous substances, *toxins*, which in turn stimulate the formation in the human body of an antibody, *antitoxin*, which circulates in the blood. These neutralize the toxins.

Immunity to disease can be produced by inoculating a person with bacteria, toxins, or viruses. Usually dead or "attenuated" cultures of organisms or minute quantities of the toxic materials are used for this purpose. For instance, if dead typhoid bacteria are injected into the body, the body responds by producing *antibodies*. These antibodies will remain in the blood for a long period and will destroy any live typhoid bacteria that enter the body, thereby rendering the individual immune to typhoid. When the number of antibodies in the blood becomes too low to render the person immune, he must receive another injection (a "booster" shot) and start the immunizing process over again. In some cases, it is possible to inject weakened bacteria and promote the development of anti-

bodies. The body generates antitoxin in the presence of weakened bacterial toxins. By injecting carefully balanced toxins and antitoxins, one may produce immunity to diphtheria, tetanus, and some other diseases. Recently, it has been discovered that toxins can be treated with chemicals to the extent that they are no longer harmful, but will still stimulate the body to produce antitoxins.

ONE-CELLED ANIMALS

In the animal kingdom, the simplest of all creatures are the single-celled organisms known as *protozoa.*

Diseases produced by amoeba-like organisms

The protozoa may be divided into four classes on the basis of their form. The first class, *Sarcodina*, contains the commonly known specimen, *amoeba*. These protozoa do not have a definite shape, but are a mass of protoplasm containing a nucleus. Amoebas move by a type of flowing motion. They engulf their food, chiefly small plants and other protozoa, into their protoplasm by literally surrounding it with their bodies. These organisms, as is the case with most protozoa, reproduce asexually by increasing in size and dividing. This process is termed *fission*. Only one or possibly two of this group of protozoa cause disease in human beings. *Endamoeba histolytica* is the cause of amoebic dysentery, a disease of the gastrointestinal tract which sometimes affects the liver and other organs. These small organisms live in the wall of the intestine, where they feed chiefly on the blood and produce varying degrees of ulceration. This causes the frequent passage of bloody and mucous stools and produces a painful condition in the lower bowels. The causative organism forms thick-walled *cysts* which enable it to survive and to infect other hosts. These cysts are resistant to some chemicals used in the purification of water, so that epidemics have been traced to water. Many people have chronic amoebic dysentery, and may become carriers. These carriers often contaminate the food and water supply, and thereby transmit the disease. Amoebic dysentery also may be spread by flies and other insects. Studies have shown that as high as 50 percent of the population in tropical American countries are infected, and as high as 10 percent in some United States communities. The disease is world-wide in distribution. (For further discussion of dysentery, see Chapter 13, "The Digestive System.")

Another amoebic type of protozoa, *Endamoeba gingivalis*, is thought to affect the mucous membranes of the mouth. This protozoan has been shown to be present in advanced cases of *pyorrhea*, a disease of the gums. While it cannot be stated definitely that the organisms are the cause of pyorrhea, they certainly are associated with it. By proper dental care and oral hygiene, most cases of pyorrhea may be prevented.

Balantidial dysentery, a rare disease of pigs and man, produces symptoms similar to those of amoebic dysentery, and is transmitted in the same manner. The organism which causes it, *Balantidium coli*, is a member of the class *Ciliata*, one of the largest groups of the protozoa. Members of this class are single cells and swim by means of the movement of hundreds of small hairlike structures (*cilia*) projecting from the surface of the cell. This is the only member of the class known to be disease-producing. The tetracycline antibiotics seem to be helpful.

Diseases caused by the flagellate protozoa

Among the protozoa is a class (*Flagellata*) whose members have long hairlike structures called *flagella*. These long, single-celled animals propel themselves through fluid by a beating motion of the flagella. Some of these organisms are plantlike, in that they produce their own food by the green pigment in their bodies. There are many free-living, nonparasitic forms, but some members of this group are parasitic.

Some of the flagellates inhabit the intestinal tract and in rare cases become so numerous that they interfere with the utilization of food by the infected person. One species, *Trichomonas vaginalis*, lives in the female genital tract and sometimes produces irritating symptoms that require medical attention. There are other flagellates that live habitually in the blood or other tissues of man.

African sleeping sickness is caused by flagellates called *trypanosomes* (*Trypanosoma gambiense, T. rhodesiense*). These are microscopic, elongated cells which swim by means of a wavy membrane ending in a flagellum. The disease is spread from animals to man by the bite of the *tsetse* fly. The trypanosomes develop in the blood and eventually invade the lymph fluid surrounding the nerves and brain, involvement of which produces the drowsiness called "sleeping sickness."

Malaria

The agents which cause malaria are protozoan parasites of the class *Sporozoa*. There are four types of human malaria. Causative agents are *Plasmodium falciparum, P. vivax, P. malariae,* and *P. ovale*. These protozoa are transmitted by *Anopheles* mosquitoes. (Malaria is discussed in detail in Chapter 24, "Tropical Diseases: Malaria.")

Other sporozoans produce diseases in man, but were presumed to be of limited geographical distribution. *Coccidiosis* is being reported more frequently in the United States, presumably because of better diagnostic methods. The symptoms are similar to those of a mild influenza at the onset followed by mild diarrhea and vague abdominal pain. The disease is self-limiting and no specific treatment is available. *Toxoplasmosis* in man is far more serious; infection of a pregnant woman leads to neonatal disease resulting in stillbirth or malformations of the infant. The protozoan *Toxoplasma gondii* is widely distributed in nature and infects a large number of animals and birds. Control and treatment of the disease have not been effectively developed.

FUNGI

Fungi are plant-like organisms which range in size from a few microns to many feet. They do not contain the green pigment *chlorophyll* which enables plants of the higher orders to manufacture their own food; therefore, fungi must live on previously produced food. If the source of food is dead organic matter, the fungus is termed a *saprophyte*; if the food is living organic matter, the fungus is called a parasite. Some fungi live on both living and nonliving organic matter.

Some fungi reproduce sexually by fusion of male and female strains of cells from the same or different colonies. They reproduce more frequently by an asexual process which consists of the formation of countless numbers of small "seeds" or spores. Each spore is identical to every other and is capable of forming a new plantlike growth exactly like that from which it came. These spores also give the sooty, green, or black appearance to spoiling fruit or bread.

Some fungi, as in the case of the yeasts and related forms, are not capable of forming a *complex* many-celled plant. Such organisms reproduce by forming buds, which after growing to a certain size, break off to form new cells.

Of the estimated 10,000 fungus species there are only 35 or 40 capable of producing disease in man. The fungi which produce disease in man are divided into two groups: those which attack only the hair, skin, and nails; and a second group which can invade deeper tissues of major internal organs to produce serious systemic diseases.

Organisms belonging to the first group produce such diseases as "athlete's foot," "jockey-strap itch," and "ringworm." These disorders are discussed at length in Chapter 8, "The Skin." In the second group of fungi, those that produce more serious systemic diseases, perhaps the most important is *Coccidioides immitis*, which produces a lung disease called *coccidioidomycosis*. In most instances, it is a mild infection of the lungs which clears spontaneously. It has been shown that from 50 to 80 percent of the people in certain areas of the southwestern United States probably have had the disease at some time during their lives.

Histoplasmosis is probably the second most important disease in this category. As with coccidioidomycosis, it was once thought to be a rare and invariably fatal disease. More recent information, however, indicates that it, too, is usually a self-limiting infection which clears spontaneously and rapidly. By testing measures similar to those used in coccidioidomycosis, it has been shown that many persons living in the central portions of the United States have had the mild form of the disease sometime in their lives. The parasitic fungus, *Histoplasma capsulatum*, which causes the infection, has also been isolated from soil, dogs, cattle, skunks, and rats. It is transmitted by inhalation of infected materials. Mild infections may involve only the skin or lungs, but the more serious types may become widely spread systemic diseases.

A yeast-like organism belonging to the genus *Candida* or *Monilia* was first associated with *thrush*, a disease involving the skin of the tongue and throat. It is now known that the organism can cause many different types of infections, ranging from relatively mild skin disorders to fatal diseases wherein the lungs, heart, and other organs may be infiltrated by the organism.

Sporotrichosis is still another mycosis which may assume many different forms. The causative agent is a small cigar-shaped organism called *Sporotrichum schenckii*. It may cause extensive ulceration of the skin and mucous membranes.

Maduromycosis is a disease seen in the tropics, where persons do not wear shoes. The disease is usually limited to the feet and is characterized by extensive ulceration and swelling. It may be caused by a wide variety of fungi. It is thought that spores of these otherwise innocuous species enter through a break in the skin to cause the infection.

There are many other types of fungus infections involving practically all parts of the body but most of these are relatively rare and will not be described here. (For further discussion of fungus diseases, see Chapter 8, "The Skin," and Chapter 24, "Tropical Diseases.")

ANIMAL PARASITES

Multicellular animals are divided into large groups on the basis of similarities in structure; each of these groups is called a phylum (plural *phyla*). Several of the phyla contain parasites that produce disease in man. Some examples of these organisms are hookworms, tapeworms, flukes, ticks, lice, and bloodsucking insects. For the purpose of this chapter, two phyla, the roundworms (*Nemathelminthes*) and the flatworms (*Platyhelminthes*) will be considered.

The roundworms

The roundworm group, called nematodes, contains many parasites. Chief among these are the hookworms. These small worms are thread-like and approximately one-half inch in length. The males have a curved or hooked tail. Each sex has a large mouth which contains many hooklike teeth. Back of the mouth is a muscular gullet. When the worm is attached to the human intestinal wall, it sucks blood into its body by contraction of the gullet. The blood is then forced into the worm's intestine. Some of the blood is digested in the worm, while much of it is passed out through the anus. Since there may be an unusually large number of worms present, the victim may experience a considerable loss of blood, resulting in anemia, lack of energy, susceptibility to disease, stunting of growth, and retarded mental development.

Each female hookworm produces about 9000 eggs each day; these pass to the outside with the feces. Should the fecal matter be deposited on the ground, the eggs hatch and the microscopic larvae crawl around on the soil. If a barefoot person comes in contact with the worms, they burrow through the skin and enter a blood vessel. By means of the blood they are carried to the lungs, where they burrow through the delicate lung tissue and migrate up the windpipe, down to the esophagus, through the stomach to the intestine. Here, they attach themselves to the intestinal wall and begin to suck blood.

Hookworm disease is widespread in the southern United States and many tropical or semi-tropical countries throughout the world. While a person seldom dies from the disease, hookworm has become a serious problem because it weakens the individual's resistance to other diseases. Likewise, the loss of blood causes the person to become lethargic and unproductive. Factors in the control of hookworm include the installation of sanitary toilets, wearing of shoes, and public education.

Trichina, a small roundworm which causes the disease *trichinosis*, requires two hosts in order that it may be transmitted. The microscopic

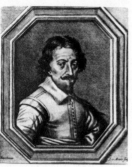

JANSSEN, Zacharias. Sixteenth century Dutch maker of spectacles. About the year 1590 he is believed to have constructed the first compound microscope. Such a microscope involves the optical principle that the alignment of two convex lenses in a row brings about a compounding of their individual magnifications. Before Janssen's time, it was impossible to see objects that were much smaller than could be observed with the unaided eye itself.

larvae become encysted in the muscle of meat-eating animals, such as the hog and the rat. Since hogs often kill and eat rats, the disease may be transmitted from rat to hog. Even more important than the eating of rats is the practice of feeding uncooked garbage to hogs, by which the hogs may contract the disease. If pork has not been sufficiently cooked and is eaten by a human being, the digestive juices dissolve the cyst or hard shell surrounding the immature worm, and the worms reach maturity within a few days. The adult male then fertilizes the female, which then burrows deep into the intestinal lining. The female produces thousands of tiny larvae which make their way by means of the blood vessels to the muscles of the body. There they coil up and secrete a thick shell to form a cyst. These cysts are likely to be more abundant in the active muscles such as the diaphragm, tongue, and eye. The worms, during their migration, produce poisons which lead to swelling and pain of the infected parts. After encystment, the calcified cysts sometimes irritate the muscle and cause muscular pains for many years. Patients may die from paralysis of the muscle during the more active phase of this disease.

All dangers of trichinosis may be avoided by cooking pork properly, since the organisms are destroyed by a temperature of 131° Fahrenheit —about the temperature at which meat loses its red color. Inspection of meat does not always reveal the presence of *Trichina*; hence, all pork must be thoroughly cooked.

During World War II, many Allied soldiers in the South Pacific were exposed to a disease known as *filariasis*. Because this disease may produce swollen limbs and a greatly enlarged scrotum, it has also been termed *elephantiasis*. It is caused by small roundworms (*filaria*) which penetrate the skin with the bite of a mosquito. These minute worms find their way into the lymphatics of the body and finally reach the lymph nodes, where they mature and mate. The young, produced periodically, migrate to the skin. Should a mosquito of the proper species bite a person having these worms in the blood, the worms enter the mosquito's body and migrate to the insect's salivary gland, where they are discharged when the mosquito bites another person. The mature worms block the lymphatic circulation, thereby producing the characteristic swelling of the tissues. The development of severe cases among the soldiers in the tropics was extremely rare. The chief method of control is to combat the mosquito carriers through the application of municipal sanitation and the individual prevention of mosquito bites.

There are other diseases caused by roundworms related to the filaria. One of these is *Loa loa*, a disease of the eyes of West Africans. This disease is characterized by the movement of the worm in the eyeball which often causes the patient to see "snakes." It is spread by the bite of a fly. In tropical America and Africa, worms known as *Onchocerca*, which are transmitted by biting flies, often form cysts as large as pigeon eggs, under the skin. From the cysts, which contain the adult worms, many small larvae make their way in the tissue just beneath the skin. This gives rise to intense pain and itching. Should the worms penetrate the eye or its nerve, they may produce blindness. The cysts may be removed surgically.

There are several species of roundworms which inhabit the intestine of man. Chief among these is *Ascaris*, the largest of the roundworms. The females of this species may reach a length of 8 to 14 inches and are from one-eighth to one-fourth inch in diameter. The males are somewhat smaller. Each female *Ascaris* may produce several million eggs, and these are deposited on the soil with fecal matter. Inside the egg shell, the young *Ascaris* undergoes development into a coiled larva. When the eggs find their way to the human mouth through unsanitary or careless habits, the parasites pass into the intestine where the shell is digested away and the larvae emerge. The larvae then make a tour of the body. They penetrate through the intestinal wall to reach a blood vessel, by which they travel to the liver, heart, and lungs. In the lungs, they leave the bloodstream and make their way up the windpipe, into the throat, down the esophagus, and finally back into the intestine, where their journey ends. There they become adults, mate, and produce eggs. The worms may be removed under medical supervision by the use of a number of drugs. Because of the construction of sanitary sewers, improvement in personal cleanliness, and the discovery of effective drugs, this organism is becoming rare in most sections of the United States.

The pinworm (*Enterobius vermicularis*) is

found throughout the world. These small worms live in the intestine near the region of the appendix. They are approximately one-half inch in length. The female migrates through the intestine to the region of the anus. During the night these worms migrate to the outside to deposit their eggs in the anal region. Their presence produces an intense itching which causes the person to scratch. From infected fingers, many objects may become contaminated, and by this means the eggs may be transferred to the mouth. A child may reinfect himself. These worms may be removed by a number of drugs, but it is difficult to prevent reinfection. The training of children in proper sanitary habits is the best means of prevention.

The flatworms

The flatworms contain two main groups, the tapeworms (*cestodes*) and the flukes (*trematodes*). The tapeworm is not an individual but a whole family of individuals arranged as segments, called *proglottids*, one behind the other; each has been produced from a common head (*scolex*). Each segment or proglottid of the tapeworm contains both the male and female reproductive apparatus but little more, since these animals absorb predigested food from the intestine of the host. The male part of the tapeworm may fertilize the female part in the same or an adjacent tapeworm segment. The fertilized eggs of the tapeworm are retained in the worm until the proglottid breaks away and passes to the outside with the feces. Should a hog eat the proglottid or the eggs, the larvae will hatch in the hog's intestine. These small larvae burrow through the intestinal wall and migrate to the other parts of the hog's body, where they develop to an encysted stage. If an individual eats improperly cooked pork containing the cyst, the human digestive juices free the larvae, which then attach themselves to the human intestine and there develop into adults. Another tapeworm more frequently found in man has a similar life cycle, except that beef cattle are the intermediate hosts. The tapeworm may be controlled by properly cooking meat, the installation of sewerage systems, and the use of specific drugs by which the adult worm may be removed from the intestine.

There are some other members of the tapeworm family that may infect man. Among these are the fish tapeworm (*Diphylobothrium*), which may produce worms 60 feet in length. These worms are obtained from raw or improperly cooked fish, and cause an anemia similar to pernicious anemia. *Echinococcus*, the adults of which are found in dogs and sheep, sometimes infects man, forming large cystlike tumors which contain thousands of small larval worms.

The worms usually can be visualized in the

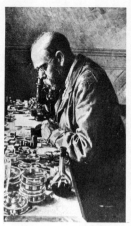

KOCH, Robert (1843-1910) German bacteriologist. He established the exact rules that must be followed in order to prove a microorganism to be the cause of some particular disease. He was a founder of modern bacteriology, and he discovered both the tubercle bacillus and the cholera vibrio. Koch also introduced many new methods into bacteriological science and in 1905 he won the Nobel prize for his numerous important contributions. *Bettmann Archive.*

ordinary light microscope. In some instances where they are difficult to find, various blood tests are made to determine their presence. Tetrachloroethylene (drug of choice for hookworm) piperazine citrate, quinacrine hydrochloride (for tapeworm), and gentian violet are all effective in worm infections. Sanitation and insect control, of course, remain the best means of preventing most of these infections.

The flukes (*trematodes*) produce a number of types of parasitic infections in man. The flukes require one and sometimes two hosts, one of which is usually a species of snail, before they reach their final destination in the bodies of man or domestic animals. Perhaps one of the best known is *Clonorchis*, the Chinese liver fluke found in many Asiatic countries. It is obtained by eating raw or improperly cooked fish. When infected fish are eaten, the young flukes migrate to the liver by way of the bile duct. There they become adults, approximately one-half inch in length. These parasites cause enlargement of the liver, jaundice, anemia, weakness, and in extreme cases, death. The adult flukes produce numerous small eggs that pass through the bile to the intestine and out with the feces. Should the eggs fall into the water, they develop into free-swimming larvae. These larvae burrow into a certain type of snail and there undergo a type of asexual reproduction in the snail's body. The larvae change eventually into free-swimming forms which penetrate the flesh of fresh water fish. In the muscle of the fish, they form cysts, which if consumed by human beings will produce infection. The installation of proper sewerage systems and the proper cooking of all fish would control this organism. The common liver fluke of cattle has a similar life history, except that the encysted stage is found in grass instead of in the fish. A similar type of human liver fluke is obtained from the encysted organism often present on aquatic vegetables, such as the water chestnut.

The blood flukes (*schistosomes*) are the cause

of a widespread blood infection affecting persons in many Asiatic countries. This parasite is regarded as the cause of much of the backwardness of many of the Asiatic populations. In Egypt, from 60 to 85 percent of the population is infected, and 10 percent of all deaths are caused directly by the disease. During World War II, many Allied soldiers were infected while in the South Pacific and Philippines. There are three species of blood flukes which infect man; all have essentially the same life cycle. The female and male are separate individuals, but remain united for most of their lives. These small threadlike worms, which are about one-half inch long, live in the larger veins of the pelvic region of the body. The spined eggs are deposited in the blood vessels; they work their way into the bladder and the intestine, where they are discharged with the urine and feces. Once outside the body and in water, they hatch and form small larvae, which penetrate certain species of snails. Within the snail's body they reproduce asexually to form thousands of free-swimming, forked-tail larvae called *cercariae*. These cercariae swim until they contact human skin or die. Should they find a host, they penetrate the skin or the membranes of the mouth; then make their way into the blood vessels, by which they are carried to the lungs and later to the liver. They spend about 20 days in the liver; then they migrate to the pelvic blood vessels where they mate and lay eggs.

The symptoms of infection with blood flukes depend upon the species of the fluke and the tissue attacked. There is usually a rash and itching where they penetrate the skin. If the flukes invade the bladder, ulceration in the wall of that organ may occur; the inflammation may extend into the ureter, causing obstruction. Or the seminal vesicle, prostate, urethra, or vagina may become involved. When the liver and spleen are infected, these organs become greatly enlarged; extreme weakness, emaciation, and death may result. Control of the disease involves treatment of infected persons with fuadin or tartar emetic, and prevention of infection by the use of chemical repellents. The poisoning of snails is also important; specific control measures have been devised for limited areas. The diagnosis of many worm infections is greatly aided by an examination of *fresh* feces for the presence of worm eggs. The parasitologist, therefore, may request such a sample for microscopic study.

(Some disease-producing organisms are discussed further in Chapter 24 "Tropical Diseases.")

5 THE RESPIRATORY SYSTEM

WHAT IT IS AND DOES

A little more than one-fifth of the air around us consists of the gas oxygen. When a substance such as coal or wood burns in air, the chemical compounds of which it is composed, mainly built up of the elements carbon, hydrogen, and oxygen, combine with the free oxygen in the air with the liberation of a great deal of energy in the form of heat. The end products of the combustion are carbon dioxide and water.

The energy which is continuously being generated in our bodies during life is ultimately derived from the foodstuffs which we eat, particularly from starch, sugars, and fats. These substances, like wood and coal, are compounds of the three chemical elements, carbon, hydrogen, and oxygen. Energy can be set free from them within the cells of the body tissues and organs by a process of combustion, but at a rate much slower than is found in a coal fire, provided that an adequate supply of free oxygen is available. Here again the end products of the combustion are carbon dioxide and water. Without free oxygen, life would be impossible, since the life processes of all the cells demand the continuous development of energy.

Breathing ensures that an adequate supply of oxygen reaches the body and that carbon dioxide resulting from the combustion is removed. Our respiratory movements, however, only bring about an interchange of gases between the interior of the lungs and the air around us. They do not conduct the needed oxygen to the remote parts of the body where it plays its role in the combustive processes. The muscles of the legs, for example, are far distant from the lungs.

The movement of oxygen from the lungs to the tissues and of carbon dioxide from the tissues back to the lungs is accomplished by the circulation of the blood, for blood constitutes the great transporting system within the body. During muscular exercise, the rate at which oxygen is used up in the muscles is greatly increased, with, of course, a corresponding increase in the production of carbon dioxide. To keep pace with this increased demand for oxygen, the rate at which the blood is circulated through the lungs and tissues must be accelerated. The rate of breathing also increases—hence the panting and increase of pulse rate when a person exercises.

The respiratory system of a human being is composed primarily of two *lungs* and the air passages which lead to them. These air passages begin at the nose and mouth, and include the windpipe and its branches which in turn divide into smaller tubes and eventually terminate in the countless tiny air sacs (*alveoli*) which are the sites for the exchange of gases between the blood and the air. The total surface area of all the alveoli within the lungs is about 100 square yards. In the walls of the alveoli, there is a close network of blood vessels which have nearly as great a total surface area. As blood passes through the lungs, it is dispersed over this vast area and is brought into close relation with air in the alveoli.

The red corpuscles in the blood contain a red pigment called *hemoglobin*. This has the property of combining with oxygen to form *oxyhemoglobin* when it is exposed to air containing a relatively high concentration of oxygen, and of yielding up oxygen when the air contains a low concentration of this gas. As the blood passes through the alveoli of the lungs, the hemoglobin therefore picks up and combines temporarily with oxygen. This blood passes through the pulmonary veins back to the heart whence it is distributed through the arteries to the tissues of the body. The cells in the tissues are continuously using up oxygen so that the concentration of this gas in them is low; as a consequence the oxyhemoglobin yields part of its oxygen to them, and when the venous blood returns to the lungs the deficiency is made good as the blood passes through the alveoli. As the tissue cells use up oxygen, they produce carbon dioxide; this passes into the bloodstream where it is carried to the lungs partly as bicarbonate of soda and partly in combination with hemoglobin. In the alveoli, the excess of carbon dioxide is liberated from the blood, passes into the air in the alveoli and is thence carried away in the expired air, so that the arterial blood leaving the lungs contains less carbon dioxide as well as more oxygen than the venous blood entering the lungs.

The mechanism of breathing

The rhythm of breathing, which alternately increases and decreases the expanded state of the lungs, begins at birth and continues throughout life. The inhalation and exhalation of the lungs is a result of changes in the capacity of the chest cavity, brought about by movement of the muscles of respiration. The most important of these muscles is the *diaphragm*, a broad sheet of muscular tissue which stretches across the bottom of the chest cavity and separates the chest cavity from the abdominal cavity. When the diaphragm moves downward, air is drawn into the lungs; when it moves upward, the air is expelled. The upward movement is a passive one of relaxation.

One complete respiration includes both an inspiration and an expiration of air. The normal number of respirations in a healthy adult human being is about 14 to 18 per minute; in children this number is higher. The respiratory rate varies with the age, the amount of activity, and state of health of the individual.

Normally, breathing is involuntary. The carbon dioxide in the blood stimulates the *respiratory center* in the brain, which in turn causes the diaphragm to move. Thus, breathing continues during sleep and is not ordinarily a conscious act, even during waking hours. However, a person can change the rate of respiration at will, and can even cease breathing for a short period. Holding of the breath results in an accumulation of carbon dioxide in the bloodstream, which acts on the brain and eventually causes a gasping for breath; consequently, it is very difficult to hold one's breath for a long time.

The nose

An intricate maze of tubes and other organs leads from the surface of the body to the lungs, permitting inspiration and expiration of air. The respiratory system begins externally with the *nose*, which is formed of bone and cartilage and covered by muscles and skin. The nose consists of two openings (*nostrils* or *nares*). Each nostril opens into its respective half of a relatively large nasal cavity (*vestibule*) which is divided into halves by the *nasal septum*. This central partition is bony in the back part and is composed of cartilage toward the front of the nose. It may deviate to one side or the other, causing a narrowing of one side of the nasal passage. When this deviation is great, obstruction of the passage may result.

Protruding from the outer wall of each half of the nasal cavity and above the roof of the mouth are three curled ridges composed of bone. These are known as the superior, the middle, and the inferior *turbinates (nasal conchae)*. The nasal cavity on each side is partially divided into three air passages by these ridges.

There is a small patch of special cells in the membrane lining the upper part of the nasal cavities which is concerned with smelling. The rest of the mucous membrane of the nose is composed of cells, the top layer of which contains short, fine hairs called *cilia* which stop dust particles. The special function of the membrane of the nose is to warm, cleanse, and moisten the air entering the nasal passages.

The paranasal sinuses

The *paranasal sinuses* are hollow spaces in the bones of the skull which connect with the nose. They may help to provide resonance, or "sounding chambers," for the voice. They also help to moisten the nasal passages with mucus. There are four such sinuses on each side of the nasal cavity. They may be described as follows: the *ethmoid sinus* on each side is found alongside the nasal cavity and below the bone forming the floor of the socket of the eye; the *frontal sinus* is located near the midline of the forehead over each eyebrow; the *sphenoid sinuses* are found back within the skull behind each nasal cavity and on a line directly above the soft palate; and the pair of *maxillary sinuses*, which are the largest, lie in the cheekbones above the molar teeth.

The pharynx

The nasal cavities connect with a larger, single cavity in the area back of the mouth, called the *pharynx*. This is an upright, almost round passage, somewhat flattened on the side

THE BREATHING MECHANISM

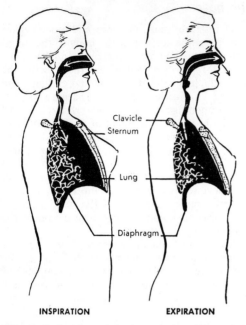

INSPIRATION   **EXPIRATION**

Changes in the sizes of the lungs and positions of the diaphragm, sternum, and clavicle during an inspiration, at left, and an expiration, at the right.

THE SINUSES

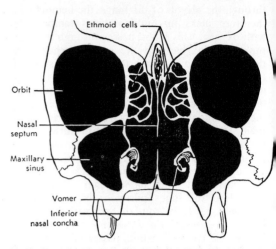

Vertical section through the skull in which the face has been removed, showing the maxillary sinuses, nasal cavity and septum, and site of ethmoid cells.

THE LARYNX

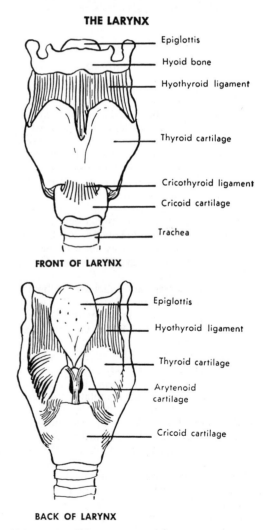

FRONT OF LARYNX

BACK OF LARYNX

Drawings depicting the front and back of the larynx, showing various anatomical parts that compose this portion of the respiratory system.

RELATIONSHIP OF PARTS OF THE RESPIRATORY SYSTEM

Cross-sectional drawing of face and neck, depicting the relationship between the nasal, oral, and tracheal portions of a normal respiratory tract.

HEART, LUNGS AND DIAPHRAGM IN RELATION TO EACH OTHER

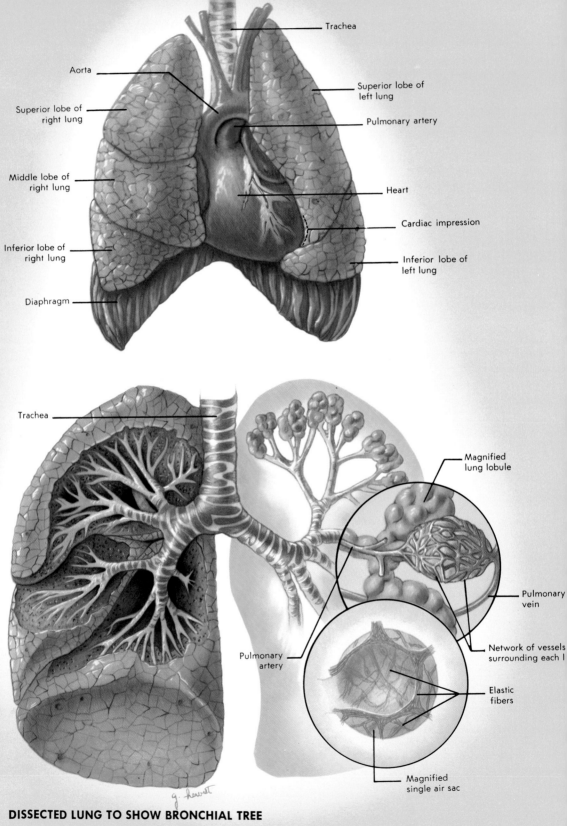

Trachea

Aorta

Superior lobe of
left lung

Superior lobe of
right lung

Pulmonary artery

Middle lobe of
right lung

Heart

Cardiac impression

Inferior lobe of
right lung

Inferior lobe of
left lung

Diaphragm

Trachea

Magnified
lung lobule

Pulmonary
vein

Network of vessels
surrounding each l

Pulmonary
artery

Elastic
fibers

Magnified
single air sac

**DISSECTED LUNG TO SHOW BRONCHIAL TREE
IN RELATION TO LUNG**

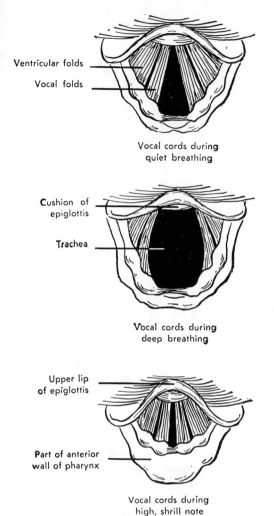

Ventricular folds

Vocal folds

Vocal cords during
quiet breathing

Cushion of
epiglottis

Trachea

Vocal cords during
deep breathing

Upper lip
of epiglottis

Part of anterior
wall of pharynx

Vocal cords during
high, shrill note

Drawings depicting position of vocal cords during quiet breathing, during deep breathing, and in position for the utterance of a high shrill note.

The entire pharynx is usually about five inches long. The nasal pharynx is widest; the oral pharynx is more narrow; and the laryngeal pharynx is the most narrow. After the incoming air enters the nostrils, it passes into the same part of the pharynx as does the food we eat. From there, the air enters a separate channel, which is the voice box. Thus, the pharynx is a common passageway of the respiratory and digestive systems. A valvelike structure at the base of the tongue, the *epiglottis*, projects backward over the larynx during swallowing, and thereby prevents food from entering the larynx.

The voice box (larynx)

The voice box, or *larynx*, is also shaped fundamentally like a tube. It is wide at the top and narrow at its lower portion. In general, it looks somewhat like a three-cornered tube with a prominent ridge on the front side. It is made up of several pieces of firm elastic tissue (*cartilage*), which are held together by muscles and ligaments. The *thyroid cartilage* is the largest cartilage of the larynx. It consists of two plates standing on end, which meet in the front of the neck and form the ridge mentioned above, the Adam's apple.

The interior of the larynx extends from the pharynx above to the windpipe (*trachea*) below. The inner tube of the larynx is divided horizontally into two parts by the projection of the muscular *vocal folds*, which contain the two *vocal cords*. These cords produce the sound which is converted into speech by the movements of the mouth and tongue.

The manner of producing the tones of the voice is interesting. When the vocal cords are tightened, the air being exhaled causes the cords to vibrate, and sounds are produced—the tighter the cords, the higher the tone. These sounds are made into words by the tongue, teeth, and lips. The degree to which a person can tighten and relax his vocal cords determines his tone range in singing or speaking. When the vocal cords are completely relaxed, no sound is made.

The windpipe (trachea) and the bronchi

After the air from the outside has passed through the larynx, it enters the windpipe (*trachea*). This is a membranous tube strengthened by rings of cartilage. It extends from the lower part of the voice box downward approximately four and one-half inches, where it divides into two other tubes known as *bronchi* (singular, *bronchus*), one going to each lung. The windpipe is almost cylindrical, but is flattened on the side nearer to the spine.

The trachea, like the nasal cavity, the nasal pharynx, and the larynx, is lined with a membrane which contains cells with small hairlike

nearest the spine. It extends downward from the base of the skull to the throat. In the back, it rests against the upper part of the spine. At the sides, it is closely associated with large blood vessels and nerves. In the front portion, the pharynx connects above with the nasal cavity, below that with the mouth cavity, and at its lowest point with the voice box (*larynx*). These three divisions of the pharynx are called, from top to bottom: the *nasal pharynx,* used for the passage of air during breathing; the *oral pharynx,* which is used both for breathing and for the passage of food; and the *laryngeal pharynx,* which has the same double function as the oral pharynx. Located in the nasal pharynx are the openings of the two *Eustachian tubes,* through which air, necessary for equalizing the pressure on both sides of the eardrum, is admitted to the middle ear.

Illustration: Anatomy of The Respiratory System . . . Grace Hewitt

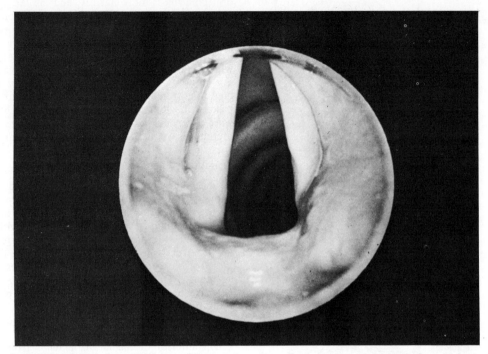

This photograph indicates the appearance of the vocal cords as they are seen in a direct view obtained with a laryngoscope during the period of an inspiration of air. *Courtesy of Paul H. Holinger, M.D., Chicago, Illinois.*

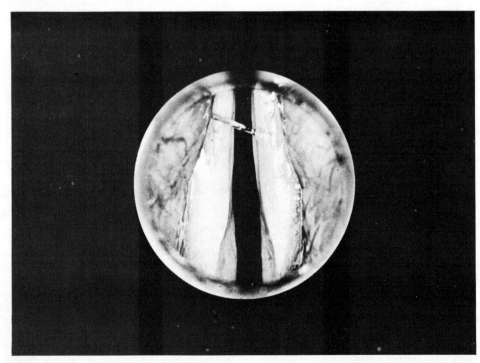

This photograph reveals how the vocal cords appear to the physician, when he views them directly through the laryngoscope, during the production of a sound. *Photo by courtesy of Paul H. Holinger, M.D., Chicago, Illinois.*

projections. These hairs beat with a rapid action which forces foreign material out of the breathing passages toward the mouth. The action of these hairs is slowed by cold, and increased by heat.

The tubes which branch off from the trachea, the bronchi, transmit air from the trachea to the lungs. The walls of the bronchi are stiff and elastic, since they are made up largely of cartilage. The right bronchus is shorter and broader than the left. This accounts for the fact that foreign bodies are more often lodged in the right than in the left bronchus. After entering the lungs, the bronchi divide into five main branches (the *lobar bronchi*) and then subdivide, finally reaching the *terminal bronchi* (or *respiratory bronchioles*). Each respiratory bronchiole communicates with a cluster of alveoli, and the bronchopulmonary unit so formed is the basic structure of all lung tissue.

The lungs

The lungs are the most important organs of respiration. They are paired structures, containing thousands of small sacs, the alveoli. The lungs are conical in shape. The right lung is composed of three lobes, the left has two. Each lobe is subdivided, in turn, into two or more *bronchopulmonary segments*, each segment representing the lung tissue supplied by one of the main branches of the lobar bronchi. In diseases such as pneumococcal pneumonia, atelectasis, and lung abscess, the lesions are typically confined to a single lobe or segment.

The lungs are soft and spongy in texture; in the adult they are gray, mottled with black, or even totally black in color, but in the infant they are pink. The dark color of the lungs of adults living in cities is the result of carbon deposits produced by the polluted atmosphere.

Sounds produced by the lungs during respiration may be heard by the physician through the use of an instrument known as the *stethoscope*. The value of listening to sounds in the chest area was known to Hippocrates, the "father of medicine," in the fifth century B.C. A nineteenth century French physician, René Laennec, endeavored to listen to lung sounds through a hollow tube of paper, one end of which was held against a patient's chest. Later, Laennec used a hollow cylinder made of wood, and employed the device in diagnosing diseases of the lungs and bronchi. The type of stethoscope in use today was invented by Doctor George Philip Cammann of New York, who died in 1863.

Each lung is covered with a membrane called the *pleura*. This membrane extends over the inner chest wall and down to the upper surface of the diaphragm. The two layers, therefore, are really a closed sac, one on either side of the chest. The space enclosed by the pleural membrane is known as the *pleural cavity*. When a person is free from disease, no real space is present. Instead, these two coverings for the lungs lie next to each other, separated only by a thin coating of fluid, which permits the surfaces to slide easily over one another during the breathing processes.

The lungs are housed in the thoracic cavity which is composed of twelve vertebrae, twelve pairs of ribs, the breastbone, muscles, and fibrous tissue. It is the expansion of this cavity, triggered by nerve impulses from the brain, that causes the lungs to expand and air to be drawn in. Conversely, it is the collapse of the thoracic cavity that causes expiration.

The diaphragm

The pleural cavity is walled off from the abdominal cavity by a sheet of muscle called the diaphragm, as previously mentioned. When a person inhales, the diaphragm moves downward toward the abdominal cavity. Conversely, it moves upward when he exhales. The up-and-down, piston-like movements of this organ account for 60 percent of the air breathed. The diaphragm is attached in the rear to the spine, at the sides to the lower six ribs, and in front to the breastbone *(sternum)*.

Function of the lungs during exercise

During strenuous exercise, the amount of oxygen used by the body increases to ten or more times that normally used. An increase in carbon dioxide also occurs in the blood. This results in a gasping for breath, a feeling of fatigue, aching muscles, and other signs of shortage of air. These symptoms appear to be caused by an inadequacy of the respiratory system, but actually

HAMBERGER, Georg Erhard (1697-1755) German physician. Hamberger is famous for his accurate description of the mechanism of the movements of respiration. He clearly recognized that the internal intercostal muscles function in inflation of the lungs, and that the external intercostal muscles function in the expiration of air from the respiratory tract. Our understanding of the mechanism of respiration was greatly advanced by these facts.

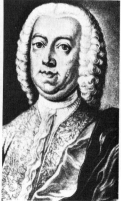

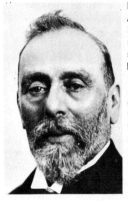

HAJEK, Markus (1861-1941) Austrian laryngologist. Hajek is known for a classic volume dealing with the accessory nasal sinuses, published in 1899. He is also noted for contributions he made to surgery of this region of the respiratory system. An operation he devised for relief of frontal sinus disease involves removal of the anterior wall of the sinus, removal of diseased tissue, and enlargement of nasal canal.

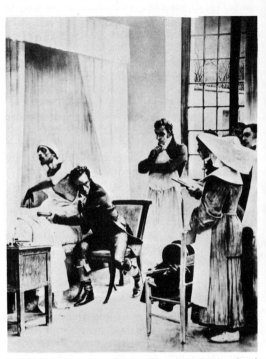

Reproduction of a painting by Chartran, showing René Laennec demonstrating the use of his newly invented stethoscope. *Bettmann Archive.*

they result from failure of the body to increase the amount of blood pumped into the heart. When the body adjusts to this condition, and panting and other symptoms cease, a "second wind" occurs.

The idea that a person completely fills his lungs with fresh air when he inhales and completely empties them of bad air when he exhales is erroneous. Only a part of the air inhaled, which is about a pint at one time, enters the lungs. The remainder stays in the passageways that lead to the lungs. This air is known as "dead air," since it does not enter into an exchange of gases in the tissues of the body.

When *respiratory failure* occurs, as in electrocution or drowning, the mechanical act of breathing often can be simulated artificially. This is referred to as *artificial respiration;* it is discussed in detail in Chapter 23: "Physical Injuries and First Aid." In many instances, if this procedure is used promptly, the life which is in danger can be saved.

Coughing and *sneezing* are normal, special protective means of preventing foreign bodies from entering the air passages. Also, coughing clears these passages of mucus, dust, bacteria, and other material brought in during inhalation of air. Because of this protective mechanism, all the lung tissue below the voice box is almost completely free of microorganisms. Should this cleansing process be interfered with, the respiratory tract would be an easy mark for invading hordes of bacteria.

Respiration is an extremely important function of the living organism. The slightest movement requires expenditure of energy, and this energy is derived in great part from combustion of oxygen and carbon. One can readily see that an adequate supply of oxygen is necessary in order to maintain life. Should the process of respiration be interfered with, the body tissues soon would stop functioning, and death would result.

RESPIRATORY DISORDERS: HAY FEVER

When a person exhibits a sensitivity to a material considered nontoxic to most other people, he is said to be *allergic* to that material. If the material is borne by the wind and produces symptoms of allergy when it comes into contact with the mucous membranes of the eyes and respiratory tract, the victim is said to have *hay fever.* There are two main types: *seasonal hay fever* is the most common and occurs during the spring and summer seasons as the result of pollen from various trees, grasses, and weeds. Weeds are the most common cause of hay fever. The other principal type is *nonseasonal* or perennial and may be caused by allergic reactions to house pets, foods, dust, and many other substances. In most cases, the causative agent is inhaled.

The reason some people react to the various allergens while others do not appears to be due in part to hereditary factors. This does not mean that hay fever is inherited; but it does suggest that some persons inherit the tendency to develop an allergic disease.

Other contributing factors include psychic stress, infections, and endocrine disturbances. Any one of these might trigger an attack. The heavily polluted atmosphere of today's cities is also associated with an increased incidence of hay fever.

The name "hay fever" is actually a misnomer since the condition is not ordinarily associated with either hay or a fever. The term was first used by an English physician named Bostock, himself a victim, in a report in 1812. The symptoms of the disease occurred during the haying season.

Seasonal hay fever

Almost all cases of seasonal hay fever are caused by pollen, which is the reproductive element of plants and is contained in the flowers of grasses, trees, and most other plants.

The pollen from many sweet-scented flowers is disseminated by insects, but that causing hay fever is usually spread by the wind. Since many plants produce large quantities of pollen, a sensitive person can easily become overexposed and experience an immediate reaction.

Although all pollen grains have the same general characteristics, the pollen of each variety of plant usually can be identified, even though the markings may vary in different plants of the same species. The grains also differ widely in size; some of them may be seen without the aid of a microscope. Pollen usually, but not always, is yellowish in color.

Seasonal hay fever can be caused by three different groups of plants, and each of these groups has a somewhat different season. First, trees produce pollen that causes hay fever during the months of April and May. The various grasses are responsible for much of the hay fever that occurs during the last half of May to the first part of July. From the middle of August to October, the weeds are active pollen-producers.

Usually, the least severe and least common form of seasonal hay fever is that which is induced by pollen from trees. Tree pollen is windborne and is easily distributed because of the height of the trees. This powdery material is light enough to allow the wind to carry it for a considerable distance, and furthermore is produced in large enough quantities to be effective as a cause of hay fever. Ten percent of all seasonal hay fever is caused by tree pollen.

Of course, an allergy to a particular tree pollen can occur only in a locale in which the tree is found in large numbers. The oak tree, the most common tree causing hay fever, is found in many sections of the United States. Three other offenders, the cottonwood, the cedar, and the poplar, grow profusely in the South and Southwest. Other trees with allergy-producing pollen include the birch, alder, hickory, black walnut, beech, maple, hackberry, sycamore, mulberry, and elm.

More common than trees as a cause of hay fever are the various grasses, which account for about 35 percent of all cases. The three most important grasses which cause hay fever are timothy, Bermuda, and June or blue grass. The greatest period of pollination for timothy, which is a northern grass, is from late June through the first week of July. Blue grass is found in many lawns in various parts of the United States, particularly in Kentucky. It is an important causative agent of hay fever during June and early July. Bermuda grass is most prevalent in the South and Southwest. There are 80 varieties of grasses found in various sections of the United States that have a common antigen; therefore a person sensitive to one type of grass is usually sensitive to all types of grasses.

Weeds are prolific pollen producers, some varieties producing more than 100,000 pollen grains from a single plant. The weeds that are most important as causative agents of hay fever include the various species of ragweed and the thistle. Other weeds causing hay fever, but not on as wide a scale as these, include the goosefoot, buckwheat, marsh elder, rabbit bush, cocklebur, hemp, and pigweed.

Ragweed, of which there are about 60 varieties, is found in one form or another all over the United States. There are six main varieties and if a person is sensitive to one type, he is usually sensitive to the others, too. Indeed, ragweed is the most significant causative factor in hay fever.

The amount of pollen found in the air is controlled by various factors, particularly wind and weather. If it rains heavily during the summer months, the plant will grow profusely and produce large quantities of pollen. Conversely, if the summer months are comparatively dry, much smaller amounts will be produced. Sunshine augments the maturing of pollen, while damp weather retards it. Rain in the early part of the day hinders the dispersal of the pollen, but does not completely stop it.

PLANTS MOST COMMONLY CAUSING HAY FEVER

The following series of photographs shows the full-grown plants that produce the pollens which are most frequently causes of pollen allergies, or hay fever. Depending upon their geographical distribution and the season of the year at

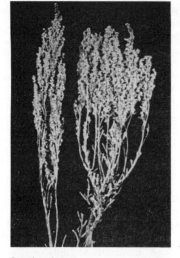

Sagebrush

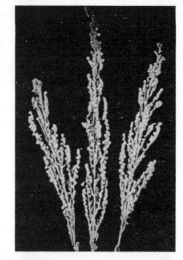

Pasture Sage

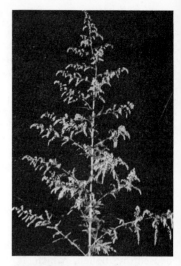

Annual Sage

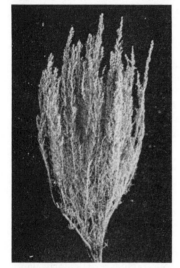

Sand Sagebrush

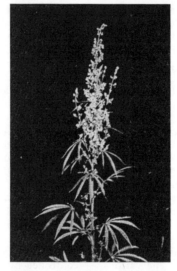

Hemp

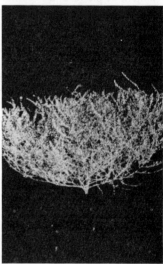

Russian Thistle

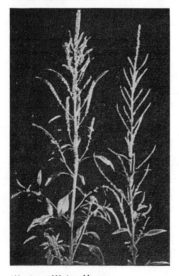

Western Water Hemp

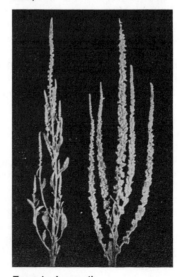

Torrey's Amaranth

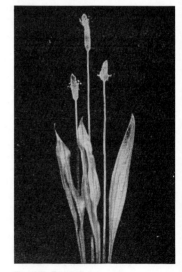

English Plantain

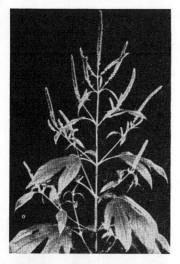

Giant Ragweed

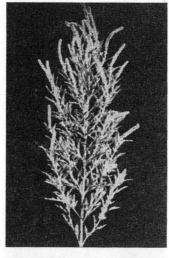

Western Ragweed

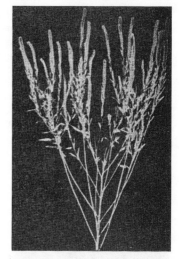

Southern Ragweed

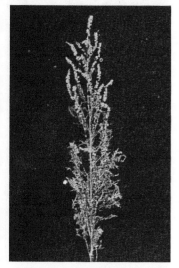

Slender False Ragweed

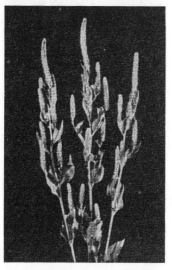

Rough Marsh Elder

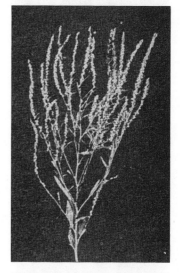

Narrow-Leaved Marsh Elder

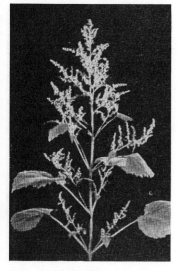

Burweed Marsh Elder

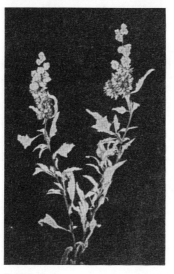

Rabbit Bush

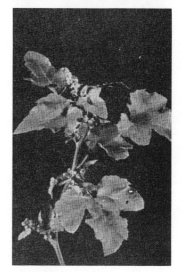

Cocklebur

which they pollinate, all of these plants are causes of this affliction. A trained allergist may, by a careful microscopic examination of the pollen grains which are floating in the air at any given time, identify which of these plants is responsible. The patient can sometimes aid his cause by becoming acquainted with the plants in his area and with their time of pollination, and making provisions to be away at that time. Page 137 shows regions of low pollen incidence. In addition to the plants shown in this series, many others, including trees and fungi, are sources of air-carried allergens. *Courtesy of Abbott Laboratories. Reproduced by permission, from the chapter "Pollens and Pollen Allergy" by Oren C. Durham in S. M. Feinberg's ALLERGY IN PRACTICE, Second Edition, 1946, The Year Book Publishers, Chicago.*

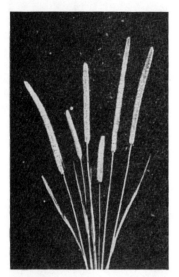

Timothy

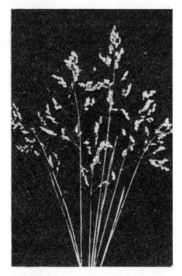

Bluegrass

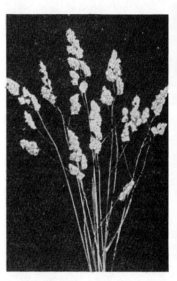

Orchard Grass

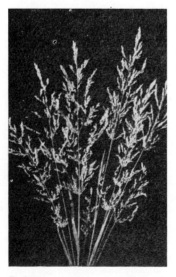

Redtop

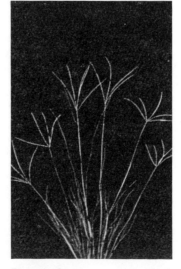

Bermuda Grass

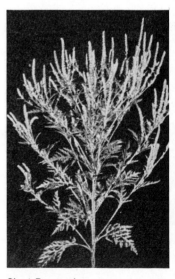

Short Ragweed

GEOGRAPHIC INCIDENCE OF
Late Summer and Fall Pollens

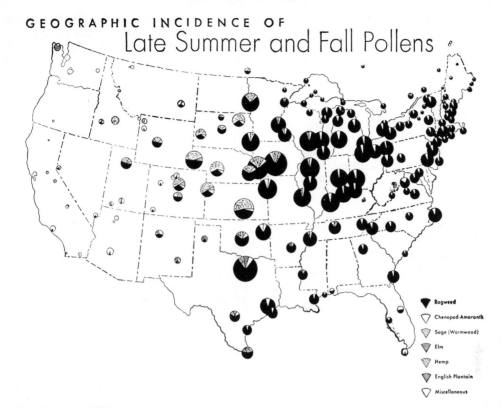

Ragweed
Chenopod-Amaranth
Sage (Wormwood)
Elm
Hemp
English Plantain
Miscellaneous

Seasonal atmospheric incidence of air-borne pollens of late summer and fall, shown in comparative seasonal totals and local proportions for typical localities. Data compiled by Oren C. Durham from studies made by members of the Pollen Survey Committee of the American Academy of Allergy in collaboration with several city and state boards of health, U.S. Weather Bureau and Canadian Meteorological Service. Revised January, 1950.

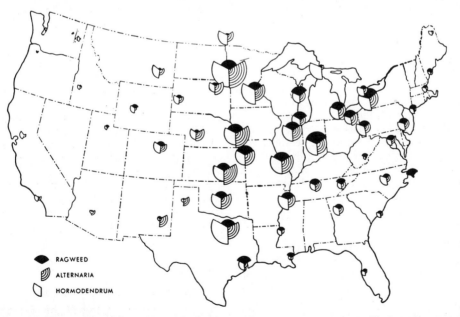

RAGWEED
ALTERNARIA
HORMODENDRUM

Atmospheric incidence of Alternaria spores and Hormodendrum spores as compared with that of ragweed pollen. The area of each segment varies according to the total number of pollen grains or spore particles found in the particular locality during one season or during the average of several seasons. The data were secured through the counting of many thousands of pollen slides exposed by the United States Weather Bureau and the Canadian Meteorological Service.

Many persons have wondered how the number of pollen grains in the atmosphere at a certain time are counted. This is a routine procedure, and the results of such a count usually are made available through the newspapers. One method of making a pollen count is to place a glass slide, one side of which is coated with oil, in a horizontal position in the atmosphere to be tested for pollen. The slide is usually left for 24 hours, and then the pollen grains collected on it are counted with the aid of a microscope. The greater the number of grains found, the greater the incidence of hay fever symptoms in the victims in that vicinity at that particular time.

Nonseasonal hay fever

The other principal type of hay fever is nonseasonal, meaning that no special seasonal pattern is involved. The allergic substances are usually inhalants, such as house dust, feathers, wool, and certain foods, which are present throughout the year.

Nonseasonal hay fever may be caused by the hair, feathers, or dander of a household or farm pet. Some persons are sensitive to the feathers in pillows or to kapok, the fibers used as filling for mattresses. House dust, especially from the bedroom, is a common causative agent. Men working in mills where wheat or corn is ground often inhale the flourlike powder, which produces irritation of the nasal mucous membranes. Reproductive cells of some fungi, when inhaled, may stimulate an allergic response.

Nonseasonal hay fever also may be caused by some kinds of foods. Many persons are sensitive to eggs, chocolate, milk, coffee, or shellfish. Some people develop hay fever after taking certain medications, such as aspirin or quinine. Nonseasonal hay fever may be continuous or spasmodic, depending upon the length of contact with the exciting factor.

The symptoms of nonseasonal hay fever tend to be less severe than those of the seasonal variety. At their mildest, they may consist of slight nasal congestion with sniffing, a tendency to an itchy nose, postnasal drip, and mouth breathing.

Symptoms

Hay fever, if mild, usually causes no permanent changes in the mucous membrane of the nose. The inner structures of the nose of a person with hay fever are the same as those of a "normal" person, except during hay fever season. During an attack, the victim's eyes usually itch and burn and are congested; there may be swelling of the mucous membranes of parts of the eye; and often the eyes show an abnormal sensitivity to light. The patient's nose itches and burns, and becomes congested; the nasal mucous membranes swell noticeably. This is accompanied by a watery, abundant nasal discharge. As the swelling of the mucous membrane of the nose increases, a partial or complete obstruction develops. When this happens, the nasal discharge thickens and becomes more mucoid in character. As soon as the passage of air through the nasal cavity is interfered with, the victim must breathe through his mouth. As a result, the mucous membranes of his soft palate, pharynx, and other respiratory organs come into more direct contact with pollen, and a vicious cycle begins.

Sneezing may relieve the symptoms of hay fever temporarily. However, violent and repeated spasms of sneezing may occur. Early morning is usually the most uncomfortable period of the day because of the increased pollen in the air at that time.

The sinuses may become infected, and thus lengthen or increase the severity of the attack. The symptoms of hay fever usually vary in severity according to the pollen count.

Recognition of hay fever

While the physician does not have difficulty in recognizing the symptoms, the actual type of hay fever is not so easily determined. A physical examination is required to rule out other diseases.

The previous history of the patient is of prime importance. As a child, did the victim show an allergic reaction to any foods? What operations, particularly on the organs of the respiratory system, were performed? Often the patient has inherited a disposition to allergy-produced diseases; consequently, an investigation of the medical history of the family is required. Minute details in the victim's living habits often lead to the discovery of the cause of an allergy. He may be questioned as to when the symptoms occur; whether they appear after changes in diet; how the victim spends his spare time, etc. These and many more questions will be raised by the physician in his effort to discover the cause of hay fever and alleviate the symptoms of the disease.

Skin tests

The physician also has objective methods of determining the causative factor. These include skin tests, and usually one of two types is used —either the *"scratch" test* or the *intracutaneous* test.

The term "scratch test" is almost as much

of a misnomer as the term "hay fever." Actually, a series of small cuts are made in the skin, without causing bleeding. A small amount of one of the suspected materials is dropped into each cut and allowed to remain there for a short time. If no reaction occurs after half an hour, the material is removed, and the reaction is regarded as negative.

The intracutaneous, or *intradermal,* test is well described by its name; sterile solutions of various allergenic agents are injected about two inches apart between the layers of the skin. After 5 to 15 minutes, the results are read.

Skin reactions in both of these tests vary from person to person, and may even vary somewhat in the same individual on different days; reactions may vary on different parts of the body. If the test is positive, a large, red, itching wheal will appear. These tests are not infallible. Some people have more sensitive skin than others; consequently, false-positive reactions are not uncommon.

A third test, used less often and not until skin testing has been completed, is the eye *(ophthalmic)* test. A drop of the same solution of pollen extract that is used for the skin tests is dropped into the eye. If the reaction is positive, a condition similar to the eye symptoms of hay fever results. The eye itches and burns. Sometimes sneezing occurs, with itching of the nose and a watery discharge, if the pollen extract has been carried into the nose.

Relief from hay fever

The inhalation of air that is free of irritating pollen will give relief from hay fever symptoms. Those who have the spring or summer type of hay fever can rarely find a climate which will give complete relief, although symptoms will be less severe in a locale in which less pollen is found. If the hay fever victim could stay aboard a ship at sea for the duration of the season, it is likely that he would experience no hay fever symptoms. Since this is impractical, the problem also may be solved by filtering and purifying the air within a room. Air conditioning is also of value.

A variety of drugs will provide relief of hay fever symptoms. Antihistamines are the most useful and will help at least four out of five patients. Ephedrine-like drugs, taken at night and either alone or in combination with antihistamines, are effective in reducing nasal congestion and lessening early morning symptoms. Corticosteroids are useful in severe cases which cannot be controlled by any of the agents mentioned above.

Another form of treatment is with the actual pollen extract which causes the hay fever. This is considered a preventive treatment, because it may cause the person's body to become acclimated to the irritant. Since the majority of patients know almost exactly when their attacks will begin, this treatment is started approximately three months prior to that time. It consists of the injection of the pollen extract at intervals of about a week. The dosage is gradually increased until the largest dose is given at about the time the symptoms usually start. From then on, the dosage remains the same until the end of the season. At the beginning of treatment, there may be a mild reaction on the spot where the injection was given; this consists of itching and swelling. Subsequent dosage is regulated by the severity of this reaction. The pollen extract treatment has been beneficial in many cases. Sometimes the physician finds it advisable to continue the injections throughout the year in order to prevent the recurrence of the symptoms in the following season. Even if the treatment is started just prior to the hay fever season, it usually must be continued from year to year.

The treatment of patients with nonseasonal hay fever consists of completely avoiding the substance or substances which cause the attack. Should contact be absolutely necessary, the physician may prescribe the allergen extract treatment, particularly if the patient's symptoms are so severe as to incapacitate him in his work.

There is much hope for the alleviation of the symptoms and the cure of the hay fever sufferer. In addition to methods now available, scientific investigations are being carried on to discover newer and better means of controlling this distressing condition.

RESPIRATORY DISORDERS: ASTHMA

Asthma is a condition wherein the patient experiences difficulty in breathing. It is caused by an obstruction to the air flow into and out of the lungs. Asthma is not a disease itself but a symptom of any one of several conditions. Diagnosis and treatment in cases of asthma imply the detection of the cause, and its elimination.

Symptoms and diagnosis

An attack of asthma is characterized by shortness of breath *(dyspnea),* wheezing, and coughing. In severe attacks, a bluish tint to the skin *(cyanosis)* can be noticed. The patient usually sits when the attack becomes severe. For the most part, exhalation is more difficult than inhalation because of the difficulty of getting air out through the contracted air passages. The attack may come on gradually or suddenly.

Asthma symptoms occur when the air entering and leaving the lungs meets a barrier of some sort. This barrier may be caused by swelling of mucous membranes and also constriction of the tubes leading from the windpipe to the lungs (the *bronchi*), brought about by allergy, emotional disturbance, or atmospheric conditions.

Although it is possible for a severe attack of asthma to result in the death of the patient, this rarely occurs. Treatment is nonetheless mandatory. If neglected or inadequately controlled, the condition can progress to a chronic, disabling, and even life-threatening disease. Distress is usually relieved in asthmatic attacks by drug injections and, if necessary, oxygen inhalation. These measures resolve the immediate symptoms, but do not cure the asthmatic condition. Until the cause is discovered and eliminated, the patient will continue to suffer asthmatic attacks.

In diagnosing asthma, the physician first takes a complete medical history, beginning with the time of the first attack. He includes in this history items regarding the patient's eating habits, health habits, and environment. Often the cause of the patient's distress is a substance to which he has been exposed for a long time. The period of sensitization varies in different individuals and also with the different allergenic materials. The physician attempts to correlate an attack with the slightest change in the patient's living routine. Perhaps wheezing began after a visit to a relative who raises rabbits, or following a visit to the beach. Perhaps he has recently "changed barbers." The patient may have had an attack after eating dessert containing chocolate or after using a vacuum cleaner. The patient's family history may reveal several relatives who have had hay fever or other respiratory or allergic types of disorders. Heredity might also be an important factor in relation to asthma.

In examining the patient suspected of having asthma, the physician will pay special attention to the nose and sinuses, the chest, teeth, and tonsils. Skin tests will determine the patient's degree of sensitivity to certain materials. These tests are discussed in the preceding section on hay fever.

Research has shown that asthma which begins before the patient is 30 years of age usually is the result of allergic sensitivity to pollens, dust, animal danders, foods, or medicines. Children are particularly prone to asthma caused by food allergies. Eggs, milk, and wheat products are among the most common causes. Of the drugs that produce allergies and cause asthma, the sulfonamides, aspirin and other coal tar products, and penicillin are the worst offenders.

Physicians have observed that emotional disturbances may precipitate or aggravate an asthmatic attack. Often asthmatic attacks are found to be incidental to family troubles or financial worries. Many times the asthmatic child or adult feels unwanted or unloved; he develops an "anxiety state," which sets off a chain reaction that ends with an attack of asthma. Then, too, a poorly adjusted mother may precipitate an attack in her child. The symptoms frequently are relieved considerably when the contributing emotional factor is eliminated. However, it is entirely possible for emotional symptoms to be the *result* of asthma, rather than the cause.

Long-term therapy

Along with attempts to identify offending allergens, some attention should be given to emotional disturbances that might be precipitating attacks of asthma.

Several drugs can also be given to control mild symptoms and prevent more serious attacks. These include ephedrine and isoproterenol. Combinations containing ephedrine, aminophylline, and phenobarbital are also of value. If none of these provides relief, minimal doses of corticosteroids can be tried.

Diet is an important consideration, too. The attending physician, acting on the basis of the results of skin tests, will advise the patient regarding foods that should be excluded from his diet. It is usually necessary to try out some foods to determine whether they can be included in the menu. A patient who is sensitive to eggs, for example, may be able to eat them well cooked, but not raw. Following the elimination of the foods to which the patient is sensitive, and the addition of those he can tolerate, a list can be made up of foods from which the patient's menu may be taken. This list should be adhered to strictly, as even the slightest deviation may result in another attack of asthma.

Adequate fluid intake is another essential in long-term therapy. Steps should be taken to insure that the asthmatic drinks large quantities of liquids every day.

Therapy during an asthmatic attack

An attack of asthma is frightening to watch and certainly is most disturbing to the patient. He will be apprehensive and should be reas-

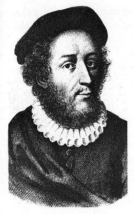

DE CHAULIAC, Guy (ca 1300-ca 1368) French surgeon. He is thought to have been the greatest surgeon of his age. The surgical text that he wrote was regarded as the best authority on surgical procedures until the time of Ambroise Paré. He emphasized the importance of other branches of medicine to surgery, and was a vigorous worker in combating the plague. He was a strong advocate of early surgery in the treatment of cancer.

sured. Someone should remain with him constantly until the arrival of the physician. The patient's main concern during an asthmatic attack is trying to get air in and out of his lungs. Usually a sitting position is best, but the patient's comfort is uppermost. Any medication previously prescribed by the attending physician for use during an attack may be given as directed. Above all, one must not alarm the patient by an anxious attitude.

When the attack is mild or moderate in severity, symptoms can generally be controlled by drugs—epinephrine, isoproterenol, or aminophylline. Sedation is also of value.

When patients experience severe attacks or *status asthmaticus*—a condition in which the attack is prolonged, with acute, severe, intractable symptoms—hospitalization is necessary. It may also be warranted for psychological reasons.

Some patients with asthma which is suspected of being emotional in origin need to have a complete change of environment and the opportunity to unburden themselves of their worries and conflicts. The privacy of the hospital room encourages both mental and physical relaxation.

In severe asthmatic attacks, the first priority is the relief of respiratory distress. Special drugs should be given even before the patient leaves home. In the hospital he will be given oxygen therapy for relief of shortness of breath. The preferred method of administration is by an intermittent positive pressure breathing apparatus which pushes oxygen into the lungs. Sedation, adequate fluid intake, and bronchodilating drugs are other essentials during the severe asthmatic attack.

Even if the patient acquires an understanding of his condition and follows the advice of his physician, he will at times experience depression and frustration because of his limited physical ability during a prolonged attack.

RESPIRATORY DISORDERS: SINUS TROUBLE

A sinus is a hollow cavity or recess in a bone. There are sinuses in most of the bones of the body, but the sinuses that occur in the skull are the ones usually thought of when a person speaks of "sinus trouble."

An understanding of the structure of the sinuses is essential to an understanding of sinus diseases. There are a number of sinuses in the facial structure. *The paranasal sinuses* are hollow cavities or recesses in the bones of the face, and are located close to the nose. They are divided into two groups. The front *(anterior)* group is composed of a *maxillary sinus* and a *frontal sinus* on each side, plus the anterior *ethmoid sinuses*. The back *(posterior)* group consists of the *sphenoid sinuses* and the posterior *ethmoid sinuses*. Both groups of paranasal sinuses have passageways leading to the nasal passages.

The sinuses are lined with a mucous membrane which is a continuation of the membrane lining the nasal cavities. The functions of the sinuses are not well understood. Some authorities believe that, like the appendix, they are an evolutionary remnant which, in many cases, may be more detrimental than useful. Others believe that the sinuses warm and moisten the air as it is inhaled. They may act as resonating chambers in the production of speech.

Larger than the others, the two *maxillary sinuses* are usually triangular in shape and are located in the cheek bones. The roof of the sinus is also the floor of the bony cavity which contains the eyeball. Roots of the molar teeth are adjacent to the floor of the sinus. The average maxillary sinus can hold approximately half an ounce of fluid. In some cases, however, it may have the capacity of an ounce.

There are two frontal sinuses: one is on the right and one is on the left in the frontal bone, just behind the eyebrow area. The partition *(septum)* which divides the two is usually no more than $\frac{1}{25}$ of an inch thick. The capacity of each of these sinuses is about one-fifth ounce.

The *sphenoid sinuses*, right and left, lie on either side of the midline in the front part of the sphenoid bone, or, more clearly, above and behind the nasal cavity on a line directly above the soft palate. Part of the roof of the sinus is formed by the bone which encases the pituitary gland. The septum seperating them is about the same thickness as the one dividing the frontal sinuses, and the size of the sphenoid sinuses is comparable to that of the frontal sinuses.

The *ethmoid sinuses* are really a series of small pockets in the ethmoid bone, located within the skull, behind and below the frontal bone

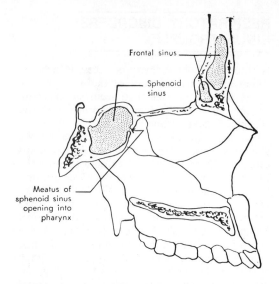

Cross-sectional side view drawing of a portion of the skull, showing location of frontal sinus, and sphenoid sinus opening into the pharynx.

and the frontal sinuses. The septa lying between the pockets are thin and may even be missing. There are usually ten of these sinuses, but the number may vary from 3 to 15 or more.

Sinusitis

Sinusitis is an inflammation of the mucous membrane lining the sinus cavity. The inflammation may be either acute, prolonged *(subacute)*, or persistent *(chronic)*.

Sinusitis may be caused by any process which interferes with the drainage and ventilation of the sinuses. It may be caused by infected teeth or by an acute infectious disease such as influenza, pneumonia, measles, or smallpox, by nasal obstruction, and by allergic reactions. In rare instances, injury to the face may be followed by sinusitis. The disease may occur in children or adults in any section of the country at any time of the year.

Acute maxillary sinusitis may create widely variable symptoms. The patient may continue his usual activities without any particular discomfort; or he may experience an elevation of temperature, pain and tenderness over the cheek, and perhaps pus in the nose accompanied by a postnasal discharge. Subacute maxillary sinusitis is a protraction of an acute attack. After repeated or lengthy attacks, the disease may become chronic. A thick nasal discharge and a postnasal drip may be present, with pus in the nose or pharynx. Sometimes the patient has a sore throat and a cough.

As in maxillary sinusitis an acute frontal sinusitis may be mild or severe. In a mild case, there is little pain and tenderness, and probably no swelling around the eye. In a severe case, however, pain around the eye comes on suddenly and is excruciating and constant. There is usually a generalized headache and swelling of the upper eyelid. The temperature of the patient may rise to 105°. It is possible for an infection of this type to extend to the bony part of the sinus. Because the frontal sinuses are close to the brain and the eyes, infection spreading in those directions may have serious consequences. Subacute frontal sinusitis is a more lasting acute attack, in which the symptoms have almost subsided, but mild discomfort persists. Chronic frontal sinusitis usually is typified by a rather heavy nasal discharge, most often from only one side of the nose. There is freedom from pain most of the time, but there may be a dull ache over the sinus during the early part of the day.

Ethmoid sinusitis, or *ethmoiditis,* in the acute phase is characterized by a dull headache, which may be moderate or intense. There may be a swelling between the inner corner of the eye and the nose. The nasal discharge may be profuse or entirely absent, depending upon whether the drainage passages are partially or completely blocked. In subacute ethmoiditis, headache may be bothersome, but the pain usually is not severe. Chronic inflammation of the ethmoid sinuses is manifested by headache, cough, a general feeling of fatigue, and a slight fever.

Acute sphenoid sinusitis occurs more frequently than is generally realized. The accompanying headache is excruciating and can be

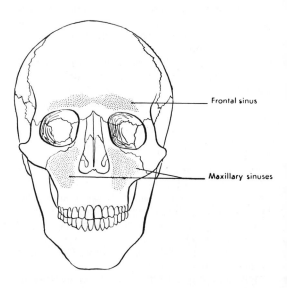

Frontal drawing of the human skull, showing the location of the frontal and maxillary sinuses which are frequent locations of common sinusitis.

relieved only partially by drugs. Symptoms of sleeplessness and a fear of choking are often present, caused by the thick discharge from the sinus. In the chronic form of the disease, the patient may experience pressure pains spreading in diverse directions. Often there is a thick, sticky postnasal drip.

The treatment of patients with any form of sinusitis must be prescribed by the physician. In the acute phases, the patient should be kept in bed in a warm, humid room until the physician arrives. Medicines to relieve pain, combat infection, and open the nasal passages may be prescribed. Drugs may be of value for patients with chronic sinusitis, but often surgical treatment is necessary to promote drainage and prevent the infection from recurring.

Tumors of the sinuses

There are two types of growths which may be found in the sinuses—malignant growths (cancer) and nonmalignant (benign) growths.

A great number of the nonmalignant growths are found in the maxillary sinuses. Two of the more common types are *polyps* and *cysts*. Polyps are inflammatory growths found inside the sinus, some of which protrude into the nose and cause a stuffy feeling or a mild headache. Polyps are encountered more frequently in this area than any other tumor. They are thought to be caused by irritation, such as that from an allergenic agent or from the drainage from the sinuses. In most cases, the polyp is best removed by a surgical operation.

A cyst in the maxillary sinus may be one of several kinds. One variety is the mucous cyst which may be either small or sufficiently large to fill the sinus. They usually do not produce symptoms except for a vague, uncomfortable feeling in the cheek. The cyst may be removed by the physician.

Whatever the disorder of the paranasal sinuses, the expert advice of a physician should be obtained promptly in order that the malady may be diagnosed and eradicated.

RESPIRATORY DISORDERS: THE COMMON COLD

The common cold is an acute inflammation of the upper respiratory tract.

Over 90 percent of the people in the United States suffer from colds each year. Nearly one-half of the persons in the United States have several colds during the year.

The common cold is contagious and spreads easily in crowded schoolrooms and business offices. It is probably the greatest cause of absenteeism among school children and workers.

Symptoms

Symptoms of the common cold include a "running" nose, frequent sneezing, sore or tickling throat, and occasionally a headache. Later, a cough and fever may develop.

Colds, although annoying, are seldom serious in the adult. However, a child with a cold should be put to bed, and a baby with a cold should have prompt medical attention. The symptoms of what is apparently a cold can be the early symptoms of many of the more serious childhood diseases, such as measles or diphtheria.

A cold takes from one to three days to develop. There are three stages of the disease. The first is the "dry" stage, which is brief. During this stage the mucous membrane of the nose feels dry and swollen. There also may be a tickling sensation in the throat, and an excessive watering of the eyes is usually present. In the next stage, a colorless, watery discharge from the nose occurs. Then follows the last stage, in which the drainage becomes thick and sticky.

Cause

The specific cause of the common cold is not known. However, it is generally believed that the infection is viral in origin. At least 30 different kinds of *rhinoviruses* and many other respiratory tract viruses are known to be causative agents. Further, it is believed that these viruses are present in the throat most of the time, but are unable to attack until body resistance is lowered. In addition, certain bacteria may be present, along with the cold virus; however, these organisms are believed to be secondary invaders and not associated with the initial attack. In other words, it is thought that cold viruses weaken the tissues and make them susceptible to infection by other organisms.

Treatment of the patient

Little progress has been made in improving the methods of treating a patient with a cold. Many of the methods used a generation or two ago are still employed. As in the past, the patient is put to bed, following a hot bath, and is given hot lemonade and other hot drinks. He is kept quiet and warmly covered and is fed a light diet. The use of some type of vaporizer also is of value in making the patient more comfortable by supplying moisture to the nose and throat.

Today, despite the innumerable varieties of cold tablets, throat sprays, medicated cough drops, medicated inhalants, and even "cold shots," the common cold usually runs its course. A truly satisfactory treatment has not been discovered. In recent years, drugs called the *anti-*

histamines have become popular cold remedies. They are widely advertised, and a number of them can be obtained without a doctor's prescription. These drugs sometimes relieve the *symptoms* of a cold in some patients, but they do not *cure* the cold. It is best to use these drugs only upon the advice of a physician, because some persons are sensitive to them.

Since at any time cold symptoms may be the first step toward a more serious condition, one should call a physician if new symptoms, such as chills or high fever, appear. A cold lasts but a few days; should the symptoms persist, there is a possibility that complications have developed.

Prevention

Health rules dictated by common sense probably help to decrease the incidence of colds. A well-balanced diet and plenty of rest and sleep will help to keep one's resistance high. Care should also be taken that rooms are not kept overheated and are well-ventilated. It is important, too, that the atmosphere of the room not be too dry. Proper humidity can be attained by keeping a pan of water near the heating apparatus.

Dressing properly helps prevent colds. The individual must avoid becoming too warm and perspiring while indoors, because it may cause him to be chilled when he goes outdoors. Adequately warm outer clothing for outdoors should be worn.

One must be careful to avoid contact with those who are infected. A sneeze in a crowded streetcar or bus can infect several people. Kissing is also a method of spreading infection. Mothers or nurses with colds should wear gauze masks while attending infants and small children.

RESPIRATORY DISORDERS: SORE THROAT

A sore throat is an inflammation or irritation of some part of the throat. The ordinary sore throat is usually the result of an infection in the area at the back of the mouth cavity (the *pharynx).* As explained in an earlier section, the pharynx is divided into three parts—the *oropharynx,* the *nasopharynx,* and the *laryngeal pharynx.* The sore throat may start in any one of these parts and extend to the others, or it may be more severe in any one of the three.

One form of sore throat *(pharyngitis)* may be a separate disease entirely or the symptom of another disease. As a disease in itself, it may be caused by invasion by infectious organisms

or by various physical agents. Foods that are too hot may irritate the mucous membrane of the pharynx. A postnasal discharge also may cause pharyngitis, by carrying disease-producing organisms down into the pharynx. Some drugs may initiate a throat disorder.

Diseases of which pharyngitis may be a symptom include the common cold, scarlet fever, influenza, tonsillitis, measles, and smallpox. It is important that the source of the pharyngitis be discovered so that proper measures can be taken if an infectious disease is present.

Pharyngitis

Acute pharyngitis usually appears rather suddenly with a feeling of dryness and soreness in the throat. There may be a constant desire to clear the throat, pain on swallowing, headache, a dry, harsh cough, and an elevation of temperature to 101° or 102°. A generalized feeling of fatigue is also present. Occasionally, there is pain in the ears; and if the infection has spread to the voice box, hoarseness will result. In children, the symptoms are more pronounced. The disease runs its course in a few days or a week.

When the doctor examines the throat, he often finds a bright red or purplish-red, swollen pharynx. A thick mucus-like exudate may cover the area. The treatment usually prescribed is similar to that for a patient with a common cold —complete bed rest, hot drinks, and aspirin to control the fever. If the pharyngitis is thought to be caused by an organism sensitive to an antibiotic or one of the sulfonamides, these drugs might be prescribed.

Chronic pharyngitis is the result of repeated attacks of acute pharyngitis. Enlarged tonsils and adenoids may cause the condition, as well as constant breathing through the mouth. It is frequently associated with chronic colds, sinusitis, and nasal infections. Probably no other area of the body is as prone to a secondary infection as is the pharynx.

There are three separate and distinct types of chronic pharyngitis—the simple or *catarrhal* type, the *hypertrophic* form, and the *atrophic* or "dry" pharyngitis.

Chronic simple pharyngitis is a persistent inflammation of the mucous membrane of the pharynx, without any complications. It is characterized by the same symptoms as an acute attack but with much less severity. There is a feeling of dryness or scratchiness in the throat. Thick, sticky mucus often fills the nasopharynx and sometimes can only be removed by suction or irrigation with saline and application of dilute silver nitrate. Extension of the inflammation to the ears may occur, causing a slight temporary deafness. Often the patient gags or vomits when a tongue depressor is placed on his tongue. The back of the pharynx may be deep red in color.

The detection of the causative agent is highly important. The physician may suggest that smoking be discontinued temporarily. If the patient habitually breathes through the mouth, he must learn to do otherwise. His occupation may be significant, if dusty materials are inhaled on the job. The doctor usually treats the patient with local medications, while the cause of the chronic pharyngitis is thoroughly investigated. Although this condition is a trying one and may last a long time, it almost always responds to treatment.

The second form of chronic pharyngitis is *hypertrophic* pharyngitis. It is also known as "clergyman's" sore throat and frequently is experienced by public speakers. This form is also a chronic inflammation of the pharynx, but it differs from the simple pharyngitis in that the lymph nodes are involved. It has the same causes as the simple form, but may be caused by the organisms of tuberculosis, syphilis, leprosy, or other diseases. Symptoms may consist of the presence of a thick secretion in the throat which is difficult to spit up. A cough is usually present. The blood vessels in the pharynx may become prominent.

A third type of sore throat is called *atrophic* or *dry pharyngitis*. Atrophy means "wasting away," which is what happens to the mucous membrane of the pharynx in this disease. In the early stage, there may be no atrophy, but only mild dryness and a shiny appearance of the pharynx. Atrophic pharyngitis often is caused by a glandular disorder, such as diabetes, or perhaps by the decreased secretions of the throat in old age.

True atrophic pharyngitis usually follows a similar disease in the nose *(atrophic rhinitis)*. The patient complains of dryness of the throat, which may be relieved by sips of water or clearing the throat. Crusts, which have a foul odor and are difficult to remove, form in the pharynx.

If the disease spreads to the larynx, hoarseness and coughing will result. Upon examination, the size of the pharyngeal tube will seem larger than usual. The surface of the pharynx appears as though it has been shellacked, and the membranes wrinkle when movement occurs. If the pharyngitis is caused by a constitutional disease, such as diabetes, the physician will endeavor to eliminate that disease.

"Strep throat"

Strep throat *(streptococcal throat)*, or septic sore throat, is a disease caused by a type of bacterium (genus *Streptococcus*) which is hemolytic —that is, destructive of red blood corpuscles. The symptoms are those of an acute pharyngitis, but much more severe. A pseudomembrane often appears in the throat. The patient's temperature may rise as high as 105°. The lymph nodes in the upper part of the neck enlarge and become sore. Many patients with strep throat develop a skin rash. Penicillin in proper dosage will usually resolve the condition, although some strains of the bacteria have developed immunity to antibiotic drugs.

Trench mouth

Trench mouth (Vincent's angina) also is characterized by a pseudomembrane, grayish or yellow-gray in appearance, and often spreading from the gums. It is an acute inflammatory disease of the gums, which may be accompanied by pain, bleeding, an offensive breath, and fever. The lymph nodes in the upper neck also may become swollen. Patients should be treated with frequent, hot mouth rinses, and drugs for pain. Antibiotics generally should not be used unless a high fever is present. For further treatment, patients with trench mouth should be referred to a dentist.

Pharyngeal diphtheria

One of the most serious of the diseases in which a false membrane covers the pharynx is pharyngeal diphtheria. In this condition, the membrane is a dirty gray in color and quite difficult to remove. When stripped off it usually leaves a bleeding, swollen surface. There is a definite, unpleasant, sweetish odor to the breath, characteristic of diphtheria. The throat is sore, the temperature rises, the lymph nodes in the neck become swollen, the back and the head ache, and the patient complains of pain on swallowing. The symptoms will vary in intensity according to the severity of the infection, which is caused by an organism known as the *Klebs-Loeffler bacillus*. Diphtheria antitoxin should be given immediately upon diagnosis. This disease is discussed in detail in Chapter 2, "The Child: *Childhood Diseases*."

Quinsy sore throat

A sore throat also may be caused by an abscess in the tissue surrounding the tonsil. This is commonly known as *quinsy sore throat (peritonsillar abscess)*. The first symptoms are those of acute pharyngitis or tonsillitis. After a few days, the pain becomes localized in one side of the throat. Swallowing becomes increasingly difficult and painful, and eventually the patient permits saliva to dribble from his mouth rather than suffer the pain caused by swallowing. or expectoration. Often the pain extends to the ear on the affected side. The patient usually holds his head somewhat tilted to that side because of inflammation of the deep muscles; for the same reason, the patient may turn his whole head and shoulders rather than the head alone. Because he can barely open his mouth, poor oral hygiene results; the breath becomes unpleasant. The lymph nodes below the angle of the jaw become enlarged and painful. The senses of smell and taste are almost lost, and speech is distorted. The tongue is heavily coated, and the patient complains of thirst. Rest in bed is necessary, and the physician will prescribe drugs to combat the infection and relieve the pain. When it is obvious that pus has accumulated, he will usually incise and drain the abscess. The infection lasts about five to ten days. Once it subsides, tonsillectomy should be done to prevent recurrences.

Syphilis

Syphilis may also occur in the throat and cause a persistent soreness. One site often invaded is the tonsils. A sore throat which lasts more than a week, accompanied by an enlarged ulcerated tonsil on one side suggests the possibility of a primary syphilitic infection. As time passes, a skin rash and enlarged lymph nodes in various parts of the body are demonstrable. There will usually be a feeling of tiredness and a fever.

The most important thing for the patient to remember about a sore throat is that the longer it lasts the more serious it can be. Any persistent or acute sore throat should be investigated promptly by a physician.

RESPIRATORY DISORDERS: LARYNGITIS

Laryngitis is an inflammation of the mucous membrane of the voice box *(larynx);* the condition is typified by hoarseness, and sometimes accompanied by a cough.

Acute laryngitis occurs frequently, often associated with the common cold. It occurs more often in the winter months than during warm weather. The condition may develop as a symptom of such diseases as measles, whooping cough, and influenza. Acute laryngitis also may follow straining of the voice, and sometimes occurs after an episode of violent weeping. Other causes of acute laryngitis are the drinking of hot liquids and the inhaling of irritating gases.

Acute laryngitis may be a contagious disease, depending upon its cause. As mentioned above, the condition frequently is associated with the common cold and diphtheria, and is thought to develop as a secondary infection. The cold is believed to be caused by a *virus* and the laryngitis by *bacteria*. The bacteria, which might have been already present, are stimulated by the cold virus. During sleep, the infectious material in the pharynx can drip into the larynx. In this way, it is possible for a chronic infection of the pharynx to cause laryngitis.

At the onset of an attack of acute laryngitis, the patient has an uncomfortable feeling of dryness in the area of the larynx. On attempting to talk, he may find that he has lost his voice, although by straining, a harsh whispering may be produced. Other than these local symptoms, the patient is not greatly distressed. He may have a slight fever and partial loss of appetite at the beginning of the attack, but recovery usually occurs within a few days. The symptoms may remain for a longer period if the patient uses his voice more than is necessary.

Acute laryngitis is more serious in children than in adults. The larynx of the young child is much smaller than that of the adult, and frequently more distressing symptoms occur. Shortness of breath *(dyspnea)* may be annoying; this may be accompanied by a bluish color *(cyanosis)* of the face and possibly by constriction *(spasm)* of the larynx. It is important to put the child in the care of a physician as soon as possible after the symptoms of acute laryngitis appear.

The patient with acute laryngitis usually is put to bed in a warm well-aired room. It is important that he rest his voice and drink liberal amounts of fluids. A vaporizer helps to relieve the patient's distress by supplying moisture to the affected area. If necessary, he may be given cough syrup or anesthetic lozenges.

Chronic laryngitis

Chronic laryngitis is a persistent inflamed condition of the mucous membrane of the voice box. It is typified chiefly by change in the voice. The chronic condition may follow

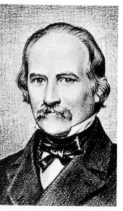

TÜRCK, Ludwig (1810-1868) Austrian laryngologist and neurologist. Türck is generally credited with first establishing the technique of laryngoscopy by virtue of his studies employing the primitive laryngoscope devised by Garcia. He is equally famous for his many investigations of the anatomy of the nervous system, and a number of nerve tracts have been named after him. A type of laryngitis that he investigated is called *Türck's trachoma.*

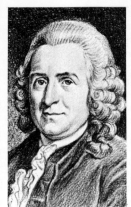

LINNAEUS, Carolus (von Linné) (1707-1778) Swedish physician and naturalist. He is said to have given the first good description of loss of speech (aphasia). Linnaeus is perhaps better known for his extensive studies on the classification of minerals, plants, and animals. His fundamental biological classification system is still in use today, and many of the species that he described are technically known by the designation that he applied to them.

an attack of acute laryngitis. Inhalations of dust and tobacco smoke also are contributing factors.

The symptoms are similar to those of acute laryngitis, but are less pronounced. In addition to voice change, the patient may "clear his throat" or cough frequently. Hoarseness, however, may also be caused by cancer of the larynx, so the patient should have a proper medical examination.

Chronic hypertrophic laryngitis

When chronic laryngitis has been present over a period of years, the mucous membranes of the larynx become thickened and tough. This condition is called *chronic hypertrophic laryngitis*. The symptoms are similar to those of chronic laryngitis but are prolonged and more severe, and there is less likelihood of regaining normal voice.

Chronic hypertrophic laryngitis can be followed by *chronic atrophic laryngitis*. In this condition, the fibrous tissue has become so thick that mucous glands have been destroyed.

Other types of laryngitis

Another type of laryngitis is *edematous laryngitis*, in which there is a swelling of the membranes of the larynx.

Myasthenic laryngitis signifies a weakness and exhaustion of the muscles in the larynx that are associated with speaking. It is a common condition among those who use their voices in their professions. This group includes singers, teachers, clergymen, train conductors, auctioneers, and others. The prevention of myasthenic laryngitis is accomplished by the use of common sense in "training" the voice. Resting the voice part of each day is important, as well as refraining from shouting, talking in a loud voice, and other unnecessary uses of the voice. In recovering from this condition, it is important that one remain completely silent if possible.

If the patient adheres to this rule, the voice has a good chance of returning to normal. There is no actual "life hazard" in this condition, but it is entirely possible to ruin a career should the condition not be properly and promptly treated.

RESPIRATORY DISORDERS: CANCER OF THE LARYNX

Cancer of the voice box *(larynx)*, like cancer elsewhere in the body, is an uncontrolled growth of cells. The disease in the larynx was mentioned in medical literature as early as 1837. Since that time, much knowledge has been acquired concerning its diagnosis and management.

Little was known about diseases in the larynx until 1854 when a singing teacher, Manuel Garcia, developed a laryngeal mirror, which provided the first satisfactory method of internal examination of the larynx. Although his discovery was received with incredulity at first, the use of the laryngeal mirror is now a common practice among physicians.

Cancer of the larynx constitutes only about two percent of all human cancers. It occurs most often in men between the ages of 40 and 60 years, although all age groups and both sexes may be affected.

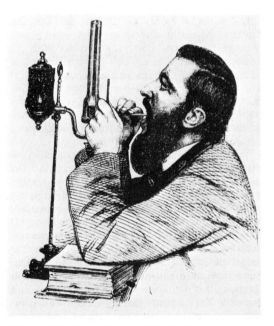

Picture of the Bohemian physiologist, Johann Czermak, conducting his studies which in 1858 first showed the value of laryngoscopy. *Bettmann Archive.*

Symptoms

The chief symptom of cancer of the larynx is hoarseness. Any voice change which lasts more than two weeks should be brought to the attention of a physician. The patient may complain of a tickling sensation in his throat, or of discomfort in his throat. Difficulty in swallowing and pain on speaking may ensue. As the disease progresses, the patient develops a cough, shortness of breath, wheezing, and halitosis. Lymph nodes in the neck may become enlarged. Occasionally the patient may spit up blood.

It is vitally important that the diagnosis of cancer of the larynx be made early. Over 80 percent of persons with cancer in this site can be cured if the growth is discovered before it spreads to nearby lymph nodes or distant body areas; however, only about 20 percent may expect to be cured after this spread has occurred. A simple examination, whereby the physician inserts a longhandled mirror at the back of the patient's mouth and looks into the mirror at the larynx, will lead to the diagnosis of most cancers in this area.

If the physician sees a growth in the mirror, a definite diagnosis of cancer cannot be made without an examination of a small piece of the suspected tissue under the microscope, to determine the presence of cancer cells. The removal and study of this tissue is called a *biopsy*.

Treatment

There are two acceptable forms of treatment which the physician may prescribe for the patient—radiation (x-ray or radium) and surgical therapy. When the disease involves a large portion of the larynx, the entire organ must be removed. While it is difficult for the patient to accept the fact that his voice box must be removed, an operation often means the difference between life and death. However, even if the patient cannot be cured, proper therapy can often prolong his life and make him much more comfortable.

If the larynx is removed, the patient's windpipe *(trachea)* is attached to the skin of the neck. Therefore, from the time of operation onward, he will no longer breathe through his nose, but through a hole in his neck instead. Consequently, he will not be able to blow his nose. Swimming should be avoided, as water entering the hole in his neck will go to the lungs, perhaps causing the patient to drown. Since the air breathed does not pass through the nose, it is no longer warmed, moistened, and cleaned. The patient, therefore, can easily inhale particles of foreign matter; he must take proper precautions to avoid this.

In spite the surgical resection that the patient has experienced, *he can learn to speak again.*

Many of these patients develop such excellent voices that their hearers are unaware that they have no voice box. In a person with a normal larynx, speech is "generated" by a column of air which is converted into sound by the vocal cords in the larynx. The larynx, therefore, merely makes the sounds—it is the tone producer. Words themselves are constructed and made intelligible by the resonating chambers (or "sounding boards") found in the head and the neck—primarily, the roof of the mouth, the tongue, the lips, and the teeth. To produce normal sounds, the vocal cords of the larynx must make certain movement. When the cords are absent, other tissues must be used in their place.

As soon as healing permits, the patient who has had his larynx removed begins taking speech lessons. In most cases, his entire class will have had their voice boxes removed, including the instructor. Although the patient may be discouraged and resentful before attending class, the fact that the teacher has no voice box, and is speaking clearly, brings new hope.

The voice teacher often tells the patient to attempt to talk even though no sounds can be made at first, in order to prevent the nerve pathways from falling into disuse. Relatives and friends can quickly learn to "hear" him by watching the movement of his lips, thus dispensing with his use of pencil and paper for communication.

It usually is necessary for the pupil to learn to speak by using the *esophageal method.* If so, the pupil is given a glass of carbonated beverage and encouraged to belch. Often this is the most difficult part of his lesson—nervousness and timidity may prevent the production of a big "burp." The teacher usually spends part of the first period putting the pupil at ease. When the pupil is able to belch at will, he is instructed to say "ba" as many times as he can with each belch. With constant repetition of this exercise, the

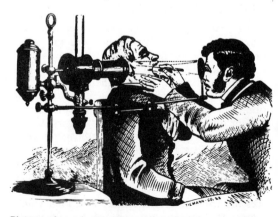

Picture of a nineteenth century physician examining a patient's larynx by the use of one of the earlier models of laryngoscope. *Bettmann Archive.*

volume gradually increases. This method is based on the fact that the student has not lost his ability to form words, but merely the power to make sound. If he can bring air up into his mouth, he can cause the column of air to vibrate against the roof of the pharynx and the adjacent structures. By constant practice, these substitute "vocal cords" will become "accustomed" to vibrating. Then the pupil is taught to say simple words each time he belches. However, esophageal speech is jerky, and the pupil should not continue this method.

In *pharyngeal speech,* the student can learn to join words and make sentences with little or no hesitation. He can carry on a conversation as well as any of his friends can. The pharyngeal method of speech is based on the fact that some air is entering the nose and mouth. This air is blocked in the pharynx with a triggerlike action of the tongue. The pupil develops the ability to expel it slowly and pronounce words as the air vibrates against his newly developed "vocal cords"—the roof of the pharynx, etc. Controlling the air as it is expelled is the main problem encountered. Rhythm and phrasing units are developed which produce smoother speech, as each word does not have to be belched up from the stomach as in the esophageal method. Few persons will be able to tell that the speaker who uses pharyngeal speech does not have a voice box, although they may mistake the rather hoarse quality of his voice for a bad cold. Whatever method of speech is used, constant practice is the most important factor.

If, despite sustained effort, the patient is unable to develop a satisfactory voice, an *artificial larynx* may be used. In early models, air exhaled through a hole in the neck passed through a reedlike mechanism producing sound, which was then conveyed to the mouth by means of a flexible tube. These models are rarely used today. Instead, patients are given battery-powered vibrators and sound producers. One highly satisfactory model consists of a small battery-powered apparatus held against the side of the throat. When activated, the device transmits vibrations to the pharynx and mouth.

Methodical, organized teaching, coupled with the cooperation of the patient, will permit almost all patients to evolve an adequate voice. The most important factor in the rehabilitation of the patient with cancer of the larynx is to catch the disease while it is still in an early stage. If the disease is diagnosed after it has become advanced, the chances of the patient's surviving are slim. Therefore, *hoarseness* of more than two weeks' duration should be investigated promptly. If the cancer is caught early, the larynx may be saved; and if the larynx must be removed, a full, vocal life can still be achieved.

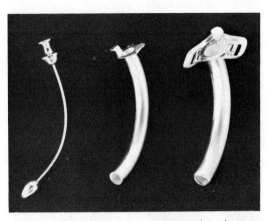

The above instruments are a set of metal tracheotomy tubes which are worn by a patient after having his larynx removed. Set includes (left to right) an obturator, inner cannula, and outer cannula.

RESPIRATORY DISORDERS: BRONCHITIS AND OTHER BRONCHIAL DISTURBANCES

Bronchitis is an inflammation of the mucous membrane of the tubes leading from the windpipe to the lungs (the *bronchi*). The condition usually affects the larger bronchi. Should the smaller bronchi be affected, the condition becomes more serious. When inflammation of the smallest bronchi, or *bronchioles,* occurs, the disease present is actually bronchial pneumonia. Acute bronchitis is found most frequently in children under three years of age and in old people, but it can occur at any age.

Many factors enter into the development of the various types of bronchitis. These include the patient's occupation, diet, and his general condition and resistance to disease. There are some occupations which create a constant hazard to the respiratory organs, and these will be discussed in detail below. Persons residing in damp and foggy climates are more apt to be victims of any type of respiratory disease.

Acute bronchitis

Acute bronchitis often is called a "chest cold." The symptoms include chest discomfort, a dry cough, fever, and loss of energy. The cough becomes more severe, and produces mucus. However, in about ten days, the symptoms will have subsided. It is possible for these symptoms to become much more severe and last for three or four weeks or even longer. Acute bronchitis often develops after the common cold.

SPEECH CLASS

Photography . . . R. A. Kolvoord.

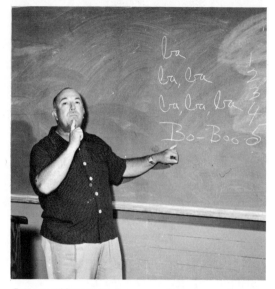

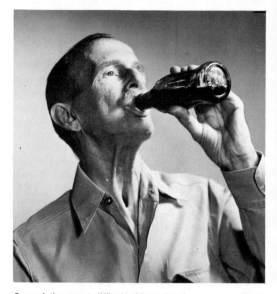

Persons without voice boxes can learn to speak again. They begin with learning to belch, and then saying the word 'ba' as many times as possible on each belch. Next, they master simple, one-syllable words, such as 'boy,' 'dog,' and 'town.' Eventually, after practice, they are able to say entire sentences with ease. This is esophageal speech.

One of the most difficult things for the person without a voice box to master is to be able to belch at will. He may need to drink soda water to achieve this. Esophageal speech is jerky. Hence, after the voice student masters the technique of this method, he studies the more difficult but much smoother technique of pharyngeal speech.

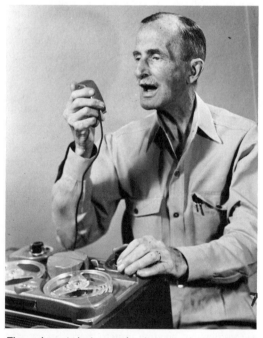

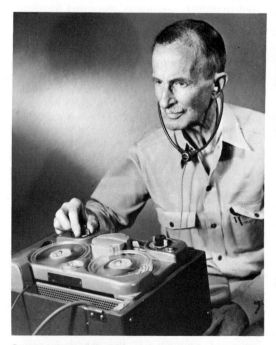

The voice student may be tense and apprehensive when he begins relearning to speak. The sound of his recorded new voice often gives him encouragement and assurance.

Some students actually do not believe they are speaking until they hear their recorded voices. Advanced students learn to correct speech defects by studying their recordings.

Acute bronchitis is usually a mild disease but may be serious in debilitated patients and those with chronic pulmonary or cardiac disease. The special danger is the development of pneumonia.

The winter months bring most of the cases of acute bronchitis. Predisposing factors are exposure, chill, fatigue, malnutrition, and rickets.

The disease can also be caused by physical and chemical irritants such as tobacco smoke, strong acid fumes, ammonia, chlorine, sulfur dioxide, or bromine.

Chronic bronchitis

In contrast to the acute form of the disease, chronic bronchitis commonly becomes a very serious condition. Its victims have a chronic cough and expectoration along with recurrent acute infections of the lower respiratory tract. The condition is especially prevalent during the winter months.

Air pollution aggravates and appears to be an important cause of chronic bronchitis. The disease is also common among heavy smokers.

Chronic bronchitis usually develops slowly over a number of years. There is a tendency for an acute upper respiratory tract infection to be followed by a persistent cough that hardly disappears before another episode occurs. Each morning the victim must devote considerable effort to expectoration of a thick, sticky sputum. Wheezing may also be present. Eventually, in a typical case of progressive bronchitis, shortness of breath develops. The final complications of the disease are strain on the heart, congestive heart failure, or an infection such as influenza or pneumonia.

A disease that is often associated with chronic bronchitis is emphysema. So frequently are the two conditions found together that some physicians question whether they are not part of the same disease entity. Emphysema is widely believed to be the usual result of prolonged bronchial irritation and hypersecretion.

The treatment for chronic bronchitis includes special attention to the patient's general health and environment. His activities should be regulated to avoid exposure and fatigue. Especially during the winter, it is desirable for him to live in a mild climate. All tobacco smoking should be stopped.

When cough and sputum persist, every effort should be made to facilitate the raising of sputum and the clearing of air passages. Expectorants, steam inhalation, and the use of vasodilators are helpful. Mucolytic agents are often effective in loosening the thick, tenacious sputum. Special medications can be prescribed for cough, bronchial spasm, if present, and acute infections. If shortness of breath is a problem, bronchodilator aerosols can be used, and in more severe cases, inhalation of oxygen by a nasal tube or an intermittent positive pressure respirator.

Bronchiectasis

Bronchiectasis refers to "dilated bronchi." This is a chronic bronchial abnormality in which the tubes, bronchi, and bronchioles are dilated and injured. A large portion of these cases are associated with abscess formation. The two main symptoms of bronchiectasis are a persistent cough and the expectoration of large amounts of sputum, sometimes foul-smelling. The condition may follow the advent of such diseases as broncho-pneumonia, tuberculosis, or lung abscess; however, the disease occurs in some patients who have no history of any prior infection. Sometimes the symptoms of bronchiectasis cannot be distinguished from the symptoms of the forerunning disease.

Occasionally, the patient spits up blood as an early symptom. As bronchiectasis progresses, some patients develop a clubbed appearance of the fingers. This condition may be present in varying degrees of intensity—from a slight inward curve of the fingernails to a noticeable bulbous enlargement of the tips of the fingers. Symptoms of advanced bronchiectasis include marked weight loss, fever, loss of appetite, and in most cases extreme weakness.

"Dry" bronchiectasis has symptoms which differ from those of simple bronchiectasis. The spitting up of blood is the chief symptom of this disease, with few if any other symptoms. Between the attacks of blood-spitting, the patient is usually asymptomatic.

A patient with bronchiectasis may live for years, although he is generally uncomfortable because of the foul odor of the sputum and his feeling of general *malaise*. If the bronchiectasis is limited to one area of the lung, the physician may advise surgical removal.

Benign bronchial tumors

The symptoms of a benign bronchial tumor may include wheezing, fever, cough, chills, the spitting of blood, and occasionally pain. However, there may be no symptoms present. These growths are detected by means of a *bronchoscopic* and x-ray examination. Bronchoscopic procedure implies the passage of a tube down the patient's throat. The physician looks through this tube to locate the tumor and also to obtain a small piece of the growth for microscopic study (biopsy). The usual treatment of patients with benign bronchial tumors is removal of the growth through the bronchoscope.

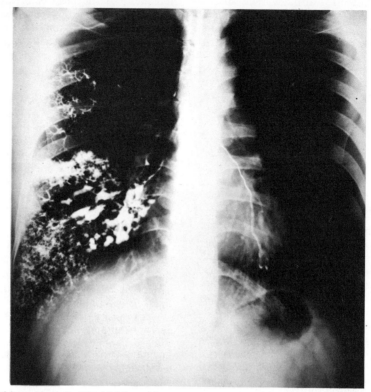

X-ray photograph of bronchiectasis. The blotchy, white patches represent pooled radiopaque material in the dilated bronchi, thereby making the diagnosis evident. *Photo by courtesy of Hermann Hospital, Houston, Texas.*

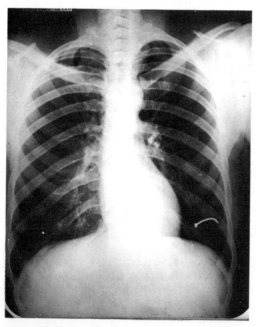

X-ray photograph of nail in lung. Patient could not account for its presence, and consulted the doctor for a chest pain. *Courtesy of Hermann Hospital.*

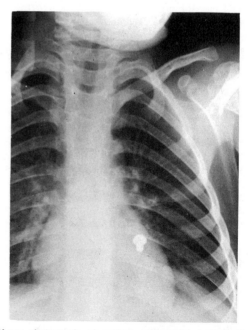

X-ray photograph of patient with metal bolt in the lung. Such pictures are great aids in removing foreign objects. *Photography by F. W. Schmidt.*

Foreign bodies in the bronchi

A foreign body can enter the bronchi: when a person is eating and the food goes down the "wrong way"; when the person carries some small object in the mouth and is suddenly jolted, causing the object to be inhaled into the bronchi; or by sucking in some foreign material unconsciously. The symptoms, if the object is high up in the tract, are sudden paroxysms of coughing, difficulty in breathing, a bluish coloring of the skin, and severe pain and discomfort. Death may result if prompt treatment is not instituted. If the object is so small as to lodge farther down in the tract, the symptoms are not especially violent. There may be a cough resulting from the irritation and fever may develop later. When inhalation of a foreign body is suspected, a physician should be called at once. In nearly every case, he will be able to have the object extracted and thereby bring about an immediate relief of all symptoms.

RESPIRATORY DISORDERS: EMPHYSEMA

One of the most common disabling disorders of the respiratory tract is *emphysema*, a condition characterized by overdistention of the lungs with air that cannot be expelled. At the microscopic level, the walls of the tiny alveoli stretch and eventually rupture, reducing the capacity of the lungs to exchange carbon dioxide and water. Chronic bronchitis of many years' duration almost always precedes the development of alveolar overdistention.

Emphysema is a progressive disease that is most common in males over 40. Its cause is unknown, but excessive smoking and atmospheric pollution may be factors.

Symptoms

Symptoms of emphysema include a long history of cough and the raising of sputum, and shortness of breath. The shortness of breath is noticeable first on exertion and later with walking and other daily activities. Bouts of wheezing are not unusual. Weakness, lethargy, anorexia, and weight loss may be present.

In patients with significant emphysema, the chest is hyperinflated and at times fixed in the inspiratory position. On inspiration the entire rib cage is lifted and accessory muscles of respiration are used. The diaphragm is flattened and hardly moves at all.

Treatment

Although changes in the lungs are irreversible, it is possible to give the emphysema patient considerable relief and to increase the functioning capacity of his lungs. The patient should be encouraged to live a moderately active life, but to avoid any exertion which might increase shortness of breath. Bed rest should be allowed only when necessary.

To control bronchospasm, patients should make regular use of bronchodilator aerosols. Thick and tenacious bronchial secretions can be thinned with sputum liquefiers, and deliberate coughing will help to bring them up. Exercises should be done to strengthen the abdominal muscles and permit more complete exhalation. Manual compression of the abdomen during expiration will aid in elevating the diaphragm. Elevating the foot of the bed will produce similar results.

Oxygen inhalation is often necessary for relief of shortness of breath, but it must be used with caution. The safest method is with the intermittent positive pressure apparatus which produces adequate ventilation and also removes carbon dioxide.

A return to normal ventilatory function cannot be expected in patients with symptomatic emphysema. The normal course of events is relentless progression; and therapy is successful if it maintains the status quo or merely slows the downward trend.

A patient with mild to moderate emphysema may live a long and comfortable life, provided all the factors producing bronchospasm and bronchial irritation are controlled. In contrast, the patient with severe emphysema has a greatly reduced life expectancy.

RESPIRATORY DISORDERS: INFLUENZA

Influenza (also called "flu" and "la grippe") is a disease of the respiratory tract caused by the influenza virus. The disease appears more frequently during the winter months. The causative agent is transmitted through discharges from respiratory tracts of persons infected with the disease.

This disease appeared centuries ago. Hippocrates described an epidemic which occurred in the year 412 B.C., presumed by authorities to have been an epidemic of influenza. Since that time, epidemics have occurred all over the world. The "flu" epidemic of 1918 spread through half the world. It is estimated that 200,000,000 individuals contracted the disease, of which at least 20,000,000 died. In the United States, approximately 20,000,000 persons came down with the flu, and 550,000 died. To some extent the severity of this pandemic can be attributed to World War I, which had devastated large sections of Europe and exposed the population to untold hardships.

The symptoms of influenza begin from one to five days after exposure to the disease. The onset is sudden. Chills and fever (ranging to 105°) are present, accompanied by headache and backache. Sore throat and a dry cough are also common symptoms, because this disease involves the throat, the trachea, and the bronchi. The infection lowers the resistance of the respiratory tract, so that it is vulnerable to attacks from other types of organisms, which may cause infection in the sinuses (*sinusitis*) or middle ear (*otitis media*), pneumonia, lung abscess, and sometimes meningitis. Encephalitis and Parkinson's syndrome sometimes develop as complications. Should influenza occur during pregnancy, the lives of both mother and child could be in danger. A patient who gives a history of loss of weight and extreme weakness following a bout of influenza should have chest x-ray and sputum examinations, in order to rule out tuberculosis. It has been found that in some cases where tuberculosis followed what was regarded as an attack of influenza, the influenza symptoms actually may have been early symptoms of tuberculosis or cancer.

A far more common complication of influenza is *influenzal pneumonia*. The symptoms include marked breathlessness and a bluish coloration of the skin, both occurring early in the course of the disease. Patients frequently cough up large amounts of blood. There is great weakness and exhaustion. This type of pneumonia usually occurs in both lungs, and the lower lobes are involved more often than the upper lobes.

The pneumonia form of influenza may be one of three types. There is the sudden, severe, often fatal type which is present from the very onset of influenza; there is the type which appears a few days after the onset of the influenza; and the type which appears after apparent recovery from the influenza. The first form is comparatively rare, and patients who develop this severe type may die within a day or two. The other two forms are similar except for the time at which the secondary infection manifests itself. The symptoms of all three may be those of bronchopneumonia or of lobar pneumonia. The sputum coughed up may be blood-tinged and mucuslike, or it may resemble pus with a pink or green tinge. A long period of convalescence often follows this disease. The patient may be left with a chronic bronchitis or bronchiectasis, and these conditions may continue throughout life.

Care of the patient

Care of the patient with influenza includes rest in bed in a room where the temperature is kept moderately high; cold air increases the tendency to cough. A daily bath in bed should be given, with care taken that the patient does not become chilled. Should the fever be high, tepid sponge baths may be given. Usually the patient is exhausted and depressed mentally as well as physically, and the person caring for him should maintain a cheerful attitude. Visitors should be excluded, not only to prevent spread of the infection, but to guard against the possibility of secondary invasion of bacteria in the patient. Nose and mouth hygiene should be carried out in the patient. The diet should include three or four quarts of fluid each day. Various drugs can be prescribed for relief of symptoms —aspirin for generalized aches and pains, phenylephrine for nasal obstruction, and a sedative mixture for cough. At all times, one should be on the alert for further symptoms, indicative of the onset of any of the complications mentioned previously.

Flu prevention

An attack of influenza will produce lasting immunity, but unfortunately the protection is only against the type of virus causing that infection. To protect against other prevalent types or at least reduce the chance of being stricken, an individual can be immunized.

If the vaccine used contains a strain of virus closely related to the one causing the most current influenza outbreak, about 70 percent of the persons immunized will be protected. Vaccination is especially important for older people, pregnant women, and patients with cardiac, pulmonary, or other chronic diseases. The length of time that immunity is effective varies from three months to one year. Immunization once a year, before the influenza season, should give maximum protection during the period of possible epidemics. Some persons are allergic to substances in the vaccine.

A number of difficulties prevent the production of a more effective influenza vaccine. Per-

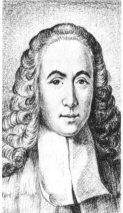

MORGAGNI, Giovanni Battista (1682-1771) Italian anatomist and pathologist. Considered the founder of pathologic anatomy, he also made original observations on many normal structures of the human body. He was the first to describe a number of anatomical structures, some of which carry his name, e.g., the *sinus of Morgagni*, which lies at the base of the skull, the *ventricle of Morgagni* which is the laryngeal ventricle, and a nasal *(Morgagni's)* concha.

haps most troublesome is the highly unstable nature of some viruses, which mutate unpredictably. In so doing they alter their antigenic properties, acquiring new armor against existing vaccines. Different antibodies are needed to neutralize the mutants, so vaccines must be changed.

Epidemics and pandemics

The difference between a pandemic and an epidemic is that a pandemic affects a great number of people over the entire world, while an epidemic is localized.

Pandemic influenza has been found to appear in three phases. The first phase affects large numbers of people, but is comparatively mild, and there are few complications. This phase lasts only a few weeks. The second phase also affects large numbers of people, but is more severe than the beginning phase. It carries with it many complications. The third phase begins more slowly and is accompanied by many severe complications, although it does not infect large numbers of people as the other phases do. The *morbidity* from influenza during a pandemic is high.

Until the pandemic of 1918, the theory generally expounded was that the bacterium, *Hemophilus influenzae*, was the specific cause of influenza. However, this idea has since given way to the virus theory. This theory has been substantiated by experiments, in which a filterable virus was isolated from patients infected with influenza. Since that time, further studies have revealed that there are three distinct types of viruses involved in the disease. The exact causative agent of pandemic influenza has not been established, and only further studies will reveal whether a distinct and separate virus is responsible. Many bacteria play the part of secondary invaders, particularly in the case of pandemic influenza.

Uncomplicated influenza shows no changes different from any other catarrhal condition of the respiratory tract. However, in the severe cases of influenza complicated with pneumonia, there are definite changes. There may be inflammation of the mucous membrane of the nose

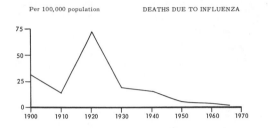
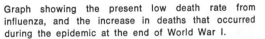

Graph showing the present low death rate from influenza, and the increase in deaths that occurred during the epidemic at the end of World War I.

(*rhinitis*), inflammation of the pharynx (*pharyngitis*), a severe tracheal and bronchial involvement (*bronchiolitis*), swelling of the small sacs in the lungs, and other changes. The paranasal sinuses may also be involved, and sometimes puslike material oozes from these sinuses.

Uncomplicated influenza accounts for about 95 percent of all cases in the first phase of a pandemic, and it is the form seen most often during epidemics of the disease. The patients usually recover promptly; they rarely experience a relapse unless complications set in; and very few of them die from influenza.

Between the simple kind of influenza and the treacherous pneumonic influenza, there is a type in which bronchitis or sinusitis or both occur, causing a prolongation of the disease. Just when the patient is expected to show signs of recovery, he begins to cough more frequently. This cough produces large amounts of sputum, which has the appearance of pus as well as mucus. These symptoms persist for about a week. The patient also may suffer from severe headaches, fever, and weakness. This type of influenza is seen in both pandemics and epidemics.

Influenza can be a mild infection, no more serious than a head cold. It can be an acute, violent plague also. No one knows when an epidemic will begin, or just how it will end. The 1918 pandemic killed about 20 million people all over the world. Records show that influenza appears regularly each winter in temperate climates; about 85 percent of flu cases occur during the cold months. Most physicians believe that the infection spreads in a mild form from person to person, until many harbor the virus. Then some combination of circumstances causes it to attack in a severe form. It was found during the 1918 attack that some healthy persons could *not* be infected with the disease, although they gargled with a solution prepared from the secretions of patients having influenza. The conclusion was, of course, that the more obvious symptoms became apparent after the most contagious stage of the disease had passed.

The riddle of influenza is still to be solved, but this generation is more fortunate than those

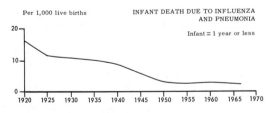

Chart depicting the decrease in the number of infant deaths reported as resulting from influenza and pneumonia in the United States, per 1,000 infant population.

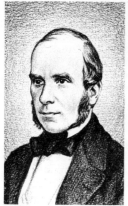

SNOW, John (1813-1858) English physician. Snow was one of the pioneers in anesthesiology, and made considerable use of both chloroform and ether in his practice, between 1848 and 1858, at a time when the use of general respiratory anesthesia had not yet achieved broad prominence. He is also famous for his study of cholera, in which he was able to demonstrate the water-borne character of this disorder, which was then poorly understood.

FRAENKEL, Albert (1848-1916) German physician. Fraenkel was the first man to show the causal relationship between pneumonia and the bacterium *Diplococcus pneumoniae*. Both Sternberg and Pasteur had isolated this organism, but the proof of its pathogenic properties awaited Fraenkel's investigations of 1886, which showed that it was responsible for a great many cases of this severe respiratory infection that until recent years was often fatal.

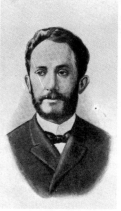

gone by. People have become educated to the fact that prompt attention to comparatively minor symptoms often averts catastrophe. Further, there is little likelihood of another pandemic. Most of the deaths of the 1918 catastrophe were caused by secondary complications, particularly pneumonia. Today's antibiotic drugs greatly reduce the danger of these complications. Thus, although influenza is still present, it is no longer the threat it once was.

RESPIRATORY DISORDERS: PNEUMONIA

Pneumonia is an inflammation involving either one or both lungs. When both lungs are infected, the condition is called *bilateral* pneumonia. Pneumonia may be caused by specific bacteria or by a virus. There are over 33 different forms of *pneumococcus (Diplococcus pneumoniae)*, one type of bacteria which may cause this infection.

In healthy individuals, the linings of the nose and throat passages are always filled with microorganisms. Given the proper conditions, these organisms can cause disease. Farther down the respiratory tract, the organisms are less profuse; and in the lower area of the lungs, they are not present at all during good health. One of the means by which organisms are cleansed from the respiratory system is by the tiny hairlike projections (*cilia*) which line the mucous membranes of the respiratory passages. These cilia sweep the infectious materials upward and thus keep them from entering the lower breathing passages. When an inflammation occurs in this area, secretions increase and inhibit the action of the cilia; thus, the respiratory system loses some of its protective function.

There are certain factors which, when present, help to pave the way for lung infections. First, infectious diseases such as influenza,

measles, and whooping cough particularly weaken the respiratory passages, so that pneumonia may develop. Also, many chronic diseases predispose the patient to pneumonia. Among these chronic conditions are heart ailments, anemia, hardening of the arteries (*arteriosclerosis*), and senility. In these cases, pneumonia is a *secondary disease* caused by disease-producing organisms already present in the respiratory tract.

History of pneumonia

This disease, with its characteristic symptoms, has been known to physicians since the time of Hippocrates, 400 B.C. However, it was not until the year 1700 that pneumonia and pleurisy were distinguished. In 1761, Leopold Auenbrugger showed how diagnosis could be facil-

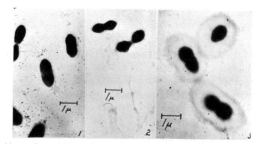

Use of antiserum in the treatment of pneumonia requires that the type of *Diplococcus pneumoniae* present be known. In the *Neufeld quellung* test, the bacterial capsule swells when it is exposed to serum from an animal previously infected with organisms of that type. Photomicrograph 1 shows type 3 organisms in water, 2 shows them in type 1 antiserum, and 3 shows the diagnostic swelling when type 1 organisms are suspended in type 1 antiserum. *Courtesy Medichrome, Clay-Adams Co., Inc., N.Y.; Dr. Stuart Mudd, Department of Microbiology, University of Pennsylvania, author; Journal of Experimental Medicine, 1943, 78: 327.*

itated by "tapping" on the chest wall in various places; this is called *percussion*. Another great aid to the diagnosis of chest diseases was the invention of the stethoscope by René Laennec in the early nineteenth century. Antipneumococcus serum was first used in 1891.

Until about 1940, pneumonia was considered one of the most serious diseases of mankind. Victims were placed in special wards, where they received serum therapy and oxygen inhalations. Even with the best of care, many died; survivors had a slow, tedious recovery. All this changed with the discovery of the sulfonamides and antibiotics. Today, pneumonia is no longer the dreaded killer of 25 to 30 years ago. Indeed, discovery of these drugs has lowered the death rate of pneumonia patients from about 33 percent to 5 percent or lower. Treatment with antibiotics (penicillin, etc.), and sulfonamides often brings the patient's temperature down to normal within a day or two. Oxygen is started early to help the patient breathe more easily.

Bacterial pneumonias

The numerous types and varieties of pneumonia are generally classified according to the causative agent—first, as either bacterial or nonbacterial (viral) and then more specifically, by the organism involved.

Of the *bacterial pneumonias*, the most common by far is *pneumococcal pneumonia,* caused by *Diplococcus pneumoniae.* Typically one or more lobes of the lung is involved, giving the disease a *lobar* distribution. This is in contrast to pneumonias in which there are scattered areas of involvement, so-called *bronchopneumonias.*

Pneumococcal pneumonia is preceded, in many instances, by an upper respiratory tract infection. The onset of pulmonary symptoms is usually sudden, with shaking chills, sharp pain in the chest, cough, expectoration of a rusty-colored sputum, fever, and headache. Shortness of breath is frequent, with rapid and often painful breathing. A peculiar expiratory grunting is also common. In pneumococcal pneumonia, the patient sweats profusely, is often cyanotic, and is acutely ill.

Pneumococcal pneumonia accounts for 90 to 95 percent of all cases of bacterial pneumonia. Other bacteria causing the disease include *staphylococci, streptococci,* and *Friedländer's bacilli.* X-ray examination of patients with these diseases often shows patchy infiltration and lack of extensive areas of consolidation, features common to bronchopneumonia. Physical signs and symptoms can be very similar, so isolation of the causative organism from sputum and blood cultures is mandatory.

Although not nearly as common as pneumococcal pneumonia, *staphylococcal pneumonia* occurs more often than the other bacterial varieties and its incidence is increasing, especially as a complication of influenza or in postsurgical or debilitated patients. Always a serious disease, it is characterized by some or all of the symptoms of pneumococcal pneumonia, *i.e.* pain in the chest, shortness of breath, cyanosis, and cough. Small lung abscesses are common, but difficult to identify by physical examination.

Streptococcal pneumonia often occurs secondary to influenza or the measles. The onset is usually gradual, with early symptoms likely to be those of bronchitis with a severe cough—dry at first, and later yielding a thin sputum. If not treated, the symptoms may become severe, with profound prostration, high fever, delirium, cyanosis, nausea, and vomiting. Inflammation of the membrane *(pleura)* covering the lungs and surface of the chest cavity is common and may lead to the collection of purulent fluid in the pleural cavity (a condition known as *empyema).*

Friedländer's pneumonia, caused by *Klebsiella pneumoniae* (better known as Friedländer's bacillus), is characteristically a disease of elderly, debilitated, or alcoholic men. The symptoms are similar to those of pneumococcal pneumonia, except that the disease progresses rapidly, leading to death within a few days if the proper therapy is not started early. Patients who recover usually do so slowly, with a persistent cough and expectoration, and chronic lung abscesses.

Viral pneumonia

"Primary atypical pneumonia," pneumonia thought to be caused by an unknown virus, was first recognized and described in about 1935. Since that time, numerous reports regarding the condition have appeared every year.

The adenovirus and the influenza virus are now recognized as causes of some cases of primary atypical pneumonia, and the organism responsible for most of the others has been identified. Surprisingly, it is not a virus at all, but a pleuro-pneumonia-like-organism (PPLO) known as *Mycoplasma pneumoniae.* Military personnel and children are the most frequent victims of *mycoplasma pneumonia.*

The diseases produced by these three organisms are similar; typically they are mild and gradual in onset. Fever, cough, malaise, headache, and sore throat are the characteristic symptoms. The most effective therapy for primary atypical pneumonia is the antibiotic tetracycline. Mortality is low even in untreated cases.

Postoperative pneumonia

More effective methods of prevention have greatly reduced the incidence of *postoperative pneumonia.* Closer attention is now paid to

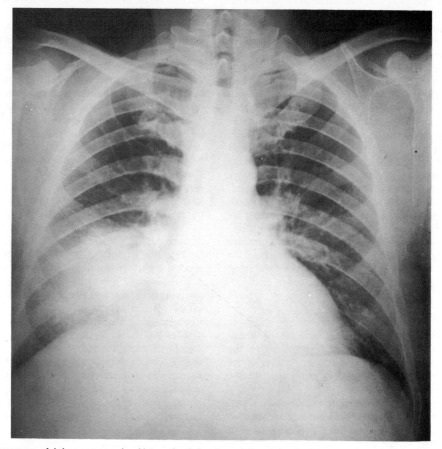

X-ray appearance of lobar pneumonia. Above the left edge of the right diaphragm, at the base of the right lung, there is a homogenous opacity (white) suggestive of pneumonia. *Photo courtesy Hermann Hospital, Houston.*

clearing the tracheobronchial tree during an operation, and to promotion of coughing and expectoration afterward. Improved methods of anesthesia have also reduced the chance of developing the disease.

If postoperative pneumonia does occur, symptoms appear early, usually on the first or second day after the operation. The symptoms include a rise in temperature and chest discomfort. A cough is often present, which causes much distress to the patient with an operative incision. Sometimes the symptoms may be of such little consequence that the condition is not detected until an x-ray examination is made, or until physical examination reveals the presence of the infection.

Patients having even a slight upper respiratory tract infection before surgery are more likely to acquire postoperative pneumonia. If routine physical examination reveals an incipient cold, it may be necessary to postpone the operation until the symptoms subside. The physician will have to decide after evaluating the various risks involved and the necessity for prompt surgery.

Aspiration pneumonia

Aspiration pneumonia results from inhaling either solid or liquid materials into the lungs. This can occur when the patient is unconscious for any reason, such as head injury, alcoholic intoxication, cerebral vascular accident, or barbiturate poisoning. The normal reflex actions which *prevent* the inhalation of foreign material have been temporarily put out of service; and when foreign material enters the lungs and bronchi, it causes an irritation of the parts concerned and brings with it the bacteria which cause the pneumonia.

Chemical pneumonia

Chemical pneumonia is caused by the inhalation of irritating and poisonous fumes—particularly such gases as chlorine, ammonia, mustard gas, methyl acetates, etc. This may occur during an accident in a factory, or in warfare. Sometimes the disease is so severe that it causes death.

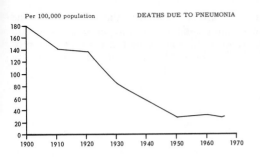

Per 100,000 population   DEATHS DUE TO PNEUMONIA

The death rate due to pneumonia consistently decreased during the first half of the twentieth century to less than 40 persons per 100,000 population.

Measles pneumonia

Measles is a common contagious disease. It starts about two weeks after the patient has been exposed to the virus which causes the infection. Its symptoms include fever, "runny" nose, loss of energy, and a cough. A rash appears a few days later. When the rash occurs, the symptoms subside. Should fever and difficult breathing continue after this phase of the disease, one might suspect *measles pneumonia*. Most of the deaths following measles are caused by this added complication. In the great majority of cases, however, recovery is rapid. (For further discussion of measles, see Chapter 2, "The Child: *Childhood Diseases*.")

Ornithosis

Ornithosis is a contagious atypical form of pneumonia transmitted to man by certain birds —principally parrots, parakeets, and lovebirds and less often poultry, pigeons, and canaries. The infective agent is a virus. Ornithosis is transmitted to man by inhalation of dust from feathers or contents of bird cages, by a bite from an infected bird, or occasionally by cough droplets from an infected patient.

The disease develops about ten days after exposure to the virus. Symptoms include loss of appetite, chills and fever, headache, and profuse sweating. Clinical signs of pneumonia, including cough and expectoration of purulent sputum, often appear. The disease usually lasts two or three weeks. The easiest way to avoid the disease is to avoid contact with potentially infectious birds.

Traumatic pneumonia

It is possible for a blow or injury to the chest, often the result of a car accident, to interfere with the functions of the lungs and to injure parts of the respiratory system. This makes it easier for the entrance of pneumonia-producing organisms. The pneumonia symptoms may be manifested immediately after the injury, or several days later.

Terminal pneumonia

Terminal pneumonia is a name given to pneumonia which develops in patients who are critically ill or dying from another condition. The patient's resistance is so low from the existing disease that the body is an easy prey to infection of the lungs. There are few outward symptoms, and the pneumonia is usually not discovered unless an autopsy is performed. Pneumonia may also be found in association with cancer of the lung and tuberculosis.

Atelectasis

Pneumonia may be associated with partial collapse of the lung *(atelectasis)*. The symptoms include a sudden attack of shortness of breath, deep bluish coloration of the skin, chest pain, and fever. The lung usually re-expands slowly within several days.

Secondary complications

Abscess and *gangrene* of the lung are secondary complications of the more severe cases of pneumonia. Usually, there are several small abscesses scattered over the affected area. The signs of lung abscess include fever, sweating, and the production of puslike sputum. Gangrene is typified by thin, brown, foul-smelling sputum.

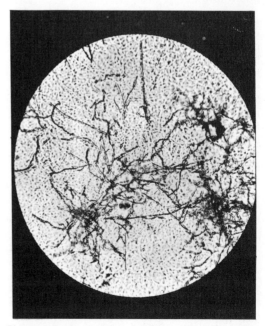

Photograph of a colony of *Streptomyces griseus*, the fungus from which the antibiotic, *streptomycin*, is made. *Courtesy Dr. Selman A. Waksman.*

Pericarditis is a serious complication of pneumonia. This condition is the inflammation and thickening of the covering of the heart (the *pericardium*). Its symptoms may be confused with pneumonia symptoms; pain in the heart area can be easily mistaken for pain in the lung area. If the pulse is extremely rapid or the blue color of the skin and shortness of breath seem more pronounced than the pneumonia suggests, there is a good possibility that pericarditis is present.

Acute pneumococcal endocarditis occurs in only about one percent of all cases of pneumonia. This condition is an inflammation of the inner lining of the heart. Middle-aged patients with a history of rheumatic infection, hardening of the arteries (*arteriosclerosis*), or syphilis are especially susceptible to this complication.

Acute otitis media, which is a middle ear infection, occurs in about two percent of pneumonia patients and affects children more often than adults. Should this condition remain undiagnosed, the infection may spread to the mastoid area or even to the brain. Inflammation of the membranes covering the brain (the *meninges*) is an extremely dangerous complication of pneumonia.

Peritonitis is an inflammation of the lining of the abdominal cavity. It occurs rarely as a complication of pneumonia. Symptoms include vomiting, diarrhea, and abdominal tenderness.

Treatment of patients with bacterial pneumonia

Antibiotics are more effective than the sulfonamides as a treatment for patients with pneumonia. Patients respond more quickly and have fewer toxic reactions to antibiotics. Penicillin is used most extensively; but other drugs —such as the tetracyclines, erythromycin, streptomycin, and chloramphenicol—are sometimes required. It was only in 1945 that a sufficient amount of penicillin was made available for general use. The drug is given to persons with acute infections by hypodermic injection. It is also given orally and breathed in as a vaporized solution (*aerosol penicillin*).

There are many forms of sulfonamides, which are also occasionally used, a few types outranking the others in efficacy. The physician usually gives the drug early in the course of the disease, in order to obtain a high level of the compound in the blood as quickly as possible.

Many patients with pneumonia require oxygen therapy to relieve cyanosis and prevent shock. It is also helpful in relieving cough and restlessness and in preventing abdominal distention. If patients are having chest pain, codeine can be given.

In addition to these specific measures, proper nursing care is essential to the well-being of the pneumonia patient. The diet must be light and easily digested, and contain a high level of proteins. Fluids should be given freely, intravenously if necessary. Care should be taken that the patient does not become constipated; enemas may be required. The patient should have his position changed frequently. It is important that he rest both physically and mentally. Care should be taken that the patient does not overexert himself in any way. He should be kept warm and dry in a room, neither too hot nor too cold. He may be propped up in bed at the angle which suits him best.

It is a wise precaution to keep the patient apart from other persons. Gauze masks should be worn by those caring for him. The dishes used by the patient should be handled separately and boiled after use. Those persons having colds or other upper respiratory conditions definitely should remain away from the patient.

After the patient has fully recovered from the pneumonia, he should have a complete physical examination by a physician. Most important in this regard is an x-ray examination of the chest.

RESPIRATORY DISORDERS: PLEURISY

Pleurisy is inflammation of the membrane which covers the lungs and the surfaces of the chest cavity (*the pleura*). The most common causes of pleurisy are pneumonia, tuberculosis, and influenza. The symptoms of pleurisy are pain which becomes severe when a deep breath is taken, cough, fever, and rapid shallow breathing.

There are three kinds of pleurisy: "dry pleurisy," "wet pleurisy," and "purulent pleurisy."

Dry pleurisy almost always follows an acute pneumonia infection. The pain which appears is usually present over the area of infection. The most reliable symptom indicating the presence of this form of pleurisy is a sound, called the "pleural friction rub," heard by the physician through his stethoscope. When the pain is moderate, it can be relieved by medication or heat application. When the underlying disease subsides, the symptoms of pleurisy disappear.

Wet pleurisy is most often associated with tuberculosis. However, lung cancer, acute rheumatic fever, pneumonia, and other diseases also may produce wet pleurisy.

Empyema is an infection of the pleural cavity in which large amounts of pus are formed. It may be acute or chronic. It is acute if it has occurred only recently and is associated with fever or other symptoms. It is considered chronic if it has been present for some time and is accompanied by few or no other symptoms.

The chronic type of empyema is seldom seen in recent times because of advances in treatment of patients in the acute stage. However, it may occur in association with tuberculosis. The appearance of the fluid from the pleural cavity in cases of empyema varies. It may be watery (*serous*) or puslike (*purulent*), or a combination of the two (*seropurulent*).

The therapy for empyema involves removal of the pus by suction, irrigation with saline, and administration of antibiotics, usually penicillin. In later stages, it may be necessary to drain the pleural cavity by surgical means. When blood can be seen in the pleural fluid, the condition is considered to be *hemorrhagic effusion*. About 75 percent of the patients with this condition have a malignant growth (cancer) of either the lung or the pleura, or both.

In any case, when the patient has reason to believe he has a "touch of pleurisy," he should consult a physician.

RESPIRATORY DISORDERS: TUBERCULOSIS

Tuberculosis is an infectious, inflammatory, contagious disease which may occur in almost any organ of the body, but occurs most frequently in the lung. It is caused by a long slender rod-shaped bacterium called the *tubercle bacillus* or *Mycobacterium tuberculosis*. This organism may live for long periods of time outside of the human body, especially in cold weather, but it is easily destroyed by sunlight and disinfectants. Three types of tubercle bacilli are known to infect man—the human, the bovine, and rarely, the avian. There has been a sharp decline in the number of cases caused by the bovine tubercle bacillus since the advent of pasteurization of milk. Current methods of testing and treating

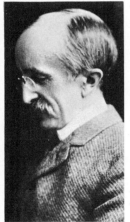

TRUDEAU, Edward Livingston (1848-1915) American physician. He was noted as the most outstanding authority on tuberculosis of his time. When stricken himself by the disorder in 1873, he went to Saranac Lake in New York, where he later established a famous sanitarium. He was an advocate of the open air method of treatment. He was responsible for extensive research on the causes and progress of the disorder, as well as on treatment. *Bettmann Archive.*

cattle with tuberculosis have also contributed to a decline in this variety.

In 1900, tuberculosis was the leading cause of death in the United States, with 200 deaths per 100,000 population. By the mid 1960s, mortality had fallen to about four deaths per 100,000. Factors responsible for this precipitous decline have been an improved standard of living, with better nutrition and housing, shorter working hours, earlier diagnosis and treatment, and the advent of drug therapy. Although the death rate in this country is now quite low, high rates still persist in poverty areas throughout the world. Even in the United States the number of new cases of tuberculosis is declining less rapidly than the number of deaths.

History of the disease

Tuberculosis is an ancient disease, as old as the history of civilization. Reference to it is made in the tablets used for writing by the Babylonians, and in old manuscripts. It was not known as tuberculosis then, as the term was not coined until 1810, but was called "consumption." Hippocrates, the "father of medicine," wrote about "consumption" in detail. Galen, a Greek physician who lived in the second century, mentioned the possibility of transmitting the disease from one person to another. Richard Morton, an English physician, published a treatise in 1689 in which he discussed the wasting away of the body; he included fear and grief among the causes of consumption.

In 1882 Robert Koch, a German physician, discovered the tubercle bacillus, and recognized it as the organism which causes tuberculosis. This discovery marked the beginning of modern methods in the attack on the disease.

Still another great contributor to our knowledge of the disease was Doctor Edward Livingston Trudeau, who was himself a victim. In 1865, when Trudeau was 17 years old, he nursed his brother through the last stages of consumption. It must have been at this time that Doctor Trudeau was infected with the disease, although symptoms did not manifest themselves until several years afterward. Then he was found to have one lung almost completely involved. First he followed his physician's advice to "go South and exercise." Finally, however, sure that death awaited him in the near future, Trudeau adjourned to the country he had always loved—the Adirondack Mountains. At that time he was an invalid with constant bouts of high fever, and his physician told him that he had only a few months to live. But he survived 42 more years and led a happy normal life. Our modern sanatoriums, so important in the management of patients with tuberculosis, and modern methods of treating tuberculous patients, are partially the results of Doctor Trudeau's experience.

"Resistance" to tuberculosis

Some species of animals seem to have more resistance to the tubercle bacillus than others. Some races may contract the disease more readily than others. And some individuals in a given race may be more susceptible or resistant than the average person of the same race. This is called "native resistance," whether it pertains to the species, the race, or the individual. Its role in the control of tuberculosis is obviously of the highest importance.

Man is more susceptible to tuberculosis than many other animals—unless the animals are taken out of their natural habitat. Monkeys confined in a zoo are more liable to contract the human type of tuberculosis than are humans.

Different breeds of animals of the same species present different levels of native resistance. For instance, the Havana rabbit contracts tuberculosis more readily than do other breeds. The same holds true among different races of men.

It is difficult to assess the amount of racial resistance because of the many uncontrolled factors involved—poverty, poor nutrition, etc. In the United States, however, some comparisons can be made. In metropolitan areas, those of Irish extraction have a higher mortality rate from tuberculosis than the average group, whereas Jewish people have a lower rate than average. Whether this is a matter of group susceptibility is difficult to say. The Negro population has a much higher death rate from tuberculosis than the Caucasian. This is not just a matter of environment, as there is evidence that the Negro is low in resistance to the tubercle bacillus. If two patients, one Caucasian and one Negro, have tuberculosis at approximately the same stage of development, and are given the same treatment and medications, the Caucasian is more likely to recover than is the Negro.

Tuberculosis *is not inherited from a parent by a child.* Nor does the fact that one of the parents develops tuberculosis necessarily mean that the child has a lowered native resistance. The parent's susceptibility may be caused by an extra large "dose" of the bacillus, or his resistance may be lowered for some other reason. More children who have tuberculous parents will develop the disease than those who have disease-free parents because of the opportunity for infection.

There is another type of resistance to tuberculosis called *acquired resistance*. This means that the body develops more immunity than was present at birth because of direct contact of the tissues with small numbers of the bacteria. *Complete immunity* to tuberculosis is not acquired, but partial resistance can be developed.

There are many factors which affect the body's resistance. Poor nutritional habits, lack of hygiene, and overcrowding all may lower the

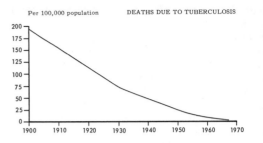

Per 100,000 population   DEATHS DUE TO TUBERCULOSIS

During the past 70 years, as methods for the detection and treatment of patients with tuberculosis have improved, death rates have declined.

natural resistance of the body. Fatigue or overwork may be inciting factors; in many patients suffering from tuberculosis, symptoms begin following overexertion. Mental strain may also decrease the body's resistance.

Acute miliary tuberculosis

When tuberculosis is disseminated throughout the body, it is called *miliary tuberculosis.* The acute form of this disease usually occurs in children and young people, although it may appear in adults occasionally. Often the patient has a healed tuberculous lesion which becomes reinfected. The lesion breaks down and many bacilli enter the bloodstream and are carried to the heart, which in turn pumps them to organs all over the body. Usually there are no preceding signs of the disease, as the patient is apparently well. Acute miliary tuberculosis is divided into three varieties—*pulmonary, meningeal,* and *generalized.*

The pulmonary type results when the germs are spread throughout the lungs. Often the patient appears to have bronchitis. The disease may start suddenly, with shortness of breath, cough, and a bluish color to the skin, accompanied by a high fever. The physician may be able to hear abnormal sounds in the chest. The pulse is rapid. The temperature may rise to 104° Fahrenheit at times.

In *meningeal miliary tuberculosis* the covering membrane of the brain is affected. The symptoms of this form of tuberculosis may be divided into three categories: (1) the prodromal stage, characterized by nausea, loss of appetite, headache, irritability, etc.; (2) the stage of irritation, characterized by vomiting, delirium, and rigidity of the neck; and (3) the paralytic stage, characterized by stupor, convulsions, and paralysis. At first the patient is fatigued and irritable. He may complain of headache, and a rise in temperature to about 100°. However, there are no symptoms referable to a definite disease in the lungs or the central nervous system. There may be vomiting, weakness, and constipation. This

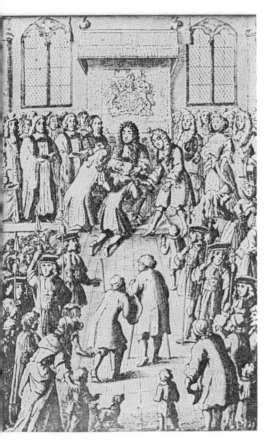

An old copper engraving depicting the supposed curative powers of the king's touch. Charles II is shown with a scrofula patient. *Bettmann Archive.*

early stage usually lasts about ten days, at which time the patient passes into the second stage characterized by increased headache, stiffening of the neck, vomiting, delirium, and other signs of pressure within the cranial cavity. After a week or ten days of these symptoms, the final stage of the disease begins. If not treated, the patient usually has convulsions and paralysis and lapses into a coma which may be followed within three or four weeks by death.

The symptoms of *generalized miliary tuberculosis* are often similar to those of typhoid fever. The disease begins rather slowly and resembles influenza or acute bronchitis. The patient complains of headache. The organs within the body may have tubercle bacilli infections disseminated throughout them. Before streptomycin was discovered, few if any patients recovered from generalized miliary tuberculosis.

Acute active pulmonary tuberculosis

Acute active pulmonary tuberculosis, called "galloping consumption," may be difficult to diagnose at the onset. The symptoms are vari-

able but loss of weight and appetite, weakness, debility, and sometimes vomiting may occur. The patient may cough up blood-stained sputum. He will probably suffer from night sweats, chills, and fever. The physician may hear rather coarse sounds in the lungs. As soon as the doctor becomes suspicious of a tuberculous lesion, he will order an x-ray picture of the chest, which is one of the best procedures for diagnosing lung diseases. He will probably have the patient's sputum examined under the microscope for the presence of the characteristic rodlike bacilli causing tuberculosis.

Chronic pulmonary tuberculosis

Chronic pulmonary tuberculosis has many and varied symptoms. The lesions cause both local and constitutional symptoms. The local signs are the same as for the acute phase—coughing and spitting up of blood. Constitutional effects are fever, fast pulse, loss of appetite, etc. Often the patient appears pale and many complain of frequently recurring colds, or of a slow and incomplete recovery from "influenza." A persistent cough is the most common symptom. At first it is usually a dry cough, but eventually a thick phlegm is brought up. The patient is short of breath, often has pain in the chest, and may spit up blood at any time during the disease.

If treatment is instituted and the response is favorable, the disease regresses; the cough and sputum decrease and finally disappear. The patient regains his lost appetite and weight, and, in general, feels much better. If the reverse is true, the disease progresses, and symptoms become more severe.

There are many complications to which the tuberculous patient is subject. Invariably the patient has pleurisy, and occasionally the lung may collapse spontaneously. Sometimes the bacillus may produce ulcers on the tongue, tonsils, pharynx, or soft palate. Inflammation of the larynx may occur. Patients in whom the disease has been present for a long period often develop intestinal lesions, perhaps as the result

LOUIS, Pierre Charles Alexandre (1787-1872) French physician. Noted for important early studies which he conducted on tuberculosis. He is generally acknowledged as having been the first to introduce statistical methods into the study of human disease (1825). Louis is also famous for his investigations of typhoid fever, and for his description of several of its most characteristic symptoms.

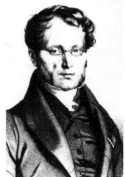

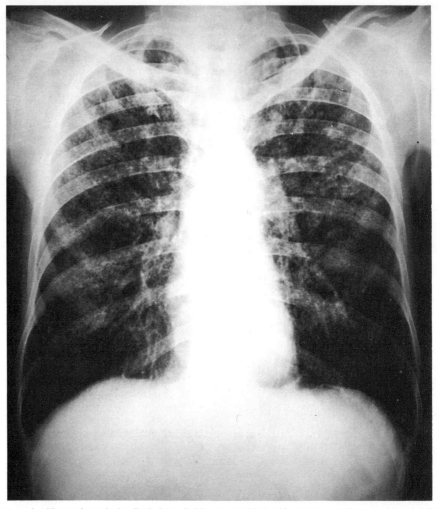

X-ray appearance of miliary tuberculosis. Both lung fields are studded with small, nodular opacities (white) which are produced by generalized, blood-borne seeding of tubercle bacilli. *Photo courtesy of Hermann Hospital, Houston.*

of swallowing sputum in which the bacteria are present. Signs of a lesion in the stomach are usually pain in the abdomen and loose stools, which have a foul odor and contain pus and mucus. Rarely, tuberculous lesions of the bone and joints may occur as a serious complication of chronic pulmonary tuberculosis.

Treatment

Drugs were used for hundreds of years in the treatment of patients with tuberculosis, but to no avail. When the sulfonamide drugs came into general use and were found to be of such great effectiveness in treating patients with infectious diseases, it was hoped that they would be of practical value in patients with tuberculosis. However, none of them proved to be of any therapeutic value. Streptomycin, an antibiotic drug, was the first effective weapon to be used against tuberculosis. Today drug therapy forms the basis for all effective treatment for tuberculosis. Of the various agents available, *isoniazid* is the most effective. It is inexpensive, easy to administer, and produces few undesirable side-effects. Since any drug given alone tends to produce resistant bacteria, combination therapy is generally advised. Isoniazid is usually combined with either streptomycin or aminosalicylic acid. Other drugs which may be used when the above agents are poorly tolerated, or when bacterial resistance has developed, include viomycin, oxytetracycline, cycloserine, and pyrazinamide. Drug therapy should be continuous, since interruption can lead to the emergence of resistant bacteria, and it should be given for 18 to 24 months.

Surgical procedures have a limited, though still important, role in the treatment of pulmonary tuberculosis. Open cavities and irreversibly diseased tissues that are well localized and persist unchanged after several months of rest and drug therapy should be surgically removed, provided the patient's general condition is good. After prolonged drug therapy, it is relatively simple to remove small wedges of lung tissue. With more extensive involvement, removal of a segment, lobe, or an entire lung may be required. Rarely *thoracoplasty,* the removal of the ribs, may be needed to decrease the size of the thoracic cavity and prevent overdistention of the remaining lung.

A prolonged period of bed rest was once considered the most important part of therapy for patients with tuberculosis. But the course of the disease has been changed so much by drug therapy that this concept has changed, too. Therapy now begins with bed rest in a sanatorium; but the patient only remains there for several months, until he is no longer infectious. When his sputum shows no evidence of tubercle bacilli, he can be released and managed with drug therapy. Sufficient rest to avoid fatigue is all that is necessary in this phase of treatment.

Prevention

Tuberculosis can be prevented. One of the main duties of the physician is to make a record or report of all patients under his care who develop a contagious disease. Laws which forbid expectorating in public places were made to prevent tuberculosis. Needless to say, removal of factors which lower native resistance—such as overcrowding, overexertion, poor nutrition, etc.—would greatly decrease the incidence of the disease.

Of great importance in the detection of tuberculosis are the periodic x-ray examinations of the chest which have become popular in recent years. Skin tests for tuberculosis are also in common use. For mass screening where ease of administration is important, a *cutaneous test* is often used. One type, the *Tine test,* utilizes a disposable unit that has four tiny prongs coated with tuberculin. Simple pressure is used to inoculate the tuberculin into the skin. When more accuracy is needed, the *intradermal skin test* is used. Material containing the toxin of the bacteria causing tuberculosis is injected between the layers of the skin, using a fine needle. A positive reaction causes reddening and inflammation of the area. Results usually can be read within 48 hours. Another skin test often used, especially in children, is the *patch test;* an ointment containing the tuberculin is put on adhesive tape and placed on the skin.

A vaccine that confers some protection against tuberculosis has been developed and used widely in some underdeveloped nations of the world. Immunization with *BCG, (Bacillus Calmette Guérin),* a weakened bovine tubercle bacillus, has been recommended for those who are likely to be exposed to tuberculosis. This would include medical personnel, relatives and close associates of known tuberculosis victims, and individuals living in the poverty areas of overcrowded cities.

Education of the public is the best way to prevent tuberculosis. Patients with the active disease must be isolated to prevent contact with well persons. Every person should have an x-ray examination of his chest and a physical examination once yearly. Tuberculosis should be suspected whenever a person presents vague symptoms such as loss of weight and appetite, nausea, persistent fever, persistent cough and expectoration, a persistent cold, and spitting of blood. When *one* person in a family is found to have tuberculosis, *every* member of the family and all close associates should be carefully checked. With the modern advances in medicine made commonly available to physicians and laymen alike, tuberculosis no longer need be a fatal disease. Indeed, as a result of such advances, it is fast becoming a scourge of the past.

RESPIRATORY DISORDERS: LUNG ABSCESS

A lung abscess is a collection of pus in the lung. This condition is known medically as *localized suppuration.* It is caused by any infection of the lungs in which bacteria or other foreign bodies stimulate the formation of pus. Inhalation of infected material is the more common method of developing this condition; it causes approximately 50 percent of all lung abscesses.

Lung abscess occurs about twice as frequently in males as in females. There seems to be no particular age group affected. There may be only one abscess present or many. The abscess may be *putrid* or *nonputrid;* the putrid lung abscess gives off an extremely foul odor.

A chronic lung abscess produces symptoms resembling those of tuberculosis, and tuberculosis is ruled out by testing the patient's sputum for tubercle bacilli. A history of recent nose or throat surgery, especially a tonsillectomy, in a patient who complains of fever, weakness, and a mucus-producing cough is most indicative of lung abscess. Another suspicious symptom is foul breath or, rather, foul odor to the sputum. Any patient complaining of these symptoms should have a thorough x-ray study and sputum examination.

The attending physician may employ nonsurgical or surgical treatment in the case of a patient with a lung abscess, depending on the individual situation. If sufficient fluids cannot be given by mouth to alleviate the dehydration incident to the high fever in these patients, fluids may be given by vein. Another helpful procedure in nonsurgical treatment is "postural drainage" in which the patient is placed in such a position that gravity drainage into the bronchial tubes will be accomplished. He is then encouraged to cough in order to bring up the material from the abscess. This may be done several times each day. Antibiotics have been found to have great value in patients with lung abscess.

If the various nonsurgical techniques do not suffice, surgical treatment is indicated. The abscess is located by means of fluoroscopy or x-ray study and surgically drained. Sometimes it is necessary to remove part of the lung, and, in fact, this is one of the most effective means of managing a chronic lung abscess. Furthermore, at least ten percent of all lung abscesses are caused by cancer of the lung; consequently, removal of the affected portion of the lung is often a necessary procedure.

RESPIRATORY DISORDERS: LUNG CANCER

Cancer may originate in either of the lungs, or it may extend to them from a malignant growth in some other part of the body.

During the last few decades, cancer of the lung has increased in incidence considerably more than that of other organs. Indeed, primary lung cancer today is the most common form of internal cancer in males. Studies are being made to determine the influence of smoking, industrial waste fumes, and car exhaust gases ("smog") on this increase. Possibly, improved diagnostic methods and today's increased life span are responsible for what seems to be an increase in incidence of the disease.

Primary cancer of the lungs is more likely to occur in men than in women. It is found more often among city dwellers than among rural people. Most of the cases appear between the ages of 40 and 70 years. The average age of occurrence varies from one study to another; usually it falls between 50 and 59 years. The disease is often found in middle-aged men who do manual labor, are heavy smokers, and are consistently exposed to dusty, irritating air. However, it has not been proved that any of these factors causes cancer. Workers in chromium mines as well as those in cobalt and uranium mines are more susceptible to cancer of the lung than is the general population. It has been thought that asbestos dust plays a part in the development of malignant disease of the lung in some persons.

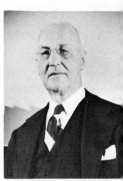

GRAHAM, Evarts Ambrose (1883-1957) American surgeon. In the year 1933, working in collaboration with J. J. Singer, Graham succeeded in the removal of an entire human lung from a patient afflicted with carcinoma. He is also noted for his introduction with W. H. Cole (1924) of *cholecystography*, a technique permitting x-ray examination of the gallbladder.

There is widespread belief that excessive cigarette smoking is a major cause of lung cancer. Reports from many different countries and population groups conclude that lung cancer develops much more often among heavy smokers than among moderate smokers or those who do not smoke at all. The risk of lung cancer is reported to be from 20 to 40 times greater among heavy smokers. But most authorities are careful to point out that this association does not necessarily prove a cause-and-effect relationship. A number of inconsistencies have been found in studies to date, and the clinical, pathologic, and experimental evidence is still controversial.

Symptoms

In about 90 percent of the patients with lung cancer, a persistent cough is the first sign of the disease. Unfortunately, the cough may be partially or entirely disregarded, and it may not appear until late in the course of the disease. The cough is usually dry or without any expectoration, although some phlegm may be coughed up. The patient may even cough up small amounts of blood, but large hemorrhages are rare. At some time during the progress of the disease, shortness of breath *(dyspnea)* will occur. This dyspnea is often out of proportion to the size of the area involved by tumor; the location of the growth has much more influence on the degree to which the respiration is affected. The patient may complain of a wheezing in one side of the chest, which is usually caused by a partial obstruction of the tube leading from the windpipe to the lung (the *bronchus*). Often there is pain in the chest, which may simulate pleurisy, or which may be felt as a dull ache behind the breastbone. As the growth advances, the patient will usually experience a loss of weight, fatigue, and sometimes hoarseness and difficulty in swallowing. He may complain of night sweats and increasing weakness. There may be a clubbed appearance of the fingers. Enlarged lymph nodes may

Another method used by the physician in the diagnosis of cancer of the lung is the *sputum test,* in which the substance coughed up is examined under the microscope. Bronchial secretions may also be examined in the same way.

Treatment

Surgical removal is the treatment of choice for patients with lung cancer. Any patient who appears to have a resectable tumor undergoes an exploratory operation. The surgeon does not usually decide how extensive the operation will need to be until he has opened the thoracic cavity. If the tumor is resectable, he will try to save as much of the lung as possible, taking out a lobe rather than an entire lung whenever he can. If the patient's lesion is too far advanced, he will probably not try to remove it.

Unfortunately, only a relatively small percentage of patients with cancer of the lung are considered operable. A cure is possible only when the patient goes to his physician before the disease has spread to other organs. Only about three percent of patients can be cured after this spread has occurred.

When surgical treatment is indicated, a preoperative "work-up" is carried out. The patient's heart and kidneys are checked. Laboratory examinations of the blood are made; if anemia is present, blood transfusions may be given. Often, antibiotic medication is given to prevent infection and to combat any infection already present. After the patient has been operated upon and returned to his room, oxygen inhalations are usually prescribed.

X-ray treatment may be advisable for a patient with cancer of the lung when the disease has reached the inoperable stage. Irradiation therapy can prolong the patient's life as well as

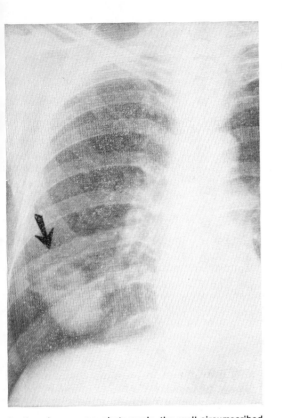

In the above x-ray photograph, the well-circumscribed opacity (white) over the lower half of the patient's right lung (arrow) is an appearance often seen in squamous cell cancer of the lung. *Photography by F. W. Schmidt.*

be found in the armpits or around the collarbone and neck. Commonly, the patient may be suspected of having pneumonia or a lung abscess; there is a good chance that any middle-aged patient who has symptoms that suggest pneumonia, for over a month, actually has lung cancer.

An x-ray picture of the chest is the most valuable asset in the early diagnosis of cancer of the lung. Long before any appreciable clinical symptoms appear, a routine chest x-ray film may show suspicious areas in the lung. If a physician believes that a lung cancer may be present, he will probably perform a *bronchoscopy.* In this procedure, a long narrow, tubular instrument with a light on the end (a *bronchoscope*) is passed into the throat; the physician can then look down this tube directly into the lung area. With this procedure the physician can determine the size and extent of the suspected cancer, and he can remove a piece of the growth for microscopic study.

Before bronchoscopy is scheduled, the patient is advised to take extra precautions in oral hygiene. Ordinarily the procedure is carried out under local anesthesia.

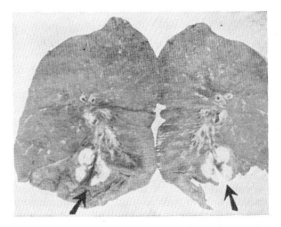

Cross-section of the lung from patient whose x-ray photograph is shown above. Arrows point to the tumor. *Photography by F. W. Schmidt.*

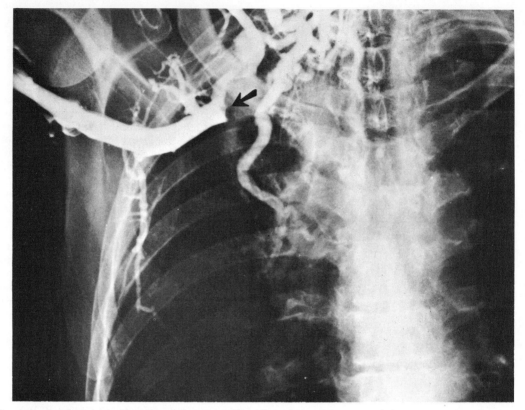

A substance injected into the veins of the arm outlines the venous system around the upper portion of the lung. The arrow points to an obstruction of a vein caused by a tumorous growth. *Photograph courtesy of Charles T. Dotter, M.D., University of Oregon Medical School, Portland, Oregon. Copyright 1952, A.M.A. Archives of Surgery.*

ease his pain. Chemotherapy, or the use of drugs, is an aid in surgical treatment, and also a means of making the patient more comfortable. The nitrogen mustard, mechlorethamine, produces transient general improvement and alleviation of distressing symptoms in some patients with advanced inoperable disease.

Cancer originating in the lung often disseminates malignant cells throughout the body. In about one third of the cases, the opposite lung is invaded. The ease with which lung cancer spreads may be caused by the fact that lungs have a rich blood and lymph supply; also the active type of cancer cells found in the lung may contribute to their spread.

The role of the patient in changing the prognosis for cancer of the lung is a vital one. If all persons with persistent coughs consult their physicians immediately and have x-ray examinations at yearly intervals, cancer, if present, will be discovered at an earlier stage and the mortality from this disease will undoubtedly decline. The annual examination is particularly desirable for all individuals over 40 years of age. Patients with lung cancer have varying degrees of impairment of pulmonary function.

This impairment varies with the location and type of tumor, coexisting emphysema and bronchitis, and the possible presence of pleural effusions. A multiprobe system is under study at present to measure regional pulmonary function in patients with bronchogenic carcinoma and metastatic lung disease. By using xenon-133 gas, this technique can determine the function of each lung and the function of different zones within each lung, providing useful information.

Lung transplantation

Many persons with advanced lung disease, especially cancer, cannot be helped with either drugs or surgical therapy. Their disease may be too extensive or involve both lungs. All that can be done at present is to keep them comfortable during the terminal phase of their illness.

One technique now being investigated as a means of saving these patients is *lung transplantation*. Unfortunately, this procedure poses even more problems than heart transplantation. It is a more complex procedure surgically, and it carries an even greater risk of failure—mainly because the lung's basic function, inhaling air from outside the body, exposes it to infection by air-borne viruses and bacteria. Dr. J. D. Hardy was the first surgeon to transplant a lung in a human being in 1963. The cancer patient with pulmonary insufficiency lived 18 days after receiving the lung from a cadaver.

RESPIRATORY DISORDERS: INDUSTRIAL DISEASES

Diseases caused by one's occupation were mentioned by Hippocrates. However, little was done to prevent these diseases until the seventeenth century, which was the period of Bernardino Ramazzini, the "patron saint of industrial medicine." Ramazzini was extremely interested in the study of the diseases of the working man. His descriptions of symptoms of various abnormal conditions have become medical classics. He pointed out the unfavorable effects on the workers' health of poor ventilation, cramped quarters, and lack of occasional rest periods. In this century, another pioneer in the field of industrial medicine was Doctor Alice Hamilton. She worked with Jane Addams of Hull House in Chicago, and traveled over the entire country investigating the many aspects of this phase of medicine. These are two of the most praiseworthy pioneers in the promotion of industrial hygiene.

In the modern plant of today, the prospective employee is subjected to a physical examination, a psychological examination, and vocational tests. Selecting personnel for specific jobs calls for special consideration. Workers who will be performing heavy manual labor should be tested for changes in the respiratory function and the heart function. A periodic recheck, if indicated, is also of great value.

In emphasizing the importance of complete physical and psychological examinations of the worker in industry, one must not overlook the necessity of the same type of examination for the executives of the organization. Regular physical examinations for this group are a part of the program of preventive medicine.

Lead poisoning

Lead poisoning is one of the oldest industrial diseases on record. The types of occupations in which workers are exposed to lead are numerous. Especially vulnerable are workers in lead smelters, those employed in refining and reclaiming lead, painters, and persons who weld or burn surfaces which contain lead. The chief method of developing lead poisoning is by inhalation of lead fumes. Another method is by

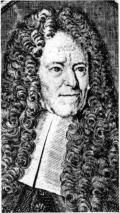

RAMAZZINI, Bernardino (1633-1714) Italian physician. He is often called the father of industrial hygiene, having devoted much of his life to the study of this subject. He described silicosis in 1700 in his important book on occupational diseases, and clearly recognized the relationship of some occupations to various respiratory disorders. He associated tuberculosis with persons who were engaged in the occupations of milling and stone cutting. *Bettmann Archive.*

swallowing the material. The greatest dangers in lead absorption is its harmful effect on the blood cells. *Anemia* often results; the lead actually changes the size and shape of the red blood cells and causes them to become brittle.

The symptoms of lead poisoning include abdominal cramping and a blue line along the gums. Abdominal cramping is usually the first symptom noticed by the patient. However, loss of appetite and *malaise* may precede other symptoms. Constipation also is frequently present, and nausea sometimes is experienced.

The first step in treating a patient with this condition is to remove him from the exposure area. In addition to medication for pain, he should be given a drug called calcium disodium edetate which forms a lead complex that is excreted in the urine. When the patient returns to work, it should be in a location where there is no possibility of further lead exposure.

Silicosis

Silicosis is a diseased condition of the lung caused by the inhalation of dust particles containing *silica* (same composition as sand). The amount of dust in the air, the length of exposure to the tainted air, and the susceptibility of the individual workman all have a direct relationship to the development of silicosis. A period of approximately ten years' exposure is needed for a marked degree of silicosis to appear. In rare instances, such occupations as sandblasting in tunnels may cause earlier development.

It is possible to develop a case of silicosis without evidence of any symptoms. The most common symptom, if symptoms are present, is shortness of breath, which gradually becomes more evident. A cough is present, but no fever. As the condition progresses, the patient notices loss of appetite, pain in the chest and high in the abdomen, and weakness. No absolute cure for silicosis has been discovered. The chief method of controlling this disease is to eliminate the hazards which promote the symptoms. Patients with silicosis are particularly susceptible to tuberculosis and other pulmonary infections.

RESPIRATORY DISORDERS: FUNGUS DISEASES OF THE LUNG

Fungus diseases of the lungs do not occur often. These yeastlike or moldlike fungi usually enter the body through the mucous membranes of the respiratory and digestive tracts. When their mode of entry is through the respiratory tract, an acute inflammation of the lungs may develop.

Actinomycosis

This is an infection caused by the fungus *Actinomyces bovis*, or "ray" fungus, which was described more than 50 years ago as the cause of "lumpy jaw" in cattle. The relationship of this fungus disease in man and cattle has not been definitely established. According to some investigators, it is possible for man to develop the condition directly from contact with cattle, but there is no conclusive evidence to uphold this theory. It is thought rather that the fungus is present in the healthy body and that loss of immunity or other conditions make it possible for the fungus to grow.

Actinomycosis of the lung is the most serious form of this particular type of fungus infection. It closely resembles tuberculosis and can easily be confused with it. However, tuberculosis can be ruled out by a sputum examination. Actinomycosis is characterized by irregular fever with abscess formation in the lung. There also may be weight loss, cough, and general loss of energy.

The treatment of patients with this condition includes x-ray therapy and surgery, as well as the use of sulfonamides and antibiotics.

Blastomycosis

Blastomycosis is an infection caused by a yeastlike fungus called *Blastomyces*. The organism can cause lesions all over the body. The lungs, however, are infected more often than other organs. This disease also resembles tuberculosis to a striking degree, and a sputum examination is necessary to distinguish between the two. The symptoms of blastomycosis include pain at the waistline, rheumatism, sore throat, difficulty in breathing, weight loss, and night sweats. However, none of these symptoms is actually conclusive. Therefore, an extensive physical examination should be made when these symptoms appear.

Coccidioidosis

Highly infectious and potentially serious is disease produced by the fungus *Coccidioides immitis*. In the United States this condition, *coccidioidosis* (or *coccidioidomycosis*), is found chiefly in the San Joaquin Valley of California and in Arizona. The infection probably occurs as a primary respiratory infection caused by inhalation of the spores of the fungus. It is also possible for the infection to develop following a skin abrasion. Public health studies have shown that members of the rodent family harbor the fungus; the rodents contaminate the soil, and thus the infection reaches man.

This disease also resembles tuberculosis. The early symptoms include chills and fever, headache, and general weakness. A cough may be present. These symptoms subside in one to two weeks, following which small "bumps" appear under the skin and then gradually disappear.

Moniliasis

The fungus *Monilia (Candida) albicans* causes the disease called moniliasis. The fungus usually invades the lungs, producing a secondary infection. This yeastlike fungus is often found in tuberculosis or cancer patients, in whom the damaged tissues offer a favorable medium for the growth of the fungus. This condition may exist as a primary infection in such diseases as thrush, middle ear infections, or infections of the vulva or vagina. This fungus has been found in dead leaves and wood and in the excreta of animals and man. The symptoms include weight loss and general weakness, fever, and cough. These symptoms may persist for several months. Sometimes, the symptoms may become more severe. However, whether symptoms are mild or severe, a physician should be consulted.

Fungus diseases are discussed further in Chapter 4, "Disease-Producing Organisms;" Chapter 8, The Skin;" and Chapter 24, "Tropical Diseases."

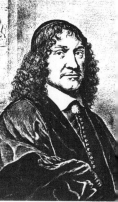

SYLVIUS, Franciscus (de la Boö) (1614-1672) Dutch physician. Sylvius' place in medical history is assured by the classic description which he wrote of pulmonary tuberculosis. He was among the earliest workers to regard digestion as a chemical process, and clearly recognized that the salivary and pancreatic secretions were important in this process. Several major anatomical areas are named after him because of his investigations in anatomy.

RESPIRATORY DISORDERS: CHEST INJURIES

Broken *(fractured)* ribs are one of the most common chest injuries. This condition probably occurs more often than is generally realized, for it may go undetected in many accident victims. Any violent blow may fracture one or more ribs, but comparatively easy blows may also cause rib breakage. Even the action of the muscles, particularly among aged persons, may break a rib. An individual with tuberculosis (or cancer) may fracture a rib with no apparent inciting factor. The most common place for breaks to occur is on the side of the chest wall at the angle of the rib, in what is called the *axillary line.*

Symptoms vary in intensity according to the severity of the break. The patient usually complains of pain when he breathes. He will often be afraid to cough because of the increased pain that coughing causes. This leads to an accumulation of secretions in the lungs, which in turn predisposes the patient to pneumonia or other respiratory diseases. If the fractured rib has injured the lung, the patient will usually cough up blood. When the rib is fractured completely, the ends rub together causing a distinctive sound called *crepitation.*

Treatment consists chiefly of prevention of pulmonary complications such as pneumonia. If the patient is confined to bed, the physician will often suggest that he assume a semisitting position. Medicines to control or prevent infection may be prescribed. The physician usually prefers that the patient abstain as much as possible from pain-killing medicines, so that the cough reflex will not be interfered with.

Strapping the chest with adhesive tape may be necessary in some injuries but should be avoided whenever possible because it tends to restrict expansion of the lung and frequently does not serve to relieve pain. In severe injuries with fractures of many ribs, a surgical operation to wire the rib ends together may be required to secure the necessary stability of the chest.

Blocking the nerves which supply the injured rib or ribs with a local anesthetic is often of value in relieving pain. It is very important in those patients who have too much pain to cough and in whom secretions tend to gather in the lungs. Injection of the nerves which supply the injured ribs will afford relief from pain and permit coughing and expectoration of accumulated secretion.

A broken rib in itself does not produce any permanent disability. An uncomplicated fracture of the rib may cause loss of full activity for a period of four to five weeks. The maximum time usually required for complete recovery, even in more complicated cases, is about eight weeks.

Fracture of the breastbone

Fracture of the breastbone *(sternum)* is a rare injury, and usually a hard blow is required to produce it. It may be caused by the pressure of the steering wheel post against the patient's chest in an automobile accident. The breastbone is protected by the elasticity of the adjacent cartilages and ribs, so the blow must usually be directly over the bone itself. When the injury sustained is severe enough to fracture the sternum, other injuries are usually inflicted as well.

The patient may complain of pain, a sense of heaviness, and shortness of breath, and may spit up blood. He may develop a bluish discoloration of the area because of injuries to the associated blood vessels. As in the case of a fractured rib, pulmonary complications must be watched for. Healing usually is completed in an uncomplicated sternal fracture in three to eight weeks.

Stab and bullet wounds

These are known as *penetrating wounds.* This type of injury during wartime may be caused by shrapnel, hand grenades, bayonets, etc. Occasionally a fishbone which catches in the throat may penetrate into the chest cavity through the esophagus. In all penetrating wounds of the chest, some internal bleeding occurs, the extent of which depends upon the severity of the injury. Air also enters the chest cavity in such a wound. Extensive bleeding from small caliber bullet wounds is not a frequent occurrence. The patient may complain of some pain when he breathes, but usually there is little discomfort or shortness of breath. It is difficult for the physician to determine the extent of the air and blood in the chest cavity by x-ray examination, although some indication is given.

FOWLER, George Ryerson (1848-1906) American surgeon. Fowler is usually credited with the introduction of the surgical operation of thoracoplasty, in the year 1893. He also devised an operation involving decortication of the lung, which was once used for the treatment of patients afflicted with chronic empyema, and was called *Fowler's operation* or *Fowler-Delorme operation.* He also made important contributions to surgical procedures on the abdomen.

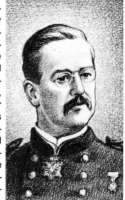

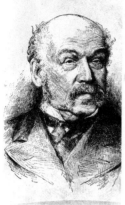

JENNER, William (1815-1898) English physician. In his extensive study on the determining causes of vesicular emphysema in 1857, he gave one of the first clear descriptions of emphysema of the lungs. He is probably best known for a study published in 1849 that clearly distinguished the differences between typhoid fever and typhus fever. Long a professor of pathological anatomy, he was one of the most eminent doctors of his time, and was one of the Queen's physicians.

Treatment consists of preventing the air passages from becoming blocked by swelling and secretions in the bronchi. Pain-killing drugs are administered only when necessary in order not to interfere with the normal cough reflex. If advisable, blood transfusion is given. The physician will usually prescribe one of the antibiotic drugs, as well as tetanus antitoxin, and oxygen may be given.

A collection of blood in the pleural cavity is called *hemothorax;* the condition may be caused by wounds in the chest, neck, or abdomen. The quantity of blood present depends to a great extent upon the type of blood vessel injured—vein, artery, or the capillaries. There may be just a few teaspoonfuls of blood or several pints present. If there is no infection in the chest, and if the blood is not clotted, the patient has few symptoms, unless the amount of blood is sufficient to press on the heart. However, if the blood should clot and if infection is present, serious complications may ensue. The formation of pus in the pleural cavity *(empyema)* or interference with the movement of the lungs *(fibrothorax)* are the two conditions which most often result.

If the amount of blood in the pleural cavity is small, it will often be absorbed in a period of two weeks to a month. If more than a very small amount is present, it should be drawn out through a needle to prevent further difficulties. If a large amount of blood is allowed to remain in the chest or if bleeding into the chest has occurred rapidly, the blood might clot and then cannot be removed through a needle. This condition is called *organized hemothorax.* Sometimes the clots can be removed by injecting a special solution to liquify them and then aspirating the liquid that results. Occasionally it is necessary to open the chest and take out the clots. The cavity is then washed out with a sterile solution and the chest closed.

If the blood should clot completely, a coating of rather tenacious material will begin to form over the pleural surfaces. This is known as a fibrinous layer. As early as ten days following the clotting, it may become strong enough to interfere with the motion of the lungs. This membrane has a grayish-red appearance. If it is abundant, it will interfere seriously with the expansion of the lung and should be removed. This can be done with ease by the surgeon three to six weeks after the injury or earlier if infection has occurred. After six weeks, the surgical procedure is more difficult. Removal of this fibrinous layer or membrane is known as *decortication.* In the treatment of patients with hemothorax, anti-infection therapy is important, and is usually continued until the chest cavity is free of blood.

Traumatic pneumothorax

Air in the pleural cavity from a chest injury *(traumatic pneumothorax)* may occur in one of three ways. There may be an "open" pneumothorax, in which air can move in and out of the pleural cavity either through an opening in the chest wall or in the lung; or a "closed" pneumothorax may develop, in which air is present in the pleural cavity but is sealed off; and finally, a pneumothorax may occur in which air enters the cavity when the patient inhales but cannot escape when he exhales.

Pneumothorax can be caused by blows which do not break a rib or make an opening into the chest cavity, if the patient already has a disease such as tuberculosis. When this happens, the lung collapses, causing a pneumothorax. This condition can occur in a person with healthy lungs, but this seldom happens. Most patients with pneumothorax following an injury which does not penetrate the inner organs have a broken rib, the ends of which rub against the lungs.

Symptoms of pneumothorax following a chest injury may include spitting up of foamy, bloody sputum, shortness of breath, and a bluish discoloration of the fingernails, lips, and perhaps the skin. An x-ray picture of the chest will show that the lung has collapsed. Treatment consists of removing the air by inserting a needle into the cavity in the same manner in which blood is *aspirated.* Usually the procedure has to be repeated several times or suction has to be applied.

Open chest wounds

Open chest wounds are those in which the tissues cannot entirely close the "hole" into the chest cavity. They may be caused by any accident which tears through the overlying tissues and rib cage into the pleural cavity. During periods of war, of course, the incidence of wounds of this type is greatly increased. The

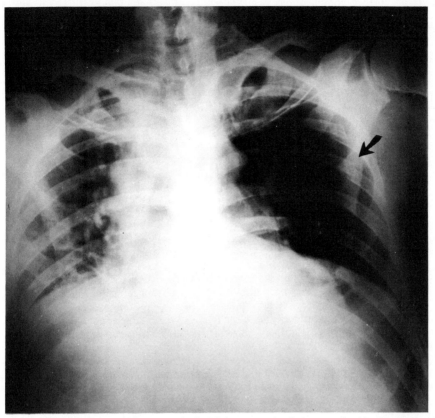

Broken ribs and a collapsed lung resulting from physical injury may clearly be seen in this chest x-ray photograph which shows the great diagnostic value of the x-ray. *Photograph by courtesy of Hermann Hospital, Houston.*

size of the opening is of prime importance in calculating its dangers; the larger the hole, the greater is the interference with the normal respiratory processes and the more likely the wound is to be fatal.

The most important step in treatment of patients with open wounds of the chest is closure of the hole. Every wound of the chest should be considered as an open wound, because it may suck air if the patient is in the proper position. A sterile gauze dressing should be firmly strapped in place over the wound, using overlapping layers of adhesive plaster. If sterile gauze is not available, the cleanest cloth available should be used under the strapping. On the battlefield, the wounded individual should cover the hole with the cleanest piece of clothing available and lie on the affected side until the aid man comes to apply the sterile dressing and the overlapping layers of adhesive plaster. This dressing need not be disturbed until the patient is in the operating room of the hospital.

As a result of open wounds in the chest cavity, the mechanics of respiration are interfered with. Because of the increased air pressure, the lung on the injured side collapses in part or completely. If one lung collapses en-

tirely, the patient's *vital lung capacity* is cut in half. The *mediastinum* is pushed toward the unaffected side by the pressure of air from the opposite side, thus exerting pressure on the "good" lung and causing it partially to collapse. Therefore the patient is unable to expand his good lung fully, and his air intake is decreased further. Sometimes the breathing ability of the patient is additionally interfered with because of the pressure of the outside air on the large veins carrying blood back to the heart.

Pneumonia

Pleurisy and acute bronchitis are often complications of a chest injury. Pneumonia, as a complication initiated by a chest injury, occurs rather seldom. *Pneumococcus* organisms are always present in the mouth and throat, and it is thought that a chest injury lowers the patient's natural resistance to the disease. If symptoms do occur, it will be within three to four days after the accident has taken place. The patient may begin to complain within 24 hours of a chill or coughing and an elevation of temperature, accompanied by a feeling of fatigue. Sometimes the patient coughs up a large amount of bloody sputum. If no further complications occur, recovery is usually uneventful.

Injury rarely can be considered an initiating factor in pulmonary tuberculosis. If signs of the disease manifest themselves within two weeks after the accident has occurred, it is possible that the injury activated the disease. X-ray films taken before the injury should be compared with later ones, and the health of the patient prior to the injury should be considered.

Mediastinitis

This is an inflammation of the wall dividing the two pleural cavities (the *mediastinum*). It occurs most often as a result of perforation of the esophagus. This can happen when a sharp foreign body becomes lodged in the esophagus, during attempts to remove it, or during examination of the organ for other reasons. *Mediastinitis* can also result from a bullet or stab wound.

The symptoms of acute mediastinitis may be violent, with severe pain under the breastbone and radiating up to the neck, chills and high fever, and difficulty in breathing and swallowing. There may also be signs of free air in the mediastinum.

A comman complication is mediastinal abscess. Sometimes the abscess opens and empties its contents into the trachea; either the patient will cough up large amounts of pus, or he may suffocate.

The treatment of acute mediastinitis includes large doses of antibiotics and surgical drainage if pus has accumulated from an abscess.

Mediastinal emphysema

Mediastinal emphysema is the introduction of air into the structures in the midchest. It can be caused by blows over the chest, by straining, or even by coughing. Puncture wounds of the same area can also cause this condition. Machines used in artificial respiration can cause *emphysema* if employed incorrectly. If the amount of air in the tissues is large enough and presses on the large blood vessels, thus interfering with the circulation to the heart and lungs, death may ensue; however, this disease usually is not a serious one.

In most patients in whom mediastinal emphysema is present, the air seeps out into the soft tissue of the neck and causes swelling of that area. Occasionally, the whole face and chest become swollen and discolored. It is in those patients who do not have a leakage of air into the soft tissues that results are more likely to be fatal, because of the pressure on the large veins.

The patient is put to bed and given sedatives if necessary. Sometimes removal of the air with a needle is indicated if the patient complains of difficulty in breathing.

Pulmonary embolism

Pulmonary embolism means obstruction of a blood vessel in the lungs. There are three different types which may occur following an injury of the chest. The first of these is the *air embolus*. For more than a century, physicians have known that the admission of air into a vein can have fatal results, though it takes much larger quantities than is commonly supposed. Automobile accidents in which the steering post crushes the patient's chest or heavy weights dropped on the chest may injure the blood vessels and allow the introduction of air. The patient complains of severe pain over the part of the chest in which the air bubble has lodged. Sometimes he may feel faint, nauseated, and may vomit.

A second type of obstruction of a blood vessel which may be caused by trauma is the *fat embolus*. The chest injury breaks the walls of the fat cells and the liquid fat escapes. Blood vessels in the same area must also be broken to allow the fat to enter the bloodstream.

The third variety of embolus which can be caused by injury is the *thromboembolism*. Injury to the blood vessels anywhere in the body can cause a blood clot to be detached and carried to the lungs. This condition is discussed in Chapter 7, "Heart and Circulation."

OTHER RESPIRATORY DISORDERS

As has been previously stated, the respiratory system is made up of the nasal passages, accessory nasal sinuses, the pharynx, the tonsils, the larynx, the trachea, the bronchi, the lungs, and the pleura. Infections or abnormalities may occur in any of these parts. Symptoms which arise from diseases of the respiratory tract frequently include cough, shortness of breath, and spitting up of mucus, blood, or pus. The spitting of blood is always a serious manifestation. The physician is greatly assisted in his diagnosis by determining the type of cough, whether dry, productive, paroxysmal, etc.; the extent of the shortness of breath; and the type of sputum spit up.

Pulmonary atelectasis

Atelectasis is the collapse of the air sacs of the lungs. Simple atelectasis has many causes. These include surgery, shock, accidents, foreign bodies in the lung, and infections. The resultant loss of function of these air sacs causes the deflation of the part of the lung affected.

In simple atelectasis, there are no symptoms if only a small part of the lung is involved. However, if a greater part of the lung tissue is affected, the patient may complain of shortness of breath (dyspnea), and a blue coloring of the skin (cyanosis) may be noticed. A rapid pulse also may be present. When a sudden and complete collapse of one or both lungs occurs, the main causes are thought to be a bronchial obstruction or the death of an area of lung tissue caused by a block in the blood supply to the area (pulmonary infarct). A complete lung collapse also may follow a chest injury. Partial lung collapse can be the result of partial blockage of the air supply. In diagnosing atelectasis, the physician will verify his diagnosis by x-ray examination, to check the position of the heart, which "leans" toward the affected side, and also the position of the diaphragm, which will be higher on the affected side. Bronchoscopy should be performed early as an aid in diagnosis and even more important, as a means of relieving bronchial obstruction.

Pulmonary fibrosis

Pulmonary fibrosis occurs when a disease process causes normal lung tissue to become scarred or fibrosed. The condition may be the result of such causes as a healing tuberculous lesion, a fungus infection, or lung injury scars. Pulmonary fibrosis is sometimes seen following bronchopneumonia or accompanying chronic bronchitis. In about one fourth of the cases, a definite cause is never established. Diagnosis is made by lung biopsy.

Pulmonary fibrosis is a chronic disease, lasting for years. The most common symptoms, when they are present, are a cough, mild dyspnea, and some cyanosis. When this condition has been present for some time, the side of the chest so affected becomes misshapen, and the shoulder is drawn downwards. The entire involved side decreases in size. Should both sides be fibrosed, the most apparent symptoms are those of chronic asthma.

In the early phase of pulmonary fibrosis, a well-balanced diet, a dry climate, and supplemental vitamins are of benefit. When fibrosis is well advanced, nothing much can be done, although the use of steroids is beneficial in some cases.

Diseases of the diaphragm

The diaphragm plays an important role in the respiratory function. One of the more common ailments of this muscle is spasm of the diaphragm. The spasm may be intermittent, with periods of relaxation (clonic), or it may be a constant tension of the muscle (tonic). Clonic spasm, or hiccup, is more common and less severe than the tonic spasm. It may be caused by swallowing air, indigestion, influenza, or more serious conditions such as a brain tumor or brain inflammation. If clonic spasm fails to respond to the simple home remedies, carbon dioxide inhalation, sedatives, tranquilizers, local anesthetics, or antispasmodics may be tried. In extreme cases, the phrenic nerve may have to be interrupted temporarily. Tonic spasm is usually the result of such diseases as lockjaw (tetanus), rabies, or epilepsy. The spasm occurs in varying degrees of intensity. Should it be of long duration, the patient may become extremely exhausted and die of asphyxiation. Tonic spasm is sometimes relieved by rubbing vigorously around the chest walls, the back, and the region over the stomach.

Paralysis of the diaphragm can occur when the phrenic nerve is involved by such diseases as poliomyelitis or diphtheria. The nerve can also be injured through a blow or other injury. An "iron lung" may be necessary to help the patient continue breathing.

Hernia of the diaphragm may be caused by an injury, by a deformity present at birth, or by a part of the stomach passing upward through the opening of the diaphragm at the esophagus. A hernia caused by injury is usually the result of severe trauma and requires surgical repair. Babies born with a large diaphragmatic hernia frequently have the contents of the abdomen in the chest (upside-down stomach) and may not survive unless the trouble is recognized and corrected surgically.

Cystic diseases of the lung have been classified into two groups: those present at birth (congenital), and those cysts acquired later in life. Congenital cysts of the lung do not occur frequently. Pulmonary cysts may be present without symptoms of any kind, or the symptoms may be profound. If necessary, they can usually be surgically excised with little risk.

Loeffler's syndrome is a name given to a group of nonspecific respiratory symptoms. These symptoms include mild fever, a cough that is slightly productive, fatigue, and occasionally breathing of an asthmatic type. There are several theories regarding the causative agent of the syndrome, but none has been proved. The treatment, after other conditions such as asthma or pneumonia have been ruled out, is bed rest.

Benign tumors of the lung

Noncancerous growths in the lung occur much less frequently than cancerous tumors.·

Most common among the benign lesions is the bronchial adenoma, which accounts for about three percent of all lung tumors. Unlike lung cancer, it usually appears before age 40 and is as common among females as among males. Symptoms, which are often similar to those of lung cancer, include the spitting of blood, cough, asthmatic wheezes, obstructive emphysema, and recurrent pneumonia.

A bronchial adenoma may be found inside the opening of the bronchus, or it may partially or completely invade the wall of the tube. On occasion, it may metastasize. The cause of this slow-growing lesion is not known.

Surgical removal is the treatment of choice. If the tumor is small, removal of a lobe may be curative. If it has spread locally, removal of a lung may be required.

There are many other tumors found in the chest cavity and chest wall. Cartilage tumors from the rib cage (*chondromas*) are rather slow-growing tumors which have a tendency to grow inward toward the important organs found in the chest. These growths may also become malignant. *Osteomas*, which are benign bone tumors, occur infrequently in the chest. They may originate in the bony structures—the breastbone, ribs, etc. They may also become cancerous and, therefore, should be removed by the physician.

Congenital abnormalities in the chest wall

Occasionally, a person is born with structural defects in the chest area. Sometimes the first rib is not attached to the breastbone; this same rib may have a joint in it; or it may even be missing altogether. These abnormalities may cause pain in the arm, back of the neck, and shoulders. If the physician discovers by x-ray examination that part of a rib is missing and the remainder is irritating a nerve, he will usually operate and remove the "stump." Often correction of posture faults will help the patient considerably. A *hernia of the lung* is said to be present when part of the lung and its covering membrane extend into an opening in the chest wall, diaphragm, or perhaps the mediastinum. This condition may be a congenital deformity, or it may occur as the result of an injury or an infection which disturbs the usual confines of the lung. The most common type of lung hernia is the one found in the space just above the collarbone. It may get smaller or even disappear when the individual inhales and reappear on exhalation and coughing. If the patient has no symptoms, the physician may decide that treatment is not indicated. If an operation is necessary, the surgeon may use the adjacent ribs to cover the opening.

Another type of congenital malformation of the chest wall is known as *pigeon breast*. The patient's breastbone is prominent, giving the appearance of a pigeon, and the chest walls are narrowed. This condition seldom occurs. Because of the change in shape of the chest, there may be some displacement of the internal organs; this results in shortness of breath, coughing, and a bluish discoloration of the skin. Individuals with this deformity may often be more susceptible to diseases of the respiratory tract. In milder forms, no treatment is necessary.

Rarely, two newborn twin babies may be found to have an attachment to each other in the region of the breastbone. This is called a *thoracopagus;* and the twins are known as *Siamese twins.* The surgeon may attempt to separate the attachment, the possibility of success depending upon the extent to which the organs of the thoracic cavity are involved.

Funnel chest (chonechondrosternon) is almost the reverse of pigeon breast in appearance. The breastbone, at its lower portion, projects inward. This, too, is a rare deformity. The patient may experience shortness of breath, bluish discoloration of the skin, and difficulty in swallowing. Surgical correction is now quite successful in properly chosen cases.

Inhalation therapy

For patients with gas exchange disorders in the heart-lung system, inhalation therapy is becoming a more and more important method of treatment. At its inception, the patient through his own breathing efforts could increase the oxygen content of his blood, although this was sometimes detrimental to carbon dioxide elimination. At present, pressure breathing devices, resuscitators, and respirators are used to administer therapeutic gases, including oxygen, helium-oxygen and carbon dioxide mixtures, thus promoting artificial ventilation and respiration, and properly balancing gas exchanges.

Indications for oxygen therapy, for example, include hypotension, hypertension, cyanosis, all acute phases of cardiopulmonary disease, during and following operation, in the unconscious patient, in severe anemia, hemorrhage, and hypovolemia, and in acidosis. In each patient, however, the need for oxygen therapy must be determined by measurement of arterial blood gases. Special problems which also may require inhalation therapy include chest injuries, intracranial lesions, myasthenia gravis, acute idiopathic polyneuritis, tetanus, and respiratory management of acute poisoning.

During many inhalation procedures, constant care must be taken by a trained inhalation therapist to avoid oxygen toxicity, respiratory obstruction, and circulatory derangements.

6 BLOOD AND BLOOD-FORMING ORGANS

WHAT THEY ARE AND DO

Blood is one of the six major forms of tissue in the body. It is liquid, and therefore mobile, and acts as a distributor of food and oxygen to the other body tissues. It also carries waste materials from the tissues to the kidneys and lungs. In addition, the blood transports *hormones* from the glands where they are secreted, to the tissues upon which they act, and it also carries cells and other substances which aid in the body's defense against infection. It assists in the maintenance of an even body temperature, and keeps the other fluids of the body in balance not only with each other, but also with the tissues.

A man of average size has a little over six quarts of blood. This blood is composed of a fluid (*plasma*) in which various cellular bodies are suspended. Among these are the red corpuscles (*erythrocytes*), the white cells (*leucocytes*), and the platelets (*thrombocytes*). The red cells are small biconcave discs about seven microns in diameter, which originate largely in bone marrow, although in fetal life they may also come from the spleen and liver. In an adult male, there are usually about five million red blood corpuscles per cubic millimeter, or about 82 billion in one cubic inch. The normal red cell count for women is usually about 4,500,000 per cubic millimeter of blood. There may be considerable normal variation. The color of these corpuscles and of blood itself is caused by a red iron-containing pigment called *hemoglobin*. Hemoglobin first combines with oxygen as the blood passes through the blood vessels of the lungs, and then it carries the oxygen to the tissues. Hemoglobin coming from the lungs is a much brighter red than that which has given up its oxygen to the tissues and is returning to the heart and lungs through the veins.

The white cells

The white cells are of several different types, irregular in shape and size, but generally larger than the red corpuscles. They differ from the red corpuscles, in that each white cell contains a *nucleus*, whereas mature red blood cells in man do not contain nuclei, having lost them before leaving the bone marrow. Adults have from 5000 to 10,000 leucocytes per cubic millimeter of blood; but in the infant the number is approximately doubled. The function of these cells is primarily that of assisting the body in its resistance to disease, but some types of leucocytes may be important in the repair of damaged tissue.

Whenever bacteria or other foreign materials enter the tissues, large numbers of white cells immediately travel through the walls of the blood vessels and to the site of disturbance. They take the bacteria and any other foreign materials into their own bodies, where they are digested. White cells are able to break up and carry away even as large an object as a splinter or thorn in the skin. They also help in carrying away dead tissue and blood clots which remain after a wound. *Pus* is largely composed of white cells which have been drawn to the infected area, as well as the dead and disintegrating tissue and bacteria. During severe infections the white cells may be increased in the blood five- or tenfold. Because of this, a white cell count is made on the blood in order to confirm diagnosis in many infections.

Blood platelets are small, colorless granules in the blood, about one-third the size of a red corpuscle. Their primary function has to do with blood clotting. When a wound occurs, a number of these platelets are attracted to the site, where they activate a substance (*thromboplastin*) which starts the clotting process. It is believed that they also help to seal off small leaks which may occur from time to time in the capillaries.

The plasma

Normal blood plasma is a clear, slightly yellowish fluid which is approximately 55 percent of the total volume of the blood. After meals, the plasma has a milky appearance, which is the result of small globules of fat suspended in it. Many laboratory tests require *clear* plasma in order to avoid errors. The patient is instructed not to eat before the blood sample is to be taken.

The plasma is a water solution in which are transported the digested food materials from the walls of the small intestine to the body tissues, as well as the waste materials from the tissues to the kidneys. Consequently, this solution contains several hundred different substances. In addition, it carries *antibodies,* which are responsible for immunity to disease, and hormones, which regulate various body activities. It also transports most of the waste carbon dioxide from the tissues back to the lungs. Aside from these substances—which occur in quite small amounts—the plasma consists of about 91 percent water, 7 percent protein material, and 0.9 percent of various mineral salts. The salts and proteins are of great importance in keeping the proper balance between the water in the tissues and in the blood; disturbances in this ratio may result in excessive water in the tissues (swelling or edema). The mineral salts in the plasma all serve other vital functions in the body and must be supplied through the diet.

Some of the blood plasma, as well as some of the white cells, filters through the walls of the blood vessels and out into the tissues. This filtered plasma (*lymph*) is a clear and colorless fluid which returns to the blood through a series of canals referred to as the *lymphatic system*. This system contains filters (*lymph nodes*) which remove bacteria and other debris from the lymph. These nodes, especially those located in the neck, armpit, and groin, may become swollen when an infection occurs in a nearby site. Blood clots do not occur normally while the blood is in the vessels. But in an injury, such as a cut finger, for example, one of the plasma proteins (*fibrin*) forms a mesh in which the blood cells are trapped, and this mesh is the clot. Blood *serum* is the yellowish fluid left after the cells and fibrin have been removed from the blood.

Manufacture and storage of blood

It has been estimated that in a healthy person about ten million red blood cells are destroyed every second. This destruction is brought about by many collisions of the cells within the blood vessels, and perhaps by other processes not yet fully understood. Four separate organs are involved in the replacement of red cells. The stimulus for production is provided by *erythropoietin*, a hormone that is apparently produced by the kidneys. The actual production is done almost entirely by the red portions of the bone marrow, but certain substances necessary for their manufacture must be supplied by the liver. Surplus red cells, needed to meet an emergency, are stored in the body, some at least being stored in the spleen. Old and worn out red cells are broken down in the spleen and the iron they contain is normally conserved.

Certain of the white cells (*granulocytes*), and the platelets are formed in the bone marrow, while the other white cells (*lymphocytes*) originate in the lymphatic system, in the spleen, and in the marrow. The proteins of the plasma are believed to be largely produced by the liver.

When a sudden loss of a large amount of blood occurs, the spleen releases large numbers of red cells to make up for the loss, and the bone marrow is stimulated to increase its rate of manufacture of blood cells. When a donor gives a pint of blood, it usually requires about seven weeks for the body reserve of red corpuscles to be replaced although the circulating red cells may be back almost to normal within

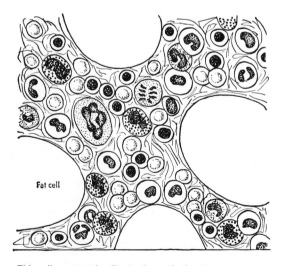

Fat cell

This diagrammatic illustration of the bone marrow enlarged about 700 times portrays the giant fat cells which make up a large part of its bulk, as well as the tremendous number of newly developing blood cells to be found within the marrow itself.

only a few hours. Repeated losses of blood within a short time may, however, easily deplete the red cell reserves.

BLOOD DISORDERS: ANEMIA

Anemia is the term applied to the many conditions that exist when the blood does not contain the number of red cells considered normal, or when the cells lack their normal amount of hemoglobin. It may be caused either by defective blood formation, cell destruction, or by an excessive loss of blood. These conditions, in turn, may be caused by a great many different types of body disorders. The physician must know exactly the type of anemia with which he is dealing before proper treatment can be instituted.

In the various anemias, the red cells frequently may be either smaller than usual (*microcytic anemia*), larger than usual (*macrocytic anemia*), or normal sized (*normocytic anemia*); they may contain too little hemoglobin (*hypochromic anemia*) or if the cells are larger than normal, they may appear to contain more than the usual amount of hemoglobin. In the hypochromic anemias, the number of red cells may be nearly normal, but the total hemoglobin in the blood is inadequate to meet the requirements of the body.

Posthemorrhagic anemias

Anemias caused by sudden blood loss as in traumatic injury are generally normocytic, that is, the cells are of normal size but reduced in number. When the blood is lost over a longer period of time from bleeding hemorrhoids, peptic ulcer, in hookworm disease, and in excessive menstrual bleeding (*menorrhagia*), a microcytic anemia may result.

Following hemorrhage, body fluids seep into the blood which restore it to its former volume; consequently, dilution of the blood occurs, and anemia may result. It may require some time for the body to manufacture the necessary red cells and other substances necessary to return the blood to normal. The symptoms of such a blood-loss anemia include a general weakness, dizziness, and faintness. In more severe cases there may be vomiting and a great thirst, the heart rate may be rapid, and the breathing weak and shallow.

The first step in the treatment of persons with a posthemorrhagic anemia is to stop the loss of blood. Blood transfusions may be given to return the blood to its proper volume before excessive dilution occurs. In milder hemorrhages, however, the body may be able to restore the lost blood without transfusion. This is often accomplished by ample rest and a good diet, including adequate amounts of the iron and protein necessary for red cell building.

Hemolytic anemias

Anemias caused by increased red blood cell destruction (*hemolytic anemias*) may be normocytic or macrocytic. Hemolysis may be caused by several different conditions. In anemias caused by hemolysis, the breakdown of red cells releases large amounts of hemoglobin end products into the plasma. These substances are converted by the liver into a number of other pigments most of which are excreted in the bile. When the production of these bile pigments is excessive, some of them appear in the body tissues, which give the skin and the whites of the eyes a yellow appearance. This condition is known as *jaundice* and is one of the symptoms of the hemolytic anemias. In *hemolytic jaundice*, the red cells are abnormally fragile and rupture easily; hence they are broken down more rapidly by the spleen than is usual. Such cells, without the interference of the spleen, are able to function normally, in spite of their fragility. Therefore, in many cases of hemolytic jaundice, the spleen is removed as a means of preventing a too-rapid de-

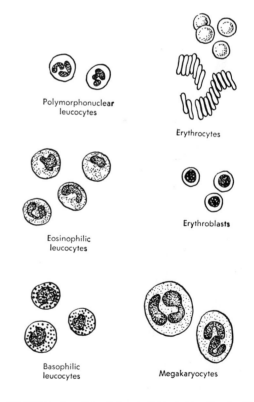

Polymorphonuclear leucocytes

Erythrocytes

Eosinophilic leucocytes

Erythroblasts

Basophilic leucocytes

Megakaryocytes

Drawings of some of the individual blood cells that may be found in human bone marrow. The cell sizes in the marrow vary greatly depending on their stage of development, most of these being enlarged about 700 times over their natural size.

struction of these cells. Some types of hemolytic anemia are inherited; others are acquired and may be associated with various systemic diseases. A variety of drugs, physical and chemical agents, and vegetable and animal poisons have been implicated as causes. In these conditions, corticosteroid therapy has proved beneficial. If there is no response to the drug, removal of the spleen is necessary.

Sickle-cell anemia is another hereditary condition in which the red blood cells are easily destroyed in the body—in this case because of their unusual sickle shape and their abnormal chemical composition. Defective hemoglobin results in misshaped red cells and an inability of the blood to carry oxygen, producing anemia. The disease is practically limited to members of the negroid races and may be accompanied by the occurrence of small ulcers about the ankles. The symptoms, as in other anemias, include a general weakness, and in severe cases, headaches, nausea, vomiting, jaundice, fever, and pains in the muscles and joints. Sickle-cell anemia is often fatal and usually at an early age; few victims live beyond the third decade. A single pair of abnormal genes, one from each parent, is responsible for the disease. Should the person inherit only one abnormal gene, he will have the sickling trait, but without the anemia; and chances are good that he will live a reasonably healthy life.

Excessive breakdown of red blood cells may also be caused by transfusion of blood of the improper type, severe burns, allergies, and leukemia.

Nutritional anemias

Anemias caused by defective blood formation may result from either nutritional deficiencies or decreased bone marrow function. Most common and least severe of these are the anemias which result when an adequate amount of iron necessary for red cell formation is not available. This results in a microcytic hypochromic anemia. Iron is essential for hemoglobin manufacture. The iron needed amounts to about 100 milligrams for one day's supply of hemoglobin. Eighty-five percent of this may be obtained from the iron released by the breakdown of older red cells. Some iron is always lost in the excretions, however, so that it must be resupplied in the diet. Moreover, where there is chronic blood loss, such as in cases of ulcers or hemorrhoids, or when the iron is not properly absorbed from the food, the need for iron may be even greater. Some common foods (milk, cereals, refined foods) contain only small amounts of iron, and many people cannot afford foods of high iron content, such as meat and leafy vegetables. Consequently, iron deficiency is not uncommon.

The symptoms of an iron-deficiency anemia vary, depending on the severity of the condition. The patient is pale, generally weak, and has a tendency to tire easily; faintness and difficulty in breathing are common. A laboratory test of the blood readily demonstrates the presence of anemia. If the patient obtains sufficient rest and a good diet, recovery is usually rapid. A common form of iron-deficiency anemia seen in young women during the last century was often called *chlorosis* or "green-sickness" because of the peculiar hue of the skin. This disease almost completely disappeared when it was discovered that the administration of iron salts would effect a cure. Another form of iron-deficiency anemia, termed *idiopathic hypochromic* anemia, is often associated with a lack of proper stomach acidity. In the absence of proper amounts of hydrochloric acid in the stomach, iron cannot be liberated from food material and converted into a form that can be absorbed. This anemia also responds rapidly to the administration of iron in the proper form.

The anemia which frequently occurs in pregnancy is in one sense not an abnormal condition, but represents an attempt on the part of the mother's body to care more efficiently for the developing baby. Because the blood must carry the necessary food, oxygen, and waste materials for two individuals instead of one, increased demands are made on the circulatory system. The need for greater blood volume results in dilution of the blood. Hence, there are relatively fewer red cells per cubic centimeter of blood during pregnancy. Increased dietary requirements or an inadequate diet may also contribute to this anemia. Vomiting in early pregnancy also may increase the danger of an iron deficiency. If the anemia of pregnancy becomes too severe, the doctor may prescribe added iron, a good protein diet, a quart of milk per day, and perhaps vitamin tablets. Such a regimen may be desirable when the anemia is of the milder form.

Usually, babies are born with adequate supplies of iron in their tissues to last several months, but infants born of a mother with an iron deficiency have low reserve stores of iron. Such infants may develop hypochromic anemias soon after birth unless their diet is supplemented with the proper amounts of iron. Milk is a poor source of iron, and infants on a diet of milk alone almost invariably develop hypochromic anemias. Anemic babies are much more subject to infections, which may in turn further increase the anemia. Therefore, these children should be treated early.

Deficiencies of a number of other raw materials necessary for hemoglobin formation also may cause hypochromic anemias. Most common of these is a protein deficiency. Such deficiencies have been known to contribute to the iron-deficiency anemias, as well as to the anemia of pregnancy.

Minute amounts of copper are required in order for the body machinery to use iron properly; and if copper is lacking from the diet, a hypochromic anemia can result. For this reason, most medical preparations containing iron now also contain small amounts of copper. Vitamin C and certain of the other vitamins are thought to be involved in the process of iron utilization and hemoglobin construction. All of these facts serve to emphasize the importance of diet in maintaining the proper health of the blood.

Bone marrow deficiency diseases

The anemias caused by impaired bone marrow function are largely of the macrocytic hyperchromic type, and they are generally of a more serious nature. The process of red cell formation in the bone marrow is a complex one that requires the cooperation of a number of other systems of the body. Consequently, it is perhaps incorrect to speak of all macrocytic anemias as originating in the bone marrow. When the red-cell-to-be first takes shape in the marrow, it is somewhat larger than it will be later on. Further, it lacks hemoglobin. Before the new cell is released into the circulation, it shrinks in size and gains hemoglobin. When something prevents proper development, or the cells are released from the marrow too early, a macrocytic anemia generally results. In order for the red cell to mature properly, the bone marrow must have adequate amounts of the growth or maturation factor, which is obtained from the liver. Most of the macrocytic anemias are caused by the inability of the bone marrow to obtain the proper supplies of this substance—which is now known to be either identical with or closely related to vitamin B_{12}. This vitamin was previously referred to as the "extrinsic factor" because it came from outside the body. An "intrinsic factor" occurs in the normal gastric juice, and is necessary for the absorption of vitamin B_{12}. Some of the macrocytic anemias are caused by an absence of the intrinsic factor in the gastric juice, and others by inadequate supplies of the maturation factor. Still other macrocytic anemias are caused by the inability of the bone marrow to make use of the maturation factor. In all but the last-mentioned type, the injection of vitamin B_{12} or a liver extract which contains the vitamin usually brings about a prompt disappearance of the anemia.

Pernicious anemia is a macrocytic anemia which seldom occurs before middle life. It is caused by the disappearance of the intrinsic factor and with it, hydrochloric acid from the gastric juices. As the disease progresses, certain changes occur in the spinal cord which result in a weakness and numbness of the limbs and finally in a complete loss of ability to control them. In addition to the weakness and pallor seen in other anemias, the symptoms of pernicious anemia may include loss of appetite, diarrhea, nausea, a sore tongue, and a yellow pigmentation of the skin. No treatment was known for pernicious anemia patients until 1926, when it was discovered that the eating of large amounts of liver would bring about a disappearance of the symptoms of the disease. Neither this treatment nor any other now known, however, is able to restore the intrinsic factor and hydrochloric acid to the gastric juice. Therefore, therapy must be continued throughout life.

Instead of eating liver, most pernicious anemia patients now receive intramuscular injections of highly concentrated liver extract or vitamin B_{12} at periodic intervals. Another of the vitamins, *folic acid*, also is effective in relieving pernicious anemia. However, it may not stop the progressive degeneration of the spinal cord. Other vitamins also may be helpful. With proper and continuous treatment, most patients with pernicious anemia are able to live normal lives.

There are a large number of other conditions in which the absorption of material from the intestine is impaired as the result of diarrhea, excess fat in the intestinal contents (*steatorrhea*), or some impairment of the intestinal wall. In these conditions (*sprue, pellagra*), there is frequently a macrocytic anemia similar to that seen in pernicious anemia. These disorders respond to liver extract, vitamin B_{12}, and folic acid. Corticosteroids have also been found useful. Infestation with the fish tapeworm, *Diphyllobothrium latum*, is common in certain areas where raw fish is eaten, and causes a macrocytic anemia in patients afflicted with this parasite. Macrocytic anemia also occurs in certain liver diseases; and improper function of the liver must be corrected before the patient can be cured of his anemic condition. In some cases of lowered

MINOT, George Richards (1885-1950) American physician. With W. P. Murphy he introduced the use of dietary liver as the specific treatment for patients suffering with pernicious anemia. With Murphy and G. H. Whipple he received a Nobel prize in 1934 for this classic work. It has since been discovered that the liver is effective in the treatment of pernicious anemia because of the large amounts of the important vitamin B_{12} that are contained in it.

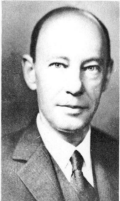

function of the thyroid gland (*myxedema*), the bone marrow is unable to utilize the maturation factor properly. This results in anemia which cannot be relieved until medication has either restored the thyroid to normal, or has supplied the thyroid hormone necessary for correct body functions. Occasionally, pregnant women contract a macrocytic anemia as the result of the heavy requirements placed on the mother's system at that time. Finally, there are other rare macrocytic anemias, the causes of which are unknown. Most of these anemias respond to liver and/or vitamin B_{12} therapy.

Perhaps the most serious of the normocytic anemias are those caused by the destruction of the bone marrow (*aplastic anemias*). All types of cells disappear from the bloodstream at a rapid rate, leaving only a small fraction of the normal number. The bone marrow is replaced by fatty tissue. What causes this chain of events is usually not known, but it can occur as a toxic reaction to x-rays, chemicals such as benzene, or drugs such as chloramphenicol and the antimetabolites. Repeated transfusions of blood are of value; and corticosteroids and the male sex hormone testosterone will produce some remissions. At times, removal of the spleen is beneficial.

In a related condition called *myelofibrosis*, the bone marrow is replaced by fibrous tissue. Patients become more and more anemic and increasingly prone to hemorrhage because of the loss of blood platelets. They also develop an enlarged spleen. The most effective treatment program appears to be androgens for the anemia and busulfan, irradiation, or surgical excision for the enlarged spleen.

All the anemias are manifested by a general tiredness and weakness, because the blood is unable to supply the tissues with adequate nourishment. The treatment of anemic patients is generally much more satisfactory and response is prompt if commenced before the disease has progressed very far or has caused permanent damage. Early detection and classification of the condition is of the greatest importance. The doctor can generally accomplish this by a laboratory examination of a sample of the patient's blood. Frequently, it may be necessary to perform certain tests on a sample of digestive juice drawn from the stomach, or upon a sample of bone marrow. In all but a few rare types of anemia, the physician can prescribe a specific substance which will bring about prompt relief, once the cause has been removed.

BLOOD DISORDERS: BLOOD POISONING

Blood poisoning (*bacteremia* or *septicemia*) is a condition in which bacteria enter the blood stream. The disease is often serious, and may result in death if not checked early. The healthy human body has the ability to keep bacteria isolated in a limited area; and the gravity of blood poisoning arises from the fact that this ability has been lost. Once bacteria get past the natural tissue barriers and into the blood stream, they can easily become established in other parts of the body. The fact that bacteria are able to enter the circulation, moreover, suggests that the patient's ability to combat infection has been weakened.

Causative agents

There are a number of different bacteria which may cause blood poisoning, but chief offenders are *streptococci* and *staphylococci*. Blood poisoning frequently begins as a local bacterial infection before spreading to the blood stream. Such infections may arise from cuts, burns, abrasions, boils, or carbuncles. All breaks in the skin, even though they seem minor, should be given careful attention because bacteria capable of causing blood poisoning may enter the body through these wounds. If a skin injury shows exaggerated signs of pus formation with severe reddening around the wound, the patient should consult a doctor at once. Early attention to such infections may prevent blood poisoning.

Blood poisoning may also follow other infections such as infections of the mastoid, tonsils, lungs, inner ears, sinuses, and genitourinary tract. When such infections are known to be present, any of the symptoms of blood poisoning should receive immediate medical attention. Bacteria may be present in the blood of persons who have typhoid fever, undulant fever, pneumonia, and other diseases. Bloodstream infections may arise from an infection around the root of a dead or damaged tooth.

Blood poisoning is the major cause of death in abortion, particularly when the operation is done by untrained persons or under unsterile

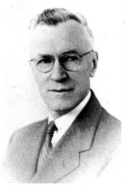

MURPHY, William Parry (1892-) American physician. With G. R. Minot, he introduced the now common dietary use of liver as an effective means of controlling the symptoms of pernicious anemia. For this important advance, he received the Nobel prize in 1934 with Minot and G. H. Whipple. Treatment with dietary liver was later replaced by the use of potent liver extract injections.

(*septic*) conditions. Septicemia resulting from abortion or from childbirth has a special name, child-bed fever (*puerperal sepsis*). This form of blood poisoning was once a major cause of death during childbirth, which frequently affected all of the obstetrical patients in a hospital. The sterile conditions found in modern delivery rooms have caused this dreaded disease to be almost a thing of the past.

Signs and symptoms

The symptoms of blood poisoning are of a general nature because the disease affects all parts of the body. There is a feeling of weakness; fever is either continuous or recurrent; and there may be periods of sweating. There may be signs of bacterial infection in distant organs such as the lungs or spleen, and heart murmurs may develop from bacterial involvement of the heart valves. The patient may develop an anemia, suffer chills similar to those of malaria, and may have severe headaches. Early recognition of blood poisoning is extremely important, since it may cause death in as short a period as two days. This rapid course is seen more frequently in children.

Treatment and prevention

Because patients suffering from septicemia may die if not treated for the condition, the physician should be notified at the first suspicion that the disease is present in the body. Many new antibiotic drugs have been discovered in recent years which greatly increase the doctor's ability to deal effectively with this blood disease. Folic acid, vitamin B_{12}, ascorbic acid, and androgens are given if the bone marrow has been damaged by the infection. Supportive blood transfusions also may be needed.

Disappearance of the symptoms is not a sufficient indication of recovery. Only repeated blood

tests, which show that the bacteria are no longer present in the blood, are proof that the infection will not flare up again.

The best means for the prevention of blood poisoning is to care for all wounds properly when they occur, and to get immediate medical care for infections of the skin, tonsils, mouth, and ear. By these two simple procedures, the chances of developing blood poisoning are kept very low.

BLOOD DISORDERS: HEMOPHILIA

The blood contains a remarkable group of substances which work together to stop bleeding from a wound by means of blood clot formation. Clotting normally occurs within five or six minutes, but in a few rare individuals this process may require hours or even days. A number of different conditions may cause such a prolonged clotting time, but the most striking is *hemophilia*.

Hemophilia, a familial blood disease, has been recognized for hundreds of years. Because of the frequency of the disease in many of the royal families of Europe, particularly those of Spain and Russia, the incidence of hemophilia has changed world history. Hemophilia in women is practically unknown; it usually affects only the male, although it is transmitted through the female. A woman may carry the genetic factor producing hemophilia, without having any of the symptoms; she might display the symptoms if each of her parents carried this factor for the disease.

Hemophilia is almost always apparent in the first year of life, and is generally recognized without difficulty because of its previous occurrence in the family. On rare occasions, it occurs in families which have no history of the condition. Therefore, unusually severe bleeding from a seemingly minor injury should always be reported to a physician. The hereditary nature of hemophilia should serve as a warning to members of families in which the disease has occurred; these persons should be on the lookout for the symptoms in themselves.

Hemophiliacs do not usually die from the first severe bleeding, because of their reserve stores of blood cells. Subsequent hemorrhage may prove fatal, however, if these stores have not been replenished. Patients who receive no medical treatment in cases of bleeding seldom live beyond their twentieth year, while those who obtain proper care have an excellent chance for a long life.

The immediate treatment of patients with hemophilia is frequently self-administered. The victim should supply himself with the special

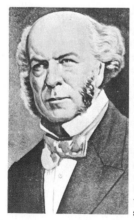

COMBE, James Scarfe (1796-1883) Scottish physician. He is famous for having given the first description of the symptoms of pernicious anemia, in the year 1824, although Addison is more frequently credited with it. While this blood disorder undoubtedly had existed long before this time, it appears to have been generally confused with a great variety of other quite unrelated conditions that had similar groups of symptoms, but no other point of similarity.

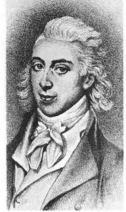

OTTO, John Conrad (1774-1844) American physician. Otto was the first man to describe accurately hemophilia and point out that this disorder does not affect women, but is nevertheless transmitted by them to their sons who are affected. Although hemophilia had been recognized long before this, and was even described in ancient medical manuscripts, it was never well understood until the report of Otto's classical investigation of this hereditary disease appeared in 1803.

clot-stimulating materials prescribed by his physician, and apply these directly to any cut or scratch. The usual methods for stopping blood flow have little or no effect.

If the patient cannot stop the bleeding himself, he may require an injection of *antihemophilic factor* (*AHF*), the special clot-forming protein that is missing from his blood. Potent doses of this protein can be prepared by freezing, thawing, and then centrifuging fresh plasma. In contrast to treatment by massive plasma transfusion which often has to be repeated and carries the risk of hepatitis, AHF concentrate can be administered quickly by syringe. It is especially valuable for the hemophiliac who needs an emergency operation.

As a general rule, the hemophiliac should avoid strenuous activities that might result in personal injury. He should be aware of the special dangers he faces. At the same time, he should not be overfearful. Over-anxiety can actually increase the frequency of bleeding.

Fortunately for the hemophilic patient, there may be remissions in his disease, during which time he may have nearly normal clotting activity for weeks or even years. A life of moderate activity with some precautions, prompt attention to bleeding, and AHF injections when necessary are the measures that will increase the life span.

Other hemorrhagic diseases

Other conditions exist in which unusually large amounts of blood may be lost. In many of such cases, bleeding may take place into the skin, as in a bruise. This symptom is referred to as *purpura*.

Essential thrombocytopenic purpura is a disease characterized by hemorrhage, and caused by a deficiency in the number of blood platelets. The spleen may be responsible for this disease by destroying the blood platelets. Corticosteroid therapy helps control the bleeding, and in most

patients is regarded as a desirable practice prior to removal of the spleen.

Still other very rare bleeding conditions occur. Purpura and excessive bleeding may occur in persons suffering from deficiency of vitamins C and K. Some newborn infants contract a hemorrhagic disease which once was frequently fatal; the victims now recover rapidly when treated with vitamin K. Purpura may occur in persons receiving antitoxin treatments, or as a symptom of snakebite poisoning, or with some types of food poisoning. The taking of certain drugs may bring about abnormal bleeding. Purpura is occasionally a symptom of such varied conditions as meningitis, scarlet fever, severe measles, chronic kidney disease, endocrine disorders, liver disease, macrocytic anemias, allergies, typhus fever, and a specific bacterial heart disease. The symptom disappears in each case when the primary cause is removed.

BLOOD DISORDERS: LEUKEMIA AND OTHER MALIGNANT DISORDERS

There are a number of diseases of the blood-forming organs which are characterized by an overproduction of blood cells. In *leukemia*, the white cells, which normally occur in a ratio of one to about 1000 red cells, may increase as much as 50- to 60-fold in some patients. This condition is extremely serious, for it is the result of a malignant process operating in the blood-producing parts of the body, particularly in the lymphatic system or the bone marrow. Mention should be made of the fact that there are a number of disorders, other than leukemia, which produce an elevated white cell count, and which occur much more frequently than leukemia.

A person with leukemia has a much brighter outlook today than he would have had a few years ago, since modern therapy may extend his life span considerably and make him much more comfortable. Furthermore, current research on leukemia is continuing to produce significant advances in our knowledge. Although no definitive cure is known as yet, the medical profession has reason to expect that more effective and more prolonged control procedures will be found. This optimism is engendered by the fact that the new syntheses and new applications of a number of chemical compounds now arrest temporarily the course of certain kinds of leukemia. Continued study of these and related substances may be expected to yield significant results.

Leukemia

There are several different kinds of leukemia. Each form differs in its symptoms and in the life

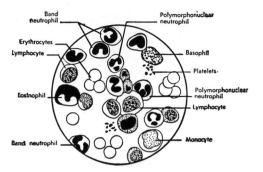

Aggregate of cells which may appear in the normal human blood; magnified about 450 times. With the exception of the *erythrocytes* and *platelets,* the various blood cells that are illustrated all represent common types of human white blood cells or *leucocytes.* Details shown appear only on staining.

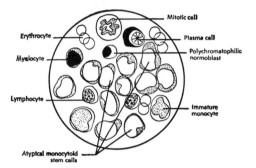

Drawing of some cells which may appear in leukemic patient's blood, magnified about 450 times. The relative numbers of the various cells shown are disproportionate but the abnormal cellular appearance may be observed by a comparison with the normal cells shown in the drawing above.

expectancy of the patient. The treatment of each individual, therefore, depends necessarily on his exact type of leukemia and on the extent and nature of the involvement of other body parts.

The leukemias in general are classified as *acute* or *chronic.* The acute forms have a sudden onset and may progress rapidly. Indeed, this type is seldom discovered until the disease has become well-advanced. The acute leukemias occur most frequently in young children; the chronic forms usually occur in persons over 35 years of age.

The onset in chronic leukemia is insidious. Sometimes the disease is discovered during a routine physical examination before symptoms have appeared. At other times, the patient consults a physician because of the persistence of relatively mild symptoms, such as discomfort in the upper abdomen, or because of the accidental discovery of a mass in this area.

Leukemia also varies with the particular type

of white cell specifically involved. Thus in *lymphocytic* leukemia, the white blood cells known as lymphocytes, which arise from the lymph nodes and spleen, are primarily involved; in *granulocytic* leukemia, one or more of the three types of granulocytes, which originate in the bone marrow, are affected. A third type, *monocytic* leukemia, is characterized by the appearance of excessive numbers of monocytes of connective tissue origin. In some acute leukemias, the total circulating white cell count may be normal or below normal (*subleukemic leukemia*), though the type of cell affected is found in excessive number in other *tissues.* Still other rarer types of leukemic cell alteration are occasionally found.

Signs and symptoms of the leukemias

The early symptoms of the different types of leukemia may be quite similar; but because of the differences in the clinical rates at which the chronic and the acute forms progress, it is most important that a prompt diagnostic differentiation be obtained. The first symptoms may be nonspecific in nature, although in the *lymphocytic* types enlarged lymph nodes may give an early clue as to the site and nature of the affliction. The patient may first notice that he is tiring readily. He may discover a heavy feeling or unusual solid resistance and distention in the abdomen caused by an enlarged spleen; he may notice oozing of blood from the gums or the nose or a purple discoloration of the skin due to spread of blood into the subcutaneous tissues. Many patients become paler as a result of the anemia which may accompany progressive leukemia, even without blood loss. Any one of these symptoms or signs may be caused, of course, by other diseases. Consequently, the ultimate diagnosis will depend upon proper laboratory studies, particularly blood and bone marrow cell interpretations.

Four findings characterize the *chronic* leukemias: (1) more or less obvious enlargement of the lymph nodes, (2) enlargement of the spleen, (3) increased numbers of white blood cells, and (4) decreased numbers of red cells (anemia). Symptoms which may be present include nervousness, loss of weight, abnormal nocturnal perspiration, and difficult breathing. The enlargement of the lymph nodes may be quite extreme in chronic lymphocytic leukemia—particularly in the areas above the collar bone, in the armpits, or in the groin. A pronounced enlargement of the spleen is more common in the chronic granulocytic type. In granulocytic or monocytic leukemia, small lumps of infiltrating cells may appear under the skin. In either acute or chronic leukemia, there may be pain in the bones and joints, or hemorrhage may occur into the brain or other vital organs.

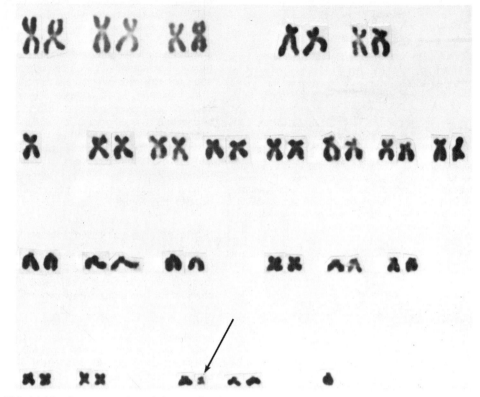

The tiny Philadelphia chromosome (arrow) is associated with chronic myelogenous leukemia. Copyright 1966 Year Book Medical Publishers, Inc., courtesy T. C. Hsu, The University of Texas M. D. Anderson Hospital, Houston.

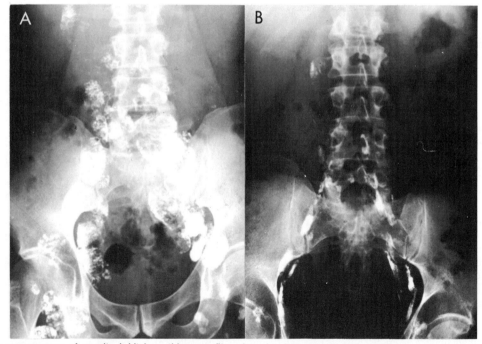

A, The coarse areas of opacity (white) on this x-ray film show involvement of pelvic and para-aortic lymph nodes by nodular lymphoma. B, Good response to therapy is shown in the later film. Copyright 1970 Year Book Medical Publishers, Inc., courtesy Sidney Wallace, The University of Texas M. D. Anderson Hospital, Houston.

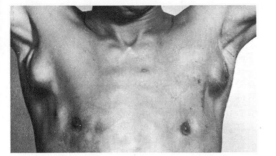

Patient with lymphoma, before treatment. Note enlarged lymph nodes in armpits, and swelling of neck nodes.

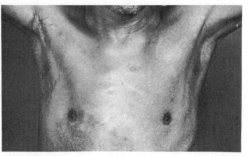

Same patient, after two months of chemotherapy. Enlarged nodes have disappeared, and patient's general health has improved.

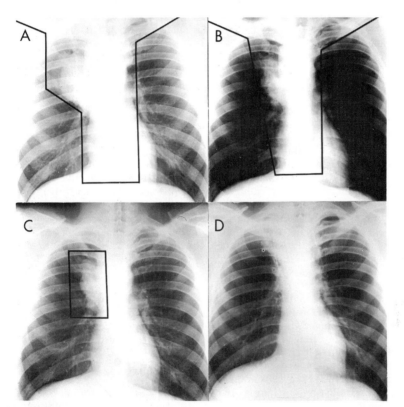

Radiotherapy for Hodgkin's disease is illustrated in these chest x-ray films. A, B, C, To spare normal lung tissues, the treatment fields were narrowed as the tumor which appears as a diffuse white area, shrank in size. D, Follow-up films revealed little remaining tumor in the area. Copyright 1970 Year Book Medical Publishers, Inc., courtesy Lillian M. Fuller et al., The University of Texas M. D. Anderson Hospital, Houston.

Acute leukemia frequently is first detected by prolonged hemorrhage following some relatively minor surgical operation, such as a tooth extraction. Fever, pain in the bones and joints, and anemia are early symptoms. An increased susceptibility to secondary infections may develop. The patient usually is weak, with fever and a rapid pulse rate. Bleeding into the skin (*purpura*), giving the appearance of a bruise, is common. In acute monocytic leukemia, the tissues of the mouth are swollen and inflamed and the gums are infiltrated and thickened, tending to obscure the teeth.

The diagnosis of leukemia is made by microscopic examination of blood and bone marrow.

Treatment of the leukemic patient

The treatment of the leukemic patient depends entirely on the type and extent of his leukemia. Leukemia is usually a progressive disease that terminates fatally after a variable period of time.

For many years, treatment of choice for this disease was irradiation. Following the introduction of the nitrogen mustards, new interest in the management of the disease was aroused and many new forms of treatment have been introduced. These have given new hope to the patient and encouragement to the investigator. Methods available now can alleviate the symptoms, and remissions can be brought about which in some cases may be so complete as to give the appearance of unqualified well-being. The remissions in the chronic leukemias may be of long duration and even in acute forms may last a number of months. With a wide variety of chemotherapeutic agents available, treatment has become relatively inexpensive, requires a minimum of hospitalization, and is relatively convenient, so that an essentially normal existence can be achieved for a time.

Patients with chronic leukemia can be treated by irradiation with either roentgen rays or radioactive phosphorous, by chemotherapy, or by a combination of both. Radioactive phosphorous is produced in an atomic pile or nuclear reactor. When the radiation is directed toward the spleen and/or lymph nodes, the organs decrease in size and the white cells decrease in number, thus relieving the pain in those areas. Smaller doses of x-rays given to the entire body strike the bone marrow also and are helpful in preventing or correcting the secondary anemias. When radioactive phosphorous enters the body, it participates in the metabolism of bone marrow and lymphoid tissues and inhibits the rapidly multiplying leukemia cells.

Some patients are initially sensitive to radiation and can stand only limited amounts; in others the leukemia cells become resistant to radiation. In either of these instances, chemotherapy is of value. Sometimes it is even the preferred method of treatment. The agents most commonly used for chronic leukemia are busulfan and chlorambucil. Busulfan is the best drug available for chronic myelocytic leukemia; it has resulted in remissions lasting as long as two years. Chlorambucil is the most satisfactory drug for chronic lymphocytic leukemia. It has no important side effects and rarely causes injury to the bone marrow. Other drugs of value in the chronic leukemias are uracil mustard and hydroxyurea.

In patients with acute leukemia, roentgen therapy is of no value, radioactive phosphorus has limited application, and the drugs used in chronic leukemia are generally ineffective. What appears to work best is the cyclic administration of another group of drugs—prednisone, amethopterin, and 6-mercaptopurine. Initial therapy is generally with steroids, usually prednisone. When a remission has been produced, administration of this agent is reduced and then stopped; and 6-mercaptopurine is introduced. When it fails, a course of steroid therapy may be given

again, followed by amethopterin. In patients who do not respond to other drugs, cyclophosphamide or vincristine sulfate may produce brief remissions. If the patient is extremely ill or has a tendency to bleed, large doses of adrenocorticotropic hormone (ACTH) or prednisone are particularly useful. New drugs are constantly being developed as a result of experimental work under the National Cancer Chemotherapy program of the National Cancer Institute.

Infection is a major complication in patients undergoing chemotherapy. To combat this problem the Life Island and the laminar air flow room have been developed. The Life Island consists of a bed enclosed by a plastic canopy with sleeves through which procedures are performed. In the laminar air flow room a bank of high-efficiency filters comprises one wall and air is distributed in a horizontal laminar flow pattern. These two units protect the patient from organisms which would reach him through the air or through physical contact with items in the environment; they provide a pathogen-free environment.

The control of anemia and *thrombocytopenic* purpura in the patient with leukemia may require supportive fresh blood transfusions until the specific medication has had opportunity and time to become effective.

Platelet replacement therapy is an effective means of preventing and controlling hemorrhage. In this technique, whole blood is drawn from a donor and spun at high speeds to separate the platelet-rich plasma from the red cells. The red cells are then returned to the donor; and the pooled platelets, which are needed for blood clotting, go to the patient. By means of this technique, one adult can furnish all the platelets that a child with leukemia needs. Granulocytes can be extracted from whole blood in a similar way and then used to help patients fight infection.

Other malignant diseases

There are other rare diseases which are similar to leukemia in their symptoms and manifestations. Two of these conditions, *Hodgkin's disease* and *lymphosarcoma,* deserve special mention.

Hodgkin's disease is a malady characterized by a painless localized enlargement of lymph nodes, usually beginning in one side of the neck. The patient may develop fever, and generalized itching or an eruption on the skin. Anemia is uncommon except in advanced cases and tests of peripheral blood have no diagnostic value. Diagnosis is made by removal of one of the affected lymph nodes for microscopic study. Surgical excision, irradiation, and chemotherapy all have a place in the treatment of patients with Hodgkin's disease. Surgical excision can be used when the condition is localized, followed perhaps by local irradiation and/or chemotherapy. X-irradiation alone is valuable for localized disease. Massive doses in the early stages can produce dramatic results, including the rapid disappearance of masses and long remissions. Nitrogen mustard is beneficial in patients with disseminated disease. Other drugs of value in treating patients with Hodgkin's disease are chlorambucil, cyclophosphamide, and vinblastine sulfate.

Lymphosarcoma similarly begins in one location, in a regional lymph node or internal organ, with or without circulating diagnostic lymphosarcoma cells in the blood. Acute lymphatic leukemia of childhood may be lymphosarcoma with the abnormal cells overflowing into the circulating blood. Whereas usually this disease is promptly fatal if untreated, when these patients receive early and proper treatment, both blood and bone marrow may revert to normal with complete restoration of health for variable periods. In lymphosarcoma, x-ray therapy is the major and most universally effective form of treatment. Chlorambucil and nitrogen mustard are effective chemotherapeutic agents in earlier stages of the disease; cyclophosphamide and vinblastine sulfate, in later stages. Prednisone may prove beneficial in patients with fever and hematologic disturbances no longer suitable for treatment with x-ray or other drugs.

Diseases caused by an overproduction of the red blood cells

On occasion, a blood study will reveal that a patient with cyanosis and fatigue has too many red blood cells, with high platelet level and leucocytosis. These findings suggest the presence of *polycythemia,* a disease in which the bone marrow shows a pronounced tendency to generalized overactivity in cell production.

The polycythemia vera patient may complain of a feeling of fullness in the head with severe headache, dizziness, and fainting. There also may be numbness or tingling sensations of the hands and feet, irritability, mental sluggishness, occasional amnesia, and ease of bruising. These various complaints arise from the effects of

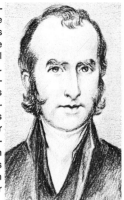

HODGKIN, Thomas (1798-1866) English physician. He is famous for the numerous contributions that he made to medicine and to normal and pathological anatomy. He contributed to the knowledge of abnormal changes that may occur in membranes, and gave what is believed to be the first clear description of aortic insufficiency. *Hodgkin's disease,* in which there is a dangerous enlargement of the lymph nodes, was named in honor of this famous investigator.

the slow viscous blood flow to the brain and to other vital tissues of the body. The spleen enlarges in its reservoir function as a storage depot for the increased marrow production of cells. *Intravascular thromboses* may occur when the platelets are very numerous.

The excess of red blood cells in polycythemia vera may be relieved by bloodletting (*venesection*), removing sufficient quantities of blood at regular intervals to maintain a normal plasma to cell-volume ratio. However, this does not control the excessive platelet and white cell levels. Radioactive phosphorus in carefully adjusted dosage is now used so that all three of the marrow elements may be controlled by central inhibition. Remissions lasting from one to three years may be induced by successive courses of P^{32} therapy. The nitrogen mustards have also been used successfully in the treatment of polycythemia vera as have the *phenylhydrazines,* but neither of these groups of agents is as effective in producing prolonged remissions as radioactive phosphorus. If these patients receive prompt and adequate P^{32} treatments, they may look forward to a long life, with hardly more complications than a normal individual of the same age would experience.

Multiple myeloma

Cancer arising in any organ of the body may spread to the blood-forming organs, and thus cause a disturbance in the blood cells. A foreign cell disorder, which appears to arise directly within the bone marrow, causing secondary changes in the blood is *plasma cell myeloma.* In later stages of the disease, the plasma cells may invade other parts of the body, including the liver, spleen, and lymph nodes, and the kidneys may suffer from depositions of abnormal proteins or *pseudoglobulins.*

One of the first signs of multiple myeloma is deep bone pain, usually in the lower back but sometimes *referred* to the chest, arms, or legs. In the beginning these pains may be vague, intermittent, or migratory; they become worse

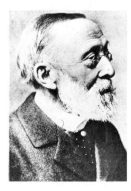

VIRCHOW, Rudolf Ludwig Karl (1821-1902) German pathologist. Virchow first described leukemia when he was but twenty-four years of age. He helped to establish the important biological principle that all living cells are derived from preexisting cells. Virchow is famous as an originator of the common modern practice of routine medical inspections and hygienic instruction for the children during the years they are attending the public and private schools.

as the disease progresses, and are particularly disturbing at night. The condition develops most commonly in men in middle age or later life. A loss of weight accompanied by mild anemia, lowering of the blood pressure, and protein in the urine *(proteinuria)* characterize the progress of the disease. One of the most formidable signs of the disease is spontaneous or pathological bone fracture. The bone in any affected area becomes greatly weakened, and appears "moth-eaten" on x-ray films. Even normal use may cause a fracture.

There are several laboratory tests which the physician may perform to aid in the diagnosis of multiple myeloma. These include microscopic examinations of the blood and the bone marrow for plasma cells. He may also make tests of the blood plasma and urine for disturbed calcium and serum *globulin metabolites,* the latter at times resulting in kidney tubule blockage leading to *uremia.* Complete skeletal x-ray pictures should be made in every suspected individual to show the exact location and extent of the bone-excavating tumors.

Although multiple myeloma, as the name implies, usually consists of numerous or multiple tumors invading the bony skeleton widely, the occasional patient shows only one localized plasma cell tumor. Surgical removal of such a single tumor may be curative. When the lesions are multiple, however, surgical excision is of no value, and only orthopedic management of pathological fractures is indicated. X-ray therapy may at times be *prophylactic* against spontaneous fractures and be pain relieving. Of all the drugs tested, melphalan appears to be the most promising. It has been associated with relief of pain, a gain in strength, and a sense of well-being. For best results, melphalan should be given in combination with four other agents— prednisone, sodium fluoride, androgen, and fluoxymesterone.

Since multiple myeloma is often a painful disease, palliative medical treatment must be directed toward measures that will control this symptom without narcotic addiction. Radioactive phosphorus may occasionally reduce the pain, though it must be used with caution so that normal blood cell formation will not be depressed. The most important aspect of the nursing care is the prevention of spontaneous fractures, particularly vertebral collapse. If fractures occur, they must be given immediate orthopedic attention. Kidney function must be conserved. Other measures directed toward increasing the life span of the patient and alleviating his suffering are the objectives of intensive research at the present time. The present rate of progress in understanding malignant diseases of the blood suggests that there will be spectacular advances in the immediate future, and offers great hope to the patient.

BLOOD DISORDERS: BENIGN BLOOD AND LYMPH DISORDERS

The large majority of changes that occur in the circulating blood cells reflect their sensitive response to disturbances in other organs of the body. There are, however, some diseases primarily involving the blood-forming organs which may be serious, but which are called *benign* to distingush them from the leukemic and malignant disorders. The cause is not always known, although viral or bacterial infections, and drug or industrial intoxications account for some.

Infectious mononucleosis

Infectious mononucleosis, sometimes called glandular fever, is a systemic disorder probably caused by a virus infection, although the causative agent is not known with certainty, and other organisms may be involved. Abnormal numbers of young, though nonleukemic, lymphocytes occur in the circulation at the expense of granulocytes. The patient has a fever and develops a swelling and tenderness, usually of all lymph nodes of the body. He may also have *pharyngitis, tonsillitis, mucous membrane ulceration,* headache, chills, sweating, abdominal pains, and a tender spleen and liver.

Although there is no specific treatment for patients with mononucleosis, and the cause has not been established, it is important that this condition be differentiated from other conditions with a more serious prognosis, but with similar symptoms and signs. Diagnosis is made by studies of the peripheral blood cells and by a serum agglutination test.

Recovery is ordinarily spontaneous, but the patient should receive antibiotic therapy for the management of superimposed infections. Rest in bed during the *febrile* stage and at least

SCHILLING, Victor (1883-1960) Austrian hematologist. Much of the work of classifying the varieties of the white blood cells was performed by Schilling. He also made important clinical observations regarding the various types of leucocytes that are present in the blood under several pathological conditions such as leukemia and certain of the acute infections. Blood counts are now a major tool in the confirmation of most medical diagnoses.

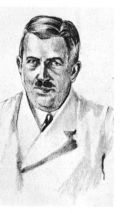

partial isolation and sterilization of eating and drinking utensils in an attempt to prevent the spread of the disease to others are important. Symptomatic remedies to ease the more unpleasant complaints experienced by the patient with infectious mononucleosis, such as fever and sore thoat, are helpful. Relapses are common, though usually no more serious than the primary episode.

Agranulocytosis

Agranulocytosis is a potentially serious *syndrome* in which the white cells may be greatly decreased or almost absent from the circulation. Because the granulocytes are important in protecting the body against infection, an individual deprived of these defensive forces for long may have an overwhelming invasion of the bloodstream and organs with dangerous disease-producing organisms. Important symptoms include general weakness, prostration, headache, shaking chills, and progressive ulcerative throat lesions. Diagnosis must be confirmed by studies of the bone marrow.

The syndrome of agranulocytosis may result from an overwhelming infection releasing toxins specifically destructive to the bone marrow and lymphatic systems. It may develop secondary to allergic sensitization to drugs with *antigenic* properties such as aminopyrine, thiouracil, some of the sulfonamides, and arsenic. Industrial toxins, particularly benzol, may damage the marrow similarly.

The patient who has agranulocytosis must be separated from contact with the causative agent; its elimination from the body must be facilitated.

Diseases of the reticuloendothelial system

The *reticuloendothelial system* of cells extends throughout the body and represents the chief source of both cellular and *humoral* antibody defense forces. These cells are found concentrated particularly in the spleen, liver, bone marrow, and lymph nodes. The reticuloendothelial system may be involved in a variety of pathologic syndromes.

Gaucher's disease is a condition in which abnormal amounts of fat are stored in the cells of the reticuloendothelial system. Diagnosis is usually readily made by direct observation of the typical cells found in the bone marrow. It is a rare disease usually manifesting its signs in childhood. The disease begins slowly, seldom producing any marrow inadequacy, the most characteristic sign being an increasing enlargement and tenderness of the abdomen caused by excessive growth of Gaucher's cells in the spleen. Either mechanical embarrassment of other intra-abdominal organic functions, or the destruction

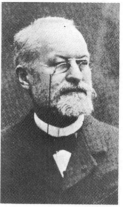

LAVERAN, Charles Louis Alphonse (1845-1922) French army physician and bacteriologist. Laveran is famous for his important discovery in the year 1880 of malarial parasites in the human red blood cells. Rupture of the cells by the parasites brings on the characteristic malarial attack, and simutaneously it also causes a hemolytic anemia. For his numerous important medical studies Laveran was awarded the Nobel prize in medicine in 1907.

of the circulating blood cells by the enlarged spleen may require removal of this organ. Removal of the spleen usually permits the resumption of a more normal life.

Niemann-Pick's disease (lipoid histiocytosis) is a rare disease of infants, occurring most often among Jewish people. Excessive quantities of a normal *phosphatide* are deposited in the reticuloendothelial cells. The patient usually shows an enlargement of liver, spleen, and lymph nodes. Malnutrition and retarded mental development and growth are common signs. No treatment is known to be effective, and such patients usually succumb at an early age from a secondary infection.

Hand-Schuller-Christian's disease (lipoid granulomatosis) is another rare reticuloendothelial disease involving *cholesterol* metabolism and occurring in the first decade of life. Among the early signs of the disease is a noticeable retardation of growth and development; later, protrusion of the eyes and the development of *diabetes insipidus* occur together with punched-out defects in the skull. Roentgen and nitrogen mustard therapy have been employed in treating patients with this disease.

Letterer-Siwe's disease (nonlipoid histiocytosis, reticuloendotheliosis) is largely limited to children under three, but does occur in adults. There is a widespread proliferation of reticuloendothelial cells. Symptoms include petechial or purpuric manifestations or a skin lesion resembling infected eczema, a persistent, spiking, low-grade fever, enlargement of spleen, liver and lymph nodes, and progressive anemia. Diagnosis is usually made by biopsy of bone marrow or lymph nodes. Therapy is primarily supportive care, antibiotics to control secondary infection, and irradiation to the skin and other areas of involvement.

Eosinophilic granuloma of the bone is a comparatively benign disorder characterized by single or multiple skeletal lesions and occurring chiefly in children or young adults. The lesions are rare in the distal ends of the extremities. Pain and swelling are common complaints and there may be mild degrees of fever. The lesions usually respond well to treatment.

BLOOD DISORDERS: AUTOIMMUNE DISEASES

Antibodies are widely acknowledged as the body's chief defense against infection. But under certain circumstances, they appear to switch roles and become the cause of disease rather than its opponent. Instead of developing antibodies against foreign substances like viruses or bacteria, victims appear to develop antibodies against their own tissues or cells. One theory is that these *autoantibodies* are formed when abnormal groups or clones of cells relinquish their normal tolerance to the host and begin to produce abnormal antibodies. Autoimmunity was first discovered in acquired hemolytic anemia and has since been suggested as a cause of numerous diseases, including idiopathic thrombocytopenic purpura, chronic leukopenia, systemic lupus erythematosus, thyroiditis, sympathetic ophthalmia, and even multiple sclerosis.

In diseases definitely established as autoimmune, chemical agents that suppress the immune response are sometimes employed. The antimetabolite 6-mercaptopurine has been used with consistent success in acquired hemolytic anemia, a disease definitely traced to autoantibodies. Results have been more spotty in systemic lupus erythematosus, a disease whose cause is still somewhat speculative.

BLOOD TRANSFUSIONS, BLOOD TYPES, AND TESTS

It was once the superstition that the blood carried certain noxious materials or spirits which were responsible for all of the ills of the body. The treatment of practically every patient, therefore, included bloodletting to rid him of these evil influences. Today the blood is known to reflect in its cellular and chemical changes many of the disorders to which mankind is heir; hence, through an understanding of the various constituents of blood, these disorders may be recognized.

Blood transfusions

Severe wounds may result in serious blood loss with consequent drop in blood pressure, so that the body tissues fail to receive the necessary

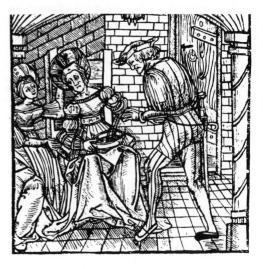

This woodcut from an old Dutch calendar portrays the custom of letting blood in order to cure a patient of some disease. This practice is described in some of the earliest historical records. The procedure was usually conducted by a barber, and was believed effective for most diseases, especially when performed at the time indicated by an astrologer as being the best. *Bettmann Archive.*

oxygen and nourishment. In such cases, blood transfusions are required to restore the circulating blood volume and replace the lost red cells. Such support is common practice also in cases of surgical shock, or during acute emergencies, following excessive blood loss at childbirth, or in hemophilia, and in medical conditions such as the leukemias and purpura.

The first recorded blood transfusion was performed in 1677 by Jean Baptiste Denys. He injected the blood of a lamb into the veins of a boy who was dying from bloodletting, and the patient "miraculously" recovered. The dangers of interspecies blood transfusions, however, prevented their further use. Today, the blood of lower animals is never transfused into human beings.

A critically ill patient may receive human blood, one of its components, such as red cells or platelets, or a "blood substitute." Whole blood is what most patients now receive; but its use is expected to decrease as techniques for extracting and storing its components are perfected. Red cells, for example, can be separated out, frozen in liquid nitrogen, and stored for years. By contrast, red cells in the whole blood form must be discarded after three weeks. Platelets, other clotting factors such as those needed by hemophilia patients, and white cells also can be extracted and used. Transfusions of plasma, once common, are now discouraged because of the danger of hepatitis and severe allergic-type reactions. Plasma substitutes, such as serum albumin, salt solutions, and synthetics like dextran are plentiful and do not carry the risk of reactions.

Human blood and blood derivatives are procured, processed, stored, and administered under strictly germ-free conditions. Furthermore, all donors are carefully questioned about past illnesses, such as malaria and infectious jaundice, and tests are performed for the presence of syphilis or other infections, before accepting the blood for therapeutic use.

In rare instances, the patient-recipient may have an unfavorable posttransfusion reaction, involving a transitory rise in temperature and slight to severe chill. The reaction may be the result of inaccurate typing and cross matching, or of foreign, contaminating substances, or of minor differences between the proteins in the blood of the patient and those in the donor.

In cases where veins are not accessible for transfusion (peripheral circulatory failure, skin burns, etc.), blood and other fluids may be given via the bone marrow. In adults, the sternum is the site of transfusion; in children, the tibia is used. This method is not attempted when veins are accessible, because infections may result; and small amounts of air are less well tolerated in the bone marrow than in the vein.

Blood types

The human blood groups were discovered around the turn of this century by Dr. Karl Landsteiner, who received the Nobel prize in 1930 for his observation of the four hereditary blood groups: namely, groups A, B, AB, and O. The proper recognition of the intergroup incompatibilities of the red cells, which result in spontaneous clumping of the cells of one group by the plasma of another, is essential to the safe and effective use of human blood transfusions.

Theoretically, blood from individuals of group O (so-called "universal donor") can be given to members of all other groups; for reasons given below, however, the use of "universal" group O blood for transfusing persons of other groups is not recommended. When he receives blood, a person of group O must have only group O blood. A person with group AB can receive blood from anyone, but can donate it only to another AB person. Group A blood may be given to group A or AB, but the group A recipient can accept only group A or O. Group B may give blood to persons with group B or AB but receive only from groups B and O.

In actual practice, it is better for the blood donor and the recipient to be of the same blood type, for two reasons: first, some universal group O bloods, when used in transfusion, react unfavorably with the blood of the recipi-

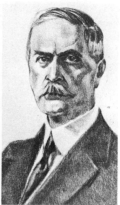

LANDSTEINER, Karl (1868-1943) American pathologist. He is world famous for having established the scientific basis of modern blood grouping, the type designations for human blood being generally known as *Landsteiner's classification*. In collaboration with A. S. Wiener in 1940 he discovered the significance of the Rh group of blood factors. His numerous contributions to the study of medicine were responsible for his winning the Nobel prize in 1930.

ent; second, type-for-type transfusion allows random sampling of the donor population to balance out with random sampling of the recipient population.

As a further precaution against unfavorable transfusion reactions, "cross-matching" is done. Prior to transfusion, small samples of the red corpuscles and *sera* of donor and recipient are mixed in the laboratory and observed with a microscope to determine whether clumping of the cells of either donor or recipient occurs in the serum of the other. If no clumping is observed during this cross-matching, the bloods are regarded as compatible, and the transfusion is done. This practice has tremendously decreased the accidents of blood transfusion.

In this country, blood groups A and O are the most common, occurring in approximately 85 percent of the population. Group AB is the rarest. In other parts of the world these relationships may differ, as for example among the aborigines of Australia, where no group B bloods have been found.

The Rh blood groups are also of great importance in transfusions and in obstetrics, but they were not recognized until 1940. Landsteiner and an associate, Wiener, found a new blood group (Rh) in human beings which was detected in the course of experiments on rhesus monkeys, hence the name Rh. Wiener and Peters soon noted that unexplained accidents in transfusion were attributable to this Rh blood group; Levine, Katzin, and Burnham correlated the Rh group with a disease of the newborn, first called *erythroblastosis fetalis*, and now generally known as *hemolytic* disease of the newborn. This disease is characterized by the breaking apart of the red blood cells.

When blood from an Rh positive donor is used for transfusion into an Rh negative recipient, the latter will develop specific antibodies which may produce a true hemolytic reaction if Rh positive cells are again introduced in a transfusion.

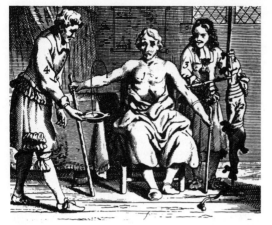

This old illustration, which dates from the year 1667, portrays both the letting of blood and also the technique of giving a blood transfusion directly from an animal into a human being. The dangerous practice of bloodletting was responsible for a great many deaths and a great saving of life resulted when this practice became outmoded. The primitive method of transfusing from an animal was also very dangerous to the patient. *Bettmann Archive.*

If an Rh negative women marries an Rh positive man and gives birth to an Rh positive child, there is a grave risk that she will become sensitized to the Rh factor in her baby's blood and begin to produce anti-Rh antibodies. The first baby is not usually affected; but with subsequent pregnancies, the mother may send enough damaging antibodies into the child's bloodstream to threaten its life. When this happens, an exchange blood transfusion with almost complete replacement of the infant's blood by Rh negative blood of the proper ABO group is necessary.

In recent years a vaccine has been developed that prevents the Rh negative woman from becoming sensitized to her baby's blood. No later than three days after a miscarriage or the birth of her first Rh positive child, the mother receives an injection of *RhoGam*. This special gamma globulin preparation curtails her production of anti-Rh antibodies and virtually eliminates any danger to future children. The injection must be repeated after each birth or miscarriage.

Human bloods may also be divided into three types called the M, N, and MN. Although these blood factors are inherited, just as are the A, B, O, and Rh factors, they have little importance in blood transfusion, nor does their presence cause any sort of disability. Since they are inherited, however, they may be used in deciding questions of disputed parentage or other medicolegal problems. Among Americans, the types occur in a ratio of approximately M, 30%; N, 20%; and MN, 50%.

Additional, less frequently occurring, and clinically less important blood types have been described which, in rare instances, can be found to be the cause of otherwise unexplained transfusion reactions and hemolytic disease in the newborn. The most important of these are known as Hr, Kell, Duffy, Lewis, Lutheran, and Kidd.

Blood tests

Since the blood performs many services for all parts of the body, it will reflect disturbances that occur as the result of many widely divergent diseases. This has led to the development of a variety of "blood tests" which the physician may perform, either to confirm a diagnosis or to follow the effectiveness of treatment in the patient.

There are two ways in which blood may be obtained for these blood tests. When only a drop or so is needed, the blood can be obtained by pricking the end of the finger, the lobe of the ear, or in the case of infants, the heel. When larger amounts are needed, the blood is taken from an appropriate vein with a hypodermic needle and syringe. The vein usually chosen is the one in the inner aspect of the elbow, but any available vein may be used when necessary.

The taking of a blood sample under *aseptic* precautions is a simple routine process in home, office, or hospital. Only slight pain is experienced when the needle enters the skin. After the needle is withdrawn, the vein will seal itself. Any bleeding from the skin puncture will be slight and will last only a few moments if slight pressure is applied to the area with sterile cotton.

There are many types of tests which the physician may desire to have performed upon the blood, and large hospital laboratories usually have separate laboratories for performing each type or group of tests. The *immunological* or *serological* tests are performed to confirm the diagnosis of selected types of infectious diseases,

INHERITANCE OF THE BLOOD GROUPS

Blood Groups of Parents	Blood Groups which may occur in Children	Blood Groups which do not occur in Children
O × O	O	A, B, AB
O × A	O, A	B, AB
A × A	O, A	B, AB
O × B	O, B	A, AB
B × B	O, B	A, AB
A × B	O, A, B, AB	—
O × AB	A, B	O, AB
A × AB	A, B, AB	O
B × AB	A, B, AB	O
AB × AB	A, B, AB	O

Copyright 1951 Laurence H. Snyder and D. C. Heath and Co.

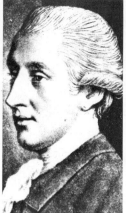

HEWSON, William (1739-1774) English surgeon. He is noted for his studies on the mechanism of blood clotting. In the year 1771 he discovered that a plasma protein known as *fibrinogen* is the particular substance that is converted into the mesh of the clot. In this process fibrinogen is converted into fibrin. He also studied the structure of the human lymphatic system, and contributed greatly to the knowledge of its physiology and anatomical arrangement.

and are based on the principle that in certain diseases there appear in the blood specific substances (antibodies) which are produced by the body in resisting invasion by specific disease-producing organisms. One of the more widely used tests is the Kolmer test for syphilis. It is routine to perform such a test on all hospital patients as a part of the concerted effort to stamp out syphilis in this country. This or a similar test is also required by law in many states for applicants for marriage licenses, and is usually ordered by the physician for pregnant women. The blood typing tests are also serological in nature. A second group of blood tests are known as *hematological.* These tests determine the number of each type of circulating blood cell (the *blood count),* the total volume of red cells in a blood sample *(hematocrit),* and the hemoglobin content of the blood. A *differential* blood count is one in which selected dyes are used to distinguish better the different kinds of white blood cells. These tests are important to the doctor in diagnosing and treating many illnesses including infections, the anemias, and the leukemias.

Still another group of tests utilizing blood samples involves *bacteriological* techniques. Blood and bone marrow samples are obtained under aseptic precautions, and introduced into a variety of artificial culture media, with subse-

quent isolation and identification of the specific microorganism responsible for the illness. Relative susceptability of the specific strain of bacteria to the available chemotherapeutic and antibiotic agents may then be determined and the effectiveness of such agents in sterilizing the blood-stream can be determined by further blood cultures.

Many *chemical* tests are performed on blood samples to determine the quantitative relationships between circulating globulins, albumin, sugar, nonprotein nitrogen, minerals, and other normal and abnormal constituents of the blood plasma. Such chemical tests are important in diabetes, kidney disease, the failing heart, and in pancreatic and liver diseases. In all of these disorders, pronounced changes in the relative amounts of the various chemical constituents of the blood occur. Not only are such chemical tests of value in confirming the physician's diagnosis of the disease, but they also help to follow the clinical course of the ailment. Chemical tests may also be performed on urine, spinal fluid, and saliva for some special purpose, and since most of these fluids are derived from the blood plasma, their chemical analysis frequently reflects changes in the blood itself. During prolonged therapy with certain drugs, it may also be desirable to measure chemically the concentration of the drug in the blood plasma.

ANDRAL, Gabriel (1797-1876) French physician. He is said to have been the originator of the term *anemia.* He was a vigorous opponent of the practice of bloodletting, once used as a treatment for many types of disorders. The term for increased circulation in a tissue area, *hyperemia,* was also proposed by Andral, who is noted for having edited the scientific writings of Laennec, the discoverer of the stethoscope and its clinical application.

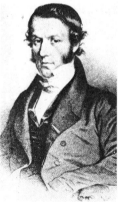

7 THE HEART AND CIRCULATION

WHAT IT IS AND DOES

The circulatory system is made up of the *heart, arteries, veins, and capillaries.* Together, they function as an intricate "pipeline" system for transporting the blood throughout the body. This pipeline has an aggregate length of tubing which reaches many miles. Some investigators have estimated that the capillary system alone would cover almost ten acres of surface.

The heart

The heart is the central pump of the circulatory system and weighs somewhat less than three-quarters of a pound, varying somewhat upon the size of the individual. The heart is essentially a hollow muscle capable of contraction like other muscles. Each contraction is designated a "heartbeat." The rate of these heartbeats can be changed by two different sets of nerves. The accelerating nerves are connected to the spinal cord and are a part of the sympathetic nervous system. The other set, which depresses the rate, is known as the *vagus nerve* and is connected to the brain stem. Starting long before birth, the beats must continue as long as life continues. The beats occur at the rate of 70 or 80 times per minute in adults, but may increase to more than 100 beats per minute during exertion or in the presence of emotional upsets. The beats continue, year after year, whether the individual is at sleep, work, or play. It has been estimated that the heart beats some three billion times during a 70-year span of human existence; this averages about 42 million beats per year. Every contraction moves a little more than two fluid ounces of blood out into the arteries. This provides a change of blood over the body about once every minute. A total of 250 million quarts of blood are moved during a lifetime of 70 years—almost enough to fill a large football stadium with blood. There are only a little over six quarts in the average human body, so that this blood requires not only rapid circulation but also a fine adjustment of controls to assure the proper and effective distribution required by the body.

The heart, by its contractions, forces the blood through the arteries to all parts of the body. The arteries end in innumerable small networks of tiny blood vessels *(capillaries),* which transfer the blood and its nutrients to the various tissues of the body. The capillaries then conduct the blood from the tissues to the veins from which it passes to the heart again. Before sending the blood back through the body, the heart shunts it up into the lungs to gather a new supply of oxygen. Then, the enriched blood returns to the heart, ready to go out again into the body.

To perform this work, the heart is divided into four chambers—two *auricles* and two *ventricles.* Blood, coming from over the body through the large veins *(venae cavae)* enters the *right* auricle. This blood has been partially depleted of its oxygen. As the lower, thick-muscled ventricles expand, this blood enters the *right* ventricle through the *tricuspid valve.* Then, the ventricle contracts and forces the blood into the pulmonary artery toward the capillaries in the lungs and is prevented from running back into the heart by the closure of the *pulmonary*

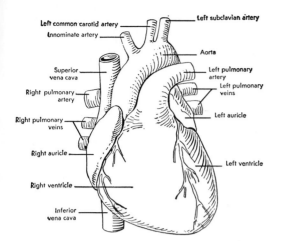

This is a drawing of the human heart as viewed from the front of the body. Many of the major anatomical characteristics of this vital organ are shown.

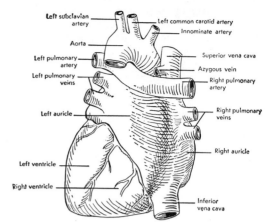

Drawing of a rear view of the normal human heart, illustrating the position of its four chambers and their relationship to the blood vessels.

valve. In the meantime, the purified blood in the *left* auricle has just arrived from the lungs through the *pulmonary veins.* From here it passes into the thick-walled *left* ventricle through the *mitral valve.* When the right ventricle forces blood out into the *pulmonary* artery, the left ventricle at the same time contracts and sends blood out into the arteries of the body, passing through the *aortic valve* into the aorta. The auricles thus act as collecting chambers, while the ventricles function as pumps. The right side of the heart collects the blood and forces it through the lungs, while the left side collects it from the lungs and forces it through the body as a whole. The four valves between the various chambers of the heart prevent the blood from flowing backward and maintain the pressure between heartbeats because of the closed system that results.

It is important that the heart muscles expand and contract at just the right time and that all the valves open and close completely at the proper time during the cycle, in order that blood can be moved forward in an orderly manner. This control is accomplished by a special structure known as the *sino-auricular node.* This is the *pacemaker* of the heart. It is not entirely dependent upon the general nervous system, and it has been known to function for some time after breathing has ceased. Sudden changes in temperature, unusual nervous stimuli, fright, a sense of impending danger, or a happy thought affect this heart center, and thereby cause speeding or slowing of the heart. Fortunately, all warm-blooded animals have such a fine adjustment that acceleration or retardation may take place within one one-hundredth of a second.

The sino-auricular node lies in the wall of the right auricle, embedded within the muscular tissue. A heavy partition extends between the left and right side of the heart, so that there is no direct connection between them except for a group of structures consisting of the *auriculo-ventricular* node, the *common bundle* and its left and right branches. The auriculo-ventricular node transmits impulses from the common bundle, also known as the *bundle of His,* thence to the two branches, and from there to a network of muscle fibers which covers the inside of each ventricle. The network extends to the outer covering of the heart. This network has been called the *Purkinje system,* and it assures an almost instantaneous response of the muscles of the ventricles once the impulse has passed into it. Although the heartbeat is not entirely independent of the general nervous system, it may carry on for some time without the ordinary nerve impulses. This is probably best shown in the heart of a rabbit which may continue to beat long after the animal has died. This automaticity of the heartbeat allows for cardiac transplantation.

The normal beating of the heart is associated with the production of electric (or better, *bio-electric*) currents in this organ. These currents are not strong, but they are carried to the surface of the body, where they may be measured by sensitive electrical instruments. With a delicate machine, the *electrocardiograph,* a chart may be made showing the current changes taking place while the heart is beating. This chart is called an *electrocardiogram.* The beat of the normal heart shows a characteristic pattern of electrical responses. An electrocardiogram showing a departure from this pattern may be used by physicians in diagnosing many heart abnormalities. The heart's action can be recorded, or monitored, without electrical connection. Hence, the heart action of the astronauts is monitored from thousands of miles out in space.

There are thousands of small muscle fibers interwoven to make up the walls of the heart. The organ also has its own circulatory system to provide the muscle with nourishment. The whole structure is sheathed with a tough sac, the *pericardium,* containing a small amount of fluid. This provides for lubrication of the rapidly moving heart.

The 70 or 80 normal heartbeats per minute do not allow much time between the expansion and contraction of the four heart chambers. The period of relaxation of the muscles, during which the heart fills, is about equal to that of contraction, when it empties. This period of relaxation permits the heart to recover fully from its work period. The contraction of the heart is called *systole;* the relaxation is called *diastole.*

For the purpose of making the blood move in only one direction, there are not only valves inside the heart, but also in the veins. In addition, in the small veins there is a constricting type of valve which helps adjust the rate of blood flow and the distribution of blood between the several organs, according to need. The capillaries act as the final speed control, by being so small that only one or two rows of

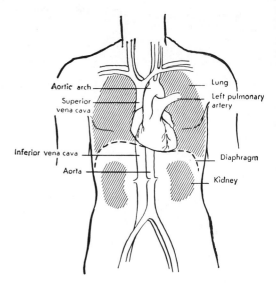

Diagram showing position of the heart and major blood vessels in relation to the kidneys, diaphragm, and lungs. Blood leaves the heart by the aorta.

blood cells may pass through at a time. Here the speed of the flow is so reduced that time is allowed for rebalancing the mineral content of the area, the exchange of oxygen for carbon dioxide and soluble food for waste materials.

Both normal wear and disease may cause undue strain upon the parts of the circulatory system. Fortunately, the make-up of the system is such that most of it may be replaced while it is being used. The smallest capillaries have a fine inner layer of plate-like cells *(endothelium)* which may be removed by circulating blood. Other cells continually grow to replace these. A second covering of muscle tissue cells permits expansion and contraction of the vessels. A third layer consists of connective tissue which is elastic, but which gives tensile strength to the vessels. All of these cells do not wear out at the same time, but the process of removing the old and replacing them with the new continues throughout life. Thus, heart muscle cells of a chicken, when nourished with the proper circulating solutions, may be grown in the laboratory for years after the chicken itself has been dead.

The problem of unloading food substances from the bloodstream at the proper places is largely one of concentration. When materials are lacking in a region just outside of the capillary, they diffuse out through the thin walls of the surrounding area, aided somewhat by the higher pressure within the blood vessels. Individual cells then absorb the nutrients needed for their maintenance and growth. This clear fluid which diffuses out of the capillaries is known as *tissue fluid.* Capillaries do not adjoin

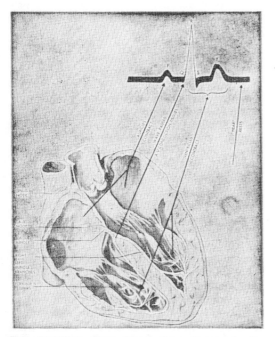

This illustration shows how various changes in the heart during a beat are recorded on the electrocardiogram. *Sharp and Dohme, SEMINAR, 1941.*

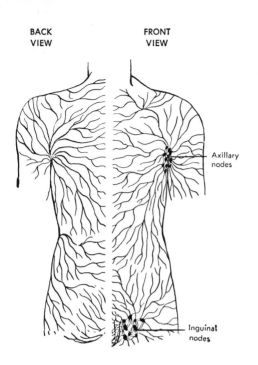

BACK
VIEW

FRONT
VIEW

Axillary
nodes

Inguinal
nodes

Schematic drawing showing the lymphatic vessels and lymphatic nodes which lie near the surface. Although a complex network of vessels exists here, the lymphatic system that lies deeper and serves the internal organs is considered more extensive.

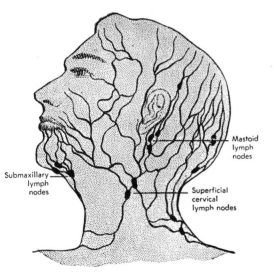

Mastoid
lymph
nodes

Submaxillary
lymph
nodes

Superficial
cervical
lymph nodes

Schematic drawing showing the location of some of the major lymphatic vessels and lymph nodes in the head and neck of man. The lymph nodes may become congested with bacteria and may be swollen in patients with certain infectious diseases.

every cell, so the tissue fluid must transport nutriment from the blood to the individual cells.

The lymphatic system

After the cells have been nourished, the excess tissue fluid, which does not re-enter the blood capillaries, is drained off by another vessel known as a *lymph duct*. It is then called *lymph*. The *lymphatic system* provides for the return of this lymph to the circulatory system. The lymph vessels join with one another to form larger and larger ones, finally forming the *thoracic* and the *right lymphatic ducts,* which lie just under the collarbone. The lymph is transported through these ducts into the blood of the right and left *subclavian* veins. Along the course of the lymph vessels are nodes or "lymph glands" which filter out infectious organisms and other debris which may have been picked up in the tissues. The lymph nodes thus serve as barriers against the spread of infection in the body. The lymph itself contains white blood cells which are able to destroy bacteria, so that it is an additional aid in the body's defenses. Most of the fat that is absorbed from the intestine first enters the lymph vessels *(lacteals)* of the intestinal wall. It is then carried by the lymph through the lymphatic system and finally into the blood. The lymph is not pumped through its system of vessels by any special organ, but is forced along by the massaging effect of other body movements.

The circulation

The beat of the heart forces a temporarily increased amount of blood into the arteries. The arterial walls are elastic, and expand to accommodate this larger volume of blood. Between beats the walls gradually contract, forcing the blood through the capillaries at an approximately constant rate. In this manner, the arteries act as a reservoir which prevents the blood from flowing through the tissues in gushes. The blood in the arteries is constantly under pressure in the same manner that the air in a balloon or rubber tire is under pressure. When the heart stops beating at death, this blood pressure causes a large portion of the blood to flow into the relatively more distensible veins. Because early anatomists found the arteries of dead persons to be nearly empty, they assumed erroneously that in life the arteries conducted air. The word *artery* is therefore derived from a Latin word which means a "windpipe."

The physician can determine the *blood pressure* within the arteries by using a device consisting of an elastic band around the arm, an air pump, and a column of mercury in a glass tube (a *manometer*). The patient's age, his activity, the composition of his blood, the secretions

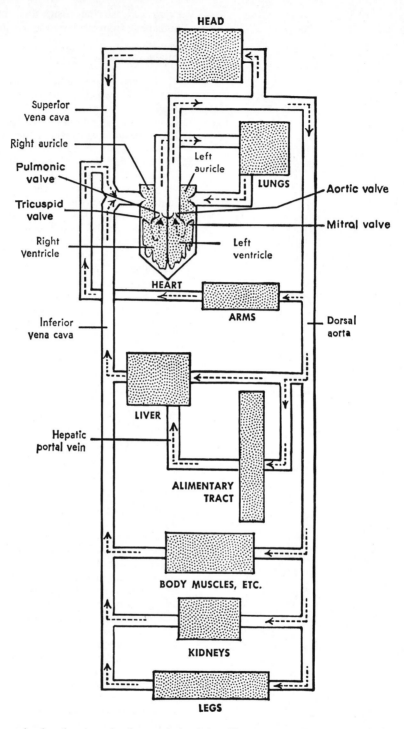

HEAD

Superior
Vena cava

Right auricle

Pulmonic
valve

Tricuspid
valve

Right
Ventricle

Left
auricle

LUNGS

Aortic valve

Mitral valve

Left
ventricle

HEART

Inferior
vena cava

ARMS

Dorsal
aorta

LIVER

Hepatic
portal vein

**ALIMENTARY
TRACT**

BODY MUSCLES, ETC.

KIDNEYS

LEGS

Schematic diagram showing the general scheme of circulation. The arrows indicate how blood leaving the left ventricle passes through various arteries to different parts of the anatomy, and how the blood returns to the heart through the veins, after which it must circulate through the lungs before leaving the left ventricle.

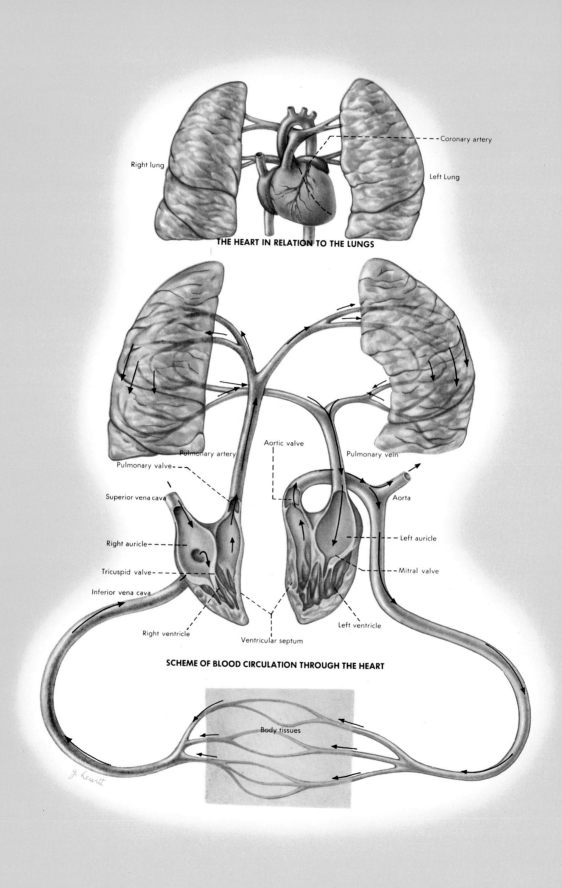

Coronary artery

Right lung

Left Lung

THE HEART IN RELATION TO THE LUNGS

Aortic valve

Pulmonary artery

Pulmonary vein

Pulmonary valve

Superior vena cava

Aorta

Right auricle

Left auricle

Tricuspid valve

Mitral valve

Inferior vena cava

Left ventricle

Right ventricle

Ventricular septum

SCHEME OF BLOOD CIRCULATION THROUGH THE HEART

Body tissues

J. Lewitt

from his adrenal glands, and the thickness of the walls of the blood vessels all have much to do with the blood pressure, which is described in greater detail elsewhere in this chapter.

Blood passing from the heart through the lungs has only about one sixth of that pressure found when the blood is forced out over the body through the *aorta*. But, it still has enough pressure to flow through the multitude of capillaries in the walls of the lungs. The lungs are composed of innumerable small sacs which have a supply of changing air. In the lung or pulmonary capillaries, the blood releases carbon dioxide and takes on oxygen.

The blood continues to flow back through the pulmonary veins and into the left auricle for distribution over the body. The loss of carbon dioxide and the assimilation of oxygen is accompanied by a change of color in the blood, from a dark to a bright red.

While the liver does not have a special connection with the heart, it acts as a storage organ for blood. Blood is carried to the liver from the stomach and intestinal tract by the *portal* vein and from the rest of the body by the *hepatic* artery. It has been estimated that the liver and portal vein drainage system may hold as much as one third of all the blood in the body. When the body is inactive and requires a smaller amount of blood, the liver and portal vein system relieves the remainder of the system by holding a large part of the excess. Some impurities are removed in the liver and excreted into the digestive tract. The hepatic vein returns the blood from the liver to the larger *vena cava* and heart for distribution over the circulatory system.

The blood supply of the heart itself is by way of special *coronary* arteries. These are necessary to supply the thick heart muscles with the large amounts of food and oxygen necessary for their continuous activity. The walls of the blood vessels themselves contain small canals through which blood is transported to nourish the cells of these tissues.

Aside from its function in the transportation of materials throughout the body, the circulatory system plays an important role in temperature regulation. This arises by virtue of the ability of the muscular walls of the blood vessels to expand or contract, thereby changing the diameter of the vessels. When the capillaries in the skin are expanded or *dilated*, a larger amount of blood flows through them. If the temperature outside of the body is below body temperature (98.6° Fahrenheit), the blood in these capillaries is cooled. This cooled blood is then transported to the interior of the body where it is able to counterbalance any tendency toward a rise in temperature. On a cold day these surface capillaries will be constricted so that the blood will not lose undue amounts of heat to the atmosphere.

Illustration: Anatomy of the Heart . . . Grace Hewitt

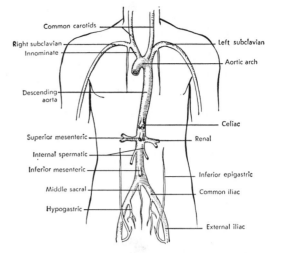

Schematic diagram illustrates the general plan of the main arteries in the body. Branching off from the aorta at various points along its length are the major arteries which conduct oxygenated blood to the many body organs and structures.

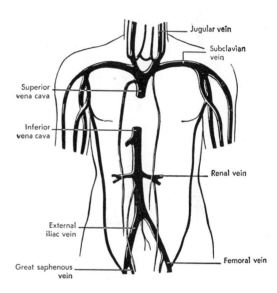

Illustration showing the plan of the main veins. The blood which has supplied the various regions of the body with food and oxygen is conducted by these veins to the superior and inferior vena cavae, which transport the blood to right auricle.

The exact sizes of the various blood vessels thus vary automatically with the particular needs of the body. Many drugs which cause a constriction of the blood vessels (*vasoconstrictors*) bring about a rise in blood pressure by causing the vessels to press more forcibly on their fixed content of blood. *Vasodilators*, by contrast, generally bring about a reduction in the blood pressure. Physiological changes in the sizes of the

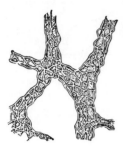

Greatly enlarged drawing of several veins, showing the intricate network (plexus) of lymphatic vessels that surround them. From these networks, the lymphatic fluid is returned by the way of larger lymphatic vessels to the blood. Without such a complex collecting system for collecting lymphatic fluid, the plasma would be lost from the blood vessels into the surrounding tissues and be left to stagnate.

blood vessels are in part under the control of vasodilators and vasoconstrictors produced naturally in the body, and partially under the control of the nervous system. Sometimes a substance that causes a constriction of the blood vessels in one tissue may dilate the vessels in another. The hormone secreted by the medulla of the adrenal glands is one example of a natural vasoconstrictor that aids in regulating the blood pressure of the body.

DISORDERS OF THE HEART AND CIRCULATION: PREVENTION

Although many advances have been made in recent years in diagnosis and therapy of the heart and circulation, the facet which in time can produce the most desired results is prevention. Accumulated data now reveal that the staggering percentage of annual deaths attributable to cardiovascular disease (over 50%) can be reduced considerably by a few simple daily rules of life, namely the avoidance of tobacco and certain foods, daily exercise, and the maintenance of proper weight.

A diet containing polyunsaturated fats (fats which are liquid at room temperature, such as

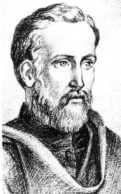

CANANO, Giovanni Battista (1515-1579) Italian anatomist. One of the greatest figures in the earlier history of modern anatomy, Canano is most noted for his very important discovery of the valves that occur in the major veins, which had previously been overlooked by the anatomists of the middle ages. A single observation such as this one was sufficient to create a major change in thinking by the medical profession regarding the circulation.

corn, cottonseed, safflower, sesame, and soybean oils) tend to lower blood-cholesterol levels and in turn lower the risk of development of certain heart diseases. Foods containing saturated fats (fats which are solid at room temperature, such as butter and cheese, whole milk, beef, pork, ham, lamb, sausage, shellfish and eggs) which are known to raise the blood-cholesterol level and the chances of strokes and heart attacks should be eaten with moderation. If either hypertension, diabetes, or a familial susceptibility to heart disease is suspected, medical advice should be sought, but other important factors, such as cigarette smoking, excessive weight and lack of regular exercise remain the problems of each individual. Any local chapter of the American Heart Association will supply menus, recipes, and further information without charge as a public service. It is entirely possible that only slight changes in the plan of daily living could be lifesaving.

DISORDERS OF THE HEART AND CIRCULATION: DIAGNOSTIC PROCEDURES

The history, obtained by the physician, and the physical examination of the patient, are often sufficient to determine the type and severity of circulatory disease present. But additional aids are of value, and will be discussed here. One of the most simple and inexpensive diagnostic procedures available to the physician is the stethoscopic examination of the heart. The only tool needed is a properly fitting stethoscope, the physician's "hearing aid." As is the case with many discoveries, the stethoscope was improvised out of pure necessity by Doctor Rene Laennec. Finding it impractical to place his ear, in the usual manner of his day, on the chest of one of his patients, because of her rather stout configuration as well as her sex, he rolled a quire of paper into a hollow tube, placed one end above the young woman's heart and placed his ear on the other end. He found, much to his delight, that he could hear the sounds of the heart much better than he ever had before. Since that day in 1816, the stethoscope has played an important role in the discovery of many defects and diseases of the heart.

In medical literature, the characteristic sounds of the beating heart are often referred to as the normal "lub-dub." Any deviation from this sound pattern may indicate some form of heart disease. In some disorders, extra noises which are called "murmurs" may be interposed with the normal heart sounds. The location of the murmur, the quality and intensity of its sound, and its timing in relation to the heartbeat help indicate to the physician the nature and degree of the disorder. For example, a harsh "machinery" type murmur heard during systole and diastole between the first and second interspaces of the ribs to the left of the sternum is a characteristic sign of *patent ductus arteriosus*, a congenital malformation which will be discussed later. A low-pitched, scarcely audible, rumbling murmur is characteristic of mitral stenosis. Murmurs during systole may indicate several different forms of heart disease, both congenital and acquired, and considerable experience is required to differentiate one from another. Many systolic murmurs, particularly in children, are of no significance and do not indicate congenital or acquired heart disease. These innocent or "functional" murmurs cause trouble only in being misinterpreted as a sign of heart disease.

Still another procedure used in the diagnosis of diseases of the chest is percussion. Percussion was first described in 1761 by Doctor Leopold Auenbrugger, who had two natural inclinations which led to the development of this diagnostic procedure. First, he was an accomplished musician, and second, he was the son of an innkeeper and so learned at an early age to estimate the amount of liquid in a barrel by listening to the sound which resulted from thumping on the outside with his fingers. The same procedure, when applied to the human chest, gives useful information on the size and shape of the heart. The duller percussion note over the solid organ, the heart, as compared to the more tympanitic sound elicited over the air-containing organ, the lung, defines the heart border.

One of the most dramatic procedures for diagnosis in use by the cardiologist today is cardiac catheterization. In this procedure, a long tube is inserted into a vein in the arm or leg and pushed slowly until the tip enters the heart. The tip of the catheter (tube) has a small opening for withdrawing samples of blood, and also contains an electrode for relaying information back to a bank of instruments and gauges for recording. Some of the most important knowledge gained by this procedure is blood pressure in the various chambers of the heart and the amount of oxygen in the blood in these chambers.

In addition, a dye which is visible to x-ray film can be injected into the bloodstream for studying the course of blood through the heart. X-ray pictures, taken at rapid intervals, will reveal the size and position of the heart chambers and great vessels. These two procedures are of particular importance in diagnosis of congenital heart disease. The dye can also be forced into the aorta through one of the arteries for studying any defects in the aorta (retrograde aortagram). After a careful evaluation of the information gained from these studies, the physician is able to ascertain the nature and severity of any defects in the valves or chambers of the heart and great vessels.

Chemical assays for certain constituents of the blood have been found useful in the diagnosis of certain disorders of the circulatory system. For instance, it has been shown that a change in the level of certain enzymes in the blood occurs when the heart muscle undergoes changes because of lack of oxygen (myocardial infarction). This information is a valuable addendum to other data obtained by the physician for evaluating the extent of myocardial damage.

DISORDERS OF THE HEART AND CIRCULATION: HARDENING OF THE ARTERIES

Arteriosclerosis, or hardening of the arteries, is a condition that exists when the walls of the blood vessels thicken and become infiltrated with excessive amounts of minerals and fatty materials. Accumulation of minerals in the human body normally is restricted to the teeth and the bones. In a number of different diseases, however, calcium salts are deposited in various other tissues. Such calcification of almost any of the soft tissues may occur in a number of rare diseases. Arteriosclerosis, however, is a common disease of middle and old age.

Vigorous, overactive people of florid countenance seem to have hardening of the arteries (and high blood pressure) more frequently than the less robust type. Arteriosclerosis occurs in all races and among people living in all climates. Alcoholics and drug addicts, contrary to popular opinion, do not seem to be unusually susceptible to the disease.

There are a number of different forms of arteriosclerosis, the names of which indicate the location of the disorder. One type is present to some extent in almost all people over 50 years of age. In this form, the hardening starts in the layer of the arterial wall most closely in contact with the blood (the *intima*). In this, and in another type in which the middle layers of the arterial walls (the *media*) are involved, the earliest and most pronounced changes are in the larger blood vessels. A third form of arteriosclerosis affects principally the smaller arteries of the kidneys, pancreas, spleen, adrenals, and certain other organs. Because this form occurs in the *arterioles*, it is called arteriolosclerosis.

The difficulties in diagnosing arteriosclerosis and the uncertainties of most remedies have perplexed the medical profession since earliest times. Both the symptoms and the required treatment vary considerably from one individual to another. The progress of the disease is slow in

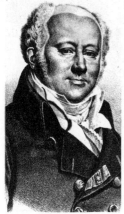

CORVISART des MARETS, Jean Nicolas (1755-1821) French clinician. He was probably the greatest heart specialist of his time, and is generally credited with the first sound exposition of the basic symptoms associated with heart disease. He was the first man to describe the exact mechanics of heart failure, and also the reason for many other relatively common types of heart disorder which up until his time had remained largely in the realm of mysticism and superstition.

most cases, and by the time first symptoms occur, the characteristic changes in the circulatory system have been developing for some time. Although gross symptoms may not develop until the sixth decade of life, loss of normal elasticity of the arteries is believed to start much earlier.

In general, the signs of arteriosclerosis are those that might be expected when the circulation is impaired. There may be a numbness or coldness in the hands and feet, and the victim may tire more readily than usual. The thinking processes may become slower and the memory, less acute. Thus, the earlier symptoms of impaired circulation of the blood induced by a slight hardening of the arteries may be those which are usually associated with advancing age.

As the condition progresses, however, the symptoms may become quite pronounced—usually in the areas of the body where the arterial hardening is most extreme. For instance, if the arteries in the extremities become hardened, cramping, aching, tingling, or sharp pains may occur upon movement of the legs or arms. There may be a decrease or complete lack of pulsation in some of the arteries, such as the *popliteal artery*, which lies just under the skin of the leg and can be examined readily by the physician. Again, if the arteries which supply blood to the brain become hardened, a partial loss of mental acuity may occur. A "stroke" (rupture or blockage of an artery) can cause a loss of memory and decreased control over normal body functions. These changes—should they occur—are not necessarily permanent.

If hardening occurs in the arteries leading to the kidneys, the symptoms may be similar to those resulting from other kidney disorders. Various types of heart disease also may occur. Other afflictions, which may have been dormant in the body for many years, frequently appear at this time.

The relationship of these many symptoms to the actual changes in the arterial walls is a complex one. The first changes in the hardened arteries are the appearance of small yellowish streaks on the inner surface of the arterial wall. These are caused by the presence of patches of newly-formed connective tissue and cells filled with fatty material. The muscle tissue in the walls slowly becomes more fibrous and less elastic, and larger amounts of fat are deposited in the surface of the blood vessel. One of the most important components of this fatty material is a substance known as *cholesterol*, the deposition of which is one of the features of arterial hardening. As new tissue is laid down in the arterial walls, part of it may project into the hollow portions of the blood vessel; this slows the flow of blood. Within the new tissue are deposited varying amounts of minerals, which bring about the hardening process. The major artery leading from the heart (the *aorta*) is frequently involved in this manner. However, this in itself seldom causes significant disease. Serious consequences may develop if a small portion of the material that clogs the vessels breaks loose and flows along in the blood stream. Such a particle is called an *embolus*, and the condition that results is known as *embolism*. The embolus may become lodged in some smaller vessel, cutting off a portion of the blood supply to some part of the body. When the brain, kidney, lung, or heart is deprived of its normal circulation in this manner, the situation is particularly dangerous. The damage to the patient depends upon the location of the occluded blood vessel. If it is in the brain, it can cause a stroke; if in the heart, a myocardial infarction (coronary thrombosis); if in the legs, pain on walking or even gangrene. Another type of arterial disease is *thromboangiitis obliterans* (Buerger's disease) which may also involve the veins. This causes gangrene but can be controlled by eliminating the cause, particularly tobacco. Other arterial diseases cause blanching of the fingers, toes, nose, and even the cheeks (Raynaud's phenomenon).

Although a mild form of arteriosclerosis occurs in most older people, there is no reason to think that this condition is a normal and unavoidable part of the aging process. While the exact causes of the disease remain largely unknown, certain factors seem to be definitely associated with the onset of arteriosclerosis. Heredity appears to play a role because the males in certain families are more prone to arterial hardening than in others. Hormones may be involved, for women seldom contract the disease before the menopause. In addition, a high cholesterol level is usually found in the patient's blood. Further, persons suffering from diabetes may develop hardening of the arteries much earlier in life than nondiabetics. Early recognition and adequate management of diabetes may forestall the development of severe arteriosclerosis.

Treatment

The seriousness of arteriosclerosis and the manner in which it is handled by the physician depend almost entirely upon the individual patient and upon the extent to which the condition has progressed. The mild form of arteriosclerosis that comes with aging is seldom accompanied by appreciable changes in the interior diameter of the arteries or by high blood pressure. For this reason, most patients are treated in such a manner as to prevent this form from becoming more severe. Almost all of the treatment rests with the patient himself, since it is he who must observe dietary precautions and find a way of life that is conducive to relaxation. Some patients may become anxious and nervous when they learn that they have a mild form of arteriosclerosis. They need not be, for actually the condition is a common one that will not seriously limit the patient in his ordinary activities.

It is now believed that methionine, inositol, and choline (fat-destroying chemicals found in plants and animals) may be even more effective in retarding the deposition of cholesterol plaques on the inner surface of the arteries.

Patients with the more severe forms of arteriosclerosis require long and careful treatment. A restful way of life, proper diet, and a healthy mental outlook are among the most important ingredients of the treatment. Since the affliction principally involves the circulatory system, the heart must be protected from overwork. Care should be taken that improperly fitting shoes or other clothing do not add a further impediment to the circulation of the blood. When the extremities are involved, one should be particularly careful to avoid exposure of the hands and feet to cold and dampness. If the disease is severe, proper care of corns, calluses, or other areas that may become infected is of great importance. A constant watch must be kept for symptoms of other diseases that may occur and complicate the condition; if any unusual symptom does appear, it should be reported at once to the physician.

A number of special treatments may be employed by the physician in cases where they seem desirable. Special diets may be prescribed which will limit the amount and type of fat that is consumed. Fish oils and vegetable oils do not contain the *saturated fatty acids* which lead to high cholesterol levels in the blood. The fats of land mammals, however, are abundant in these substances and so are usually forbidden in the patient's diet.

An interesting new scientific approach to an old proverb came to light when an investigation by Ancel Keys showed that 15 grams of pectin per day would also lower the level of unwanted fatty substances in the blood. Thus, the familiar old adage, "An apple a day keeps the doctor away" at last found scientific verification since 15 grams is the amount of pectin found in two ripe apples. (Further information may be found in Chapter 21, "Nutrition" and in "Prevention of Cardiovascular Disease" in this chapter.) Massage and heat should only be applied by the physician.

There are certain drugs known to reduce the blood levels of cholesterol. Among these are certain analogues or precursors of the hormone of the thyroid gland (triiodothyropropionic acid). These along with proper diet may prove useful in preventing arteriosclerosis.

In some instances when the disease has progressed to a considerable degree, parts of the afflicted areas may have to be removed surgically and circulation restored with a Dacron graft (see "How an Artery is Transplanted" in this chapter). Occasionally, the artery can just be reamed out surgically with a process known as *endarterectomy*. Such steps are of great value in improving the comfort of the patient. Surgical treatment may also be necessary if the circulation in an afflicted portion of the body is so curtailed that the tissues in that area die. This condition, known as *gangrene*, requires immediate treatment if the limb, and perhaps the life of the patient, is to be saved.

In cases of *pulmonary embolism*, where clots have occurred in the vessels of the lungs, the heart-lung by-pass machine using sugar and water instead of whole blood for the primer, which reduces the time required to find the right type of blood and allows the surgeon immediate access to the diseased vessels, has been lifesaving in many instances.

DISORDERS OF THE HEART AND CIRCULATION: VARICOSE VEINS

Varicose veins are veins that have lost their elasticity and as a consequence are irregularly enlarged and swollen; they have a dilated, lumpy, twisted and tortuous appearance. The overlying skin may be affected with ulcers. Varicose veins are most often seen in the legs of middle-aged and older persons, although certain conditions, such as pregnancy, may cause them to appear in younger adults. The dilation of the veins results from the inability of the weakened venous walls to withstand the pressure of the blood within the veins.

If the veins were simply continuous tubes running from the legs to the heart, the weight of a column of blood carried this high would press out on the leg veins when the individual stood erect. Normally, the column of blood is broken by the presence of valves which prevent the full weight of the blood from causing a pressure on the veins in the leg. If a vein loses its elasticity, it will become distended, and the valves will fail

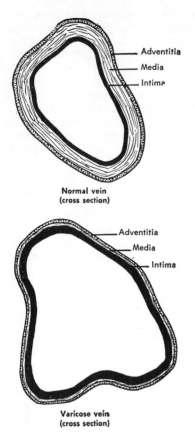

Normal vein
(cross section)

Adventitia
Media
Intima

Adventitia
Media
Intima

Varicose vein
(cross section)

Diagrammatic drawings of normal and varicose veins, showing thickened *intima* in the latter which results in loss of elasticity and increased size.

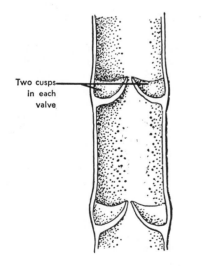

Two cusps in each valve

This drawing of a larger vein portrays how valves composed of two cusps occur along the vein and prevent the backflow of blood in these vessels.

to close completely and function properly. The weight of the blood in that vein then presses out on walls of the vein, causing even more distention; and a reversal of the flow of blood in that vein may occur. The veins also may become swollen when a venous constriction prevents the normal emptying of the blood.

Symptoms

The symptoms of varicose veins depend upon the cause of the condition, its duration, location, and severity. Since the leg veins are normally somewhat distended when an individual is in a standing position, the condition may not be noticed when it first appears. Often the change in the veins is slow, progressing over many years. This is particularly true when the situation results from standing for long periods of time. In such cases, the first suggestion of the disease that an individual may have is a sensation of heaviness or fatigue in the legs. The patient may notice that he develops cramps in his legs at night. There may be a dull ache in the feet and legs, and the ankles may swell more than is usual after a day's work. All such symptoms can result from other conditions, so they are not conclusive evidence of varicose veins.

The classical sign of varicose veins is the actual appearance in the legs of swollen, tortuous blue veins. The enlargement may affect a short segment of a single vein, or nearly all of the veins in the entire leg. When a systemic disease is responsible for the disorder, it usually appears in both legs to an equal degree. A *phlebitis*, constriction, injury, or obstruction in the veins in one leg, however, will cause varicose veins in only that leg.

Aside from their disfiguring nature, varicose veins can cause appreciable physical discomfort. Both dull and stabbing pains may be felt, and the entire limb may become quite swollen. When the condition has existed for some time, the veins sometimes become toughened and thick, so that they feel firm to the touch. More often, however, they are soft and elastic, except at the hard knotty swellings which occur in the regions of the valves. Ulceration and bleeding may leave large black and blue areas beneath the skin.

In men a type of varicosity may occur in which the veins in the scrotum are affected. In this condition, known as *varicocele*, the scrotum contains a soft tumor-like mass of swollen venous material. Likewise, varicosity of the veins in the rectum is known as *hemorrhoids* or *piles*. This condition is discussed in detail in Chapter 13, "The Digestive System."

Prevention

Persons from families with histories of varicose veins should give considerable thought to

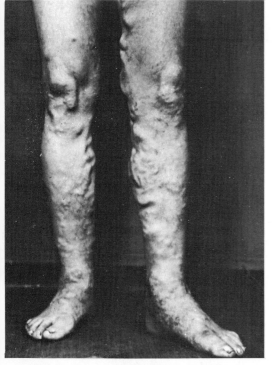

Great saphenous vein varicoses on both legs.

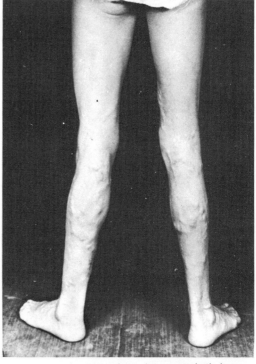

Lesser saphenous vein varicoses on both legs.

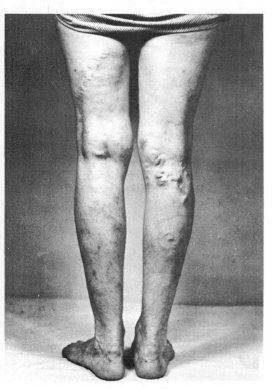

Greater and lesser saphenous vein varicoses.

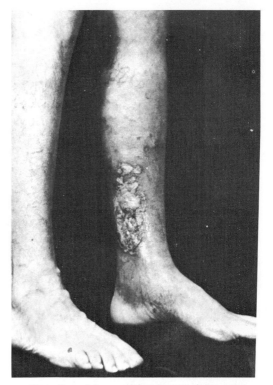

Ulceration of leg resulting from varicose veins.

Photographs from Eger, Sherman A., M.D.; and Wagner, Frederick B., Jr., M.D.; Varicose Veins, GP, Sept. 1951, Vol. 4, No. 3., 32–39. Copyright American Academy of General Practice.

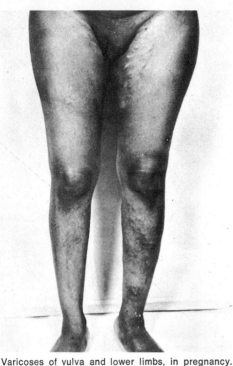 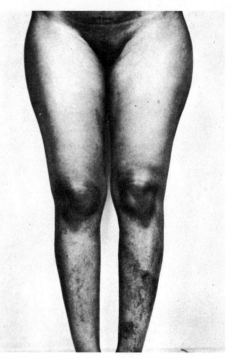

Varicoses of vulva and lower limbs, in pregnancy.   Varicoses of vulva and leg recede after delivery.

Photographs from Eger, Sherman A., M.D.; and Wagner, Frederick B., Jr., M.D.; Varicose Veins, GP, Sept. 1951, Vol. 4, No. 3., 32–39. Copyright American Academy of General Practice.

the simple measures that can be used to lessen the probability of their having this venous disorder. They should attempt to follow occupations which do not involve long hours of standing. When resting, such persons should practice elevating the legs on a footstool or in some other manner, so that the venous pressure in the legs is minimized. During long automobile, airplane, or train trips, they should take frequent opportunities to get up and walk about. Clothing should be loose. Garters, girdles, elastic waistbands, and tight-fitting shoes should be avoided. Both occupational and avocational pursuits should be those in which the dangers of blows to the legs are minimized. During pregnancy, a regular time should be spent in a reclining position, and the signs of any unusual symptom in the legs should be reported to the obstetrician.

Treatment

Determination of the cause of varicose veins must precede any positive steps toward alleviating the condition. When varicosity develops suddenly, there is probably a sudden increase in pressure or a temporary obstruction of the venous flow above the level of the varicosity. Such circulatory obstructions may disappear in

a short time, so that little treatment is needed. Usually the condition is slowly progressive.

Some cases may require no more care than an increase in the amount of time that the patient keeps the legs elevated. Stockings of elastic yarn or mercerized silk often are used for supporting the veins in the legs. Rubber and adhesive tape bandages are also effective but are more trouble to apply. Supporting stockings should be made to measure, and worn only under medical supervision. The leg dressing must exert uniform pressure without constricting veins at a higher level.

Elevation of the legs above the heart level will permit easy emptying of the veins and relieve swelling and pain. Bathing the limb in lukewarm water also may be helpful if infected leg ulcers are not present.

One of the oldest and best known methods for treating patients with varicosities involves the use of solutions which harden or *sclerose* those veins most severely afflicted. The invention and development of the hypodermic syringe by the French physician Pravaz in 1853 was followed almost immediately by his demonstration that the injection of veins with iron chloride solutions caused them to harden and ultimately to become less painful. Since that time, a great many improvements have been made in the injection technique and in the materials that may be used for this purpose. Many considerations enter into the decision as to whether this technique is suitable for use in any particular case. These include the size and location of the varicosities, the age and general health of the patient, and his economic ability to afford other, generally more expensive, but better, methods of treatment.

Injection treatment of the patient is generally conducted in the physician's office, and on repeated trips small amounts of sclerosing solution are injected into the varicosity at different points along its length. In a few hours after the injection, the vein becomes tender, hard and painful, and the tissues around it may be red and swollen. The pain subsides after a few days, however, and in a few weeks the injected portion of the vein becomes a hard cord, which withers and disappears after about two months.

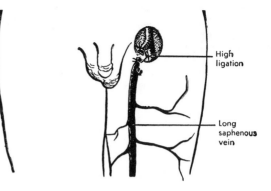

This drawing illustrates the position at which the saphenous vein may be ligated to relieve its distention in patients suffering with varicose veins.

The blood, which previously passed through it, is transported by alternate circulatory pathways in an efficient manner. In some cases, however, these pathways over a period of years also may become varicose, and require subsequent medical attention.

In many cases, the disorder may progress so that the varicose veins get increasingly dilated and tortuous. Hence, it may be necessary to remove portions of a vein that are particularly bothersome or even strip out the entire varicosed vein. In milder cases, it may be necessary merely to tie off (*ligate*) the varicose veins to relieve the pressure. These treatments add greatly to the patient's comfort. Occasionally, a combination of an operation and sclerosing solutions which close off small veins is necessary. Such surgical measures are quite common and are most often likely to afford complete and lasting relief.

Patients with varicose veins must observe the same precautions that are used to prevent the occurrence of the condition. Ample rest with the legs in a horizontal position is of paramount importance. Occupations should be found that do

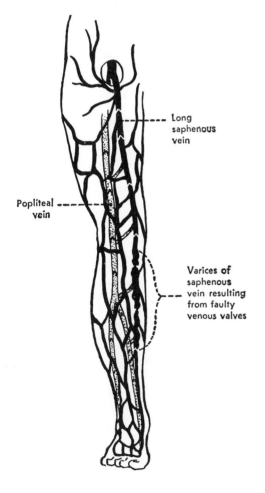

This drawing shows the anatomical distribution of the deep and superficial leg veins and how faulty venous valves may result in varicose veins.

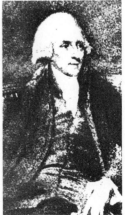

WITHERING, William (1741-1799) English physician. His most famous discovery and the one that changed the entire course of treatment of patients suffering from heart disease was the introduction of the use of digitalis into medical practice during the years 1783-1785. He obtained the secret of this important drug from an old woman versed in the use of herbs and put it to immediate use in the treatment of dropsy. He was also the author of a treatise on scarlet fever.

not demand prolonged periods of standing. Apparel which might constrict the veins and interfere with their normal flow must be avoided. None of these measures will cure the condition, but under competent medical attention, most patients with varicose veins may expect to enjoy a normal span of life with little suffering from their affliction.

DISORDERS OF THE HEART AND CIRCULATION: ANEURYSM

Any weakness in the wall of an artery may bring about distention or the formation of a sac or pouch which protrudes from the wall of the artery, and is called an *aneurysm*.

There are a number of different types of aneurysms. In a *true* aneurysm, the wall of the sac consists of at least one of the layers of tissue that make up the wall of the blood vessel. *False* aneurysms exist when all of the layers of the artery have ruptured, but the blood is still retained by the surrounding tissues. In some cases, the blood may be forced by its pressure between the layers of the arterial wall, causing the layers to separate and form a dissecting aneurysm. Occasionally, an artery and vein may be connected in such a manner that a continuing flow of blood passes from the artery to the vein. Such *arteriovenous* communications result from wounds, aneurysms, or congenital connections between the vessels.

Aneurysms may occur in any artery, the most common site being the large artery leading from the heart (*the aorta*). Small aneurysms sometimes develop in blood vessels as the result of injuries. The rupture of even a small aneurysm in the brain, heart, or other vital organ can be fatal.

Today the most common cause of aortic aneurysm is atherosclerosis (hardening of the arteries). Further, any injury to an arterial wall may leave it so weakened that an aneurysm eventually may occur. Infected (*mycotic*) aneurysms result from destruction of arterial walls by an infectious agent. Pneumonia, streptococcal infections, and gonorrhea are typical diseases that may leave such a weakened blood vessel. Aneurysms of the aorta formerly were common as the result of a previous syphilitic infection, but now are very rare. The most frequent cause of aneurysm is the weakening of the blood vessel wall caused by inflammation and calcium deposition, as in atherosclerosis.

An aneurysm may exist at any site along the aorta, but most common aneurysms seen today are in the abdominal aorta. The symptoms that result are, for the most part, dependent upon the size of the sac and the parts of the body upon which it exerts pressure. These sacs frequently become large, sometimes larger than an orange, and cause severe crowding of the chest or abdominal cavity. There may be a bulging of the area above the collar bone when the aneurysm is near the top of the aorta. Pressure may also be exerted against the ribs, in which case a pulsation may be felt or even seen in this area. Aneurysms are sometimes painful. The pain may be located in the center of the chest, or may radiate into the arms. When aneurysms press against the ribs, the spine, or other bones, the bone may become eroded; pain is particularly great in such instances.

Difficulty in breathing (*dyspnea*) is another common symptom, and may cause more discomfort than actual pain. Dyspnea results from pressure on the windpipe or smaller air passages leading to the lungs. A "brassy" cough is another frequent symptom of aortic aneurysm in the chest.

Aneurysms may cause headaches, abdominal distress, or swelling in various parts of the body, depending on their location. However, many are so symptomless that they are discovered only when careful abdominal examination is done or an x-ray examination is made for some other reason. Most of the symptoms that have been described may also appear as the result of many other diseases. Moreover, many persons have a slight enlargement of the aorta without having an aneurysm. Hence, an x-ray examination is usually necessary to establish that an aneurysm is present. In recent years, angiography, in which contrast material is introduced into the blood vessels, followed by x-ray examination, has become a valuable diagnostic aid.

Treatment

Many aneurysms remain small and never require special treatment, but generally aneurysms tend to grow larger and may progress to rupture. Until recent years, the treatment of such patients centered around alleviating the symptoms and preventing rupture of the sac. The treatment of choice now is complete surgical excision of the aneurysm with subsequent restoration of circulation with an implanted, pleated artificial graft. If the artery is small, the graft may be a segment of vein from the patient. The consensus is that the longer the delay in instigation of surgical therapy, the greater the risk of rupture or the development of more hazardous problems.

Aneurysms in some smaller blood vessels which supply nonvital areas of the body may be tied off and obliterated by special techniques so that the blood no longer passes through the distended area. Other arteries then take over the work of the closed-off vessel.

The size and location of the aneurysm, as well as the general health of the patient, are major

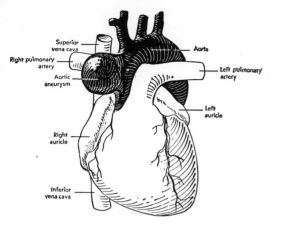

Superior vena cava
Aorta
Right pulmonary artery
Left pulmonary artery
Aortic aneurysm
Left auricle
Right auricle
Inferior vena cava

Illustration of the appearance of an aortic aneurysm, one of the most frequent types of partial rupture of the muscular walls of blood vessels.

determining factors in the physician's choice of treatment. In certain cases, an aneurysm may be complicated; but it is remarkable how minimal the risk is when operating on an abdominal aortic aneurysm. In other instances, the aneurysm may not be sufficiently dangerous to warrant undertaking a complex surgical procedure.

Since the advent of tough, resilient plastic materials such as Dacron and Teflon, the most common treatment is surgical removal followed by replacement of the excised portion with an artificial graft. The vessel is first clamped on each side of the existing aneurysm and the sac is opened. The synthetic tube is then grafted to the vessel with multiple sutures and the blood allowed to resume its flow. In time the intima or inner layer of the blood vessels begins to grow into the synthetic graft, thus completely incorporating it into the vascular system. In recent years, probably no facet of cardiovascular surgery has become so refined as the surgical removal of diseased arteries with subsequent transplantation of a synthetic graft.

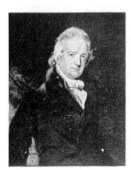

ABERNETHY, John (1764-1831) English surgeon. Abernethy is best remembered in the realm of surgery for the operation that he devised for the relief of patients endangered by an aneurysm, in which the external iliac artery is ligated. Although the procedure involved was a complex one in view of general surgical progress at that time (1796), the operation was sufficiently successful that it bore his name for many years after his death and is still a well-recognized one.

The mental attitude of the patient has a great deal to do with the outlook for his future. Excitement is undesirable. While the patient must be carefully instructed as to the limitations placed on his physical activities, he should not be alarmed. It should be emphasized that the period of invalidism after the appearance of an aneurysm may be followed by a renewal of many of the patient's former activities. Indeed, many patients with aneurysms live for a great number of years after the condition develops, and often work at a gainful employment.

DISORDERS OF THE HEART AND CIRCULATION: HIGH AND LOW BLOOD PRESSURE

Blood pressure refers to the amount of pressure exerted by the blood on the walls of the arteries. When the left *ventricle* of the heart contracts, it forces blood out into the arteries; this causes the major arteries to expand to receive the oncoming blood. The muscular lining of the arteries resists this pressure, and the blood is squeezed out into the smaller vessels of the body. Thus, blood pressure is that amount of pressure the blood is under as a result of the pumping of the heart, the resistance of the arterial walls, and the closing of the heart valves.

The maximum pressure in the arteries is related to the contraction of the left ventricle, and is referred to as the *systolic* pressure. The minimum pressure, which exists just before the heartbeat which follows, is the *diastolic* pressure. The pressure of the blood in the smaller *arterioles* and in the capillaries is much less than in the arteries.

The first demonstration of blood pressure was made over 200 years ago by the English clergyman and scientist, Stephen Hales. A brass tube was inserted in the artery of a horse; the other end of the tube was connected to a long glass tube, using as the connecting link the trachea of a goose (rubber tubing had not been invented). By this means it was possible to observe that the blood rushed into the upright glass tube and eventually rose by repeated pulsations to a height of eight feet and three inches. The top of the column of blood then continued to pulse back and forth a short distance below and above this point. From this observation, the experimenter concluded that the blood pressure of the horse was such that it would support or counterbalance the weight of a column of blood over eight feet high.

Hales' original method of measuring blood pressure was both inconvenient and inaccurate, because the long glass tube greatly increased the volume of the arterial system. Physicians today use a device known as a *sphygmomanometer*. This consists of a flat rubber bag which is connected to a column of mercury. The bag may be inflated with air by a small hand pump or bulb. The height of the column of mercury indicates the pressure of the air in the rubber bag. If this bag is wound around the arm and then inflated with air, it will become so tight that it cuts off the circulation of the arteries in the arm. Under these circumstances, there will cease to be any pulse in the arm beyond the point at which the circulation is cut off. If now the pressure in the arm band is gradually released, it will eventually come down to some point at which the maximum systolic pressure is just able to force the blood through the arteries under the rubber arm band. This pressure may be detected by listening to the arteries with a special instrument made to conduct such sounds, a *stethoscope*. At this point, the pressure of the air in the cuff equals the systolic pressure, and may be read from the height of the column of mercury as the sounds are heard. When the pressure in the cuff is further released, a point will be reached at which the blood will be able to flow through the constricted artery under its lower, or diastolic pressure. The reading on the column of mercury at the moment the last distinct sounds are heard, is the diastolic pressure. Since mercury is about 13.5 times as heavy as water or blood, the pressure in terms of the height of a column of mercury is less than one-thirteenth as high as it would be in terms of a column of water—or blood, as in Hales' experiment. The value is usually stated in millimeters of mercury rather than in inches.

The average systolic blood pressure in young adult men is about 120 millimeters (about five inches) of mercury. The diastolic pressure is about 80 millimeters of mercury. These figures are frequently stated as 120/80, or 120 over 80. Pressures in this range usually are able to provide the body with an adequately circulating supply of blood without placing any undue strain

on the walls of the blood vessels. Considerable *normal* variations from these values may occur, and values as much as 20 millimeters below those stated may be encountered in healthy individuals. At birth, the systolic pressure is between 20 and 60 millimeters, and it does not reach 120 until about the seventeenth year. With age, the pressure gradually rises until at 60 years it is about 140/87. These are average values, and one should not be alarmed if his pressure varies from those here presented. In women, the systolic pressure remains about four to five millimeters lower than that of men of the same age. Digestion, exercise, posture, and emotional states may all cause transient variations in the normal pressure. Overweight persons frequently have a higher blood pressure than do individuals who are of normal weight.

A number of factors must work together to maintain the blood pressure within normal limits. The pumping action of the heart itself, of course, is of major importance as is the competency of the heart valves in closing so that no leakage occurs back from the arteries into the heart chambers. The elasticity of the arterial walls also influences the pressure. The resistance that the blood meets in the smaller blood vessels causes considerable variation. The amount of blood in the circulatory system and its thickness (*viscosity*) are also factors. When any of these variables change markedly, the blood pressure may be increased or decreased. These pressure changes, in turn, may produce abnormalities in the structure and function of the heart and blood vessels. The most common variation in the blood pressure is an increase in its magnitude, which is referred to as *hypertension* or high blood pressure.

Hypertension

When a person under conditions of rest consistently has a blood pressure that exceeds 145/90 millimeters of mercury, he is said to have high blood pressure or hypertension. This disorder of the circulation is said to account for 15 to 20 percent of all deaths in the United States in people over 50 years of age. There is evidence that some degree of high blood pressure exists in over 80 percent of all persons over 70 years of age. In some cases, the conditions may result from nervous tension, disturbances of the adrenal glands, kidney disease, vascular disorders, particularly those relating to a narrowing of the renal artery, and a variety of other conditions that are relatively rare. The most common form, however, is caused by factors which are only partially known, and is referred to as *essential hypertension*. In many patients, hypertension is a relatively benign condition existing for years without the development of a critical episode, such as a myocardial infarction,

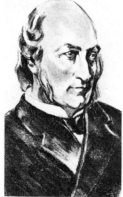

POTAIN, Pierre Carl Edouard (1825-1901) French physician. Most noted for his many important studies on the diseases of the heart, lungs, and stomach, he was also the inventor of the air sphygmomanometer in the year 1889. By this device, the measurement of human blood pressures was greatly facilitated in routine medical practice. He is remembered for his abilities in identifying groups of symptoms that might be indicative of specific diseases.

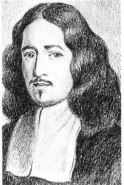

MALPIGHI, Marcello (1628-1694) Italian anatomist and pioneer histologist. Malpighi was the first individual to observe the capillary circulation. He discovered and described a great many of the finer anatomic details of the kidneys, lungs, secretory glands, and nervous system. The glomerulus is often referred to as the Malpighi capsule. He is considered by many as the founder of modern microscopic anatomy.

heart failure, or stroke. However, the actuarial statistics show that the disability and mortality rates of such patients are higher each year than those for persons with normal blood pressure. This has important implications in terms of the decision regarding therapy. In other patients, the course of this disease is rapid and malignant from the beginning, producing a wide variety of serious complications and early death. In young persons and those without evidence of arteriosclerosis, it is imperative to determine whether hypertension is the result of decreased blood supply to the kidney, narrowing (congenital) of the aorta or to tumor or hypersecretion of the adrenal glands.

The increased blood pressure in essential hypertension is caused by an increase in the resistance offered to the flow of the blood through the smaller vessels of the circulatory system. The cause of the constriction of these vessels is unknown. Nervous strain may play an important role. Hereditary factors probably are involved to some extent. Total abstinence from tobacco use is imperative because nicotine causes not only spasms of the small arteries and thus increases resistance to the passage of blood but also favors the development of arteriosclerosis.

Symptoms

High blood pressure itself produces few symptoms, most cases being discovered by accident or through complications which it may produce. The only typical change is the increase in the blood pressure itself. Changes in the smaller blood vessels may cause a number of symptoms. Palpitation of the heart, headache, dizziness, flushing of the face and distended temporal and facial vessels, and fatigue are often noted. In more severe cases, hypertension leads to degenerative changes in the heart and circulation which may present a wide variety of symptoms.

In many cases, it is now known that an impoverished blood supply to one or both of the kidneys can produce what is referred to as renal

hypertension. If either or both of the arteries supplying blood to the kidneys is blocked by a clot, the patient's blood pressure will rise remarkably. This condition can be diagnosed by the study of radioactive or radiopaque materials injected into the bloodstream. Surgical removal of the thrombus brings immediate relief.

Treatment

The outlook for the hypertensive patient depends upon the extent to which the disease has progressed, its rate of progress, and the persistence with which the physician's instructions are followed. In the majority of cases, high blood pressure does not present a serious threat to the life and happiness of the patient. An exception is when the patient becomes unduly anxious and nervous about his condition. He must understand that, with care, his condition may be neither a great handicap nor a danger. A complete physical and functional evaluation by a competent physician may determine if disease or malfunction of one of the organs of the body is producing the elevated pressure and might be corrected surgically. Frequently the kidney is involved, or one of several types of tumors may be present.

In mild cases, bed rest is desirable for a brief period of time, since it usually helps to alleviate any symptoms that may have developed. Following this initial rest period, the patient should seek an occupation at which there is little hard physical labor, and in which he will have considerable time free for rest and relaxation. He should have at least nine hours of sleep each night. Mental and physical stress must be eliminated. Overexertion should be avoided. Obese persons should reduce their weight. Smaller meals are beneficial.

When it is desired to lower the blood pressure within a short period of time, special diets which are low in sodium have been found to be beneficial as an addendum to drug therapy. Salt is the usual source of sodium in a normal diet. A sodium-free diet generally contains rice cooked in unsalted water, sugar, fruit, fruit juices, and other fluids. After the blood pressure has dropped, the diet may be modified to include other items that make it more attractive. Close adherence to these diets, even though they may not be pleasant, is necessary in order to insure their effectiveness.

Within recent years, an entire battery of antihypertensive agents, drugs which lower the blood pressure, have been discovered and are now in clinical use. Derivatives of extracts from Rauwolfia serpentina, a plant commonly known as snake root, and probably used as a medicine in India hundreds of years ago, have now become very popular in the treatment of patients with hypertension. Other drugs such as hex-

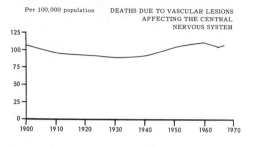

Per 100,000 population   DEATHS DUE TO VASCULAR LESIONS AFFECTING THE CENTRAL NERVOUS SYSTEM

This graph shows the consistently high rate of death in the United States resulting from circulatory lesions that affect the central nervous system.

amethonium compounds, spiralactone, methyldopa, guanethidine, and chlorothiazides can also produce a dramatic decrease in blood pressure. The most attentive surveillance by the physician is required to establish the correct dosage for the patient, as there is an ever-present danger of side effects. In many patients, it is desirable for them to learn to take their own blood pressure at home and so determine whether treatment is effective.

Many patients with extremely high blood pressure have been known to live for years. In many cases, however, consistently high blood pressure will cause secondary changes in the body. Often, these occur in the heart, which must work much harder to pump the blood against the increased pressure in the arteries. Continued overworking of the heart may result in heart failure. In other patients, the hypertension may cause a rupture or thrombus of the blood vessels in the brain. In a few cases, the kidneys may be damaged. Treatment of advanced cases of high blood pressure usually is directed toward preventing these crises. A woman with hypertension should consult her physician before endeavoring to become pregnant, for the chances of her having a normal pregnancy might be reduced, depending on the severity and cause of the hypertension.

Hypotension

When the systolic arterial pressure is consistently below 100 millimeters of mercury, low blood pressure (*hypotension*) is said to exist. Many perfectly healthy individuals have a blood pressure that is somewhat below the average. A moderately low value is usually considered conducive to a longer life. When no cause for the low pressure can be found, the condition is known as *essential hypotension*. The condition usually results in no untoward symptoms.

When a person moves from a reclining to a sitting or standing position, changes occur in the circulatory system which keep the blood pressure at a value normal for that person. In *orthostatic* or postural hypotension, the regulatory

mechanism does not operate properly, so that standing causes a drop in blood pressure which may result in unconsciousness. Most normal individuals occasionally may experience a slight giddiness when they stand up quickly, but the severe changes in postural hypotension are sufficient to be called to the attention of the physician.

A number of unrelated diseases, largely degenerative in nature, may bring about hypotension as a secondary symptom. Acute fevers, heart failure, Addison's disease, hypothyroidism, malnutrition, anemia, and hyperinsulinism may all produce this symptom. Internal hemorrhage, shock, fainting, and anesthesia are associated with transient hypotension. In each of these cases, the blood pressure usually becomes normal as soon as the original causative condition disappears. Often, the symptoms of hypotension are obscured by signs of the disease that brings it about. In a few extreme cases, weakness, dizziness, and faintness may give indications of inadequate circulation in the brain. However, a sufficient blood supply to the tissues usually is maintained despite a considerable drop in arterial pressure. Indeed, hypotension is really of significance only when the pressure drops below that necessary to produce adequate filtration through the kidneys.

DISORDERS OF THE HEART AND CIRCULATION: CORONARY THROMBOSIS

A typical "heart attack" is often the result of myocardial infarction (muscle damage caused by interference with the blood supply), which is usually the result of coronary thrombosis or coronary occlusions. These latter terms are used interchangeably. The victim may experience a great deal of fear when he has such an attack. Actually, about 80 percent of persons with a myocardial infarction survive the initial attack.

Mechanism of attack

An understanding of the mechanism of coronary thrombosis will enable the patient and his relatives to cooperate more effectively with the physician. As discussed earlier, the heart has two *coronary arteries* which supply the heart muscle with blood. If one of these arteries becomes clogged, the blood supply of a portion of the heart is shut off, and the tissue in the affected area will immediately begin to degenerate and die. The effect is the same as if the heart were actually wounded. A normal coronary artery may become plugged by a clot

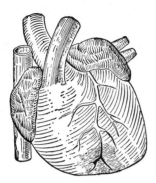

The heart after an attack of coronary thrombosis. A clot has blocked off (occluded) one of the coronary arteries, shutting off the blood supply to a portion of the heart. The shaded area represents the region which is no longer receiving blood. In this region scar tissue must form if the patient is to recover. Meanwhile, the second coronary artery will take up the work of the occluded artery.

(thrombus), but more frequently the clot will plug a hardened (or *sclerotic)* artery, because the passageway for blood in such an artery is already narrow. When one coronary artery becomes clogged, the smaller branches of the other artery gradually, over a period of weeks, begin to take up the work of the occluded artery. After a length of time, the healthy artery and its branches will be supplying blood to most of the areas which have been cut off. This is called *collateral circulation.* Meanwhile, the wounded muscle heals and a scar forms over the area. If the second artery can carry the load for both, the victim lives. If it cannot, he dies. Fortunately, in most cases the unplugged artery can do the task—that is, if the heart can be spared from all strain until collateral circulation is established and the scar tissue formed.

In some patients, the attack of coronary thrombosis occurs immediately after unusual physical exertion, mental strain, emotional upset, exposure to extreme cold, the eating of a heavy meal, a surgical operation, and other situations where the heart is called upon to do a larger job than usual. It is not proved that these actions *cause* coronary thrombosis, but there does seem to be some sort of relationship. However, there are many cases in which the victims experienced their heart attacks while at rest or asleep.

It is estimated that at least 22,000,000 persons in America suffer from some form of heart or vascular disease, and that there are approximately 570,000 deaths from "heart attack" each year. In three out of four cases, the victim is a man, and his age is usually between 50 and 70 years. However, coronary thrombosis has occurred in persons under 20. The former concept, however, that coronary heart disease is an "executive disease" has been largely abandoned. Studies in large corporations now show that the high-ranking personnel have less heart attacks than the clerical help or those performing more menial tasks. The typical victim of this disease is an aggressive, high-keyed, and active individual and usually a smoker.

Symptoms

The symptoms of coronary thrombosis usually follow a more or less regular pattern. The most predominant symptom is a constricting or crushing pain felt in the region beneath the breastbone *(sternum).* Onset of the pain is usually abrupt, but in a few cases it is gradual at the beginning, and then increases until it becomes severe. Most often the pain is continuous, but it can be intermittent. Although the heart region, beneath the sternum, is the eventual site of the pain, it may not be the first place in which the ache is felt. Instead, the pain may be noted initially in the arms, neck, or very likely the left shoulder. It may radiate to the jaws, teeth and arms, particularly the left arm. Along with the pain, there will be extreme sweating and shortness of breath. When the attack is but a few minutes old, the patient may become pale and appear to be in a state of shock. The patient's hands often feel cold to the touch, and his lips may be blue. The pulse becomes rapid, but may be so weak that it cannot be felt. In nearly every case, the heart beats much faster than normal. Many patients complain that they are dizzy and nauseated. The majority later report that they experienced a feeling of impending death throughout the first stages of the attack.

Before diagnosticians knew what a coronary thrombosis was, the condition was often attributed to "acute indigestion." This was because many patients reported that the pain was in the stomach region, and that there was accompanying nausea and vomiting. Even today, many persons with these symptoms do not call in a physician; they believe that they are only having a bout of "acute indigestion." This can be a fatal error. Only the doctor can make the distinction correctly.

What to do

If a person is suffering an attack of severe chest pain, which might be coronary thrombosis, the first thing to do is to *call a doctor!* If the patient survives the acute attack, his chances for living are greatly increased. But he is by no means out of danger. On the first or second day after the attack, his temperature may reach 104°. This will probably subside in a week or so. During the second and third weeks, the damaged muscle tissue will begin to be replaced with scar tissue. Throughout this period, it is imperative that the patient be under constant medical supervision.

When the doctor first sees the patient, he will probably give him an injection of morphine, or some related drug, to control the intense pain. As soon as possible, the patient will be allowed to breathe oxygen from a tank or in an oxygen tent. The oxygen makes breathing easier and helps to relieve the burden on the heart. Also, this will supply more oxygen to the capillaries and tissues around the injured area.

Treatment with drugs

The physician may prescribe an anticoagulant, a compound which prevents the clotting of the blood. Any of several derivatives of coumarin and heparin have been found useful in the prevention of clotting in patients with coronary disease. However, because of the possibility of hemorrhage, some patients are bad risks for this type of therapy, and in those treated, the dosage must be carefully regulated. The patient should be constantly monitored by the physician with the electrocardiograph, and other vital signs should be carefully observed.

The history of the discovery of one of these drugs, coumarin, indicates the potential danger involved in their use. Great numbers of cattle died each year in Wisconsin from uncontrolled hemorrhage. After several years of study, it was discovered that spoiled red clover was destroying the clotting mechanism in the blood of these cattle. In 1938 Doctor Karl Paul Link isolated the compound, coumarin, from the clover. The result was dicumarol. Doctor Link concluded that this compound might be of use in the prevention and treatment of coronary thrombosis. He suspected that dicumarol, if administered in the proper amounts, would prevent a clot from forming in the blood stream of human beings. The first trials were made on human patients in 1940, and physicians were enthusiastic over the results. In one series of 1000 patients with heart disease, the number

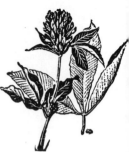

Drawing of red clover (Trifolium) illustrating details of the flower, bud, and leaves of this ordinary but valuable plant. From the spoiled clover may be isolated coumarin, a potent substance which has found extensive use in treating patients threatened with venous thrombosis. Coumarin acts as an anti-coagulant, prolonging the clotting time. It is now manufactured synthetically, rather than from the red clover.

of deaths that normally could have been expected was cut in half following the administration of dicumarol. The anticoagulant of choice for long-term therapy is heparin. Anticoagulant use in coronary thrombosis has become the preferred treatment because many physicians believe that this form of treatment is worth the slight risk of hemorrhage. If hemorrhage does occur, the prothrombin time may be restored to therapeutic levels in four hours by administration of vitamin K_1. Studies by the U.S. Veterans Administration and others have shown that anticoagulant drugs, when used in adequate doses, may be of value in lessening the risk of complications for some years after an attack. Other studies in which too low dosages of these drugs were used have failed to demonstrate benefit.

Important for the victim's recovery as any drug is that he have rest for a time during the healing period. Depending upon the decision of the physician, in severe cases, the length of convalescence may be several weeks. However, mild exercise is permitted as soon as it seems feasible. Comfort is an important item, because discomfort causes restlessness; and the purpose of all the imposed rest is defeated by restlessness. The patient may be propped up slightly in the bed; he must refrain entirely from smoking.

The rest must be mental as well as physical during the first seven to ten days. It is best to keep from the patient anything that will excite him, even disturbing topics of conversation.

The average survivor of an attack of coronary thrombosis can resume nearly normal habits within about three months. He should work toward this goal gradually, slowly building up to the point where he can work a two-hour day, then four, then six hours a day, until an eight-hour day is attained. In more severe cases, patients must curtail their return to work for as much as a year.

A former coronary thrombosis patient will be in danger of a second attack as long as he

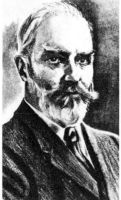

CUSHNY, Arthur Robertson (1866-1926) Scottish physician and pharmacologist. Noted for his numerous important studies on the action of digitalis on the human heart, as well as his recognition with Edmunds in 1901 of the condition of auricular fibrillation in the human heart. He also contributed to the development of our modern understanding of urine formation by filtration and selective reabsorption in the tubules of the human kidneys.

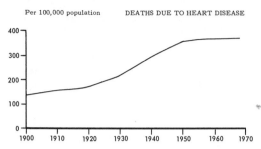

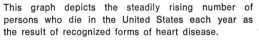

Per 100,000 population   DEATHS DUE TO HEART DISEASE

This graph depicts the steadily rising number of persons who die in the United States each year as the result of recognized forms of heart disease.

lives; but, so is everyone in relative danger of an attack, first or second. He who has experienced heart disease is less likely to do the things which will bring about an attack than are his "healthy" associates. Overeating and obesity are always to be avoided, especially during convalescence. Strenuous activity and competitive sports are forbidden. If the patient is overweight, it is a good idea to reduce by dieting; however, he must avoid steam baths and even forego hot baths in his own tub. Alcohol is not harmful if taken in moderate quantities. Continued abstinence from the use of tobacco is imperative.

From the first few minutes of the initial attack of coronary thrombosis through the remainder of the victim's life, the patient is acutely aware that sudden death is a definite possibility, and much tact is necessary to allay his fears. Fear itself can bring about a return of symptoms. Oversolicitousness is not necessary; understanding is.

The patient's associates must realize that he can return to a nearly normal life by gradual stages, just as they realize that a danger always exists. As one medical writer says: "No case of coronary occlusion, no matter how serious it may appear, should be considered hopeless; and no mild case should be considered entirely safe."

Surgical treatment

Among the numerous surgical procedures which have been tried are the implantation of the mammary arteries in the heart muscle, excision of the infarcted area of heart muscle, and the cleaning out of the obstruction from the affected coronary artery. These are advanced technical procedures and are not widely used at present, but they may have considerable potential for the future. During the acute attack, a common cause of death is the development of irregularity (arrhythmias) of the heart. Today most modern hospitals have coronary care units to give intensive care to these patients. Probably their most important function is the rapid hand-

ling of these arrhythmias and complete heart stoppage—by means of shock therapy and numerous appropriate drugs.

DISORDERS OF THE HEART AND CIRCULATION: BACTERIAL ENDOCARDITIS

Bacterial endocarditis is a bacterial infection of the *endocardium,* the thin *serous* membrane lining the cavities of the heart. It accounts for 2 percent of all organic heart disease. A patient with bacterial endocarditis has an excellent chance for survival if he receives prompt treatment. Various medicines, when properly administered, lead to recovery.

Several different types of bacteria can cause bacterial endocarditis. It has been known for a long time that bacteria occasionally gain access to the blood *vascular* system of the body. Usually these invaders are quickly destroyed by the *leucocytes,* or white cells, of the blood. However, if the bacteria appear in the blood as the result of an infection elsewhere in the body (blood poisoning or *septicemia*), they may be present in very large numbers. Should invading bacteria become attached to the inside of the heart, to one of the valves of the heart, or to the inner wall of one of the major blood vessels, the result is termed bacterial *endocarditis* (affecting the heart) or *endoarteritis* (affecting an artery).

This condition is especially serious because the circulatory tissues are poorly equipped for combating infection. Whereas other tissues of the body may literally wall up an infection so that it can be destroyed by the white cells, the heart and arterial tissues have no such ability to isolate an infection.

A large proportion of persons who have bacterial endocarditis have had a previous heart disability. The heart may have some congenital structural defect, or the endocarditis may have resulted from a disease of the heart, such as rheumatic fever. Affected persons usually are young adults, although the disease may attack in any age group.

Signs and symptoms

The two forms of bacterial endocarditis are the *acute* and the *subacute.* The acute form arises suddenly and is characterized by rapid appearance and continuing presence of the symptoms. Unless treatment is instituted at once, death results within a few days.

Subacute bacterial endocarditis begins slowly,

and the patient may live without treatment for some time, although death is almost inevitable within a few months, or occasionally within a year or two, if the patient is not treated medically. The sooner treatment is instituted, however, the greater are the chances of complete recovery.

One of the most characteristic signs of bacterial endocarditis is fever. This is always the case with the acute form, but persons with the subacute form of the disease may suffer only intermittent fevers. The onset of the fever is almost always a result of the presence of free bacteria in the blood stream. The physician may withdraw a sample of blood during a *febrile* period for culture of the organism. The patient also suffers from *anemia,* which is partly caused by the destruction of red blood cells by the bacteria.

Embolism is also a complication of bacterial endocarditis. An embolism occurs when a foreign or other abnormal particle *(embolus)* circulates within the blood stream and blocks the passage of blood through a vessel. It is frequently a portion of a thrombus (clot) which breaks loose from the wall of a blood vessel or the heart, and is carried to another part of the body by the flow of the blood. Emboli in bacterial endocarditis are formed when small bits of the bacterial growths and the surrounding material become loosened from their attachment at the point of infection. They flow on with the blood until they reach a vessel too small for them to pass through; they plug the vessel, and disrupt the circulation.

Emboli which develop because of the disease may cause *Osler's nodes* in the skin. These are small, raised, reddened areas found most often on the inside of the fingers and toes. They may be somewhat tender, but usually disappear within a few days. Larger and much more painful lumps may appear on the limbs, beneath the skin; usually they remain about a week. Sometimes these are caused by hemorrhage.

When a bacterial embolus lodges within an artery, it may cause a bulging sac from the wall of the artery called a *mycotic aneurysm.* These aneurysms usually appear in the smaller arteries, such as those that supply the skin; however, they may occur elsewhere. Aneurysms are considered in great detail elsewhere in this chapter.

When emboli become lodged within the blood vessels of the lungs, they produce symptoms similar to those of *hemorrhagic bronchopneumonia.* Emboli affecting the kidneys will cause many of the signs and symptoms of kidney malfunction, but rarely cause fatal *nephritis.* An embolus lodging in the brain may result in widespread damage to nervous tissue by cutting off the blood supply to nerve centers. Probably because of toxins manufactured by the bacteria, the smaller blood vessels (the *capillaries*) often become unusually fragile. The rupture of the walls of these tiny vessels causes a hemorrhage; the resulting symptoms depend upon the location of the capillaries affected. When capillaries in the skin are affected by the toxins, numerous small, purplish spots appear in the skin. They may be seen almost anywhere in the skin or mucous membrane. When they appear under the nails, the spots often resemble splinters. There may be capillary ruptures on the surface of internal organs, notably the heart and kidneys. In addition to these signs, the spleen usually becomes enlarged, and may feel tender to the touch.

An individual suffering from bacterial endocarditis may not exhibit all of the symptoms and signs which have been discussed. The physician can sometimes predict the appearance of certain signs, based on his knowledge of the patient's heart. He can do this because he knows that the areas of the body immediately supplied by the infected region of the circulatory system will be the most affected. Thus, an individual having an infection of the right side of the heart might well exhibit signs in the lungs, since they are supplied with blood by the right side of the heart. Conversely, an individual who has an infection of the left side of the heart, the *aorta,* or the *mitral valve,* will be more likely to have systemic symptoms—emboli in the skin and organs, kidney involvement, enlargement of the spleen, and aneurysms.

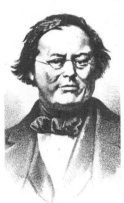

ROKITANSKY, Carl von (1804-1878) Austrian pathologic anatomist. Generally recognized as one of the greatest pathologists of all time, his many classic descriptions of various abnormalities of the internal organs contributed in an important manner to the advances that were made in medical science during the mid-nineteenth century. The procedures and approaches that he developed for the study of human pathology remain the basis of many modern practices.

Treatment

In almost all cases, the infection can be controlled by one or more of the various antibiotic drugs, particularly penicillin, streptomycin, and chloromycetin. However, the dosages must be large and prolonged to insure that the drugs destroy the bacteria. The usual period for antibiotic administration is about one month. In most cases, blood tests will show that the bac-

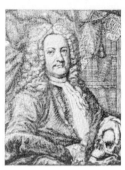

THEBESIUS, Adam Christian (1686-1732) German physician. Thebesius was noted as one of the great physiological investigators of his period in Europe, and principal among his observations was the description that he gave of the coronary valves, which had not previously been recognized by anatomists. His studies of details of the circulatory system contributed greatly to the eighteenth century advances in understanding of its disorders.

DISORDERS OF THE HEART AND CIRCULATION: RHEUMATIC FEVER

Rheumatic fever is a systemic disease which usually affects young people. The disease may result in serious and permanent injury to the heart. Many cases of rheumatic fever are not detected because the symptoms of the disease itself are often slight and go unnoticed. However, the heart may be injured permanently in these cases, although the injury may not be discovered until later in life.

Although bacteria of the *Streptococcus* group play a definite causative role in this disease, the mechanism by which they do it is not understood. The most popular theory is that of an allergic response on the part of the patient (host) to the Streptococcus (invading organism). Nearly all cases of rheumatic fever follow an infection by a Streptococcus, such as "strep" throat, tonsillitis, nose infection, scarlet fever, or *erysipelas*. Early and adequate treatment prevent development of later cardiac damage in most instances. Physicians now give large prophylactic doses of penicillin to children with streptococcal throat infections.

teria are resistant to one or more types of antibiotic, so that the treatment may be even longer. In such cases, larger doses of the drug, or a change to another antibiotic usually will be effective.

Many of the symptoms which are caused by emboli and toxins disappear eventually, and will not recur after the infection is removed. Important exceptions to this are kidney involvement and certain heart diseases. When these conditions occur, they require special treatment over and above that given for the original infection. Kidney malfunction caused by bacterial endocarditis may be permanent, restricting the patient to reduced activity throughout the rest of his life. Heart and kidney symptoms can be reduced or prevented in most cases if the patient seeks medical treatment promptly.

Prevention

Preventive measures against bacterial endocarditis are important for those individuals predisposed to the condition. Persons having heart defects should learn from their doctor the possibility of their contracting the disease.

The individual with chronic heart disease should discuss this with his dentist or surgeon before he undergoes tooth extraction or simple ear, nose, or throat operations, such as tonsillectomy. These procedures may be especially dangerous for him, since bacteria from a throat infection or tooth abscess enter the blood stream in large numbers and, consequently, infect damaged areas of the heart. Under these circumstances, the physician or dentist will perform the operation only after giving large amounts of penicillin or other antibiotic over a period of a day or two.

When an individual unusually susceptible to bacterial endocarditis suffers from any infectious disease, the physician usually prescribes a vigorous course of treatment to prevent the possible development of bacterial endocarditis.

Who is susceptible to rheumatic fever?

Everyone contracting a streptococcal infection does not develop rheumatic fever. One reason is that, apparently, only one type of Streptococcus *(Group A hemolytic Streptococcus)* can cause rheumatic fever, although several other types are responsible for throat and nose infections. Laboratory study of the organism causing the infection usually indicates whether the infection is capable of producing rheumatic fever later on.

Another reason why rheumatic fever is much less common than streptococcal infections is that probably not everyone is susceptible. The susceptibility may have a hereditary basis. Furthermore, susceptibility depends to a great extent upon age. Individuals between 6 and 19 years of age are most frequently affected, while persons older or younger than this are not so likely to contract the disease. Older persons with rheumatic fever usually escape much of the heart involvement, although the arthritic symptoms may be more pronounced.

There is an effective means of preventing the development of rheumatic fever. All respiratory infections, especially during the winter months, should receive early attention by a physician. The administration of penicillin in the proper amounts for streptococcal respiratory infections nearly always arrests the onset of rheumatic fever. However, antibiotics are not indicated for virus infections that cause the common cold.

Subclinical rheumatic fever

Often the symptoms of rheumatic fever may be so slight that they are completely overlooked by the patient. The physician may recognize the condition, however, by a routine examination, which enables him to treat the patient properly and thus prevent subsequent intensity of the disease. One of the most common features of a slight attack of rheumatic fever in children is what is sometimes called "growing pains." Although these indefinite aches also may be indicative of other conditions, they justify a trip to the doctor's office for thorough examination. The pains associated with rheumatic fever usually occur in the joints, particularly the knee and elbow. Parents should bear in mind that although rheumatic fever usually follows a streptococcal infection by one to four weeks, the infection may have been so slight as to have escaped notice completely.

Course of the disease

After the initial streptococcal infection, which may or may not have been noticed, there is usually a "latent" period of one to four weeks in which the patient feels quite well, or only slightly ill. During this period the physician may be able to detect changes in the heart, if that organ has been affected. The onset of rheumatic fever, following the latent period, may be sudden (*acute*) or it may progress slowly (*chronic*). The course of the disease is seldom exactly the same for any two patients, but certain generalizations can be made. As the name implies, rheumatic fever is usually characterized

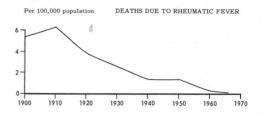
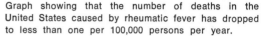

Graph showing that the number of deaths in the United States caused by rheumatic fever has dropped to less than one per 100,000 persons per year.

by a fever and rheumatism of the joints. In acute cases, the fever may be as high as 104° by the second day. It may continue high for many weeks, but usually lasts only ten to 14 days.

The joint manifestations of rheumatic fever include swelling, redness, tenderness, and mild to extreme pain. The larger joints usually are affected first. A bizarre symptom of this rheumatism is its migratory nature. The inflammation may spread to other joints as previously affected joints return to normal. A joint often remains painful and inflamed for about four to ten days, but usually shows no permanent after-effects.

Skin reactions occur frequently. Most often they are reddish areas which may spread and coalesce. The rashes seldom cause the patient any discomfort since they are not painful and usually do not itch.

Another manifestation is the development of lumps beneath the skin. When this happens, it indicates a more serious form of the disease. Consequently, the physician usually makes a thorough investigation by feeling the skin over joints and muscles. These nodules sometimes occur in the scalp.

Children suffering from rheumatic fever may show the symptoms of St. Vitus' dance (*chorea*), which may be accompanied by mental hallucinations.

Heart and circulatory involvements

Heart involvement is one of the most common and the most serious aspect of rheumatic fever. The valves of the heart may be affected and thus interfere with the normal function of the heart. Permanent damage to the valve may develop resulting in mitral incompetence (leakage) or mitral stenosis (obstruction) or both. Mitral incompetence has only recently been corrected by surgeons. The chances of success are greater in mitral stenosis which has been successfully treated surgically during the past decade. Two techniques are used. In the simpler one, the surgeon sticks his finger into the pa-

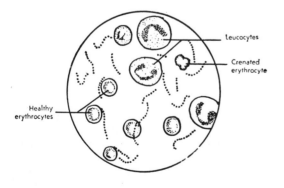

Chains of round bacteria and numbers of disrupted red cells are typical of the microscopic appearance of blood infected by hemolytic streptococci.

tient's heart and either fractures the structured valve or cuts it to open it. The other requires the use of the heart-lung machine, but permits the operative exposure and correction or even replacement of the diseased valve. Although the operations appear to be dangerous, they are nearly always successful when conducted by a skilled surgeon. People with this affliction can now be much improved by these new surgical techniques. The aortic valve and the tricuspid valve have also been replaced surgically. The first artificial valve used clinically was the aortic valve developed by Charles Hufnagel and W. P. Harvey.

To detect heart involvement, the physician must see the patient frequently in order that he may listen for unusual sounds (murmurs) in the heartbeat and unusual rhythms in the pulse. When the heart is affected, the patient must receive special consideration, not only during the illness and the convalescent period, but occasionally even after recovery seems complete.

Treatment and care of the patient

In order to reduce the fever and alleviate the rheumatic pains, the physician generally administers various forms of *salicylates,* one of which is aspirin. However, the level of these drugs must be high to be effective. Therefore, untrained persons administering them to the patient must be extremely careful in following the doctor's directions. Too little will have no result, while too much may poison the patient. Signs of poisoning by the salicylates include ringing in the ears or deafness, nausea, and vomiting. Stomach discomfort may follow the taking of the drugs, so that other medications may have to be given simultaneously. Some persons seem unable to tolerate the salicylates and must take other drugs. *Aminopyrine* is an effective drug, but may produce serious side

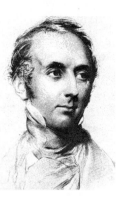

KEY, Charles Ashton (1793-1849) English surgeon. Noted for the surgical procedures that he introduced into the treatment of patients suffering from cardiac disorders. He developed methods for the ligation of the external iliac artery for femoral aneurysm and ligation of the subclavian for axillary aneurysm. The two surgical methods were the standard for these conditions for years, and set an approach by which improvements in the treatment of aneurysm were developed.

effects which limit or prevent its use. *Morphine* or *codeine* may be used occasionally for relief of severe pain in patients who are not relieved by the administration of other drugs.

The physician, from time to time, may discontinue the administration of the pain-relieving drugs in order to determine whether the pain has disappeared, diminished, spread in area, or increased. Withholding the drugs may cause the patient some discomfort, but the physician must have the information gained thereby. The care which the patient receives during and after his illness may determine whether he will recover and return to a normal life by preventing major permanent damage to the heart valves. This is particularly true in the more acute cases.

In most cases, the patient should be hospitalized for as long as the physician deems necessary. In the hospital he will receive constant attention from trained persons. Daily visits by the physician are sometimes necessary. In severe cases, the progress of the disease and the effects of the drugs are determined by frequent checks on the patient's temperature, heartbeat, pulse rate, and by laboratory examinations of blood and urine.

Early in the course of the disease the patient is not permitted to leave his bed. The position which he maintains is also of great importance. In many cases, the heart works most easily when the patient's legs are lower than the head, although some patients must recline at all times. The position also has some effect on the pain.

The length of the convalescent period depends upon the severity of the disease. A person only slightly affected may be able to be up and about within a month, providing the fever and other symptoms have disappeared. The more severely affected patient must remain in bed many weeks, sometimes months. After long periods of confinement, the change to a more active life must be made slowly. When symptoms disappear, the patient may begin by sitting

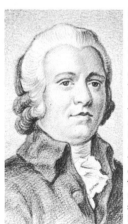

DESAULT, Pierre Joseph (1744-1795) French surgeon. Contributed to many fields of surgery, including the modern techniques of surgery of the circulatory system. He developed the method for ligating blood vessels for the treatment of aneurysms, published after his death in 1801, and made a great many important contributions to the knowledge of fractures and dislocations, including their adjustment. Many dressings and splints were first described in Desault's work.

up for a short time each day, and increase the time gradually until he is able to sit four or five hours daily. At this point, the patient may be helped to his feet and permitted to take a few steps. Progress continues at such a pace until he is able to return to normal routines.

Relapse and recurrence

During the period of convalescence or shortly after it, the patient may experience a sudden return of symptoms (a *relapse*). This may be brought on by a reinfection, by getting out of bed too soon, by engaging in excessive exertion, or by a strong emotional experience. A relapse greatly increases the possibility of permanent heart damage, valve thickening and leakage, or scarred heart muscle with damaged conduction mechanism leading to cardiac irregularities.

Recurrence of rheumatic fever was formerly quite common. It is brought on by a second streptococcal infection. For this reason, a person once having had rheumatic fever must realize that he may contract it again. He must avoid exposure to streptococcal infections in other individuals and consult his physician for all streptococcal respiratory infections. Physicians now recommend the administration of penicillin or sulfonamides as a prophylactic measure for several years for children who are especially susceptible to streptococcal infections.

The future for the rheumatic fever patient

The patient's attitude toward his heart is important after recovery from rheumatic fever. Frequently, individuals who have had minor or no heart complications may develop anxiety concerning their hearts. This is partly caused by the long period of illness and convalescence, during which the heart received a great deal of attention. In patients having no heart involvement, rapid and unusual heartbeats may develop in later years as a result of this mental attitude. The patient and his family must face facts and cease to worry about the heart, if there has been no heart damage. The same considerations may also hold true for those individuals who have sustained heart damage as a result of the disease. Overattention to the damaged heart may bring on further complications which may render the patient incompetent to carry on a normal life. Only the physician who has studied the individual during and after the disease is able to determine the extent of the damage and the limitations to be placed upon the patient. If the physician recommends a quiet way of life, the patient should find out exactly what is meant. Permanent invalidism rarely results from rheumatic fever. However, the patient may be

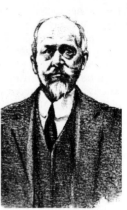

FANO, Giulio (1856-1930) Italian physiologist. One of the greatest students of the physiology of the circulatory system, he made major contributions to the medical knowledge of the electrical impulses of the heart, which later proved to be of the greatest importance from the standpoint of the development of modern electrocardiography. The development of this diagnostic tool was based on the previous work of several brilliant physiologists.

advised to seek a profession and hobbies which do not require an unusual expenditure of energy.

Tales told by well-meaning but uninformed persons should be ignored. A healthy mental attitude along with an occasional check up should permit the patient to lead a fairly active life.

Rheumatic heart disease

Rheumatic heart disease may result from rheumatic fever, and is responsible for over 90 percent of all heart disorders that occur in patients under 30. It is the second most common form of heart disease in adults. It may be active or inactive; in the latter case, the infection has ceased, but leaves the heart with scars that may produce difficulty at a later date. About 50 percent of the patients with rheumatic fever develop some heart complications. Rheumatic heart disease is often a predisposing factor in renal infarction.

Rheumatic heart disease most commonly affects the thick muscular wall (*myocardium*) and the valves of the heart. The disorder may be manifest in the form of various irregularities in the heartbeat, which may or may not be readily apparent to the patient. There is seldom any pain in the heart region, although in some cases there may be some difficulty in breathing. In many patients, the condition may subside spontaneously, and then recur at a later date. Since recurrent attacks may further damage the heart, the patient must be alert for a return of the symptoms.

The treatment of patients with rheumatic heart disease is largely the same as that described for those with rheumatic fever. Among the major problems that occur are those associated with the inactive form of the disease. While the disease subsides, in most cases, after a relatively short time, it may leave scars on the heart, particularly on the valves. Years later, this scarring may cause interference with the action of the heart. Treatment of patients with inactive forms of the disease is directed toward the prevention of later complications. Both medicine and surgery are of value in correcting these conditions. Recent advances have made it possible for many patients with rheumatic heart defects to lead long and useful lives. Replacement of the diseased mitral valve with an artificial valve has become rather commonplace and the results are usually highly successful.

OTHER CARDIOVASCULAR DISORDERS

Circulatory disorders account for over 90 percent of all heart disease. Many forms of circulatory trouble are compound in nature; that is, a number of conditions can exist simultaneously. The frequent appearance of hardening of the arteries in combination with high blood pressure is an example. In addition, many situations, such as "heart failure," may result from involvement of the heart with any one of several other disorders. Hence, heart failure should be considered as a symptom of heart disease, rather than a disease itself. Circulatory disorders may be present at birth, or they may arise as a result of events that occur later in life. In the latter case, however, they may be caused by an hereditary predisposition to the condition.

Congenital disorders

Most congenital disorders of the circulatory system appear in the embryo as the result of some defect in development, usually between the fifth and eighth week of pregnancy. An infection in the mother during pregnancy, such as German measles (rubella), may be responsible for the abnormality. In some cases, the heart may be located in the right side of the body, although this seldom causes any difficulty and may not be noticed. More serious defects are those which involve the size and development of the chambers of the heart, its valves, and connecting vessels. In some patients, such congenital defects may manifest themselves only after many years, and cause nothing more than a slight discomfort in breathing. In other instances, the defects may be such as to inhibit seriously the flow of blood through the heart and lungs.

In one of the malformations *(patent ductus arteriosus)*, a small duct connecting the aorta and the pulmonary artery fails to close at birth. Since the pressure is higher in the aorta, blood will flow from this vessel to the pulmonary artery and back to the lungs, from which it had just come. This means that even when the lungs are working at full capacity, all the oxygenated blood is not being circulated to the body. Difficulty in breathing and palpitation are outstanding symptoms. Once it is discovered, this defect can be repaired surgically by tying or dividing and sewing the open ends of the duct.

Perhaps because of newer and better methods of diagnosis, cardiologists are now finding cases of coronary heart disease (once believed to be the bane of the middle aged) in infants.

If defects exist which allow a mixing of arterial and venous blood, the patient frequently has a bluish or *cyanotic* appearance. This condition, if not corrected, may limit the life of the patient to a relatively few years. Best known of the cyanotic congenital heart defects are those that are found in "blue babies." One of the most common conditions causing blue babies is really a combination of four malformations *(tetralogy of Fallot)*. In this disorder, the prenatal partition *(septum)* between the two pumping chambers *(ventricles)* of the heart has failed to close at birth. In addition, the major artery (the *aorta*) leading from the heart is slightly out of place, and the artery leading from the heart to the lungs is constricted. The right ventricle, therefore, not only must pump blood through the lungs, but also must work directly against pressure from the left, so that the ventricle becomes enlarged because of the extra work. Blood which has been through the lungs becomes mixed with that which has not. An increase in the number of red blood cells may occur to compensate for the circulatory insufficiency. The child's fingers may be club-shaped, and there may be a failure on the part of the child to develop physically in a normal manner. Because of breathlessness, such children may adopt a squatting position for ease in breathing.

Formerly, the treatment of blue babies was limited, and consisted in preventing infection and overactivity of the child. Under the best of conditions, the span of life was short. This situation changed greatly as the result of an ingenious surgical operation devised by Doctors Alfred Blalock and Helen Taussig. The operation is designed to increase the circulation of blood, and is a technique which can be used for several different conditions. One of the arteries —the *aorta, common carotid, subclavian,* or *innominate*—is connected to the pulmonary artery. There is then an increase of the blood flow to the lungs sufficient to permit the patient maximum activity without placing undue strain on the heart. This operation, when needed, is usually performed before the baby is four years old. This operation corrects the blueness and allows the baby to thrive and grow. At a later date, the child can then be totally corrected with a second operation, utilizing the heart-lung machine. This machine enables the surgeon to work within the heart and thereby correct the intracardiac defects. Many of the former "blue babies" receiving the Blalock operation have gone on to adulthood and given birth to children (some normal and some with heart malformations).

Congenital anomalies

Each of the four valves of the heart (considered here in the order of blood flow) may have congenital anomalies. The *tricuspid valve* may have a deformity of the leaflets, known as *Ebstein's malformation of the tricuspid valve*. Or there may be *tricuspid atresia*, in which the valve never forms, preventing the normal flow of blood from the right auricle into the right ventricle. Instead, it flows from the right auricle into the left auricle through a hole in the wall between the two upper chambers of the heart. The *pulmonary valve* cusps are partially fused in some individuals and prevent the proper flow of blood, *pulmonary stenosis*. This condition can be caused by narrowing of the orifice leading to the valve or fusion of the leaves of the valve itself. In the normal heart the systolic pressure is the same on both sides of the valve. If the pressure is found to be lower in the pulmonary artery than in the right ventricle, the physician knows that *pulmonary stenosis* exists. The *mitral valve*, the next valve in order, may have *atresia*, *incompetence*, or *stenosis*, although isolated cases of these conditions are rare. The *aortic valve*, the last valve in the heart, may have a congenital narrowing of the orifice or fusion of the cusps, known as *aortic stenosis*. Most of these abnormalities of the heart valves can be corrected surgically.

The most common congenital malformation occurring as a single lesion is *ventricular septal defect*, in which there is a hole in the wall between the left and right ventricles. Following diagnosis, this abnormality can be corrected surgically by sewing a patch composed of a tough, resilient plastic material over the opening. A hole between the two auricles, *atrial septal defect*, allows blood to flow from the left side of the heart as the result of pressure differences. This defect can be corrected by directly suturing the edges of the defect.

A more complicated group of defects occurs when there is a hole between both the upper chambers (atria) and lower chambers (ventrica) with malformed intervening tissue and one or both valves between the atria and ventrica. These most difficult lesions can be corrected with the use of the heart-lung machine and always require the use of a patch and often a prosthetic valve.

In some cases, the oxygenated blood from the lungs returns partially or totally to the right side

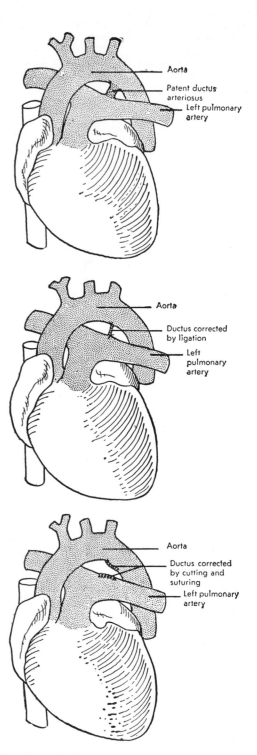

The three drawings show, from top to bottom, a *ductus arteriosus* between the aorta and pulmonary artery that has not closed at birth in the usual manner, the method by which this connecting tube is tied off, or cut and sutured. This is but one of several surgical procedures widely used today for correction of congenital circulatory defects.

of the heart instead of draining into the left auricle. This type of malformation, *anomalous drainage of pulmonary veins*, is characterized by a very abnormal condition—the same amount of oxygen being present in all the chambers of the heart, the pulmonary artery, and the aorta. This condition can be corrected by various surgical procedures in which the anomalous drainage is redirected into the correct left auricle.

In *coarctation of the aorta*, another rather common congenital heart defect, the main artery leaving the heart is constricted to such an extent that the flow of blood to all parts of the body is restricted. When the diagnosis of this condition has been confirmed, the constriction can be removed surgically and the ends of the aorta reunited or the defect bridged with a synthetic vessel, thus allowing the blood to flow freely.

One of the most outstanding achievements within recent years, in the treatment of patients with malformations of the heart and great vessels, is the development by John Gibbon of a mechanical device to take the place of the heart and lungs during surgical treatment. This artificial heart and lung apparatus allows the surgeon to operate on the heart for long periods of time in a dry, bloodless field, under direct vision. The machine consists of a pump to draw the blood from the vena cavae, through tubes which are connected to these veins before they enter the heart. The blood is pumped under controlled pressure and flow to an "artificial lung," usually a plastic, membranous bag where it is allowed to contact a steady stream of oxygen. The oxygenated blood is then pumped through another tube into the arterial system. The oxygen content, temperature, degree of alkalinity or acidity, rate of flow, and pressure must all be carefully regulated throughout the entire surgical procedure. Checks on the circulation in the extremities are made constantly during the by-pass of the heart and lungs to prevent the death of tissues because of inadequate blood supply.

Prevention

An important step has been taken with the development of rubella vaccine, which should be administered to all young females before pregnancy. However, the physician should be certain that there is no chance that the patient is pregnant. If given during pregnancy, it may produce congenital defects like those caused by rubella. The recognition that some drugs, notably thalidomide, may produce congenital defects should also alert the physician to the need for minimizing the use of drugs and keeping careful records of all drugs taken by the pregnant patient.

Carditis

The heart is subject to a number of other infectious and inflammatory conditions. Diphtheria may bring about both a collapse in the circulation throughout the body and changes in the heart itself *(toxic diphtheric myocarditis)*. The same type of disturbances may result from pneumonia and other infections. Inflammation of the muscular walls of the heart *(myocarditis)* may occur without any apparent cause. Myocarditis also may result from poisoning by certain drugs. Acute inflammation of the kidneys may produce a severe carditis. The treatment in each of these cases not only involves control of the original source of the inflammation, when known, but also involves steps to prevent the heart from becoming incompetent. Any form of carditis is serious and requires continued and careful medical attention.

Pericarditis is an inflammation of the *pericardium,* the membrane covering the heart. This condition is often caused by infections in the heart or other parts of the body, or may originate from a wound or tumor of the heart. Pericarditis may appear in a number of forms, most of which respond well to prompt treatment. In *dry* or *fibrinous* pericarditis, pain may occur in the region of the heart or shoulders, and the physician can usually hear distinct sounds of friction when he listens to the heartbeat. In other cases, the pericardium may become filled with fluid, causing pain, discomfort in breathing, and disturbances in the heartbeat and blood pressure. In *chronic constrictive* pericarditis, the pericardium may become so fibrinous or even calcified as literally to encase the heart in "stone" and restrict its movements. Sometimes such calcified material can be successfully removed by surgery. Adherent pericarditis is caused by an anchoring of the heart to the surrounding tissues, caused by new tissue *(adhesions)* following an inflammation.

Angina pectoris

Because the heart is an extremely active muscle, it requires a continuous and adequate supply of oxygen from the blood. Any impediment in the arteries supplying the heart muscle may impair the cardiac blood supply. Lack of oxygen in the blood *(anoxemia)* also may cause an inadequate supply of oxygen to the heart muscle. Under such circumstances, persons who exert themselves to only a limited extent may suffer from pain in the chest or the area below the collar bones. Such pain, frequently excruciating, is referred to as *angina pectoris*. It usually occurs in persons over 40 years of age, and its alleviation depends upon the cause of the heart condition; in other words, angina pectoris is not, properly speaking, a disease, but rather a symptom associated with temporary anoxia of the heart muscle (*myocardial anoxia*). The physician has various drugs and surgical measures available. Today, various operations can increase blood supply to the heart muscle, either by direct or by indirect means. Surgical procedures are frequently helpful in relieving the pain.

Other heart conditions

A number of heart conditions result from disturbances in the lungs. Most common of these is *pulmonary embolism,* in which a clot forming in one of the veins becomes lodged in the pulmonary artery, which it partially plugs, thus decreasing the flow of blood through the lungs. This can be fatal, although many patients recover completely if they have immediate medical attention. Proper care for bedridden patients greatly decreases the likelihood of the formation of such a clot. By using sugar and water to prime the pump of the heart-lung bypass machine instead of the 15 or 20 pints of properly matched blood formerly required, many defects of the heart, such as congenital valvular anomalies, septal defects, and piercing wounds, are now readily corrected. Surgery has been unusually successful also in increasing the flow of blood to the brain in *stroke* victims and to the kidneys in renal hypertension either by reaming out the arteries or by replacing them with new artificial grafts.

Thyrotoxic heart disease is caused by the stress placed upon the heart and circulatory system from an overactive thyroid gland. The condition is not serious in younger patients, but may become so at middle age or beyond. Treatment directed toward the underlying thyroid condition usually causes a disappearance of the cardiac symptoms.

Emphysema, a form of fibrosis of the lung, is a common cause of heart strain and enlargement. One of the major causes of this condition is smoking.

Heart failure means that the heart or some of its chambers fail to discharge their contents properly. The exact mechanism of the disease producing this is often not completely understood, and may be due to a variety of diseases in which there is heart muscle failure. When the left ventricle fails, the pressure rises in the left auricle and in the pulmonary veins. Heart failure is not necessarily fatal, and many persons who at one time have suffered from it may live for many years.

Symptoms of heart failure include difficulty in breathing and generalized enlargement of the veins caused by increased pressure in the right auricle and the veins. The liver becomes enlarged and fluids accumulate in the tissues with marked swelling (*edema,* commonly referred to as *dropsy*) of areas such as the feet and ankles. The dropsy can usually be corrected by a low salt diet and *diuretics,* a group of drugs which stimulate the kidneys to excrete water and sodium.

Peripheral vascular disease occurs in a large number of individuals past the age of 50. The blood vessels in the arms and legs become hardened and decrease the flow of blood to those areas. If the blood supply is diminished extensively, ulcerations and gangrene may occur. Treatment is concerned with increasing the blood supply and the prevention of clotting. The patient must totally abstain from smoking.

Some of the diseases of the heart and circulation are related to disturbances of the normal rhythm of the heartbeat. These disorders, known as *arrhythmias,* may express themselves in different ways. *Premature beats,* sudden increase of heartbeat (*paroxysmal tachycardia*), slow heartbeat (*bradycardia*), and heart block are some of the manifestations of temporary toxic conditions or permanent organic damage which may be associated with coronary heart disease.

Premature beats are often benign, and although they are frequently found in the elderly, they are not uncommon in young people and even children. When these extra beats are not associated with other signs of heart disease, they are of no consequence and are only annoying to the patient. A drug to reduce the sensitivity of the heart muscle, such as quinidine or procaine amide often is successful in removing the premature beats.

Attacks of paroxysmal tachycardia (fast heart beat unrelated to exercise, anxiety, fever, or infection) can be treated with digitalis or quinidine, under close supervision of the physician. Frequently, the irregularities are due to more serious states such as atrial fibrillation and atrial flutter. These require careful control by the physician.

A very slow heart rate results from complete heart block. Rates of 30-40 beats per minute may occur without any symptoms. A few patients, however, with these slow rates will faint (Adams-Stokes attack) for a few seconds or minutes. Isopropyl norepinephrine, under the tongue, may relieve or reduce the attacks. When episodes of arrhythmia become unusually severe or frequent and medical treatment fails to be therapeutic, a pacemaker is used to regulate the beating of the heart. This small, battery-operated device is implanted below the surface of the skin, usually in the abdominal area. Wire leads carry electronic impulses to the heart muscle inducing a steady rhythmic beat. Thousands of individuals currently enjoy normal activities with these battery-operated "tickers."

TRANSPLANTATION OF THE HUMAN HEART

After the problems surrounding transplantation of human arteries had been resolved, the next big step in surgical reparation of a diseased cardiovascular system was replacement of a failing heart by a donor heart in good condition; but many problems faced the team of surgeons and cardiologists attempting this feat. Carrel and Guthrie performed the first experimental heart transplantation in 1907. In this early work the heart was usually transplanted into the animal's neck. Further work suggested that the additional heart act as an auxiliary pump when inserted into the animal's chest. The Mann technique, described in 1933, has served as the basis for heart transplants with modifications by many investigators, including Lillehei. A major breakthrough was made in 1960, when Lower and Shumway reported eight homotransplantations after which five of the animals lived from 6 to 21 days. With technical and physiological problems studied and minimized, work was conducted to combat the immune response with immunosuppressive drugs. Then, in 1964 Hardy attempted to transplant the heart of a large chimpanzee into a 68-year-old man, using Shumway's technique. About one hour after the operation the heart was judged incapable of supporting the circulation of a large man. On December 3, 1967, the first human heart transplantation was performed by Dr.Christiaan Barnard in Cape Town, South Africa. Within a year, more than 140 persons had undergone heart transplant over the world, with varying survival results ranging from only a few hours to more than a year. While some patients enjoyed only a few weeks of relative good health following the transplantation, others survived from six months to a year before dying from infection or rejection. Advanced surgical techniques in the hands of skilled cardiovascular surgeons have virtually assured the success of the transplant itself, but the postoperative course has been complicated by one of the body's immune defense mechanisms, automatically triggered to reject foreign proteins. A regimen of intensive and sophisticated medical treatment must be employed in all heart transplant patients in an effort to negate rejection. Experimental work is underway with drugs, such as the purinethiols, and antilymphocyte serum as immunosuppressive agents. This treatment, however, increases the patient's susceptibility to an infection, which might result in death even before rejection occurs.

An important medicolegal aspect of heart transplantation has been a new definition of death. This resulted from the need for determination of the time of death of donors used for heart transplantation. In order to be qualified as a potential heart donor, the patient must have suffered irreversible brain death, and yet have a beating heart. A totally-flat electroencephalogram is the indication of brain death. Even though this has occurred, the heart and respiration may be maintained artificially long enough to transport the donor to the hospital where the transplant team and recipient are waiting. Thus, a beating heart is no longer the major legal criterion for life.

It has been found that the closer the match between the tissue and blood of the donor and the recipient, the greater is the chance of the patient accepting his new heart. This histocompatibility (cellular acceptance of cells foreign to the organism) is of prime importance in the longevity of a patient with any transplanted organ.

Because of the problem of biological rejection to foreign protein, leaders in the field of cardiovascular surgery have considered for years the possibility of a totally artificial heart. Dr. Michael E. DeBakey and his associates in Houston, Texas, and other investigators have conducted extensive experiments, using various animal and plastic cardiac models, in attempting to develop a satisfactory artificial heart. On April 4, 1969, the first implantation of an artificial heart into a human being was performed in Houston, Texas, by Doctor Denton A. Cooley. This device sustained life for 64 hours, after which it was replaced by a donor heart. Still to be solved at that time were the problems of red cell destruction, kidney damage, and a portable, internal power source.

HOW AN ARTERY IS TRANSPLANTED

One of the great advances in surgery of the heart and blood vessels is the development of the technique of arterial transplantation. Originally, sections of arteries were obtained from the bodies of healthy individuals who had died suddenly. However, because these transplanted arteries rapidly underwent arteriosclerotic changes, they are not now used. They have been replaced by the use of artificial vessels composed of Teflon or Dacron. These vessels are almost indestructible, are readily available, and have proved most satisfactory. They do not cause the reaction (shock) that occurs in an individual when a part from another human or animal is placed inside his body. More recently, there has been an increased tendency for surgeons to use pieces of vein from the patient himself, for this provides an even better

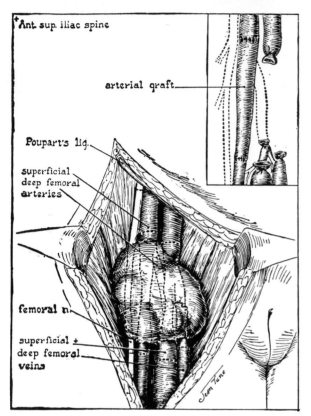

Ant. sup. iliac spine

arterial graft

Poupart's lig.

superficial
deep femoral
arteries

femoral n.

superficial ±
deep femoral
veins

Jean Fane

1. Sketch showing a tumor in a woman's leg, which required removal of over three inches of the femoral artery. Succeeding figures show how new artery was transplanted.

chance of long-term good results. The following picture series illustrates the surgical procedure. *Copyright 1951, A.M.A. Archives of Surgery. Courtesy Henry Swan, M.D., and H. Mason Morfit, M.D.*

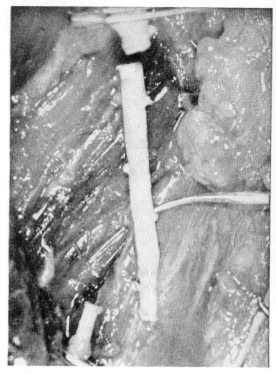

2. A section of another artery which is approximately the same length and caliber of the femoral artery is inserted into the gap that resulted from the operation.

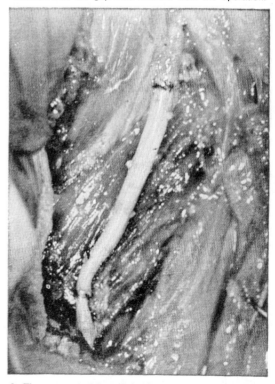

3. The new arterial graft is then sewed to both ends of the severed artery. The clamps shown at the top and bottom of Fig. 2 are now removed and the blood flow resumes.

8 THE SKIN

WHAT IT IS AND DOES

The skin is the largest organ of the body and provides the body surface with a protective covering. In addition, it performs numerous other important and essential services. The skin helps to regulate the body temperature. It cooperates with the kidneys and lungs in the vital process of excretion of waste materials. It serves as a waterproof covering to prevent loss of critical body fluids, as well as to keep external fluids from passing into the tissues. The skin is also an important sensory organ, detecting such external conditions as heat and cold. Through the sensation of pain, nerves in the skin notify the brain of any injury to the body.

Aside from these purely biological aspects of its functions, the skin plays an important social role in everyday life. The initial impression that one often makes in social contacts depends to a considerable extent upon the appearance of the skin, and an unhealthy skin may prove a handicap. Further, the skin provides a means of judging a person's age, and it may tell much about the kind of life that one has led.

Fingernails and toenails are actually modifications of the skin. Another modified form of the skin is found in the body cavities, the mouth, the nose, the digestive tract, and the eyes. This "internal skin" is referred to as *mucous membrane* and differs from the outer skin in many ways, particularly in its ability to secrete a sticky liquid called *mucus*. The mucous membranes are much thinner than the external skin, as they lack the horny layer or *cutis;* hence, mucous membranes often appear pink because

the blood vessels can be seen more easily through them. The internal membranes also lack sweat glands and hair. Their ability to detect heat, cold, touch, and pain is different from that of the skin proper. Like the outer skin, however, they perform specialized services for the parts of the body in which they are located.

The appearance of the skin

The visible surface of the skin is a tough material which is composed largely of dead cells. These cells are constantly and inconspicuously being sloughed off, and in this manner the surface of smooth skin is gradually being renewed. Healthy skin has a somewhat velvety appearance because of the openings of the many glands of the skin *(pores)*. These pores form small diamond-shaped patterns which can be seen most easily at the joints. The skin may have a waxy or greasy appearance because of the oily fluid secreted by the *sebaceous glands* located within it. Almost all of the body is covered by hair, which grows from pits or *follicles* within the skin.

The color of the skin is governed largely by the presence of a brown to black pigment called *melanin*. Melanin is produced by special cells *(melanocytes)* in a complex series of biochemical reactions. The process must begin with the oxidation of tyrosine, an important amino acid, and is catalyzed by *tyrosinase,* an enzyme found in both human beings and lower animals. How much melanin is produced in this way depends primarily on hereditary factors; under certain conditions, it may be greater than normal or missing entirely. In some persons, melanin is

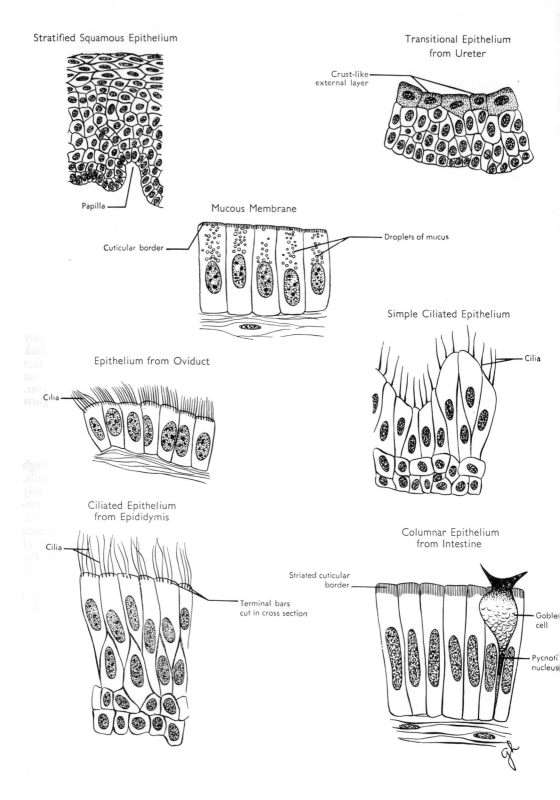

Stratified Squamous Epithelium

Papilla

Transitional Epithelium
from Ureter

Crust-like
external layer

Mucous Membrane

Cuticular border

Droplets of mucus

Simple Ciliated Epithelium

Cilia

Epithelium from Oviduct

Cilia

Ciliated Epithelium
from Epididymis

Cilia

Terminal bars
cut in cross section

Columnar Epithelium
from Intestine

Striated cuticular
border

Goblet
cell

Pycnotic
nucleus

Various Types of Epithelium

unevenly distributed, being entirely absent in patches or large areas of skin.

Exposure to sunlight stimulates greater production of melanin in the skin, resulting in a "tan" if distribution is even, or freckles if it is uneven. This is nature's way of protecting sensitive skin cells, since the melanin pigment absorbs much of the harmful radiation. Biochemically, the sun's rays affect tyrosinase activity. They remove the inhibitors that normally restrain this enzyme, and hence more melanin is produced. A suntan fades away when the melanin gradually migrates with the epidermal cells toward the skin's surface and is sloughed off. However, chemical reactions within the skin also destroy some of the pigment.

Skin with a small amount of melanin has a pink color, given to the skin by the blood in the numerous, small, superficial blood vessels *(capillaries)* which supply it with food and oxygen. Such a person suffering from anemia may appear pale because the blood in these vessels does not contain sufficient red corpuscles or sufficient *hemoglobin;* hence, it is not as red as it should be. In the emotional state of embarrassment accompanied by blushing, the amount of blood in the capillaries may be increased and the individual will appear ruddy.

The skin may receive a yellowish tinge from *carotene,* a pigment found in many vegetables and closely related to vitamin A. When excessive amounts of food containing vitamin A are eaten (carrots, for instance), the skin may take on an abnormally yellow color; this condition is called *carotenemia.* It disappears when the vitamin A in the diet is reduced to normal amounts. Further, the skin may become discolored from a large number of unnatural causes. *Jaundice,* for example, which results from diseases of certain internal organs, causes the skin to appear more yellow.

To the experienced eye, changes in the color and texture of the skin may be indicative of systemic disease. The normal appearance of the skin changes with age. The skin of an infant is soft and elastic. With advancing age, the skin becomes thick and more yellow. It loses its elasticity and may become dry, wrinkled, and translucent. The aging of the skin often is speeded up by constant irritation or by prolonged exposure to sunlight and wind.

Structure of the skin

The skin of an adult of average size weighs from six to seven and one-half pounds, or about twice the weight of the liver; it has a surface area of approximately two square yards. In thickness, it varies from $1/32$ of an inch to $1/8$ of an inch.

The skin is composed of several layers of specialized skin cells, as well as numerous glands, nerves, hairs and hair follicles, and blood vessels. The outer portion of the skin is called the *epidermis.* This represents only a small part of the thickness of the skin, and normally contains no blood vessels or nerves. The outer layer of this epidermis, called the *cornified layer,* or *stratum corneum,* contains the dead cells which are constantly being flaked off. It is tough because it contains a hornlike material called *keratin.* The outer layer of the epidermis also contains a large amount of fatty material.

There is a second and lighter layer, the *stratum lucidum,* located directly below the horny layer of the epidermis, especially prominent on the palms and soles.

The innermost layer of the epidermis, the *stratum mucosum,* contains most of the melanin pigment of the skin. There is no blood supply to this stratum, so it must obtain its food from a fluid *(lymph)* which filters out of the blood and flows among the cells. Consequently, when wounds of the skin do not penetrate deeper than the epidermis, there is no bleeding, but there may be an oozing of a clear liquid, which is lymph.

The epidermis grows continually in order to replace cells of the outer layer which are being lost. This growth takes place in the inner portion of the epidermis, the stratum mucosum. The cells of this layer grow and multiply, pushing older cells outward. As the cells are forced toward the outer layer, they change in appearance; melanin pigmentation is lost, and the cells become tougher. The outward growth of the epidermis is responsible for the fact that when splinters or other small particles are embedded in the skin, they eventually work their way to the surface.

The *dermis* is the layer of the skin which lies just below the epidermis. Most of the structures from which the hairs grow *(hair follicles)* are found in this layer. There is a system of blood vessels throughout the dermis. The dermis also contains a complex network of elastic fibers running in all directions. These fibers are responsible for the elasticity of the skin. Also, the numerous nerves and nerve endings which are responsible for the sensations of the skin are located in the dermis. Certain of these nerves act in maintaining proper conditions in the skin, and in modifying those conditions in emergencies, such as exposure to heat and cold. Nerve endings located in all parts of the dermis notify the body of external dangers, such as changes in temperature, and injuries. The nerve endings responsible for touch sensation are more numerous than heat- or cold-sensation nerves.

The dermis is not a smooth layer of cells; rather, it has innumerable small projections which extend into the epidermis, and cause an interlocking of the two layers. Because these projections are arranged in rows, they appear as

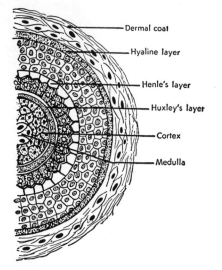

Greatly enlarged cross-sectional diagram illustrating the various layers of which an ordinary hair follicle is composed. Only the cortex and medulla layers are portions of the hair shaft itself, the other layers making up the surrounding wall of the follicle from which the shaft develops and emerges.

ridges in the skin, particularly on the inside tips of the fingers; these ridges constitute the patterns of the fingertips, and are made use of in finger-printing.

The third major layer of the skin is located beneath the dermis. It is called the *subdermis,* and consists mostly of fatty tissue. This layer is responsible for most of the insulating ability of the skin. However, the fat layer is missing from some parts of the body, such as the eyelids. The subdermis varies in depth.

The hair

There are several different kinds of hair on the body. Its appearance depends on age and body location. The so-called *lanugo* is that hair which develops on the unborn child. Usually, it is shed before birth, or within the first few months after birth. The lanugo is immediately replaced by *secondary hair* which is fine and soft and is often referred to as "baby hair." The coarser hair of later life is called *tertiary hair.* Hairs are continually lost from all parts of the body throughout life, and those which replace them often are coarser than their predecessors. As a result, the body and scalp hair of older persons may be exceedingly coarse. With increasing age, hair may also lose its pigment (*melanin*) and become gray or white.

There are about 125,000 hairs on the scalp of the average person. Dark persons usually have fewer scalp hairs than blonds. Hair is sparser on others parts of the body; there are

Illustration: Anatomy of the Skin . . . Grace Hewitt

about 200 to 300 hairs per square inch on the chin and 100 to 130 per square inch on the black of the hand. Scalp hair usually grows from three to five inches in a year and may become as long as two to three feet, or even longer.

The hairs of the body originate from *hair follicles* embedded in the skin. The lower part of the follicle extends into the dermis where it is supplied with blood vessels. As a rule, only one hair grows from a single follicle. That part of the hair beneath the surface of the skin is called the *root,* while the part extending outward from the skin is termed the *shaft.* The sebaceous glands of the skin have their openings in the hair follicles. These glands secrete a substance *(sebum)* which is responsible for the oily appearance of the skin or scalp. Persons with oily skin possess overactive sebaceous glands. When the hair follicle becomes plugged, the sebum collects within it, turns dark at the surface, and becomes a "blackhead."

Minute muscles *(erectors pilorum)* are connected to the hair follicle. When these muscles contract, they temporarily displace the entire follicle, causing the hair to "stand on end." The skin surrounding the hair is also elevated by the contraction of these muscles; the result is a prickled appearance of the skin, sometimes called "goose pimples." Contraction of the muscles also exerts pressure on the sebaceous

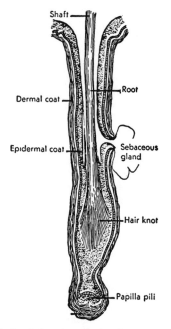

This hair is at the stage in its development at which it will shortly fall out. The root is hardened and the hair has separated at the papilla, leaving the papilla pili. The follicle is constricted at its base. A new papilla will bud out from the old follicle wall.

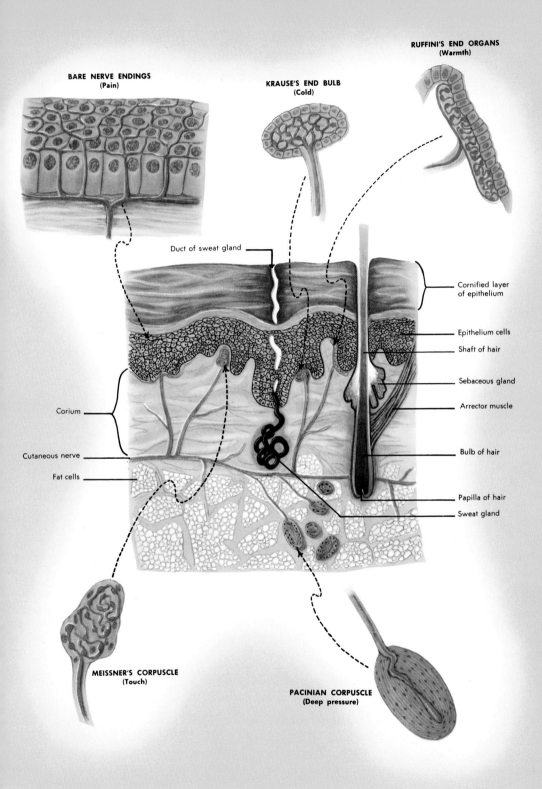

BARE NERVE ENDINGS
(Pain)

KRAUSE'S END BULB
(Cold)

RUFFINI'S END ORGANS
(Warmth)

Duct of sweat gland

Cornified layer
of epithelium

Epithelium cells

Shaft of hair

Corium

Sebaceous gland

Arrector muscle

Cutaneous nerve

Bulb of hair

Fat cells

Papilla of hair

Sweat gland

MEISSNER'S CORPUSCLE
(Touch)

PACINIAN CORPUSCLE
(Deep pressure)

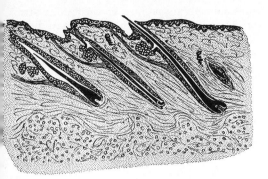

This cross-sectional diagram of the human scalp shows how the hair follicles may grow at an angle which allows the hair shaft to lie flat upon the head. A contraction of the small muscle lying just below the sebaceous gland can cause the hair to become erect and can also cause goose pimples to develop.

glands, causing the emission of extra amounts of sebum. Thus, this set of reactions is an added aid in protecting the body from sudden cold; the hairs form a better insulation when standing erect and the sebum coats the skin with a further barrier against the cold.

Sweat glands

There are two types of sweat glands, the more numerous being the *eccrine* glands. These are distributed over the entire surface of the body. They are located in the dermis of the skin, but their secretions are carried to the surface by tiny ducts, or pores. The secretions of these glands consist of a watery solution containing small amounts of salts, vitamins, amino acids, and fatty acids. They also contain small amounts of waste products. The main function of the eccrine glands is to cool the body. Sweat evaporates from the surface of the skin, and this evaporation cools the skin and the blood in the vessels of the dermis. Then, when the cooled blood flows back to the interior of the body, it cools the other body areas. Cooling is essential, since the cells of the body emit large amounts of heat during their normal activities.

The sweat glands also aid the body in keeping out infection, because some of the substances in perspiration have antibacterial properties. Consequently, persons with dry skins often are more susceptible to certain diseases.

The *apocrine* glands are the second major type of sweat glands. These glands are found only in certain regions of the body, particularly under the arms, around the nipples, on the abdomen, and around the anus and genitalia. Apocrine glands develop after puberty and are associated with the follicles of hairs which develop at puberty. These are the sweat glands that produce a secretion, the odor of which is regarded by

many persons as unpleasant. Women have about twice as many apocrine glands as men. The milk-producing glands of a woman's breasts are modifications of the apocrine sweat glands.

The nails

The nails are special structures growing from the skin and are made up of cells containing large amounts of the tough material of the skin, keratin. At its base and part of the way along its sides, the nail is embedded in the skin. The skin beneath the nail is similar to ordinary skin except that it contains elastic fibers which are connected to the nail to hold it firmly.

The nails themselves are thin, hard, translucent plaques. They are made up of dead cells from the stratum lucidum of the epidermis. At the point of their origin at the roots beneath the skin and extending out into the visible part of the nail, the nails are very thin. This area of growth is white in appearance, and has the shape of a semicircle or half moon. It is called the *lunule*. The fingernails grow about two inches a year. At this rate, it requires about one week for material at the root of the nail to become visible at the cuticle.

Disorders of the skin

Diseases of the skin may be very serious. However, the vast majority of skin disorders do not endanger life if they are given prompt and proper attention. The various manifestations of skin diseases depend to a large extent upon which part of the skin is involved. Thus, there are diseases of the individual layers of the epidermis and dermis, of the hair or hair follicles, of the blood or nerve supplies of the skin and of the sweat glands. Furthermore, diseases may be general, affecting large areas of skin, or they may be localized, affecting perhaps only one pore. Many skin diseases are secondary to internal diseases, such as infections.

Because of the important role of the skin in protection, in sensation, and in excretion, it deserves especial care. Such attention does much to make for a healthy, happy, and attractive individual.

SKIN DISORDERS: ALLERGIES

The term *allergy* is applied to any condition in which a person reacts in a hypersensitive or unusual manner to any substance or agent. People may become allergic to various foods, drugs, dusts, pollens, fabrics, plants, bacteria, animals, heat, sunlight, or many other things. The symptoms that result from an allergy may be of many different kinds, but most generally affect the skin and mucous membranes. Such a hypersensitive condition of the skin is caused by changes that take place throughout the body.

Whenever foreign material invades the tissues, the body reacts to combat the intruder. In some cases, white blood cells may attack, devour, and digest the material. When the invading material is protein in nature, it is called an *antigen*. In the presence of an invading antigen, the body makes certain other specific protein materials called *antibodies* which are able to combine with the *specific* antigen for which they were formed and render it harmless. Such antibodies are then stored for future use in the event that the same antigen may again invade the tissues. The normal existence of such antibodies in the body confers on it *immunity* to the specific materials. Thus when a virus enters the body and causes chickenpox, the body reacts by making antibodies to the chickenpox virus and storing them away, so that at a later date if the virus invades the tissues, the antibodies can combine immediately with the virus protein and render it harmless before the disease can occur. Antibodies may be gained by having a disease, by having some milder form of it, or of a closely related disease, or receiving serum from some other person or animal that has the antibodies.

Small amounts of protein materials (plant and animal tissues or cells) other than disease-producing organisms may also gain entry into the body. Most proteins that are consumed in the food are broken up in the digestive system, but small amounts of certain types from specific foods may pass through the intestinal wall and into the blood. Pollen and small particles of dust may pass into or through the mucous membranes of the nasal passages, lungs, or throat. Occasionally, minute particles may also pass through the skin. Certain drugs and poisons which are not proteins may enter the body also. If these substances combine with one of the body proteins, then they acquire a protein nature. Heat, cold, sunlight, and x-rays may cause changes in some body proteins making them foreign to the body, in a sense. In all of these cases, the foreign protein acts as an antigen, and the body may produce antibodies to it. When this happens, a person is said to be sensitized to that antigen or substance. Such allergy-producing antigens are frequently referred to as *allergens*.

The antibodies remain free in the circulation for a while, but eventually become attached to various tissue surfaces where they are ready for use when needed. When a substance to which the person is sensitized again enters the body, these antibodies are believed to be torn away from the body tissues, and engaged in an attack on the invading substance. This almost imperceptible tissue damage is believed to cause the release of small amounts of a chemical substance called *histamine*. Histamine is then carried by the circulation to the skin and mucous membranes where it produces the characteristic symptoms of allergy—various skin disorders, sneezing, etc.

Two things, therefore, are necessary for an allergic reaction to occur. There must first be an initial sensitization to some specific substance. This first exposure may never be noticed by the person in any way, so that allergy patients frequently find it hard to believe that they have been previously sensitized. There then must be a second exposure to the same substance, and at this time the typical symptoms of the allergy will become apparent. The reaction time (time between exposure to the allergen and the appearance of symptoms) is usually 24-48 hours, but occasionally it is less than 12 or more than 90. Although severe reactions may require two or three weeks to subside completely, the allergic symptoms generally disappear rapidly following removal of the substance to which the person is hypersensitive. However, they will return again whenever there is a further exposure.

When only a small patch of the skin is exposed to the substance to which a person is sensitive, there frequently may be only a small localized skin reaction. When the exposure is greater, or the antigen enters the system through the mucous membranes or the gastrointestinal tract, the reaction may be generalized and affect the entire body. Sometimes one portion of the body may show a more extreme reaction than the others because tissues in that area are more sensitive to the effects of the histamine.

While many of the facts concerning allergy are only partially understood, there is sound evidence that the explanation given is essentially the correct one. The reasons for the appearance of some specific allergy in one individual but not in most others are complex in nature, and probably involve specific structural or functional weaknesses. This is borne out by the fact that, in some cases at least, allergies may be inherited. Inherited or acquired weaknesses in the tissues may make it easier for some antigens to enter the body of certain persons. Furthermore, there is reason to believe that the adrenal glands are involved in some unknown manner in the production of symptoms of allergy, and differences in the adrenal glands of various individuals may influence their susceptibility to become allergic. Mental attitudes also are known to play a part in the production of allergies in some people. (For further discussion of the effects of the mind on the body see Chapter 19, "The Mind.")

Symptoms

Allergies may cause a wide variety of different symptoms. Many of these symptoms also may occur as the result of other quite different disorders. This is particularly true of the great variety of skin symptoms. In other sections of this chapter, numerous conditions are described in which there is an inflammation of the skin (*dermatitis*) caused by factors other than allergy. In these nonallergic conditions, the skin changes are often identical with those observed in persons who have an allergy. Therefore, the diagnosis of an allergy may be particularly difficult, and in many cases requires that the physician perform various special tests upon the patient. Often, however, the results of these tests are conflicting and nondecisive.

A number of relatively common allergic diseases are more manifest in other parts of the body than in the skin. *Hay fever*, for instance, affects the mucous membranes of the nose, eyes, and upper respiratory tract. In *asthma* the lower portions of the respiratory system are most prominently involved. (For further discussion of these subjects see Chapter 5, "The Respiratory System: *Hay Fever* and *Asthma*.") In some allergic conditions there also may be upsets of the digestive system, and occasionally severe headaches may result. In all of these cases there may be some accompanying change in the skin, but in other commonly encountered allergies the skin changes constitute about the only symptoms. The specific skin symptom may bear very little relation to the cause of the allergy; a particular antigen produces varying types of response in the skin of different individuals.

One of the most common skin changes associated with allergy is simply a reddening (*erythema* or *hyperemia*), caused by increased amounts of blood in the lower layers of the skin due to localized capillary dilatation. Reddened areas of this type may be restricted to a small area of the body, or may be general over its surface. They turn white when subjected to pressure from a finger, seldom are long-lasting, and either disappear within a few days or progress into some other type of symptom.

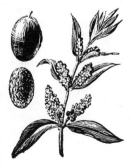

Illustration of a branch and the familiar fruit of the European olive tree, *Olea europaea*. Although the purified oil of this plant is frequently employed as a lubricant for dry and scaly skins, some individuals unfortunately become sensitized to it, so that even bland olive oil may on rare occasions cause a severe allergy.

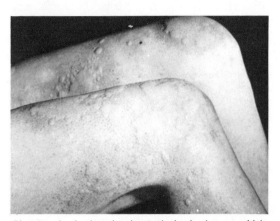

Photograph of a leg showing typical raised areas which constitute the most usual sign of hives or urticaria. *Courtesy Mayo Clinic, Paul A. O'Leary, M.D.*

Hives (*urticaria*) is another common skin condition in which whitish or reddish, slightly elevated areas of the skin appear. These *wheals* may be small, like pimples (*papules*), or much larger patches or streaks *(welts)*. They generally cover the entire body, being most common on the areas covered by clothing. They are frequently accompanied by prickling, itching, or burning sensations. Hives are caused by the accumulation of tissue fluids (*edema*) beneath the epidermis in areas seen as wheals. The condition generally arises rapidly, may last for an hour or so, and then disappears as quickly as it came, if its cause has been removed. *Papular urticaria* occurs almost entirely in children between the ages of two and seven, and is characterized by small red patches, in the middle of which is a small red pimple. The patch frequently disappears soon after its appearance, while the papule may persist for days or even weeks. This disorder usually appears at night, and is most common on the outer surfaces of the arms, legs, and buttocks, and on the face.

A third type of symptom frequently associated with allergy is known as *eczema*. There is a reddening of the skin, followed by the appearance of minute blisters or *vesicles*. These vesicles become larger and are generally accompanied by an intense itching. In acute cases, these blisters break and exude a fluid which forms a crust on the skin. The crust then flakes off, frequently as the result of a secondary inflammation of the skin. Such a series of events may continue to recur, and may become more complex as the result of secondary infections that arise in the damaged skin. Eczema may cover any area of the body, and is one of the most severe of all allergic symptoms. Eczema-type reactions of the skin also may result from some infections and as the result of various nervous conditions.

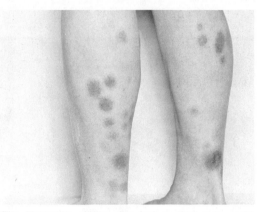

The illustration shows skin lesions that may occur from hypersensitivity resulting from exposure to barbiturates. *Courtesy of Department of Dermatology, Mayo Clinic, Paul A. O'Leary M.D.*

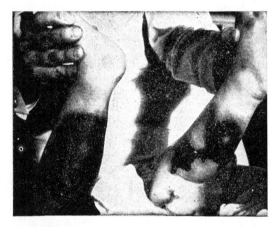

Photograph depicting the severity of the symptoms that in certain cases may develop from hypersensitivity to some drugs, in this case a sulfonamide. *Courtesy of Ashton L. Welsh, M.D.*

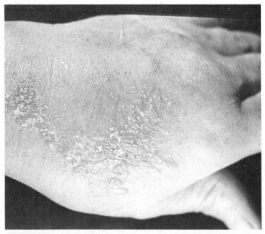

This blistered hand is typical of the dermatitis that may occur from contact with some toxic substance, or as the result of allergy to some often nontoxic substance. *Courtesy of Ashton L. Welsh, M.D.*

Other symptoms that are occasionally seen as the result of an allergy include *nodules,* which are small hard bodies beneath the skin, and large blisters (*blebs* or *bullae*). As the result of the various skin changes which occur, *secondary lesions* eventually may develop. These include abrasions or erosions, fissures or cracks, ulcers, and scars. These secondary lesions are seldom encountered when the patient receives prompt treatment and the cause of the allergy is determined and removed.

Allergy-producing agents

Food allergies: Hypersensitivity to specific foods is relatively uncommon, contrary to popular belief. Such allergies are almost invariably caused by protein in the food. Milk, eggs, peas, beans, and shellfish are most frequent causes of such conditions, and they usually produce hives. Shellfish are also a common cause of giant urticaria, in which there is an unusually large amount of swelling of the lips, eyelids, ear lobes, tongue, external genitalia, and other areas.

Food allergies in infants frequently result in a severe eczema, and are most often caused by egg white, milk, wheat, oats, barley, and corn. Since eczema may result the first time an infant eats egg white or some other of these foods, it seems possible that sensitization of a child may have occurred while it was receiving its nourishment through the placenta—that is, before it was born. Infantile eczema most often appears in the second or third month of life, and may disappear spontaneously by the end of the second year, with no remaining signs of the food hypersensitivity. The condition may appear again or become worse following vaccination, colds, or eruption of the teeth. Although infantile eczema occurs in well-fed and healthy infants, the nervous irritability which it causes so interferes with sleep that the general health of the child eventually may be impaired. Malnutrition, diarrhea, and other generalized disturbances may be indirect results of the condition.

Sensitivity to egg, wheat, and milk usually occurs less frequently with increasing age, and disappears almost completely between the fourth and twelfth years. The skin eruptions in older children are less crusty and oozing than in infants, and tend to be drier and more pimply. The itching is severe, however, and scratching of the eruption causes thickening of the skin, which results in further itching. The danger of infection of scratches so obtained is one of the more serious aspects of childhood eczema.

Drug allergies: A large number of chemical substances when taken into the body or applied to the body's surface are capable of producing severe allergic symptoms. Not only are such skin conditions encountered as the result of some medicine to which the body has become sensitized, but they also occur as the result of contact with various industrial chemicals. A great many chemical substances are capable of producing a hypersensitivity in the body, and the list of materials that have produced such manifestations is therefore a very long one.

Skin eruptions caused by drugs differ somewhat from other allergies in that they frequently manifest brighter colors, appear suddenly, occur symmetrically on the body, are frequently extensive, and do not generally produce other body disturbances. Most symptoms disappear after administration of the drug is stopped. Skin eruptions caused by iodides and bromides disappear more slowly, however, and those caused by arsenic hypersensitivity may *appear* long after the drug has been taken and may last indefinitely. Hypersensitivity to phenolphthalein, which is used as a laxative, also may produce an inflammation which lasts long after administration of the drug has been stopped. The detective work of the physician is sometimes complicated when cross-sensitivity occurs. In such instances, the patient is allergic not only to one drug, but also to its close chemical relatives. Thus, an individual with a primary sensitivity to procaine may be unable to tolerate the sulfonamides and other related compounds, as well. Allergies have been seen in nursing babies whose mothers were taking some drug, but aside from this instance, drug allergies are relatively rare in infants.

The nature of the skin eruptions which result from drug allergies is varied. Occasionally, the symptoms may be accompanied by a rise in temperature, cramps, ringing in the ears, nausea, a sore throat or sneezing, and pains in the arms and legs. The changes in the skin may be those of eczema, hives, or erythema. Occasionally, these may be accompanied by hemorrhagic changes in the skin, thickening of the skin, blisters, and boil-like eruptions. Among the more common drugs that may cause eruptions might be listed acetanilide, amidopyrine, antipyrine, arsenic compounds, aspirin, atabrine, barbituric acid derivatives, benzoic acid, benzocaine, bismuth, bromides, digitalis, insulin, iodides, ipecac, liver extract, opium and morphine, penicillin, phenobarbital, phenolphthalein, quinine, salicylic acid, sulfonamides, and turpentine. Over 200 other less widely used substances also have been reported as effective in producing a hypersensitivity. Except for reactions to penicillin, it is evident that allergy to any one of these drugs is a relatively rare condition, when one considers the number of persons to whom they are administered without ill effects.

Included among the various medicinal preparations which are capable of producing allergies should be mentioned the various serums and other animal products. When various immunizing serums, such as tetanus antitoxin, are repeatedly injected into an individual, they occa-

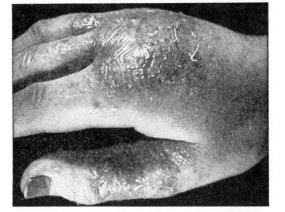

The dermatitis shown in this photograph resulted from contact with a soap. Many persons are sensitive to soap, which is a frequent cause of skin eruptions. *Courtesy of Ashton L. Welsh, M.D.*

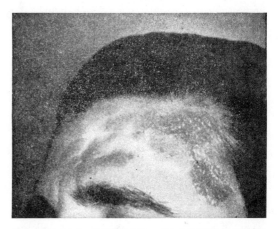

The leather of a hat band was the causative agent for the dermatitis shown in this photograph. This condition is a quite common one but is easily prevented. *Courtesy of Ashton L. Welsh, M.D.*

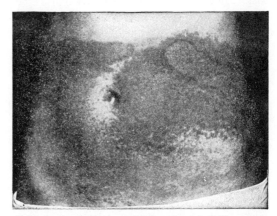

Vulcanized rubber in a girdle stimulated the severe dermatitis shown in this photograph of the area that was exposed. *Courtesy Department of Dermatology, Mayo Clinic, Paul A. O'Leary, M.D.*

sionally produce a sensitive condition as the result of the development of antibodies against the proteins in that serum. In some acute cases, the entire body may react violently to a further administration of the same serum. The dangerous condition which occurs within a few moments in such cases is known as *shock*. Sometimes a single large dose of serum from another individual or animal may cause *serum sickness* a week or so after the serum was administered. Modern methods of preparing the sera for injection have caused a marked decrease in the incidence of this condition.

Other chemical allergens

Persons engaged in occupations in which they are constantly exposed to some chemical substance are prone to develop a hypersensitivity to such materials. Airplane workers may develop allergies to glues, bakers to flour, barbers to quinine, dentists to Novocaine, and painters to linseed oil. In many cases, the distribution of the symptoms follows the parts of the body most exposed to the allergens, but if the patient is highly sensitive or is exposed to large amounts of the antigenic substance, the entire body surface may become affected.

Various soaps and detergents are also common allergens, although these agents are more often responsible for *primary irritant dermatitis*, a condition easily confused with true allergy. True allergy to soaps and detergents is usually due to additives, such as perfumes, included in the manufacturer's formula to enhance the product's appeal. However, excessive use of cleaning agents which are not in themselves allergens often lays the groundwork for skin allergy because it promotes penetration of allergens by breaking down nature's protective barriers. Housewives, domestic workers, and restaurant employees are especially susceptible. When harsh soaps or detergents dissolve the fatty film of the skin, extract important water-holding substances, and break down skin protein, allergens are much more easily absorbed through the entire thickness of skin.

Toilet preparations and cosmetics also are allergens for some persons. Nail polish is a common offender most often affecting the face and neck. A mother's nail polish may sensitize the skin of her child. Lipstick, lacquers, hair dyes, hair-waving solution, and perfumes have been known to produce allergies. Hairdressers are particularly prone to develop such sensitivities. Mild outbreaks or eruptions following the use of any of these preparations generally subside as soon as the particular offending article is removed. When perfume is placed behind the ear and a transitory reddening appears in that area, the use of that particular perfume should be stopped; even such mild forms of allergy may become

severe. Sensitivity to lanolin or wool fat, which is frequently incorporated in cold creams, is of common occurrence.

Clothing: Articles of clothing, watchbands, plastic frames for glasses, and jewelry may also produce severe eruptions of the skin in certain hypersensitized persons. Allergies caused by clothing may be engendered by the fabric itself, or by some substance in the fabric. Dyes and preservatives which are incorporated into many fabrics are particularly active in this regard. Leather, furs, silk, cotton, wool, and feathers are prominent among the materials that cause clothing allergies. Substances added to rubber, plastics, and leather to improve their physical properties are also common causes of skin eruptions. Many individuals who are hypersensitive to some particular fur are not affected by fur from some other species of animal. Furthermore, dyes and preservatives used in treating the fur are common irritants and may cause some confusion as to the actual cause of the allergy. In a great many cases, the cause of a clothing allergy may be detected by observing the distribution of the symptoms, which approximate that portion of the body with which the article of apparel comes in contact. Occasionally, the symptoms are more generalized, and may include a reddening of the entire body, sneezing, and headache.

Allergies caused by specific fabrics are among the most frequent that occur during childhood. Allergies to wool and various dyed fabrics manifest themselves in the form of itching eczema-like eruptions similar in many ways to those caused by food hypersensitivities. Wool allergy is largely seasonal, being more common in the winter months when woolen clothing is used. It is usually restricted to the portions of the skin exposed to the clothing, and is worse when profuse sweating occurs. Wool from different types of sheep or wool treated in different ways may cause different symptoms. Following prolonged periods of freedom from contact with the wool, the hypersensitivity may disappear entirely.

Dusts and pollens: Various microscopic particles borne in the wind come in contact with the mucous membranes of the eyes and respiratory tract and produce symptoms characteristic of allergy in these organs. When the affliction is seasonal, it probably is caused by pollen from plants, and is called hay fever or allergic *coryza*. (For further discussion see Chapter 5, "The Respiratory System: *Hay Fever*.")

Plants and animals: Hypersensitivity to plants is among the most common causes of skin allergies. So many persons develop a severe skin eruption when exposed to poison ivy that this condition is seldom thought of as an allergy. However, about one person in five is not subject to ivy poisoning in any way. Prior contact with the plant or with dust from it is necessary

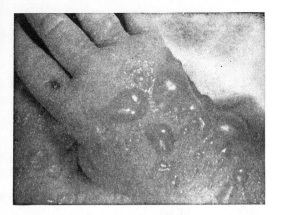

These blisters are typical of those which are seen in patients who have come in contact with poison ivy, or other noxious plants which grow wild in this country. *Courtesy of Ashton L. Welsh, M.D.*

for a subsequent exposure to produce ivy poisoning, and newborn infants and others who have never had such a prior contact are not affected by the plant. The allergy is caused by a chemical substance in the ivy leaves that is held in contact with the skin by its containing resin; this same type of substance is also responsible for allergy to poison oak and poison sumac.

The symptoms of ivy poisoning usually develop from several hours to several days after exposure. They commence as a reddening on the hands, wrists, neck, face, and other exposed parts. There may be a generalized swelling of the skin, and small vesicles form which later coalesce into larger blisters. Contrary to popular belief, the fluid contained in these blisters does not produce further symptoms of ivy poisoning when it comes in contact with unaffected portions of the body. Serum eventually exudes from the blisters, and the skin becomes crusty and dry. After a period of time the symptoms generally disappear spontaneously. Allergic reactions to poison sumac, oak, dogwood, and primrose may remain at the erythema or reddening stage, and less frequently produce blistering.

A variety of other plants including primrose and chrysanthemum are occasionally active in sensitizing some individuals who have come in contact with them. Exposure of allergic persons to these plants produces symptoms similar to those occurring from ivy poisoning. Furthermore, many of these plants actually contain poisonous chemicals in them or in fine hairs on their leaves, which are toxic for all persons, and which produce symptoms because of their toxicity rather than because of an allergy. In addition, a number of other plant materials are able to sensitize the skin to light, so that the skin changes occur only after exposure to the sun

or other strong radiation. Among these might be mentioned limes, parsnips, figs, bergamot, and rue.

Lower members of the plant family, such as bacteria and fungi, are also able to produce allergic skin changes. Such reactions may be primary or secondary. Many of the less typical forms of common infectious diseases are believed to be caused by secondary symptoms which are produced because of a hypersensitivity to the disease-producing organism.

Insect bite hypersensitivity is common. In some individuals, a simple mosquito bite may produce a large and painful swelling out of all proportion to that seen in most other persons. Bites or stings by bees, wasps, bedbugs, lice, fleas, gnats, caterpillars, and various marine fishes and other animals may produce extreme reactions in some few individuals who have previously been sensitized to the allergenic materials of the particular species.

Heat, cold, and light: Heat, cold, and light may be the direct cause of burns, chapping, and sunburn, but in some sensitive persons they may produce allergic skin changes. These usually take the form of hives. In most cases, the symptoms subside rapidly after the cause has been removed. Hives caused by cold are seen on the hands, feet, ankles, neck, face, and ears of sensitive persons who go outside in cold weather. A piece of ice placed on the skin of a normal person produces only a reddening; while in cold-sensitive persons, it causes a wheal that may extend beyond the contact point of the ice. Such persons should remain indoors during winter or live in warm climates if possible. The symptoms of allergy to heat are much the same as those to cold. Ordinary light sensitivity is also similar, but there are some rarer forms of this condition that differ greatly. In *summer prurigo* or *solar eczema,* the lesions caused by the sun include pimples, wheals, and reddening. They are quite persistent and recur each spring, generally disappearing in the fall. Sensitization

Drawing of a branch of poison ivy (*Rhus toxicodendron*), illustrating the typical triple notched leaves, and the flowers and fruit, which are less commonly observed. The plant grows near the ground, or may climb up the side of trees or into bushes. The dermatitis which results from it is usually more severe than the dermatitis caused by other plants, and is typified by progressive reddening which eventually progresses to an extensive blistering.

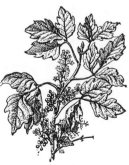

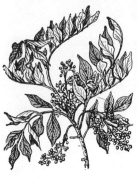

This drawing of a branch from a poison sumac *(Rhus vernix)* shows the very characteristic shape of the leaves and the berries. The severe dermatitis which results from contact with the plant is of an allergic nature, and may be prevented, when necessary, by desensitization treatments. Poison sumac is but one of a number of common plants that prove a hazard to most people who go about in underbrush or other uncleared areas.

to light may be produced by the ingestion of a variety of drugs, particularly the sulfonamides and the phenothiazines.

Psychosomatic factors: Occasionally allergic symptoms appear which cannot be attributed to any of the various agents already discussed. These symptoms do not disappear when various foodstuffs are eliminated from the diet, when clothing is changed, or by any of the usual methods for disposing of an allergy. Many such symptoms are believed to be caused by mental influences upon the body. The mechanism by which these allergic symptoms arise is not well understood, but it is thought that strong emotions cause a release of various chemical substances into the blood stream—substances which are capable of sensitizing the body and which act as allergens. Subsequent emotional disturbances bring about another release of these substances, with the result that an allergic reaction such as hives develops. These effects are particularly troublesome to women during the menopause. Often the family physician or a psychiatrist, after making a thorough study of the emotional background of such patients, can aid the patient in getting relief from these symptoms.

The symptoms of mentally-induced skin afflictions are much the same as those of other skin disorders, and are greatly varied as to type and severity. In many cases, they are accompanied by other body disturbances. The skin disease usually disappears when the mental problem is solved. In many cases, such conditions arise as the result of emotional conflicts of which the patient is not consciously aware. Typical causative problems include economic insecurity, changes in environment, unbalanced or changed family relationships, sexual maladjustment, social insecurity, and feelings of guilt. Any strong emotional reaction such as fear, jealousy, or hatred may evoke such a response. To say that such conditions are "all in the mind" is both true and false, for although their removal is only through the mind, the ability for a person to recognize this may be absent. (For a more detailed discussion of the relation of mental disturbance to physical disease, see Chapter 19, "The Mind: *Psychosomatic Disorders.*")

Determination of the cause of allergies

The exact nature of the substance to which an individual is hypersensitive must be ascertained before a person with an allergy can be properly treated. The causative agent is sometimes quite obvious, but more often it can only be detected by careful examination, inquiry, and testing of the allergic individual by a physician. There are a number of methods that the doctor may employ to help him in this search for the allergen, and all of them require the closest cooperation of the patient.

A case history is most important, for by finding the age at which an allergic dermatitis first occurred, and the circumstances surrounding the daily life of the individual, the doctor may be able to draw some important conclusions as to the probable cause. He may take a careful look into the dietary habits, the brands of cosmetics, and other seemingly trivial things concerning the patient. The patient must be most thorough in answering these questions, because some minor item that might be overlooked could be the cause of the allergy. The physician may ask for samples of various things, even of dust from the house in which the patient resides. He will undoubtedly perform a careful physical examination in order to detect possible signs of the allergy that have not as yet become apparent to the patient.

Perhaps the most helpful of all of the means at the physician's disposal are the skin tests, in which the patient's skin actually is exposed to a large number of different possible allergens. A positive reaction to an allergen consists of a reddening or a small wheal or blisters at the site

PIRQUET, von Cesenatico, Clemens Peter (1874-1929) Austrian physician and pediatrician. In the year 1907, he first introduced the application of a simple tuberculin skin test as a method for the diagnosis of human tuberculosis. He is noted for first suggesting the use of the term *allergy.* He also made studies on serum sickness, and contributed a number of important medical investigations concerning the fundamental nature and causes of cancerous growths found in the human body.

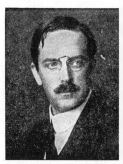

of contact with the test substance. It is possible to test a number of potential allergens in this manner on a small area of the skin. One of the most commonly used tests is the *patch* test.

The conditions of the patch test are made to simulate those caused by actual contact of the skin with the offending agent. The test substance is applied to the skin; if in a day or two no change occurs in the skin, the reaction is said to be negative; but if itching occurs and there is a skin reaction, it seems likely that the offending substance has been found. Patch tests are dangerous when conducted by untrained persons, since only minute amounts of test material can be used safely without provoking a severe skin reaction.

The treatment of any allergic patient is apt to be difficult. In some cases, the physician may even think it necessary to refer a patient to a specialist such as an allergist or a dermatologist. The first and most important step in the treatment is the discovery of the offending substance, and the second step is to avoid that substance as much as possible. In some cases, this is not so easy as it may seem. It is not possible for most people to leave the area in which they live when hay fever season arrives, for instance, nor is it always possible to change one's occupation. For that reason, it may be necessary for a physician to undertake further steps in prevention of the allergic conditions.

It is sometimes possible to "desensitize" a person to some material to which he is allergic, although desensitization of a person for a skin allergy usually is impractical. Furthermore, such a procedure may have little effect or only temporary value. Desensitization usually is undertaken only when other measures have failed.

A group of drugs known as *antihistamines* are of major importance in the treatment of many allergic patients. When taken under medical supervision, they frequently are effective in alleviating symptoms of allergy, and in preventing a recurrence of the symptoms, even in the presence of the allergen. The doctor may also prescribe various powders, lotions, and ointments to soothe the skin and ease the patient. Because many materials are able to irritate a skin that is already aggravated by an allergic condition, it is important that the patient use great care in what he allows to come in contact with the affected skin. Such substances should be limited to those approved by the physician.

Cortisone or ACTH are powerful hormonal agents which are sometimes used internally in the control of the symptoms of allergic disorders. In cases of dermatitis, preparations of cortisone ointments are commonly applied to the skin. Since improper use of these compounds can produce undesirable side effects, they should be employed only by patients under strict medical supervision.

SKIN DISORDERS: DERMATITIS

Dermatitis is defined as an inflammation of the skin. The term is frequently used erroneously as a synonym for *dermatosis,* which means skin disease. Seemingly, there are an unlimited number of disorders which may affect the skin, so that the field in medicine concerned with the skin and its diseases, or *dermatology,* is broad and complex.

Many skin disorders are so exceedingly rare that most physicians have never seen them. Such rare disorders are not given detailed consideration in this volume. Others are so common, or important, that they are discussed in separate sections in this chapter. In the present section consideration is given those conditions which occur with a reasonable degree of frequency, but which do not merit separate extended discussions. A number of tropical diseases which manifest themselves by skin disorders are discussed separately in Chapter 24, "Tropical Diseases."

The symptoms of a dermatitis are varied, and include reddening *(erythema),* small blisters, crusting, oozing of fluids, scaliness, cracking or fissuring, and other secondary changes from the normal appearance. The causes of these conditions are many, and include burns, physical irritants, infections, plant and insect poisons, strong chemicals (industrial), nutritional deficiency, disturbances of other parts of the body, and systemic diseases. The dry skin of the elderly is often worse in winter.

A similar set of skin changes may be caused by a number of different disease-producing agents, so that the accurate diagnosis of skin conditions is difficult. Nevertheless, the treatment of a person with a skin disorder largely depends upon its cause. The discussion of dermatitis, therefore, is arranged primarily according to the conditions causing the different forms of skin disease. Some forms of dermatitis are resistant to treatment, and require long periods of careful medical attention before they can be overcome. Consequently, one should see that any dermatitis that may appear upon his body receives prompt medical attention. Self-diagnosis and self-treatment are not only ineffective in most cases, but can lead to severe and dangerous complications.

Dermatitis resulting from physical and mechanical factors

Heat, cold, chaffing, and scratching may produce a number of common forms of dermatitis. Sunburn, for instance, is caused by the ultraviolet rays from the sun. These rays can be filtered out by certain sun-screening agents or

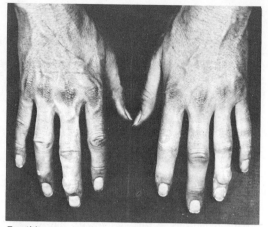

Frostbite may produce several other severe and grave consequences, in addition to the blisters shown here. *Courtesy of Department of Dermatology, Mayo Clinic, Paul A. O'Leary, M.D.*

by opaque chemicals tinted to skin color. Such compounds are of especial value for light-sensitive persons and remain effective for about three to four hours after application, depending upon the extent of exposure to moisture, perspiration, and rubbing. In this connection, lotions and creams that produce an "artificial tan" or a "double tan" have become highly popular over the last decade. They contain dihydroxyacetone, a chemical capable of reacting with elements of the skin to bring about "tanning" within a few hour of application. The resulting skin color often has undesirable yellow overtones, however. Dihydroxyacetone confers no protection against actual sunburn. Furthermore, while the compound appears innocuous so far, some dermatologists have expressed concern over its possible long-term side effects.

Severe sunburn is a more serious condition than is generally thought. This is because the severe irritation caused by the rays greatly interferes with the performance of the many functions of the skin. In a typical sunburn, the initial reddening (*erythema*) is followed by the appearance of minute blisters (*vesicles*) which may grow together to form larger blisters. The intense itching experienced during this period usually disappears after several days, or about the time that the outer layer of the skin peels off. Chronic overexposure to the sun may produce more serious changes. (For a further discussion of sunburn see Chapter 23, "Physical Injuries and First Aid: *Sunburn and Other Burns.*") Burns may also be caused by prolonged exposure to x-rays or radium rays; and many physicians, particularly radiologists, have been seriously burned by these rays.

Prickly heat (*miliaria rubra*) occurs in warm climates among certain persons who sweat profusely or dress too warmly. It is caused by the retention of sweat as a result of clogging of the pores. The eruption takes the form of minute pimples and blisters which burn and itch intensely, but disappear spontaneously in a few days, if cared for properly. Frequent baths, light and loose clothing, and avoidance of soap are all helpful in controlling the itching. If these measures are not successful, a physician can generally prescribe a drug to be applied to the skin which will make the patient comfortable.

Chilblain and frostbite are two common dermatoses occurring as the result of overexposure to cold. Chilblain is characterized by a reddening of the face, ears, hands, and feet with accompanying itching or burning. The symptoms are more severe than the ordinary discomfort experienced by most persons during cold weather, and result largely from poor circulation. Exercise, improvement of the diet, and warm clothing are helpful in the prevention and control of the condition, but severe cases require medical attention. In frostbite, the flesh of the fingers, toes, ears, nose, cheeks, and other parts become so cold that the circulation in the area is seriously impaired. The symptoms vary with the degree of cold and the length of exposure to it. With increasing severity there is reddening, swelling, blisters, and death of the tissue (*gangrene*). Rubbing or application of warm or hot pads to the frozen part is to be *avoided,* and medical attention is imperative in order to avoid serious consequences—even possibly the loss of some part of an extremity.

Other skin changes may result from scratching or picking at the skin with fingernails or other objects, or from irritation of the skin by the chaffing of clothing. Bedsores on invalids are caused by such mechanical irritation, and can be prevented by proper nursing techniques. Rubbing the skin over a long period of time may cause it to assume a permanent thickened and leathery appearance. When two surfaces of the

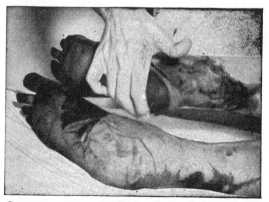

Gangrene occurs most frequently in the extremities, as shown in this picture in which the feet and ankles are affected by this exceedingly dangerous and often fatal disease. *Photo F. W. Schmidt.*

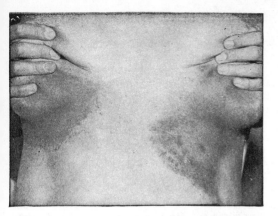

Intertrigo affects the areas of the body that are subject to friction, such as the area below the breasts, and the areas between fingers and toes. *Photo F. W. Schmidt.*

skin touch each other such as between the thighs, and cause friction, a resulting inflammation may develop. This condition is known as *intertrigo,* and may be accompanied by cracking, oozing, burning, and itching. Such lesions frequently are complicated by infection, either by yeasts, bacteria, or both, and require attention.

Corns are hard, cone-shaped, thickened areas of the skin which usually appear on the toes as the result of friction or pressure from improperly fitting shoes or socks. The inner portion of the corn is pointed, so that external pressure forces the point of the corn into the underlying tissues with a painful effect. The sufferer can buy "corn plasters," which may be treatment enough. However, if the corn persists or becomes infected, a physician should be consulted. Proper footwear following treatment usually results in a complete cure. Calluses resemble corns, except that they cover larger areas and have no pointed central core. Frequently, they disappear when proper care is given the feet.

Dermatitis resulting from viruses, bacteria, and molds

Many cases of dermatitis are caused by an infectious agent which either infects the skin or invades the body as a whole and causes symptoms of dermatitis. The source of these disorders determines whether the skin itself is the site toward which attention is directed, or whether medical care must be given to the body as a whole. The symptoms of both types of skin diseases may be similar, although generalized infections usually attack a greater area of the skin. In either case, the dermatitis may be contagious, so that the additional problem of isolation exists in caring for the patient.

Fever blisters or cold sores *(herpes simplex)*

are among the most common infections of man. Occurring most frequently in children of the one-to-five age group, this condition is caused by a large virus, and the lesions usually appear as an itching group of small blisters on the lips. The base of these blisters may be reddened. At other times, the eruption may occur on the nose, face, ears, genitals, or any mucous membrane. A fluid exudes from the sores and forms a crust; eventually this flakes off. There occasionally may be a swelling of the lymph nodes in the areas near the sore, but the disease usually disappears spontaneously within a week or two. The virus is thought to remain dormant in body tissues, becoming active only in the presence of "trigger mechanisms": upper respiratory tract infections, fever, menstrual periods, other physical or emotional stress, overexposure to sunlight, and perhaps the use of certain foods, or drugs. Although the infection is seldom severe, herpes simplex of the cornea of the eye, if not properly treated, can result in impaired vision or blindness. When the lesions are troublesome or recurrent, the physician can sometimes elicit the initiating factor from a detailed history, and preventive measures can be taken. Otherwise, supportive measures are helpful. For example, cold sores in the mouth may be soothed and cleaned by a 10 percent salt solution. Since moisture aggravates inflammation, drying lotions or liquids, such as camphor spirit, may be applied to oozing lesions. For secondary infections, the physician may prescribe topical or systemic antibiotics, depending on the severity of the condition. Steroids are sometimes given, but never

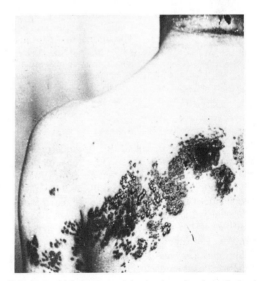

Shingles, which is caused by a virus, is characterized by blisters, such as those shown here broadly distributed along a band on one side of the patient's back. *Courtesy of Ashton L. Welsh, M.D.*

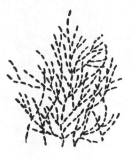

This drawing of the causative agent of actinomycosis, *Actinomyces bovis,* has been magnified approximately 1.5 thousand times. The fungus grows in the form of branching white filaments, which may infect the lungs or other important internal organs. When the skin is infected, the resulting dermatitis is usually secondary to invasion of some of the underlying tissues by this dangerous member of the *Actinomyces* family.

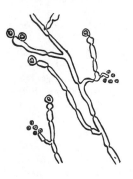

Drawing of the fungus which produces both thrush and moniliasis, *Monilia albicans,* magnified by about 165 times. This dangerous organism is closely related to the common yeasts, and although it may grow in filaments, it also forms buds at the ends of these branches. These may then break off and grow into another plant. Several of the other species of *Monilia* are also known to cause extremely severe infections that heal slowly.

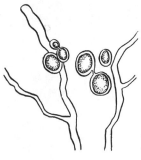

Illustration of the causative agent of human blastomycosis, a species of *Blastomyces,* magnified nearly 300 times. The organism is very closely related to the common baker's yeast, which, however, is not considered pathogenic to man. Blastomycosis is one of the most unpleasant kinds of infectious skin diseases, although it is uncommon in most civilized countries and non-tropical areas.

for eye lesions, because this medication may actually induce blindness. Other agents which have proven useful in selected cases are iododeoxyuridine and vitamin B. Smallpox vaccination, once widely used, is now believed worthless as a preventive measure for herpes simplex. However, work is underway to develop a herpes simplex vaccine.

Shingles *(herpes zoster)* is another relatively common virus disease characterized by the appearance of small patches of blisters the size of a matchhead, on a red base. It almost always appears on only one side of the body. The disease occurs most often in spring and autumn, chiefly in adults. It appears suddenly, preceded by severe pain in the affected area, and sometimes fever. The pain varies greatly in intensity, and although the skin symptoms usually subside a few weeks after the initial attack, the pain may last for several months. Proper soothing medicines usually permit a patient to remain active; but in old people the condition may be disabling. While shingles is not generally regarded as a dangerous disease, the possibility that it may affect nerves leading to the eyes or to other important organs is great. If it is suspected that the disease is present, therefore, a physician should be called. A number of other virus diseases also produce skin eruptions, and are discussed elsewhere. (See Chapter 2, "The Child.")

A large number of skin diseases of varying severity are caused by molds or fungi. Two of such diseases, ringworm and athlete's foot, are discussed in separate sections in this chapter. Many of the others are less common and merit only passing mention. Most of these diseases are named after the particular species of fungus which is the causative agent of the disease. *Moniliasis* is a skin disease caused by a yeast-like fungus, which may also affect the mucous membrane of the mouth, and cause a condition commonly known as *thrush.* More severe fungus infections include *blastomycosis, coccidioidomycosis, torulosis,* and *sporotrichosis.* Each of these serious conditions is rather rare and requires highly specialized diagnostic ability and treatment in order to restore the patient to health.

Pityriasis versicolor or *chromophytosis* is a rather common fungus infection in which there appear fawn-colored patches on the trunk and limbs. It is most common in young adults. The colored patches that occur in chromophytosis actually may be lighter than the surrounding skin in dark-complexioned persons. In any patient, the patches may be accompanied by inflammation and itching. Medical attention effects a prompt cure.

Actinomycosis is caused by a mold which ordinarily affects the respiratory system. When it infects the skin, it generally involves the mouth, jaw, neck, shoulders, or back. Red swollen areas slowly develop and exude a pus-like material. The involvement of the skin is usually secondary to an infection of the underlying tissues. Acintomycosis is a dangerous condition, but it responds to modern drugs when it has not become too advanced before medical attention is given.

The dermatitis of bacterial infections may be caused by: bacteria which are located in the skin itself; bacteria which are distributed in the skin and the other parts of the body; or bacteria which are solely in other parts of the body. In many rather common infectious diseases—such as scarlet fever, brucellosis, pneumonia, typhoid fever, rheumatic fever, and meningitis—an eruption or rash may appear on the skin which is not caused by the bacteria but by secondary effects which the organisms produce. Treatment of patients with these conditions involves the destruction of the bacteria which have invaded the body as a whole. Most of the dermatitis caused by bacterial infection of the body in general are discussed in detail in other chapters of this book. The characteristic changes which occur in the skin of patients with the various types of venereal disease are likewise discussed in Chapter 15, "The Reproductive System: *Venereal Diseases*." The bacterial dermatoses discussed in the present chapter are, with a few exceptions, those in which the bacteria principally affect the skin.

Most common of the bacterial skin infections are boils *(furuncles)*. These are round, tender, reddened elevations on the skin which contain a central core filled with pus and bacteria, usually staphylococci. Some boils come to a "head" and exude the central core before they regress and disappear; other boils recede spontaneously without rupturing. Boils may result from small wounds such as are caused by a sliver, irritation, scratching, or friction, or by any disease or process which allows the bacteria to gain entrance into the skin. Persons with other forms of dermatitis, as well as persons who suffer from diabetes, anemia, and many other conditions, may show a predisposition to have boils. Such eruptions may be spread by contact from one area of the skin to another, or in some severe cases they may spread via the blood and lymph.

Boils should *not* be squeezed, since this procedure may cause the infection to escape into the surrounding tissues or even to be transferred to other sites. Boils should be kept as clean as possible and covered to prevent spread of the infection, and to avoid friction. When a healthy person has a single, small boil, it usually heals spontaneously; but if severe or multiple, medical attention is extremely desirable to prevent an extension of the disease. Multiple boils may require treatment with antibiotics or special vaccinations. Boils appearing on the eyelids, nose, ears, genitals, lips, or mucous membranes also require special attention, as they are more prone to be followed by complications.

Carbuncles are deep, grouped boils. They are large, reddened swellings appearing most often on the back of the neck. They may have a number of perforations, ooze pus-like material, crust over, and slough off. Carbuncles are dangerous and require prompt medical attention. They are almost always scar-forming. Their management involves the use of antibiotics, x-rays, and rarely surgery.

A number of other pus-forming eruptions of the skin are not uncommon. Barber's itch or *sycosis vulgaris* is a typical example, and is

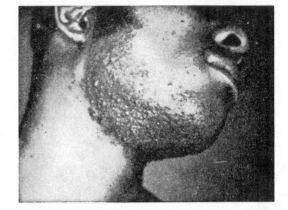

Sycosis vulgaris is a disease involving infection of the hair follicles. It usually occurs in the bearded area as shown. *Courtesy Ashton L. Welsh, M.D.*

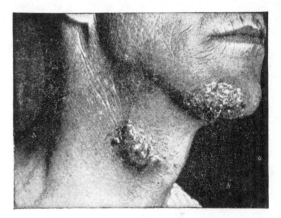

This man suffers from tinea barbae or ringworm of the bearded region. *Courtesy Dept. of Dermatology, Mayo Clinic, Paul A. O'Leary, M.D.*

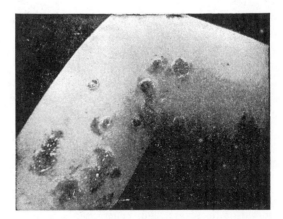

The skin lesions shown are quite characteristic of impetigo, childhood disease caused by infection of the skin. *Courtesy Ashton L. Welsh, M.D.*

caused by an infection with staphylococci. The initial symptom may be a reddened area below the nose, accompanied by burning and itching. This may be followed by several small, pus-filled swellings on the reddened area. Each of these swellings is characteristically pierced by a hair, since the disease attacks primarily the hair follicles. In this manner the disease gradually spreads until it eventually may affect the entire bearded region. The condition must be distinguished from another form of barber's itch (tinea barbae), which affects the lower bearded regions below the jaw, and which is, in reality, ringworm. Laws governing sanitation in barber shops have largely eliminated this source of dermatitis. Proper treatment of patients with the condition varies between careful hygienic measures, externally applied fungicides, and occasionally more drastic procedures.

Impetigo is a common disease of childhood, but also occurs in adults. It is caused by staphylococci and streptococci and is characterized by the appearance of a number of small blisters on the skin. Usually, the blisters become pus-filled and then rupture, forming a crust that continues to build up and spread by continuous oozing. While the condition may remain localized, impetigo can also be spread by the fingers to other parts of the body. Impetigo is highly contagious only in infants and young children, but adults may also transmit the disease. Poor personal hygiene, the use of public swimming pools, beauty and barber shops, and contact with infected pets are all sources of impetigo. Medical care is essential to remedy the disorder. Treatment usually consists of appropriate topical antibiotics and instructions for careful, regular home care. Sometimes an oral broad-spectrum antibiotic is prescribed for a few days, since acute kidney disease has occasionally been attributed to impetigo. Much of the success of the treatment depends upon the patient's care to prevent spread. Regular cleansing, particularly of the hands, and the use of paper towels are particularly important. Some physicians advocate the use of special antiseptic soaps containing hexachlorophene or other bacteriostatic agents.

Ecythema (ulcerative impetigo) may, for practical purposes, be considered synonymous with primary impetigo, since the treatment and symptoms are almost identical. Ecythema usually represents a recurrence or extension of primary impetigo. In children, the condition frequently develops following insect bites or trauma, especially on the lower legs. The protection of newborn infants from persons carrying either infection is essential. *Impetigo neonatorum* is a severe and generalized systemic disease requiring the immediate attention of a physician in order to prevent a rapidly fatal outcome. Epidemics in hospital nurseries are becoming an increasing problem as antibiotic-resistant strains of staphylococci continue to proliferate.

Erysipelas, or St. Anthony's Fire, is a particularly severe streptococcal infection of the skin and subcutaneous tissues. This condition is accompanied by headache, vomiting, chills and fever, pain in the joints, and prostration. Most of the symptoms are caused by a poison (toxin) given off by the bacteria. The affected skin area is red, swollen, and warm to the touch; it is separated from the surrounding skin by being sharply demarcated and hot. In some cases, there may be blisters or other eruptions, in addition to the reddened area. The lesions become larger by simply spreading from the margins, and sometimes while they grow larger in one area, they recede in another. Since the disease may be fatal—particularly in the very young and in the aged—it is most essential that a doctor be consulted immediately. Furthermore, the patient should be confined to bed. Antibiotics can be used to suppress the infection and the symptoms. Erysipelas usually clears up in a relatively short time when the patient is properly treated.

A number of diseases which primarily affect domestic animals occasionally are transmitted to human beings. *Erysipeloid,* which is caused by the bacillus (*Erysipelothrix rhusiopathiae*) that produces swine erysipelas, is characterized by a bluish, inflamed, marginated swelling, usually on the hands, but other areas may be affected. The disease may be acquired from either healthy or sick swine, from other animal species, from injuries by articles which have previously been in contact with animals, and even from fish. Medical treatment is required even though the disorder usually disappears spontaneously after a few weeks. *Glanders,* caused by infection with *Malleomyces mallei* is contracted by persons working with horses or cattle, and is a dangerous but rare disease. The skin eruptions that occur are ulcerative in nature and may spread to other parts of the body. Surgery, antitoxins, and antibiotics are all usually necessary in effecting a cure. *Anthrax,* the cause of which is *Bacillus anthracis,* is generally contracted from infected animals, as well as from unsterilized shaving brushes and leather goods. It is a relatively rare condition that usually starts like a carbuncle and may end fatally. The carbuncle-like lesion spreads and affects the entire body. Rapid treatment with the proper antibiotics and serum provides the best outlook for patients with anthrax. This disease is of great historical importance because the anthrax bacillus was the first microorganism proved definitely to be the cause of an infectious disease. *Tularemia,* caused by *Pasteurella tularensis,* is transmitted to man by infected wild rabbits, squirrels, and other small animals, and by the

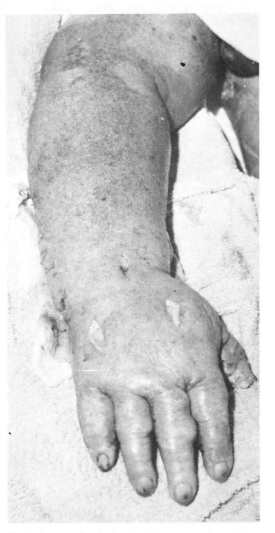

Erysipelas, or St. Anthony's Fire, is a severe infectious skin disease. *Courtesy Department of Dermatology, Mayo Clinic, Paul A. O'Leary, M.D.*

Diphtheria of the skin is rare, and in most cases is caused by infection of some pre-existing wound with the diphtheria organism, *Corynebacterium diphtheriae*. The usual symptoms are a false membrane and gray ulceration around the swollen edges of the infected area. Such infections, although they are quite small in extent, are almost invariably fatal if not given prompt medical care. Diphtheria immunization is helpful in preventing the occurrence of the disease. (For further discussion of diphtheria see Chapter 2, "The Child.")

Tuberculosis of the skin is more common in Europe than in North America. There are two distinct varieties of this disease. In one, the tubercle bacillus *(Mycobacterium tuberculosis)* can be found in the eruptions. This is true tuberculosis of the skin. The other form *(tuberculids)* has many of the characteristics of the true tuberculosis, but the bacillus usually does not occur in the sores. Tuberculin or tuberculin-like substances probably cause this allergic reaction. This condition may appear after an injection of tuberculin or may be secondary to an internal focal infection of tuberculosis. The tuberculous eruptions may take several forms—widespread pimples, ulcerations, nodules, or areas of fungus-like granulation.

The treatment of patients with tuberculosis of the skin, like the treatment given those with tuberculosis of other parts of the body, is most effective when the disease has not progressed to a late stage. In some cases, small tuberculous areas may be removed surgically, while in other cases various forms of radiation are helpful. Recently, a number of modern drugs have made the treatment of patients with this disease more effective. In many cases, skin tuberculosis is accompanied by lung tuberculosis. (For a discussion of tuberculosis of the lungs, see Chapter 5, "The Respiratory System: *Tuberculosis*.")

When deep wounds or lesions become infected with certain types of bacteria, or when the circulation to some tissue is interrupted, *gangrene* may develop. Whereas gangrene is usually

bite of infected ticks and deerflies. It is probably observed most frequently among hunters, who acquire the disease while dressing rabbits or other game; the bacteria gain admission to the body through a minor abrasion, hangnail, or small wound. This disease almost always is accompanied by chills and fever, headache, and other constitutional symptoms. When the site of infection is on the face or hands, a small pimple develops and eventually becomes ulcerated and infected. When the bacteria apparently do not enter through a wound, the symptoms are less distinctive, and may simulate a number of other forms of dermatitis. The disease is a dangerous one, and requires prompt treatment with antibiotics.

This drawing of the causative bacterium of erysipeloid, *Erysipelothrix rhusiopathiae,* is magnified about 1,200 times. This same small bacterium is also the cause of swine erysipelas. Erysipeloid is a relatively mild disorder that generally clears up in a short time spontaneously. It is but one of several types of moderately infectious dermatitis that are common among those persons who are in constant daily contact with livestock.

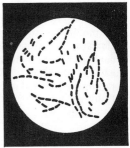

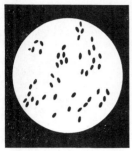

This drawing of the causative agent of human glanders, *Malleomyces mallei,* is magnified about 300 times. The dread affliction is almost entirely restricted to those persons who work with horses and with cattle, and is a very dangerous although quite rare infection. It is another example of a once extremely fatal disease that now responds very favorably to the proper administration of several of the more modern antibiotics.

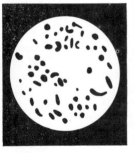

This drawing of the causative agent of anthrax, *Bacillus anthracis,* has been magnified about 1,200 times. This dangerous bacterium is contracted most frequently by persons who are working with livestock or some animal products. Although anthrax commences as a dermatitic sore, its later symptoms may frequently be severe. Modern antibiotics have done much to change the outlook for those persons who contract anthrax.

This drawing of the causative agent of tularemia, *Pasteurella tularensis,* has been magnified about 1,800 times. This dangerous bacterium is carried in both insects and in several higher animals, but it is not spread directly from man to man. Wild rabbits, deerflies, and also ticks are among the most frequent carriers, and these virulent microorganisms may be easily transmitted through the tick eggs for many generations of ticks.

dermatitis, the disease starts with blisters which become infected. These blisters fill with pus, and eventually result in a crusted, oozing, itchy condition. Such symptoms are believed to be caused by a secondary infection on the underlying eczema. In another disorder called *nodular erythema* or *erythema nodosum,* a number of small nodular swellings occur on the shins and other parts of the legs. The reddened swellings, which seem to be below the surface of the skin, are tender for some time, but frequently recede spontaneously. Such a condition usually indicates there is an allergic response of the blood vessels of the skin to some bacterial infection. In young women, such swellings occasionally appear in the spring and autumn without any apparent cause. In most other cases, however, the cause may be any of several conditions such as streptococcal infection, tuberculosis, rheumatism, septic sore throat, or sensitivity to drugs.

Pityriasis rosea is a dermatosis that appears to be feebly infectious, although the organism which causes it is unknown. It is usually mild, and is manifested by small salmon-colored patches which eventually coalesce to cause larger pigmented areas. This condition largely affects the trunk, and is more prevalent in young adults during the spring and summer months. It may disappear spontaneously within a few weeks, but requires careful medical attention to distinguish it from a number of other more severe skin disorders. Lotions which normally have a soothing effect on the skin may be irritating in this disease, so only properly prescribed materials should be employed to ease the itching.

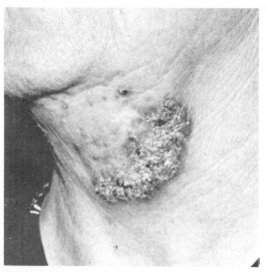

Tuberculosis cutis, or tuberculosis of the skin, is shown here in one typical form. There are many types of this disease. *Courtesy Department of Dermatology, Mayo Clinic, Paul A. O'Leary, M.D.*

thought of as affecting the fingers, toes, or limbs, it may be restricted to the skin. The word "gangrene" implies that the afflicted area is dying or dead; consequently, the condition causes marked changes in the body as a whole. Symptoms include fever, headache, pain, darkening of the affected area, and an unpleasant odor. Only prompt treatment can save the affected area from amputation and, possibly, even the patient's life.

Aside from these well-recognized bacterial causes of dermatitis, many other skin disorders are the indirect result of bacterial infections. In a condition known as *infectious eczemoid*

Dermatitis resulting from plants and animals

The skin disorders which result from contact with various green plants are largely allergic in nature, and are discussed in the previous section. Only in a few rare cases do plants cause a dermatitis by direct action. A variety of minute animals, however, cause severe skin eruptions by bites, stings, or by burrowing into the skin itself. A dermatitis of this type is seldom serious, but its cure may present a number of problems. Details of the control of such skin parasites are presented in Chapter 25, "Sanitation."

Scabies, or itch, results from infection of the skin by small mites about one fiftieth of an inch long (*Acarus scabiei*). These mites live on the surface of the skin, but the female burrows into the skin to lay its eggs. During this process the mite may remain under the skin for some time, traveling along and creating an extended tunnel in which the eggs are laid. The young develop in a few days, and then come directly to the surface where they spend their lives until they, in turn, are ready to lay eggs. The typical sign of scabies is the short, winding burrow in the skin which most often occurs between the fingers or toes. In children this may be accompanied by tiny

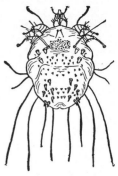

This drawing of the common scabies mite, *Sarcoptes* or *Acarus scabiei*, is magnified about 50 times. While the mite normally lives principally upon the skin, the female usually lays her eggs underneath the surface. About a month after one has been infested with these mites, his body becomes sensitive to them, and this fact accounts for the very intense itching that is associated with the presence of scabies on the skin.

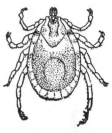

This drawing of the common dog tick, *Dermacentor andersoni*, is magnified about 7 times. Bites by these ticks may cause headaches, abdominal pain, vomiting, chills, and fever, but these symptoms will pass in about 12-36 hours. Some ticks may also carry the organisms of such highly dangerous infections as Rocky Mountain spotted fever, and are able to transmit these diseases to whatever individual they may happen to feed upon.

blisters on the surface of the skin near the burrow. In this stage of the dermatitis, there is very little itching. Later, the skin may develop an allergy or hypersensitivity to the mite, which causes the severe itching associated with scabies. Consequently, by the time the disease is first noticed, the mite usually has spread over a large portion of the body. The treatment of a patient with scabies is entirely a matter of ridding him of the mites. Underwear and bedclothing must be changed daily for a week or two or until all the eggs are hatched out, and care must be taken to avoid infecting other persons with whom the patient is associated. Daily baths and the use of a sulfur ointment, benzoate emulsion, and other recently developed drugs, such as gamma benzene hexachloride and crotamiton, frequently discourage any further activity of the mite on the skin. The use of these compounds requires a physician's advice, not only to make the medication effective, but also to prevent reactions in those individuals who cannot tolerate them.

A number of *ticks* of varying kinds and sizes also may infect the skin and cause severe eruptions. These are picked up frequently in brushy areas or by contact with dogs or other animals that carry them. The female tick attaches itself to the skin by its nose and draws blood for food from the underlying vessels. After several hours or days, the tick will become filled with blood

This photograph shows salmon-colored patches which appear on patients with pityriasis rosea. The patches may grow and coalesce, but eventually disappear. *Courtesy of Ashton L. Welsh, M.D.*

and drop from the skin. If pulled off by force, the "nose" or, more properly, the *proboscis* may be left in the skin and cause an infected sore.

A tick may remain attached to the skin for several hours without being noticed; its bite may cause headaches, abdominal pain, vomiting, and chills and fever. The symptoms disappear in from 12 to 36 hours after the tick is removed. The greatest danger from ticks is the possibility that the tick may carry some infectious microorganism and transmit it to the person it feeds upon. *Rocky Mountain spotted fever* is one such severe infection carried by certain ticks (*Dermacentor andersoni*). Any unusual symptoms following a tick bite should receive prompt medical attention.

One type of *chigger* bite results from small mites or red bugs (*Trombicula irritans*). These mites secrete a keratolytic agent which dissolves the outer layer of skin on which the animal feeds, and causes a red and intensely itching, swollen area. The mites are picked up from grasses and brush, and consequently affect the legs and lower portions of the body more than the upper areas. They accumulate usually underneath garters and belts and in other areas where tight clothing restricts their movement. A physician can prescribe an ointment which will destroy the chigger and relieve the itching. Scratching of insect bites may result in secondary infection which is difficult to cure. Chigger bites can be prevented by rubbing wet "sulfur-foam" impreg-

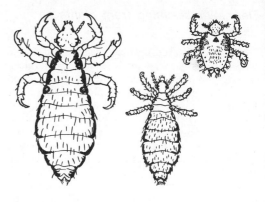

Drawing of the body louse (*Pediculus corporis*), the head louse (*Pediculus capitis*) and the pubic or crab louse (*Phthirius pubis*), all magnified about 12 times. These three parasites can be carriers of various infectious diseases including typhus fever.

nated material on the extremities before going into areas where chiggers are abundant; also, on returning from the country, a good preventive measure is to shower, with liberal use of soap. Control of chiggers is discussed in Chapter 25, "Environmental Health and Sanitation." A number of mites carried by fowls, other animals, or grain also may cause similar symptoms and require like treatment.

Pediculosis is caused by infestation of the skin by lice (*Pediculidae*) which live on the blood that they suck from the body. The bite of the louse causes an itching dermatitis which is aggravated and infected by scratching. There are three major varieties of lice: the head louse, the body louse, and the pubic or crab louse. In addition to making their victims uncomfortable, lice can be carriers of severe diseases such as typhus fever. Consequently, they should be eradicated immediately. Eradication requires thorough washing and disinfestation of clothing, and application to the patient's skin of a suitable ointment which will kill the lice. Many effective delousing agents are available; some of them are irritating to the skin and should only be used when they have been prescribed by a physician. During epidemics, DDT has been used effectively as a delousing powder.

Bedbugs are small, odorous, wingless bugs (*Cimicidae*) that feed on the blood in a manner similar to that of lice. The reaction to bedbug bites varies among different individuals, but generally consists of a small, red puncture spot surrounded by a swollen, inflamed area. In severe cases, these swellings may be painful, and the reddening of the skin involve a considerable area. The use of soothing ointments to prevent scratching frequently causes the inflammation to subside in a short time. A house that contains bedbugs requires fumigation in order to destroy them completely, because bedbugs live during

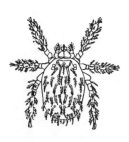

This drawing of the ordinary chigger or harvest bug, *Trombicula irritans,* has been magnified about 35 times. The typical swollen, itching and inflamed bites often produced by this red mite are easily confused with those inflicted by the larger reddish colored sand flea. Chiggers are generally picked up while walking in tall grass or in brush, and therefore they affect the lower extremities of those that they attack.

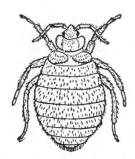

This drawing of a common bedbug, *Cimex lectularius,* has been magnified about 10 times. This smelly little animal may cause extremely painful bites in some persons who may be quite sensitive to it, and it is an exceedingly difficult creature to drive from a dwelling once it has been able to establish itself. Bedbugs may be taken as a sign that places which they inhabit may also harbor other obnoxious parasites.

the daytime in crevices in the floors and walls and in furniture, and are difficult to find. Fumigation may be accomplished with hydrocyanic acid gas (a deadly poison), or fumes of sulfur, formol, or other vapors. (For a further discussion on the control of insects, see Chapter 25, "Sanitation: *Control of Lice and Other Insects.*")

Fleas (*Siphonaptera*) live, for the most part, on lower animals, but occasionally infest human beings, as well. They feed on blood, and leave swollen, reddened areas on the skin that may be severe to a sensitive skin. Such diseases as typhus and plague are carried by rat fleas. Infested animals should be treated with various dusting powders, and houses can be cleared of fleas by spraying or scrubbing with disinfectants. *Sand fleas* burrow into the skin in order to deposit their eggs. They live in dry sandy soil in warm climates, and most often affect the feet, ankles, and legs. The reddened swelling which they cause may become the size of a pea, or larger, and is susceptible to secondary infection by bacteria. A bath with strong soap followed by the application of soothing ointments helps to relieve the itching. However, the lesion disappears much more rapidly if a physician removes the flea and its "cocoon" from the skin.

The bites of most spiders and centipedes are relatively harmless, unless they result in secondary infection. Other than the immediate pain, they usually produce only an itching, swollen area on the skin surrounded by some degree of reddening. However, a particularly poisonous variety, the *black widow* spider (*Lactrodectus mactans*), may cause severe systemic symptoms that require immediate medical attention. First aid in these cases is discussed in Chapter 23, "Physical Injuries and First Aid."

Hookworm is a small, parasitic worm (*Ancylostoma duodenale* or *Necator americanus*) which is regarded primarily as an intestinal parasite, although it produces characteristic skin symptoms. The dermatosis is caused by an invasion of the skin by the young, or *larvae*, of the worm, and occurs several months before the general systemic symptoms become pronounced. The earliest signs are in the soles of the feet, since it is through the soles that the worm originally enters the body from the soil. Small, reddened pimples develop into blisters which may eventually become pus-filled. The disease is a serious one and requires prompt medical attention. In *sandworm disease*, which is generally caused by hookworms carried by cats or dogs, the larvae may cause extensive winding burrows in the skin. The condition is frequently referred to as *creeping eruption.*

A variety of other parasites also may cause some form of dermatitis in man. *Swimmers' itch* is thought to be caused by a small aquatic worm which invades the skin of persons who swim or wade in contaminated water. Reddened itching

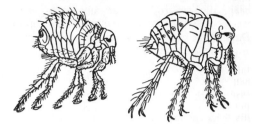

Drawing of the common sand flea *(Tunga penetrans)* and the human flea *(Pulex irritans)*, both magnified approximately 39 times. Fleas may transmit such dread diseases as plague and typhus fever, and an infection of their bites may result in severe ulceration of the skin in the affected area.

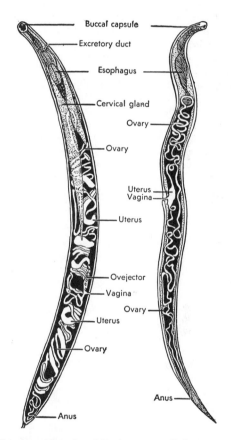

Buccal capsule

Excretory duct

Esophagus

Cervical gland

Ovary

Ovary

Uterus
Vagina

Uterus

Ovejector

Vagina

Ovary

Uterus

Ovary

Anus

Anus

Drawing of females of the two worms that are generally the cause of hookworm, *Ancylostoma duodenale* and *Necator americanus,* each magnified about 10 times. The females produce about 9,000 eggs each day. Of the two, *Necator americanus* is the more common form in North, South and Central America, where it is believed to have been introduced through slaves from Central Africa.

pimples or patches develop a day or two after the exposure. The disease may be prevented by thoroughly bathing with soap and rubbing the skin with a towel after exposure. *Taenia*, or pork tapeworm infection, may cause painful nodules in the skin which disappear only when the general body infection is remedied. Skin eruptions also may be caused by stings from such common insects as mosquitoes, ants, gnats, bees, wasps, beetles, scorpions, and caterpillars.

Dermatitis caused by chemicals

When chemical substances have a direct irritating effect upon the skin, the phenomenon is called *primary irritant dermatitis*, and does not result from allergic sensitivity. Sufficient exposure will bring about the dermatitis in all individuals, although the threshold of sensitivity may vary from person to person. Acids, alkalis, petroleum products, and mineral dusts are among the worst offenders in this regard. The symptoms of a mild chemical dermatitis are almost invariably limited to a reddening or erythema of the areas of the skin that have come in contact with the injurious substance. More severe cases manifest blistering or chemical burns, oozing, crusting, and symptoms of other forms of dermatitis. Although the eczematous nature of primary irritant dermatitis often mimics that of an allergic response, the former is less often intermittent and the reaction time (time between exposure to the irritant and first appearance of symptoms) is much shorter. Treatment in every case starts with avoidance of exposure to the irritant; in most instances, the skin will return to its normal state of health without further aid.

Chemical dermatitis may occur in the home; "dishpan hands" is a skin disorder which is caused by the use of strong soaps or detergents (see also "other chemical allergens," page 238). However, most severe cases of chemical dermatitis result from exposure in the pursuit of some occupation. The incidence of occupational skin disorders, per capita, has greatly decreased during recent years because of better hygienic practices in most industries. Safety devices, protective clothing, ventilating systems, adequate bathing facilities, medical inspections, and training of

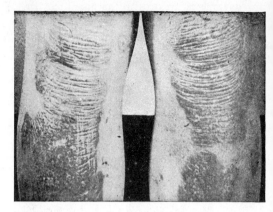

Psoriasis, a skin disease of unknown cause, is shown here in a typical location as reddened areas covered by white scales. The extremities, elbows, knees, trunk and scalp are all affected by the disorder, and only the mucous membranes of the body seem to be immune. The condition occurs in many forms, but is not generally believed to be contagious, as are many other dermatoses that resemble it. *Courtesy of Ashton L. Welsh, M.D.*

workers all have been important measures in this improvement.

Dermatitis resulting from malnutrition

Dermatitis is occasionally a symptom of malnutrition. In vitamin A deficiency, the skin becomes dry, scaly, and develops small, spiny lesions. Vitamin A is believed to have an important role in maintaining the health of the skin. Indeed, vitamin A has been found to bring about an alleviation of the symptoms of skin disorders resulting from other causes. Dermatitis caused by a deficiency of vitamin B_2 (*riboflavin*) is manifest by oily scaling about the ears and nose, and by cracking at the corners of the lips. The symptoms usually are complicated by those of other nutritional deficiencies.

In *pellagra*, a disease caused by a nicotinic acid deficiency, the dermatitis is found on the parts of the body exposed to sunlight, particularly the face and hands. The condition is seen as an intense redness which terminates abruptly where the clothing commences. There is a drying and pigmentation of the skin and a dry red tongue. The cure of patients with these conditions is effected by an adequate diet. Dermatoses caused by deficiencies of other vitamins, fats, and proteins may occur, and are more difficult to recognize.

Dermatitis resulting from organic disorders

A number of forms of dermatitis are caused by disturbances in one or more of the organs of

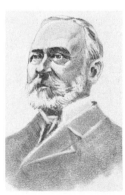

WHITE, James Clarke (1833-1916), American dermatologist. He was an outstanding pioneer in the field of dermatology, and was the first person in the United States ever to be appointed as a professor of dermatology, a position now recognized as essential for all schools of medicine. He contributed a large share of our knowledge concerning many skin diseases. He was the first to describe keratosis follicularis, which is also commonly known as *White's disease*.

the body, and therefore can be remedied only by resolving the primary organic disorder. Insufficient thyroid function (*myxedema*) is frequently accompanied by a swelling of the skin. The skin also may have a dry and waxy appearance. In a number of other conditions, various fatty and protein materials may infiltrate the skin and give it a lumpy or nodular appearance. In other cases, the skin may become highly elastic (*India rubber skin*), or its attachment to the underlying tissues may become so loose that it hangs in folds from the body.

Porphyria is the name given to a small group of organic diseases caused by a metabolic abnormality. In several forms of porphyria, dermatitis may be the only or the most important symptom. The basic organic defect involves the metabolism or *porphyrins*, compounds from which plant and animal respiratory pigments are made. The green chlorophyll of plants is perhaps best known of the porphyrins. In human beings afflicted with porphyria, porphyrins are produced in excess and deposited in the skin and other anatomical areas.

Variegate and *cutaneous porphyria* are congenital disorders in which the skin is highly sensitive to trauma on sun-exposed surfaces. Redness, blisters, and open sores appear with little provocation and heal only slowly, leaving darkened scars. Abdominal pain and nervous system disturbances often accompany the dermatitis of variegate porphyria. In cutaneous porphyria, skin symptoms predominate, and excessive growth of body hair and deepened skin pigmentation may also occur. Acute attacks of both forms of porphyria may, in some patients, be precipitated by one or more of the following: barbiturates, sulfonamides, general anesthesia, chloroquine, griseofulvin, estrogens, and alcohol. Treatment is largely prophylactic, consisting of avoidance of direct sunlight when possible, protection of the skin from trauma, and abstinence from drugs known to bring on attacks. In variegate porphyria, acute attacks are associated with a 25 percent mortality rate. Otherwise, both forms are rarely life-threatening.

Congenital photosensitive porphyria is an extremely rare variety of porphyria, in which sensitivity to sunlight is so pronounced that many patients cannot venture outdoors during daylight. Despite the most elaborate precautions, these individuals are subject to painful, incapacitating dermatitis unless they live an indoors existence.

A localized area of skin occasionally may commence to grow at an unusually rapid rate, and after a short time return to its normal rate of growth. To distinguish these areas from malignant tumors (*cancer*), the growths are termed *benign tumors*. Such tumors require expert medical diagnosis. Identification is of extreme importance because of the precancerous nature

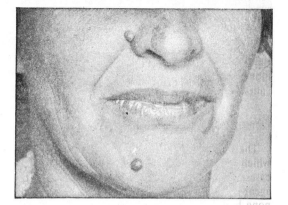

These facial moles are examples of nonpigmented types. They are raised and have other typical characteristics. *Photography F. W. Schmidt.*

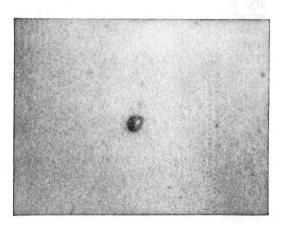

Photograph of a raised pigmented mole or nevus. It will probably never become malignant, unless unduly irritated. *Photography F. W. Schmidt.*

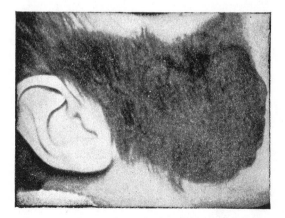

The unusually large, hairy nevus or mole on the face of this infant can be successfully removed by a surgical operation. *Photography F. W. Schmidt.*

of some of these skin growths. Common types of benign growths, some of which may involve the skin, include: *fibroma*, in which connective tissue is involved; *lipoma*, in which fatty tissue is involved; *neuroma*, which involves nerve tissue; *leiomyoma* or *myoma* which are smooth muscle tumors; and others. If these growths are removed early in their development, they seldom cause lasting damage.

Dermatitis of unknown cause

There are a large number of dermatoses for which no cause is known. In many of these cases, there is a possibility that an infectious agent is responsible for the disorder, even though none has yet been demonstrated.

Psoriasis, afflicting two to three percent of the adult white population (but rarely Negroes), is the most common dermatosis of unknown origin. The lesions consist of rounded, reddish, dry, scaly patches covered by grayish-white, mica-like scales. These patches may spread and become extensive. The disorder is recurrent, tending to disappear during the summer in temperate climates. In general, psoriasis is most prevalent on the scalp, nails, lower back, knees, and elbows. Although the cause is unknown, heredity is thought to be a factor. The medical histories of about one third of psoriasis patients show a familial incidence. Secondary factors include infection, local trauma, disturbances in body chemistry, and psychosomatic influences.

Since psoriasis is a disease of infinite variety, the advice of a physician is essential. Because of the almost inevitable recurrences, the patient's best psychological insurance is an acceptance of his condition and the integration of it into his self-image. Therapeutic measures include daily removal of scales, application of prescribed ointments, and in severe cases, oral steroids. Recent research into a group of drugs called folic acid antagonists has also shown promising results. Methotrexate, one of these compounds, produced marked improvement in over half of a large number of cases reviewed in the professional medical literature. Because of its dangerous side effects, however, this drug is usually reserved for severe or intractable forms of the disease. Supportive measures consist of adequate diet, rest, care of intercurrent disease, removal of possible infections, and, occasionally, psychotherapy. Acute attacks usually subside, but permanent cure is rare. Although the lesions are troublesome, they seldom cause lasting physiological harm.

Lichen planus, lupus erythematosus, and *scleroderma* are three other skin diseases of unknown cause. These are relatively uncommon, and the patient having them will require the services of a physician. A more rare condition in which there are large numbers of blisters is known as *pemphigus*; it likewise requires medical attention.

SKIN DISORDERS: MOLES, WARTS, AND BLEMISHES

Moles which are present at birth, or develop shortly after birth, are referred to as *nevi* (singular: *nevus*). Another word for nevus is "birthmark." Brown or black moles are common forms for nevi, although red, blue, and colorless nevi are not unusual. The cause of nevi is not known, and a method of preventing their appearance has not been discovered. They definitely are *not* caused by frightening or otherwise exciting experiences of the mother before the birth of the child. If left alone, birthmarks rarely cause any serious physical difficulty.

Location and classification of moles

Almost everyone has at least one mole, and it is not uncommon to find persons with scores of them. Moles can appear on almost any part of the skin, including the scalp. They may vary greatly in their appearance, depending on the layer of the skin responsible for their origin. Although most moles develop before or shortly after birth, some do not appear until puberty. The most important medical aspect of moles is the possibility of their transformation into a cancerous growth (*malignant melanoma*). Malignant melanoma is a relatively rare disease; and although it arises from some types of moles, most persons who have moles have no reason to fear it.

Moles have considerable cosmetic importance. An occasional mole on the face is often referred to as a "beauty spot." Unfortunately, however, some moles may be very large and unsightly, covered with hair, or located in a conspicuous area of the skin. When such a mole detracts from the appearance, it can be removed, often without a trace of scar. Occasionally, hairs may grow out of elevated moles. They may be quite small and smooth, or much more rarely, they may be extremely large and cover an extensive area of the skin. The term "bathing-trunk" nevus is used in describing such a mole when it covers almost the entire waist and buttock area, giving the appearance of bathing trunks. The cause of such extensive mole formation is not known.

Blue moles are much less common than the brown varieties. They are not actually blue, but appear so because the brown pigment is deeply buried in the skin and seems blue when viewed through the epidermis. White moles (*amelanotic nevi*) may assume the characteristics of colored moles, but are colorless because they lack mel-

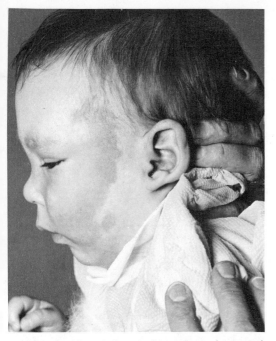

This infant, with typical *port-wine* nevi can be treated best in childhood. *Courtesy Dept. of Dermatology, Mayo Clinic, Paul A. O'Leary, M.D.*

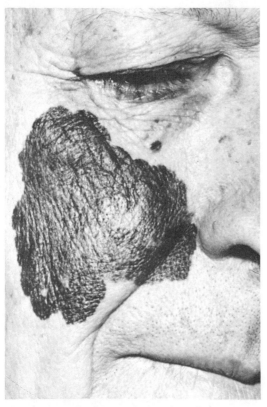

This photograph shows a large pigmented nevus or mole on the cheek. *Courtesy Dept. of Dermatology, Mayo Clinic, Paul A. O'Leary, M.D.*

anin, the normal pigment of the skin. Cancer seldom develops from these growths.

Sebaceous moles are yellow, soft growths with a rough-appearing surface. These lesions occur singly or in groups. They are the result of an unusual growth of the sebaceous or oil-producing glands of the skin. The edge of this type of mole may be pitted and pimply. When sebaceous moles occur in the scalp, they usually do not permit normal hair growth, so that the area is partially bald. Yellow moles, which often develop shortly after birth, are rarely precancerous.

A *linear* nevus is the term applied to the rare condition in which moles appear in streaks, or cover large patches of skin. The streak may be made up of any type of mole. It may be raised, flat, smooth, or rough in appearance. Surgical removal usually gives good results.

Management of moles

Since most moles never cause any serious disturbance, they are best left alone, unless, of course, they are seriously disfiguring or are located in an area in which they might be subject to frequent irritation or injury. Moles on the soles of the feet, palms of the hands, collar line of the neck, belt line of the waist, and on the genitals are especially liable to frequent irritation or injury. These should be removed just before the onset of puberty. Cancerous changes in moles are practically never seen before the onset of puberty. Any mole which shows rapid increase in size, change of color, scaling, itching, or bleeding requires that the entire area should be surgically removed immediately. This must be done by a physician and the specimen examined microscopically by a pathologist to determine whether it has become malignant. An "electric needle" must never be used. Nor should any mole be removed by a cosmetician, barber or beauty shop employee or by anyone not licensed to practice medicine. Improper removal of a mole may aggravate a malignant tendency; hence, moles should be removed only by a physician.

Hemangioma

Hemangiomas are reddish or purplish structures or stains of the skin which are present at birth or develop shortly thereafter. They are an unusual formation of blood vessels, predominantly composed of small capillaries at the surface of the skin. There are three major types of hemangiomas: the "port-wine" stain, the "strawberry" or "raspberry" mark, and the greatly elevated type called *hemangioma cavernosum*. In all forms, the blemishes sometimes disappear without treatment, although scarring may result. Scarring may result, however, after even the most careful medical removal, so that the parents of an affected child should consider the possibility of scarring before having such blemishes removed.

Strawberry or raspberry marks appear at birth or shortly thereafter as raised, flat areas ranging in color from bright red to purple. These blemishes may be small, or may cover large areas. They are most often found on the face, scalp, neck, or shoulders. Many authorities believe that treatment of persons with this type of blemish should be carried out early in life, perhaps within the first year. Delay of therapy until maturity may cause the treatment to be less effective or may increase the amount of scarring. Although many persons prefer to have these blemishes removed by injection of chemicals, application of "dry ice," x-ray or radium therapy, the least scarring and best cosmetic results often are attained by surgical excision.

Often, the treatment of patients with these hemangiomas is limited to concealment by cosmetics. It is also possible to conceal the coloration by tatooing the blemish the color of the surrounding skin. There is a more direct method for complete removal of the blemish, carried out by surgically scraping the skin. This procedure *cannot* be done by anyone but a physician familiar with the technique, since there is always bleeding.

Cavernous hemangiomas appear as rounded, red or purple, spongy masses, usually found on the head and neck. They may be small and not become a problem. If a cavernous hemangioma is large and located where it is in danger of injury, however, it is best that medical attention be sought. Injury which results in bleeding can lead to a serious blood loss.

Freckles

Freckles are small skin blemishes caused by exposure to ultraviolet rays, either in sunshine or from artificial sources. They are found most frequently in persons with blond hair and fair skins. As a rule, freckles do not appear until about the seventh or eighth year of life, but they usually remain for the rest of one's life. However, freckles often fade slightly during the winter months or when carefully protected from sunlight.

Freckles may be confined to certain exposed areas of the skin, or they may occur all over the skin. Lotions and ointments designed to bleach freckles have little effect, although sunburn lotions may minimize freckle formation.

There are many cosmetics which may be used to conceal freckles, if their presence is not desired. In case a freckled person suffers mentally from his appearance, the physician may use chemicals to remove the outer portion of the skin and thereby the freckles. The procedure is dangerous when attempted by unskilled persons,

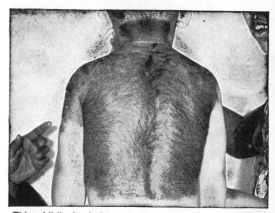

This child's back is covered by a large hairy raised nevus. The condition can probably be eliminated through surgery. *Photography F. W. Schmidt.*

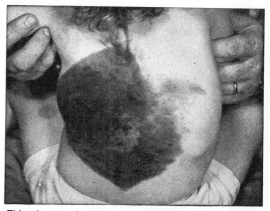

This photograph shows a large dark nevus growing in the skin of the back. Nevi of this size are seldom encountered. *Photography F. W. Schmidt.*

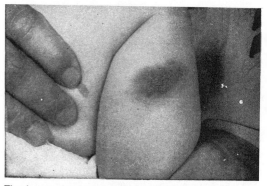

The hemangioma shown here on the leg of an infant can be removed, with little scarring, by proper medical treatment. *Photography F. W. Schmidt.*

and does not eliminate the freckles permanently. The patient must avoid exposure to the sun to minimize subsequent appearance of freckles.

Warts

Warts are small, benign epithelial tumors caused by viruses and found most frequently on the skin of children. Characteristically, the wart consists of a clearly demarcated, raised area of skin which is rough or pitted on the surface. It is most often flesh-colored, but may be slightly darker than the normal skin. Because warts are caused by a virus, and are infectious, they may occur in large numbers and spread locally, especially on sites exposed to trauma. Often new warts appear along scratch lines passed through older warts. Most warts disappear spontaneously after a year or two, but occasionally they spread or continue indefinitely. When constant pressure is exerted upon a wart, particularly those on the palms or soles, serious difficulty may arise from a secondary bacterial infection or from formation of a hard structure resembling a corn or callus.

Removal of warts can be accomplished by a variety of methods, but since the causative virus often remains behind, recurrence at the same or new sites is probable. For this reason, many physicians elect to leave sparse, "silent" warts alone. In certain cases, electrodessication (destruction by electric current) is employed under local anesthesia. Wart tissue may also be destroyed by application of various topical agents, by freezing with liquid nitrogen (performed by a specialist), or by surgical excision. The psychogenic component of this condition has made treatment difficult to assess. X-ray therapy has generally fallen into disuse because of the attending radiation risks.

Chloasma

Chloasma is a disease which usually affects only women. It results in "moth patches," or

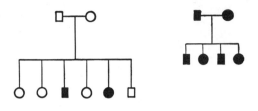

These charts represent the pedigrees of two families of albinos. Squares represent men, circles indicate women, and darkened figures are those persons who were albinos. Both brother and sister were afflicted in the first family, but every person was an albino in the second family pedigree.

patches of darkened skin found chiefly on the face, the nipple, and the external genitalia. The condition frequently occurs in pregnant women, in which cases it disappears after the pregnancy ends. Chloasma may also appear during the menopause and accompany abnormal conditions of the ovaries and female reproductive organs. In many cases, however, the disease may occur without such internal complications. The physician often is able to prescribe treatment to be carried out by the patient. This treatment may include special methods for washing the affected areas of skin such as nightly washing without removal of the soap until morning—with the use of certain astringents, and perhaps a bleaching ointment.

Albinism

Albinism is a rare inherited condition in which the skin, hair, and eyes lack the melanin pigment normally present. It results from a biochemical deficiency in which specialized skin cells called melanocytes are unable to synthesize melanin from the amino acid tyrosine (see page 229). The melanocytes of albinos lack tyrosinase, the enzyme necessary to carry forward the pigment-making reaction. Albinism has no treatment. Victims have an abnormally white, translucent skin, even when they are of Negro ancestry. The hair is white and the eyes appear pink from the reflection of blood vessels through the pupil, the surrounding iris of which does not contain pigment. Because the skin is thin and lacks pigment, the albino, whenever possible, should avoid any direct exposure to the sun, since he is abnormally sensitive to sunlight.

Albinism always occurs in children if both their parents are albinos. When the families of the normal-appearing parents include one or more albinos, the children of these, or the third generation, may or may not be albino. The physician, if he knows there is albinism in the family of a patient, can usually give a fairly accurate estimate of the chances of the appearance of the disease in succeeding generations.

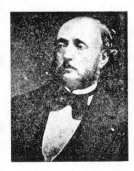

OLLIER, Leopold Louis Xavier Edouard (1830-1900), French surgeon. He is most famous for the method of skin grafting which he first introduced in 1872. It involves the use of pieces of skin of intermediate thickness consisting of the epidermis alone, or of all the skin elements. Moreover he devised a number of special surgical operations for amputations at the knee, elbow and shoulder. Each of these operations was at one time known as *Ollier's operation*.

Vitiligo

Vitiligo (leukoderma), sometimes undesirably termed "Piebald skin," is a condition in which white patches appear on the skin due to absence of pigmentation. Over one third of the patients have a family history of vitiligo, and it afflicts at least 1% of the white population. Among darker races, it occurs less frequently. Loss of pigment usually begins in the second decade of life, with no systemic symptoms. The disorder is purely cosmetic. Where hair growth occurs on involved skin, the hair, too, is usually without pigment (i.e., white). Unlike albinism, vitiligo is never associated with loss of eye pigment. The affected areas are especially sensitive to sunlight. Commonly involved anatomical sites are the hands, underarms, neck, around the eyes, and the genital regions. In about half of the patients, some partial and temporary repigmentation can be seen during the summer months.

Since treatment methods remain largely unsatisfactory, most patients are advised simply to

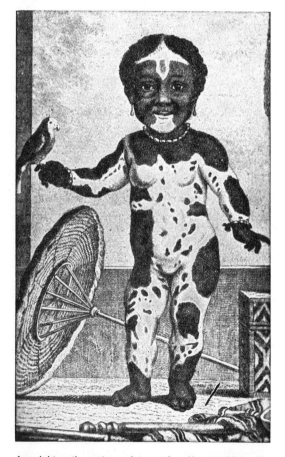

An eighteenth century picture of a Negro child with vitiligo. This depigmenting disease of the skin occurs in numerous forms and in all degrees of severity. It is not generally considered to be dangerous, although it is often badly disfiguring. *Bettmann Archive.*

camouflage their defect with specially prepared cosmetic pastes and lotions and also to protect the sensitive areas from sunlight with appropriate ointments. A few selected patients, in whom some melanin-producing potential can still be biochemically demonstrated in the affected areas, are given methoxypsoralen with good temporary results. However, the drug is sometimes poorly tolerated, the appearance of pigment is slow, and the effect is rarely sustained over 18 months. Complete spontaneous cure is rare.

Tattoos

Tattoos, accidental or intentional, consist of the introduction of various insoluble substances beneath the epidermis. Accidental tattoos are frequently seen in automobile accidents when dirt or other foreign matter is ground into skin abrasions. "Colliers' stripes" in coal-miners appear as bluish-gray stripes on exposed skin where coal dust has penetrated abrasions. Decorative tattoos, deriving from primitive religious and fertility rites, still flourish under more acceptable guises in certain groups in Western culture, notably among men in the armed forces and among members of some teen-age gangs.

The tattoo artist introduces particles of pigment into the dermis with an electric needle. While various outbreaks of infection have been traced to this procedure, the most common hazard is allergic sensitivity to one of the pigments used. Since the pigment is insoluble and therefore permanently implanted, excision of the offending area is usually recommended when allergy develops. Trials with laser beams have proven promising for tattoo removal, but the procedure is still experimental. Other local complications which require tattoo removal are syphilitic lesions, lichen planus, or psoriasis appearing in tattoo sites. All of these conditions seem to show a predilection for tattooed areas. Most often, however, the individual seeks to eradicate a decorative tattoo on purely esthetic grounds. Depending upon the location and size of the tattoo, simple excision, dermabrasion, or chemosurgery may be employed. Subsequent skin grafting depends upon the extent of the resulting defect and cosmetic considerations.

SKIN DISORDERS: BLACKHEADS AND PIMPLES

Blackheads and pimples are common forms of skin eruptions which may cause widespread unsightliness, especially if they become numerous. Both conditions most often originate in the hair follicles, where the *sebaceous glands* deposit their secretions. *Sebum,* the secretion of the sebaceous glands, is an oily material containing

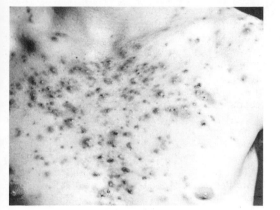

A case of acne vulgaris which has assumed cystic form on the chest. Usually acne vulgaris responds well to treatment. *Courtesy Department of Dermatology, Mayo Clinic, Paul A. O'Leary, M.D.*

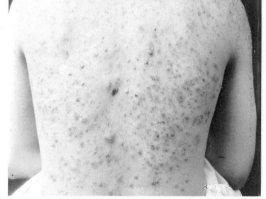

Back of a patient suffering from a typical cystic type of acne vulgaris. Cleanliness is a major aspect of treatment. *Courtesy Department of Dermatology, Mayo Clinic, Paul A. O'Leary, M.D.*

microscopic particles of waste material. When a hair follicle becomes plugged, the sebum collects within the follicle. At the pore opening on the surface of the skin, sebum becomes oxidized by exposure to the oxygen of the air and takes on a black discoloration. Such a blemish is referred to as a blackhead because of the blackened area at the surface.

Blackheads may occur almost anywhere on the body, but are most common to those areas where the sebaceous glands are more numerous and more active. Consequently, they usually are seen on the face, particularly about the nose, on the chest, and on the upper part of the back. Persons with noticeably oily skin usually have more blackheads than those with dry skin. Frequent and continual removal of the oil by soap and water or with cosmetics often prevents blackheads from forming, or keeps their formation at a minimum.

Pimples are small raised areas of the skin which often have yellow centers caused by the accumulation of pus. The surrounding skin is reddened and the pimple may be tender. Pimples can occur on almost any area of the skin.

The cause of pimples is not so easily explained as that of blackheads. These unsightly lesions may result from many conditions, but they frequently represent a blackhead which has become infected or inflamed.

Development of pimples may indicate an improper diet, an imbalance of endocrine function, or minute skin infections. They also may be the forerunners of more serious skin disorders, or a manifestation of a generalized disease of the entire body. Consequently, when pimples become numerous, the patient should consult his physician to determine the reasons for the pimples rather than try to eliminate the disorder himself. If the cause is internal, medication applied to the pimples may have little effect, and may possibly result in permanent damage to the skin.

Pimples should not be squeezed, since this provides an excellent opportunity for invasion of the area by the bacteria which are always present on and in the skin. When an occasional pimple occurs on the face, it can be concealed almost completely by cosmetics which can be purchased for use by both men and women. If a pimple persists for a week or two, the patient should become suspicious of a more serious condition, and seek medical advice. When pimples recur frequently, the patient should visit a doctor, who often is able to suggest a simple procedure, sometimes a change in the diet, which will eliminate the trouble.

Chronic forms

Acne vulgaris is probably the most common disorder associated with blackheads and pimples. It is characterized by blackheads, pustules, cysts, and nodules appearing most frequently on the face, but occasionally involving the back, chest, and arms. The disorder has no sex preference, but is so common at puberty that it affects well over half of all teenagers to some degree. Ordinarily, it persists at least a year, sometimes to college age, and infrequently to middle age. There seems to be a familial predisposition to acne. Many possible causative factors have been implicated: diet, drugs, hormonal imbalance, local irritation, climate, and psychological tensions. Often bacteria are found in the pustules, but they probably represent a secondary infection and not a primary cause.

Acne follows a definite pattern. The sebaceous glands, generally on the cheeks, become overactive. A blackhead is formed in the pores with a semi-solid core of sebum. This inflames the surrounding tissue, producing a nodule. The lesion then begins to develop pus. If the superficial layer of skin breaks, an open pustule will be formed; if not, the lesion will become a cyst.

The two most serious effects, barring infection, are scarring of the skin and psychologic reactions to the cosmetic handicap. If severe scarring results, special make-up may be purchased to cover permanent skin imperfections. Or, the physician may refer the patient to a specialist for possible dermabrasion, a procedure in which the skin is ground down so that the epidermal cells can regenerate an external layer of skin smoother than that previously present. When an adolescent has psychologic problems over his appearance which seem disproportionate to the extent of the skin eruption, it may be that he is using his condition as an unconscious excuse to avoid difficult but necessary personal adjustments. Therapy is therefore important for both medical and psychological reasons. The adolescent who is made to realize that the disease responds to treatment, and generally results in no permanent disfigurement, is less likely to become withdrawn and nervous. Since faithful adherence to the treatment program is essential for as long as the process persists, one or both parents should accompany a teen-ager on his first visit to the physician.

Depending on the state and severity of the lesions, the physician may prescribe one or more of the following: drying lotions, topical steroid preparations, topical antibiotics, x-ray therapy (although many dermatologists have abandoned its use), or oral antibiotics. Hormones may be given to correct an imbalance. Moving to a warm, sunny climate with low humidity, while infeasible for many patients, is sometimes more effective than any other treatment. Since certain foods apparently aggravate acne, dietary restrictions may also help: abstinence from chocolate, nuts, cola drinks, and certain seafoods, along with limitation of milk intake. The physician may recommend elimination of suspected foods, one at a time, until the offender is discovered. Bromides and iodides, known to bring on acnelike eruptions, should also be avoided.

The acne patient helps himself best by keeping his skin clean, and by refraining from scratching, picking, rubbing, or otherwise injuring the lesions. Infection can be spread. Cleanliness is essential. All grease, dirt, and cosmetics should be removed twice daily by bland castile soap, and a mild antiseptic lotion should be used. Most cases of acne are improved by an intelligently conducted treatment program. Because the condition varies so from person to person, the patient should put himself under the guidance of a physician. Properly administered antibiotics will bring the chronic infection under control so that with continued proper hygiene the infection should remain in a reduced or quiescent state until the patient is well past puberty.

Another peculiar form of acne, termed *acne excoriée*, is caused by constant squeezing or otherwise irritating blackheads or pimples. This constant irritation of the facial tissues may result in infection and scarring. This disorder is observed more often among nervous, "high-strung" individuals who give their skin too much attention. Hence, the physician should be aware of such a background of the patient. He may recommend that the patient consult a psychiatrist, if some serious emotional basis appears to be responsible for the scratching.

Seborrheic dermatitis is another chronic disease of the skin involving overactive sebaceous glands. The skin of patients with this condition continually looks greasy. The disorder usually appears during adolescence, and may or may not be accompanied by blackhead formation, or acne. The face, particularly the nose and forehead, and the scalp are most seriously affected, although the entire body generally is involved to some extent. Seborrhea of the scalp is called *dandruff*, which is discussed later in this chapter. Treatment lies chiefly in frequent cleansing of the affected skin. Various special astringents and ointments are also valuable. When there is scaling or crusting of the skin, as well as the abnormal oiliness, it is possible there may be an infection present, or the patient may be malnourished.

Rosacea is a chronic skin disease similar to acne. It is thought to be of internal origin, and appears as a result of any disorder which causes persistent flushing of the face. The skin becomes bright red and oily. The sores differ from those of acne in that often they are not so deep and are less pointed. Sometimes, the eyes may become involved. Women are more susceptible to this condition than men. The physician can recommend a diet which may be successful in clearing the face. This diet varies with the severity of the disease, but most often excludes such items as alcohol, coffee, tea, dairy products, nuts, eggs, extremely hot or cold foods, highly seasoned or rich food, and vitamin A-containing foods.

CARDANUS, Hieronymus (1501-1576), Italian physician and mathematician. He was justly famous as one of the greatest clinicians of this period in history. One remarkable volume of his that was published in the year 1550 contained over 800 illustrations of the human face. Because of the hallucinations from which he suffered, he made early studies on the nature of mental diseases. His mathematical treatises are also quite famous.

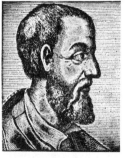

SKIN DISORDERS: SMALLPOX

Smallpox (*variola*) is a generalized disease, but its severest visible manifestations are found on the skin. It is caused by a virus and is highly communicable, with an incubation period of one to two weeks. The onset of smallpox is abrupt, with fever, chills, and rapid pulse and respiration. Other symptoms may include violent headache, back and muscle pains, nausea, and vomiting. Because of this, it is often mistaken for influenza. Not until the third or fourth day of active disease does the skin rash appear. This begins as raised, reddened areas which become pimple-like within a few hours. About the fifth day these become small blisters filled with pus.

The rash usually appears first on the forehead and wrists. Then it spreads to the rest of the face and arms, as well as to the soles of the feet. All parts of the skin, including the mucous membrane, may become involved. The skin lesions begin to dry up about eight or nine days after their first appearance, but it usually requires a month or more before they have completely disappeared.

Permanent scarring nearly always takes place. The extent and depth of the scars depend upon the severity of the disease. Scarring may be increased by damage to the sores, often self-inflicted by the patient, and also by secondary infection of the sores by bacteria. Scarring, particularly of the face, may be exceptionally pronounced in *confluent* smallpox, in which the eruptions, rather than appearing as separate sores are so closely grouped as to coalesce.

Care of the patient

The diagnosis of smallpox requires the services of an experienced physician. Frequently, the diagnosis is not made for some days after symptoms appear, because the disease is mistaken for less serious ailments such as chicken pox, or other dermatoses. Such delay increases the possibility of disfigurement, and decreases the patient's chances of survival.

An important aspect in the care of the patient is isolation and quarantine. Smallpox is one of the most contagious diseases known. Contagion begins 24–48 hours before the onset of any symptoms and persists until the last crusts have disappeared from the sores during convalescence. Throughout this period, it can be transmitted by food utensils, bed sheets, and other objects which have been in contact with the patient. Since the virus is also airborne for limited distances, no one should be allowed near the patient unless the presence of the healthy person is necessary and he is known to be immune because of recent vaccination or having had the disease himself.

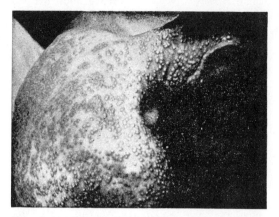

This photograph of a patient with smallpox was taken at a time when the typical skin eruptions were in a stage of peak development. In severe cases, such as the one shown here, the lesions generally leave permanent pits or "pock marks" in the skin. *Courtesy Ashton L. Welsh, M.D.*

Regarding the patient himself, one of the main considerations is the possible infection of the skin eruptions by bacteria. To minimize this danger, the physician will administer drugs to prevent itching which might lead to scratching, and thereby to secondary infection. As an added precaution, the patient's fingers and other body surfaces which might rub against the lesions should be kept scrupulously clean. Bed linens and clothing must be changed regularly and sterilized. Penicillin or broad-spectrum antibiotics are usually prescribed to prevent secondary bacterial infection. Patients with very severe smallpox, especially children, may refuse food and fluids to the extent that kidney and circulatory function are endangered. In such cases, fluids are injected intravenously or given by a tube which is passed through the nose down into the stomach. The eyes may require special care, with application of prescribed solutions or ointments, if swelling and inflammation are severe. Crusts which form on the skin lesions should never be forcibly removed, since this increases scarring and risk of infection.

Prevention of smallpox

It has been known for centuries that once a person has had smallpox, he is immune to the disease and will not contract it again. Vaccination is a deliberate infection of the patient with a disease—not actually smallpox itself, but one which is able to produce immunity to smallpox. The virus used may be obtained from lesions produced in calves or rabbits that have been infected with smallpox virus. Such passage through one of these animals causes the virus to lose its ability to cause the natural disease in man. However, when it is rubbed into the epidermis, the weakened virus causes a local sore which lends immunity to the dangerous form of smallpox for five to seven years. *Cowpox* virus, while causing a serious disease in cattle, may be used for vaccination of human beings. The material used for vaccination is called *vaccine*, and is specially prepared so that it contains no infectious microorganisms other than the particular virus.

The area of the body chosen as the site for the vaccination most often is the upper arm or thigh. It should be an area relatively free from friction by clothing or other parts of the body.

Vaccination is usually carried out by placing a drop of vaccine upon the cleansed skin. The physician then gently rubs a needle against the skin underlying the drop of vaccine. Only the outermost layer of the skin is punctured, so that there is no bleeding, although lymph is exuded from the wound and mixes with the vaccine. The lymph-vaccine mixture is allowed to dry on the skin. It is not necessary to bandage the vaccination unless the patient attempts to scratch the area, or unless there is a possibility of irritation from clothing.

A wheal, or slightly raised area, develops at the site of the vaccination almost immediately, but soon disappears. A day or so later the area becomes reddened and small blisters of pinpoint size appear within this reddish region. In the following days the red area enlarges and the blisters fuse to form a single and larger blister. The fluid within the blister is clear at first but gradually becomes cloudy and later pus-like. During this period the patient may exhibit a fever, and during the eighth or ninth day following the vaccination he may be ill. From the ninth to the twelfth days, the red area increases in size and the skin around it becomes hard and

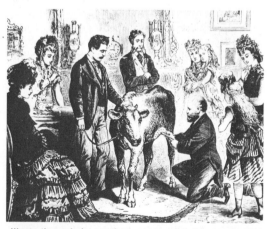

Illustration of the method once used for vaccinating patients for smallpox by transferring the virus directly to them from its bovine source. Although inconvenient, it was effective. *Bettmann Archive.*

thickened. After the twelfth day, the sore begins to heal; and the blister disappears, leaving a black scab which begins to shrink. This scab becomes loose around the edges at first, and eventually falls off. The skin under the crust then is red and slightly pitted. The redness disappears slowly, and a slight scar may remain.

The scratching of a fresh vaccination, followed by scratching of other parts of the body, must be avoided, because vaccination lesions can be transferred to any part of the skin in this way.

The immunity to smallpox gained by vaccination is not permanent. Consequently, vaccinations must be repeated, usually in five to seven years, to insure continued safety. Doctors frequently recommend that vaccination be made during the first year of life. When the second or subsequent vaccinations do not "take"—that is, they heal within a few days, or do not form the customary lesion—the patient is said to have an *immune reaction*. This implies that the immunity from the previous vaccination has not been lost. When an individual vaccinated many years before does contact the disease, it is likely to be mild.

Certain precautions should attend smallpox vaccination. No person with general illness or extensive skin eruptions should be vaccinated, particularly an infant or child with eczema or impetigo. Furthermore, any child with such a skin rash should be kept away from recently vaccinated persons. *Eczema vaccinatum,* which may follow such exposure, is uncommon, but carries a high mortality rate. Women known to be pregnant should also avoid smallpox vaccination unless there are compelling reasons, since fatal infection of the fetus sometimes occurs. Smallpox vaccination is especially hazardous for adult patients with cancer who are being treated with steroids, nitrogen mustard, or radiation therapy. The therapeutic impairment of their natural immune mechanisms may allow the vaccinia virus to multiply dangerously, to the point where the patient's life is threatened. Finally, one should not receive yellow fever vaccination simultaneously, because both vaccines employ live viruses.

For persons exposed to smallpox, revaccination is usually performed immediately. Hyperimmune serum is also employed for prophylaxis. Trials of a drug called thiosemicarbazone (or methisazone) have been relatively successful in preventing active disease in susceptible contacts. The drug has reduced the expected incidence of smallpox by 94 percent, compared with 75 percent for immune globulin, although troublesome side reactions may occur.

Permanent eradication of smallpox as a disease of man is possible. Since the human body provides the principal natural reservoir for the virus, elimination of the disease by vaccination in endemic areas (chiefly Africa and Asia) could accomplish this. Through the World Health Organization, progress has been made over the last decade, but it has been slow. In this age of high-speed travel, disease spread may be unexpected and disastrous, as it has already proven in Britain, where compulsory immunization programs have relaxed and smallpox imported from abroad has caused several serious outbreaks.

Edward Jenner

Vaccination had its beginnings in the last part of the eighteenth century. A rural English physician, Edward Jenner, learned from a milkmaid that contraction of cowpox would make one immune to smallpox. In 1796, Jenner inoculated a young boy with cowpox virus, and then attempted to cause the child to contract smallpox. The child remained healthy, and Jenner reported the experiment in a private publication; medical journals refused to print his findings. For some years, the public ridiculed Jenner. There was a rumor that vaccination would cause one to grow the horns and tail of a cow. However, the method finally was accepted and employed freely. As a result, smallpox, which during the Middle Ages killed 25 to 30 percent of the European population in a single epidemic, now has become a relatively rare disease in all countries with high medical standards. Modern treatment saves the lives of most persons with the disease.

SKIN DISORDERS: RINGWORM

Ringworm *(tinea)* is a common disease of the skin, scalp, or nails caused by infection by a fungus (usually of the genera *Microsporum, Trichophyton,* or *Epidermophyton).* Ringworm generally takes the form of one or several raised, round sores on the skin which seem to heal in the center while the edges continue to grow outward. Occasionally, the healed centers become reinfected, and a second "ring" develops and grows within the original one. In some types of ringworm, there is no healing of the center and the lesion continues to grow. The sores of ringworm begin as small, slightly raised areas with a reddish color. As they enlarge, they become redder, and often contain one or many blistered areas. There may be a slight itching or burning sensation.

A less common type of ringworm appears most frequently in the crotch or under the arms. Called "jockey-strap itch," dhobie itch, or *tinea cruris,* it does not heal in the center, and may cover large areas of the skin. This type of ringworm lacks the circular appearance of the com-

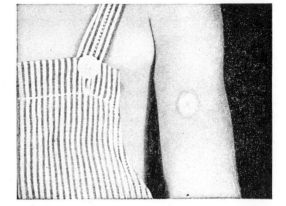

This child has a typical ringworm lesion on the upper arm. The outer ring shows active infection while the center of the sore heals. Ringworm is highly contagious. *Courtesy Ashton L. Welsh, M.D.*

mon disease but often resembles butterfly wings when the sore spreads over the inner surface of both legs.

Ringworm of the scalp is common among children, but relatively rare in adults. It produces areas of partial baldness, which are usually temporary. Because children are highly susceptible to this type of ringworm, outbreaks sometimes occur in schools.

The patient with ringworm is usually treated with griseofulvin, an antibiotic compound which is especially effective against certain fungus infections and is derived from a species of *Penicillium* mold. The drug is generally taken orally for several weeks, but in refractory cases must be taken for four months or more. A few types of ringworm infection do not respond to griseofulvin, in which case other medication may be prescribed. Secondary treatment measures help prevent spread of the fungus and injury to the lesions. Specifically, all sores should be kept clean, dry, and protected, even from the irritation of clothing. Fungi thrive on damp, warm skin, especially in areas such as the crotch, where perspiration is unable to evaporate readily. In ringworm of the scalp, hairs over the infected site should be clipped to avoid transmitting the fungus to other individuals.

Ringworm is a highly contagious disease. It can be spread by animals, as well as by human beings. Dogs and cats that are not bathed frequently are common sources of human infection. Ringworm may be acquired by direct contact with the infection, or it may spread to other areas on the skin of a single individual. Objects handled by infected individuals also carry the fungus. Occasional sources of infection are the backs and arms of theater chairs, combs, and brushes.

To prevent the acquiring of the disease, all known contact with infected persons should

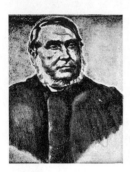

DEVERGIE, Marie Guillaume Alphonse (1798-1879). French dermatologist. He is famous for being the first man to be able to demonstrate clearly the fungus origin of *tinea cruris*. He was also universally noted for his lucid description of *pityriasis rubra* which at one time was known as *Devergie's disease*. The scientific basis of dermatology was established by Devergie and other investigators who conducted their fundamental studies during the midnineteenth century.

be avoided whenever possible; combs and personal effects belonging to another must not be used, and articles furnished for public use in washrooms, theaters, or wherever the public congregates, should be shunned.

Early recognition of a ringworm infection and adequate immediate treatment of the patient usually prevents spread of the disease to other parts of the body and eradicates the fungus growth in the areas already affected.

SKIN DISORDERS: ATHLETE'S FOOT

Athlete's foot, a fungus infection of the foot, is said to be a penalty of civilization. Among primitive peoples unaccustomed to wearing shoes it is rare. Contrary to general opinion, athlete's foot seems not to be easily transmitted from one person to another by the use of communal showers or any other shared facility. Individual susceptibility and foot hygiene appear to be more important. When the skin remains warm and moist for long periods, fungi of the genus *Trichophyton* find optimum conditions to invade the dead outer layer *(stratum corneum)* and begin to grow. In general, there is a painful itching or burning sensation in the infected areas. Symptoms vary somewhat depending on which of two species of *Trichophyton* fungus is responsible.

Types of athlete's foot

Two major types of athlete's foot can be distinguished. In the more common forms, called *intertriginous,* a crack or fissure appears in the skin, usually at the base of the fifth toe or between the fourth and fifth toes. In most cases, there is also a visible mass of loose dead skin clinging between the toes. When this loose skin is removed, the skin beneath appears reddened and shiny. The second, or *squamous-hyperkeratotic* type begins with a reddening and subsequent scaling and thickening of the skin, usually also between the toes. Sometimes areas with increased amounts of the hornlike material of the skin *(keratin)* are observed and these may resemble calluses. Both types of athlete's foot may spread to cover part or all of the soles. Both feet may be involved, but more frequently attacks occur to a greater extent on one foot than on the other. The hands are only rarely affected, more often in "hypersensitive" individuals in whom allergic reactions are common; the infection is confined largely to the back of the hand and the fingers. The small blisterlike pimples which arise on the hands of patients with athlete's foot are not infected lesions, but possibly are allergic reactions to the same fungus that has attacked the feet.

There are several other diseases which can cause lesions similar to those of athlete's foot. Since the treatment prescribed depends upon the type of infection present, the physician may perform a microscopic examination of scrapings of the infected areas before he begins treatment. Many preparations which the patient might himself select in the hope of alleviating his discomfort can have undesirable effects if the disease is not athlete's foot. It is apparent, therefore, that management of this or other similar diseases should always be under the supervision of a physician.

Athlete's foot affects men more often than women. The condition usually is chronic but may clear up during the colder months of the year. This is probably because in winter the feet are not moist and warm, conditions which stimulate the growth of the fungus. When the infection flourishes throughout the winter, or increases in intensity, the physician should be notified, for the disease may not be athlete's foot, but something more serious.

CARTER, Henry Vandyke (1831-1897), English physician working in India. He is famous for his description of an infection of the foot which resembles actinomycosis and is known as *mycetoma,* and also as *madura foot,* because it occurs with great frequency in Madura, in the south of India. He also described relapsing fever and in 1882 produced the disease in the laboratory in monkeys. He discovered the organism which causes rat bite fever.

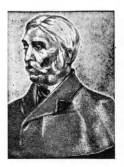

Drawing of one of the causative agents of athlete's foot, a species of *Trichophyton*, magnified 300 times. This fungus infection of the human skin is a very common one that occurs universally. Some cases of athlete's foot may also result from infections with the fungus *Epidermophyton*. A careful microscopic examination for the organism within the skin may be necessary in order to arrive at the correct diagnosis of the causative agent.

This drawing is of the causative agent of dhobie or jockey-strap itch, *Epidermophyton inguinale*, magnified approximately 275 times. The organism causes an eruption on the inner and upper surfaces of the leg, and is actually an exceedingly close relative of the common ringworm-producing organism. Although cleanliness helps to prevent fungus infections, medical treatment is usually required to arrest them completely.

Drawing of the usual causative agent of ringworm of the human scalp, *Microsporum audouini*, here magnified approximately 500 times. Species of *Microsporum*, along with a very few other related organisms, are also the cause of ringworm on other parts of the human body. Ringworm is commonest among city children, and is generally considered to be spread through personal contact, although pets may also transport it.

Treatment

Some mild cases of athlete's foot require no treatment, but will disappear as soon as cool weather arrives. Nevertheless, it is advisable to employ measures which will forestall the development of a more serious condition. The feet should be kept clean and dry. The skin between the toes must be dried thoroughly after bathing and any softened, loose epidermis gently rubbed away. Cotton pads may be inserted between the toes to absorb moisture. Bland, drying dusting powder may be sprinkled on all foot surfaces and into the socks. Light, permeable shoes or sandals are recommended during warm weather. For many patients, the condition improves when they go barefoot whenever possible.

Certain topical medications are also useful in mild or moderate cases, although one must avoid preparations which might result in irritation or sensitization. Tolnaftate, an antifungal drug, has been found to be especially useful in athlete's foot. It is generally prescribed in liquid

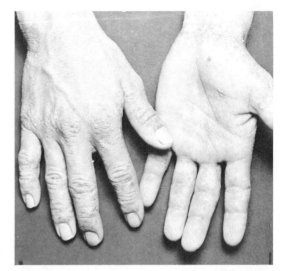

While athlete's foot may also affect the hands, many of the lesions such as those shown in the above photograph are in reality an allergic reaction on the hands to a more severe and longstanding foot infection. *Courtesy Dept. of Dermatology, Mayo Clinic, Paul A. O'Leary, M.D.*

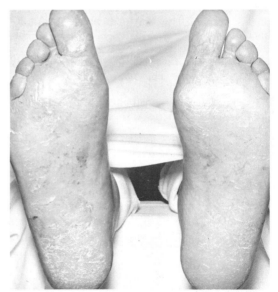

This photograph shows the dermatitis that occurs in many cases of athlete's foot. The skin between and underneath the toes is generally the most severely infected, and one foot may be affected much worse than the other. *Courtesy Dept. of Dermatology, Mayo Clinic, Paul A. O'Leary, M.D.*

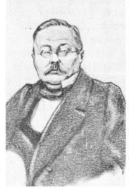

HEBRA, Ferdinand von (1816-1880), Austrian dermatologist and founder of modern dermatology. In 1845 he published a classification of skin diseases based on changes they bring about in the skin. He established the nature of a number of skin diseases that are caused by parasites. He is credited with first describing such diseases as pityriasis rubra *(Hebra's pityriasis)*, tinea cruris *(Hebra's eczema)*, impetigo herpetiformis, and many others.

or powder form. Other antifungal agents, such as salicylic acid and benzoic acid, may be suggested by the physician. Sometimes a topical steroid preparation is of value. Generally, heavy or greasy ointments are contraindicated because they tend to retain moisture at the skin surface, and thus aggravate the condition.

During acute flare-ups, when inflammation is relatively severe, professional advice should be sought. The patient should not attempt to treat himself. The physician will institute measures to counteract the inflammation before antifungal medications are given. Usually, this consists of foot soaks in certain solutions, application of a steroid or calamine lotion, and, in disabling cases, short-term administration of oral steroids. In such instances, adequate rest is essential. The patient should remain off his feet as much as possible. Griseofulvin, an antifungal drug which is taken orally, is sometimes useful for certain forms of athlete's foot (particularly chronic infections caused by *Trichophyton rubrum),* but recurrence is likely unless the all-important hygienic and supportive measures are observed.

Any patient with chronic, recurring, or severe athlete's foot should consult his physician. Incorrect self-diagnosis or ill-advised self-treatment may cause more damage than the original disorder.

SKIN DISORDERS: PRECANCER AND CANCER OF THE SKIN

Cancer of the skin is usually apparent from its very beginning; hence, it is possible for the patient to receive treatment while the disease is in an early stage of development. Since most cancer is curable when detected early, the outlook for most persons with skin cancer is excellent. This favorable prospect is even further enhanced by the fact that skin cancer is often preceded by other types of skin lesions, known as precancerous lesions, which warn the patient and his physician that treatment is required. In

this way, the cancer can be prevented even before it develops.

Precancer of the skin

A precancerous lesion of the skin is *not necessarily* the forerunner of cancer. The term is applied to certain conditions of the skin which are more apt to become cancerous than when the skin is normal. However, since there is a definite possibility that these conditions may ultimately terminate in cancer, it is especially important that they be recognized and that proper treatment be given.

Senile atrophy is the term used to describe a condition in the skin of older people. The skin becomes dry; sometimes there is chapping or scaling, and it loses its elasticity. It assumes a grayish color, and body hairs disappear or become more sparse. This condition may also be found in those people who have been exposed chronically to the sun's rays for long periods, especially blonds. Such changes in the skin of young people are referred to as "farmer's skin" or "sailor's skin," since in these two occupations this skin condition often develops on parts of the body that are continuously exposed to sunlight. The hands, face, and neck are involved most frequently. The prevention of senile atrophy by individuals exposed to wind, sun, and weather can readily be accomplished by the use of protective ointments on the exposed skin and mucous membranes such as the lips. Any bland ointment such as vaseline or lanolin generously applied to the exposed areas at frequent intervals will alleviate but not prevent the senile atrophy. Treatment of the patient includes the application of lotions to decrease the dryness, and also protection from sunlight by clothing, including wide-brimmed hats, and special ointments. It is important that ointments used for this purpose contain the necessary ingredients to filter out the harmful ultraviolet rays of the sun. The use of such special protective ointments will allow the skin to tan without producing a sunburn. Since farmer's skin is a precancerous condition, the appearance in the affected skin of a pimple or ulcer which remains for several weeks should receive medical attention, for it may indicate the beginning of a cancer.

Senile keratosis of the skin is a condition in which one or more wart-like growths appear on the face, arms, or other parts exposed to sun and wind. It is a common disease of older people, but is also found occasionally among younger persons. The lesions sometimes become as large as a pea, may be either rounded or flat, and are usually dark gray or brownish, but sometimes black. The surface may be scaly or rough. These lesions grow slowly, do not disappear spontaneously, and gradually increase in

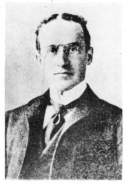

BOWEN, John Templeton (1857-1941), American dermatologist. It was through his investigations that attention was first drawn to certain important types of precancerous skin conditions. Years of careful clinical observation were required to establish those dermatoses which are now known to have precancerous potentialities. By the early recognition of such forms it is now readily possible to prevent many cases of skin cancer that are difficult to cure.

number. Because senile keratosis may develop into skin cancer, the physician generally advises removal, either by surgical, electrocautery, or chemotherapeutical methods. Surgical or electrocautery are simple procedures. Recent use of the newer chemicals in properly selected cases allows the patient to apply the prescribed medication which gradually destroys the keratosis. Any lesion of this type which develops soreness, becomes red or ulcerated, turns black, or causes the surrounding skin to become red should be removed at once.

Seborrheic keratosis of the skin consists of one or many wart-like lesions ranging from the size of a pea to that of a large coin. This disease is also more common in older people. The lesions are generally found on the back, chest, and temples. They have a greasy appearance, and may range in color from yellowish-brown to grayish-black. The lesions usually develop slowly and do not disappear spontaneously. The physician can readily remove them.

Arsenical keratosis is similar in appearance to senile keratosis. The lesions are wart-like growths of the skin, most frequently found on the palms, fingers, and soles. The condition is caused in some persons by exposure to arsenic over a considerable time, either from having taken drugs containing arsenic or as the result of occupational exposure to the chemical. Since these lesions may develop into cancers, they should receive medical attention. The physician frequently can see signs of such transformation long before the patient can recognize any change in his skin. Early recognition of cancer permits removal of the cancerous area; late recognition sometimes leaves no alternative except amputation of the affected part.

Occupational dermatoses are frequently of a precancerous nature. They are found as skin irritations in persons working with certain materials *(carcinogens)* capable of causing cancer. The most common offenders are products of tar and coal distillation. The prevention of this type of cancer is accomplished largely in the elimina-

tion of the occupational hazards, chiefly by special means of protection for workers. An occupational dermatitis usually can be recognized if it appears after continued contact, becomes chronic, and is then alleviated by a vacation from the job. The condition is most frequently seen in the hands, feet, and parts of the body most likely to come into direct contact with the irritating material. The original dermatitis generally can be cleared up by a change of job or by the institution of protective devices. Proper medication of the affected areas with lotions and ointments also may be necessary. Individuals developing skin difficulties suspected of being the result of their profession or job should determine the cause by consultation with a doctor. If necessary, affected persons should change jobs rather than risk chronic occupational dermatitis with the chance of cancer.

Scars from extensive burns occasionally develop into skin cancer. For this reason, they should be watched closely for warning signs. Deep burns covering large areas of the body are particularly likely to give rise to cancer in the scar tissue. Usually, any malignant change in a scar takes many years to develop. Plastic surgery for severe burn scars is a great aid in eliminating the possibility of subsequent cancer.

Occasionally, patients who have received x-ray or radium therapy show evidence of skin changes at the site of the treatment. Such changes are classed as precancerous conditions and should be carefully watched for any unusual changes which might indicate a conversion to a cancerous lesion.

Areas of the skin which are chronically exposed to irritation or heat are sometimes susceptible to cancer. This holds true for cancer of the lip, found most frequently among men who have smoked pipes for a long time.

Xeroderma pigmentosum is a relatively rare hereditary disease developing in early childhood. The initial symptom usually is the appearance of red spots on parts of the skin exposed to the sun's rays. The spots disappear, leaving areas

REVERDIN, Jacques L. (1842-1908), Swiss surgeon. He is best known for the methods of skin grafting which he introduced. *Reverdin's method* involves the transplantation of small pieces of skin to the skinless area. These transplanted pieces will then grow to form new and larger areas of skin. He also carried out experiments on myxedema, and he was able to prove that the disease could be produced by the surgical removal of the thyroid gland.

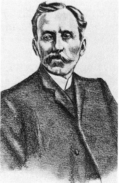

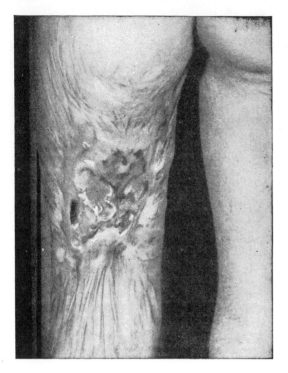

This picture of a large ulcerated burn scar shows the type that is likely to develop into cancer if not given adequate medical attention. Deep burns are more dangerous than superficial ones, and scars from them may require removal for safety.

of darker pigmentation. As the disease progresses, new crops of lesions appear, as well as numerous white patches, which give the skin a very blotchy appearance. Dark wart-like structures also are seen. The disease is rather serious because of the likelihood of skin cancer developing from it. Treatment of the patient involves protection from sunlight, and the use of various ointments and salves to relieve the discomfort.

Leukoplakia is a chronic disease of the mucous membranes characterized by the appearance of white patches. These may eventually grow together forming larger patches, or may take the form of wart-like structures or ulcers. The female genitals, the inner aspect of the lips, the mucosa of the mouth, the tongue, and the gums are the most common sites of leukoplakia. Often this condition can be corrected by removing any source of constant physical or chemical irritation to the affected region. Improperly fitted dentures, for instance, may provide sufficient irritation to cause leukoplakia. Surgical removal of the area frequently is desirable, and is a relatively simple procedure. The condition definitely requires medical attention because of the possibility that cancer might ultimately develop in the affected area.

Kraurosis vulvae is a disease of the mucous membrane of the vulva which resembles leukoplakia. The membranes itch and become dry, shriveled, and sometimes discolored. The condition has many causes, and sometimes requires surgery for complete alleviation, in order to eliminate the possibility of cancer. A similar disease of the penis, *kraurosis penis,* is evidenced by ivory-colored lesions or a mottled appearance caused by white plaques. It is an extremely rare disease.

Probably the most common of all precancerous conditions of the skin are some types of pigmented moles. Cancer developing from a mole is called *malignant melanoma.* Those moles most likely to become malignant are the round, flat, or slightly raised dark bluish moles which have smooth surfaces and contain no hair. The physician may deem it desirable to remove them before any symptoms of cancer appear. However, any mole should be removed promptly if it shows signs of growth, bleeding, color change, inflammation, or if it itches. Removal should be performed only by a physician. Improper removal of moles by nonmedical persons is apt to lead to more trouble than leaving the mole alone!

If a mole is exposed to constant irritation— as it is when located where clothing is apt to rub against it—it should be removed, or at least constantly watched for unusual signs. Cancer formation from moles is rare in all age groups, and is particularly rare before puberty. When cancer does develop in a mole, it is likely to be in a very dangerous form.

Some *benign tumors* may be considered precancerous in that they may ultimately change to cancerous growths and spread to the internal organs of the body. Tumors are rather common occurrences, but the patient should never accept them as benign without consulting a physician.

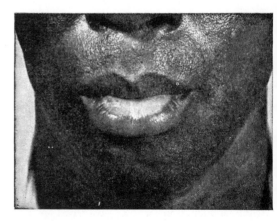

This photograph of a patient with leukoplakia shows the characteristic white patches on the mucous membrane of the mouth. These are potentially precancerous lesions requiring removal.

The causes of many tumors are unknown; some types appear with unusually high frequency in some families, and consequently, heredity is thought to play a role in their development. Still others undoubtedly result from infections by a variety of microorganisms or from chronic irritation of an area of the body. Often, treatment depends upon the cause of the tumor. Even though a doctor may judge a skin tumor to be benign, he will warn the patient to be continually observant in order to detect any changes in its size or consistency.

Cancer of the skin

Cancer of the skin, as of other tissues of the body, is characterized by the continued growth of tissue in an abnormal and uncontrolled manner. Whereas benign tumors of the skin may attain a certain size and then cease growth, a cancer will continue growing indefinitely, although its rate of growth may range from slow to rapid and may vary through the years. An important feature of a cancer is its ability to *metastasize*. A metastasizing cancer is one which spreads to other regions and tissues of the body. A cancer is frequently referred to as a malignant tumor to distinguish it from a benign tumor, which does not spread to distant parts of the body.

Uncontrolled skin cancer may eventually cause the death of the patient. The growth may become so large that it can destroy the nearby blood vessels supplying other parts of the body. It may also metastasize to more vital organs which, in turn, may be so damaged that the patient dies.

Most persons with skin cancer can be treated successfully if a physician is consulted early enough. *Self-diagnosis of skin cancer is an impossibility.* Even the experienced doctor may

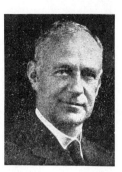

DAVIS, John Staige (1872-1946), American surgeon. Famous for his numerous and highly ingenious contributions to plastic surgery, particularly of the human face. He also devised a number of novel methods for the repair of facial defects and one special type of skin graft has been named after him. It principally is because of the efforts of plastic surgeons that much cancer surgery is no longer scar-forming and disfiguring, as it most frequently was until quite recent times.

have difficulty in diagnosing it because of its similarity to other skin diseases. In order to complete his diagnosis and to classify the exact type of skin cancer, he almost invariably performs a preliminary *biopsy*. This procedure entails the removal of a small bit of tissue from the suspected growth for microscopic study. In most cases, the patient cannot receive treatment until the biopsy is performed, since treatment depends upon the exact type of cancer present.

Even though diagnosis is difficult, the patient may have certain clues as to whether a skin sore may be a cancer. In the first place, he should be familiar with the various precancerous conditions of the skin, particularly if he knows that any of them exist on his own skin. However, skin cancers can arise in an area of skin not known to have had any previous disease or unusual irritation. In all cases, any sore or growth which persists for more than two or three weeks, should be regarded with suspicion. If the sore or lump shows signs of rapid growth or spread or fails to heal completely, the patient should not hesitate to consult a doctor immediately. Even though most chronic or rapidly spreading skin disorders are not cancer, they are sufficiently serious to merit professional attention.

Treatment

Skin cancer patients are treated surgically, by x-irradiation, or with locally administered chemotherapeutic agents. Treatment depends on the type of cancer involved, its location, the rate of growth, the time since its inception, and the possibility of metastasis. Patients who receive treatment early may require only x-irradiation or chemotherapy, whereas the same cancer might require extensive surgery or amputation if neglected too long. Patients with slowly growing skin cancer sometimes wait years before going to a doctor, at which time they may find that metastases exist.

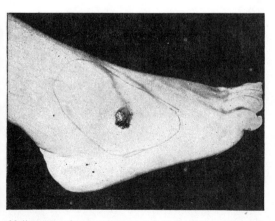

Malignant melanoma may appear in the form of a small dark growth on the skin, as in this case, and the lesion demands immediate removal, along with much adjoining tissue for complete safety.

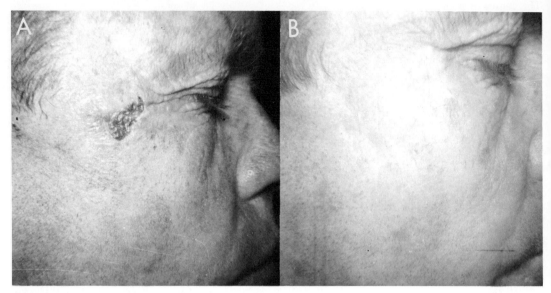

A, Relatively innocuous-appearing, ulcerous skin cancer that had invaded the underlying nerve. B, Therapy included removal of the tumor and use of a skin graft. Copyright 1964 Year Book Medical Publishers, Inc., courtesy A. J. Ballantyne, The University of Texas M. D. Anderson Hospital, Houston.

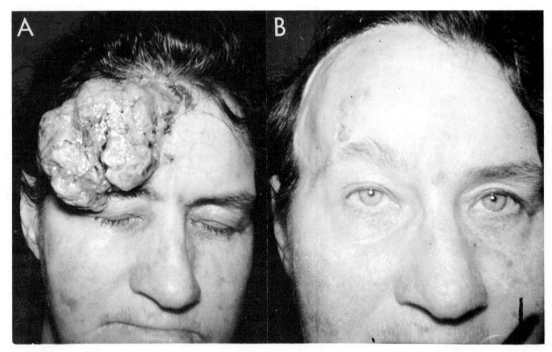

A, Despite the formidable appearance of the large, basal cell carcinoma, it remained localized on surface structures. B, Appearance after removal of the tumor. Copyright 1964 Year Book Medical Publishers, Inc., courtesy A. J. Ballantyne, The University of Texas M. D. Anderson Hospital, Houston.

Classification of skin cancer

Cancer of the skin is classified according to the type of skin cells which are involved. The chief form of skin cancer is called *carcinoma*. Carcinoma of the skin occurs most frequently among fairskinned persons who spend much time outdoors, especially in a dry, sunny climate. Although individual predisposition is known to play a role, it is now generally conceded that excessive exposure to sunlight is a major factor in producing most carcinoma of the skin. The malignant process begins in the cells of the epidermis, or outer half of the skin. There are two major types which are designated as *basal cell* carcinoma and *squamous cell* carcinoma; this distinction is made by microscopic examination.

Basal cell carcinoma. This type of carcinoma accounts for well over half of all cases of skin cancer. It is made up largely of cells resembling those of the innermost cells of the *stratum mucosum,* the deepest layer of the epidermis. The growths occur more frequently on the face than on other areas of the body. A typical basal cell carcinoma is a hard pinkish or waxy growth, which may spread slowly or show signs of healing with formation of a tight cluster of similar nodules around it. Its appearance is usually altered by accidental injury, bleeding, and scaling. Basal cell carcinomas may become pigmented, so that they appear more like a dark malignant mole.

Squamous cell carcinoma: This type of skin cancer begins in the cells of the outermost layer or the stratum mucosum. In its early stages, a squamous cell carcinoma looks much like a basal cell carcinoma. Skin cancer of this type is most frequently found in persons who have been long exposed to the sun and the wind. As might be expected, the growths usually are encountered on the face, the ears, and the backs of the hands. Squamous cell carcinomas vary greatly in their behavior; some grow rapidly, others slowly. Occasionally, a slowly developing lesion will suddenly be accelerated in its spread, for no apparent reason. Squamous cell lesions usually grow faster than the basal cell variety and also have the tendency to metastasize. There are two general types of squamous cell carcinoma: the *ulcerating* type, and the *papillary* type. The latter can best be described as cauliflowerlike in shape and structure.

Metatypical carcinomas: These are skin carcinomas which microscopically appear to contain both basal and squamous cells. Many carcinomas of the skin are mixed to a certain extent, but one type or the other is usually predominant.

Intraepidermal and superficial carcinomas of the skin are those in which the cancerous nature of the growths may remain confined to the skin for many years without metastasis or damages to nearby tissue. There are several specific diseases which belong to this group, in particular: Bowen's disease, Queyrat's erythroplasia, Paget's disease, and multiple flat superficial epitheliomas. With the possible exception of Paget's disease, in which a cancer develops in the area of the nipple, these diseases are all slow in their course, and respond well to treatment.

Metastatic carcinoma of the skin: When cancers in internal areas of the body metastasize, they may spread to the skin. Secondary skin cancers are usually found on the chest, under the arms, on the abdomen, or around the genitals. The nodules, which may range in color from ivory to red, sometimes grow quite rapidly.

Treatment of the skin carcinoma patient: The patient whose skin condition is diagnosed as carcinoma is usually treated by surgical excision, some form of radiation therapy, or chemotherapy. When the physician believes that surgical removal will be the most effective way to eradicate the disease, the incision must be wider and deeper than the carcinoma if regrowth is to be prevented. Skin-grafting may be employed if a large defect is left. Recent trials with locally applied chemotherapeutic agents have yielded good results, especially for basal cell carcinoma, and these are coming into use. Podophyllin resin, fluorouracil, colcemid, and methotrexate are among the compounds which appear to selectively destroy some kinds of carcinomas, while leaving the surrounding skin intact.

Malignant melanoma: Treatment of persons with early malignant melanoma demands extensive removal of the growth and the skin surrounding it, as well as the lymph glands that drain the involved area. Early treatment is essential, since this type of carcinoma spreads more quickly than other forms of skin cancer. Perfusion with chemotherapeutic agents is now being done as a research method, with the hope of controlling the widespread metastases of this virulent disease.

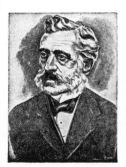

LANGENBECK, Bernhard Rudolph Konrad von (1810-1887), German surgeon. He is noted for having made many important contributions to the early development of plastic surgery. He modified an earlier existing method for plastic surgery of the nose, and he also devised a special method for the surgical care of cleft palate. Many operations need no longer be so disfiguring as a result of recent advances that have been made in the field of plastic surgery, especially of the face.

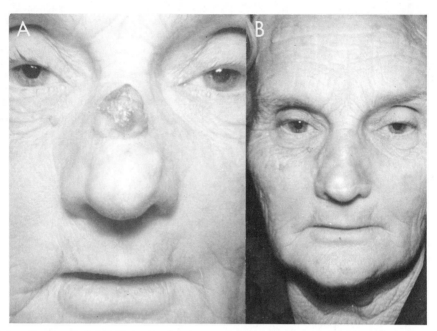

A, Tumor before therapy. B, A full thickness of skin was grafted onto the nose of this patient after removal of the tumor and surrounding calluses, giving a very satisfactory cosmetic result. Copyright 1964 Year Book Medical Publishers, Inc., courtesy R. H. Jesse, The University of Texas, M. D. Anderson Hospital, Houston.

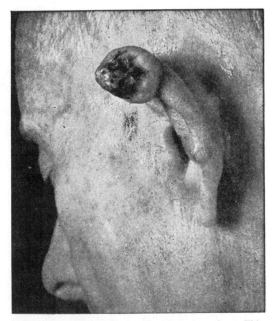

Picture of a patient with a typical cutaneous horn. This type of lesion usually appears in persons past 60 years of age, and is a potentially precancerous one. Cutaneous horns should be removed surgically at the very earliest possible moment. Procrastination in this can have serious consequences.

Sarcoma of the skin: Cancer arising in the skin from layers below the epidermis is termed *sarcoma.* Unlike carcinoma, the sarcomas of the skin occur in young persons. The different types of sarcoma are named in accordance with the type of cells primarily involved. *Fibrosarcoma,* for example, involves fibrous connective tissue and *fibroneurosarcoma* is comprised chiefly of nerve cells. Sarcomas may also arise from muscle, blood and lymph tissue, fat, and other tissues.

Treatment of patients with sarcoma of the skin is largely surgical, since most of these lesions are resistant to irradiation. Early surgical treatment may result in cure.

SKIN DISORDERS: CYSTS

A cyst is a collection of liquid or semiliquid material in or immediately beneath the skin and generally contained in a limiting sac or membrane. There are many small glands in the skin which may become plugged and retain their secretions, which result in a cyst. Cysts may form around a foreign body. The cause cannot

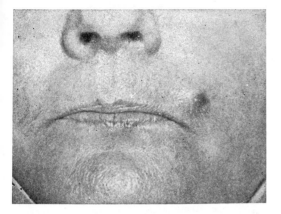

A sebaceous cyst on the face. Such a cyst, although rarely malignant, may be removed by a physician for cosmetic purposes. It may also be desirable to excise one when it appears on the body in areas that are subject to chafing or in areas that are rubbed by clothing. *Photography F. W. Schmidt.*

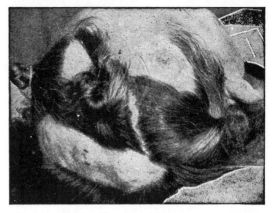

In this photograph the patient's head has been shaved in some areas to reveal the presence of a number of very large sebaceous cysts. Such cysts may appear singly or in number, as in this case, but usually are smaller than those shown. Removal is quite simple. *Photography F. W. Schmidt.*

always be determined, and treatment may or may not be necessary, depending upon medical evaluation. Cysts usually appear as lumps beneath otherwise normal skin or mucous membrane. Occasionally the skin itself may appear slightly altered. Whereas tumors seem to be firmly attached to the underlying tissue, a cyst usually can be moved about slightly without displacing the tissue beneath or the skin above.

Sebaceous cysts

Sebaceous glands are tiny structures connected with the root of a hair, which secrete an oil or grease. The commonest examples of a sebaceous cyst are whiteheads and blackheads, which are discussed elsewhere in this chapter. Large sebaceous cysts may occur, and on almost any part of the body except the soles and palms, which have no sebaceous glands. Such cysts often appear on the scalp, back, and scrotum, where they may be marble-sized swellings attached to the overlying normal skin by a narrow connective strip of tissue; these are called *wens*. A cyst on the eyelid is called a *chalazion*.

Treatment consists of removing the cyst along with all of its retaining sac, as a minor surgical procedure. Self-treatment is unsuccessful in most cases, for the cysts will return after being simply opened if the contents are allowed to escape without removal of the sac. It may also be dangerous, because bacteria have an opportunity to enter the area and cause infection. Chalazia must be treated differently from most other sebaceous cysts because of their location. (For further discussion see Chapter 17, "The Eye.")

Mucous cysts generally occur in the mouth as the result of plugging of one of the small glands that secrete mucous material. Such cysts on the lower lip seldom become larger than a large pea, but on the tongue they may reach the size of a hen's egg. These cysts are generally painless, and may be readily evacuated and the cyst wall removed by a physician.

Multiple benign cystic epithelioma is a condition in which a number of pinhead-size, smooth, shiny, rounded, pimple-like cysts appear on the face, neck, or chest. The condition usually is not considered serious but may require medical attention, both as a safety precaution and to improve the patient's appearance.

Traumatic epithelial cysts occur when a small amount of skin or foreign material becomes lodged beneath the skin and becomes enclosed in a thick, horny layer of skin. They generally result from accidents, and seldom have any greater significance than being annoying if they become too large. They are easily removed.

SKIN DISORDERS: NAIL DISORDERS

Disorders of the finger- and toenails may result from infections, injuries, general metabolic disorders, or hereditary defects. Most disturbances caused by injury or infection heal readily. The nail is restored to normal, provided that the tissue from which the nail is derived is not permanently damaged. Hereditary defects of the nails are seldom severe. The simple hangnail causes concern to some persons, but its only medical importance is that it may offer an opening for bacterial infection. It does not signify any specific systemic disorder or vitamin deficiency. The only treatment necessary is to clip off the hangnail and apply an antiseptic. Occasionally, malignant growths occur about the nails. Consequently, any lump or sore in that area which does not heal in a reasonable length of time should be brought to the attention of a physician.

Nail disorders are classified according to their location and appearance, but their correction depends, to a considerable extent, on the causative factor. Nail infections are similar to infections of other parts of the body. The same bacteria and fungi which cause inflammation of the skin are responsible for similar symptoms under and around the edges of the nails.

The term *onychia* designates an inflammation of the nail bed, as contrasted with an inflammation of the skin surrounding the nail, which is called *paronychia*. When conditions permit, such as a penetrating injury or bruise, large numbers of microorganisms can grow under the nail and produce a painful and disfiguring disorder. Staphylococci are among the most common of these organisms, and infections with the fungi which cause ringworm are not unusual. When pigment-forming microorganisms are the cause of the disease, the nail may become discolored. *Green nails* are the result of infection by green pigment-producing bacteria. Both psoriasis and fungus infections may cause whitish or yellowish discoloration of the nails, and may be accompanied by thickening, with formation of crumbling, dry material beneath the nails and eventual separation of them from underlying tissues. Both of these conditions may occur in the nails, alone, or be associated with lesions on the skin due to the same causes. These disorders necessitate the attention of a physician.

Paronychia is a relatively common condition characterized by a shiny, red, tender, swollen area surrounding the nail. In most instances, this disorder is mild and disappears spontaneously, but in some cases, the inflammation may spread under the nail into adjoining parts of the finger or toe. Staphylococci and streptococci are the bacteria most frequently encountered as infectious agents. *Monilia albicans* is a yeast that frequently infects the tissue around the nails. These organisms may invade the area by way of a wound or a hangnail. In severe cases, the nail may be cast off, but will grow again if the tissues at the base of the nail have not been destroyed or too severely scarred. Paronychia may also be caused by other microorganisms, such as those responsible for tuberculosis, syphilis, and diphtheria. Skin eruptions on the hands which result from athlete's foot, psoriasis, and other conditions may all interfere with the health of the nails.

Onychia may be caused by agents other than

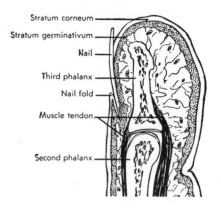

Longitudinal section of finger tip, showing manner in which the fingernail is imbedded. Nails grow only in the halfmoon-shaped *lunule*. The average rate of growth is about two inches each year.

infectious ones. When nail inflammations occur frequently, there is a probability that a systemic condition may be a contributing factor. Allergy is one of these contributing conditions.

Distortion of the nails occurs by extension of skin eruptions from the surrounding skin to the nail bed. *Contact dermatitis* is frequently found in workers in industries in which they are exposed, by contact, to certain chemicals and other materials that irritate the nails and skin. In all of these conditions, the nails may become separated from the nail bed, a condition known as *onycholysis*, and may divide into two or more layers, or be completely lost. When the tissue from which the nail grows is permanently scarred, a new nail may not develop; or, if there is but a small amount of scarring, the new nail may be deformed. Shedding of the nails (*onychomadesis*) occurs without local inflammation. It is generally associated with some systemic disease of a vascular, nervous, or nutritive origin. Local treatment involves measures to pre-

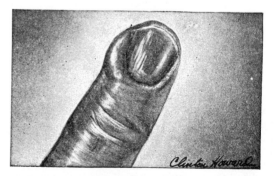

This illustration portrays the typical inflamed swollen appearance of the skin surrounding the nail in a case of paronychia, a relatively common dermatitis frequently caused by staphylococci.

vent infection, but the initiating factor must be managed in order to stop the condition.

Injuries are common causes of nail disorders. For example, burns and frostbite may damage or destroy the nails, and may sometimes sufficiently injure the nail bed so that the possibility of further growth is eliminated. Overexposure to radium or x-ray may cause the nails to become brittle and fragile, or to split transversely. X-ray, administered by an expert, will not produce any change in the nails. Other cases of undue brittleness, hardness or splitting may result from infections, nutritional disorders, circulatory or glandular disorders.

The constant pressure placed on the nail bed and roots by nail biting (*onychophagia*) may cause a permanent shortening of the nail. This shortening may become extreme, leaving the nails so short that they are useless for picking up small objects. Nails which are bitten or cut too short are not only ineffective, unsightly, and painful, but are an invitation to permanently scarring infections.

One of the commonest forms of nail disorders is the ingrown toenail. Ingrown toenails occur most frequently on the great toes. The condition is caused by a combination of improperly fitting shoes and incorrect cutting of the nails. Sometimes shoes are too narrow or too short, or high heels force the toes into a wedge at the front of the shoe, causing ingrown nails. When the corners of the nails are cut rounded, rather than trimmed straight across, the edges may be forced into the marginal tissues. The constant pressure exerted by the nail on the surrounding tissues, plus secondary infection which sooner or later occurs, cause the painful irritation associated with this disorder. In severe cases, the infection may spread beneath the nail, extend into the lymphatic vessels and eventually, the bloodstream. Hence, ingrown nails may lead to serious conditions. Ingrown nails generally disappear when well-fitting shoes are worn, and when the nails are trimmed straight across. However,

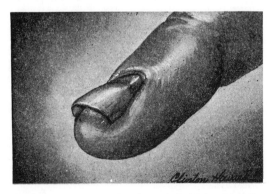

Drawing of a typical case of onycholysis, in which the nail is separated from its bed. The nail may be lost, in which case a new one often develops.

simple surgical procedures may be necessary to relieve the discomfort.

Peeling off of the nails at the tips is a common and mild form of a condition in which the nails separate into layers (*onychoschizia*). When nails are allowed to become too long, they are unduly subject to shocks, and peeling is probably a result of mechanical damage to the nails. The condition is more frequent among typists and pianists, because of the constant hammering on the nails in these occupations. The use of nail enamel may cause changes in the nails by increasing their fragility and encouraging peeling. Diseases, nutritional disturbances, organic disorders, and hereditary weaknesses in nail structure all may be causative factors in peeling of the nails. Keeping the nails cut reasonably short improves the condition, in most cases. Severe peeling should be called to the attention of a physician.

A great many characteristics of normal fingernails are inherited. Long slender nails, or shorter broad nails, for instance, may be a family characteristic. In rare cases, the nails may be missing entirely at birth, or they may be unusually thick or grow in some other unusual manner.

The appearance of scattered white spots on the nails (*leukonychia*) is normal, but may be more pronounced in some persons than in others. These spots may occur because of some minor injury or from pressures exerted during manicuring. In some cases, these spots appear as white lines. The entire nail may be white in rare instances. These whitened areas have no significance from the standpoint of health, and there is no treatment known which will make them disappear.

SKIN DISORDERS: DANDRUFF

Dandruff is the most common disease of the scalp, and is characterized by the presence of small flakes on the scalp and in the hair. This condition in the scalp is termed *seborrheic dermatitis*. Much evidence points to a low-grade infection as the cause of this condition, but this point has not yet been proved. Dandruff is almost always accompanied by overactivity of the *sebaceous glands*, connected to the roots of the hairs. These glands produce an oily material called *sebum*. This oily substance makes the scales greasy. In acute cases of dandruff, the flakes may be exceedingly greasy and the scalp itches and becomes red and sore.

Dandruff is sometimes accompanied by an increased number of bacteria or fungi normally found on the scalp. It is most generally thought that they have little effect on the dandruff. They may complicate the condition by producing secondary infection. Thus, when dandruff is accompanied by intense itching, the patient may scratch the scalp. The fingernails thereby deposit germs into the broken areas and these areas may become infected. Such infections complicate the management of the dandruff. They frequently cease to occur as soon as the dandruff is under control.

The seborrheic process may spread to the skin back of the ears, conchae of the ears, eyebrows, eyelids and nasal creases, and even over the sternum. In these areas, the skin becomes red, and is covered by a greasy scale. Lesions respond to the same chemicals that are used to treat the same process on the scalp.

Treatment

Frequent washing of the hair and thorough massages help to remove the excess oil and flakes. This may be all the treatment required for mild cases, although various preparations for the scalp are helpful in controlling the dandruff, and preventing secondary infections.

In advanced cases of dandruff accompanied by intense itching or soreness, soap and water may be irritating. Persons whose scalps are thus involved require the attention of a physician, who may prescribe special medication to bring the condition under control. More important, the doctor can determine by a microscopic examination of the scalp the exact type of the trouble. There are other diseases which simulate dandruff, but which require different treatment.

SKIN DISORDERS: BALDNESS

Baldness, involving either total or partial loss of scalp hair, is a common condition found much more frequently in men than in women. Whether baldness can be prevented or whether the hair can be restored when lost depends almost entirely on the cause of the baldness. For this reason, baldness must be considered from the standpoint of its cause.

Hereditary baldness

Pattern baldness is one of the most frequently encountered forms of baldness. It usually begins relatively early in life, appearing first at the temples, and then at the vertex of the scalp. Hair loss may be slow or rapid. The process commonly extends until only a ring of hair, on the back and sides of the scalp, remains. This is particularly true in males. In females, hair loss usually extends until only a very sparse growth remains on the crown of the head. Since this type of baldness is inherited, it is probably the most difficult type of baldness with which to cope. At best, treatments only postpone the loss of hair.

The inheritance of pattern baldness is influenced by sex. A typical pedigree is shown in the accompanying diagram. It will be noted that pattern baldness appears in all the sons of a woman who carries the gene. Further, the trait can appear in a man when neither of his parents has it; in this case, the woman carries the gene for the trait but, since it is influenced by sex, the gene does not express itself. The trait will show up in about one half of the sons of a man who has pattern baldness.

When the gene for baldness is present in both parents of a woman, she may or may not become bald; and if she does, the chances are that she will not lose nearly so much hair as will a man who is so afflicted. This, too, suggests the influence of sex on the trait. When a man inherits the condition from both his parents, all of his sons will be bald; and the sons of all his daughters will have, at least, a fifty-fifty chance of becoming bald.

It is difficult to tell whether a woman with a full head of hair is able to pass the condition on to her sons and grandsons. Some idea of the possibility of such a condition can be obtained from a consideration of her parents and grandparents.

Once pattern baldness appears, there is little that the individual or his physician can do to prevent its further development. There are two approaches to the situation, one of which will usually serve the patient. First, the individual may learn to accept and live with his condition. If he recognizes that he is not alone, and that other men do not suffer socially or economically by their loss of hair, he is on the way to conquering his problem. He must recognize that baldness is an hereditary condition over which no one has control. It does not indicate that he is intelligent or dull; in fact, it indicates only that he is losing his hair.

A second possibility for the bald man is the purchase of a wig or toupee. Women who discover large losses of hair almost invariably resort to this measure. It has been estimated that six women out of every 100 in this country will eventually suffer from partial baldness.

Premature baldness is also found most commonly in men. It generally begins after the twenty-fifth year, but may appear earlier. Failure to maintain adequate hygienic care of the scalp may play a part in bringing on premature baldness. An imbalance of the sex hormones, with no other apparent effects, may be partially responsible. Prompt initiation of proper scalp care may be somewhat effective in delaying the progress of the baldness. Ultraviolet irradiation administered by an expert may also help temporarily.

Hypotrichosis is a rare disease characterized by an almost complete absence of body hair from birth. It occurs with equal frequency in males and females, and treatment is of little or no avail. There is no serious impairment of bodily health.

Symptomatic baldness

Baldness sometimes appears as a symptom of infections or other conditions, and frequently is followed by a natural return of hair when the health is normal again. The new hair is often lighter in color, and may be curly even though the original hair was dark and straight. Such peculiarities are usually temporary, and the hair eventually regains its normal appearance.

Sudden loss of hair can result from typhoid fever or scarlet fever, in which case not only scalp but also body hair, eyebrows, and pubic hair may be lost. Pneumonia, influenza, and other serious or extensive infections of the respiratory tract may also occasionally cause sudden hair loss. Baldness resulting from these diseases is almost invariably temporary and requires no special treatment. Syphilis may cause patches of baldness or loss of hair on some areas of the body. Leprosy sometimes causes loss of the hairs of the eyebrows and eyelashes. Diffuse hair loss may occur during pregnancy. Regrowth, usually, follows delivery. If regrowth does not occur in three or four months, medical attention should be sought.

A gradual loss or thinning of the hair may be caused by severe nutritional deficiencies and certain wasting diseases such as cancer and tuberculosis. A slow diffuse loss of hair also may be observed in some diseases involving the endocrine glands, particularly the pituitary and thyroid glands. An alteration in the function of the sex glands after childbirth may have a similar result.

The internal use of certain drugs, such as thallium acetate, may cause a temporary loss of hair, but it will return after the use of the drug is discontinued. Such drugs are occasionally

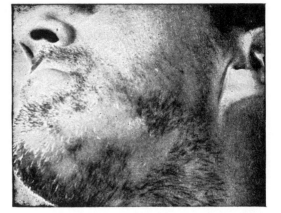

Alopecia areata of "area baldness" is shown here as affecting the bearded region. It can occur almost anywhere on the body and may disappear spontaneously. *Courtesy Ashton L. Welsh, M.D.*

used in the treatment of patients with certain kinds of scalp ringworm in which the presence of the hair is detrimental to treatment.

"Area" baldness (*alopecia areata*) is characterized by sudden losses of hair, which result in one or more bald patches on the scalp or on other parts of the body. The cause of this condition is not known. The bald patches may remain for a considerable time, but there is usually a return of the hair, even without treatment. The disease tends to recur from year to year, appearing most often during the winter. It attacks men more frequently than women, and generally starts between the ages of 20 and 30. When it appears in children, the final result may be total baldness.

In area baldness, the scalp usually remains normal in appearance. The patches of baldness may be single or numerous, and two or more patches may gradually increase in size and coalesce until they form one larger patch. The fact that the baldness disappears within a few weeks usually leads the patient to believe that medical treatment is not needed. In many cases, this is true. Should the disease return too frequently, however, or cover unusually large areas of the scalp, damage may result to the hair follicles, those organs of the skin from which the hairs grow. The only acceptable medical treatment, other than good care of the hair and scalp, involves the careful irritation of the bald areas. Light rays or chemical irritants may be used, but because of the great danger of severe burns or other damage to the hair follicles or the scalp, the patient should not attempt self-treatment. The physician can decide from the history and nature of the disturbance whether such treatments are necessary or desirable, and he then can carry them out with complete safety.

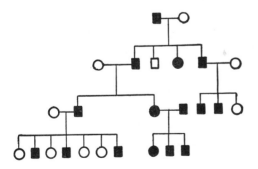

This pedigree of baldness in a family indicates how the characteristic was passed along by the great grandfather to three of his children, five grandchildren, and six great grandchildren. Note that twelve of the fifteen bald persons were males. (Square symbols, males; black, bald persons.)

The fact that hair often returns spontaneously in area baldness has been exploited by many cosmeticians and "hair experts," who claim that they can cure baldness. Actually they seldom cure baldness of any kind; area baldness may disappear and hereditary baldness will remain in spite of what the patient or cosmetician does. Certain other diseases, systemic or local, which are associated with scarring, may produce area baldness. These include systemic diseases such as lupus erythematosus and scleroderma, and such local diseases as lupus vulgaris, deep fungus infections, folliculitis decalvans, and the like. The sites of hair loss in all of these conditions also show scarring of the skin.

There are other scalp disorders that may lead to temporary or permanent losses of the hair. Injury to the scalp, burns, some forms of dermatitis of the scalp—such as acne, herpes, pus-forming infections, and ringworm—are among the most frequent scalp conditions causing baldness. Occasionally, areas of baldness may be caused by overexposure to x-rays. In any of these cases, prevention of baldness is possible only by seeking proper medical aid.

OTHER SKIN DISORDERS

All the skin disorders that have been discussed in this chapter are characterized by some visible change in the outer layer of the skin (the epidermis). In addition to these diseases, there are a number of skin conditions in which some change takes place in the sensations within the skin. These disorders usually are not accompanied by any apparent sores or blemishes. However, sensory disturbances of the skin may occur in a few cases where the dermatitis that usually accompanies them has not yet had time to appear, or is not severe enough to be readily apparent.

Such irregularities of sensation are caused primarily by abnormal behavior of the nervous system. The defect may result from changes in the nerves of the skin, or of the larger nerves that transport impulses from the skin to the brain. In some cases, the disorder may involve the brain itself, and may indicate an unhealthy mental or emotional condition.

The treatment of patients with these disorders differs greatly from the methods used with the other skin diseases, since the application of lotions or other skin medicines can seldom be expected to improve the underlying nervous disorder.

Nervous disorders of the skin are called *cutaneous neuroses*. They may include either increased or decreased sensitivity of the skin. Vitamin deficiencies may cause various types of hyperesthesias. In some cases of vitamin B_1

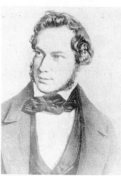

HENLE, Friedrich Gustav Jakob (1809-1885), German anatomist. He was the first person to describe the construction of the various outer layers of the skin and intestinal tract and to point out their great significance. He is also known for his discovery and description of the portion of the nephron unit now known as Henle's loop. *Courtesy N.Y. Academy of Medicine.*

(*thiamine*) deficiency, the soles of the feet become so sensitive that walking is most difficult, and even stroking the soles with the finger produces extreme pain. With other nervous disorders, there may be a pronounced feeling of prickling, tingling, or creeping (*paresthesia*) on the skin without any visible cause. Any of these symptoms may occur for brief periods in apparently healthy individuals; but when they remain for more than a few hours, a serious internal condition may be present.

Localized areas of the skin may suddenly become painful (*dermatalgia*) for no apparent reason. Dermatalgia may be caused by a disease of some of the nerve pathways. Also, patients with severe emotional or mental disturbances sometimes experience this symptom, and psychotherapy is required to relieve the condition. The variety of skin sensations reported by hysterical or neurotic patients is great. Some mental patients feel that the skin is actually infected by a disease-producing organism, and attempt a treatment which is designed in their mind to remedy the situation. Other persons have uncontrollable urges to pick or scratch the skin or to pull out hairs. Occasionally, neurotic individuals may inflict wounds upon their skin to simulate some dermatitis or injury in order to invoke sympathy. In all of these cases, the services of a competent physician or psychiatrist are essential, since such behavior may lead to grave consequences. Indeed, the common unconscious habit that many persons have of rubbing or picking on their skin may cause a dermatosis.

Sensations of warmth and coolness in the skin may be caused by circulatory disturbances as well as by nervous disorders. A number of irregularities of the smaller blood vessels may produce a change in the amount of blood flowing to and from the skin, causing abnormalities in temperature sensation. When burning pain and general hyperesthesia of the skin result from a nerve injury, the condition is known as *causalgia*. This usually occurs in one of the arms or on the hands, and is aggravated by any motion of the affected part. The skin may become cold, and have a shiny, wet appearance. In some instances, immersion of the afflicted part in hot water will relieve the unpleasant sensation. But in more severe cases, the injured nerve may require special therapy. In general, any severe or prolonged sensory disturbance of the skin merits medical attention.

Diabetes, leukemia, tuberculosis, and cancer may all cause itching in their early stages, although no visible skin lesions are present. Thyroid disorders, gout, jaundice, and reactions to certain drugs are also capable of producing itching without a skin eruption. Allergies are among the most frequent causes of such itching; however, in most cases, an allergy develops rapidly into more advanced stages in which there are pronounced sores and blemishes of the skin. Because of the variety of possible causative agents, any person with a persistent itching without visible skin symptoms should consult his physician.

SKIN-GRAFTING

Whenever important areas of skin are lost, destroyed, or disfigured by disease, accident, or surgery, skin-grafting may be considered. Although this procedure is most extensively used for burned patients, it is commonly employed for other defects, as well. There are three basic types of skin grafts: *autografts, homografts,* and *heterografts.* An autograft consists of skin taken from one site on a patient and grafted onto another site. A homograft is tissue taken from one individual and grafted onto another. A heterograft is skin removed from an animal and grafted onto a human.

Only autografted skin survives transplantation permanently, a fact which many persons find surprising in this age of transplantation miracles. The few rare exceptions include grafting of skin from one to another of a pair of identical twins (because they share an identical genetic background). In other patients, rejection of homografts or heterografts eventually occurs; the body's immune mechanisms will not tolerate the foreign protein. Homografts and heterografts do serve a useful function, however. They provide temporary skin cover until autografting is later feasible. In severely burned patients, for example, this protects the underlying tissue, prevents critical heat and fluid loss, and safeguards against massive infection. These advantages are often life-saving. The skin of recently deceased cadavers has proved quite suitable for homografts. Pig skin, with its gross and microscopic resemblance to human skin, is an example of a heterograft which offers good temporary coverage.

9 THE SKELETON AND MUSCLES

WHAT THEY ARE AND DO

Man's highly developed ability to make many and complex movements is made possible by the skeleton and muscles of his body. He can stand, bend, walk; he can acquire skills in motion, as in sports, arts, and occupations. He exercises more control over his environment than any other animal, and he can mobilize his physical forces for defense, work, or amusement. This magnificent physical independence can be curtailed or lost the moment a bone is broken, a joint is dislocated, or one or more groups of muscles are paralyzed. Such an event makes him dependent upon others to a greater or lesser degree. The skeletal system alone is the framework on which the rest of the body is built.

Bone and bones

Bone is a tissue; *bones* are organs. Bone is derived from connective tissue cells which become specialized in function. Bone tissue consists of two permanent components: the *osteocytes*, which are the specialized cells of the bone, and the surrounding *matrix*, which is composed of minute fibers and a cementing substance. This cementing substance contains mineral salts, mainly calcium phosphate. Similar to bone, and comprising a portion of the skeleton is *cartilage*. Cartilage is much more elastic than bone; it is often referred to as "gristle." Some bone may begin as cartilage which is later replaced by bone tissue.

Mature bone of mammals is *lamellated*; that is, it is made up of thin plates (*lamellae*) of bone tissue. The plates occur in bundles; this arrangement offers increased resistance to shearing forces. The shape and arrangement of the lamellae differ in the two major types of mature bone—*spongy* and *compact*. In spongy bone, the matrix consists of a lamellated network of interlacing walls resembling the structure of a sponge; this form can be found in the skull and ribs. In compact bone, the bundles of lamellae are arranged in vertical cylinders around a central canal; this bone is found in the long bones of the arms and legs. The blood vessels and nerves run through the central canals of compact bone and send minute extensions into the bone substance. Great numbers of these vertical cylinders are needed to make up the thickness of a typical bone.

Bone grows by the addition of new bone to old. In spongy bone, new bone is deposited upon the old within the meshes of the lamellated network. In compact bone, new bone is primarily laid down on the outer surface. In both types, the bone is first laid down as immature (soft) bone which gradually becomes mature bone, hard and rigid with calcification. Long, hollow bones—such as those in the arm or leg—are made from compact bone. They grow in circumference by the deposition of bone on the outer surface of the shaft. At the same time, the inner cavity becomes enlarged by the resorption or eating away of bone tissue. The ends of long bones are not hollow, but consist of a spongelike section of bone covered by a layer of compact bone and capped by cartilage on the joint surface where one bone moves against another.

The structure of the cartilage, which caps the ends of bones that rub against one another in joints, is adapted to bear the strain of pressure and to facilitate the smooth gliding of the opposing surfaces during motion.

Long bones provide an example of the principle that a hollow tube is stronger than a solid one. A long bone such as the thighbone (*femur*) is subjected to enormous stresses in the form of bending forces and in weight-bearing. It gains maximal strength with a minimal amount of material by increasing the size of the hollow center while adding to the tissue on the outer surface at the same time.

Lengthening of long bones is accomplished by the development of bone at the ends. Between the spongelike bone ends and the shaft of the bone is an area of growth called the *epiphysis* or *epiphyseal cartilage*. Growth in length takes place only in this zone. The older cartilage becomes bone in the area next to the shaft, while new epiphyseal cartilage continues to form in the area next to the cap. When the epiphyseal area is completely replaced by bone tissue, the bone ceases to grow in length. Normally, in the human being, such growth is completed at about the age of 25; but physiologic disturbances may accelerate, retard, stop, or prolong growth. Hormones play an important part in the "sealing" of the epiphyses.

In infants and children, bones are softer than in adults, and yield readily to pressure or injury. This accounts for malformations, distortions in posture, foot defects, and so on. Certain primitive tribes take advantage of the softness of skull bones in infants to mold the heads by binding. Young bones bend before breaking, and socalled "greenstick fractures" are common in children. In such a fracture, the shaft bends; and when the force is great enough, the bone on the convex surface breaks, much as a green twig may splinter along one side, remaining intact on the other.

A deficiency of bone-making materials or disturbed processes of utilization of these materials may increase the softness and porous condition of bone. In the vitamin deficiency disease, rickets (lack of vitamin D), the shafts of long bones bend under strain, such as weight-bearing; consequently, the patient may have curved long bones throughout his life. When vitamin C is inadequate, changes may occur at the ends of the long bones in the line between the shaft and the epiphysis and under the periosteum as a result of hemorrhages, in growing children. In the adult, only the periosteal changes occur. Older persons have bones which are more porous because their bodies are not able to utilize bonemaking material adequately, while absorption of bone matrix continues.

Bone is covered by a membrane called the *periosteum*, which contains the vessels for supplying some of the nourishment to the bones. The periosteum is composed of two layers of

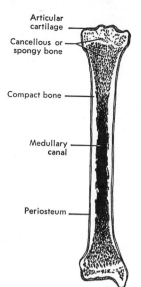

Drawing of a longitudinal section through the tibia. The red marrow is in the cancellous bone and the yellow marrow in the medullary canal. The periosteum is a layer that provides a smooth protective covering around the outer surface.

connective tissue. The outer layer is a compact arrangement of specialized fibers liberally supplied with blood vessels and nerves. Because of its nerve supply, the periosteum is sensitive and accounts for any pain or pressure felt in the bone. The structure of the inner layer of the periosteum (*cambium*) is less compact and has fewer blood vessels of its own. The periosteum adheres to the bone by means of fibers of connective tissue which anchor themselves in the bone tissue. The periosteum varies in thickness, being thinnest where the tendons of muscles are attached to bone, and thickest along the hollow portion of long bones.

Before birth and during infancy, *red marrow* is present in the long bones and in the network of spongy bones. Red marrow is one site of manufacture of the red blood cells. Blood vessels are threaded through the marrow, bringing oxygen and nutrients and taking away the waste products. The newly-made red blood cells enter the circulation by way of these vessels. When a person is about six years old, changes begin to take place in the red marrow. *Yellow marrow*, or fatty marrow, is formed, replacing the bloodmaking marrow; and most of the marrow cells change into fat cells. With these changes, the color of the marrow changes to yellow.

Yellow marrow is present in mature hollow bones. The formation of yellow marrow to replace red marrow takes place in regular order, beginning in the bones of the lower leg, followed by the thighbone, bones of the forearm, and finally in the bone of the upper arm. This replacement process also occurs in the epiphyses. In the adult, the formation of red blood cells takes place only in the spongy flat bones of the skull, the ribs and pelvis, the bone of the spine, and the breastbone.

Blood vessels and nerves

Without blood, most tissues die. The arteries bring to bone the elements necessary for the maintenance of life, and the veins carry away the waste products. The blood supply of bone is of major importance during the growing years, but also has a bearing in adults on the development of inflammations, on destruction of bone tissue, on the localizing of secondary tumors, and on the processes of repair.

In spongy bone, the blood vessels form a network within the substance of the bone marrow. In compact bones, the vessels run in the longitudinal canals in the center of the bundles of lamellae, with branches penetrating into the bone substance. The arteries become smaller and less numerous as the red marrow changes to yellow marrow, because the bone is no longer growing and in need of abundant nutrient materials. This reduction in the number of blood vessels becomes intensified with advancing years and is the foundation of the popular belief that old bones are brittle and do not heal well.

Arteries entering bone and marrow are accompanied by nerves, some of which are anchored to the blood vessel walls by nerve extensions.

The skeleton

The pattern of support provided by the skeleton of a human being is called *axial* and *appendicular*; the head and spinal column form the axial portion, and the arms and legs are the appendages. Two bony girdles connect the axis and appendages; these are the shoulder girdle, and the pelvic girdle. These four elements comprise the skeleton.

The central, and perhaps most important, of these elements is the spinal column—literally and figuratively, the backbone of the body. The spinal column is composed of small, movable bones, called the *vertebrae*. The pattern of the spinal column (or vertebral column) permits flexibility in bending forward, to either side, and, to a limited extent, backward; rotation also is afforded by the ability to twist the body as on a spindle in the regions of the lower back and neck.

The vertebrae of the spinal column have different functions. They are designated according to location as: the seven *cervical* vertebrae in the neck; the twelve *thoracic* vertebrae in the chest area; and five movable *lumbar* vertebrae in the midsection of the lower part of the back.

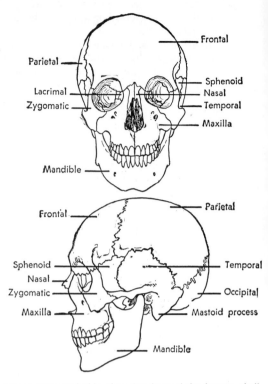

These front and side view drawings of the human skull show the location of the individual bones that fuse to form the skeletal portion of the head.

These make a total of 24 movable vertebrae. The spinal column also contains five vertebrae which are fused into a single bone, the *sacrum*, and four more fused into the single *coccyx*. The vertebrae increase in size downward, the cervical being smallest and the lumbar largest.

Each vertebra is an irregular bone, the component parts of which are: the body; the hollow inside (*neural arch*), through which passes the spinal cord; the *spinous process*, which projects from the vertebral body at the crest of the neural arch, and is one of the tips that can be felt by running a finger up or down the spine; and lateral projections on each side of the spinous process. These bony projections afford a site of attachment for the strong muscles and ligaments of the back, giving them a mechanical advantage in movement and control of the back. They also serve as a braking system against exaggerated bending of the body which might endanger the spinal cord. In some persons, the two sides of the neural arch do not fuse, with the result that a hernial sac, containing nervous tissue and cerebrospinal fluid, protrudes into adjacent tissues. This condition is known as spina bifida, and is congenital.

The vertebral joints have cartilage on the contacting surfaces and are provided with a joint capsule. In addition, a structure called the

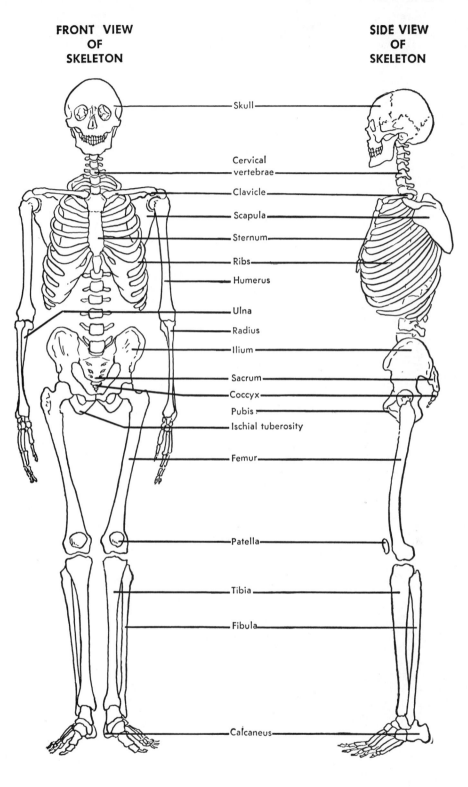

FRONT VIEW
OF
SKELETON

SIDE VIEW
OF
SKELETON

Skull

Cervical
vertebrae

Clavicle

Scapula

Sternum

Ribs

Humerus

Ulna

Radius

Ilium

Sacrum

Coccyx

Pubis

Ischial tuberosity

Femur

Patella

Tibia

Fibula

Calcaneus

THE HUMAN SKELETON

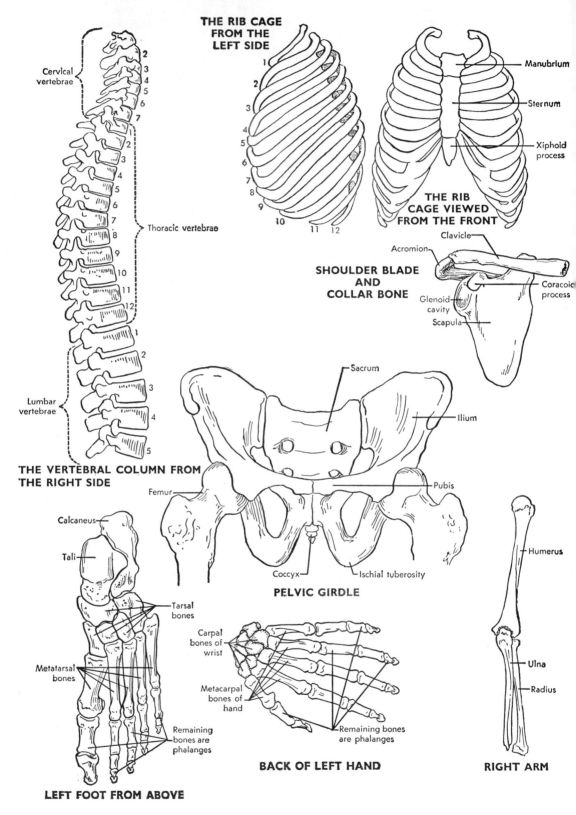

Cervical vertebrae

**THE RIB CAGE
FROM THE
LEFT SIDE**

Thoracic vertebrae

Lumbar vertebrae

**THE VERTEBRAL COLUMN FROM
THE RIGHT SIDE**

Manubrium

Sternum

Xiphoid process

**THE RIB
CAGE VIEWED
FROM THE FRONT**

**SHOULDER BLADE
AND
COLLAR BONE**

Clavicle

Acromion

Coracoid process

Glenoid cavity

Scapula

Sacrum

Ilium

Femur

Pubis

Calcaneus

Tali

Coccyx

Ischial tuberosity

PELVIC GIRDLE

Humerus

Tarsal bones

Carpal bones of wrist

Metatarsal bones

Metacarpal bones of hand

Ulna

Radius

Remaining bones are phalanges

Remaining bones are phalanges

BACK OF LEFT HAND

RIGHT ARM

LEFT FOOT FROM ABOVE

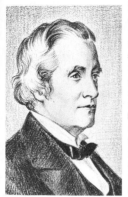

BOWMAN, William (1816-1892) English anatomist and ophthalmologist. Famous for his classic descriptions of the renal corpuscle and the striped muscle. Because of his work in ophthalmic surgery, many physicians regard him as most responsible for its advancement in England. Bowman's corneal membrane and Bowman's capsule in the kidney are named after him. In 1842 the Royal Society presented him their medal for his work in physiology.

intervertebral disc lies between each of two movable vertebral bodies. The disc is composed of cartilaginous plates above and below the *nucleus pulposus*, a highly elastic and semifluid tissue, which is held in place by many fibers running from various portions of the cartilaginous plates at the edges of each vertebra. The disc serves as a buffer, taking up the shocks and strains to which the spinal column is subjected. It acts as a cushion, flattening out under pressure and shifting its position in accommodation to changes in direction of motion. Exaggerated motions or strain may damage the discs. "Slipped disc" occurs with moderate frequency, and is found more often in laborers.

The *thoracic cage* is closely related to the spinal column. It is formed by the twelve pairs of *ribs*. The ribs are important in the inflation and deflation of the lungs for breathing. These flat bones are attached at the back to the thoracic vertebrae and curve toward the front. The upper seven opposing pairs of ribs are attached in front to the breastbone (*sternum*). Each rib of the succeeding three pairs is attached by cartilage to the rib immediately above it. The last two pairs of ribs are unattached at the front; these are known as the "floating" ribs.

At the top of the spinal column and attached to the first cervical vertebra is the skull. The skull is made up of the *cranium*, which houses the brain, and the bones of the face. The facial bones include framing for the eyes, ears, nose, and jaws—two bones on each side which comprise the upper jaw (the *maxilla*), and the lower jaw (the *mandible*).

The appendicular portion of the skeleton is bilateral, and facilitates locomotion and elaboration of movements. In the appendages, beginning at shoulder and hip, the bones decrease progressively in size while increasing in number, as noted in fingers and toes. Strength is afforded by a single large bone in each upper arm (*humerus*) and a similar such bone in each thigh (*femur*). The forearms and lower legs each have

two bones; in the forearm, these are the *radius* and the *ulna*; and in the lower leg they are called the *tibia* and *fibula*. These double rows of bones in each appendage make it possible for rotation of the particular appendage outward (*supination*) and inward (*pronation*) on the long axis.

There are eight bones in each wrist. The seven similar bones of the lower extremity are considered to be in the foot; each foot and hand has five additional bones. There is a total of 14 bones in all of the fingers or toes of any one extremity. What these numerous smaller bones lack in strength they compensate for in flexibility and intricacy of movement.

The shoulder girdle is composed of the shoulder blade (*scapula*) on each side at the back, and the collarbone (*clavicle*) in front. At the outer end of the scapula is a cartilage-lined socket in which is fitted the cartilage-covered head of the humerus of the arm; this forms the shoulder joint. The bones of the shoulder girdle are loosely assembled, but they are held in place by strong muscles and tendons.

The pelvic girdle is more firmly assembled, making it more capable of answering the greater demands upon it for weight-bearing and other functions. Its two halves are lowest at the front portion and are united there by cartilage and ligaments. At the back, each half of the pelvis is united to the sacrum by ligaments, all of which form the two *sacroiliac* joints. On each outer side of the pelvis, the bone is shaped into a cartilage-lined socket in which is fitted the head of the femur of the thigh; this forms the *hip joint*. The entire pelvis acts as a sort of basin which supports the abdominal organs. During pregnancy and childbirth, the pelvis has a particularly important function.

Joints

Without joints, the skeleton would be a stiff, immovable set of bones. Some joints have no motion (they are *fixed*); some have limited motion, while others have wide motion. In the adult, the joints of the cranium are fixed; the tooth-like edges of adjoining pieces, which are capable of sliding over one another to minimize the size of the baby's head during birth, become closely united and calcified early in life. The joints which have the most freedom of motion are the ball-and-socket joints of the shoulder and hip. The spinal column could be considered as a series of joints.

A typical joint is the knee. The cartilage-covered ends of the femur of the thigh and the tibia of the lower leg are bound into contact by strong, tough bands of fibrous tissue called *ligaments*. Enveloping these bone ends and fibrous bands is a collar formed by ligaments, and this encloses the joint like a sac. This is known as the *joint capsule*. It is lined with a thin membrane (the *synovia*), which secretes a lubricating fluid, called the *synovial fluid*. The cartilage on the bone ends provides a surface for smooth gliding motion, and the synovial fluid is the lubricant.

Muscle and muscles

The skeleton, with all its complex bones and joints, cannot move without muscles. The striated muscles, which control skeletal movement, are called "voluntary" muscles because they are controlled by the will. The smooth muscles such as those of the stomach and intestine are called "involuntary" because the individual exercises no conscious control over them.

The components of skeletal muscles are the elongated muscle fibers and the surrounding, containing *matrix*, a connective tissue called the *perimysium*. Upon stimulation, the muscle fiber contracts lengthwise, thereby shortening itself. When all the fibers within a single muscle group contract, the muscle shortens and thickens. All skeletal muscle is called *striated muscle*, the term being derived from the transversely striped appearance of the tissue under the microscope. The muscle fiber as a whole contains *sarcoplasm* which is composed of a multitude of parallel-arranged *fibrils* which are the working or contractile elements of muscle fibers. These muscle fibers are contained within a sheath of *muscle cells*. Bundles of muscle fibers are usually compartmented in sheaths of fibrous connective tissue which is called the perimysium. A collection of such muscle fiber bundles into a functional unit forms the discrete, easily-visible muscle groups which are the named "muscles" of the body, for example, the biceps. The connective tissue which binds the fibers together can readily be seen in dried beef. The muscle fibers can be pulled apart lengthwise in well-cooked beef; this "stringiness" of skeletal muscle is so well recognized that in carving meat the cut is made "across the grain."

Muscle tissue is richly supplied with blood vessels, because this tissue requires a more rapid turnover of food materials than any other body tissue. Muscle tissue also is well-supplied with nerves—motor nerves for movement and sensory nerves for sensation. A muscle moves because of impulses transmitted to it along a motor nerve. Hence, any interference in the nerve supply of a skeletal muscle deprives that muscle of the power of movement. If the nerve is regenerated and again becomes functionally competent, the muscle's power to contract returns. If the nerve is not repaired, the muscle shrinks and wastes away. Muscle loss occurs in diseases such as infantile paralysis (*poliomyelitis*) and progressive muscular atrophy, in which the nerves that affect the muscles degenerate. Muscle loss from nonuse occurs in persons confined to bed for long periods. The condition also is common to aged persons and to persons who have a period of total inactivity of specific muscles.

About 500 muscles of various sizes are present in deep and surface layers of the human body, from the scalp and face to the toes. These muscles act in unison. For example, when one muscle group pulls the forearm upward (*flexion*), another set of muscles is available to pull it outward again (*extension*). This balanced system of opposing muscle groups exists for every motion of which the body is capable. Grace in movement is the outward expression of harmony in the synchronized action of muscles; awkwardness suggests disharmony or faulty synchronization.

The principal function of skeletal muscle tissue is to contract. Contraction entails the expenditure of energy, and energy comes from the combustion (or *oxidation*) of foodstuffs. In muscle, as in other organs, this combustion leaves waste products which must be eliminated. The *lactic acid* which is formed may be the cause for the feeling of tiredness which follows strenuous exercise. If a stimulus to a muscle is perpetuated beyond the limits it can normally endure, the waste products of combustion accumulate faster than they can be eliminated. Consequently, the muscle becomes tired and, if overexercised, reaches the point where it will no longer obey a stimulus to act. This is known as muscle fatigue. A period of rest serves to restore normal muscle activity. Another function of muscles is to give a sense of bodily position through proprioceptors, as discussed in Chapter 11, "The Brain and Nervous System."

Therapeutic exercises have been designed for management of certain types of diseases and malfunctions of muscle groups. Some of them produce movement in a limb while in others, the limb is held rigid. These exercises assist

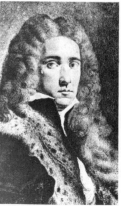

SANTORINI, Giovanni Domenico (1681-1737) Italian anatomist. Regarded as one of the great dissecting anatomists of his time. He published valuable anatomical observations on the musculature of the face, larynx, and penis. His name is associated with many structures, among them the muscles of the external ear, and the one for which he is best remembered, the accessory pancreatic duct. His anatomical drawings are regarded as masterpieces.

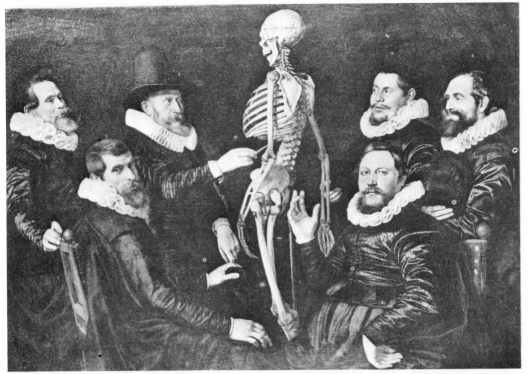

Reproduction of the famous Dutch painting, *Anatomical Lesson of Dr. Sebastian Egbertsz in 1619,* by Thomas de Keyser, which hangs in the Ryks Museum in Amsterdam. Physicians of this period were more thoroughly versed in the structure of the skeleton and muscles than they were in physiology or other parts of the anatomy.

in the development of muscles that have degenerated or become paralyzed. This special branch of medicine is called *kinesiology* and is practiced by trained personnel who are familiar with the exact type of muscular action required for restoring any particular set of muscles. Muscular tone and co-ordination, stabilization of joints, and normal appearance and function of muscles can often be restored by the kinesiologist when these qualities have been lost because of injury or disease.

Tendons

Skeletal muscles are attached to their respective bones by *tendons*. Tendons are specialized extensions of muscle. The connective tissue which binds the bundles of striated muscle fibers together extends beyond the muscle and forms a tough, inelastic cord with few nerves and blood vessels; this is the tendon. Tendons anchor muscles to bone by means of connective tissue fibers which enter the bone structure. Some tendons are located so near the surface that they can easily be identified, as for example, the "hamstring" tendons at the back of the knee, and the "Achilles" tendon above the heel. Injury to tendons impairs motion. Their improper

development causes various physical defects. Most such conditions respond well to treatment.

Together, the skeleton and muscles have more component parts than any other body system. They also have a large share of responsibility in body function. Every movement made by an individual—be it smiling or lifting a great weight—depends upon these systems. Ingestion of foods and waste elimination from the body are greatly aided by the bones and muscle. The heart itself is a specialized muscle. The skeleton and muscles are some of the structures which distinguish the independent animal, including man, from the stationary plant.

DISORDERS OF THE SKELETON AND MUSCLES: TRICHINOSIS

The disease *trichinosis* is named for the parasitic worm that causes it, *Trichina spiralis.* In the larval stage of the worm's life cycle, it lies embedded in a cyst in the muscle tissue of animals, mainly hogs. Human beings acquire the disease by eating undercooked or uncooked pork or pork products made from pigs infested with Trichinae.

FRONT VIEW

BACK VIEW

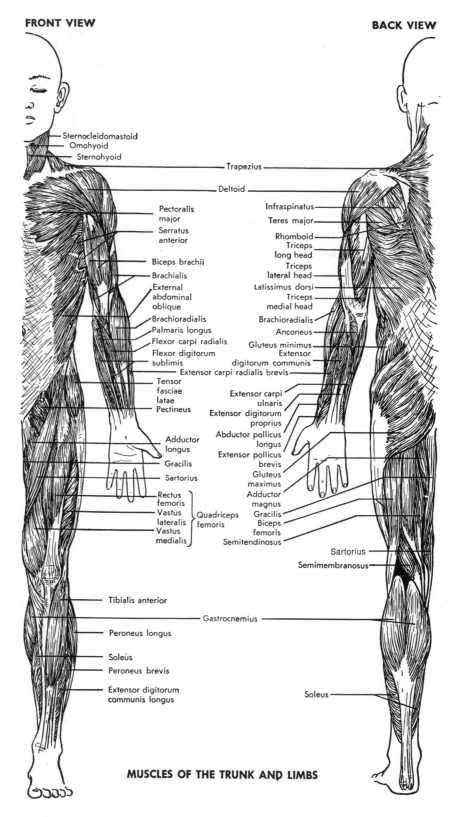

Sternocleidomastoid
Omohyoid
Sternohyoid

Trapezius

Deltoid

Pectoralis major
Serratus anterior

Biceps brachii
Brachialis
External abdominal oblique
Brachioradialis
Palmaris longus
Flexor carpi radialis
Flexor digitorum sublimis

Tensor fasciae latae
Pectineus

Adductor longus
Gracilis
Sartorius

Rectus femoris
Vastus lateralis
Vastus medialis

Quadriceps femoris

Tibialis anterior

Peroneus longus

Soleus
Peroneus brevis

Extensor digitorum communis longus

Infraspinatus
Teres major
Rhomboid
Triceps long head
Triceps lateral head
Latissimus dorsi
Triceps medial head
Brachioradialis
Anconeus
Gluteus minimus
Extensor digitorum communis
Extensor carpi radialis brevis
Extensor carpi ulnaris
Extensor digitorum proprius
Abductor pollicus longus
Extensor pollicus brevis
Gluteus maximus
Adductor magnus
Gracilis
Biceps femoris
Semitendinosus
Sartorius
Semimembranosus

Gastrocnemius

Soleus

MUSCLES OF THE TRUNK AND LIMBS

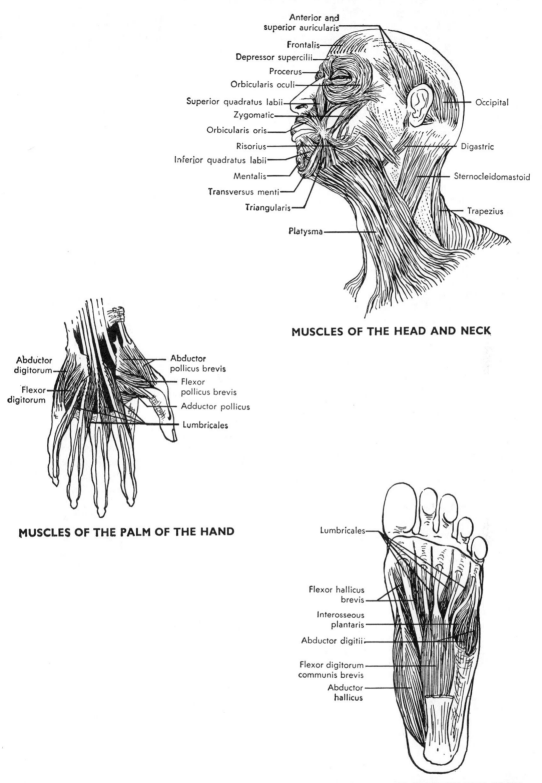

MUSCLES OF THE HEAD AND NECK

MUSCLES OF THE PALM OF THE HAND

MUSCLES OF THE SOLE OF THE FOOT

After the meat has been eaten, the life cycle of the parasite resumes its course. In the stomach and intestines of man, the processes of digestion break down the meat fibers around the encysted larvae, liberating them. The larvae promptly attach themselves to the inner lining of the small intestine where, under the stimulus of abundant nourishment, they mature quickly. The females produce living young (in contrast to egg-producing parasites), and these young are deposited in the lymph vessels of the intestine. They are carried by the lymphatic system to nearby lymph nodes; from the nodes they enter the blood and are on their way to the lungs and heart, and eventually the entire body.

At each stage of their travels, the parasites produce symptoms of invasion. There may be diarrhea, nausea, abdominal pain, and fever. In the lungs, the symptoms may suggest pneumonia. The larvae may coil themselves in the muscle walls of the heart and thereby affect the function of that organ. By invading the brain and its membranes, they may produce inflammation. Eventually the larvae reach the skeletal muscles. There they settle down, coiled in the typical spiral from which they derive their name, *spiralis,* and begin the encysted stage of their lives. At this stage, the patient complains of stiffness, pain, and swelling in the muscles; fever, sweating, and insomnia may also be experienced.

Before inspection of meats and packing plants became universal, epidemics of trichinosis were not uncommon. Today, epidemics are rare. The disease may crop up locally when the meat of an infected animal has been purchased from a source outside the customary channels of inspection. Sporadic cases may cause such slight clinical symptoms as to be difficult to diagnose. In fact, many persons carry encysted Trichina larvae in their muscles throughout life, with symptoms so vague as to provoke no complaints warranting investigation. Diagnosis has been materially aided by the development of certain

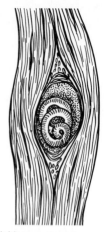

Drawing of *Trichina,* a round worm that frequently parasitizes man, hogs, and other mammals, shown encysted in muscle fiber of a hog.

laboratory methods now available to the physician.

The individual has two ways to help prevent trichinosis: pork or pork products should be purchased only from reliable sources which are under proper inspection; and pork, whether purchased or home-grown, should be cooked at a temperature and for a length of time sufficient to destroy any Trichina larvae that may be present. In home kitchens this means, for pork roasts, an oven temperature of 350° Fahrenheit and roasting time of 35 minutes per pound of fresh pork; the internal temperature of the meat itself, taken by a meat thermometer, should be at least 185°, especially for thick pieces such as hams and shoulders. Processed hams which are pre-tenderized may be cooked at an oven temperature of 300° and an internal temperature of 150°, allowing a roasting time of 20 to 30 minutes per pound. Cured hams from a reliable packer are safer than smoked ham from an obscure source. For fresh pork, a good rule is to consider meat cooked until gray in color safer than white, and white in color safer than "pink pork," which is definitely unsafe. Pork products, especially pork frankfurters, are dangerous because they often are eaten uncooked.

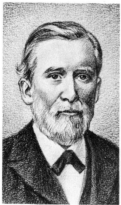

ZENKER, Friedrich Albert (1825-1898) German pathologist. Described a paralysis of certain body areas served by the peroneal nerve, and a degenerative disease which liquifies the striated muscle fibers, both diseases bearing his name. He identified the genus Trichina as the cause of trichinosis, a disease contracted by ingesting uncooked pork containing the organisms; he also described the muscular and intestinal forms which are found in man.

DISORDERS OF THE SKELETON AND MUSCLES: MUSCLE CANCER

Malignant tumors that originate in skeletal muscle tissue are a type of cancer known as *sarcoma*. Secondary cancers may migrate to muscle tissue from a primary cancer (either sarcomatous or carcinomatous type) elsewhere in the body. The primary form usually is first manifested by the presence of a "lump" in the

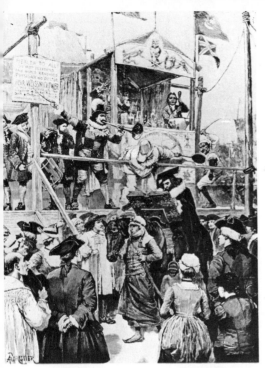

An old engraving showing a quack peddling his wares. Persons with cancer have always provided a fertile field for the quack. *Bettman Archive.*

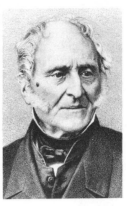

CRUVEILHIER, Jean (1791-1874) French pathologist. Wrote one of the greatest works of its kind, his *Human Pathological Anatomy* (1829--42), for which he is internationally famous. He was the first to describe disseminated sclerosis, and gave an early and accurate account of progressive muscular atrophy, called *Cruveilhier's disease.* Other diseases to which his name has been given include a form of stomach ulcer, and congenital cirrhosis of the liver.

muscle. Later in the disease, groups of cancer cells break away from the parent growth, enter the pathways of the blood stream, and migrate to distant organs where they set up secondary cancer "colonies." The cells may settle in the lungs, bones, skins, kidneys, pancreas, ovaries, or brain.

Even though it is one of the most highly malignant forms of cancer, patients with primary muscle cancer can be cured. The most important single factor in the survival from any form of cancer is *early diagnosis.* To this rule, cancer of muscle is no exception. If given proper treatment before the disease has spread to the lungs and other areas, a large percentage of patients can be cured; but cure is rarely possible after spread has occurred. Early diagnosis of this disease should be possible because the tumors are externally apparent. However, they are easily overlooked or their potential danger is ignored. In many cases, a lump or mass is present for months or longer, but is ignored because its presence causes no disability. There is no pain, unless the growth impinges upon a nerve, and there is seldom any interference with movement. *No lump in a muscle should be disregarded until it has been thoroughly investigated by a physician.*

Most of the known facts about cancer of skeletal muscle are of a negative character. As a rule, a history of injury is lacking. There is no

age preference; the growth has been found in the newborn, as well as in the octogenarian. It shows no conspicuous sex preference. Muscle cancer can grow slowly and almost imperceptibly, or with extreme rapidity. Untreated, it may kill in a matter of months, or after years. The one positive characteristic of the disease is the frequency with which it arises in the muscles of the thigh; but it is found also, in order of frequency, in the muscles of the leg and foot, arm, forearm, hand, trunk, head and neck. When the growth occurs in an extremity, the patient may best be treated surgically. This may include amputation. In muscles such as those of the head and neck, tumors often cannot be adequately removed surgically. Radiation therapy or anticancer drugs may be used in such cases. Even when the muscle cancer seems to be under control, recurrences may appear several years later. Patients are asked to return for frequent periodic check-ups over a long period so that any recurrences may be detected.

DISORDERS OF THE SKELETON, MUSCLES, AND TENDONS: SPRAINS, RUPTURES, FRACTURES, AND DISLOCATIONS

The bones of the human body are relatively strong and resistant to injury. However, sprains, fractures, and dislocations occur frequently. Most common of these are sprains. In a *sprain* the tough bands of fibrous tissue which bind two bones together at their joint (the *ligaments*) are stretched beyond functional limits and some of their fibers torn. In range of severity, sprains can imply mild strains of the ligaments, even tearing of a few fibers. Ruptures may be partial, incomplete, or complete, involving the ligaments, joint capsule, muscles, tendons, blood vessels, and nerves depending on the extent of the injury. The tearing of blood vessels causes blood to escape into the surrounding area and is responsible for the rainbow effects that may be seen. Swelling may be great, and pain often is severe. When a severe sprain occurs, the injured part should be immobilized by a splint or other means; then, the patient should be taken to a physician for treatment. Complete ruptures require surgical repair.

The cause of sprain may be a slip or twist that is trivial in relation to the damage caused. Sometimes no such injury is recalled. Stepping onto or off a curb or bus, a twist on uneven pavement, or a slip on a waxed floor can cause sprained ankles. A heel caught on a step, wrenching the foot forward violently, can cause severe sprain of foot and toe ligaments. Women at housework and men shoveling snow have sustained sprains of the ligaments of the *lumbosacral* and *sacroiliac* joints.

Whiplash injuries of the neck are usually caused when an automobile is struck from behind. The occupant's head is abruptly and forcefully extended and then flexed, with associated stretching and tearing of the muscles and ligaments of the neck, sometimes accompanied by hemorrhage and damage to the nerve roots. Proper treatment usually brings complete relief of symptoms.

When whiplash symptoms cannot be medically verified, they may be considered to be self-delusion or even strong psychological reactions to a blow from the rear. However, experimentally induced whiplash injuries in monkeys have caused bruises and hemorrhages in the brains of some animals. The brain damage was not apparent until autopsy. Many neurologists now think that whiplash may sometimes produce undetected brain injury in human beings.

At times, sprains are very painful, but often they are dismissed lightly, faith being put in self-healing. However, authorities maintain that in a great many cases a sprained ankle is accompanied by subluxation, or incomplete dislocation. The spontaneous return of the bones to their position does not minimize the after-effects. The relaxation of ligaments, joint capsule tendons, and muscles after severe strains, mild rupture, and dislocations are the cause of much chronic pain and disability. Further, there is always a possibility that a fracture may have occurred, and this can only be determined by x-ray studies. *Every* sprain should receive medical attention.

Painful feet

The long arch, stretching on the inside border of the foot from heel to toes, is the elastic spring upon which the entire weight is placed. The arch, made up of numerous bones, is held together by muscles and ligaments. The integrity of the arch as a spring depends upon the integrity of the "spring" ligament *(inferior calcaneoscaphoid ligament)*, which is the principal inside support.

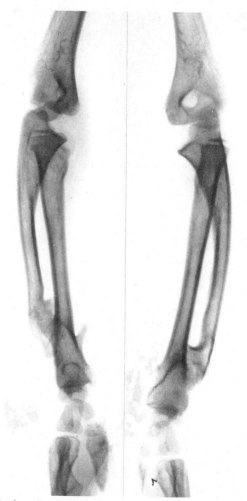

An hereditary type of bone disorder, chondrodysplasia, causes bending, shortening, and other deformities of the bones. Copyright 1965 Year Book Medical Publishers, Inc., courtesy M. M. Copeland, The University of Texas M. D. Anderson Hospital, Houston.

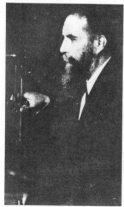

ROENTGEN, Wilhelm Konrad (1845-1923) German physicist. In 1895 Roentgen discovered x-rays, thereby providing the means by which opaque objects within the body may be photographed. X-rays are often referred to as *roentgen* rays, and the field of medicine involved with their use in diagnosis and treatment is known as *roentgenology*. Long active as a professor of physics in the leading universities of Germany, he received the Nobel prize in the year 1901.

Chronic strain is the most common cause of painful feet. Foot strain may be caused by: long periods of standing, walking, or running, especially by those unaccustomed to such activities; overweight; badly-fitting shoes; stockings that are too short; poor posture; "knock-knees"; curvature of the spine; and other factors. The constant wearing of high heels is a source of pain, because high heels frequently lead to a shortening of the calf muscles which decreases the range of dorsiflexion of the foot.

Flat foot is a common foot disorder. Flat foot may be the result of occupation, obesity, disease, injury, or paralysis. It may be based on inborn weakness of the foot arch or may be be acquired through overstrain and poor position in walking or standing. Poorly-fitted shoes or debilitating illnesses contribute to the condition by promoting relaxation of the ligaments which normally bind the arch into a flexible spring. The ligaments stretch, relax, and become incapable of returning to their original condition. When this occurs the bones lose their normal position, and the arch flattens. Idiopathic or congenital flat foot is rarely symptomatic.

If the flat foot is still flexible, much can be done to correct the condition by proper shoes, arch supports, pads, strapping, training in proper foot position, and strengthening of muscles and other structures by appropriate exercises. All these should be carried out under expert direction. Once a flat foot has become rigid, it may be necessary to break up the fibrous adhesions which have formed, possibly by the use of a cast or even surgical intervention. In any case, such procedures should be decided upon by the physician.

Dislocations

When a bone is dislocated, it is moved partially or completely out of its normal relationship to the surrounding structures of a joint. The integrity of a joint depends upon the ligamentous structures and the muscles which support the bones forming the joint. In some individuals, the joint structures are a more loosely held aggregate, and dislocation and recurrent dislocation take place more easily.

Dislocation occurs when the bones are in a position in which muscle support is at a minimum. For example, a direct blow against the shoulder finds the joint in its most vulnerable position. The head of the bone of the upper arm (the *humerus)* is thrust against the joint capsule where muscle support is lacking. The head bursts through the capsule and is dislocated. In "dashboard dislocation" of the hip, as occurs in automobile accidents, the sitting position of the victim is a contributing factor; the force thrusts the hipbone backward out of its

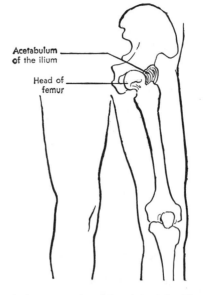

Acetabulum of the ilium

Head of femur

A typical, low anterior dislocation of the hip, showing how the head of the femur is displaced from its socket (acetabulum) located in the ilium.

socket. In a hinge joint like the knee or elbow, twisting or forcible extension beyond the normal range of the extended leg or arm tears the ligaments, ruptures the joint capsule, and displaces the bones. Dislocation of spinal vertebrae from twists or blows endangers the spinal cord by compression. No joint is immune from dislocation, and bizarre accidents account for many.

Dislocation causes pain and limitation of movement. Nerves may also be severely injured. In shoulder dislocations, for instance, the drag on nerves may cause paralysis of muscles of arm or hand. The displaced head of the humerus may press upon blood vessels, impeding circulation with the result that the hand is blue and cold. In hip dislocations, the major motor nerve may be paralyzed; and if nutrient-supplying blood vessels are torn, the head of the thighbone may become necrotic, soft, and die, or osteoarthritis may develop. Such side effects are typical of the share other structures have in *traumatic* dislocations.

Spontaneous dislocations take place in joints which have been the site of paralysis or have infections that cause spasm of muscles. *Recurrent* dislocation results from a number of causes. Such dislocation has followed the incomplete or improper healing of a torn ligament in a weight-bearing joint. Anatomical defects or the use of ill-fitting shoes which impair muscles and tendons are among the causes of recurrent dislocation. Recurrent dislocations of the shoulder are common in athletes in whom the first dislocation makes the joint more susceptible

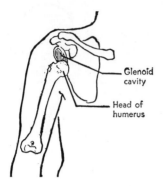

This drawing shows a subglenoid dislocation at the shoulder, with the head of humerus displaced anteriorly from its place in the glenoid cavity.

to successive ones. Surgical procedures may be used to correct recurrent dislocations.

Sudden locking, or sudden giving way of the joint, constitutes the principal symptoms of *internal derangements of the knee*. The condition is common in athletes and is precipitated by a sudden twisting which tears ligaments, or injures or displaces other internal knee structures. Such an injury is common in football players. Fat tags in the knee structure may become pinched, bruised, or swollen, causing locking; this occurs in skiers. Locking of the knee joint causes immediate disability, but may disappear with a snap or manipulation. Recurrence is common. Loose bodies in the knee are a result of inflammation of the synovial membrane and occur in patients with arthritis or tuberculosis of the bone. Carefully chosen surgical treatment followed by appropriate physical therapy and rehabilitation can usually correct this condition.

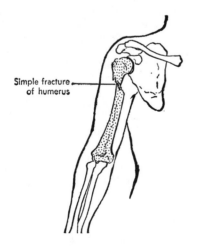

This drawing illustrates the appearance of a simple fracture of the humerus; the surrounding tissues of the arm have remained relatively free of injury.

Congenital dislocation of the hip, caused by improper development during the fetal life, is thought by many to be a heritable condition. Females are much more likely to be afflicted than males, and the dislocation may be of one or both hips. This condition is often difficult to diagnose before the child begins to walk, although, unfortunately, it is during infancy that treatment is most useful. The first symptoms may be a more pronounced rotation of the femur than in normal infants. When only one hip is affected, the creases in the infant's thigh may not be symmetrical. As the child begins to walk, she may develop a limp and marked lordosis. Later, there is always a shortening of the thigh and a wide space between the thighs when the child stands with feet together. There is no pain associated with the dislocation until adulthood and this is usually a low back pain resulting from lordosis. Treatment involves a long tedious procedure employing casts and weights to gradually correct the dislocation. Surgical treatment may be required if soft tissues have developed in the space to which the head of the femur is to be restored.

When any type of dislocation occurs, no one but a physician should attempt to put the injured joint back in place. There is great danger of further injury to the tendons, muscles, blood vessels, and nerves. Until the doctor arrives, the patient should be made as comfortable as possible and kept warm. If cold compresses are applied to the injured joint, they may relieve pain, contract the blood vessels, and prevent swelling.

Fractures

A fractured bone is a broken bone. The structural lines of stress of bones will absorb most of the shocks of normal motion. Force that imposes an overload of stress, or is applied in a direction counter to that of normal position, causes bones to break. Common causes of broken bones are falls and twists. Direct blows can dislocate and fracture the shoulder or ribs, and "dashboard dislocation" and fracture of the hip occur often in automobile collisions. If there is any reason to suspect that a person has sustained a fracture, a doctor should be notified immediately. In extensive injuries, it is best not to move the patient before the physician arrives.

Fractures are classed as *primary fractures,* which occur in healthy persons as the result of trauma, and *pathologic fractures,* which occur in persons with diseased or weakened bones.

Primary fractures are divided into two main groups: simple and open (old term *compound*). A *simple fracture* implies a break in the bone without subsequent tearing of the muscles and skin. An *open fracture* implies a break in the bone which causes a wound to the outside,

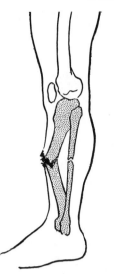

Drawing which illustrates an open (compound) fracture of the tibia, showing how the surrounding tissues of the leg have been subjected to severe damage.

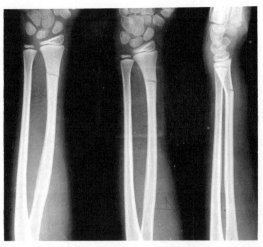

These three x-ray photographs show the appearance of the "green-stick" type of fracture, which occurs frequently in children. *Courtesy of Hermann Hospital, Houston.*

either from a splintered piece of bone or an entire bone breaking through the skin. Because open fractures carry the added danger of infection and torn tissue, they constitute the more serious type of broken bones. Another, less common type is the sprain-fracture, in which the force that tears the fibers of the ligaments also chips off a piece of bone. Similarly, fracture-dislocation occurs when the bone, or bones, have been broken and dislocated, sometimes accompanied by rupture of the joint structures; shoulder, knee, wrist, and and ankle joints are common sites of fracture-dislocations.

Special fractures

Automobile accidents are responsible for 58 percent of the cases of broken neck (*fracture of the cervical vertebrae*). The mobility of the cervical spine increases its vulnerability to the application of sudden and violent forward force. A sudden jerk, a sudden bump against the top of the car, or diving into a shallow pool are types of forces that cause a broken or dislocated neck. The injury often causes compression of the spinal cord, which may cause the death of the victim.

Spontaneous fractures occur without appreciable trauma in fragile bones of aged persons. These breaks can occur also in younger, normal bones. An example of this is the so-called "march fractures" in soldiers, in which the small bones of the feet are broken. In such cases, the fracture has been ascribed to overfatigue of muscles during long marches, with the result that the bones are deprived of the protective action of muscles.

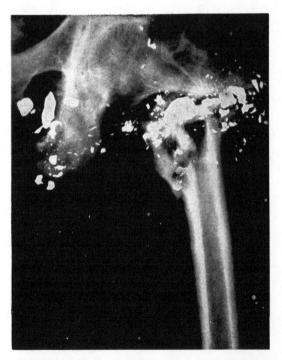

A shotgun fracture of the pelvis and upper femur can be studied in detail by the orthopedist with the aid of x-ray photography. *Courtesy of Hermann Hospital, Houston.*

Pathologic fractures occur in diseased bone. Persons with primary or secondary bone tumors may experience this type of bone breaks. Other conditions which predispose the individual to fracture are bone cysts, and generalized condi-

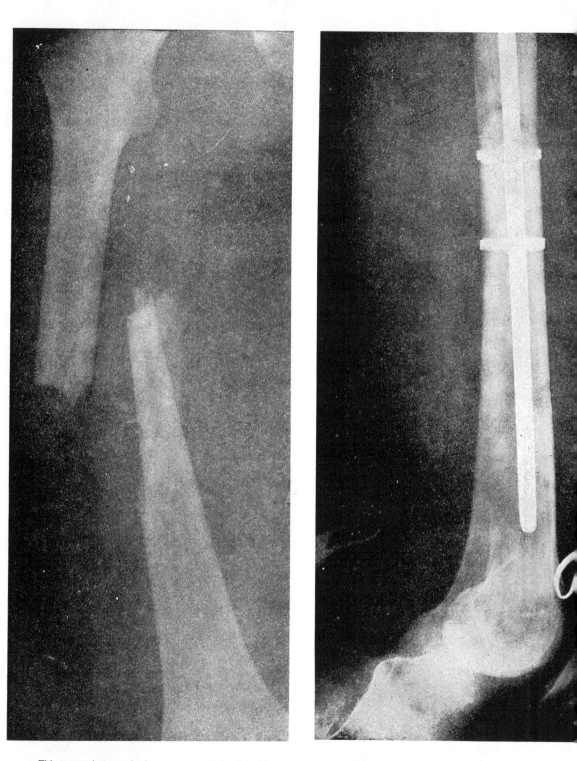

This x-ray photograph shows a severely fractured femur with the broken ends completely separated from each other. *Photo Courtesy of Hermann Hospital, Houston.*

The fractured femur shown in this x-ray photograph has been repaired; it is supported by an intramedullary rod. *Photo Courtesy of Hermann Hospital, Houston, Texas.*

tions such as rickets. In these instances, the bone is easily fractured from the slightest trauma or from none at all. Ribs are frequently involved in pathologic fractures; coughing may cause a rib to fracture.

As healing proceeds, the primary *callus* is converted into bone. As time passes, this bone organizes itself into compact and cancellous bony tissue. Parallel changes take place in the marrow space and other areas. Healing normally is completed in eight to twelve weeks in the larger bones, but fractures do not always heal in the expected length of time. *Delayed union* may be caused by: interposition of soft parts between fractured ends, preventing them from coming together; other factors, such as infection; circulatory impairment, which may delay union until the formation of new blood vessels can revitalize dying fragments; defective initial blood clot such as may result from crush injury that damages the local circulation, thus retarding the healing process; excessive motion of bone fragments due to resorption of post-injury swelling in the initial cast; systemic conditions, such as found in older persons in whom the speed of bone absorption exceeds that of bone formation; and the malalignment of fragments.

Other factors also may delay healing of a fracture. Digestive disturbances in old age interfere with the utilization of necessary calcium and vitamin D. A decreased local blood supply may result from senile changes in the blood system. In particular, a deficiency of protein impairs bone metabolism, and as a result, breakdown of bone exceeds build-up. In some cases, bones may fail to unite. The causes of this failure usually are of a mechanical nature.

Great advances have been made in the management and treatment of patients with fractures, including fractures which do not unite. The use of live bone grafts from another person has proved successful. Also, good results have been obtained by the insertion of nails, screws, and plates of inert metals; these hold the bone together temporarily until it heals, or permanently in some cases. *Intramedullary rods* have been used, especially in the treatment of fractures of the larger long bones, and often have shortened the time the patient spends in the hospital. Operating room techniques have improved, and better instruments have been developed. Today's patient with a broken bone can have confidence in the probability that he will not be permanently crippled.

HOW A FRACTURED HIP IS REPAIRED

One of the most spectacular advances in orthopedic surgery during recent years has been employment of various types of internal splints, pins, wires, and other devices for the fixation of fractures. A great variety of techniques have been developed to modify such internal splints to fit almost every type of fracture. While various materials are employed, stainless steel,

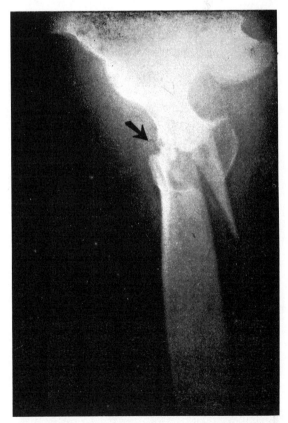

1. This x-ray photograph clearly shows the severe break in the femur at the point of the arrow. Proximity to the pelvis means a large plaster cast will be needed or surgical reduction and internal fixation by means of nails, plates and screws.

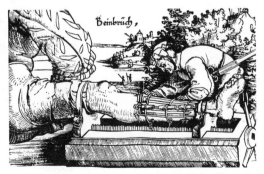

This sixteenth century woodcut by Wechtlin illustrates the technique employed during that period for splinting a fracture. *Bettmann Archive.*

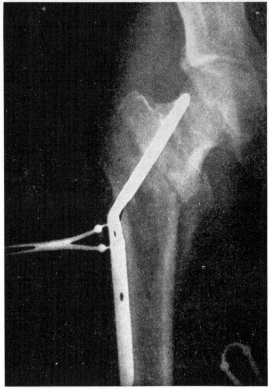

2. Metal splint to be used must be properly shaped so it will fit along shaft of the femur, while one end penetrates fractured area and passes into head of the bone.

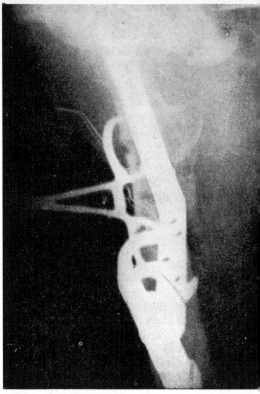

3. The end of the metal plate that passes through fracture line thus serves as a nail to fix permanently the two broken ends together whether or not they ever heal.

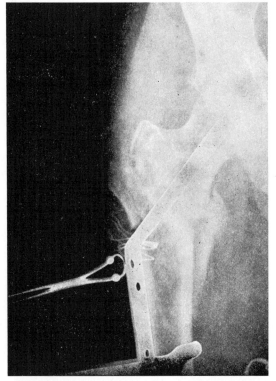

4. With metal pin inserted, other end fits flush along the bone to which it will then be secured by screws, thus preventing the splint from working out of bone.

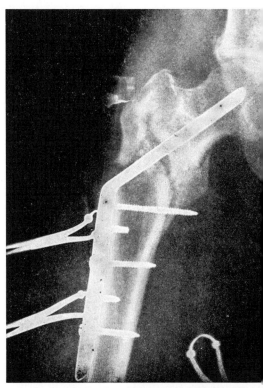

5. In the x-ray photograph the metal plate has been securely screwed into the bone, and instruments may now be removed and the wound will be permanently closed.

Teflon, polyethylene, and vitallium are in most general use. These devices prove less cumbersome to the patient than external splints, and permit earlier use of the fractured member. When properly inserted, they seldom cause any difficulty to the patient. In the accompanying series of x-ray photographs, a fractured femur is repaired by the use of one special kind of metal splint. Although the process requires surgery for the insertion of the support, the inconvenience involved is small by comparison with that which normally attends the use of an external plaster cast for the fixation of the fracture. Many other fractures require only pins or screws. *Pictures by courtesy Hermann Hospital, Houston.*

DISORDERS OF THE SKELETON AND MUSCLES: RUPTURE

Hernia, or "rupture," results when any organ or tissue pushes through an opening in the cavity in which it is confined. By common usage, however, the term "hernia" has come to mean the protrusion of some portion of the abdominal contents through an opening in the abdominal wall.

A hernia consists of a *sac*, the contents of the sac, and the layers of tissue of which the sac is composed.

Hernias are of two main classes: *congenital* hernia in which the sac was present before birth; and *acquired* hernia in which the sac is formed after birth and pushes through an opening in the muscle wall which failed to close at birth, or that was formed following an incision. A large percentage of acquired hernias result from injury or strain, such as those hernias which occur when a person lifts a heavy object. Hernias may occur in the groin, the navel, the membrane separating the abdominal and chest cavities *(diaphragm)*, in surgical incisions, and elsewhere.

All herniation takes place through a normal opening, or through an opening that should have been eliminated at some period of development, or through an opening which had closed and then reopened in later life.

The hernial sac has a mouth, a neck, and a body. The mouth connects with the abdominal cavity and is called the *hernial ring;* the body is the pouch or sac that projects outside the abdominal wall; and the neck connects the mouth and body of the sac.

The contents of the sac might be any of the abdominal organs, in whole or part; loops of the intestine are commonly found in hernias. The sac and its contents are subject to injury which can lead to serious complications. The skin surface is vulnerable to blows, falls, pres-

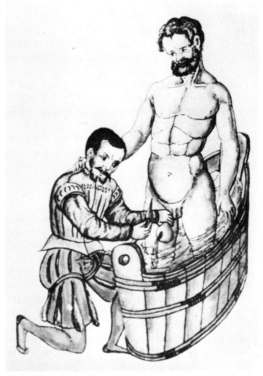

Illustration from the sixteenth century in which the physician is tapping a patient to relieve pressure on a hydrocoele. *Bettmann Archive.*

sure, irritation from binders or trusses, or may become inflamed, infected, or abscessed. From within, the contents of the sac are prone to strangulation when the blood supply is cut off by a narrow or constricted hernial ring; gangrene and death may follow, in rare instances, unless treatment is sought promptly.

Hernias are spoken of as being *reducible* or *irreducible.* Reduction may be spontaneous; for example, sac contents may return unaided to the abdominal cavity when the patient lies flat on his back. If the patient remains untreated, however, a reducible hernia may become irreducible; that is, the contents of the sac can no longer be returned to the abdominal cavity. Irreducibility may be caused by increased size of the hernia, formation of adhesions, or development of a small or constricted hernial ring. Hernias of enormous size, hanging down to the knees, have been reported. An irreducible hernia is a constant source of danger.

Hernias occurring in the groin are either *inguinal* hernias or *femoral* hernias. Inguinal hernias account for 92 percent of all hernias. Superficially, inguinal and femoral hernias look alike, because the bulge is in the groin. Anatomically they differ. Inguinal hernias slip through the normal openings for the passage of nerves or organs of the reproductive system. Femoral hernias occur through the passageway for nerves and vessels to the thigh.

Normally, the deep and shallow layers of muscles and ligaments on the abdominal wall protect these normal openings against herniation. As intra-abdominal tension rises—as by straining, coughing, or lifting—the muscles contract and flatten like a shutter across the openings. But when the muscles, or other protective structures of these openings, are weak, the shutter action fails; an increase of intra-abdominal tension may push part of the abdominal organs through the opening into the preformed sac, and a hernia is begun. Successive incidents of tension increase the size of the sac by forcing more and more intra-abdominal tissue into it.

Hernias of the navel are called *umbilical* hernias. The navel is an opening that should close in the process of development. After birth, it is a scar formed of interlaced muscle fibers of the contracted *umbilical ring*. Sometimes a defect occurring before birth prevents its closing, and the baby is born with a hernia, or may soon acquire one. During infancy, when scarring is not yet firm, whooping cough, a fall, or other strain placed upon the area may cause herniation. In adults between 25 and 40 years of age, obesity and pregnancy are the most common predisposing causes of this form of hernia.

Obese women are the most frequent subjects of hernia in the site of a surgical incision. Some incisional hernias are caused by failure of the layers of deep muscle and *fascia* to knit firmly after surgery. Blood clot, infection, exudate, and swelling in the line of incision, as well as increased intra-abdominal tension, also are factors favoring herniation. But deep wound disruption should not be confused with the breaking apart of the skin edges after removal of stitches. Such superficial opening is not serious.

The neck of the incisional hernia is a firm ring of scar tissue. Because of the large hernial ring, these hernias are difficult to control by a truss. Large incisional hernias may cause invalidism, unless surgical relief is obtained.

Treatment

The treatment of a hernia patient can be accomplished by a mechanical device (truss), or surgery. Most authorities agree that a truss is a makeshift which is acceptable only when surgery would be hazardous. If a truss must be worn, it should be worn on advice of a physician, and should be fitted by him.

The advances in surgical treatment of hernia have kept pace with the advances in other fields of surgery. Better techniques have made possible the surgical repair of hernias which not so many decades ago would have been irreparable. It is often necessary to close the opening with a fascial graft or an inert foreign material such as Marlex (polypropylene) mesh.

DISORDERS OF THE SKELETON AND MUSCLES: ARTHRITIS

Arthritis is a name applied to a great variety of diseases. In 1963, the American Rheumatism Association adopted a tentative classification of arthritis and rheumatism. Of the more than 80 diseases and syndromes included, the only feature common to all was that at some stage they involve the joints or adjacent tissues.

Arthritis has existed for millions of years. Bones of many prehistoric reptiles and mammals have been found to have characteristic arthritic markings. Obviously, the disease is neither new nor original to man. The bones of *Pithecanthropus erectus,* one of the earliest types of man, have revealed arthritic lesions; Neanderthal man also had arthritis, as did the ancient Egyptians and the pre-Columbian Indians of North America.

Most forms of arthritis fall into one of the following categories: infectious (caused by a specific microorganism), possibly infectious (of unknown origin), degenerative, traumatic, metabolic, or nonarticular (such as bursitis, tendinitis).

Degenerative arthritis and *rheumatoid arthritis* (popularly referred to as *rheumatism*) are the most common types of arthritis. The two disorders are vastly different in nature, development, and treatment required. Degenerative arthritis is the form of the disease in which the aging process is involved; rheumatoid arthritis is the inflammatory and crippling type of the disease. This discussion will be limited to these two classes of arthritis.

Degenerative arthritis is characterized by an absence of the positive signs typical of rheumatoid arthritis. In a patient with degenerative arthritis, there is no fever, no anemia, no loss of weight, no general joint stiffening or deformity, and no inflammation of the joint membrane.

Degenerative arthritis is a disease of advancing years, commonly becoming apparent after 40. In bones, the process of aging begins early, although symptomatic evidence may not appear until the later decades of life. Microscopic examination of knee joints following amputation has shown that degenerative changes start as early as the second decade of life, and that they continue progressively into the later years. Hence, it appears that joints remain normal for only a short time following maturity, and that degeneration starts early, although the expression of the damage sustained may be late.

The degenerative process first attacks the cartilage, particularly the center of the cap on the bone; the gliding surface of that cartilage is flaked off. The degenerative process then destroys the binding material that holds together the bundles of cartilage fibers, leaving them erect like the pile of a carpet. In weight-bearing joints, these fibers soon are worn off, and fissures and pits appear. Ultimately, all the cartilage is worn away, the joint space disappears, and the bone surfaces are in direct contact. The cartilage is the shock absorber of joints, and with its loss, arthritic changes become more obvious.

The cause of the degenerative process is unknown. Innumerable theories have been proposed and have been discarded. Apparently, degenerative arthritis fundamentally is an aging process, although what sets it in motion and why it takes place faster in some individuals have never been determined.

It is conceded that degenerative changes take place in the joint cartilage as a result of wear and tear, and various forms of injury (trauma), both great and small. Why this is so is not known. It is assumed, however, that a constitutional predisposition may be a factor. In other words, there are some persons who are born with cartilage that wears out faster under the strains and stresses of living than does the cartilage of other people. In some persons, the cartilage will have worn thin by middle age, while in others at 80 it seems to have sustained comparatively little damage. This is called the "wearing capacity" of cartilage.

Age and trauma hold first place as predisposing factors. Age plays its role here as it does in other organ systems. Trauma takes a variety of forms. Careful studies and reports of groups of cases ascribe the arthritis in men at heavy labor to the trauma of their work; conversely, other reports, probably just as carefully prepared, have shown that the same degenerative changes have been found in the same age groups of persons who had done little or no hard work. Nevertheless, a traumatizing element of causation is conceded. Fractures, torn ligaments, and other injuries involving joints become predisposing factors, because the impaired tissue is more vulnerable to the effect of subsequent wear and tear of ordinary function, due to malalignment and support. The degenerative arthritis that results is called traumatic arthritis.

Poor posture is a traumatizing factor because it violates the principles of good body mechanics. The contact surfaces of bones in joints are constructed to bear the load of stress and weight-bearing. Poor posture shifts the points of contact and causes strains, throwing a burden upon portions of bones and joints not meant to bear it. The degenerative arthritis so engendered is called "static," and photographs of victims are available showing how they started in poor posture and were "frozen" in it by stiffening of the joints. Knock-knees and bowlegs, flat feet with turned ankles and strained ligaments, and a distortion of the normal curves of the spine contribute to the development of degenerative arthritis.

Symptoms and signs

In the early years when the disease process is starting, x-ray films fail to reveal bone changes. After the age of 50, however, practically all people have x-ray evidence of bone changes, although only 5 percent of these have any arthritic symptoms. It has been estimated that about 24 million Americans have demonstrable degenerative arthritis, but only a small proportion of this number have any appreciable complaints.

The principal symptom is either stiffness or pain. These symptoms occur during motion, and rest gives relief. Patients do not experience muscular spasm, wasting, or flexion deformities, in contrast to the patient with rheumatoid arthritis. True bony stiffening is rare.

The principal sign typical of degenerative arthritis is the appearance of knobs at the end joints of the first and second fingers. These are called Heberden's nodes. These nodes are an overgrowth (hypertrophy) of bone at the margins of the joint. They differ from those of gout by being immovable, because they are attached to the bone, whereas those of gout are freely movable and contain urate crystals. The nodes differ from those of rheumatoid arthritis, because in the latter the middle joint is attacked and the swelling is spindle-shaped; and usually the joint is hot and shiny.

Heberden's nodes on the fingers are nine times as common in women as in men. They worry patients because of their unsightliness rather than because of any functional difficulty, which is rare. The nodes occur in men following trauma.

The joints most frequently involved in degenerative arthritis are the end joints of the fingers, the lumbar vertebrae, knees, sacroiliac, lower cervical vertebrae, hips, and shoulders. This type of arthritis practically never affects the wrists, elbows, knuckles, or feet.

Degenerative disease of the knee is one of the most troublesome forms. Usually it manifests itself between ages 40 and 50 with pain, stiffness, and creaking on motion. These symptoms are most pronounced after sitting or a night's rest, or when going up or down stairs. The joint limbers up after it has been in motion. Pain and tenderness may be present, especially around the kneecap.

In women, the most common place for degenerative change is the end (terminal) joints of of the fingers. In men, the lower spine is most frequently involved. It has been estimated that

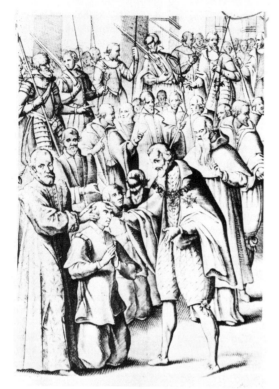

Engraving which portrays King Henry IV exercising the alleged divine power of monarchs to heal diseased or injured individuals. *Bettmann Archive.*

body, or complain that they cannot raise their arms to the head or back of the neck. If nerves in the thoracic area are affected, the pain may circle the chest and be confused with the pain of heart disease. In the lumbar region, the nerve distribution will give rise to pain down the legs, often called *sciatica.*

Normally, the strong ligaments attached at the sacroiliac joint prevent much motion, but when they are relaxed, symptoms may appear. Low back pain, pain down the legs or in the groin, and localized muscle spasm are the principal subjective evidences of degenerative arthritis in this joint.

Half a dozen names have been given degenerative disease of the hip joint, the most disabling form of the disease. Pain begins so insidiously that it is almost unnoticed, and the patient limps slightly. Pain passes along the nerve pathways to the groin and down the leg, and patients frequently complain of sciatica. As in knee joint disease, the hip stiffens after sitting. At times the pain may interfere with sleep. With a wearing away of the hip joint cartilage, the joint space is narrowed or lost; this becomes particularly apparent in the weight-bearing portion where the head of the thighbone fits into its socket. There is abundant bone spur formation around the margins. As a rule the patient with degenerative arthritis of the hip is otherwise in excellent physical condition.

Degenerative arthritis may attack other joints as well, including the ribs. The ribs are never still, moving continuously with the motion of the chest in respiration. Spinal nerves make their exit from the vertebrae close to the ribs, and corresponding symptoms occur with irritation of these nerves. Normally, the position of the ribs is in a slightly downward slant. In poor posture, this downward sag is greatly increased, with corresponding strain on muscles and ligaments. The articulation of rib and vertebra acts as a fulcrum, twisting the rib, and, if continued, this may lead to arthritic change.

Treatment

Medical science has not discovered a means of remaking cartilage once it is destroyed. The changes that take place in degenerative diseases are not reversible. However, a most reassuring fact is that degenerative arthritis does not force the individual into a status of helpless invalidism. Creaking, stiffness, and mild pain suffered by the great majority of victims may be a nuisance, but not a calamity. The nodes on the fingers may be unsightly, but they do not seriously impair function.

The physician should arrange for a complete program of therapy to suit the needs of the individual arthritic patient. Such a plan provides for rest, avoidance of strain or trauma, weight

degenerative arthritis of the spine is present in practically all persons over the age of 50, although not all complain of pain or other symptoms.

The spinal type of arthritis is a reaction to the loss of buffer action of the intervertebral discs as they become thinned, less elastic and less firm, dehydrated, torn, and distorted from a combination of factors including age and continued trauma. The loss of buffer action increases the mobility of the vertebral joints upon one another, and speeds degenerative arthritic changes in the posterior portions of the joints, while bony outgrowths (*exostoses*) develop from the margins. If these are great enough to press upon one another, the friction may cause their fusion, and with the fusion stiffening takes place. A fused, stiff spine does not occur frequently in patients with degenerative arthritis.

Postural defects have been found to be common in patients with degenerative arthritis of the spine.

In addition to local pain caused by the bone changes, arthritis of the spine may cause pain along the nerves which come out from the nerve roots along the spine. In the cervical region, the pain is of cervical distribution. Patients suffer sharp pain from jarring of the reduction if necessary to decrease the burden upon the knees, heat applied in various ways, massage, exercise, promotion of good posture, foot care for posture and support, and orthopedic appliances when required. The only drugs of any value in degenerative arthritis are those for the relief of pain.

Rest is of particular importance. When the hip or knee is involved, there should be daily rest periods in the recumbent position. Wage earners are urged to take a rest at noon, and an hour's rest after the evening meal is recommended for all. As a rule, complete bed rest is not required.

The notion that continuous and diligent exercise will force motion into the joints should be discouraged. Exercise is important to improve circulation and prevent fibrous adhesions and other changes. But overexercise does more harm than good. Exercise that leaves discomfort lasting more than two hours is too strenuous. The general slowing down of body processes in advancing years, manifested as it is in all organ systems of the body, should be met by a slowing down of the pace of younger years.

Physical therapy is a source of comfort to arthritic patients. Various types of baths are available in most cities, and these can be arranged by the physician. Massage following application of heat helps to improve circulation, reduce spasm, and prevent further degeneration.

Abdominal supports may be needed by obese patients. This relieves the drag on back muscles which pulls the spinal curves out of alignment.

In general, the arthritic patient is simply a person whose joints have grown old. With proper care, he may grow old with relative comfort.

DISORDERS OF THE SKELETON AND MUSCLES: RHEUMATISM

Chronic rheumatoid arthritis, popularly known as rheumatism, is a systemic disease, the principal feature of which is inflammation of joints and associated structures. It is characterized by periods of improvement which may raise the false hope of recovery. Attacks of pain and disability do recur. The disease is progressive in course; changes take place in the joint structures which increasingly impair and limit motion. Unless the progress of the disease can be checked, it is only a matter of time before crippling deformities become permanently fixed, and the patient is totally disabled. Over 3,000,000 Americans suffer from this chronic disabling disease. Together with other forms of arthritis, it is responsible for 16 percent of the long-term disability in this country. Only heart disease exceeds this percentage (17 percent).

Rheumatoid arthritis first attacks the membrane which lines the joint (*synovial membrane*), causing inflammation of the membrane. The synovial membrane enlarges rapidly; this process is called *proliferation*. The membrane formed by this synovial activity, called the *pannus*, covers the joint. Extensions of this membrane eat into the underlying cartilage which normally forms the gliding surfaces of the joint. At the same time, changes are taking place in the bony substance below the cartilage. The bone loses its mineral components and becomes fibrous; this degeneration also spreads to the cartilage. In time, this two-way attack, from bone and from joint, on the cartilage converts it into bloodless fibrous tissue. The result is a stiffening (*ankylosis*) of the joint. The ankylosis, which was fibrous, may become bony. Once this has taken place, the end of the process is signaled by the end of pain and motion, and the patient is permanently crippled.

While these changes are taking place within the joint, parallel events are taking place in the joint's supporting structures. Because motion causes pain, the muscles go into spasm as a protective mechanism to immobilize the joint. The flexor muscles being stronger than the extensors, their contraction bends the joints (*flexion*), and the contracted muscles and tendons hold the joint in the flexed position. The opposing muscles (the *extensors*) wither away from disuse. Ultimately, the flexor muscles also degenerate. Because fibrous and bony changes take place simultaneously within the joint, the flexion deformities which are typical of rheumatoid arthritis develop. These combined changes create the spindle-shaped swelling of rheumatoid arthritis.

Although many theories have been advanced, the cause of rheumatoid arthritis remains unknown. When the adrenal hormone *cortisone* was found successful in relieving the symptoms of this disease, the possibility of adrenal deficiency as a causative factor was considered. No such evidence has been found.

Currently under investigation is the theory that rheumatoid arthritis may be an autoimmune disease, that is, a disease in which the body becomes allergic to part of itself. Certain abnormal substances in the blood characterize this disease, as well as other diseases, such as lupus erythematosus. This type of inclusion (called the "rheumatoid factor") is seen in about 80 percent of the patients who have had the disease for some time. Investigations are under way to determine whether this "rheumatoid factor" in the blood (which resembles some known antibodies) could be an autoantibody. The role of this substance in the mechanism of rheumatoid arthritis is not known.

The most popular theory has been that this disease is caused by infection. Yet no infectious agent has been found. However, new experimental evidence proves that some actual active agent (perhaps a virus) does occur in the tissues of rheumatoid arthritis patients. This agent has been transmitted to mice (both directly and congenitally). Pregnant female mice were injected with material surgically removed from the joints of patients with chronic rheumatoid arthritis. Later, their newborn offspring received similar injections. In five generations of the mice, almost half of the animals developed joint disorders which resembled human rheumatoid arthritis. Such reactions occurred in at least two generations of mice which were not injected. These initial findings may indicate that rheumatoid arthritis is a "slow-virus" disease, in which symptoms do not appear until long after the infection by a virus takes place. If a causative virus can be isolated, a vaccine against rheumatoid arthritis may eventually be developed.

Clinical features

No set pattern characterizes the beginning and course of rheumatoid arthritis. While it is most common in persons between the ages of 20 and 40, it has developed after 50 and has been found in infants and children. Women are affected by this disease three times more frequently than are men. It may begin in a variety of ways, and precipitating factors are equally varied. It may follow an acute or chronic respiratory infection. It may occur after emotional stress or overexposure to cold and damp. Some persons may have a constitutional predisposition to chronic rheumatoid arthritis. People between the ages of 20 and 40, who are thin, lacking in bodily vigor, have a tendency to a sagging of internal organs (*ptosis*), and often become overfatigued, are the typical patients having this disease. However, not all patients fit this description. Overfatigue becomes a precipitating factor, setting in motion a train of events which is difficult and sometimes impossible to stop.

This disease may begin with fever, pain, and swelling in one or more joints. Its development

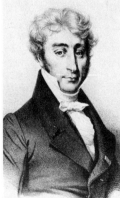

DELPECH, Jacques Mathieu (1777-1832) French orthopedic surgeon. One of the few orthopedists of his day deserving the name. He, with Larrey, Lisfranc, Dupuytren, and Roux developed orthopedic surgery in France, and was one of the first surgeons to practice subcutaneous section of the Achilles tendon in treating patients with clubfoot (1816). He was one of the first to identify the tuberculous nature of the spinal caries constituting Pott's disease.

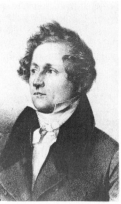

DIEFENBACH, Johann Friedrich (1792-1847) German surgeon. With other surgeons of German and Viennese schools, he placed orthopedic surgery on a firm foundation for growth in German-speaking countries. Also a specialist in other branches of surgery, he is distinguished for his work in plastic surgery, especially rhinoplasty. In 1842, he treated strabismus successfully by myotomy for the first time, though poor results caused its abandonment.

may go unnoticed over a period of months, with the patient complaining of fatigue, numbness and tingling in the extremities, and loss of weight. The joint pains may be fleeting, or they may be migratory, subsiding in one joint before starting in another. The characteristic points of attack are the *middle* joints of the fingers, which become warm, painful, and swollen. In time, this swelling takes on the characteristic spindle shape of rheumatoid arthritis. This contour is brought about by the simultaneous thickening and swelling of joint structures and the wasting of muscles. At this stage, motion causes pain. The condition may subside, only to return in weeks or months, with greater intensity. Occasionally, the disease begins as an acute inflammation of many joints (*polyarthritis*) and suggests acute rheumatic fever.

While this clinical description applies to the majority of patients, statistics show that in about 15 percent of them, the development and course of the disease are not typical. The joint involvement may vary in extent and degree and from one joint to another. Or there may be symmetrical involvement of small or large joints.

In rheumatoid arthritis, the order of frequency of joint involvement is as follows: the middle joints of the fingers, joints of the hands, toes, wrists, knees, elbows, shoulders, and hips. No joint is immune; the joint formed by the jawbone at the temple is not an unusual point of attack. Muscular weakness and wasting are common. Nodules under the skin sometimes appear below the elbow. Skin changes are frequent. The hands usually are cold and clammy, and the skin over the diseased portions is wasted, smooth, and shiny. Flexion deformities develop, as described. Constitutional symptoms become more pronounced with advance of the disease.

The muscular wasting is not limited to the muscles around the involved joints. Muscles of the extremities may degenerate, and sometimes over-all loss of body weight is extreme. Small muscles of the hands are particular targets for the wasting process.

Rheumatoid arthritis of the spine

Rheumatoid arthritis of the spine is not as common as the disease in other joints. However, it is exceedingly disabling. The earliest x-ray finding is sclerosis, or even fusion, of the sacroiliac joints. The disease begins in the synovial membrane of the small posterior intervertebral joints. As a rule, the disease starts in the lower lumbar vertebrae and progresses upward, although sometimes the cervical vertebrae are the first to be involved. Constitutional symptoms are severe. Ultimately, the spine is stiffened by a bony bridge across the intervertebral spaces, which deprives the joints of motion. To this is added a calcification or hardening of the longitudinal ligaments along the spine; when this happens, the patient is said to have a "bamboo spine." When this stiffening process has taken place with the spine in poor postural position, the entire body posture is distorted and the disability is severe.

Treatment

The course of rheumatoid arthritis is unpredictable, and every patient constitutes an individual problem for the physician.

The treatment of patients with rheumatoid arthritis has passed through the stages experienced by all diseases of which the cause is unknown. Through the years, the unhappy victims have hoped for a magic pill that would reverse the progress of their disease, end their misery, and restore their well-being. The patients easily become the victims of clever quacks, old wives' tales, private formulas, and miscellaneous "cures" obtained in various ways. Even the doctor has had discouraging results of treatment prescribed, because often what benefited one patient has no effect on another.

A new era of hope opened in April, 1949, when Doctors Philip S. Hench and Edward C. Kendall of the Mayo Clinic announced the encouraging results that had been achieved in patients with rheumatoid arthritis by the administration of *cortisone*, a hormone from the adrenal gland. Crippled arthritics, who had been confined to bed, were able to walk again.

The history of the relation of these hormones to rheumatoid arthritis began in 1925 when Hench observed that these patients commonly suffer from weakness, fatigue, and low blood pressure. Subsequently it was observed that men with rheumatoid arthritis improved after an attack of jaundice, and that arthritic women were relieved during pregnancy. This suggested that a hormone common to both sexes had some unknown effect on the disease processes. Hench believed that the adrenal gland was the source of this common hormone.

Compound E, as cortisone was first called, was isolated in the laboratory in 1935. It was first tested clinically in May, 1948, when it was administered to a patient with disease of the adrenal glands. Because of their inability to produce the drug in quantity, the manufacturers were able to supply the men at the Mayo Clinic with only enough additional cortisone to treat a single patient with severe rheumatoid arthritis. Cortisone was administered to this patient for the first time on September 21, 1948. The remarkable symptomatic relief achieved in this case marked a milestone in therapy for patients with this disease.

The drug *ACTH* is derived from the pituitary gland; this hormone stimulates the adrenal to secrete its own cortisone. The letters making the name "ACTH" are a contraction of the first letters of the name of the hormone—*adreno-cortico-tropic hormone*. The effect of ACTH on rheumatoid arthritis had not been suspected by earlier workers who had been isolating hormones from the pituitary glands. To Hench and his associates, the results of cortisone suggested that an attempt should be made to determine the possible value of ACTH in patients with rheumatoid arthritis. On February 8, 1949, ACTH was used clinically for the first time on a volunteer rheumatoid arthritic patient. In a few days, it became apparent that the clinical effect of ACTH upon the arthritic symptoms was similar to that produced by cortisone.

Based on these discoveries, several compounds with similar effects have been developed and are clinically available. Cortisone, ACTH, and similar compounds give relief *only* of symptoms; they do not cure. When treatment is stopped, symptoms return. Experience with long-term therapy by corticoid hormones has proved that serious complications may result from such use. At present, other anti-inflammatory drugs are more commonly used. Indomethacin, a relatively new drug, is proving to be more effective than aspirin or phenylbutazone for control of fever and joint inflammation and swelling.

Gold salts have been given patients with rheumatoid arthritis. It is the opinion of most medical authorities that gold salts are not the ideal drug for these patients. The salts are toxic; all patients do not respond to the treatment; and the disease frequently returns after cessation of treatment. There is no way of learning in advance how a given patient will react to gold salts.

Patients suffering from rheumatoid arthritis derive much comfort and benefit from other forms of treatment which have been firmly established on a clinical basis. Among these measures are rest, both physical and mental; occupational therapy; physical therapy including heat, massage, and exercise; orthopedic treatment; a diet supplying all the accessory food factors necessary for good nutrition; drugs as

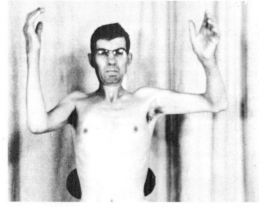

1. Photograph of an untreated patient who is suffering from subacute rheumatoid arthritis, showing the limit to which he was able to raise his arms. Pain expressed in patient's face was caused by this limited amount of movement.

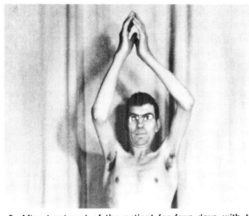

2. After treatment of the patient for four days with the drug cortisone, he was able to raise his arms considerably higher because of the greatly decreased stiffness. The patient also experienced a pronounced reduction of pain.

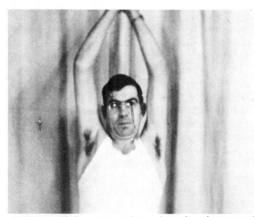

3. Picture of the same patient taken after three months of treatment with cortisone showing his return to relative normalcy with accompanying improvement of his general physical status. He has also gained considerable weight.

prescribed by the physician; avoidance of cold, dampness, and drafts.

Exercise is prescribed by the physician. The proper exercises, although they may be painful, help to prevent permanent fixation of joints. Sometimes the doctor splints the joint; splinting aids in retarding the development of deformities. This is particularly necessary when the disease is in the knees, hips, or spine. A joint, when permitted to remain in a contracted state too long, develops irreversible changes in the tissues which no amount of subsequent stretching will be able to correct.

Surgical procedures may become necessary to improve function in severely crippled joints. An experimental operation has been devised to replace finger joints which are badly crippled by rheumatoid arthritis. Stainless steel as well as silicone rubber implants have been substituted for the diseased knuckle and middle joints. Initial results have been encouraging.

The physician is able to plan a course of treatment and management that is best for the individual patient. The patient's co-operation in that plan serves his own interest.

DISORDERS OF THE SKELETON AND MUSCLES: GOUT

Gout is a metabolic disease in which high levels of *uric acid* in the blood are characteristic. It is not known whether these levels result from an excessive production of uric acid or from its inadequate excretion by the kidneys, or from both factors.

Hippocrates described the classic symptoms of this disease as it appeared among the ancient Greeks. One of the oldest therapeutic agents is colchicine (meadow saffron or autumn crocus) which has been used to control the pain of gout since the fifth century. Many distinguished persons in history, including Frederick the Great and Benjamin Franklin, had bouts with the severe pain of gout.

The onset of the first acute attack of gout is marked by sudden and excruciating pain in a joint. Within hours, the affected joint is hot, red, swollen, and extremely tender. In 70 percent of the cases, the large toe is affected by the initial attack. In subsequent attacks, an increasing number of joints are involved, especially those of the knees, ankles, feet, hips, shoulders, elbows, wrists, and hands. The disease more commonly attacks joints of the lower extremities.

The acute phase lasts only a short time (days or weeks) and then disappears completely until the next attack. This characteristic sets gout apart from other joint diseases. The severity of

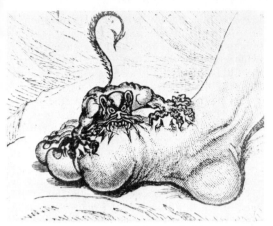

The gout. By Gillray, 1799. *Bettmann Archive.*

the first attack and the length of the remission period are variable.

Colchicine is still widely used for the symptomatic relief of acute gout. How this drug controls the pain of gout is not understood. Phenylbutazone or other anti-inflammatory agents may be prescribed as alternatives.

In advanced stages of gout, about 50 percent of the patients develop knobby deformities beneath the skin. Containing urate deposits, these masses occur in or adjacent to cartilage at joints or in the ears. Eventually these deposits may become large and contribute to severe joint damage.

When the acute phase of an attack subsides, drugs are given to prevent joint destruction. Medicine which increases the excretion of uric acid in the urine (*uricosuric drugs*) is prescribed. Probenecid is often used for this purpose. A new drug, allopurinol, has a similar effect by blocking the production of uric acid. Although more clinical experience is needed, the agent is effective for patients who do not respond well to the uricosuric drugs.

Excesses in food (especially those with high purine content) and drink were once thought to cause attacks of gout. Diet is no longer considered a significant factor in the management of the disease. Drugs are much more effective than low-purine diets for reducing uric acid levels in the blood.

Since gout is often genetically related, close relatives of persons with the disease should have tests to determine their blood uric acid levels. If they have significant elevations, preventive therapy with drugs may be started.

Just what is wrong with the enzyme systems of gout patients is not known. In all documented cases of the Lesch-Nyhan syndrome, a very rare hereditary disease only recently described, one certain enzyme is missing from the blood. This same missing enzyme was shown to be the cause of a few cases of gout. Thus, gout is not a disorder with a single cause. Perhaps other enzyme deficiencies will be found which explain additional occurrences.

In a group of university professors given physical and psychological tests, those who had high levels of uric acid in the blood often seemed to rate higher in traits such as drive, leadership qualities, and achievement. In another series, corporation executives had higher mean levels of uric acid in the blood than did the craftsmen. Further studies may show whether uric acid has any effect upon the reasoning centers of the brain which might explain these statistical observations.

DISORDERS OF THE SKELETON AND MUSCLES: LOW BACK PAIN

Low back pain is a symptom, not a disease. It is one of the complaints heard most frequently by the physician. It constitutes one of the largest problems of the industrial and military surgeon.

The causes of backache are legion. These causes are divided roughly into classes: mechanical, traumatic, disease-produced, and present-at-birth (*congenital*). Among the mechanical causes are faulty posture, obesity, faulty body mechanics, and occupational strains such as the bent-over positions assumed for clerical work. Any injury or sprain of the vertebrae, their ligaments, muscles, or nerves can produce low back pain. Some of the diseases which can result in this symptom are: lumbago, rheumatoid arthritis, tuberculosis, syphilis, osteomyelitis, undulant fever, rickets, gout and many others. As for congenital defects, some investigators believe that these arise because man's spine is still undergoing evolution to accommodate itself to the upright posture. Consequently, a larger number of persons than is generally realized are born with slightly defective spinal columns, and these may give rise to backache later in life.

The low back region has four principal areas in which pain can originate. Pain localized around one of these areas becomes one element in a larger syndrome made up of composite symptoms and signs.

Sciatica

The term "sciatica" has been a wastebasket for every condition that might be called backache, although there may be no connection between the symptoms and the sciatic nerve. The sciatic nerve is both large and long. Flat as a ribbon at its origin from the lumbrosacral plexus, it courses down the entire length of the leg, sending its branches and subdivisions into the thigh, lower leg, and foot. All along its course, it is subject to irritation or compression.

True sciatica—that is, *sciatic neuritis*, or inflammation of the sciatic nerve—is comparatively rare. It may be caused by lead poisoning or alcoholism. Sciatic pain accompanies a variety of conditions.

The sciatic nerve sometimes experiences the pain of other nerves. Such an action is called a *referred pain*. In referred sciatic pain, there is no irritation of the nerve roots of the sciatic nerve; the pain centers in the back report to pain centers in the spinal cord which, by a relay system, report the pain in the form of sciatic pain. For instance, the patient submits to the doctor's probing finger on his back until the finger presses on a "trigger point"; then the patient reacts with pain. A trigger point, under pressure, reproduces the local or radiating pain. The trigger points of tenderness in the lower back aid in distinguishing the source of the pain and its distribution. The muscles and ligaments involved most often are those that span the vertebral spines, bind the vertebrae together, and form the muscular supporting structures of the lower back. The muscles receive their innervation from nerves that have no immediate connection with the sciatic nerve, and the "sciatic pain" is referred in nature.

Through the exchange along nerve pathways, diseases and disorders within the abdominal cavity can cause sciatic pain by referral—that is, the pain is referred to another body area than that which, in reality, causes the pain. Among these conditions are colitis, ulcer, cancer, adhesions, hernia, chronic constipation, sagging of the abdominal organs (*ptosis*), prostatitis, relaxation of supporting pelvic structures after childbirth, and certain diseases of the anus, rectum, and sigmoid colon. The genitourinary system is a frequent source of low back pain by referral over nerve pathways. In the male, prostatic infection ranks high as a cause; cancer of the prostate may produce pain in the back, hips, and legs. In the female, the old diagnosis of "tipped or fallen uterus" has been outmoded by better knowledge. In women who have borne children, referred low back pain is more likely to be caused by relaxed supporting structures within the pelvis; but an increase in the curve of the lower spine (*lordosis* or sway-back) occurs frequently, and causes backache. Sway-back in either sex, associated with a heavy pendulous abdomen which places a drag on the muscles and ligaments of the back, is a common source of pain.

The largest of the nerve roots of the sciatic nerve is the fifth lumbar nerve root. Conversely, the smallest of the openings at its exit from the spine is that of the fifth lumbar. At its source, therefore, this nerve is subject to being squeezed as it passes through its small opening; also, it may be affected by twists or compression if bony abnormalities exist, by stretching, and by inflammation from neighboring disease. Clinical evidence points to the lumbosacral junction and the fifth lumbar nerve, as being the areas most frequently implicated in sciatic pain.

Having passed this first hazard, the sciatic nerve passes over the *ischial spine* of the pelvis, where it again is subject to pressure upon the bone, from overlying muscles. It then courses downward, over the hip, and down the back of the thigh, between a number of heavy muscle groups.

Characteristically, sciatic pain is felt at the back of the thigh, somewhat toward the outside of the leg. The pain distribution follows the distribution of the nerve and its branches to muscles of the thigh and lower leg.

There may be aching, soreness, or pain, all of which movement may aggravate. Or there may be numbness, tingling, or other abnormal sensations of the skin surface. Sneezing, coughing, and straining may intensify sciatic pain. Sciatic symptoms are intensified before a storm.

Sciatic patients are more comfortable in warm climates than in cold and in dry weather rather than damp; and if they must live in a cold climate, they are more comfortable in northern sections with "dry" cold than in northeastern sections where cold, moist winds prevail.

Fifth lumbar vertebra

The *sacrum*—which is a bone formed from the fusing of the sacral vertebrae—and *pelvis* are the rigid structures upon which is imposed the flexible spine. The fifth lumbar vertebra is the shock absorber of the spine. The transverse processes of this vertebra should be thick and short, and their positions are such as to afford ligamentous anchorage upon the sacrum. Imperfections of function based on anatomic abnormalities are responsible for many of the symptoms from this area. Sometimes the only means of giving relief is by operation which permanently stiffens the unstable joint.

Lumbosacral syndrome

The small opening through which the fifth lumbar nerve must pass has been mentioned as a cause of sciatic pain. The junction of the fifth lumbar vertebra with the sacrum (the *lumbosacral area*) also is a site of low back pain. Nerves from the sacral openings may be compressed in the *intervertebral canal*, located vertically in the center of the vertebrae. Symptoms are referred along the distribution of these nerves as far as the upper and lower surfaces of the foot, the great toe, and the heel.

Men engaged in heavy physical labor while in bent-over or twisted positions, and especially those exposed to damp weather, are the most frequent victims of backache of lumbosacral origin. A sharp attack of "lumbago" may stretch into a period of chronic sciatic pain. Muscle spasm may hold the lumbosacral region rigid. The victim can bend from the hips, lumbar, and thoracic regions, but forward bending from the lumbosacral joint is limited by pain. Sometimes a protective lateral curvature of the spine is assumed by the patient for relief. Duration of these attacks may be long, and they are aggravated by faulty posture, repeated traumatic incidents, inclement weather, infections, or metabolic disorders. The pain is intensified by coughing, sneezing, movement, or certain positions. Arthritis may be superimposed on a chronic lumbosacral syndrome.

Slipped vertebra (spondylolisthesis)

Spondylolisthesis is an exaggerated lumbar curve (sway-back), with the fifth lumbar vertebra being the focal point which robs the lower spine of stability because of its extreme forward position. Defective ossification of the *neural arch*, located at the back of the vertebra, is the fundamental defect; cartilage and fibrous tissue form an inadequate substitute for normal bone as a supporting structure at this point of strain. The softer, more flexible tissue establishes a discontinuity between the vertebral body and the arch. This abnormality has been found in ten percent of the skeletons examined. Mechanically, the body of the fifth lumbar vertebra slips forward toward the front of the body until it is warped over the sacrum; strain is thus placed upon the weakest link—the fibrous tissue in the neural arch, instead of normal bone.

The backache from slipped vertebra disappears during rest and reappears on exertion. The pain is referred down the thigh and leg.

Intervertebral disc syndrome

Low back pain may be caused by injury to the *intervertebral discs*, which are the pads of cartilage between the vertebrae. Protrusion of the disc is directly related to the *nucleus pulposus*, which is the central portion of the disc and gives "bounce" to the flexible spinal column. Like the bubble in a spirit level or a freewheeling ball bearing, the nucleus pulposus accommodates itself to the force of gravity by shifting its position with the position of the spine. When the spine is bent in forward position, the nucleus pulposus moves to the back; in backward position, it rides forward. In lateral flexion, it shifts to the opposite side. If there is severe compression of the nucleus pulposus between the cartilaginous disc plates, it may be forced out of its bed, and portions of the cartilage of the disc may go with it. Such compression is exerted by falls, jumps, or straining efforts in the bent-over position. Lifting, bending, twisting, or slipping often precipitate repeated attacks of pain.

The discs most frequently extruded are those between the fourth and fifth lumbar vertebrae and the fifth lumbar and sacrum. If it is the fifth lumbar disc that is extruded, pain of sciatic type and distribution is caused. If the third or fourth lumbar discs are extruded, the pain distribution is down the inner front surface of the thigh.

A complex of symptoms—low back pain, sciatic pain intensified by sneezing or coughing, and intermittency of attacks—is typical of disc protrusion.

The pain can usually be trigger-pointed. Sciatic pain down one side occurs in about 80 percent of the patients, down both sides in 16 percent, and is not typical in the remainder. Numbness or tingling in the outer border of the leg and foot is present in 65 percent of patients. In the supine position, most skeletal muscles of the back normally are relaxed, and leg-raising from the horizontal puts the stretch on the sciatic nerve. If compression is present, this maneuver causes pain.

A protruded disc may complicate a case of slipped vertebra. The intervertebral disc is subject also to degenerative changes like those taking place in other bones and cartilages. It may be destroyed or fractured in compression injuries or by falls. In either, the disc space is destroyed, bringing the vertebral surfaces closer together; symptoms of nerve pressure and functional disabilities result.

Calcification of the entire disc or the nucleus pulposus may occur, or it may be destroyed by tuberculosis of the spine. Cancer rarely attacks the disc.

Sacroiliac syndrome

The *sacroiliac* is a true joint. Shaped like a narrow slit, it is formed by the sacrum and ilium on each side. It is capable only of slight motion. The joint is enmeshed by strong ligaments which extend to the spinous processes of the sacrum and portions of the pelvis. The fibers of the joint capsule are interwoven with the sacroiliac ligaments, making for greater strength. The *sacral plexus* of nerves lies directly on the bone of the sacrum, unprotected by muscular padding.

The oblique slits of the sacroiliac joints form the slanting sides upon which the sacrum wedges like a keystone. Great thrusting and leverage forces are brought to bear upon the sacroiliac joints, and the strength of the ligaments supports them. The legs and pelvis push upward against the keystone junction from below. The trunk and spinal column push downward from above, adding leverage demands by turns, twists, and pulls.

Most of the pain from sacroiliac joints is caused by injury. These injuries consist of twists, sprains, and strains. Anything that requires twisting to one side, forward, and downward, while leverage is exerted through the hamstring muscles of the opposite side, may cause sacroiliac injury. Shoveling snow is a common cause of sacroiliac strain, especially in people unaccustomed to such work. Attempting to raise a "stuck" window almost equals snow-shoveling as a cause. Raising the corner of a desk while trying to shove under a corner of a rug is another force that may result in sacroiliac strain. Housewives twisting downward to dust baseboards or wipe windows so injure themselves; men standing with legs astraddle and lifting heavy objects from one side to the other, or even playing with a child while in this position, sustain the injury in the same way. In fact, the list of movements that can evoke sacroiliac strain can be extended almost infinitely.

Painful spots can be trigger-pointed on the back. Pain is distributed from the *sacrosciatic notch (superior gluteal nerve)*, down the back of the thigh and outer border of the thigh and leg. In some patients, it is focused on the hip and lower back.

Motion of the lower back is limited, and stiffness is constant. The victim sits on the buttock opposite the strained sacroiliac, walks upstairs one step at a time, dragging the painful leg from step to step, and limps because he cannot bear weight on the affected side. In bed, it is difficult to find a comfortable position, and usually the victim lies on the unaffected side. Sometimes, tucking a pillow or cushion under the affected sacroiliac brings some comfort in bed.

The sacroiliac joints are subject also to arthritis, infection, inflammation, tuberculosis, and osteomyelitis.

Many investigators believe that the lumbosacral joint, rather than the sacroiliac joint is responsible for many of the so-called sacroiliac complaints.

Other low back conditions

Strain of the *iliolumbar ligaments*, located in the small triangle formed by the midline of the lower spine and the rear portion of the *iliac crest*, is caused by the same forces that cause sacroiliac strain. One of these ligaments, the *ligamentum flavum*, may become enlarged and impinge upon the nerve roots in the vertebral canal, causing sciatic pain.

Lumbago, *myositis*, and *fibrositis* are conditions popularly called "muscular rheumatism," all of which produce backache. Sudden pain in the back or in another involved muscle group is the first symptom. The causes of this group of conditions remain completely unknown.

The "locked back" syndrome implies an attack of violent pain, usually occurring in middle-aged men who have been overworked mentally and physically. The attack of back pain is so severe that hospitalization may be necessary.

Treatment

Treatment of patients with low back pain is either conservative or surgical. Nonsurgical measures are preferred, and are successful in 90 percent of cases; but when they fail, surgical intervention becomes necessary. Practically all of these patients need some type of posture training and proper exercise; some need bed rest, and others need supports of some kind.

Early treatment is of utmost importance, and the patient should seek the help of a physician when the pain is first noted. Procrastination can cause the establishment of a chronic condition with possible repercussions in the form of arthritis. Chronic back conditions are extremely difficult to manage successfully. They can be prevented easier than they can be cured.

Nonsurgical measures include rest; protection of the injured part; physical therapy with heat, baths, diathermy, radiant light, or ultrasound; supports of adhesive strapping; local injections of anesthetic drugs; relaxing drugs, by mouth; and traction, splints, belts, braces, corsets, and other mechanical aids. The careful use of active exercises as prescribed by a physician is frequently helpful. Efforts are made to improve the patient's general physical condition. Some measures can be carried out at home under the physician's instructions. Very often the patient is placed in a hospital for prompt and efficient treatment, which in many cases reduces the period of inactivity considerably.

Orthopedic surgeons always keep in mind the rule that for these patients physical and psychological rest must be obtained where "fatigue is the warning, pain the monitor, infection the punishment, and rest the cure." Surgery to remove the herniation of the disk and possible fixation of the lumbar spine is dependent on the history and findings of the individual patient.

DISORDERS OF THE SKELETON AND MUSCLES: BONE INFLAMMATION

Infection and inflammation of the bones or joints may be acute or chronic. Acute infection of a joint in which pus is produced is called acute *pyogenic arthritis*; of bone, acute *pyogenic osteomyelitis*. The word pyogenic refers to pus.

Infection reaches these structures by way of the blood stream, although joints may be invaded by disease-producing organisms from a nearby infection. Infection may be acquired from open wounds, especially battle wounds in which bones become inoculated with disease-producing bacteria.

The most common organisms found in acute pyogenic arthritis are staphylococci, which occur in 90 percent of the cases. The local infection in the bone or joint and the body's attempt to combat it cause swelling and pain. Sometimes the joint capsule ruptures spontaneously.

In bone, infection takes place when clumps of disease-producing organisms are deposited by the blood from a nutrient artery. The marrow portion (*metaphysis*) of long bones and the outer membrane (*periosteum*) are often involved, because these structures are so abundantly supplied with blood vessels of small size. At the spot where the virulent bacteria are deposited, they destroy a minute piece of the bone. The bone, in turn, is defended by the arrival of large numbers of red and white blood cells. The white blood cells perform their customary function of destroying the invading bacteria. If they succeed, the bone heals. If they fail, the bacteria continue to multiply, causing more destruction and forming large amounts of pus. The pus is channeled along the bone canals and reaches the bone surface, where it spreads between the periosteum and the bone. This causes intense pain, which is relieved as soon as the periosteum ruptures or is incised and drained.

Chronic osteomyelitis

The organisms of tuberculosis, actinomycosis, as well as parasites and disease-producing yeasts may cause chronic bone infection (*osteomyelitis*). The response of the bone is related to the type of organism which has invaded it, the defensive ability of the invaded tissue, and the constitutional ability to repair damage. The common reaction is for the bone to become active in laying down membranous tissue; however, the formation of the new bone is haphazard, and it is not laid down in the normal lines of stress. This is known as *involucrum* formation. If the infection is controlled and the dead tissues are absorbed or eliminated, the involucrum is replaced gradually by normal bone, laid down in the lines of functional stress.

When a piece of bone dies and loses continuity with its parent bone, it is called a *sequestrum*. Small sequestra created by osteomyelitis may be absorbed by the healthy bone or eliminated by the blood stream. Sequestra may degenerate into small pieces which escape from the area through sinus tracts, but a large sequestrum may be trapped and require surgical removal. The total process of elimination may take months or years.

The spinal column and sacroiliac joints are also subject to these infections. Destruction of the spongy portion of the vertebral bodies causes their collapse, thereby destroying the upright integrity of the spine and resulting in the deformity known as "humpback" (*kyphosis*). The most common cause of this deformity is tuberculosis.

Despite new drugs that fight infection, surgery remains the ultimate resource for the removal of dead bone and correction of deformities.

Osteitis fibrosa

In the disease, *osteitis fibrosa*, x-ray photographs reveal scattered areas that appear as cysts in the bones, but they are filled with fibrous tissue and a network of poorly calcified fibrous bone. The cause of this condition is not known, but it has been suggested that there is an upset of the bonemaking activity. It appears during childhood, and is associated with pigmentation on the skin. Pathologic fractures may occur.

In *generalized* osteitis fibrosa (*parathyroid osteodystrophy*), all bones are involved. The cause of this condition is an overfunction of the *parathyroid* glands or a functioning tumor of the glands. As the disease progresses, bone is resorbed and is replaced by overgrowths of fibrous tissue, fluid, gelatinous or fibrous masses, or material resembling the structure of "giant cell" tumors. There is a rapid loss of calcium, and grotesque physical deformities are conspicuous—"humpback," bending of the long bones, or telescoping with resultant shortening of the bones. The withdrawal of calcium from the bones causes a higher calcium level in the circulating blood. This, in turn, causes weakness, muscular fatigue, constipation, vomiting, abdominal pain, formation of urinary calculi, and excessive urination. The severity of the symptoms is correlated with the amount of parathyroid hormone secreted.

Unless the patient is treated, the disease may be fatal within a few years; but if a parathyroid tumor is present and is removed before much damage has been sustained, recovery can be expected. Bone abnormalities are permanent. See Chapter 10, "The Endocrine System: *The Parathyroids*."

Paget's disease (osteitis deformans)

This progressive disease begins in the spongy bone marrow and spreads thence to other portions in a process of bone destruction and bone formation which gives the bones a mottled appearance in x-ray pictures. New bone is not laid down in the normal lines of stress. Long bones become greatly thickened, sometimes twice their normal size. The skull enlarges. Sacrum, skull, pelvis, and the lower extremities are most extensively involved.

The cause is unknown. The disease occurs after 40 years of age and predominates in the sixth decade. If pain is present, it usually is over the long bones of the legs, or the spine; if in the skull, it takes the form of headache. Recent reports suggest the experimental drug, mithramycin, can suppress the activity of Paget's disease. However, porcine or salmon thyrocalcitonin may prove more effective and safer.

The disease is not fatal, but the patient often succumbs to complications such as spontaneous fractures, secondary anemia, circulatory disturbances, or bone sarcoma.

Osteochondritis dissecans

This disorder results when areas of bone and cartilage separate from the articular surface, because of trauma or blockage of circulation to the area. The ends of the femur or the lower end of the humerus are most commonly affected. It is seen most often in adolescents. Usual symptoms are mild pain and stiffness; often it is detected while the patient is being examined for some other complaint. Since the lesion usually does not heal, treatment consists of surgical removal of the affected area. Otherwise the detached material will remain as a source of chronic pain and irritation. Results of treatment are usually excellent.

Another form of osteochondritis, known as Legg-Calvé-Perthes disease or osteochrondritis of the hip, in which the head of the femur is involved, occurs most commonly in children between the ages of three and ten. This disorder, which probably results from interference with the blood supply, causes a degeneration and eventual replacement of the bony tissues of the capital epiphysis of the femur. The disease runs its course in from two to six years. Usually, the earlier the onset the more severe the disease will be, and greater residual damage will result. The aim of treatment is to protect from pressure of weight bearing and preserve the normal contour of the femoral head. Surgical treatment in some patients is required to partially correct the residual deformities after complete replacement of the bony tissues.

Rheumatoid spondylitis

A disease which affects young males in particular. It is also known as Marie-Strumpell disease. In this form of spondylitis, inflammation of the sacroiliac, intervertebral and costo-vertebral joints produce pain and stiffness. Complete rigidity of the spine and thorax may result from paraspinal calcification, with ossification and ankylosis of the spinal joints. The cause of this systemic illness is unknown.

Letterer-Siwe disease

This disease is largely limited to young children under three years of age with occasional cases occurring in young adults. This blood disease of unknown cause is marked by a proliferation of histiocytes in body organs. Resulting skeletal lesions cause localized areas of bone destruction. This disease is usually fatal. Similar though milder diseases are Schuller-Christian disease and eosinophilic granuloma.

DISORDERS OF THE SKELETON AND MUSCLES: BONE CANCER

Cancer which originates in bone tissue is called *sarcoma*. Bones are also invaded by malignant tumors (usually of the *carcinoma* type) which tian disease and eosinophilic granuloma.

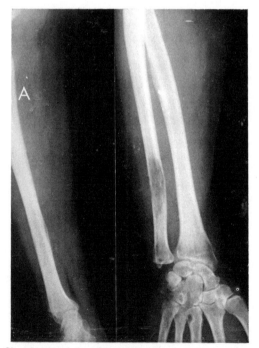

Chondroma of the ulna appears as a dark area on an x-ray film. Symptoms include recurrent, usually mild, soreness in an affected bone. Copyright 1965 Year Book Medical Publishers, Inc., courtesy M. M. Copeland, The University of Texas M. D. Anderson Hospital, Houston.

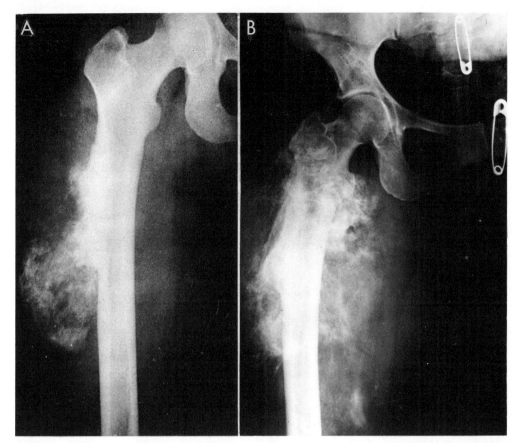

X-ray films of a bone tumor of the upper femur. The tumor tissue appears as a diffuse white area around the bone. The patient had noted soreness and swelling of the upper thigh. Copyright 1965 Year Book Medical Publishers, Inc., courtesy M. M. Copeland, The University of Texas M. D. Anderson Hospital, Houston.

breast, lung, prostate, kidney, or thyroid. Cancers which have spread from one organ to another are said to be *metastatic*.

As with all forms of cancer, the cause of primary bone cancer is unknown. Some believe that injury to the bone is a precipitating factor, but there is little chance that this is true.

The most common types of primary bone cancers are osteosarcomas, Ewing's sarcomas, reticulum cell sarcomas, myelomas, and giant cell tumors.

Osteosarcomas most often affect persons in the age group from 10 to 25, males more often than females. This sarcoma shows a preference for the femur, tibia, and humerus. Osteosarcomas tend to spread to the lungs at an early stage. For this reason, it is often impossible to control even early tumors of this type.

Perhaps two thirds of the persons who develop Ewing's sarcoma are under 20 years of age. These tumors commonly affect the trunk bones or the long limb bones.

Reticulum cell sarcoma, which is malignant

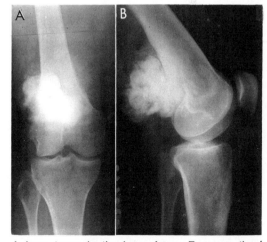

A bone tumor in the lower femur. Tumorous tissue appears as a diffuse white area around the bone. Copyright 1965 Year Book Medical Publishers, Inc., courtesy M. M. Copeland, The University of Texas M. D. Anderson Hospital, Houston.

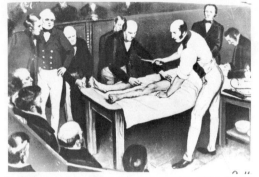

Dr. Robert Liston performing an operation while Joseph Lister, extreme left, looks on. Liston introduced ether anesthesia in Europe; Lister founded antiseptic surgery. *Bettmann Archive.*

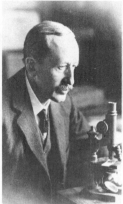

EWING, James (1866-1943) American pathologist. He was one of the foremost authorities on tumors, and was widely acclaimed for his evaluation of different varieties, in a masterly work published in 1919. He described a form of bone sarcoma involving the shaft of the long bones, characterized by cells of endothelial type, and seen most frequently before the twentieth year; to this type of tumor Ewing's name has been applied.

lymphoma in bones, tends to spread to regional lymph nodes. This cancer type, which seems more common in males, is least common in patients under 20.

Myelomas may ultimately involve many bones of the body, although they may be confined to one bone for long periods. They are seen most often in the 40 to 60 age group, and more often in males than in females.

The nature of the giant cell tumors is often very puzzling. Sometimes even microscopic studies of cells from these tumors do not indicate with certainty whether they are benign or malignant. Various grades of giant cell tumors are identifiable. Many of these tumors tend to recur after they are surgically removed. They have a higher incidence among the 20 to 40 age group, and may be found in females more often than in males.

The cells of bone sarcoma are spread in the body by way of the blood stream; the most frequent place for secondary deposits is the lungs, from which the malignant cells are again distributed to the brain or abdominal organs. Before the disease has spread, proper treatment may effect a cure in some patients with bone cancer. However, after the disease has spread, cure is rarely possibly.

The bones most frequently invaded by tumors from other organs are the vertebrae, pelvis, femur, ribs, sternum, humerus, and skull. For patients with this form of the disease, therapy is designed to relieve pain and prolong life.

Pain is the first symptom of bone cancer. The onset may be insidious, the early symptoms suggesting a mild arthritis or neuritis. Fairly early in the disease, a hard, painful lump may be noted over which the skin moves freely. The temperature of the skin over the lump may be elevated slightly. As the disease progresses, the pain becomes continual and boring in character; it is aggravated by weight bearing or motion of nearby joints. The pain reaches its peak during the night. The pain in Ewing's

sarcoma in children is moderate in early stages, coming and going and sometimes stopping altogether for a period, then returning. Moderate fever is present early, later rising to 103° or 104°; there may be an accompanying anemia and a high white cell count.

Diagnosis of bone cancer is suggested by x-ray films. Final confirmation of diagnosis is made by studying a small piece of the tumor under a microscope.

Treatment

Amputation, carried out well above the level of the growth, is the preferred treatment in most cases in which the tumor is in the long bones. If present in less accessible areas—pelvis or skull—wide excision must be done. Irradiation therapy is generally preferred in the management of Ewing's sarcomas, reticulum cell sarcomas, and giant cell tumors. In some cases of reticulum cell sarcoma, radical surgical procedures are used if there is no apparent spread of disease and if the involved bone is accessible. If so, the regional lymph nodes may also be irradiated to prevent tumor spread. Some surgeons recommend irradiation of primary osteogenic sarcomas before an operation. X-ray therapy is also used to relieve pain of metastatic bone cancer. In certain cases, hormone therapy may have temporary benefits.

Benign tumors

Rarely, tumors which are not cancerous originate in bone tissue. The most common type is the osteochondromas. Occasionally, these tumors become malignant.

Symptoms of these tumors may resemble those of bone cancer. Careful diagnostic tests are necessary to distinguish between them.

Surgical and nonsurgical procedures may be required. If the tumors are of the type that may become cancerous, periodic x-ray examinations will detect any such alteration.

DISORDERS OF THE SKELETON AND MUSCLES: SCOLIOSIS

Scoliosis, or curvature of the spine, may range in symptoms from mild postural asymmetry to the pronounced "hunch-back" or "razor back." Postural scoliosis can be corrected by voluntary muscular effort. However, more serious and debilitating curvature may be caused by improper muscle action along the spine when the individual has no control. In a few cases, this condition can be traced to paralytic disease, but most commonly, no cause is known and it is therefore termed *idiopathic* scoliosis.

The bones of the spine and the ribs show no evidence of malformation on x-ray films. Rather, the vertebrae are displaced to form a curved line along one region of the spinal column. When two regions are affected, an S-shaped curvature results. The "razor back" deformity is caused by accompanying rotation of the spinal column in such a way that the rib cage is also rotated.

Infantile idiopathic scoliosis occurs in both sexes with about equal frequency. The curvature is most often to the left and in the thoracic region. The condition will often progress from the time of its discovery, usually within the first year of life, to a severe deformity. In rare cases, the condition has been known to correct itself without treatment, but only during infancy.

Adolescent idiopathic scoliosis is more common than the infantile form. This condition is most often noticed around the age of eleven or twelve. Females are affected about nine times more frequently than males. Early symptoms may be asymmetry of the hips or unevenness of the shoulders. This asymmetry, and any visible curvature, will not disappear when the individual stands on one leg or sits, as with simple postural laxness.

It is difficult for the physician to predict the ultimate stage to which scoliosis will advance. In general, however, it can be said that the earlier the age of onset, the more severe the deformity is likely to be. The deformity will no longer increase after the growth of the spine is complete, around the age of fifteen for girls and seventeen for boys.

Various means are possible in the treatment of scoliosis. The simplest involves remedial exercises, which may result in marked improvement. Special braces may be employed to prevent increase in deformity. Application of a turnbuckle cast, followed by fusion of the vertebrae, may bring about a true correction of the condition. In a recent surgical innovation, the curved spine is first straightened, then stabilized in the corrected position by metal rods fastened to the spine with metal hooks.

DISORDERS OF THE SKELETON AND MUSCLES: MUSCULAR DYSTROPHY

Muscular dystrophy is actually a group of hereditary diseases in which muscle fibers undergo progressive damage and eventual destruction. Of the eight variants of dystrophy which are known, the two most common are the Duchenne types, named for the French neurologist who first described them in 1858. The less serious Duchenne dystrophy often affects adults. The aggressive form is the most serious and the most commonly known form of muscular dystrophy. Occurring almost exclusively in males, the disease becomes evident usually within the first five years of life. Symptoms may include frequent falls, difficulty in rising from the floor and in climbing stairs, and enlargement of the calf muscles. Manual muscle tests, blood tests to measure the levels of certain enzymes, and muscle biopsy are used in diagnosing this disorder.

In early stages of this type of dystrophy, high levels of certain enzymes are almost always found in the blood. Creatine phosphokinase (CPK) is the enzyme which indicates both the active disease and carriers of the disease. Sisters of patients with known Duchenne muscular dystrophy or mothers of one child with the disease often also have high levels of CPK in their blood. Such women, with no clinical evidence of the disease, are carriers of this dystrophy. Half of the carrier's sons will have the disease and half of her daughters will also be carriers. Known carriers, at least two thirds of whom can be detected by measuring the level of CPK in their blood, should be advised not to have children. The incidence of this disease could be decreased if such genetic counseling is followed.

No specific treatment is yet available for muscular dystrophy patients. However, early diagnosis, a careful program of physical therapy, and braces can extend independent ambulation for several years. The family should be aware of the slowly progressive nature of the disease and of the patient's total needs. Parents can be trained to assist in physical therapy designed to maintain maximal, symmetrical muscular strength and to delay functional deterioration. Also, weight gain and physical inactivity must be avoided. When the patient can no longer walk without assistance, long leg braces may be used for periods of up to two years.

Although mild to moderate mental retardation usually occurs in this disease, there is no progressive mental deterioration. Also, these children often become depressed and uncommunicative. A normal school environment is important as long as possible to prevent social isolation.

AMPUTATIONS AND ARTIFICIAL REPLACEMENTS

Writers of antiquity described artificial limbs (*prostheses*), and the written records have been substantiated by the actual finding of these appliances. The Royal College of Surgeons in London has on display an artificial lower leg consisting of metal plates surrounding a wooden core; it is estimated to date to 300 B.C. Probably the most famous artificial limb was the metal hand with jointed fingers made for a warrior, Götz von Berlichingen, in the sixteenth century. The structural features of the hand testify to the craftsmanship of the time.

Loss of limbs reached enormous proportions during the Middle Ages. Not only had the invention and use of cannon shot added to the brutality of war, but the civilian population lost limbs to the official axman, because amputation had become the accepted form of judicial punishment. In addition, widespread diseases such as leprosy accounted for further losses.

Surgeons have followed in the wake of warmakers to remake the bodies that battle marred. Improvements in surgical techniques often have been born as the aftermath of war. In the matter of amputations, surgeons have learned to prepare a stump that will not only bear weight but will also salvage the functional capacities of remaining muscles and put them to use in the manipulation of the artificial replacement. The limb maker, on his part, has become adept in the fitting of limbs to the individual's particular requirement, as well as making the limbs of maximum usefulness.

War veterans are not, however, the only customers for artificial limbs. The limbs lost in peace-time exceed the number lost in warfare. Each year there are about 75,000 amputations in the civilian population and of these 40,000 are of sufficient magnitude to require artificial replacement. At least half of these amputations are made necessary by accidents, with disease and congenital defect or other causes accounting for the remainder. About one million amputees, including women and children, are in the United States today.

Rejoined limbs

Initial enthusiasm has given way to guarded optimism concerning the replantation of completely severed limbs. On May 23, 1962, the completely severed right arm of a 12-year-old boy was successfully rejoined by a surgical team at the Massachusetts General Hospital. One year later, the boy had some sensation in the fingers, but faced many additional months of therapy.

Step by step in this complicated process, the surgeon rejoins the bone; restores circulation through the veins, arteries, and lymph vessels, at least partially repairs the nerves, and finally, repairs the soft tissue. Problems can occur with any of these steps. Also, the time of disability is longer than when amputation is followed by fitting with a prosthesis. A series of rehabilitative operations are necessary. Since nerve damage may be more severe than initially recognized, unsatisfactory function and sensation may be obtained. It is now generally agreed that replantation should be considered only for patients who would benefit more from having their own limb, even if its function is impaired, than from a prosthesis. Ideal candidates would be patients under 30 with a cleanly severed limb.

The stump

Surgeon and limb maker co-operate in solving the amputee's problem. The surgeon prepares a stump, which is suitable for a prosthesis, to retain muscular function and a good weight-bearing end. The limb maker undertakes the proper fitting, shaping, and alignment of the artificial limb so that it will be functionally adequate for the amputee's needs. At times, reamputation at a later date may become necessary, especially when the first amputation was done under conditions of emergency. At the second operation, the functional aspects receive the consideration they deserve. The length of the stump is governed by a number of factors, not the least being the amputee's occupation, and his ability and willingness to learn to use the artificial limb to best advantage. As a rule, amputation through a joint is less satisfactory from a functional point of view than through the long bones at prescribed levels.

Complications

Leg stumps sometimes are subject to complications. A period of tenderness is to be expected until the tissues have become adapted to pressure and friction. But at times, tenderness persists for a period longer than normal. This may be caused by low-grade infection with congestion and swelling. A blood clot may become infected, or the cut nerves may be the site of pain. Circulation of the blood may be impaired with swelling, coldness, and pain as a result. The scar, too, may be a source of pain when it adheres to underlying soft tissue, causing drag on nerves, or a pull on muscles attached to the scar. A sac (*bursa*) may form where there is pressure or irritation over a bony point,

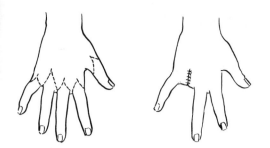

Method for the amputation of a finger, illustrating on the left the lines of incision which would be made, and on the right the sutured wound.

but it disappears when the artificial limb has been readjusted to proper fit.

The development of skin disorders in a stump is common, and is caused by a combination of uncleanliness and a poorly fitting artificial limb. Among such conditions are infected hair follicles, boils, skin eruptions, and maceration.

As a rule, the phenomenon of experiencing sensation within a limb that has been amputated (*phantom limb*) disappears within a reasonable time. In psychically predisposed individuals, however, the sensations persist as an illusion or psychic projection. This condition is little understood and difficult to manage.

Stump hygiene

Knitted stump socks should be changed daily, washed with mild soaps, rinsed thoroughly, and hung out to dry with the open end down. When the artificial limb is not being used, the stump should be unclothed, and, if possible, exposed to fresh air and sunshine. Daily bathing of the stump is of the greatest importance; particular attention should be given to skin folds where maceration otherwise will develop. Nonirritating soaps and washcloths should be employed. Daily care improves skin tone. Nonmedicated talcum powder should precede the drawing on of the stump sock.

Materials in artificial replacements

Wood, especially that from a willow tree, possesses the advantages of lightness, firmness, resiliency, and permanent form, once it has been shaped. Consequently, it is most often used in artificial limbs. In a wood socket, the stump can be protected against pressure. The wood socket can be treated so that it is perspiration proof and free from friction. It can be thin, hence light in weight. Wood can be cut, sawed, carved, glued, and doweled. Its size can be adjusted to accommodate shrinkage of the stump, or quickly lengthened for growing chil-

dren without loss of strength or durability. It can be shaped to suitable form for women. The thin parchment rawhide with which wooden limbs are covered adds strength and the ability to withstand hard usage.

Aluminum or duralumin is used for replacements where lightness is of particular importance. Hence, it is employed for the debilitated and the aged amputee, and for some individuals with thigh amputations. The fitting and functional alignment of metal limbs are somewhat more difficult than for those made of wood.

In recent years, research has developed extensive use of plastics in the manufacture of prostheses especially for replacement of the upper extremity. Techniques have been developed to secure snug molds of the stump contours. With these sockets, inserts of sponge rubber provide a softer weight bearing surface, for below-the-knee amputees.

Research in the area of earlier fitting of prostheses has reached the stage of immediate postsurgical fitting. This has helped to preserve the whole body image for the patient psychologically and has prevented postsurgical swelling. The older patient has been able to be mobilized earlier and more rapidly postamputation, as he is able to maintain his balance better with the second leg while on crutches.

Webbing is used usually for control straps and belts, while leather is used mainly for foot coverings, high corsets, and molded sockets. Leather has the advantage of "breathing," contouring to the shape of the stump, and is of lightweight. It has disadvantages in that it is

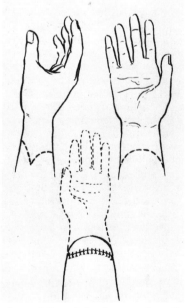

Method of amputation of the forearm above the wrist. Dotted lines show location and type of incision. Stump is closed by interrupted sutures.

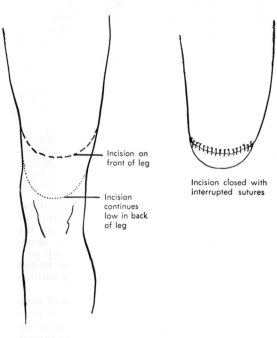

Method of amputation of a leg above the knee, showing line of incision around leg to provide closure flap, and closure with interrupted sutures.

unsanitary, does not resist perspiration, is hot and heavy, and stretches out of shape with long use unless heavily reinforced.

Legs

In an artificial lower limb, the most important portions are the socket, the ankle, and the knee. Fitting of the socket has a direct bearing upon the usefulness of the limb and the ability to walk with a normal gait. Experts believe that simple U-bolt joints are the best, for they afford stability and strength while permitting as much motion as the amputee will be likely to need or use. Some limb makers eliminate the ankle joint entirely, firmly affixing a vulcanized rubber foot directly to the skin. The fixed-axis knee joint has been found to be the most practical.

Good stability of the knee is established by aligning the center of gravity in the artificial limb in a plane slightly behind that in the natural leg. Given a reasonable length of stump, and strength in the muscles of stump and hip, walking with a more natural gait becomes possible without mechanical aids and controls. In the final analysis, the manner in which an amputee walks on an artificial leg depends upon his willingness and ability to learn to do so, granted that the alignment has been good. Learning to use the muscles of thigh and hip to move the leg makes the difference between a natural gait or walking with dependence upon control straps,

locks, and other mechanical means. Some persons never use such aids and even accomplish the difficult feat of walking up and down stairs. Often physiotherapy is helpful in strengthening the muscles of the stump. An understanding of the physiologic mechanics of walking—a constant falling forward with constant self-recovery —helps in learning to walk on one or two artificial legs.

Immediate postoperative prostheses

In 1963, Dr. Marian Weiss of Poland startled surgeons with his report of fitting patients with temporary plaster and metal prostheses immediately after below-the-knee amputations. Until recently, pain and discomfort associated with lower extremity prostheses made several months necessary for healing before such devices were fitted. As a result of research and clinical testing, over 700 patients in the United States had had some type of immediate postsurgical fitting routine by June of 1967.

The physical and psychological benefits of this routine are significant. The rigid plaster dressing which is used provides physiological protection of the wound and minimizes swelling in the stump. Usually on the day after the amputation, the patient is permitted to stand and exercises are begun early. This uninterrupted activity decreases the incidence of complications such as pulmonary embolisms. Also, these patients have less pain and muscle atrophy than other amputees.

High morale results from the shorter hospital stay, the lower total cost of rehabilitation, and the shortened period of inactivity. Most patients whose stumps heal properly can be fitted with a definitive socket and prosthesis within 25 to 35 days after the amputation.

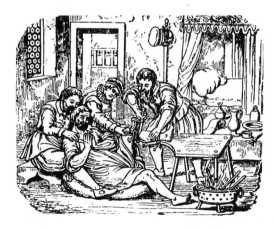

Old engraving depicting an early technique for amputation of a leg. Cauteries to stop the blood flow are heated in the stove. *Bettmann Archive.*

Arms

Upper limb replacements have been greatly improved cosmetically and functionally in recent years so that they are being used much more extensively by the patients than in the past. However, replacements are cumbersome, awkward, and offer too little benefit to bother with much of the time. Legs are needed for getting about, but a hand is used to perform a myriad of intricate combinations of motion and function. No mechanical hand could possibly do what a normal hand does. This discovery proves to be frustrating to amputees until they realize that full range of motion is not needed, and that a few necessary motions that can be well-performed serve them adequately. The selection of the particular arm replacement for the particular needs of the amputee requires good judgment. The amputee needs a tool that will help him do his particular work as well as to help himself. A banker can get along with a dress arm since he uses his hands relatively little. But the worker in a steel mill needs a tool that will help him lift and hold heavy weights. Between these extremes ranges a wide assortment of occupations which require less or more hand action. The old "pirate's hook" has been replaced by functional hooks designed with particular occupations in mind. While at first sight the hook may offend the amputee, this feeling can become submerged in the pride of accomplishment when he discovers how much he can do for himself. Amputees are capable of feeding, dressing, and otherwise helping themselves with a single hand; with a functional artificial replacement, they may continue in their former occupations or others equally productive.

The voluntary-muscle-control hand is closed by control from the opposite shoulder. The springtension hand is held closed by a strong spring within the hand, the fingers and thumb are forced apart by a pull from the opposite shoulder. Hands are also fitted with locking devices in closed positions. With a voluntary-control hand, a pencil can be used, a glass held lightly, a tie tied, or a heavy suitcase carried.

Utility appliances are available in wide variety from which a selection may be made for a particular need. These can be attached to the threaded wrist connection. With such a utility device, steelworkers can return to the job, carpenters resume their craft, using chisels, files, saws, and hammers, and farmers use devices fitted over shovel or pitchfork handles.

In actual practice, the utility hook has been found to be the most useful appliance, and amputees find that it meets their requirements. In fact, double arm amputees, equipped with such appliances, are engaged in almost every kind of occupation, including piloting airplanes, farming, mechanical engineering, and all kinds of industrial work.

In selected cases the *cineplastic* type of replacement is useful. In this type, the remaining arm muscles are put to work for extension and contraction by activating them with ivory pins to which the appliance is attached. This form of link is unsuited where strength is required, but is useful in sedentary occupations where skill and motion are needed.

Myo-electric arms

Minute electrical impulses from the brain move along nerves to activate the body's muscles. Using this familiar principle, Russian scientists developed a compact and sophisticated type of artificial arm. The unique myo-electric device they first described in 1960 is controlled by the greatly amplified electrical impulses of the patient's own nerves.

After amputation, forearm stump muscles continue to receive these impulses. As the amputee uses the muscles, this electronic prosthesis relays amplified signals to the artificial hand, which is then able to grasp and release as directed by the wearer's own nerves. Weighing less than three pounds, the device consists of a hand with a drive mechanism, an amplifier, a power supply unit, a current-tapping device, and a battery charger. Research and development on variations of this type of prosthesis are now under way in the United States.

Replacements in children

The fitting of artificial replacements to children has been taken out of the realm of emotionalism. The time is passing when a child, born without one or more limbs, or losing them through disease or accident, is condemned to a narrowed existence. Doctors urge the early amputation of malformed or diseased limbs and the fitting of artificial replacements. It has been

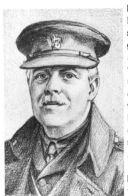

JONES, Robert (1858-1933). English orthopedic surgeon. Numbered among the outstanding orthopedic surgeons of World War I. His attempts to give back to the wounded the effective use of their bodies developed into pioneer work in tendon transplanting and bone grafting. Like other surgeons of his era, Jones made improvements on available aids to the surgeon, including a splint, named for him, and designed for fractures of the humerus.

demonstrated that children adjust themselves much more quickly and normally than adults to the use of artificial limbs; and for the sake of even, parallel growth and development, it is extremely important that a young child be equipped with artificial limbs and learn to use them as he grows. A natural leg, not used because of partial deformity or disease, becomes wasted and useless; whereas if amputated, and an artificial leg attached, normal development of muscles takes place in the stump. A child of eleven months, fitted with an artificial leg, learns to walk and run as well as a child with two normal legs, and muscle development in the hips and stump is not retarded. Children born with thighs missing (the leg below the knee articulating at the hip) can be fitted with two artificial limbs with or without amputation of the feet. The feet are retained wherever possible to allow the patient greater freedom at night or in emergencies. Children learn to use these replacements well, and when dressed maintain the normal appearance of their contemporaries.

Young people are sensitive to deformities and often welcome amputation and a replacement which enables them to walk with a normal gait and which does not engage the attention that a twisted and shortened limb does. There are many instances on record in which children have been fitted in early age with artificial limbs and have grown up normally to lead useful lives. A boy of 16, with amputation of both forearms and both legs below the knees, was equipped with replacements and utility hooks and has been able to support himself by driving a school bus and as a farm helper. A man who had been born without forearms or legs has reached middle age, using artificial legs but no devices on his forearms. He farms extensively, drives a car and tractor, rides horseback, walks up and down stairs, and since childhood has looked after his personal needs such as dressing and feeding himself. Extensive research is being directed to the patient with congenital bilateral hip disarticulation. Progress has been made so that with the patient sitting in a bucket-type socket, by alternately rocking the pelvis from side to side, he can throw the weight on the everted foot of that side; then, by a rotary motion of the pelvis, he can cause the opposite extremity to make a small forward step. Even this small step is very gratifying to the young patient. Further improvements are still being sought for these severe limb-deficient individuals to make them independent.

In children, adjustments in length are needed for every half inch of growth. Fitted at one year, new adjustments are needed between the ages of two and one-half and three years; the next adjustment is needed two or three years later; and thereafter an adjustment is needed not oftener than every three to five years until full growth is reached. The cost is small when weighed against the great benefits the child derives from the normal physical development it permits and from the psychologic effect of not being shut out from the companionship and activity of other children.

Factors in rehabilitation

Rehabilitation of the amputee is a fourfold problem: he must resume the routines of daily living; he must learn to care for his personal hygiene; he must acquire the ability to transport himself; and he must acquire the ability to make a living, whether in his former occupation or in a newly learned one.

The majority of amputees make rapid and satisfactory adjustments. They maintain a hopeful outlook, and make an eager and determined effort to learn to use their new limbs to best advantage. A small number, however, become more severely handicapped by emotional problems caused by their physical disability.

Most amputees take pride and pleasure in overcoming a handicap and demonstrating the marvels they can accomplish which the average person takes as a matter of course. Alexander de Seversky, aeronautical engineer, claimed that the loss of his right leg in World War I "awakened powers and aptitudes . . . which were dormant. It focused mental energies which otherwise would probably have been dissipated."

A number of voluntary agencies serve the physically handicapped. Some of these are:

American Federation of the Physically Handicapped, Inc.

National Society for Crippled Children and Adults, Inc.

National Council of Rehabilitation

The National Foundation

Shriners Hospital for Crippled Children

Office of Vocational Rehabilitation of the Department of Health, Education and Welfare

Children's Bureau of the Department of Health, Education and Welfare

Veterans Administration, and under it, the Prosthetic Appliances Service.

In addition, a number of civic clubs, such as Rotary, Lions, and Kiwanis, and various religious organizations have programs of service dedicated to the aid of physically handicapped persons.

The Vocational Rehabilitation Act of 1954 increased the programs for securing employment for the handicapped. The law is administered by an agency of the federal government, but actual services for the handicapped are provided by state agencies.

The United States government is the country's biggest employer of the handicapped. The Civil Service Commission practices selective place-

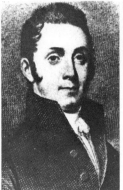

MOTT, Valentine (1785-1865) American surgeon. He was internationally famous for his surgery of the skeletal system and his operations on major blood vessels. In 1824 he performed a successful amputation at the hip joint, and in the years 1818-1827 he performed therapeutic ligations of the innominate artery, the carotid artery, the common iliac artery, and the subclavian. For many years he was a professor of surgery.

ment of the disabled. Their capabilities are matched with the actual requirements of jobs.

Reconstructive surgery of the face

Defects of the face may be inborn *(congenital)* or acquired. Most inborn defects can be corrected by *plastic surgery*, which implies the correction of defects by the use of tissue from other parts of the patient's body. But some congenital defects may be so extensive as to rank with the severe losses of bone, muscle, and skin caused by war injuries, cancer, or accidents. In these, *reconstructive surgery* becomes necessary to restore normal facial contours. Reconstructive surgery replaces lost tissues by means of artificial implants constructed to the form of the lost tissue.

From the beginning, the problem of reconstructive surgery was to find a substitute material which would permit restoration of the normal facial contours, yet be nonirritating to the tissues, and hold its shape and place. Most of the earlier methods failed because the "fillers" did not stay in place or retain their shape. Copper, paraffin, and soft plastics irritate the tissue; celluloid disintegrates; gelatin is too friable; ivory and synthetic materials cannot be molded to shape.

The difference between earlier and recent methods is that the modern replacement is sculptured, and these replacements remain in place because they fit one specific area and will not shrink or irritate tissue. The materials most successfully used are silver and latex. Silver is beaten to shape; latex is poured.

If silver is used, a negative mold of plaster of Paris is made of the defect. From the negative, a positive is cast which serves as a working basis for the making of a silver replacement, the thin sheet of silver being worked over the mold with horn mallets and burnishers. The silver then is painted to match the skin tone of the wearer. Small or large defects can be corrected by the silver method. If loss of an eye socket is involved, a hole is cut in the silver mold, and an artificial eye, matching the normal eye, is inserted.

When latex is used, molds are made as in the silver method. But the latex is then poured into a mold and vulcanized for 24 hours at high temperature. The latex is trimmed, and again vulcanized. When applied to the patient, latex replacements are held in place by the use of adhesive preparations. Additional fillers and coloring material must be used to match the individual complexion. With properly made replacements, even large defects become unnoticeable; and most patients, realizing that no one pays attention to the replacement, lose much of their sensitivity to their defect.

More recently, injectable silicone fluids have been used to correct severe facial deformity. Patients showed no complications in follow-ups over three years. These substances are heat-stable, do not deteriorate, do not drift, and cause minimal tissue reaction. Clinical use of the silicone fluids has been suspended until additional data are available. Requirements of the Food and Drug Administration must be met since the fluids are injected and thus are considered "drugs."

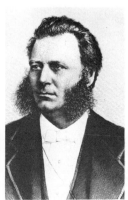

SAYRE, Lewis Albert (1820-1900) American surgeon. First professor of orthopedic surgery in the U.S. Renowned for his work in this field, he performed the first hip resection for hip-joint disease (1855). Developing an original treatment for lateral curvature of the spine, he applied a plaster of Paris jacket for its support. For this purpose he suspended the patient with his own invention, a device known as *Sayre's apparatus.*

HOW ARTIFICIAL REPLACEMENTS ARE MADE AND USED

The various hands and hooks shown on the following pages are of two basic types. The first is purely cosmetic, and is not intended to give functional service. The second is used as a tool. Since a complete functioning hand cannot be reproduced, the most important feature of our hands, the opposition of the thumb with the fingers, is the one incorporated in the hooks. Although the hook does not seem very useful at first glance, close inspection will reveal that the principle of opposition is present in each.

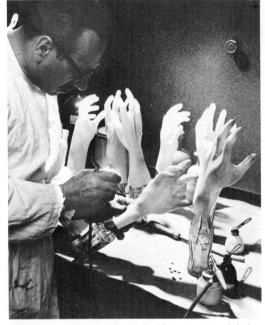

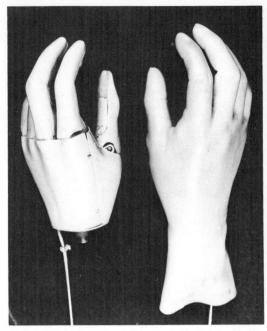

These are cosmetic gloves in the process of being tinted to match the normal skin tones of the wearer. The gloves fit over the artificial hand and appear very life-like.

This is a photograph of the prosthetic hand with the cosmetic glove developed by the Army, for use of amputees. This hand has two fingers and thumb which are functional.

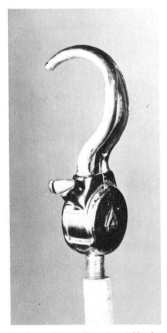

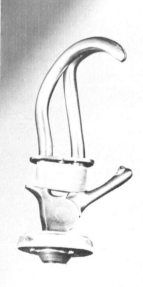

Northrop-Sierra Two Load Hook
This hook was devised to obtain an effective grip without the use of rubber bands. The grip may be varied simply by moving a lever.

Dorrance Hook
This is an all-purpose hook, which employs rubber bands to provide its gripping power. Grip may be increased by adding more bands.

David Hook
This hook is similar to Dorrance hook except that the clamping surface is changed. The hook uses a spring in place of rubber bands.

Courtesy, Prosthetic and Sensory Aids Service, Veterans Administration, New York.

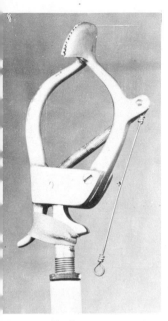

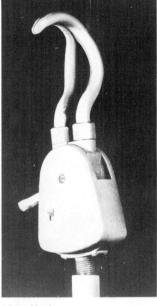

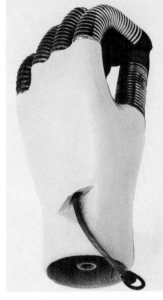

Trautman Hook
Although this hook can be used to grasp round objects, it also is provided with an extension for handling smaller, flat-surfaced objects.

APRL Hook
This hook is an Army development. It incorporates with ease a wide range of pressures, from 50 pounds down to one-half ounce.

Becker Hand
The Becker hand is usually covered with a cosmetic glove, and has some usable movement. The thumb and the forefinger are opposable.

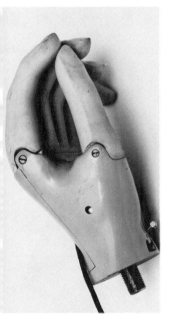

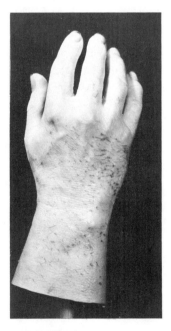

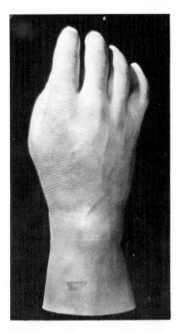

Miracle Hand
The miracle hand combines cosmetic value with some usefulness. Forefinger and thumb are opposable, but not as strong as the hook.

Bettinger Hand
The Bettinger hand is purely a cosmetic device. The fingers may be pre-set into any desired position; the hand offers some support.

Tenenbaum Hand
This hand is very similar to the Bettinger hand and it too is employed for cosmetic purposes exclusively, but offers some support.

Courtesy, Prosthetic and Sensory Aids Service, Veterans Administration, New York.

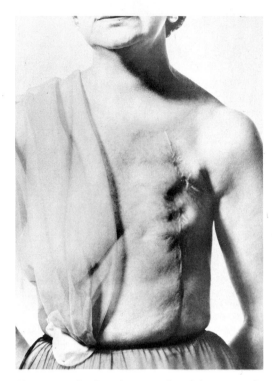

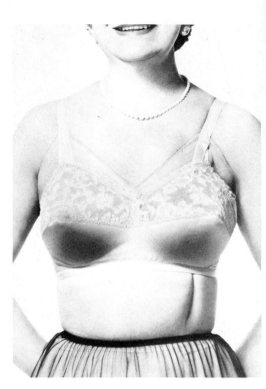

Mastectomy involves large portions of a woman's musculature, and retraining in arm use is frequently necessary. This series of three pictures shows a woman who underwent a simple mastectomy. *Courtesy Identical Form, Inc.*

On the left, the mastectomy scar is shown and on the right is shown the prosthetic bra used to provide the cosmetic build-up so necessary to the patient's feeling of well-being and confidence. *Courtesy Identical Form, Inc.*

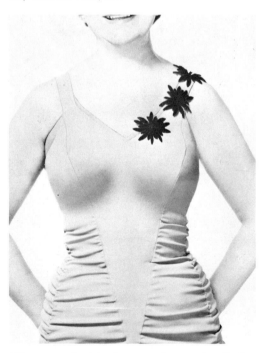

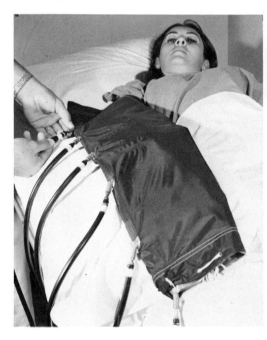

This same patient is shown wearing a swimsuit after her mastectomy. With the prosthetic bra in place it is impossible to see that she has had a breast removed. *Courtesy Identical Form, Inc.*

A patient is undergoing pneumomassage to help prevent lymphedema, a frequent complication of mastectomies in which swelling of tissues limits the freedom of movement of the arm. *Courtesy The University of Texas M. D. Anderson Hospital.*

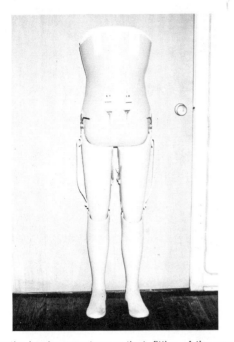

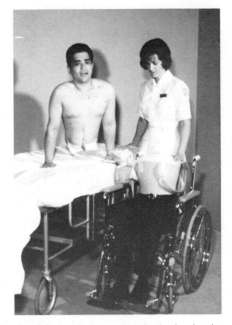

For the hemicorporectomy patient, fitting of the prosthesis is essential, even if only to allow the patient to sit in a wheel chair. The patient can sometimes ambulate using crutches and a swing-through gait.

On the left is shown a prosthesis for hemicorporectomy with full body jacket, hip and knee joints with positive locks, and SACH feet. On the right a patient with hemicorporectomy is preparing to enter his prosthesis.

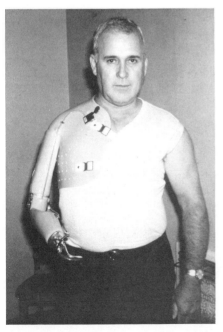

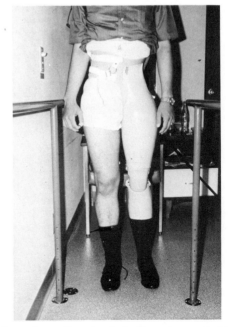

This functional prosthesis for interscapular thoracic amputees has chest control of forearm lift, nudge control elbow lock, passive shoulder abduction, and opposite shoulder movement to control terminal device.

The patient with a hemipelvectomy has no ischium, thus making it necessary for him to carry his weight on soft tissue, which provides very poor stability. The prosthesis for this patient has a free hip and knee joint.

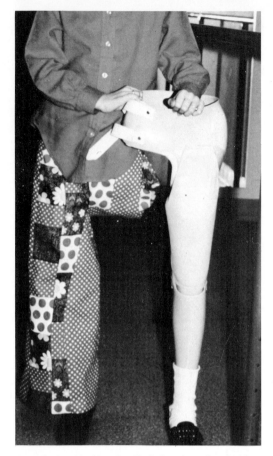

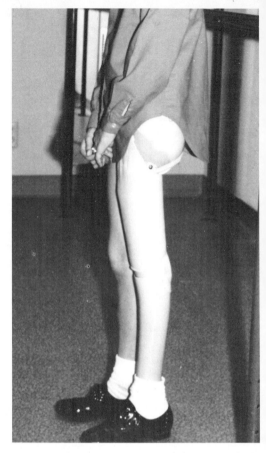

A patient with hip disarticulation has the ischium remaining to provide a good weight-bearing surface and good stability. In the first photograph, the patient is shown with the hip disarticulation prosthesis with free hip and knee joint. In the second photo-graph, the patient is shown wearing her prosthesis for hip disarticulation. *Pictures on this and the preceding page courtesy of The University of Texas M. D. Anderson Hospital, Houston, Texas.*

The average finger tip pressure which can be exerted by the normal hand is around 20 pounds. The hooks, by adding or removing rubber bands or springs, can range from a few ounces to 40 or 50 pounds. The majority of the hooks are operated by a shoulder harness which opens the hook with a shrugging movement of the shoulder; the spring or rubber band closes it on the object to be grasped. Recently, however, some patients have been fitted with hooks designed to be operated by a muscle of the chest or arm. In this method, the muscle chosen is isolated by surgery, and then covered by skin, so that a loop of muscle is outside the body. This operation is known as *cineplasty*. A plastic hook can be slipped under this loop of muscle and the prosthetic device is operated by contraction of the muscle. Many persons using this system report that a much greater range of pressures may be used because the patient can "feel" what the device is doing. Ordinarily, the patient tends to crush small objects such as a match box, because he cannot judge the amount of pressure required to hold it gently but firmly. In 1945, the Army started a research program to develop a functional hand which would also have good cosmetic value, and have had encouraging success with this project. Some of the hands are shown on succeeding pages, together with additional photographs of the hands in everyday use. The reader will note that while the degree of normal hand function recovered with the use of these prosthetic devices is often amazing, there is every reason to believe that continuing research will develop appliances with a much wider range of movement, greater ease of control, and improved appearance.

10 THE ENDOCRINE SYSTEM

WHAT IT IS AND DOES

The endocrine system is made up of several organs situated in various parts of the body, all of which are characterized by their ability to produce active chemical substances called *hormones*. The organs of the endocrine system are called "glands of internal secretion" because, as the name implies, they secrete the products of their activities directly into the blood stream to be distributed throughout the body. The endocrine glands are the pituitary, the hypothalamus, the thyroid, the parathyroids, the testes, the ovaries, the adrenals, the thymus, part of the pancreas, and possibly the pineal body. In addition, during pregnancy, the placenta (the spongy structure in the uterus through which the fetus is nourished) also secretes hormones. The pituitary occupies a central position of control over a considerable portion of the endocrine system and is often referred to as the master gland.

The glands of internal secretion, or *endocrines* as they are often called, are different from certain other glands of the body, such as the salivary or sweat glands, which discharge the products of their activities to the external surfaces of the body by means of ducts (the digestive tract is considered "external" in that it is a cavity which passes through the body). Some endocrine glands also perform other activities; the pancreas produces a digestive secretion which is passed into the small intestine through a system of ducts, and the testes and ovaries are involved in reproduction. Only the endocrine functions will be discussed in this chapter.

Functions

Hormones fall into two general categories, "messengers" and "managers." Most of the endocrine glands produce one or more of each type. The messengers are those hormones which act upon tissues and organs outside of the endocrine system to speed or slow their normal functions. The managers also carry messages, but always within the endocrine system. They are important in maintaining balanced function within the system. They are responsible for the fact that some endocrine actions occur constantly; some occur periodically; some during certain years only; and some occur only once during the life of the individual.

The reproductive system is especially affected by hormones. The growth and maturation of the organs of this system are directly dependent upon endocrine activity. After puberty, the production of the reproductive germ cells is influenced by hormones. In the female, hormones regulate the processes concerned with menstruation, and should pregnancy occur, they operate to prevent menstruation and further the development of the embryo in many ways. Towards the end of pregnancy, hormones act upon the breast to stimulate milk production; and finally, certain hormones set off muscle contractions in the uterus, which mark the beginning of labor.

The endocrine system is responsible for a great many other regulatory activities of the body. The rate of growth and final size of the body, the body contour, distribution of hair, total weight, and the masculine or feminine aspect of the body are all influenced by the

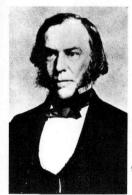

BROWN-SÉQUARD, C. E. (1817-1894) British physiologist in France. Regarded as one of the founders of endocrinology, and successor to Claude Bernard, who first conceived the doctrine of the internal secretions of certain ductless glands. His work on animal adrenal glands and use of testicular and other organ extracts led to the development of modern organotherapy. His experiments on the nervous system were priceless to physiology.

hormones. Internally, the hormones regulate the amount of urine produced, the body temperature, the rate of metabolism, the calcium and sugar levels in the blood, and many other chemical activities. The endocrine system is also a great factor in the personality; and, conversely, the personality can affect the function of the endocrine system.

Relation to the nervous system

One of the principal functions of the nervous system is to correlate all the parts of the body so that they may function harmoniously as a unit. In achieving this harmony, the nervous system is supplemented by the endocrine system; the two systems mutually affect each other. Mental strain, fear, anger, or any emotional state affects the activities of the endocrine glands. The accelerated production of a hormone of the adrenals (adrenalin) in a state of rage or fear is a well-known phenomenon. It has been considered a "defense mechanism" when an emergency calls for greater than usual amounts of energy. More subtle changes occur constantly in the endocrine system, elicited by some form of nervous stimulation. In some instances, the changes in endocrine activity are reflected in perceptible acts; in others they remain imperceptible. The crying spells, hot flashes, and irritability sometimes seen in women during premenstrual tension or menopause illustrate this point well.

The hypothalamus, located at the base of the brain, immediately above the pituitary, is part of both the nervous system and the endocrine system. The nerves connecting it to the pituitary as well as to the centers of neurosecretion permit a direction and indirect influence by the nervous system upon its endocrine counterpart. This influence is all the greater because the pituitary in turn has definite influence over the other endocrine glands. The hypothalamus also produces hormones which stimulate and which inhibit the pituitary gland.

Placenta

The placenta, that mysterious body of tissue which forms during pregnancy to nourish and protect the fetus, is a hormone-producing organ. However, the full extent of its secretory activity has not been established with certainty. The placenta was long believed to be an autonomous endocrine structure since its functional activity is not stimulated by the pituitary or other endocrine glands. However, recent evidence indicates that the placenta is, in some respects, an incomplete endocrine organ, since it merely synthesizes some of the hormones from elements made elsewhere, in either the fetus or the mother.

There are some hormones that are known to be made in the placenta. These include *chorionic gonadotrophin,* on which several tests for pregnancy are based; *placental lactogen,* which acts on the breasts to induce lactation; and *relaxin,* which produces relaxation of supporting pelvic structures so that their positions change to support the growing fetus and, finally, to allow birth. Other hormones, which are ordinarily produced in other endocrine glands, are also believed to be secreted by the placenta during pregnancy. The complete role of the placenta in pregnancy is discussed in Chapter 2, "Life Begins."

Hormone production by nonendocrine tumors

At times, neoplastic tumors arising in nonendocrine organs may secrete hormones and produce endocrine-like disease states. The reason for this is a source of some puzzlement and has not been explained to date.

In some cases, an excess of calcium in the blood is caused, even though the action of the parathyroid glands is normal. This is the result of the secretion of a substance with parathyroid hormone-like activity. In other cases, Cushing's syndrome occurs in patients with tumors of the thymus, pancreas, ovary, thyroid, or other organs. Cushing's syndrome ordinarily results from an excess of adrenocorticotrophic hormone (ACTH), which is secreted by the pituitary. A diabetes-like condition may occur in some patients with mesenchymal or hepatic tumors, even though there is no disturbance of the pancreas.

Such cases as these are rare, however. Treatment consists of removal of the tumor, following which the endocrine symptoms disappear. Where removal is impossible or incomplete, or if the tumor recurs, treatment with drugs or irradiation may result in disappearance of the tumor and the endocrine symptoms.

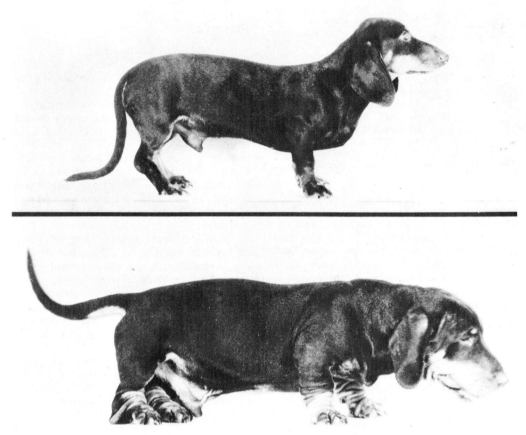

Many of the effects of hormones have been learned by observing their effects on lower animals. The top picture shows a normal dachshund; below is shown one treated with growth hormone extracted from the pituitary gland. *Photographs by courtesy of Dr. Herbert M. Evans. Copyright 1933, University of California.*

THE PITUITARY

The pituitary gland is an endocrine gland that plays a predominant role in the control of many body functions. Formerly, it was believed that this organ, located just below the brain, was the source of mucus which was secreted into the nasal cavity. Indeed, the name is derived from the word "pituita," which means nasal mucus. This erroneous concept has been dispelled, but the name pituitary continues to be applied to this organ. The word *hypophysis* which means undergrowth is also used to denote this gland, and it is preferred by many scientists.

Only within recent years has the role of this important organ become known; some of its functions still remain unrevealed. The pituitary gland is the most important organ in the regulation of growth, milk production, and in the control of many other endocrine glands. In turn, the pituitary is regulated to some extent by many of the other endocrine glands, as well as by the hypothalamus which lies immediately above it.

It has long been known that such severe pituitary disturbances as tumors influence the function of other endocrine glands. It has now been shown that tumors of the pituitary can upset the body's hormone balance so severely as to cause mental illness also. The tumors can usually be removed surgically, with good chances of relieving the emotional disturbances of which they are the indirect cause.

Too, physical disorders caused by pituitary overactivity may be managed by surgical removal of the pituitary or by the implantation of minute "seeds" of radioactive yttrium or gold into the sella turcica (the portion of the sphenoid bone surrounding the pituitary gland). In the future, cryogenic techniques (treatment with very low temperatures) will probably be used for pituitary overactivity.

In addition to all the functions discussed, the pituitary exhibits numerous activities for which no individual hormones have been detected.

Anatomy

The pituitary gland in the human being is a small organ the size of an average pea, and it weighs about the same. It is larger in women than in men, particularly in those women who have borne children. It is joined to the undersurface of the brain by a thin stalk and is protected by a bony structure that surrounds the gland. Because of its shape, the bony structure is called the "turkish saddle" (*sella turcica*).

The pituitary is made up chiefly of two distinct parts called *lobes*—an *anterior lobe* and a *posterior lobe*. There is also a middle portion, the *pars intermedia*, that constitutes only a minor fraction of the entire gland. Under the microscope, this simple division of the pituitary appears far more complex.

The supply of incoming nerve fibers is large; it has been estimated that approximately 50,000 nerve fibers enter into this organ, being confined almost exclusively to the posterior lobe. The blood supply, which is arranged in a circular pattern to avoid even the smallest temporary breakdown, is also extensive. It serves the gland by bringing food, gases, and hormones and by conveying the secretions of the pituitary to other parts of the body.

The pituitary produces a number of hormones, each endowed with the ability to produce some specific effect in one or more organs of the body, especially other endocrine organs. The hormones produced by the anterior lobe are different from those produced by the pars intermedia. Most of the pituitary hormones are protein in nature.

The functions controlled by each part of the pituitary are entirely different. The largest number of hormones are produced by the anterior lobe; hence, it performs most of the functions of the whole gland. The posterior lobe does not in itself manufacture any hormones, although it does receive and store hormones made by the hypothalamus.

Hormones regulating other endocrines

The pituitary has been called the "master gland" since it is believed to be the endocrinological headquarters. The anterior lobe of the pituitary regulates the growth and proper functioning of other endocrine organs by complicated processes. For example, it produces a hormone called the thyrotrophic hormone which acts on the thyroid to stimulate its production of thyroid hormone. When the thyroid hormone reaches the proper level in the blood, the pituitary is affected to the point of reducing or stopping its production of thyrotrophic hormone. When the blood level falls again, the pituitary goes once more into action, causing the thyroid to resume function. This is known as

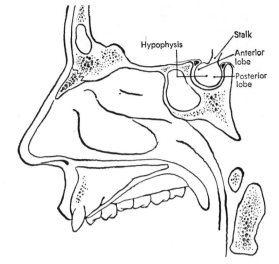

Sagittal section through the human skull showing the location of the pituitary gland, or hypophysis, at the base of the skull, and its major parts.

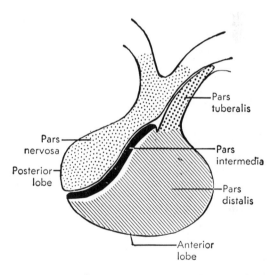

Drawing of the human pituitary gland, illustrating how its tissues are divided so as to form several anatomically and functionally distinct parts.

the feedback regulating mechanism. By this means the thyroid hormone is maintained at a constant level at all times.

Similar checks and balances exist between the pituitary and other glands, either to maintain constant blood levels of hormone, or to bring about a sudden increase when desirable and a subsequent decrease when the immediate need is past. This push-and-pull principle thus permits the body to adapt quickly to sudden stresses or unusual situations. However, it complicates the picture when an apparent malfunction of one of the glands occurs. In the disorder known as *cretinism,* which is characterized by retarded physical and mental development in children, the thyroid fails to produce sufficient hormone. However, the ultimate cause of the disease may in fact lie in the failure of the pituitary to produce its thyrotrophic hormone.

In addition to the thyrotrophic hormone, the anterior pituitary is believed to secrete several other hormones. These include the adrenocorticotrophic hormone (ACTH), the follicle-stimulating and luteinizing components which make up the gonadotrophic hormone, the luteotrophic hormone, or lactogenic hormone, and the growth hormone. Several of these will be discussed in the following paragraphs.

Gonadotrophic hormone

The anterior lobe also produces active principles that are effective stimulators of the *gonads.* The hormones that act on the sex organs (*gonads*) are called *gonadotrophic hormones.* The sexual organs in both male and female have a double function, reproduction and the production of sex hormones. The anterior lobe of the pituitary, by manufacturing and secreting the gonadotrophic hormones, controls the production of these hormones in the ovaries and the testes. In addition to these functions, the gonadotrophins, directly and indirectly, stimulate the development of the sex organs and the maintenance of their structure.

The testes, under the influence of the gonadotrophins, manufacture the male hormones. These in turn exert their action on the other parts of the body, chiefly the organs of reproduction. When the testicular tubules have developed under the influence of the male hormones, maturation of the spermatozoa also is stimulated by the gonadotrophin from the anterior lobe of the pituitary. Failure to produce male hormones results in immature appearance and lack of development of the accessory sex organs; in the previously normal adult, loss of the male hormones results in changes in appearance and degeneration of the accessory sex organs.

In women, the ovaries, under control of the hormones from the anterior lobe of the pituitary, produce the female hormones. The maturation of ova in the ovaries is stimulated by the gonadotrophins from the pituitary. The female hormones act on the reproductive organs and are responsible for the proper growth and function of the uterus, vagina, and other reproductive organs. It is not uncommon to observe disturbance in sexual characteristics of individuals with defective pituitary function.

Deficient pituitary activity is in many cases reflected in lack of development of the sex organs, which may remain infantile. When accompanied by obesity, the condition is known as the *adiposogenital syndrome.* Other disturbances

in the sexual functions of both women and men arise when the anterior lobe of the pituitary fails to produce the proper amount of hormones.

The rate of production of gonadotrophins by the pituitary is influenced by the production of sex hormones by the ovaries and testes. The effects are mutual, and the two glands—the pituitary gland and the ovaries in the female and the testes in the male—maintain an exact balance in the production of hormones.

Adrenocorticotrophic hormone

The anterior lobe of the pituitary produces at least one hormone which acts on the adrenal glands, a substance called *adrenocorticotrophic hormone.* This name is usually abbreviated to *ACTH.* The adrenals are two small organs located near the upper portion of the kidneys. They are discussed in detail later in this chapter. In the *cortex,* or outer layer of these glands, a large number of hormones are produced. These hormones of the adrenal cortex are controlled by the anterior lobe of the pituitary in the same manner as are the secretions of the gonads. ACTH stimulates the production of most of the cortical hormones, but especially

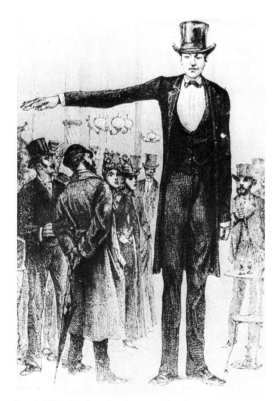

Josef Winkelmaier, the famous Austrian pituitary giant, attained the height of 8 feet 9 inches at the time of his death at 22 in 1887. *Bettmann Archive.*

the well-known *hydrocortisone*. If the production of ACTH is below normal, the adrenal cortex diminishes in size, and the production of most cortical hormones falls to low levels.

Methods to measure ACTH directly are poor, so one must measure the ability of the pituitary to secrete ACTH by indirect means. A metabolic test has been devised which can delineate the levels of ACTH present in the urine. Metopirone, an enzyme inhibitor, is given to a patient. Within three days, test results indicate whether ACTH is being formed within an individual, and thus, whether his pituitary function is intact.

In recent years, ACTH has been isolated from pituitaries of cattle and pigs, and is now available in pure form. In addition, ACTH can now be synthesized (constructed) in the laboratory in two different forms. One type, which uses only 19 amino acids (the building blocks of ACTH), rather than the 39 which are found in naturally occurring ACTH, may find use in special situations in which only selected aspects of the action of ACTH are desired. The other type of ACTH which can be synthesized contains 23 amino acids and is believed to be capable of all the biological activities of naturally occurring ACTH.

ACTH has been found useful as therapy for a variety of disorders, as well as for the diagnosis of some conditions. Although the principal effect of ACTH is to stimulate the adrenal cortex to greater secretion, it also may perform some of the functions of the adrenal glands when the adrenals are absent.

Therapeutically, ACTH may be used to supplement or replace corticoids in the various collagen diseases; it maintains adrenocortical activity in patients in whom ACTH secretion has been suppressed as a result of corticoid therapy. ACTH is effective in the management of certain hematologic diseases, as well as in conditions of stress. It can be used in the treatment for certain spasms involving the head, trunk, and arms of infants. It can also be used for treating young children subject to convulsions caused by diabetes.

ACTH may be employed in the treatment for severe allergic manifestations associated with dermatitis. Despite the effectiveness of ACTH, however, allergic reactions to the hormones may occur. The reactions result from the animal protein associated with the preparation, not from the ACTH itself. Such reactions do not occur in previously ACTH-sensitized patients treated with synthetic preparations. In the future, the use of synthetic ACTH only should prevent such reactions from occurring.

Diagnostically, ACTH may be used to differentiate primary from secondary adrenal insufficiency, or to determine the capacity of the adrenal glands to respond to trophic stimulation.

It has been employed to determine the presence or absence of functions of the adrenal gland and to differentiate between hyperplasia and neoplasia. Increased adrenocortical responsiveness to ACTH occurs in patients with Cushing's syndrome.

Regulation of metabolism

The chemistry of the body is represented by a series of reactions that transform food into various forms of energy. The transformation is smooth and well-controlled, so that sufficient amounts of energy may be delivered in cases of stress, or excess energy stored in times of rest. This perfect balance of the many chemical transformations is regulated in part by the nervous system and in part by the endocrine system. Of the endocrine glands, the pituitary plays the major role in the regulation of metabolism. It regulates metabolism either directly or by regulating other endocrine glands. By acting on the thyroid gland, the anterior lobe regulates the amount of oxygen that the body tissues consume. The tissues are constantly burning food, and like any other type of combustion, the burning of food needs oxygen. The amount of oxygen consumed is a good measure of the amount of food burned. Even if the body is at rest, food continues to be burned at a fairly constant rate to keep the body alive. The minimum amount of combustion that takes place in a resting body is called the *basal metabolic rate* and represents an over-all effect of all the chemical changes. The basal metabolic rate is usually constant; it is controlled directly by the thyroid and indirectly by the anterior lobe of the pituitary. Deficient production of the thyroid-stimulating or *thyrotrophic* hormone results in a decreased basal metabolic rate. Conversely, an increased production of the thyroid-stimulating hormone induces the thyroid to speed up combustion, increasing the basal metabolic rate.

Basal metabolism is only an end result of many intermediary reactions that occur in the body. The food which the body uses undergoes many transformations, so that part may be used as raw materials for the formation of new tissue, and part may be burned as fuel. Proteins constitute an important portion of the food and represent, with the exception of water, the major ingredient of which tissues are made. But proteins as they are present in food are different from the proteins of the tissues, and food proteins have to be transformed into tissue proteins. The deposition of proteins and their reconstruction to form new tissue is partly controlled by the anterior lobe of the pituitary gland.

The amount of protein ingested in an ordinary diet is usually in excess of the protein needed for the formation of new tissue. The body converts the excess protein into other compounds, mostly sugar, that can be burned to yield energy. The transformation of protein into sugar for fuel is also a process controlled indirectly by the anterior lobe of the pituitary through its action on the adrenal cortex. Excess sugar and starches that have not been burned or stored in the liver and muscles as glycogen (which means "sugar former") are eventually converted into body fat and stored in other parts of the body as reserve food. If the function of the pituitary is deficient, fat storage suffers and emaciation may result.

The main source of energy in the body comes from the combustion of sugars and starches (*carbohydrates*). The utilization of sugars and starches is profoundly influenced by the secretions from the anterior lobe of the pituitary, either directly or by action upon other endocrine glands.

The pars intermedia

The anterior lobe of the pituitary produces most of the active principles of the gland and regulates the largest number of functions. However, the middle portion, the *pars intermedia*, produces active principles of which little is known. The hormones of the pars intermedia are known to be concerned with the regulation of changes in pigmentation in fish and frogs. Since this is a minor function in man, there is a smaller intermediate lobe in the human pituitary. In man, as in lower forms of life, the degree of pigmentation is determined to a considerable extent by *intermedin*.

The posterior lobe and the hypothalamus

Although the posterior lobe of the pituitary is now thought to produce no hormones, it receives and stores several active hormones which are produced in the hypothalamus, that part of the brain which lies directly above the gland. Two of the hormones produced in the hypothalamus and stored in the posterior part of the pituitary are *vasopressin*, which has an antidiuretic effect, and *oxytocin*, which induces uterine contractions.

Growth disorders

Like any other organ of the body, the pituitary is susceptible to the growth of tumors that may make the gland overactive or underactive, depending on the type of tumor. When the tumor is made up of active glandular cells, the increase in mass of the gland is reflected in an overproduction of hormones. However, tumors with inactive cells may grow and exert pressure upon the other portions of the pituitary gland, causing damage and destruction of active glan-

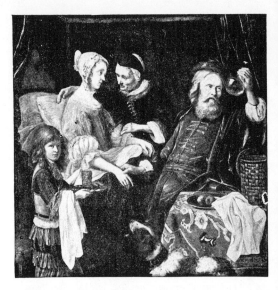

Old painting by the artist, Torenvliet, entitled *Visit of the Doctor*. Even in the seventeenth century, examination of a urine specimen was a common practice. It appears in many old paintings.

dular tissue; this results in a deficient production of hormones. In both instances, the net result is a series of derangements that take many different forms.

Decreased function of the pituitary results in retarded growth. The growth hormone, or *somatotrophic* hormone, exerts its major effect upon the size of the organs and the skeleton, which in cases of decreased pituitary function remains small. The condition that results is called *pituitary dwarfism* or *infantilism*. Teeth grow slowly if insufficient growth hormone is produced, and the development of permanent teeth is considerably delayed. Untreated pituitary dwarfs do not grow over three or four feet in height and remain sexually immature.

Specific therapy for such patients is the administration of pituitary growth hormone of primate or human origin. However, even with human growth hormone, refractory states may develop, resulting in poor growth.

At first, the growth rate for children treated with human growth hormone is at least three times as great as without treatment, or about three inches per year. In subsequent years, the growth rate declines. Weight increases proportionately to height, and bone age advances normally.

Pituitary dwarfs never achieve normal endocrine function. For dwarfed girls to develop breast tissue and to menstruate, they must be treated with estrogen. However, treatment with estrogen may stop growth of the bones before the patient has attained acceptable height. Therefore, it is wise to delay therapy with the female sex hormones as long as possible.

Although many forms of dwarfism are the result of pituitary or thyroid insufficiency, some are genetically determined. A most remarkable example of this can be seen in the Amish community of Pennsylvania. The Amish people now number more than 44,000; however, all are descended from the same group of about 200 immigrants. Since 1860, 49 cases of a dwarfism known as the Ellis-van Creveld syndrome have been verified in this community. All of these dwarfs were descended, directly or indirectly, from a single man and wife.

This type of dwarfism is different from that discussed earlier. Ellis-van Creveld dwarfs range in height from 40 to 60 inches. They have six fingers on each hand, the extra one on the outside beyond the little finger. Sometimes there is a sixth toe. Many of the babies have heart abnormalities and a weakness or deficiency of cartilage in the chest. One fourth of dwarfed children with such defects die within two weeks of birth; however, many others achieve near normal life spans. There is no mental retardation or loss of intelligence.

The most familiar form of dwarfism is called *achondroplasia.* Persons afflicted with this type have large heads with saddle or scooped-out noses, short extremities, and sway backs.

Hormones of high molecular weight are usually active only in closely related species. This is true of growth hormone. Therefore, the desirability of having human growth hormone for treating human beings is paramount. It takes the hormone from 150 or more glands to treat for one year a child with the type of deformity which will respond to therapy. Human growth hormone is obtained by extraction from the pituitaries of recently deceased human beings. Pituitary "banks" have been established in several medical centers to store the hormone in order that portions large enough for treatment may be accumulated. It is hoped that, with new techniques such as tissue culture of pituitary cells or even the chemical synthesis of human somatotrophin, a sufficient amount of material may be made available for wide use.

Sometimes, the anterior lobe or the entire pituitary gland may become enlarged and the production of hormones may increase above the normal range, as when active tumor develops in the gland. The production of excessive amounts of growth hormone may cause exaggerated growth. If the condition develops while the bones are in the process of growing, the result is *giantism*; individuals with this condition may grow to over eight feet in height.

The prevention of giantism, however, is relatively simple if diagnosis is made early. To close the epiphyses (open ends of the bones, which are still growing) of probable giants, estrogen is used in girls; both estrogen and testosterone are employed in boys. This treatment does not affect later gonadal function adversely. The epiphyses of these patients should be studied at four- to six-month intervals to determine whether growth is stopping and if therapy can be discontinued. An x-ray film of the hands and wrist is often used since this is simple to obtain and since the epiphyses in the wrists are the last ones to close.

In later life, when the bones have ceased to grow in length, an overactive pituitary causes excessive stimulation of the growth centers which results in the disease known as *acromegaly*. The name implies large extremities. It is a disease characterized by an abnormal development of the feet and hands. The jaw is prominent and large, as are the bones of the skull. The face may become angular and irregular, and the general appearance is that of a primitive man. The fully developed disease is readily discerned by the layman; the early disease is difficult to detect.

Patients with acromegaly usually have enlargement of the pituitary gland caused by a tumor. Steroid therapy is given, depending in part on the extent of the condition and the level of circulating growth hormone in the blood. During therapy, the patient should be watched carefully with regard to diminution of the visual field. If there is a change in visual acuity, this should be reported to the physician immediately.

Acromegaly also occurs to a slight degree in some women during pregnancy, but regresses after delivery.

Cushing's disease and Cushing's syndrome

Rarely, a tumor made up of special cells develops in the anterior lobe of the pituitary, and a number of characteristic changes occur in the body. The disease was first described by Doctor Harvey Cushing, and is called Cushing's disease. The condition is recognized by obesity of the abdomen, face, and buttocks, but not of the limbs. The skin about the face and hands is redder than normal. Hair grows profusely, and women may grow mustaches and beards. Bones become brittle and suffer a considerable loss of the mineral components. Sexual functions may fall to a low level or become suppressed altogether.

When the manifestations of Cushing's disease occur in patients with excessive production of adrenal cortical hormones of the adrenal glands, the condition is called *Cushing's syndrome* (see discussion on overactivity in section on the adrenal glands, later in this chapter). The adrenal hormone production is excessive also in Cushing's disease, as a result of overstimulation of the adrenals by pituitary hormone (ACTH) produced in excess by the tumor.

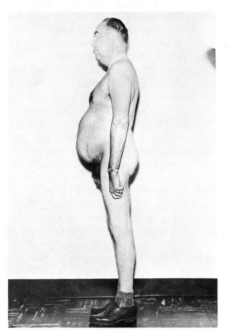

This picture shows a man afflicted with Cushing's syndrome. Padded abdomen and purple streaks are characteristic. A tumor of the pituitary was removed, correcting the symptoms. In some cases the syndrome may also be produced by excessive secretion of hormone by the adrenal cortex. *Courtesy of G. J. Hamwi, M.D., Department of Medicine, Division of Endocrine and Metabolic Disease, Ohio State University, Columbus, Ohio.*

Atrophy and Fröhlich's syndrome

Atrophy or degeneration of the anterior lobe in adults results in a disease sometimes known as *Simmonds'* or *Simmonds-Sheehan disease*. This disorder is characterized by an extreme appearance of aging. Axillary and pubic hair are lost, there is a loss of teeth, and hair of the head becomes gray and sparse. The skin is wrinkled and the face has a wizened appearance. All the metabolic functions of the body are affected, and eventually the mental functions decline. The notion that there is an excessive weight loss in this disease persists despite much evidence to the contrary. Patients usually have a normal distribution of body weight.

This condition occurs most often in women and nearly always arises after postpartum hemorrhage or shock and excessive loss of blood. The condition gradually deteriorates over a period of years. The pituitary atrophy is now believed to be the result of anoxia, or lack of oxygen reaching the gland during the shortage of blood.

Simmonds-Sheehan disease is sometimes confused with *anorexia nervosa*. This is a serious nervous condition, emotional in etiology, in which a patient eats little food and is greatly emaciated. Patients with anorexia nervosa, generally adolescent or young adult females, have a history of aversion to food and other evidence of severe neurosis. These patients are very active rather than apathetic, and they do not lose body hair or skin pigmentation, as women with Simmonds-Sheehan disease. Amenorrhea is a constant feature of Simmonds-Sheehan disease, but is not always present in anorexia nervosa. Although there was much confusion about the two disorders in the past, a metabolic test called the Metapirone test can now distinguish between the two conditions. Hormonal treatment in anorexia nervosa is secondary to psychiatric and dietary treatment.

In some instances, a lesion of the hypothalamus affects the anterior lobe and results in a disease known as the *Fröhlich's syndrome* or *dystrophia adiposogenitalis*. The latter name is derived from the fact that patients suffering from this disease are excessively fat, and their sexual organs are infantile. The disease takes different forms, depending on the age of the patient. In early childhood, the disease causes dwarfism, and in children before puberty the condition is typified by the "fat boy." The victims are mentally lazy and possess voracious appetites. Their sexual organs are underdeveloped, and they are sexually indifferent. When the disease develops in adulthood, male patients become effeminate, with soft skin and feminine distribution of fat in the breast region and thighs. In female patients, the obesity is extreme; it is not uncommon to see patients with this disorder weighing 300 pounds.

The obesity itself is not a direct result of tumor in the pituitary. The pituitary gland has no relationship to obesity, although many people believe so. The obesity is actually a result of the same tumor's affecting the adjacent hypothalamus. True Fröhlich's syndrome, then, consists of tumor, in the hypothalamus, perhaps extending to the pituitary. Pituitary insufficiencies result in the immaturity of the sexual organs. Hypothalamic disease results in a disturbance of the "appetite control center" with resulting obesity.

This disease should not be confused with the typical obesity of childhood and adolescence. Fröhlich's syndrome is very rare, and most fat children do not have this condition nor any detectable glandular disturbance; instead, they are obese because of bad dietary habits.

HYPOTHALAMUS

The hypothalamus is part of the diencephalon, the central portion of the brain. The hypothalamus is intimately concerned with the regulation of many autonomic functions, including body temperature, sleep, behavior, appetite, and emotional response. In addition, it is now evident that the hypothalamus has important endocrine functions. It secretes the neurohypophyseal hormones, *oxytocin* and *vasopressin*, and to a considerable degree governs the hormonal activity of the posterior part of the pituitary gland. The hypothalamus is regarded, therefore, as a neuroendocrine structure, the cells of which combine the characteristics of nerve cells and glandular cells.

Hypothalamic hormones

One of the hormones made in the hypothalamus and stored in the posterior lobe of the pituitary is *vasopressin*. The release of this hormone brings about an anti-diuretic effect, that is, it slows down the rate of urine formation. When the posterior lobe is damaged, the patient may suffer from a condition called *diabetes insipidus*. This disease is characterized by excessive urine production, usually two to three gallons daily. The patient is constantly thirsty and must drink large amounts of water day and night to replace fluid losses. Administration of vasopressin or of an extract of the posterior pituitary lobe will check the flow of urine.

Oxytocin is another hormone formed by the hypothalamus and stored in the posterior lobe of the pituitary. At the end of pregnancy, release of this hormone brings about uterine contraction and signals the beginning of labor. Under certain special conditions, oxytocin may be administered to induce labor.

In 1954, 58 years after the first demonstration of the vasopressor potency in pituitary extracts, a team led by the biochemist Vincent du Vigneaud discovered the structure of vasopressin and oxytocin and synthesized oxytocin. This achievement was a milestone in endocrinology, because for the first time a biologically active peptide hormone had been synthesized.

Hypothalamic releasing factors

Separate neurohumors regulating the secretion and release of anterior pituitary hormones have been demonstrated or postulated for adrenocorticotrophic hormone (ACTH), thyrotrophic hormone (TSH), the luteinizing gonadotrophic hormone (LH), and the follicle-stimulating gonadotrophic hormone (FSH).

These neuroendocrine mediators are generally referred to as releasing factors. There is some evidence suggesting that there are anatomically distinct areas concerned with the secretion or release of each releasing factor, but this is not certain. The precise chemical composition of the factors has not yet been established, although recent studies suggest that they are water-soluble polypeptides similar to vasopressin.

Hypothalamic-related endocrine disorders

The proportion of cases in which endocrine dysfunction can be attributed to a demonstrable hypothalamic lesion is relatively small. However, it is common knowledge that a disturbance of one endocrine gland may influence other members of the endocrine system to varying degrees. Although many factors are involved in these endocrine interrelationships, the hypothalamus plays a major role in transmitting the influence of disordered hormonal function from one gland to another.

Other factors which influence endocrine function via the hypothalamus include environmental elements such as light, odors, temperature, and altitude, some peripheral stimuli, central nervous system lesions, and psychogenic (emotional) factors.

Endocrine disorders resulting from hypothalamic lesions include diabetes insipidus, sexual precocity, hypogonadism, obesity, galactorrhea, and impaired thyroid and adrenal function.

Disorders of gonadal function are the most common manifestations of endocrine dysfunction in patients with lesions involving the hypothalamus. Presumably, these are mediated by disturbance in the hypothalamic regulation of the pituitary gonadotrophic hormones, causing either increased or diminished secretion, depending upon the location and extent of the lesion. With increased secretion in children, premature sexual maturation commonly occurs. In some instances, other manifestations of hypothalamic involvement may be evident also, for instance excessive hunger and thirst, impairment of temperature control, sleep disturbances, and emotional outbursts.

Sexual infantilism in children or gonadal failure in adults may also result from hypothalamic lesions causing low excretion of gonadotrophic hormone by the pituitary. In women, cessation of the menses is usually the first complaint, while in men, loss of libido and sexual potency are early manifestations. In children, growth may be stunted if the pituitary is involved. Obesity or diabetes insipidus may be present, and visual disturbances are frequently noted.

The type of obesity associated with hypothalamic lesions results from disturbance in the appetite center leading to uncontrolled food intake. Obesity of this kind occurring in association with sexual infantilism is known as Fröhlich's syndrome. Diabetes insipidus and stunted growth may also be present.

THE THYROID

The thyroid is an endocrine gland located in the neck. How it got its name is something of a

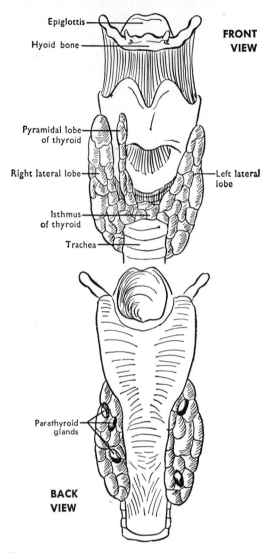

Epiglottis

Hyoid bone

FRONT VIEW

Pyramidal lobe of thyroid

Right lateral lobe

Left lateral lobe

Isthmus of thyroid

Trachea

Parathyroid glands

BACK VIEW

Front and rear drawings of the thyroid gland, showing the relationship to the other organs of the neck and their close location to the parathyroids.

it can neither be seen as a bulge nor felt as a distinct organ.

The thyroid has a brownish red, pulpy appearance and has one of the most copious blood supplies of any organ in the body. The average adult possesses approximately five quarts of blood, an amount which passes through the thyroid gland once an hour. The rapid flow, which brings both thyrotrophic hormone (a thyroid-stimulating hormone of the anterior pituitary gland) and iodide (for building thyroid hormones), exerts a considerable influence on thyroid activity.

Viewed through a microscope, the thyroid is seen to be composed of a great many small, hollow, ball-like units known as *follicles*. The average diameter of each follicle is about 1/100 of an inch, although there is considerable variation in size in the healthy gland, and even greater variation when certain diseases are present. The functional cells of the thyroid (*acinar cells*) make up these follicles, the walls of which are one cell thick. Each follicle has its own small artery that supplies blood to a network of *capillaries* which themselves subsequently reunite to form a small vein.

Inside each follicle is a jelly-like material composed of thyroglobulin and called *colloid*. The raw materials for hormone production are brought to the thyroid cells by the blood, and the finished products, known as *thyroxine* and *triiodothyronine* are carried away by the blood through the veins of the thyroid. The thyroid provides storage of hormone that is not immediately required. The excess hormone is stored in the colloid material which fills the follicles.

Another hormone produced in the thyroid is *thyrocalcitonin (calcitonin)*, which functions in conjunction with parathyroid hormone to regulate the level of calcium in the blood. The activity of thyrocalcitonin is discussed in the section on parathyroid.

The thyroid gland synthesizes, stores, and secretes the thyroid hormones. These hormones, *thyroxine* and *triiodothyronine*, are necessary for growth, development, and metabolism.

The metabolism of iodine is centrally involved in thyroid physiology. The daily ration of iodine is absorbed into the blood from the gastrointestinal tract as *iodide*. Iodide circulating in the blood enters the thyroid by a mechanism known as the *"iodide trap,"* which concentrates iodide to a level 25 times that in the blood. The thyroid then builds the hormones triiodothyronine and thyroxine which are stored in the thyroid colloid for release as necessary.

In response to the stimulus of a center in the brain, thyroxine and triiodothyronine are released into the blood stream. A small portion of the thyroxine is "free" in the blood stream (only free thyroxine can enter the cells of the body), but most of it is chemically bound to a

mystery. The original Greek word for thyroid means "shield." However, it is actually shaped more like a butterfly than like a traditional shield. It is one of the largest endocrine glands in the body, averaging 0.7 ounce in weight. It is the first gland to develop both in the individual and in the evolution of the species. It is situated in the front of the neck where the latter joins the chest. The "wings" of the butterfly lie on either side of the windpipe and are known as lobes. The body of the butterfly is represented by a small bridge (*isthmus*) which passes in front of the windpipe, and connects the wings.

The normal thyroid is packed so neatly between other adjoining structures in the neck that

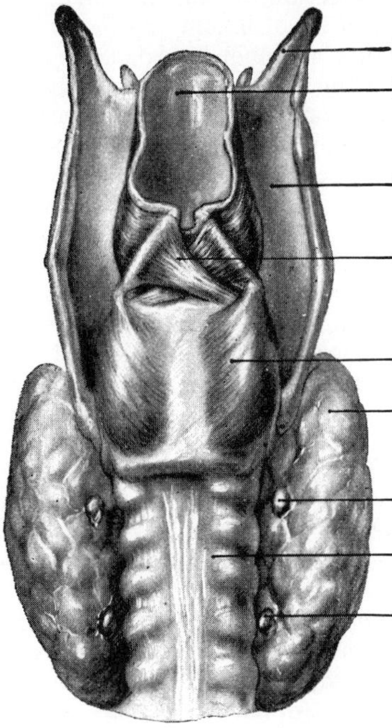
Hyoid bone
Epiglottis
Thyroid cartilage
Arytenoideus muscle
Posterior crico-arytenoideus muscle
Thyroid gland
Right superior parathyroid gland
Trachea
Right inferior parathyroid gland

Posterior view of the organs of the human neck, showing the relationship of the thyroid and parathyroid glands to the trachea and the larynx.

protein. Triiodothyronine is less closely bound to protein. Probably more than 80 percent of the iodine in the blood is in the form of thyroxine; the rest in triiodothyronine. Protein-bound thyroid hormone normally is greatly increased during pregnancy and during treatment with estrogen.

The two thyroid hormones have the same effects on the body qualitatively, but quantitatively there are differences. Their function is to stimulate the metabolism of nearly all cells except those of the brain, thyroid, testis, spleen, and uterus. The effect of thyroxine is not observed until one or more days after administration, but the effect is maintained and is lost only after several days. The response to triiodothyronine may occur within six hours after administration, and by 36 to 48 hours the response has disappeared.

Regulation

The growth and function of the thyroid are under the control of the *thyrotrophic hormone* secreted by the anterior pituitary. These cells in turn vary their secretion rate in response to amount of thyroid hormone in the blood. Thus, a fall in the amount of thyroid hormone in the blood is countered by an increased secretion of thyrotrophin, which stimulates the thyroid to increase the production of hormones. This "feedback" system maintains a balance in thyroid activity. The role of pituitary in this system is at least partly controlled by stimulation from the hypothalamus.

The exact means by which the thyroid hormone influences the cells of the body are not clearly understood. One of the most striking effects, however, is upon the consumption of oxygen by living cells. As has been described elsewhere, the tissues of the body derive energy for their various specialized tasks through the slow regulated "burning" of certain ingredients taken in as food. Just as oxygen is required for the burning of a candle, so is it also required for the utilization of food. One of the main tasks of the thyroid hormone appears to be the maintenance of the burning process (called *metabolism*) at an optimal level. In this connection, the quantity of thyroid hormone is small but powerful. A single ounce of blood from a healthy person contains less than one millionth of an ounce of thyroid hormone. Even in the severest form of hyperthyroidism, the amount is increased to only about seven millionths of an ounce per ounce of blood.

Tests of thyroid function

As stated, one of the main tasks of the thyroid hormone appears to be the maintenance of metabolism at an optimal level. The *basal metabolic rate* is the name given to the minimum rate of energy production required to keep a body functioning when completely at rest. Rest is only a relative term; the heart, of course, beats; the kidneys function; body cells are replaced; and breathing, intestinal activity, and other functions continue. When these activities are minimal, the amount of oxygen required for energy production is likewise minimal. If the body is strenuously engaged in labor or other activity, much more oxygen is required.

Several machines have been devised to measure the amount of oxygen consumed by individuals at rest. Appropriate calculations relating this amount of oxygen to the body surface area give a figure known as the basal metabolic rate (abbreviated BMR). The numbers obtained by such measurements are expressed as plus or minus values, the assumption being that zero is normal. Actually, however, most authorities agree that anything from minus 15 to plus 15 may be regarded as normal. Occasionally, values in an even wider range than this are found in individuals who appear to be perfectly healthy. Persons with insufficient thyroid hormone in the blood and tissues have low basal metabolic rates; in the complete absence of the thyroid, the BMR may be as low as minus 40. In patients with diseases caused by excessive amounts of thyroid hormone, the basal metabolic rate may be more than plus 100.

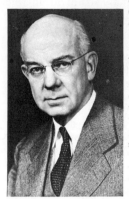

KENDALL, Edward Calvin (1886-) American physiologist and chemist. Isolated in crystalline form the active agent in the secretions of the thyroid gland, which he has called "thyroxin." This discovery has proved to be of prime importance in establishing the chemical nature of the agent and for providing a basis for future study. With other investigators, he also isolated certain active steroids which are found in hormones produced by the adrenal cortex.

In order for the physician to interpret the basal metabolic rate properly, the patient must comply rigidly with certain requirements. The measurements are usually made in the morning, preferably after a good night's sleep. There must be neither excitement nor recent exercise, and the intestinal tract must be at rest. It is most important that no food be eaten after the preceding evening meal.

Properly done, measurement of the basal metabolic rate is a useful test, but there are newer ones which are of great assistance in the diagnosis of overactivity or underactivity of the thyroid gland. One of the newer methods depends upon the actual measurement by chemical means, of the quantity of thyroid hormone in the patient's blood. This measurement is among the most delicate employed in medical work, and, because of its delicacy, it is subject to certain errors.

These measurements are called the *PBI test* (because it measures protein-bound iodine) and the *BEI test* (because it measures butanol-extractable iodine). As indicated by their names, both these tests determine the amount of hormone in the blood by measuring the amount of iodine present. Thus, the results of the two tests can be altered by the presence in the body of any other source of iodine or by some medications. To perform these tests, about one-third of an ounce of blood is obtained from one of the veins in the arm, and in this quantity of fluid there are only a few billionths of an ounce of iodine. Because this is a very small amount, the measurements may, as mentioned, be greatly complicated if the patient has unusual amounts of iodine from other sources in his blood. Most common sources of interfering iodine are iodine antiseptics, iodine-containing medications including some vitamin preparations and weight-control products, and x-ray examinations involving the use of radiopaque materials containing iodine. Exposure of the patient to mercury or mercurial medications will also interfere with the measurement of thyroid hormone, since mercury has the effect of binding up the iodine in such a way that it cannot be detected.

The measurement of free thyroxine actually gives a more accurate determination, because this test eliminates the contamination by iodine. Recently, several methods have been developed which measure thyroxine separate from contaminating iodinated materials. The methods measure thyroxine accurately even in the presence of high concentrations of contaminating materials, including x-ray contrast media, and are of great assistance when other iodinated materials are present in the blood.

Radioactive iodine

Tests of thyroid function which employ *radioactive iodine* (^{131}I) are now widely available. The one most frequently employed is measurement of the amount of radioactivated iodine absorbed by the thyroid. Chemically, radioactive iodine is the same as ordinary nonradioactive iodine; therefore, thyroid cells utilize one type as readily as the other. When a patient takes a drink of water containing a minute amount of radioactive iodine, the radioactive iodine is absorbed from the stomach and intestines into the blood. Thyroid cells collect the radioactive iodine from the blood and use it as a building block in making thyroxine and triiodothyronine. (An underactive thyroid gland shows little affinity for collecting and utilizing this radioactive iodine whereas an overactive gland exhibits a great affinity for it and will collect nearly all the radioactive atoms.) The hormone produced is then stored in the colloid for later distribution throughout the body.

When a patient is given a dose of ^{131}I in water, the amount that accumulates in the neck

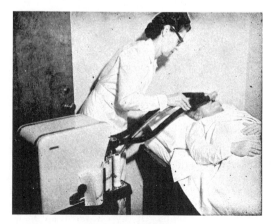

In the basal metabolism test, shown here, the inhaled and exhaled gases are measured in a test apparatus. *Courtesy of Hermann Hospital, Houston.*

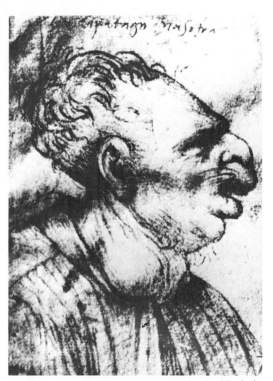

Goiterous figure attributed to Leonardo da Vinci, in the Ambrosina in Milano. *Bettmann Archive.*

is measured 24 hours later. Normally, the thyroid accumulates between 15 and 50 percent of an administered does of ^{131}I within 24 hours. Values above 55 to 60 percent are seen in patients with thyrotoxicosis, patients with prolonged iodine deficiency, and those on certain medications. Thyroid uptake values below 15 percent occur in hypothyroid states. The rate of appearance of protein-bound radioactive iodine in the blood also is used as an index of thyroid function.

Within the body, each small particle, or *atom*, of radioactive iodine emits waves known as *beta rays* and *gamma rays*. About 85 percent of this radiation is in the form of beta rays, which penetrate only one or two millimeters into body tissue. However, the gamma rays, like the better known x-rays, can penetrate tissue further and can be detected by such devices as a Geiger counter or scintillation crystal.

Much information regarding the configuration of the thyroid gland and the nature of nodules contained in it may be obtained by "scanning" with a detecting device after administration of [131]I. A scanning unit held close to the neck can record a "picture" of the thyroid gland by differential shading which indicates the distribution of the radioactive iodine. This allows for comparisons in terms of activity between different areas of the thyroid gland. This procedure is quite helpful in the study of nodules or cysts.

In general, a nodule showing no activity ("cold") is more likely to be cancerous than is a nodule showing increased activity.

Diseases of the thyroid

The thyroid is subject to a great variety of diseases, other than under- and overactivity. The gland may become greatly enlarged for a number of reasons; it may become infected with either viruses or bacteria; and it may give rise to the development of several types of cancer.

The most common disease of the thyroid is goiter. The term, goiter, means enlargement of the thyroid. The degree of enlargement is not always related to the degree of function; in fact the largest goiters seldom produce excessive thyroid hormone. The most common variety of goiter, *endemic goiter*, occurs most frequently in those areas of the world where the supply of iodine in the soil is low. If, for example, the iodine has been washed out of the soil, as often occurs in mountainous areas, the plants which grow there contain little of this important substance. Since plants serve either directly or indirectly as the major source of food for the inhabitants of such areas, their bodies soon become deficient in iodine, without which it is impossible to make thyroxin. In these cases, the thyroid gland becomes larger, seemingly to compensate for underproduction of hormone, caused by the lack of iodine. Sometimes the compensation is successful; sometimes it is not. The outcome depends almost entirely upon the amount of iodine available to the gland. No degree of enlargement will compensate fully if there is an absolute deficiency of iodine. Later, if adequate quantities of iodine become available, there may be some slight decrease in the size of the goiter, but usually the gland does not shrink back to normal size. Individuals affected with this kind of goiter are likely to have low basal metabolic rates. If the condition exists during infancy, there is a serious interference with normal growth and development, and the resulting individual is known as a *cretin*.

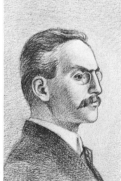

MAGNUS-LEVY, Adolf (1865-1955) German clinical physiologist in the United States. Demonstrated in the course of his researches into the intermediate products of metabolism that deficient production of thyroid hormone is associated with reduced metabolism; he also discovered that this hormonal imbalance may be restored by administering dried thyroid. In other studies on diabetic coma, he attempted to elucidate the nature of diabetes.

Some idea of the great degree of depletion of iodine from the soil in goiter areas can be gained by considering the minute quantities of iodine which are needed by the average normal adult. The entire body probably does not contain more than 20 milligrams—approximately one fifteen-hundredth of an ounce—of iodine. This quantity corresponds roughly to the amount of iodine contained in two drops of tincture of iodine. The daily requirement in the diet is much smaller, since the body uses much of the iodine over and over again. The thyroid gland contains roughly one third of all the iodine in the body. Some of this is present in the hormone which is being stored; the remainder is being processed into new hormone for immediate delivery. To replace the amount of iodine which is lost from the body, as little as one two-millionth of an ounce per day would be sufficient. Smelling the cork of a tincture of iodine bottle would be almost sufficient to supply the body with this amount. In many mountainous, and a few nonmountainous areas of the world, even this tiny quantity is not available in either diet or drinking water. There has been a remarkable decrease in the occurrence of goiters in such areas after public health laws demanded that iodine be added to table salt. In the case of those goiters, however, which have gone beyond the stage at which they may be made to return to normal size by the administration of iodine, surgical removal is now a safe and effective means of freeing the patient from these unsightly, inconvenient, and sometimes dangerous growths.

Lack of iodine in the diet is not the only circumstance which may lead to the development of goiter, although it is the most common. A large number of vegetables have a goiter-producing quality. Cabbage, Brussels sprouts, cauliflower, turnips, rutabaga, and soy beans, if taken daily into the body over long periods, may lead to the development of goiters. This does not mean that these foods are unsuitable or dangerous for human use; quite the contrary is true.

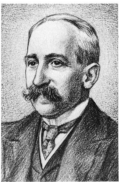

SEMON, Felix (1849-1921) English laryngologist. Made some very penetrating observations on myxedema and cretinism, and on the relationship between them (1883). In his studies of cancerous thyroid glands he noticed the disease's paralytic effect on the vocal cords; this immobility has been named *Semon's symptom. Semon's law* largely limits progressive organic lesions of the motor laryngeal nerves to abductor muscles of the vocal cords.

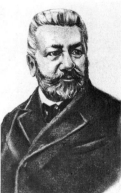

LANNELONGUE, Odilon Marc (1840-1911) French surgeon. He was the first to transplant the thyroid gland of an animal, in this case a sheep, to a human being to restore the normal flow of thyroid hormone. Lannelongue was concerned especially with the diseases and surgery of the bones. He is known as the originator of several operations including a craniectomy, bearing his name, for relief of excess pressure on the brain.

Only great amounts and high frequency of use of these foods need be avoided. The quantity of goiter-producing material in these various foods varies from season to season. For example, cabbage that is grown in the fall or winter months may cause goiter, whereas that grown during the spring and summer months cannot do so even if it constitutes the whole diet. There are few authentic cases on record of patients who ingested sufficiently large amounts of any of these foods to cause serious difficulty.

There are certain factors within the body itself which influence to some extent the development of goiter, how soon it shall develop, and how large it is to become. Women appear to be more susceptible than men to the development of goiter, at least in "low iodine" areas of the world. Not only do goiters develop more frequently among women, but the growths also develop earlier, become larger and are somewhat less apt to return to normal size spontaneously than are similar enlargements in men. During pregnancy a goiter may become larger, and although at the termination of pregnancy there is usually some regression in size, the thyroid frequently does not resume its former dimension. Hence, if pregnancy is repeated often, there may be considerable additional enlargement of the goiter.

Fortunately, the systematic consumption of iodized table salt has largely done away with the endemic goiter problem in the United States and to a considerable degree in other traditional goiter belts of the world. In Switzerland for example, the problem was very serious. The number of cretins born within the borders of that country was so great that special farms had to be provided and maintained by the government for the care of these mentally and physically deficient individuals. The number has decreased remarkably in recent years.

In addition to endemic goiters caused by iodine deficiency, there are growths called *simple goiters* which are not related to the pres-

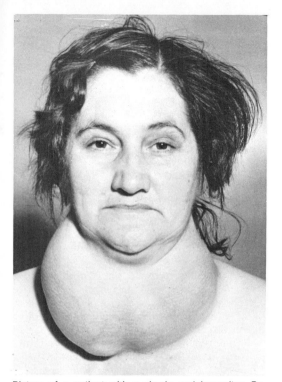

Picture of a patient with a simple nodular goiter. Patient showed no symptoms other than enlargement of thyroid gland. *Photograph by courtesy George J. Hamwi, Ohio State University.*

in the normal thyroid tissue, in which the adenoma is growing, go into a resting phase. Even this shutdown is not sufficient to prevent the blood level of thyroid hormone from becoming too high. It is usually necessary for the patient's welfare to remove the offending nodule or adenoma, after which the resting normal thyroid tissue once again resumes its usual rate of secretion of thyroid hormone.

Although cancer of the thyroid is to be discussed later in this chapter, it is appropriate to mention here that a significant number of single nodules in the normally active thyroid gland prove to be malignant *(cancer).* The incidence of cancer is much lower if more than one nodule, or adenoma, exists in the thyroid gland, or if the thyroid is overactive. The possibility that a nodule in this organ is a cancer is even greater if the patient is in the younger age groups. It is imperative therefore that *every* enlargement in the region of the thyroid gland be examined carefully by a physician, particularly if the patient is young. Cancer of the thyroid gland is often curable by surgical means if treatment is started promptly.

ence of iodine. The cause of simple goiter is largely unknown. Since some foods are known to inhibit the production of thyroid hormone, it has been thought that dietary factors might be responsible for cases of simple goiter. Also, since simple goiter is most often seen in adolescent girls, endocrine factors have been suggested, and the fact that simple goiter seems to run in families suggests that genetically determined factors may play a role.

Nodular goiter

There is another kind of lump development in the thyroid which is not related to the presence of iodine. Single or multiple lumps (or nodules) may develop in an otherwise normal thyroid gland. Most often, such nodules occur in older individuals. Sometimes women who had thyroid enlargement as adolescents develop the nodules in their fifties and sixties. Many of the nodules, if examined under the microscope, strongly resemble the embryonic thyroid gland. Some produce no thyroid hormone; others produce no more per gram of tissue than the surrounding normal thyroid gland itself produces; and still others (known as *hyperfunctioning adenomas*) produce abnormally large quantities of thyroid hormone. In the latter event, the cells

Graves' disease (hyperthyroidism)

Overactivity of the thyroid (hyperthyroidism) is a disease which has many names and several forms. The most spectacular type is frequently known as *exophthalmic goiter* or *Graves' disease.* In the fully developed case, patients begin to notice increased nervousness and irritability, often crying over trivial incidents which previously they would have ignored. There is a great increase in appetite; food may be taken almost constantly throughout the day and part of the night. There may be a tendency toward insomnia or restless sleep. The heart beats rapidly and forcibly. Sometimes each beat visibly shakes the whole body. Despite increased intake of food, there is constant loss of weight. Perspiration increases, and the affected individual feels uncomfortably warm under circumstances which are pleasant for normal persons. The person wears a minimum of clothing, even in cold weather, and may still complain of the heat. The skin becomes hot, moist, and smooth, almost velvety. The nails are thin, concave, and may actually separate from the tissues of the finger or toe for some distance from their free margin. The hair becomes silky. A tremor is present. If the hands are extended from the body with the fingers spread, there is an uncontrollable trembling. As weight loss increases, weakness becomes pronounced, and the patient may be unable to rise from a chair without assistance.

One or both eyes may protrude from their sockets *(exophthalmos),* in serious cases to such a degree that the eyelids cannot be closed, and even in sleep the eyes may remain open. The lids and "white" of the eyes become puffy; the latter may become excessively dry and ulcerated. Because of the protrusion of the eyes, the face has the appearance of fright or anger.

The eye symptoms in patients with hyperthyroidism vary in degree from minimal to very severe exophthalmos. Fortunately, in most patients the eye symptoms are mild; they are characterized by a retraction of the lids, resulting in a stare or a wide-eyed look. The patient also may blink frequently. It is of interest that two other findings in Graves' disease, localized swelling and breast enlargement, are much more common in patients with severe exophthalmos than in those not so afflicted.

In these patients, the thyroid gland enlarges and the rate of blood flow through the organ is considerably increased. With the aid of a stethoscope, a whooshing noise can be heard therein in association with each heartbeat. The emotional stability may be seriously affected in some individuals. In advanced cases, there may be persistent diarrhea, and the output of urine may be small. In women with advanced hyperthyroidism, there may be enlargement of the breasts and the menses may cease.

Typically, the basal metabolic rate is elevated in patients with Graves' disease and the degree of elevation correlates with the severity of the syndrome of hyperthyroidism. The thyroid gland is usually two and one-half to four times the normal size. In extreme situations, it may be as much as ten or more times normal size. The *colloid* is usually completely lost and the thyroid *acinar cells* lose their normal appearance.

One or all of these signs and symptoms may be present. Furthermore, other diseases can be responsible for one or more of the symptoms. In fact, some of these symptoms may exist in perfectly healthy individuals. Prominent eyes, for example, may be nothing more than a family characteristic.

Most of the difficulty seen in Graves' disease

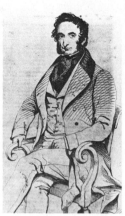

GRAVES, Robert James (1797-1853) Irish physician. In 1835, Graves gave the first satisfactory description of exophthalmic goiter. This disorder is now sometimes called Graves' disease. Exophthalmic goiter is a form of thyroid disorder marked by an enlargement of the thyroid gland, with an abnormal protrusion of the eyeballs. Symptoms include acceleration of the pulse, psychic disturbance, and increased basal metabolism. Graves is also credited with discarding the practice of starving fever patients.

can be traced directly to the abnormally high level of hormone circulating in the blood, or to some abnormality in the secretion itself. Everything is speeded up; more food is burned; more heat is produced; the sweat glands secrete faster; the heart beats faster; the muscles move faster; and the brain thinks faster. The human body, while capable of responding in emergencies, is not designed for continuous operation at the highest possible speed. It is hardly surprising, therefore, that unchecked hyperthyroidism materially shortens life, just as operating a gasoline motor or other mechanical device at peak rate will cause it to wear out more quickly.

The cause of hyperthyroidism is unknown; however, there does seem to be a genetic relationship involved. In one study of a group of relatives of patients suffering from Graves' disease, it was found that 50 percent of the relatives had a change in thyroid function. There is also the interesting fact that patients with this disorder often relate the beginning of their symptoms to major emotional or traumatic crises in their lives. It has yet to be proved that these factors are more than precipitating factors, or indeed that they are more than coincidental. Many endocrinologists believe, however, that Graves' disease is basically a familial condition in which the full-blown affliction is merely triggered into existence by emotional or physical stress.

An additional theory which as yet lacks any sound proof is that Graves' disease is somehow a manifestation of an autoimmune disorder in the body's defense system.

Treatment

Great progress has been made in the treatment of patients with Graves' disease in the past few years. The primary purpose of treat-

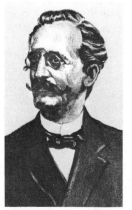

BAUMANN, Eugen (1846-1896) German physician and biochemist. He was the first man to demonstrate the presence in the thyroid gland of iodine in organic combination. Previous to this work it was recognized that iodine was deficient in the soil in areas where goiter was endemic, but the physiological role of iodine was unknown. Baumann's discovery in 1895 was followed by Kendall's isolation in 1914 of the iodine-containing thyroid hormone, thyroxin.

ment is to reduce the rate of production of thyroid hormone. In many patients, the overactivity of the thyroid gland can be controlled by treatment with antithyroid drugs or iodide. For others, removal of the thyroid gland is a practical and fairly simple operation; however, patients with hyperthyroidism are poor surgical risks unless certain steps are taken to control their disease before the thyroid gland is removed. Several such methods of control are now available to the surgeon. Treatment with iodine causes the thyroid activity to subside somewhat. Most of the symptoms mentioned, except for those involving the eyes, may be relieved either partially or completely, by the use of iodine. A few cases are known in which iodine is without any effect. The beneficial effects of iodine in this disease are not usually lasting. Therefore, there is often a limited time during which the patient so treated must be subjected to a more permanent treatment. If one waits too long, the disease may become active again in spite of continued iodine treatment, and surgery again becomes a risky procedure.

If the disease has not been permitted to run too long a course, the surgical removal of most, but not all, of the diseased thyroid gland usually results in restoration of good health and relief of symptoms. The eyes, however, may not return to normal. Usually, there is some improvement, although in many instances the eyes continue to bulge slightly when all other evidence of the disease has disappeared. Rarely, the eyes become worse in spite of treatment, and a separate procedure may be required in an attempt to restore them to their normal position.

It will be recalled that certain foodstuffs are known to produce goiter. The chemicals which are responsible for this action can be produced synthetically and may be useful in the treatment of patients with hyperthyroidism. These substances, *thiouracils*, have made possible improvement in the medical treatment of patients with Graves' disease during the past few years. A certain number of patients respond satisfactorily without the need of surgery; even those who do need surgical treatment can be much better prepared for their operations if these chemicals are given either separately or with iodine.

Radioactive iodine

The newest and most spectacular treatment for patients with hyperthyroidism is radioactive iodine. The rays which are discharged from the radioactive iodine atoms have the ability to kill living material under appropriate circumstances. If sufficient amounts of radioactive iodine are given to a patient with hyperthyroidism, many of the thyroid cells are thereby destroyed. After

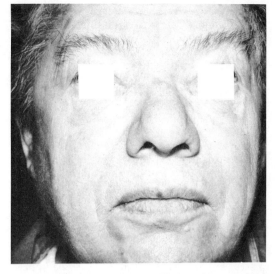

This photograph of a patient suffering with myxedema shows characteristic coarse features typical of this disorder and which give the impression that the patient is almost completely lacking in emotional response. *Courtesy Dr. J. B. Trunnell.*

oral ingestion, radioactive iodine reaches a concentration in the thyroid at least 10,000 times greater than in other tissues. Thus, great effect on the thyroid can be achieved without damage to surrounding structures. The patient will experience little inconvenience beyond a burning sensation in the throat which may persist for several days.

Treatment with radioactive iodine has become common since it was first used in 1942. However, it is customary in most treatment centers to limit radioiodine therapy to patients beyond the age of 25. Younger patients are treated surgically unless there are specific reasons to avoid an operation. For example, radioiodine is used in young patients who have complicating heart disease or who have had thyroid surgery in the past and in whom repeated operation might carry an added risk. In general, however, radioactive iodine treatment has found considerable use because of its simplicity and safety.

Hypothyroidism and myxedema

If for any reason the thyroid gland is absent, or is unable to produce adequate quantities of thyroid hormone, a condition known as hypothyroidism (or in its extreme form, myxedema) develops. Hypothyroid patients may be classified as having *adult myxedema, juvenile myxedema,* or *cretinism* (very young children). In many respects, this state is the opposite of that encountered in hyperthyroidism. A majority of the body tissues become infiltrated with a mucuslike fluid which causes puffiness of the skin and may even cause interference with the normal function of certain of the internal organs. The skin becomes excessively dry; the hair is brittle, falls out, and is difficult to comb or to curl; the fingernails are brittle; and the loose tissues of the face become characteristically puffy, with the result that the affected individual appears to be wearing a mask. The skin may become slightly tinged with yellow as a result of inability of the body to convert *carotene*, a yellow material present in vegetables, to vitamin A. Subsequently, the deficiency of vitamin A leads to roughening of the skin on certain areas of the body, notably those around the elbows. The tongue enlarges and in extreme cases prevents closure of the mouth. The vocal cords are affected in such a way as to produce a peculiar huskiness or hoarseness and deepening of the voice. The ability to think is usually not impaired, but the speed of thinking may be noticeably slowed. Patients with myxdema tire easily and usually feel sleepy most of the time. Instances are known in which sleep overcame the patient while taking a cold shower. Ordinarily, however, patients with myxedema avoid cold environments, inasmuch as their bodies produce less heat than the average person, so that they feel cold most of the time. This may be true even in warm weather.

Heavy clothing is preferred. There is an authentic record of a couple who were on the point of obtaining a divorce because the hus-

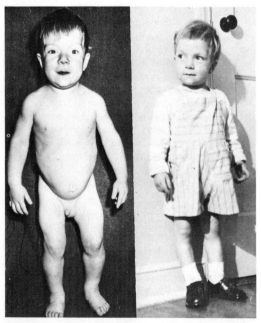

Photograph of a child suffering from cretinism as a result of congenital absence of thyroid gland. On right is same child after four months of therapy. *Courtesy Rita S. Finkler, M. D. Copyright Cyclopedia of Medicine, Surgery, F. A. Davis Co. 1950.*

band had hyperthyroidism and wanted no covers while in bed, while his wife had hypothyroidism and demanded several blankets. The divorce was averted by removing the man's thyroid gland and by administering dried thyroid substance by mouth to his wife. Each then became reasonably normal.

The heart may become enlarged, and in prolonged cases may fail as a result of interference with its normal function. As in the case of hyperthyroidism, there may be accentuation of already present mental weakness, in which case severe mental disturbances can occur. This type of mental illness is known as *myxedema madness* and can usually be overcome in a most dramatic fashion by the oral administration of dried thyroid substance obtained from cattle. Recently, synthetic thyroxine has been used in preference to thyroid extract. Occasionally, correction of the condition is brought about by triiodothyronine.

When hypothyroidism exists in early life, a disease state known as *cretinism* is produced. Many of the signs and symptoms described for the adult form of hypothyroidism appear, but in addition there is a remarkable stunting of growth and failure of development of mental processes beyond the age of two or three years. It is unfortunate that, unlike the adult form, treatment with dried thyroid material is not successful in reversing these latter alterations, unless the disease is recognized at an early age and treatment begun promptly. The increasing availability of radioactive iodine may eventually make the early testing and recognition of this disorder a simpler and surer procedure.

Juvenile myxedema differs from cretinism in that there is no permanent retardation of mental development. The disease begins in childhood—it is not present at birth. In most cases, it is attributable to destruction of the thyroid gland during the early years by unknown causes, but it sometimes is the result of failure to produce sufficient thyroid hormone as growth progresses.

Tumors of the thyroid

Some tumors of the thyroid are benign, while others are malignant. The term, benign, is applied to those tumors which, although they may grow to considerable size, do not spread to other parts of the body *(metastasize)*. Malignant tumors, or cancers, do have this ability to colonize elsewhere in the body.

Among the benign tumors, two further subdivisions may be recognized. Some do not produce unusually large quantities of thyroid hormone, whereas others do. Reference has already been made to the state of hyperthyroidism which can be produced by the latter. The tendency for some of the benign tumors to change into malignant tumors also is observed in the thyroid gland. Hence, it is usually recommended when a nodule or small tumor is discovered in the thyroid that the mass be removed surgically and examined under a microscope in order that its type be determined. If cancer is found to be present, a more extensive operation must be carried out.

There is a wide spectrum of activity or aggressiveness on the part of cancers arising in the thyroid gland. One of the least malignant and also one of the most malignant cancers affecting man may arise in this organ. Fortunately, the latter type is rare and a rather large number of patients with thyroid cancer live for long periods.

Although the reason is not known, it is unusual for patients with extensive thyroid cancer to have hyperthyroidism. A number of patients with thyroid cancer, however, have been studied carefully and have been found to contain literally several pounds of thyroid cancer tissue. Even under these circumstances, no hyperthyroidism existed until, in the course of treatment with radioactive iodine, the hormone which the cancer had been producing and storing was released to the circulating blood. These experiences suggest that thyroid cancer can produce hormone as does the normal thyroid but has difficulty in releasing the substance.

Cancer of the thyroid gland can occur at any age. There is a sudden increase in the rate of occurrence at about the time of puberty.

The best treatment for most types of thyroid cancer is early, thorough removal by surgery. If untreated, the spread of the tumor is limited for a time to the lymph nodes in the neck; secondary tumors may then appear in all tissues of the body, the lungs and bones being frequent sites. It is estimated that about 60 percent of cases treated by adequate surgical methods have no further trouble. X-ray and radium therapy also have been useful in some patients for suppressing the growth of those tumors which extend beyond the reach of surgery.

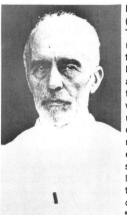

KOCHER, Emil Theodor (1841-1917) Swiss surgeon. The first to remove the thyroid gland as a treatment for thyrotoxic goiter in man. Kocher performed this operation on thousands of patients, at a time when it was regarded as one of the most difficult of surgical procedures, yet the mortality rate among his patients was extremely low. He also made significant studies on coagulation of the blood, and on the physiology and anatomy of the brain and nervous system.

Since 1940, radioactive iodine has been successful in partially and temporarily controlling certain secondary tumors from the thyroid. Radioactive iodine is of value because of the tendency of some forms of thyroid cancer to soak up the radioactive iodine atoms which are circulating in the blood after the patient has been given a drink of the material. Each atom then behaves as a tiny x-ray machine, operating directly inside the malignant tissue. The advantage of this type of treatment is that the skin overlying the cancer tissue does not need to be damaged by x-rays as they pass from the x-ray tube to the interior of the body en route to the tumor cells. Consequently, much larger doses of radiant energy can be delivered to the tumor cells without damage to normal tissues. The goal of cancer treatment is "selective damage," i.e., death of cancer cells and no injury to noncancer cells. However, this type of treatment must be restricted to selected types of cancer, since normal thyroid cells also soak up the radioactive atoms. Therefore, a number of serious difficulties remain to be worked out. The percentage of cases actually benefited remains small.

Thyroiditis

Essentially, every tissue of the body is susceptible to inflammatory infection. The thyroid gland is no exception. *Thyroiditis* is the name given to the inflammation of this gland regardless of the mechanism involved. As in the case of most inflammatory processes, there are pain and tenderness in the tissues affected. In acute cases, the usual signs and symptoms of infection are also present; these include chills and fever, perspiration, generalized weakness, and malaise.

If the infection has been caused by a germ which is susceptible to one of the modern drugs, the treatment of patients with thyroiditis is relatively simple. The majority of patients with thyroiditis are thought to suffer from infection by small viruslike particles which are not harmed by such agents as penicillin, aureomycin, etc. This common type of thyroiditis occasionally gives evidence of being contagious.

The best treatment appears to be administration of a substance called *prednisone*, a compound related to the hormones of the adrenal cortex. The swelling of the gland is often quickly relieved and with it the discomfort which the patient experienced before treatment. Hydrocortisone, ACTH, and a small amount of x-ray therapy may also be used.

There are several noninfectious diseases of the thyroid which are not well understood. Among these are Hashimoto's struma and Riedel's struma. Hashimoto's struma, which is seen more frequently than Riedel's struma, usually occurs before middle life and affects women much more frequently than men. The gland becomes moderately enlarged and has been compared in consistency to the granular structure of an apple. The process often requires a long time to develop, but the eventual effect may be destruction of the thyroid gland followed by hypothyroidism. Administration of desiccated or synthetic thyroid substance may cause the enlargement to subside remarkably. There is usually no interference with breathing; hence, surgical removal is unnecessary unless there are pressure symptoms or the enlargement is very unattractive.

Riedel's struma, or Riedel's thyroiditis, usually occurs after middle life and is found chiefly in middle-aged women. Its cause is unknown. The effect on the thyroid gland is one of great disorganization and destruction of the functional architecture which was described earlier. Somehow, the thyroid manages in spite of the destruction to produce enough hormone to prevent the average person from developing serious hypothyroidism or myxedema. The gland may become sufficiently enlarged, however, to cause pressure on the windpipe, thereby necessitating removal of most of it.

Recent progress in the understanding of the thyroid gland has been rapid. The organ has been and is being studied intensively, not only for a better understanding of its own activities, but also to gain knowledge of how other endocrine organs influence those activities. Lessons learned in the study of this gland have often been of value in understanding diseases of entirely different organs.

THE PARATHYROIDS

The parathyroid glands in man, although four in number, have a combined size scarcely greater than that of a large pea. Nevertheless, their removal is followed by death unless proper treatment is given.

Normally, the parathyroid glands are adherent to, or even imbedded within, the back part of the thyroid gland. All of these structures lie in the lower front portion of the neck. The main purpose of the parathyroid glands appears to be their secretion of one or more hormones which are responsible for the maintenance of normal concentrations of calcium and phosphorus in many of the body tissues. If there is insufficient parathyroid hormone, the concentration of calcium in the blood becomes too low; this causes a condition called *tetany*, the symptoms of which are a type of muscle spasm and convulsion, together with other body changes which will be described later. If there is too much parathyroid hormone, the level of calcium in the

body fluids increases greatly. Since this extra calcium has been withdrawn from the bones, the latter structures become soft and can no longer maintain the body in a sufficiently rigid condition for normal functioning. This disease is known as *osteitis fibrosa*, and is usually caused by a functioning tumor of the parathyroids. If the serum concentration of calcium is consistently too high, masses of calcium (stones) may be deposited in tissues. These are particularly dangerous in the kidney where they cause obstruction and hemorrhage leading eventually to kidney failure.

Infrequently, there are either more or fewer than the standard four parathyroid glands. Occasionally, though, these are not all in the usual location, some of them being as far away as the upper part of the chest. Should one of the tissues in this latter location become overactive it may be difficult for the surgeon to find it and to remove it.

How the parathyroid works

Most (99 percent) of the calcium in the body is deposited in the bones, giving them their characteristic hardness and rigidity. It is combined there with phosphorous and other minerals. There is, however, a certain amount of calcium in the blood and other body fluids, and ordinarily this level is stable. Every 100 cc of blood contains between 9.5 and 10.5 thousandths of a gram of calcium and about four thousandths of a gram of phosphorus. In the average healthy individual, these values change little throughout life. The parathyroid hormone and one other appear to be chiefly responsible for preserving this finely balanced equilibrium.

The controlled secretion of a hormone from the parathyroid glands (called, simply, parathyroid hormone) is partly responsible for maintaining the constant normal level of blood calcium. This hormone brings about an elevation of blood calcium by two mechanisms: (1) it causes bone to release calcium into the blood stream and (2) it causes the kidney to increase the excretion of phosphate, thereby indirectly raising the blood calcium level by decreasing the blood phosphate concentration.

Another hormone, calcitonin or thyrocalcitonin, is released when the calcium level in blood passing through the thyroid and parathyroid glands is high. This second hormone lowers blood calcium and blocks the action of the first parathyroid hormone.

In other words, the calcium level in the blood is controlled by a feedback mechanism. Passage through the parathyroid of blood low in calcium brings about the release of parathyroid hormone, which acts to increase the calcium level, as described. When blood high in calcium passes through the glands, calcitonin (thyrocalcitonin) is released, resulting in a lowering of blood calcium content.

The second hormone is a product of the thyroid gland. When the hormone was first found in 1961, it was believed to originate in the parathyroid. However, subsequent research has shown that passage of blood high in calcium through the thyroid elicits the same release of hormone. Whatever the source, its mechanism of action in regulating the level of calcium is clear.

Diseases of the parathyroid gland

Hypoparathyroidism: The term hypoparathyroidism means subnormal parathyroid function. Rarely, the condition may occur in newborn infants as a result of hemorrhage which partially destroys the parathyroid gland. It is most common in adults who have undergone surgical removal of these tissues as an occasional consequence of removal of diseased thyroid tissue.

If the parathyroids are completely removed, tetany occurs quite rapidly. The most common symptom is a tightening and a spasm of the muscles, most evident in the position assumed by the fingers and toes. The name *carpopedal spasm* has been applied to inability to straighten the fingers and toes. There is usually considerable apprehension in the form of a sense of impending doom or disaster. There may be difficulty in inhalation, spasm of muscles in the larynx (voice box), vomiting, and abdominal pain. Injection of a solution of calcium will cause all of the symptoms to cease temporarily within less than a minute. There are other medications which are used to maintain such individuals at a normal calcium balance indefinitely. One of these is the parathyroid hormone. There are other substances which can be taken indefinitely. One of these is known as *A.T. 10 (antitetanic substances 10)*. A few drops a day, together with a slightly increased calcium content of the diet, will suffice to maintain most patients who have been deprived of their parathyroid glands. More recently, *vitamin D₂* has been found to provide the same benefits at a lower cost.

It is usually important to pay attention to the dietary intake of phosphorus, which should be as low as possible. The main foods to be avoided are dairy products. These same foods are the best sources of calcium. Many patients, therefore, require supplementary calcium in the form of tablets.

Hyperparathyroidism: The term, hyperparathyroidism, implies that excessive quantities of parathyroid hormone are being introduced into the body fluids of the patient. The condition is known as *von Recklinghausen's disease or osteitis fibrosa cystica.* The usual cause for the condition is the development of a small benign tumor (*adenoma*) in one of the parathyroid glands. Not only are there more parathyroid cells than are required, but these cells secrete more parathyroid hormone than the body can accommodate. Calcium is withdrawn from the bones, a fact which explains the high levels seen in the blood. There is usually some deformity or bowing of the bones. The muscles become weak and ineffective. Bones may break easily as a result of slight jarring or twisting. X-rays of such patients indicate an unusual transparency of most of the bones. Areas of extra calcium deposits or stones may be seen in the skin, muscles, kidneys, and many other tissues as well. Perhaps the greatest danger in this disease results from the obstruction and interference with kidney function by such stones. Unless these patients are treated adequately, a series of complications—weakness, loss of appetite, poor nutrition, infection and loss of kidney function—will result in a fatal outcome. If the diagnosis is made early, however, removal of the adenoma will cause most of the symptoms to disappear.

Occasionally there is no tumor, but only a uniform enlargement of one or all of the parathyroid glands. Under these conditions, removal of all affected tissue must be carried out, and the patient will then require treatment with vitamin D₂ and calcium, as described under the section about hypoparathyroidism.

Cancer of the parathyroid gland is exceedingly rare. Surgery is the preferred form of treatment if it can be instituted early in the course of the disease.

THE GONADS

Gonad is the name applied to the ovary of the female and the testis of the male. Not only are they the fundamental organs of reproduction, but they also produce several hormones as well. The two testes are made up of tissues that specialize in producing the male germ cells and tissues that manufacture the male hormone. The two ovaries provide the egg (*ovum*) and several hormones that are involved in the regulation of sexual function. Because the ovaries and testes produce hormones, they are considered endocrine glands. Collectively, these male and female hormones are called *gonadal* hormones.

The hormones produced by the ovaries are called "female hormones." The name female or male hormone does not imply that these substances are produced exclusively by either sex, but that they are produced predominantly by one sex. Thus, certain structures in males, especially the adrenals, can and do produce female hormones that are excreted in the urine. Women also produce male hormones, and in some instances, where the balance is disturbed by disease, the effects of overproduction of male hormone become evident. In such instances, women develop signs of masculinity. Changes in gonadal structure and tissues can cause changes in the functioning of the organs. For example, radiation to the ovaries or testes can lessen or completely destroy the ability of these organs to produce hormones.

The anatomy, much of the physiology, and the diseases of the reproductive system are discussed in Chapter 15, "The Reproductive System." The discussion in this chapter is limited to the endocrinological aspects of the gonads.

Functions of the hormones

Sex hormones act primarily upon the reproductive system, which in both men and women is made up of the gonads and the accessory or secondary sex organs. The proper development and functioning of the accessory sex organs are dependent upon the production of sex hormones. In women the accessory sex organs are the breast, the womb (*uterus*), Fallopian tubes, vagina, vulva, and clitoris; each serves a particular function in the complex process of reproduction. In men the secondary or accessory sex organs are represented by a series of tubes, or ducts, that convey the germ cells from the testes through the penis to the outside of the body, plus several glands located at different points. These glands are the prostate glands, the seminal vesicles, and Cowper's glands. Again, each performs a particular function, and each is dependent on the male hormone for its proper functioning. Castration results in a decrease in size of all these structures, and eventually they cease to function. This effect is the result of removing the source of male hormone.

Secondary sex characteristics

Male and female hormones are poured into the blood like all other hormones, and exert different actions on different parts of the body, imparting qualities that are typical of each sex. Thus, the distribution of hair on the body, particularly pubic hair, varies greatly. In women pubic hair often is limited above by a horizontal line, and the hair may grow in a triangular zone. In men the growth of pubic hair may extend from the navel to the anus. The hair on other parts of the body, namely the face, chest, legs, and arms, is more abundant in men. The female voice is high pitched, and the larynx is less developed than in the male. Other qualities, such as breast development, shape of the pelvis, and

distribution of fat, are also different in the sexes as a result of different sex hormone production.

Extraction of hormones

Both male and female sex hormones belong to the group of chemical substances called *steroids* to which also belong the hormones produced by the adrenal cortex. Steroids are naturally occurring substances that are found largely in vegetable oils, from which they can be extracted in pure form. The steroids obtained from these reasonably cheap sources serve as raw materials for the synthesis of several hormones. Some of the female sex hormones, however, are still obtained from animal sources by means of extensive and complicated extraction procedures.

Pregnant women excrete large quantities of certain sex hormones in their urine. In the past, urine from pregnant women was used as a source of a female sex hormone (*estrone*). Pregnant mares also eliminate large amounts of estrone in their urine, which now is used as a major source of that substance. It is indeed fortunate that the sex hormones produced by animals are identical with those produced by human beings, because this allows sufficient quantities of these rare substances to be available for research and for the treatment of patients. In the last few years, urine obtained from postmenopausal women has been utilized on an industrial scale to obtain a hormone that stimulates the gonads. It is called "human menopausal gonadotrophin."

The male gonads: testes

The endocrine function of the testes has been recognized for centuries, although unexplained; animals have long been castrated in order to tame them or to modify their flesh and increase its value as foodstuff. In 1849, the German scientist Arnold Adolf Berthold experimented with chickens and observed that castrated cocks will not undergo the typical changes that follow castration if the testes are implanted in other parts of the body. By so doing, he demonstrated that the testes produce a substance which is responsible for maintaining the male characteristics.

The discovery did not impress many scientists until 20 years later when the famous French physician Charles Edouard Brown-Séquard, at the age of 72 injected himself with extracts of testes. He reported that he felt younger and more active. His report may have been colored by his own fantasy, but the fact remains that his experiment stimulated scientists all over the world to investigate the nature of this mysterious substance. Finally, the male hormone (androgen) was isolated in pure form in 1935 and named testosterone. Later, other hormones were found in the urine and were also isolated in pure form, but their potency was much less than the potency of testosterone obtained from the testes.

The quantity of hormone present either in testes or urine is so small that it requires gallons of urine or many pounds of testes to isolate a few grains of pure material. The potency of these substances is so great that extremely minute quantities suffice to elicit amazing effects. However, male hormone is constantly being produced in certain cells of the testes, poured into the blood stream, and delivered to other parts of the body. The levels of hormone concentration in blood are minute and relatively constant, because as new male hormone enters the blood, some is excreted in the urine. In the liver, the male hormone is converted into other compounds with less potency. Thus the liver helps to maintain a proper balance; when the liver is diseased, as in cirrhosis, hormone imbalance in the male can result in breast enlargement and loss of sperm production.

Some endocrinologists believe that the testicular system secretes another hormone, inhibin, which acts on the pituitary gland to control the release of gonadotrophic hormone which, in turn, causes the testes to make testosterone. This would fit the concept of feedback control for amount of testosterone produced; however, the existence of such a substance has not been established.

The male sex hormone is produced after complete development of the testes. At puberty, the secondary sexual characteristics make their appearance rapidly. There are wide variations in the age of onset, duration, and the sequence of the events that characterize the biological pattern of male puberty. In normal boys, signs of puberty may appear at any age between 10 and 17 years. The average age of onset is 12 to 13 years. Once initiated, the major changes are usually completed or well-advanced in three to four years; in a small percentage of normal persons, adult maturity is not attained until the age of 21.

The sequence of events that marks the pubertal period is initiated by an acceleration in the growth of the testes and scrotum. Following this, there is an increase in the size of the penis, the appearance of pubic hair, and gradual enlargement of the prostate and other accessory organs and glands. Concomitantly, an acceleration of growth takes place in the skeleton and muscles. The adolescent growth spurt is completed in about three years and, in boys, accounts for an average increment in height of about 8 inches (4 to 12 inches) and a gain in weight of about 40 pounds.

Occasionally, maturation is delayed beyond the age of 17 years. Although this is not usually a health problem, it may be a severe psychological handicap to a young man and a source of anxiety to his parents. In such an event, a physician may elect to use medical treatment to speed the maturation process.

A related problem in the development of sexual characteristics in boys is *cryptorchidism,* or undescended testes. This problem is discussed in Chapter 15 in the section on the male organs of reproduction.

The reverse phenomenon, early sexual development or sexual precocity, occurs three times more frequently in girls than in boys. The main cause of this in boys is tumors; these may be cerebral (affecting the pituitary), adrenocortical, testicular, or nonendocrine hormone-secreting tumors. The tumors cause the untimely release of testosterone, and precocious puberty begins. The help of a physician should be obtained to determine the cause of precocious sexual development. In some cases, treatment is needed.

In instances when the output of male hormone is excessive, symptoms develop that are usually the opposite of the symptoms elicited by an insufficient output of hormone. It is believed that in adults, excessive hormone may be reflected in an excessive sexual drive and exaggerated masculine body characteristics. There is little reason to believe that female homosexual tendencies are produced by excesses of male hormone.

When the output of male hormone is less than normal, a condition known as hypogonadism develops. A patient who is of adolescent age or younger may develop symptoms characterized by effeminate traits and retarded development of the sexual organs. There will be scant growth of facial hair and a female distribution of pubic hair. In men who have attained maturity, the signs of androgen deficiency are less conspicuous. The most common events are reduction in prostatic size, diminished growth of the beard and body hair, the appearance of fine wrinkles around the eyes, and a pasty, sallow complexion. Also, semen volume is reduced.

A common form of hypogonadism is known as Klinefelter's syndrome. Feminine characteristics and infertility may exist. Patients with this condition are often tall with disproportionately long lower extremities. Mental retardation and psychopathic behavior are not uncommon, and men with this syndrome are often poorly adapted socially.

In 1956, it was discovered that Klinefelter's syndrome is the result of a genetically determined defect. Treatment for patients with Klinefelter's syndrome must be closely supervised by a physician, as the use of hormones is usually involved.

In the male, with age, sexual activity declines gradually. The "change of life" or climacteric in men is not as conspicuous as it is in women, and the age at which it occurs varies over a wider range. At the time of the male climacteric, sexual activity declines to a low level. The changes that follow this stage of a man's life are mostly changes in temperament, but there are other changes related to the blood vessels. Men can be helped in the transition from an active to an inactive sexual life by the administration of small doses of testosterone; however, the need for such help is generally not great.

Tumors of the testes are uncommon. The greatest incidence occurs in men in their twenties and thirties. The most common testicular tumor is called seminoma. Generally, this tumor is relatively slow growing and responds well to radiotherapy. Other tumors of 'the testes may grow more quickly and may require surgical removal.

The female gonads: ovaries

The ovaries are two almond-shaped organs, one of which is located on each side of the womb. Each is about the size of a walnut. They were recognized long ago and believed to be "female testes."

The ovaries, unlike the testes, produce several hormones. These are called by different names, but grouped together under the term "female sex hormones" because they are chiefly, but not exclusively, produced in the female. The female hormones regulate various functions of the body, but their major duty is regulation of the female reproductive system. The sexual characteristics of women, such as body shape, development of

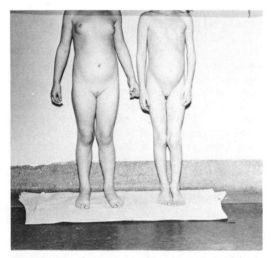

Of these two five-year-old girls, the one at right is normal, while the one at left shows premature sexual development resulting from an ovarian tumor. Surgical removal restored her to normalcy. *Courtesy George J. Hamwi, Ohio State University.*

breasts, distribution of hair, voice, etc., are controlled by some of the female sex hormones. In the regulation of the menstrual cycle in women, all of the ovarian hormones participate, in addition to some of the hormones from the pituitary gland. Two chemically determined types of ovarian hormones are: the estrogenic steroids or *estrogens* (*estradiol, estrone,* etc.) and *progestagens* (*progesterone,* etc.). Within recent years, it has been possible to produce these hormones synthetically.

The control that ovarian hormones exert upon the reproductive system is not limited to the accessory or secondary sex organs—i.e., the womb, Fallopian tubes, vagina, vulva, and clitoris. In an indirect sense, the ovaries themselves are affected by their own secretions, since a reciprocal ovary-pituitary relationship is of importance in the regulation of the ovaries. The maturation of the eggs, ovulation, and other changes that occur in the ovaries are dependent, then, to some degree, on the hormones from the ovaries.

The sexual cycle in women is well-regulated as long as the production and secretion of both the gonadotrophic hormones of the pituitary gland and the sex hormones from the ovaries are normal. This happens most of the time, but occasionally the pituitary gland, the ovaries, or both may vary in their production of hormones. When the pituitary gland becomes underactive as a result of disease, the production of all the pituitary homones is affected. Among those hormones are included those that stimulate the growth of the ovaries and regulate their function. In the absence of a sufficient quantity of sex hormones from the pituitary gland, the ovaries will not grow properly, and they will produce insufficient amounts of ovarian hormones. The result of hormone deficiency is eventually reflected in a series of disturbances in various parts of the body. The most notable disturbance is in the menstrual cycle. In adult women, the menstrual flow may cease as a result of insufficient hormone production, or it may become irregular. In girls, puberty may be delayed considerably, and the development of their accessory sex organs may be retarded or arrested. Underdevelopment of the breasts is often the result of insufficient production of hormones. Sometimes the breast may be insensitive to the hormones and fail to respond.

The ovaries can also become overactive and produce larger than normal quantities of hormones. The overactivity of the ovaries may be the result of an excessive production of hormones from the pituitary gland. In some instances, the production of gonadotrophic hormones from the pituitary may be premature, and as a result, the ovaries mature early in life. Children affected by this form of precocious puberty may become fertile at an unusually early

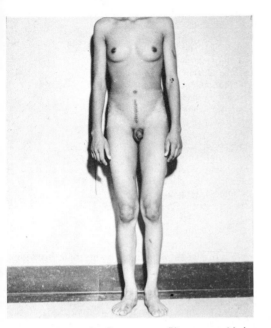

This true hermaphrodite was a fifteen-year-old boy whose gonads contained both male and female parts. Normal male characteristics were restored by surgical removal of the ovarian tissue. *Courtesy of George J. Hamwi, Ohio State University.*

age. A case was known in a small Peruvian village where a girl of five years and eight months gave birth to a healthy and apparently normal child. This mother had *Albright's syndrome*. Characteristics of this disorder include bone disorders, patches of brown pigment on the skin, and true sexual precocity.

Ninety percent of girls with sexual precocity have the type caused by early production of hormones. However, any girl who is sexually precocious should be examined by a physician so that any possibility of a brain tumor or rare ovarian or adrenal disease can be excluded.

In adult women, overproduction of sex hormones from the ovaries results in many conditions that affect mostly, but not exclusively, the accessory sex organs. The breasts are also sensitive to the action of hormones from the ovaries and respond to some of the hormones by increasing in size. At puberty, the breasts become larger and in most women remain so throughout life. A more detailed discussion of the breasts and the manner in which they are affected by puberty, pregnancy, and lactation may be found in Chapter 16, "The Breast."

Ovulation

The ovaries of young females contain innumerable little "nests," each a potential source of an egg. At birth, there are nearly half a million such nests in the ovaries, but the number decreases with age. The eggs develop from these nests in a series of stages until they reach full maturity and are ready to be discharged. While the egg is undergoing all these changes, the nest becomes a blister which is relatively large. Such blisters were recognized as early as the seventeenth century by the Dutch physician, de Graaf, who described them, and they now bear his name (*Graafian follicles*). When the egg has fully matured, the follicle ruptures and the egg is released; this process is called *ovulation*. The egg is then conveyed from the ovary to the Fallopian tube.

At some stage in the process of egg maturation, some special cells inside the follicle begin to produce one of the estrogens. This substance is poured into the blood stream and conveyed to all the organs of the body. The estrogen acts upon the pituitary to augment other hormones produced by the pituitary, called gonadotrophins. There are several gonadotrophins, one of which stimulates the follicles, but only those follicles that have been rendered sensitive by the action of estrogen. The process occurs in women approximately once a month; and usually only one follicle is affected by the hormone from the pituitary, so that only one egg—in rare occasions, two eggs—reaches maturity in a month. Thus, the ovary by producing various hormones controls the process involved in the maturation of the egg and the final release from the follicle.

This is only part of the sexual cycle in women, however, and other events occur following the

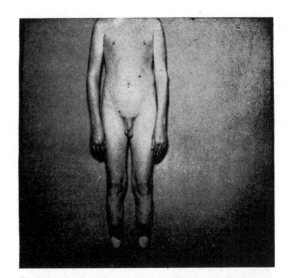

Photograph of a 19-year-old boy whose growth stopped at 14 years due to the presence of a pituitary tumor. Normal body hair is largely absent. The tumor caused a serious deficiency of thyroid and sex hormones. *Photograph by courtesy of Dr. George J. Hamwi, Ohio State University.*

rupture of the follicle. Conditions are different if the egg is fertilized, and changes in the uterus are necessary for it to maintain the fertilized ovum. If the ovum is not fertilized, it disintegrates and a new cycle begins. This cycle occurs with singular regularity, and its control is largely the result of hormonal action.

Other hormones become predominant after ovulation, and they finish the task initiated by the estrogens. These hormones are produced by cells of the "yellow body" or corpus luteum, which is the endocrine structure that develops like a scar in the ovary in the site of the ruptured follicle, after the egg has been released. The corpus luteum is stimulated by a second hormone from the pituitary gland to manufacture both estrogen and a second hormone called *progestin* (*progesterone*), sometimes called the pregnancy hormone.

Progesterone is most important during pregnancy, but it also has some valuable functions in the preparation of the uterus to receive the fertilized egg. Progesterone is presumably produced to some extent even before the egg has been released from the follicle, which is in the middle of the menstrual cycle. At this time, progesterone acts on the uterus, which undergoes a series of changes that will be discussed later. The changes in the womb condition the walls so that they are capable of holding the fertilized egg and furnish the necessary nourishment. If the egg is not fertilized it will not be retained by the womb; then, the corpus luteum in the ovary disintegrates. Menstruation follows, and a new cycle begins.

If pregnancy occurs, progesterone acts to protect the embryo. Abortion may result in the first three or four months of pregnancy if the corpus luteum is damaged. If progesterone is injected into a pregnant woman who is threatened with abortion, pregnancy is often prolonged, and the birth of a premature child may be averted in some instances.

The breasts of the pregnant woman are stimulated by both estrogen and progesterone action. They become well-developed and conditioned so that they are capable of secreting milk. Both estrogen and progesterone affect ovulation and menstruation and prepare the various accessory reproductive organs for a successful pregnancy. Thus, the most outstanding events in the female cycle, ovulation and menstruation, are regulated in large measure by both pituitary and ovarian hormones. Many irregularities in the cycle are the results of disturbances in the hormonal balance, which can have many causes.

The most important hormones produced by the ovaries, estrogen and progesterone, are not limited in their action to the regulation of the sexual cycle. They exert other effects in other parts of the body. Estrogens are responsible for the development of the secondary sexual charac-

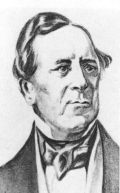

RATHKE, Martin H. (1793-1860) German anatomist. Known best for his early description of the pituitary gland, the small organ which is, to use Cushing's apt image, "the conductor of the endocrine orchestra." Other organs to which Rathke's name has been given, include a portion of a paramesonephric duct which may persist after birth, and the craniobuccal pouch in the embryo which ultimately forms the anterior lobe of the hypophysis in the child.

teristics of the female. Just as the male hormone tends to masculinize, estrogen tends to feminize the individual. The hormone is partly destroyed by the liver when it passes through the organ and partly converted to other compounds, which eventually are excreted in the urine. Consequently, the level maintained in the body is usually fairly constant.

Several of the estrogens have been made available to the physician in suitable preparations that are used on many occasions. Injections of estrogens in men repress the function of the testes and the formation of male hormone, which in turn controls the growth of the prostate gland and all other structures of the male reproductive system. On the basis of this knowledge, estrogens are given to patients suffering from cancer of the prostate gland in order to diminish their pain and actually reduce the size of the tumor. Patients undergoing this treatment may become impotent; if the doses are large, their mammary glands may enlarge sometimes to the size of the female mammary glands. However, this condition disappears immediately just as soon as the hormone therapy is discontinued.

The menstrual cycle

The sexual cycle in women is a more or less regular occurrence punctuated approximately every 28 days by *menstruation*. Menstruation is the name applied to the process of discharging the lining of the womb after disintegration; it normally occurs from puberty to menopause except when pregnancy intervenes. The lining of the womb (*endometrium*) is a mucous membrane that is constantly changing from a thin membrane into a thicker, more glandular type of structure that eventually may serve as a nest for the fertilized egg. At the end of the sexual cycle, if conception has not taken place, the endometrium degenerates, the blood vessels undergo changes, and menstruation ensues.

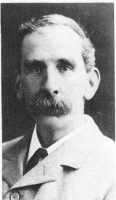

HORSLEY, Victor A. H. (1857-1916) English surgeon. Contributed to the development of neurosurgery and surgery of the endocrine glands. His experimental surgery showed the causal relationship of thyroid deficiency to cretinism and myxedema (1884). In 1886 he cut away some cerebral cortex in a successful treatment for traumatic epilepsy, and in 1888 with the Englishman, Gowers, he effectively removed a tumor from the spinal column.

In some societies menstruation has been the subject of much superstition and fear. The ancients ascribed the regularity of appearance of the menstrual flow to the planets because the menstrual cycle corresponds to that of the moon, and even believed that menstruation was evil. The menstruating woman was the object of scorn and fear, and sexual intercourse was avoided on the basis of superstition. Today, the attitude towards menstruation has changed, although many mistaken ideas remain. Menstruation is a normal and healthy physiological process, albeit somewhat inconvenient.

The lining of the womb is sensitive to the action of sex hormones produced by the ovary, which in turn is sensitive to some of the hormones of the pituitary gland. Sex hormones regulate menstruation, and the entire sexual cycle in women is regulated by a complex hormonal mechanism of checks and balances.

The menstrual cycle is the time interval which extends from the onset of one period of uterine bleeding to the onset of the following period. The menstrual cycle is divided into several stages which are determined by the condition of the *endometrium*, or lining of the womb. The first part of the cycle, the period of menstruation or actual bleeding, usually last about 5 days, although this varies in individuals. When the menstrual discharge ceases, the second stage begins in which the lining of the womb increases in thickness. This second period is called the proliferative or growing stage and lasts for approximately 7 to 10 days. Ovulation occurs at the end of the second period and before the start of the third period. The third period of the cycle is called the *secretory* or *progestational* stage and extends over the last 12 to 14 days of the cycle. The changes in the lining of the womb are controlled by the ovarian hormones. The lining during this period contains actively-secreting glands, many thick folds, and an increased blood supply. The uterus is now ready to receive a fertilized egg. However, if a fertilized egg is not implanted in the uterus, the uterine lining disintegrates and menstruation occurs again.

At about the 14th day before the beginning of the menstrual flow the egg is discharged from the ovary (*ovulation*). At the time of ovulation, the changes in the uterus (now in the secretory stage) depend upon the action of estrogen and a *progestogen* called *progesterone*. Progesterone is produced by the "shell" from which the egg erupted in the ovary, the *corpus luteum*. As stated, progesterone prepares the uterine wall for pregnancy, by conditioning the cells to hold the fertilized egg and furnish the necessary nourishment. If pregnancy does not occur, the corpus luteum in the ovary disintegrates and the production of progesterone ceases. If pregnancy does not occur, the corpus luteum in the ovary disintegrates and the production of progesterone ceases. If pregnancy does occur, the placenta also gradually acquires the ability to produce progesterone, thereby aiding the corpus luteum of pregnancy in this task. During the entire period of development of the embryo, the process of menstruation is, of course, inhibited.

If pregnancy does not occur, the production of estrogens is reduced soon after the egg has been delivered to the tube. The estrogen in the blood falls to low levels; the lining of the uterus receives no stimulus and begins to become thinner; the blood circulation slows considerably in this region; and later the blood vessels contract for a few hours. Following this contraction, the vessels dilate, and bleeding begins.

The menstrual blood is not like ordinary blood although it is similar. The main difference is that menstrual blood does not clot as readily as ordinary blood, but clots are not rare. The flow lasts three to seven days in most women, but there are great variations depending on the individual. The menstrual flow appears every 27 or 28 days, but again there is considerable variation in different women. It varies anywhere from every 18 days to as long as every 35 to 40 days. In rare instances, the cycle may be even longer. The relationship of the various phases of the menstrual and ovulatory cycle to female fertility and sterility is discussed at length in Chapter 15, "The Reproductive System."

The amount of blood lost during menstruation can sometimes be significant. It may be the cause of anemia in some women because the amount of iron lost is greater than that taken in the ordinary diet; hence, there is need for medical observation and medication.

Usually, some personality and bodily changes precede the menstrual flow. The breasts become firmer, heavier, and somewhat tender. Menstruation affects the nervous system to some degree; and the nervous system, in turn, can alter menstrual habits considerably. Nervous stimulation is a major factor in modern times when women participate in nearly all types of activities and are exposed constantly to the many vicissitudes of modern life. The tensions of the premenstrual period can often be eased or removed with diuretics, drugs which bring about a temporary reduction in stored fluid of the body. Fear, particularly fear of pregnancy when pregnancy is not desired, is a common cause of menstrual irregularities. An intense desire to become pregnant may also delay menstruation. Under emotional strain, a woman may fail to menstruate. Anger, worries, and other emotional states are known to delay menstruation. In other instances, menstrual irregularities may be the result of disease, in which case the physician must ascertain the cause.

Menstrual disorders are common, and sometimes it is difficult to decide what is a disorder and what is not. If for no particular reason a woman who menstruates regularly fails to do so, or if menstruation becomes painful, scant, or profuse, she should seek medical advice. However, if the menstrual flow has never appeared regularly, a delay of several days usually has little or no significance.

Pain in menstruation

Occasionally menstruation is accompanied by pain. The condition of painful menstruation, *menorrhalgia* (also called *dysmenorrhea*), is not to be confused with the normal discomfort in the pelvis that usually accompanies menstruation. The essential cause of pain is excessive tension in the womb or contractions of the womb to expel the torn lining. The pain in the womb has also been ascribed to a deficient supply of blood to the womb during menstruation. The causes vary greatly and may be an anatomical malformation, such as an underdeveloped womb, or disturbances in hormone balance, in which case the patient may respond well to treatment with various hormone preparations. The pain occurs only at the time of menstruation and is localized in the lower abdomen but may extend to the back and down the legs. The patient may become irritable, suffer headaches, and feel uncomfortable. In cases of excessive pain, nausea and vomiting may ensue. When the pain is tolerable, the patient usually carries on her daily duties but takes mild drugs to soothe her pain and relieve the contractions of the womb. The pain, however, may be severe, and the patient may become bedridden for several days.

To alleviate the pain, the doctor ascertains the underlying cause and administers accordingly. Hormone therapy to prevent ovulation temporarily will often prevent the pain of menstruation. A fullterm pregnancy frequently corrects most of the irregularities of menstruation.

Other disorders

Painful menstruation is only one of several disorders that are associated with the menstrual flow. Occasionally, the bleeding becomes scant or ceases to appear altogether in women that have previously menstruated; or sometimes menstruation fails to appear in the adolescent girl. This condition is called *amenorrhea,* but the term includes also the disorder characterized by unusually long intervals between periods. The cause in both cases may be associated with an underdeveloped womb and ovaries, or may be the result of other diseases like anemia or tuberculosis. Malnutrition and "reducing diets" lead to all types of nutritional deficiencies that can cause amenorrhea. Like many disorders associated with the menstrual cycle, amenorrhea may respond well to a change in habits from sedentary to out-of-door activities; physical exercises to develop the muscular and circulatory systems are also helpful.

Excessive flow of blood or frequent bleeding is an abnormal condition and is associated with disturbances in the reproductive or endocrine system. Often the bleeding becomes so profuse that anemia may follow if the condition is not controlled. Abnormal functioning of the thyroid gland is sometimes the cause of this condition, and good response is obtained by correcting the function of the thyroid gland by means of hormone preparations. In other cases, bleeding results from nervous stimulation, fright, fatigue, tumors, cancer of uterus or ovaries, etc. A careful examination by the doctor will establish the underlying cause of this condition which may not only be annoying, but may also be the cause of ill health and a symptom of more severe underlying disturbances.

The menopause

The *menopause* is that period in a woman's life when ovarian function declines to a low level. At this time, menstrual and reproductive functions also lessen and eventually cease. The average age of a woman in the "change of life," as it is also called, is 47 years. However, it may occur anywhere between 30 and 55 years of age. In some cases, the menopause is induced artificially—either by surgery or x-rays—for various diseased conditions.

The period of the menopause lasts from six months to three years, depending upon the individual. In general, this is a period of readjustment which must be made within the woman's body as a result of the decline of ovarian function. The first notable change is concerned with menstruation. In the majority of menopausal women, there is less bleeding with each period, and the periods are farther apart. However, there may be a complete cessation of bleeding in one month's time in some patients. Concurrently with the lessening of menstruation, there is a shrinkage of the woman's internal reproductive organs.

Symptoms of the menopause

Most women pass through the menopause with few or no untoward symptoms. In about 15 percent of all women the symptoms are troublesome. There may be magnification of physical ailments already present. Usually, however, symptoms are limited to hot flashes during the day and often at night, headache, dizziness, nervousness, irritability, and loss of appetite. Psychological symptoms are also manifested; the patient may experience "crying spells," a feeling of depression, and general listlessness. The menopause may be a trying period to the marital and family harmony.

As stated above, the average woman experiences less bleeding, and finally no bleeding, during the menopause. In some cases, there may be excessive bleeding occurring at the regular intervals. Most likely this is a harmless event; however, a physician should be consulted, because in this period of life there are other serious causes of vaginal bleeding, among them cancer.

Bleeding may occur between the periods, either as a frank flow of blood or in the form of "spotting." Investigation of this type of bleeding is extremely urgent because a small percentage of women with this symptom have cancer.

Postmenopausal bleeding—that bleeding that occurs six months or longer after menstruation has definitely ceased—has an even more serious significance. This symptom *is not a normal event of the change of life,* as many women have been led to believe. Approximately 50 percent of women with this symptom have cancer. Indeed, the false idea that all symptoms occurring at this time are related to the menopause is the chief reason for delayed recognition of cancer during this period. And delay in the diagnosis of cancer can be fatal.

Most women go through the menopause with no need for treatment of any kind. For the more extreme symptoms, the physician may prescribe the female hormone as a replacement for the hormone which is no longer produced. If the symptoms are only mildly troublesome, the physician may suggest some sort of mild sedative.

For women who do experience excessive symptoms of menopause as a result of insufficient estrogen, the physician may choose to use estrogen replacement therapy. This means that estrogen, often synthetic, is prescribed to replace the estrogen that is no longer being produced by the ovaries. The administration of estrogen must be evaluated carefully, as some women will require more of the replacement hormone than will others. Also, some women will require estrogen in combination with a progestogen.

Estrogen is usually administered in cycles; for example, a small tablet containing estrogen, or estrogen and progestogen, may be taken each day for three weeks. Then the tablet is not taken for one week. Women who take the estrogen during and even following menopause continue to experience the regular menstrual flow at about the same 28-day cycle interval. Longer cycles than 28 days may be established. Some physicians recommend that the tablet be taken daily for up to 40 days; then no pill is taken for 10 days (allowing menstruation to occur), thus establishing a 50-day cycle. The stimulation of the estrogen or estrogen and progestogen on the uterine lining causes the lining to build a thick blood-engorged layer which sloughs off at the end of the medication. With the beginning of another series of estrogen-containing tablets, another cycle begins.

Many physicians believe that the administration of replacement estrogen has other benefits besides the obvious one of alleviating the symptoms of menopause and prescribe it for menopausal and postmenopausal women without symptoms. For example, the incidence of heart attacks in postmenopausal women approaches that in men, but the rate of heart attacks in women taking estrogen remains low, as in premenopausal women who have sufficient estrogen. Estrogen also contributes to keeping the bones strong and hard, the breasts firm, and the skin supple and relatively wrinkle-free. In some older women, the external genital organs become thin, irritated, and itchy, and sexual activity becomes difficult and even painful; estrogen therapy can prevent this. Urinary tract tissues also have an estrogen dependence, and urinary tract dysfunctions which may develop following menopause can be avoided with estrogen therapy.

Many superstitions and false ideas exist concerning the menopause. For instance, postmenopausal women are said to become fat and lose their beauty. This is not so; any gain in weight at this time is usually moderate, and other bodily changes noted are caused by increasing age rather than by the menopause.

Further, the menopause does not imply an end to sexual activities. The woman usually desires and is able to experience sexual intercourse as often as she did before. Some women will have more desire for intercourse because they no longer fear pregnancy.

Above all, "change of life" does not mean that the woman should expect any particular change or readjustment of her activities and interests. Her health will continue to be good if it was good in the years before. Her family and social life should continue in the same patterns. All adjustments are internal and normal. Any abnormality is probably caused by some other factor and should be checked by her physician.

THE ADRENAL GLANDS

Just above each kidney there is a gland known as the *adrenal*. In ancient times, these small organs were believed to be the source of *black bile*. The anatomists who first studied the adrenal glands believed them to be capsules containing fluid but this was later proved to be erroneous. The fluid found inside the adrenal glands usually resulted from decomposition of the internal structure after death; in those days, autopsies were performed secretly, and often the bodies were not opened until several weeks after death. As the attitude of the people toward anatomists became more tolerant, a more careful study of the human body became possible, and the erroneous concepts that the adrenal glands were capsules containing fluid or that they produced black bile were disproved. The name *adrenal* means "near the kidney." Because in human beings the adrenals are located near the top of the kidneys, they are sometimes called *suprarenal glands*.

The over-all activity of the adrenal cortex is under the control of the pituitary hormone adrenocorticotrophin (ACTH). The pituitary releases ACTH in response to stimulation by a corticotrophin-releasing factor (CRF) formed in the hypothalamus. Release of CRF is inhibited by corticosteroids in the blood, forming a negative feedback system that stabilizes adrenal activity. This system oscillates slowly, with maximal activity late at night and minimal activity late in the afternoon. CRF is also released during stress, without regard to the blood corticoid concentration.

The glands are relatively small, and the average weight of each is about five grams. Each gland consists of two parts, which differ not only in origin and structure, but also in function. One part, the inner portion of the gland, is the medulla and produces, so far as is known, one active hormone called *adrenalin* or *epinephrine*. The outer layer of the gland is the *cortex* and produces a large variety of hormones—some possessing different types of activities and some a single type of activity. At present, 28 of these hormones have been isolated.

Adrenalin

Adrenalin, the hormone from the medulla, may be produced as a result of emotional stimulation of the nervous system and is one of the few hormones that is directly influenced by the nervous system. Adrenalin increases blood pressure, speeds up the respiration and the heartbeat, augments the amount of sugar in the blood, and in stressful situations, gives the individual a feeling of added strength and aggressiveness. When adrenalin is poured into the blood by the adrenal glands—as happens in cases of fear, rage, and other circumstances of stress—the sugar level in the blood increases rapidly at the expense of stored sugar in the liver and muscles. Surprising as it may seem, rage makes a person's blood "sweet" and not "sour." The result is a type of defense mechanism in times of stress which gives the individual added fuel for increased activity.

Noradrenalin, which is chemically very similar to adrenalin, is also produced by the adrenal medulla. However, its effects are not the same, in some cases are even opposite. Noradrenalin is also found in nerve cells throughout the body, where it functions as a transmitter of nerve impulses from one nerve cell to the next.

Hormones of the cortex

The outer layer, or cortex, of the adrenal is vital, and obliteration can result in death. Under specific circumstances, surgical removal of the cortex becomes necessary; these patients are given extracts from the adrenals of animals or purified hormones to maintain an adequate balance of body functions.

The adrenal glands, like all other endocrine organs, are under the control of the pituitary gland which produces a hormone that exerts a stimulatory action on the cortex. The hormone of the pituitary gland, ACTH *(adrenocorticotrophic hormone),* is effective in quite small

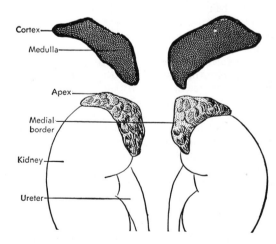

Drawing of a cross section through the adrenal or suprarenal glands; the lower drawing illustrates their location on the upper part of the kidneys.

amounts in stimulating the cortex. One of the 50 or more steroids produced by the adrenals is *hydrocortisone,* which eventually acts on the pituitary to inhibit the production of ACTH—a sort of check and balance system.

The action of ACTH is not upon the production of a single hormone, but upon the production of all the hormones from the adrenal cortex. Small as this part of the gland may seem, it is one of the most active tissues in the body, constantly making a large variety of complex chemical substances that are poured into the blood and delivered to the liver, muscles, sex organs, and many other parts of the body. Once they arrive at their destination, these complex chemical substances perform many functions, most of which consist of regulating the chemical transformations that go on constantly in all the tissues.

Hydrocortisone

Hydrocortisone, the best known of the "cortical hormones"—so called because they are produced in the cortex—is used today in patients with rheumatoid arthritis, rheumatic fever, and many other diseases. The temporary improvements which have been obtained in patients with rheumatoid arthritis are spectacular.

Hydrocortisone is used in the treatment of patients with a large variety of disorders, including skin diseases, malignant blood diseases and anemia, allergies, diseases of the eye, and even emotional disturbances. Prednisone is another adrenocortical steroid. It is a synthetic hormone developed chemically with the purpose of obtaining a more potent anti-inflammatory hormone than hydrocortisone. In addition, newer synthetic steroids are available including some with practically no salt-retaining activity and even greater anti-inflammatory effect.

Aldosterone

Insufficient production of aldosterone (the salt-retaining hormone) by the adrenals results in a disturbance in the distribution of water and salt in the body. Normally, the amount of water surrounding the tissues and the amount of water inside the cells is well-balanced with the water in the blood, so that there is always a constant amount in all regions. When the adrenal glands are damaged or the production of aldosterone diminishes, there is a profound change in the water distribution that begins with an excessive loss of water and salt in the urine. The loss of salt occurs at the expense of salt from the blood, and the water lost in the urine is at the expense of water surrounding the tissues. The body becomes dehydrated, and water must pass from the blood into the surrounding areas of tissues

to maintain the necessary amount of fluid in the cells. The blood becomes thick because of the excessive loss of water; and a state of shock may be established. The administration of water and salt as well as extracts from adrenals of animals or purified aldosterone corrects the condition.

Aldosteronism (lack of salt-retaining hormone) may occur in either sex from childhood to old age, but is found most commonly in individuals in their thirties and forties. It may occur in individuals with high blood pressure, especially if they have one or more of the following symptoms: severe "bursting" central headache, muscle weakness or cramps, fatigue, increased thirst, and change in bladder habits.

Other cortical hormones

Hydrocortisone is a powerful hormone and the effects produced in the body are numerous. But hydrocortisone represents only one of the several hormones that are manufactured by the adrenals. All resemble each other chemically, but are different in their activities. Adrenal hormones regulate the chemical transformations of sugars, starches, and proteins in the liver, muscles, and other parts of the body; still others control to a degree the growth of hair and proper development of sexual characteristics. The molecules of which these hormones are made are similar to the molecules of male and female sex hormones, and so they share both properties; some make the body "masculine," and others make it "feminine" in appearance. Normally, the production of both types is balanced and never changes a man's personality or physical characteristics into those of a woman or vice versa. However, under extraordinary circumstances, as when an active tumor develops in the outer layer of the adrenals, some of these hormones are produced in excess; and the result is striking, particularly in women. They assume a mannish appearance, with an exaggerated growth of hair all over the body, and there may be a mustache and beard growth. The condition influences all the sexual characteristics of the woman so afflicted to the point that recognition as a woman becomes difficult. Upon removal of the tumor by surgical operation, the subject usually returns to the original state of normalcy.

The important role of the adrenal glands in the body economy may be better appreciated when certain animal experiments are cited. Laboratory animals from which the two adrenal glands have been removed by surgical operation will not live long after the operation if salt is omitted from their drinking water; but they will live for several months if salt is given to them with the water they drink. Moreover, the animals suffer unduly from changes in temperature or inappropriate feeding. They have no resistance. Failure to receive adequate nourishment for only a short time may be fatal, because the blood sugar level drops to a dangerous point. If animals in which the adrenals have been removed are given adrenal extracts from other animals or purified hormones, together with an appropriate diet, most of the symptoms disappear. The animals are normal in appearance and actions and, except that they have no adrenal glands, they are indistinguishable from normal animals.

Addison's disease

Addison's disease is characterized by deficient functioning of the adrenals. Although in many instances the cause is not known, many cases are believed to result from an autoimmune disorder, i.e., an immune reaction by the body against some stimulus naturally present within itself. The glands degenerate and fail to function properly. Sometimes it is caused by involvement of the glands by tuberculosis. Adrenal insufficiency may also result from insufficient pituitary ACTH. The course of the disease follows a definite pattern, characterized by the multiplicity of disturbances that occur in the chemistry of the body. The patient is usually fatigued both mentally and physically; his blood pressure is low; and his digestion becomes impaired. There may be vomiting, diarrhea, loss of body weight, and many changes in the constituents of the blood. The skin becomes pigmented, one of the most obvious features of the disease. The membranes of the mouth become pigmented also.

Some time ago, patients with Addison's disease did not live long, but with the advent of modern hormonal treatment, over 70 percent of these patients survive. The usual form of treatment for a person with Addison's disease is the administration of cortisol or cortisone, usually supplemented by a sodium-retaining hormone to maintain the salt level in the body. The existence of purified hormones simplifies the treatment, and each symptom can be alleviated with a corresponding hormone. Thus, there is available in pure form one of the hormones responsible for maintaining the water and salt balance in the body, and when this substance is given, water and salt balance is restored. Again, like hydrocortisone, this particular hormone controlling water balance is a powerful drug, and its proper dosage and control are of great importance. The weight and physical condition of the patient must be checked constantly, and any increase in weight may be the result of improper dosages of the drug.

Patients suffering a crisis caused by adrenal insufficiency must receive large quantities of salt and sugar solution intravenously and large doses of cortisone. Meals must be at frequent intervals and consist of abundant amounts of starches.

Overactivity

The adrenal glands also can become overactive and produce a larger amount of hormones than normal. In some instances, the overproduction of hormones may be the result of an active tumor that secretes ACTH, thereby stimulating the adrenal cortex. In other cases, the outer layer of the adrenal glands receives excessive ACTH from the pituitary gland. An excess of ACTH forces the adrenal glands to work excessively and to produce overabundant amounts of adrenal hormones. Indirectly, when the pituitary suffers, so do the adrenals, and the result is the same as if the adrenals themselves had become defective. Whatever the cause, the end result is too many hormones in the body, a condition reflected in a variety of symptoms.

In some patients with overactive adrenals, there is an excessive development of fat, accompanied by sexual disturbances. The symptoms vary according to the age and sex of the patient. If the disease develops during fetal life and the child is a female, a form of *hermaphroditism,* or "dual sexuality," may result, in which the clitoris is enlarged and resembles the penis. Other signs of masculinization accompany this condition. Among children, the disease takes a different form, usually making the child obese with great muscular development, and giving him the appearance of a "little Hercules." Young boys suffering from overactive adrenals may develop all the sexual characteristics of men, and they look like men. In girls and adult women, the symptoms of excessive production of adrenal hormones are characterized by a trend towards masculinization. Girls develop a masculine appearance with an abnormal development of the clitoris and hair. In adult females, the transformation is more spectacular and, as previously discussed, they change their appearance to the extent that they are almost indistinguishable from men. This condition is called the *adrenogenital syndrome.* Hair grows abundantly over the body, the skin becomes rough, and the body build resembles that of a man, with broad shoulders and strong muscles. The breasts become small, and menstruation is irregular or absent. These symptoms disappear if the cause, usually a tumor of the adrenals, can be removed.

Cushing's syndrome is the disorder caused by excessive secretion of glucocorticoids by the adrenal cortex. Adrenal hyperactivity may be produced by excessive stimulation of the adrenal gland as a result of a tumor of the pituitary secreting too much ACTH; by abnormal functioning of the corticotrophine-releasing factor; by an ACTH-like substance produced by a tumor elsewhere in the body; or by a benign or malignant tumor in the adrenal gland.

The true Cushing's syndrome occurs rarely and affects more women than men; however, mild degrees of abnormality are now being recognized fairly often with improved diagnostic techniques, so the disease may be more widespread than formerly believed.

The disease usually begins so subtly that the exact date of onset is unknown; however, if a tumor is present, the onset may be comparatively rapid. The first changes are usually weight gain in the trunk, alteration or cessation of menses, muscle weakness, and rounding of the face. The face and upper chest become sated with blood and the skin is oily; acne and florid infection are common. Bone weakening may cause backache, and even vertebral collapse may occur. The skin bruises easily and cuts heal poorly. High blood pressure is common and may lead to congestive heart failure. The patient is usually depressed and may become psychotic.

If clear-cut evidence of an adrenal tumor exists, surgical excision followed by corticosteroid medication is essential. If a pituitary tumor is the cause, irradiation or surgical procedures may be used to correct the problem.

Other types of tumors may also produce Cushing's syndrome, as described in the section on the pituitary gland.

The adrenal glands have become the subject of active medical investigation; and within recent years several new regulatory functions have been attributed to these small glands. Situations of stress, excessive cold, disease, and many other emergencies set in motion an alarm reaction in the adrenal glands, and a prompt action follows. The exact mechanism of this action is not known, but it is probably an adjustment of the production of hormones by the glands to restore the balance of all the chemical reactions of the body. The versatility of cortisone in the management of many ills repre-

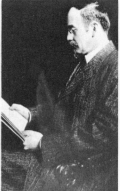

ABEL, John Jacob (1857-1938) American pharmacologist. First (1898) to isolate the active principle of the adrenal glands, naming it epinephrine. By discovering the exclusive discharge of phenolsulfonphthalein by the kidney, he made possible the measurement of its excretory power, and was first to test organ efficiency with dye-indicators. With Cushny he founded and edited the *Journal of Pharmacology and Experimental Therapeutics.*

sents perhaps the best example of the manner in which the adrenal glands, by producing many hormones, maintain the body in health and keep it resistant to the impact of stresses both from without and within.

THE THYMUS GLAND

The thymus is an organ situated within the chest cavity, close to the heart. It has been known for centuries and was believed to be the seat of courage and affection in ancient times because it is situated close to the heart. The word, thymus, is derived from a Greek word which has two meanings: "courage" and "thyme." The shape of this organ resembles the leaves of the thyme plant.

The thymus is not always the same size, and it does not grow progressively as most organs do. From the day of birth to the age of twelve or thereabouts, the thymus grows gradually until it reaches a maximum size and weight; at this time, the organ is the size of a small egg and weights about the same. At about the age of 15, the thymus begins to diminish in size and weight, until in old age it is practically nonexistent. During pregnancy, the thymus usually becomes smaller than normal, but recovers its original size after delivery. Infectious diseases, x-rays, and hormones act on the thymus in such a way that the gland becomes smaller.

For many years, the function of the thymus gland was unknown. It was even believed that men could live without the thymus and suffer no particular ill effects. Recent studies on experimental animals, however, have shown that this is not so. The thymus has a central role in establishing the immunological capacities of the body. In mice whose thymus glands were removed immediately after birth, the spleens never grew to full adult size and most of the lymphoid tissues (in which protective white cells, or lymphocytes, are made) were degenerated. The

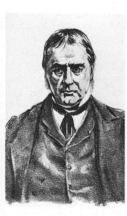

GULL, William Whitey (1816-1890) English physician. Noted for his important studies on the effects of partial and complete thyroidectomy, which created widespread recognition of the important role of the thyroid in physiology. He was among the first to recognize the cause of myxedema. When the latter disorder results from atrophy of the thyroid, it is called *Gull's disease.* Gull made other important contributions to pathology aside from his major thyroid gland studies.

animals could not resist infections, i.e., they could not produce antibodies to combat bacteria or other infectious elements in their bodies which were making them sick.

The same is true in man. The thymus apparently elaborates a hormone which is responsible for the production of cells with the capacity to make antibodies and reject foreign elements. During the first weeks of life, the thymus produces the basic cells that are then distributed throughout the body to other lymphocyte "factories," the lymph nodes and spleen. At short notice, these organs can mass-produce lymphocytes and carry on the production of antibodies, which protect the body against invading microbes or foreign tissues.

Once the mature cells have been distributed, the thymus seems to have done its main job. In adult life, and even in later childhood, the gland can be removed with little apparent effect. Perhaps it eventually does become useless, despite its vital early role.

In 1966, biochemists reported the identification of the thymus hormone. This hormone, which was named *thymosin,* is believed to bring about the maturation, proliferation, and immunological competence of the lymphocytes. Further studies are now in progress to determine the method of action of thymosin and to outline what its exact effects are on the human organism.

The dependence of the thymus on other endocrine glands and its sensitivity to their secretions is intriguing.

The hormones from the adrenal cortex and the sex hormones act on the thymus and inhibit its function. But the hormone from the thyroid gland has a stimulating effect on this organ. The pituitary gland, by acting on the adrenals and gonads, inhibits the thymus; by acting on the thyroid, it stimulates the thymus.

The thymus on some occasions may become larger than normal, and the condition usually is associated with disturbances in other endocrine glands. In cases of adrenal insufficiency, the thymus and other lymphoid organs increase in size; similar effects are observed when the thyroid gland becomes overactive. This enlargement is thought to be in rare instances associated in some way with the cause of sudden death in apparently healthy children or young adults exposed to some stress, such as surgery.

The thymus, like all organs of the body, may be the site of tumor formation. There are several types of tumors that may develop in the thymus gland, some rare and others more common. Whatever the type of tumor, the symptoms manifest themselves by local pressure, difficulty in breathing, and bluish coloration of the skin. The symptoms are probably the result of pressure by the tumor upon the windpipe and upon nerves in the chest. Tumors of the thymus are removed surgically, or if surgery is not possible, they may be destroyed by the action of x-rays. When surgery is done early in the course of development of the tumor, it often effects permanent cure.

The thymus has been found to be enlarged in many cases of *myasthenia gravis.* This is a disease of the muscles and is characterized by extreme muscular weakness. The patient is usually constantly fatigued or becomes fatigued upon minor exertion. The muscles of the face and neck are the main targets of this disease, and the result is reflected in a sad and sleepy expression. The cause of this disease is unknown. Some patients suffering from myasthenia gravis have been benefited by a removal of the enlarged thymus.

THE PINEAL GLAND

The functions of the pineal body are still obscure; in particular, the debate as to whether the pineal is or is not an endocrine gland has fluctuated for many years. Much of the discussion has centered around the question of whether hormonal effects associated with lesions of the pineal may not result from pressure or involvement of the hypothalamus and other neighboring structures. However, recent studies support the view that the pineal contains and probably secretes certain humoral substances and may influence the secretion of others.

The pineal gland is about the size of a small vitamin capsule and is located in the central part of the brain, as is the pituitary gland, but a little higher up.

In man, extensive calcification of the pineal body begins during the second decade of life, and by the sixth decade, over 70 percent of all pineals show x-ray evidence of calcification. However, this does not necessarily imply loss of functional activity, since recent evidence indicates that the human pineal may retain functional activity throughout the entire life span.

The product of the secretion of the pineal gland is a hormone known as melatonin. Melatonin causes marked skin blanching or lightening by its action on the pigment cells; this effect is the opposite of that produced by the pituitary melanocyte-stimulating hormone.

Ancient physicians were impressed by the location of the gland and ascribed to this organ the function of thinking. The French philosopher, René Descartes, also was impressed by the location of the gland and expressed the view that the pineal body must be the "seat of the soul." Later, some writers considered the pineal body as the remnants of a

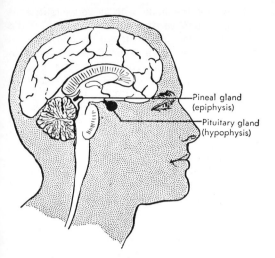

This cross-section of a human head shows the location of the pineal gland (epiphysis) and the pituitary gland (hypophysis) and their relationship.

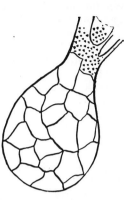

Drawing of the gross appearance of the human pineal gland which seems to be made up of large cells filled with a crystalline chemical material.

"third eye" similar to that found in reptiles and amphibians. In these creatures, the third or parietal eye serves as a light-receptive organ. Interestingly, there is recent evidence to indicate that the function of the pineal gland in man may be influenced indirectly by the stimulation of light. When rats are placed in continuous light, the capacity of the pineal to synthesize melatonin is increased. The increase varies according to a diurnal cycle, depending upon the environmental lighting. These observations suggest that the pineal may serve as a "biological clock" which helps to regulate certain endocrine rhythms.

Pineal tumors are among the rarest tumors. Processes destroying the pineal gland are characterized by precocious sexual development in a manner that is suggestive of an overactive pituitary gland. A different situation arises if the tumor is truly a pineal neoplasm (*pinealoma*). In this case, there may be a depression of gonadal function. It is interesting that the precocious sexual development that results from pineal destruction appears to be limited to boys about two or three years old. The boys manifest definite signs of adult masculinity. The sex organs become adult in size and function, and pubic hair appears similar to that of a mature man. There has been no satisfactory explanation of why nearly all cases of sexual precocity associated with pineal tumors have occurred in boys. In adult men with true pineal tumors, indeed a different situation, there may be degeneration of the testes.

The surgical removal of pineal tumors is not often advisable, because of the high mortality rate. Radiation therapy may result in a temporary cure. These tumors are so rare that the physician seldom suspects them except in cases where the symptoms are clearly defined, as in children with precocious sexual development. In adults, the symptoms may be the result of cranial pressure. These include headaches, vomiting, neck rigidity, and muscular weakness. The eyesight may be affected, and loss of vision occurs gradually because of destruction of the optic nerves. Permanent cures may be obtained by surgical removal of the tumor in some cases.

THE PANCREAS

The pancreas is an organ situated in the abdomen and connected to the digestive system by means of a duct that shares its opening with the gallbladder. The normal, average pancreas is the size of an open hand and is grayish-pink in color. The pancreas is, in fact, two glands, one of which is unequivocally endocrine, because some elements that make up this organ produce three different hormones known as insulin, glucagon, and gastrin. Of the cells in the pancreas, very few are for endocrine secretion. The major portion of this gland produces a complex fluid, the *pancreatic juice,* that is poured into the small intestine to aid in the digestion of food. This fact was known to ancient physicians, and they surmised that the pancreas must be like a salivary gland; thus the name "abdominal salivary gland" was given to this organ.

About a century ago, Paul Langerhans made a careful study of the pancreas and discovered the existence of cell accumulations that resemble little islands among the other cells of this organ. A few years later, the cell accumulations were described again, and the name *islets of Langer-*

hans was given to these structures. There are about a million of these islets in an average pancreas, and they are distributed throughout this organ. Recently, three types of islet cells have been differentiated and designated as alpha, beta, and D-cells of the islet. The beta cells produce insulin, the alpha cells form a hormone called *glucagon,* and the D-cells secrete gastrin.

Insulin and glucagon are both important in the regulation of sugar levels in the blood; their actions, however, are opposite. Insulin permits the absorption of sugar *(glucose)* by various cells of the body, following which the sugar molecules are linked together to form glycogen, a storage form for sugar. Insulin also speeds up the conversion of glucose into energy and heat. In contrast glucagon brings about the breakdown of stored glycogen in the liver.

At risk of oversimplification, it could be stated that the lack of insulin activity causes the symptoms of the disease known as *diabetes mellitus.* Besides insulin and glucagon, other factors are also involved in the regulation of blood sugar levels, particularly adrenalin from the adrenals and certain other substances, one of which (growth hormone) is produced by the pituitary gland. These factors regulate the sugar level to a large extent with the mediation of the liver and the muscles, both of which store glycogen until it is released into the blood, depending on the need. There are many types of sugars in nature, of which glucose is the most important to the human body. Glucose occurs in fruits and is not so sweet as ordinary table sugar (sucrose). Glucose is also the basic material in starches and is a constituent of many other types of food which, like sucrose, are broken down by the action of digestive juices

and provide the body with large quantities of glucose. Much of the glucose obtained from food enters the blood stream to be conveyed to the liver, where it is temporarily stored in the form of glycogen. The liver supplies glucose to the blood as needed, to be distributed throughout the body. Normally, the quantity of glucose being utilized by the tissues and the amount of glucose poured into the blood by the liver is maintained in equilibrium, so that the level remains the same. This process is similar to the maintenance of a constant level of water in a swimming pool by regulating the amount of water entering and the amount leaving the pool.

The name *insulin* was given first to a substance, the existence of which was suspected but not yet discovered and which was presumed to come from the islets of Langerhans. The name was derived from the word, *insula,* which means "an island." One role of the pancreas, and more precisely of the islets of Langerhans, was discovered in the latter part of the nineteenth century by two scientists who were experimenting with dogs. They observed that after the pancreas was removed surgically the animal developed a condition similar to diabetes in human beings. In 1921, Sir Frederick G. Banting and his assistant, Charles Best, were able to devise a method for the isolation of insulin from the pancreas. Banting had been a practicing physician in a small community in Canada until his interest was aroused by some articles he had read in medical journals concerning the pancreas. The pancreas was thought to produce an active principle necessary for the proper burning of sugar by the tissues, but the active principle had not been isolated in spite of many

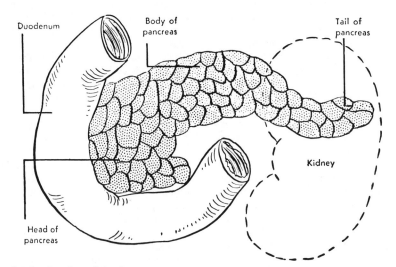

Drawing showing location of the human pancreas and its relationship to the kidney and duodenum.

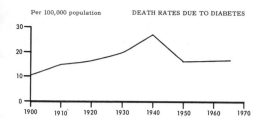

Per 100,000 population   DEATH RATES DUE TO DIABETES

This chart depicts the considerable increase in the number of persons in the United States dying from diabetes mellitus during the first half of the twentieth century. A major portion of this increase may be attributed to the fact that more people now live to the age at which diabetes appears. Probably because of better care and understanding of the disease, death rates now are leveling.

efforts. Banting conceived the idea that he might isolate insulin more readily from the islets of Langerhans if the remainder of the pancreas could be destroyed. He reasoned that such destruction might be accomplished by tying the ducts of the pancreas since this had been shown to damage the digestive part of the gland more than the islets. He could not easily translate his idea into action unless he could be provided with the necessary facilities and help. He sought advice and found it at the University of Toronto, from Professor J. J. R. McLeod. He was given the necessary facilities and began his work with the help of Charles Best, then a recent graduate in physiology and biochemistry. In less than nine months, Banting's greatest expectations had been realized. As he had hoped, insulin could be extracted from the remnants of the degenerated pancreas made up almost solely of islets of Langerhans. The two scientists proceeded to make extracts of this tissue and injected it into dogs. The experiment proved successful, so without further delay the extracts were given to diabetic patients who responded rapidly to the treatment. Today, insulin is a relatively inexpensive commodity available to all diabetic patients, thanks to the efforts of Banting and Best and to the improved methods devised for the extraction and purification of insulin on a large scale.

Disorders of the islet cells

Under certain conditions, the islet cells are destroyed or partially damaged by disease or influenced so that the quantity of insulin produced is inadequate for the normal regulation of the level of blood sugar. This occurs in diabetes; and patients suffering from this disease excrete significant amounts of sugar in their urine.

The islets of Langerhans may also be the site of tumor formation, resulting in an increase in the number of active cells. One clinical disorder resulting from this overactivity caused by *islet cell tumors* is *hyperinsulinism*. In hyperinsulinism, which is caused by overactivity of the beta cells, there is an excess production of insulin. The excess insulin may cause the blood sugar to fall to dangerous levels, but the patient will respond to the administration of sugar in the form of candy, fruit juices, or other sweets. Beta cell tumors must be removed surgically.

A tumor involving the D-cells of the islets of Langerhans is called the D-cell adenoma. This tumor causes a condition known as the *Zollinger-Ellison syndrome*. In this syndrome, the D-cells secrete an excessive amount of gastrin. This, in turn, stimulates the parietal cells of the stomach to produce an increased volume of gastric juices. The gastric hyperactivity can lead to severe peptic ulcer sometimes accompanied by excessive diarrhea. The D-cell adenoma may be either malignant or benign, but it must be removed surgically to relieve the symptoms. Of interest, the presence of a D-cell adenoma also causes an increase in insulin secretion by the beta cells.

Diabetes mellitus

In the patient with diabetes mellitus, there is either no insulin present or the insulin is insufficient for the patient's needs. As a result, glucose (sugar) enters the cells of the body only with difficulty. The liver, however, continues to dispense glucose into the blood stream at a normal level. The amount of sugar in the blood then rises to abnormally high levels and "spills over" into the urine and is carried out of the body. Thus, the body is deprived of the glucose necessary for proper functioning.

Diabetes mellitus, then, is characterized by the presence of excessive quantities of sugar in the blood and by its excretion into the urine. The name, *diabetes mellitus,* is used in contradistinction to a second type of diabetes, called *diabetes insipidus*. Mellitus means honey-like, and the name was applied to this type of diabetes because of the sweetness of the urine. Diabetes insipidus, conversely, is a disease characterized by the excessive elimination of urine, but the urine in this case is insipid or tasteless. This latter condition is associated with disturbances in a part of the hypothalamic-hypophyseal system.

Diabetes mellitus has been believed to be associated with a faulty function of the islets of Langerhans; however, there is evidence now that adequate insulin may be present in one type of diabetes. In this type of diabetes, similar amounts of free insulin appear in the splenic vein (which leads from the pancreas) of diabetics as in normal subjects. However, in the hepatic vein (which leads from the liver), diabetics have no free insulin whereas normal subjects do. This suggests that in some patients, the disease may result from an hepatic rather than a pancreatic disturbance.

Diabetes, therefore, takes two forms, one of which is most commonly found in children and the other in adults. In the juvenile type, the pancreas is usually depleted of insulin. However, in the adult type, there is usually adequate insulin present in the pancreas, but it is not being utilized.

The course of diabetes also takes two forms. In some patients, the disease is readily controlled; these patients are said to have "stable" disease. Other patients have rapid and unpredictable swings from very low to very high blood sugar levels (both of which may be dangerous) and are said to have "brittle" or unstable diabetes. Patients with stable diabetes generally have little difficulty in controlling their disease. Patients with unstable disease, however, must pay closer attention to medications, diet, and exercise and must be on the alert for the possible development of complications. Under some circumstances, unstable diabetes may become stable, and vice versa. Brittle diabetes is seen most often in children, but is found in some adults.

Many factors are known to cause the appearance of diabetes. Any form of physical stress, particularly infection and trauma (accidental or even a surgical procedure), may unmask or aggravate the disease. Emotional stress or other endocrine diseases may cause eruption of the diabetic state. Also, the incidence of diabetes is higher in the older age brackets and in obese people. (In these two latter groups, however, the disease can be controlled simply by weight reduction and proper diet.)

Many geneticists believe that diabetes is heritable, but others disagree because an acceptable pattern for the inheritance of the disease has not been presented. Diabetes rarely occurs in newborn infants, but appears with increasing frequency in individuals in the older age brackets. It has been estimated that the over-all prevalence of diabetes is 1.4 to 1.7 percent of the total population. However, in those over the age of 60 years, the prevalence may be as high as 10 percent. There is no apparent predilection for any nationality or race. In the United States, diabetes occurs more in women than in men until after the child-bearing age, and occurs more frequently in women who have had many children.

For convenience, diabetes is sometimes divided into three phases: (1) the *latent phase,* when no disease can be demonstrated; (2) the *preclinical phase,* when biochemical abnormalities are demonstrable, but no clinically apparent symptoms are present; and (3) the *clinical phase,* when symptoms become apparent.

As with many diseases, the treatment for diabetes is most effective if started when the disease is still in an early stage. The earlier treatment is begun, the less is the likelihood that the effects of the disease throughout the body will become serious. A person with diabetes in the preclinical phase can often control the disease with careful diet alone. Should the disease advance, the person may take insulin or an oral hypoglycemic agent.

The tests for diabetes are simple and easy, and may be included in any physical examination. Those individuals who might be especially prone to develop this disease should be tested for diabetes regularly. These would include relatives of patients with diabetes, women who have had increased blood sugar levels during pregnancy, and women who have given birth to exceptionally large babies.

Apart from the high blood sugar and the presence of sugar in the urine, the diabetic patient exhibits many other symptoms. He is frequently thirsty and drinks large volumes of water. Other symptoms are excessive urination, increased frequency in urination, excessive appetite, loss of weight, and general weakness. In addition to these symptoms, it is not uncommon to observe itching of the skin, constipation, drowsiness, and muscular pains. In older patients, complications associated with changes in blood vessels and the nervous system are often observed. As a result of these complications, a series of other conditions may result such as nervousness, neuralgias, neuritis, cataracts, and gangrene of the feet or hands.

The disease attacks the young and the old, women and men, and in each case it follows a somewhat different course. In nearly all patients, the first obvious sign of diabetes is the presence of sugar in the urine and a high level of blood sugar. Sudden changes in weight may be suspicious, particularly when there is a rapid decrease in weight for no apparent reason. In some cases before the onset of other symptoms, the patient may become nervous and irritable without cause. The appearance of sugar in the urine may be delayed considerably after the first symptoms appear, and constitutes the first obvious sign. In some instances, sugar may be found in the urine of persons who are not diabetic—for example, pregnant women.

In the more advanced cases of diabetes, *acid intoxication* may result and is characterized by such symptoms as weakness, loss of appetite, nausea, increased breathing, skin flushes, and a typical acetone odor of the breath. The odor of acetone on the breath may be mistaken for that of alcohol. This has led many police agencies to adopt chemical alcohol intoxication tests to prevent unjust and possibly fatal incarceration of diabetics. When the acetone intoxication is extreme, loss of consciousness *(coma)* and even death may result. The patient who suffers from acid intoxication must be under constant observation, and his care must be carefully planned by the physician.

Treatment

Cure of diabetes mellitus is impossible at present, but the goal of life-long control can be obtained. The main aims of treatment for this disease, then, are to prevent acid intoxication, to avoid complications of the disease, and to maintain as well-balanced and well-regulated an existence as is possible.

The most obvious form of therapy, of course, is supplying the blood stream with the insulin which is not being provided by the body. Since the discoveries of Banting and Best, this has been possible. Insulin is now available in fast- and slow-acting forms, and the type, amount, and schedule of administration can be tailored to fit the individual. Insulin must be administered by injection. (The proper method for insulin injection is discussed in more detail later in this chapter.) Insulin cannot be taken orally because it is destroyed by the digestive processes. However, methods for synthesizing (making) insulin in the laboratory are now available, and it is hoped that a form can be developed which can be ingested by mouth.

Within the past 10 years, another form of medication has become widely used for some types of diabetes. The oral hypoglycemic agents, as they are called, are often useful in individuals with the adult type of diabetes who developed the disease after the age of 40 and who do not require more than 40 units of insulin per day.

Oral hypoglycemic agents are of two types, the *sulfonylureas* and the *diguanides.* The sulfonylureas act by stimulating the pancreas to produce more insulin or by triggering the release of insulin bound in chemical combinations. Obviously, these drugs are effective only in those patients whose pancreatic beta cells are still capable of responding. The diguanides act by allowing more effective use of the insulin already available.

At times, sulfonylureas will cease to be effective in patients who have previously responded well to them. These patients often can then be adequately treated with a combination of the sulfonylureas and diguanides. All patients whose diabetes cannot be adequately controlled with oral drugs or diet, of course, must use insulin.

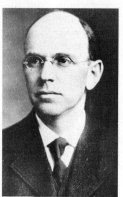

JOSLIN, Elliott Proctor (1869-1962) American physician. Regarded as one of the great authorities on the subject of diabetes, especially on diabetes mellitus. His investigations into the causes and treatment of this disease have brought out the observation that it is related to obesity in adulthood, with about 50 percent of all diabetes occurring between the ages of 40 and 60. He has stressed fasting and food restrictions in treating diabetic patients.

It is possible that many older persons who develop diabetes could have their disease regulated with a strict diet alone, but many prefer more liberal diets even at the cost of daily oral medication.

Insulin shock

Insulin is used not as a cure but as a replacement. Insulin is made available in well-standardized doses so that the patient may learn to use it without danger, but occasionally the patient may take too much insulin and develop a state of shock because of a marked reduction in the level of blood sugar. In such instances, the patient becomes nervous, sweats profusely, becomes weak, and faints. When the reaction is more intense, the subject exhibits emotional symptoms—laughing, crying, fright, excitement, negativism, and even loss of memory. The symptoms may culminate in muscular spasms. The pulse is usually elevated, and the patient in an unconscious state has dilated pupils. Insulin shock seldom results in death when the shock is not complicated by other factors. The reaction ordinarily occurs two to four hours after the administration of unmodified insulin and before mealtime.

If the insulin has been administered and not followed by a meal, the reaction may occur within one hour. Mild insulin reactions disappear rapidly after the ingestion of orange juice, sugar, or some other sweet. The diabetic patient always carries with him some candy or sweet to be used as an antidote when insulin shock is impending. In severe cases of insulin reaction, the patient may not be conscious enough to ingest sugar or its equivalent; attempts to feed him should not be made, for he may inhale the food and choke. If the individual loses .consciousness, glucagon may be injected beneath the skin, and the patient will recover consciousness within a few moments. After the patient is conscious, fruit juices and sugar can be offered. Sometimes, the patient does not respond to glucagon, and the physician must resort to the administration of glucose given by vein.

In succeeding sections, a discussion is given of the proper methods of insulin administration, the amount and types of exercise recommended, dieting factors, and the specific physical hygiene necessary. All of these are required for the diabetic patient to live a long, healthy life. Statistics demonstrate that, with proper self-care, the diabetic patient may live as long as or longer than many normal persons.

Aside from diabetes, there are other disorders of the pancreas such as infections, cancer, etc. These conditions are discussed in detail in Chapter 13, "The Digestive System: *Intestinal disorders.*"

Complications

In patients with diabetes, certain complications occur with great frequency and are considered part of the disease. Diabetic patients also have some of the same complications which occur with other degenerative diseases, but these occur in the diabetic at an earlier age and with greater frequency. Those complications which occur specifically in diabetics include arteriosclerosis, kidney ailments, disorders of the eye, and complications of the nervous system. All these appear to have a common basis, which is referred to as the *microangiopathy of diabetes mellitus.*

Microangiopathy of diabetes is an accumulation of a substance called hyalin in and around the walls of small blood-carrying vessels. Such changes have a predilection for the vessels of the kidney, retina, skin, and nerves.

Severe and advanced arteriosclerosis (hardening and thickening of the small blood vessels) may occur in diabetics. Involvement of the coronary arteries and of the arteries of the legs is perhaps of the greatest significance. Coronary arteriosclerosis with angina attacks and thrombosis of coronary arteries with subsequent myocardial infarction occur more commonly in diabetics than in nondiabetics. (For a detailed discussion on these conditions, see Chapter 7, "The Heart and Circulation.") Further, arteriosclerotic changes in the vessels of the brain account for the high incidence of cerebrovascular disorders in diabetics.

Symptoms suggesting advanced arteriosclerosis in the leg include coldness, a sensation of numbness, and intermittent lameness. Inadequacy of the circulation may become apparent during exercise or exposure to cold or after burns or infections, i.e., under conditions requiring an increased blood supply. Gangrene is the most dangerous and dreaded complication of arteriosclerosis of the extremities. Diabetic gangrene can be brought about by local infections (e.g., ingrown toenails, mistreated corns) or by minor cuts and abrasions.

Arteriosclerosis of the large renal arteries may cause varying degrees of *kidney failure.* Microangiopathy of the kidney is responsible for three types of glomerular lesions that occur in the kidneys of diabetic patients. Renal failure is the most common cause of death in these patients.

Microangiopathy of the eye—conjunctiva, lens, and retina—may occur in patients with diabetes. In the retina, deep hemorrhages occur; in late stages, waxy exudates may be present. Severe impairment of vision or blindness may result. Occasionally, these changes begin before diabetes is diagnosed; the first time the disease is suspected is when the patient visits the ophthalmologist because of impaired vision.

Nervous disorders are common in diabetics over 40 years of age. Again, this appears to result from deposition of hyaline material (microangiopathy) in the walls of blood vessels leading to the nerves, interfering with the blood supply. The symptoms are the same as those encountered in other secondary nervous disorders and include pain, muscle tenderness and weakness, diminished or absent tendon reflexes, numbness at the skin surface, diminished vibratory sense, and in advanced stages, atrophy of the muscles.

Although the above conditions can improve with treatment of the diabetes, slowly progressive numbness of the hands and feet is extremely common after many years of diabetes and is almost never reversible. The patient should avoid injury to numb areas, for cure is difficult when the circulation is impaired.

Patients with uncontrolled diabetes have decreased "natural resistance" to infectious agents. In fact, they even seem to have heightened susceptibility to staphylococcal skin infections. Furuncles often occur in crops rather than singly; these should be treated with care lest they develop into carbuncles. Carbuncles are most common in the neck in men and in the vulvar region in women. Although they are a serious complication of diabetes, the use of antibiotics is lessening the danger from them. Naturally, the practice of manipulating or squeezing pimples or boils must be strictly avoided.

The presence of diabetes renders infections more severe by lowering resistance in some way. Moreover, the presence of infection aggravates the diabetes. In extreme cases, response to insulin is diminished so that relatively enormous quantities are sometimes required. This vicious circle can be broken only by energetic and appropriate treatment for both the diabetes and the infection.

Despite all the complications, however, many patients who have been diabetic for 30 years or more have escaped these problems. Usually, these are the patients who have taken fastidious care of themselves over the years and have never gone long with more than minimal insulin reactions, indicating a definite attempt at diabetic regulation.

Self-care of the diabetic patient

Less than 50 years ago, a diabetic patient's life depended upon the severity of his disease. If his diabetes was mild, he lived; if it was not, he died. There existed no effective medical treatment. Since the discovery of insulin, however, the outlook for diabetics has changed to one of hope.

There are three major factors in the care of the diabetic: proper administration of insulin or oral hypoglycemic agents, body hygiene, and correct dieting. It is important that a balance be maintained between food intake, amount of exercise, and quantity of insulin injected. The blood sugar level may be elevated by a meal, or lowered by exercise, which causes sugar to be consumed as energy. Thus, more insulin is needed after a meal, and less after exercise.

One of the best methods of holding the blood sugar level at reasonable values is to make frequent checks on the amount of sugar that has "spilled over" into the urine. Various commercial products are available with which the diabetic may test his own urine. The simplest ones involve incorporation of chemicals into a tablet or absorbent paper. Sugar in the urine will cause changes in the color of the tablet or paper which indicate how much if any sugar is present.

The amount of insulin taken and the manner in which it is administered will depend upon the kind of insulin prescribed by the physician. *Regular insulin*, which is injected under the skin,

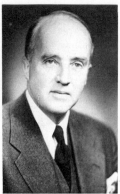

BEST, Charles Herbert (1899-) Canadian physiologist and physician. Famed for his work with Banting and Macleod which resulted in the discovery of insulin in 1922. Applied the use of the anticoagulant, heparin, to the prevention of threatened thrombosis. Made numerous other important contributions to physiology and medicine. Dr. Best is also noted as the coauthor of a widely used textbook of physiology, along with Taylor. *Photographer: Ashley and Crippen.*

is effective for about 6 to 8 hours after injection. It is prompt in beginning to work and is the form which should be used in emergencies. *Globin insulin* is effective for 8 to 16 hours. If the physician prescribes *protamine-zinc* insulin, the patient probably will have to take a maximum of one injection each day because protamine-zinc is absorbed more slowly by the blood from the site of injection. NPH, a specially modified insulin, has a duration of action intermediate between the unmodified or regular and protamine-zinc insulin. Lente insulins are newer preparations and consist of regular insulin modified with zinc.

Two methods of self-care are essential: administration of insulin (or oral hypoglycemic agent) and analysis of the urine. Both are necessary if the diabetic is to have a long and comfortable life. The patient with diabetes is far more responsible for his own care than is a person with nearly any other disease. Whether or not he lives a long, healthy life is greatly dependent upon the daily routine he sets up for himself and upon the manner in which he follows that routine.

It is vital that the diabetic patient carefully plan his day to allow sufficient time for exercise and meals, scheduled at specific hours. He must further allow time to attend to physical hygiene and regular bowel elimination; he must take out time for sufficient rest and sleep. Body cleanliness is absolutely necessary because any type of infection is far more serious in the diabetic than it is in other persons. The hands should be washed several times a day, particularly before meals. Small cuts or hangnails must be cared for immediately to forestall infection. Shaving should be performed with care to guard against cuts which could become sites of infection. Dental hygiene must be meticulous to prevent tooth or gum infections.

Of all the patient's body, the feet probably should receive the most attention. As mentioned in earlier sections, there is likely to be a de-

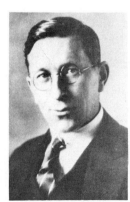

BANTING, Frederick G. (1891-1941) Canadian physician. In collaboration with C. H. Best and J. J. R. Macleod he discovered insulin in 1922, and he was subsequently among the investigators that first applied it to the control of diabetes mellitus. Became professor of medical research at Toronto, which position he held for many years during which he contributed to physiology and medicine. He was knighted and in 1923 received the Nobel prize along with Doctor Macleod.

creased flow of blood to the feet of a diabetic patient; consequently, the possibility of infection in this area is increased. To improve circulation of the feet, the patient should wear warm stockings in cold weather, as well as woolen bed socks; hot water bottles or electrical heating pads are to be avoided as they may cause burns. Circulation will be further improved if the patient does not cross his legs when sitting. He should also get off of his feet for at least five minutes of every hour during the day and elevate his feet at this time, if possible. *Contrast* baths (alternating warm and cool water) that begin and end with warm water are helpful, as is daily massage of the feet and legs. Foot exercises are of value in maintaining circulation to the feet; the physician will recommend the time, length, and frequency of these exercises.

Shoes must be selected carefully so that they will not cut off circulation. Stockings should be one-half inch longer than the length of the foot. Circular garters, rolled stockings, and all other constricting articles of clothing are to be avoided.

The feet must be bathed daily. Gentle washing between the toes is advised. Afterward, the feet should be thoroughly dried. The area between the toes should be wiped gently until dry, and foot powder should then be applied. When the feet are dry and scaly, the patient should rub them with lanolin, except for the area between the toes. When the feet perspire and remain moist, they should be rubbed with alcohol.

The toenails should be cut straight across, but they must never be cut shorter than the end of the toe. Any corns or similar growths on the feet must be cared for by the physician. The patient must never use a corn remedy or cut into a corn.

Gangrene of the feet is a serious complication of diabetes, but it can be avoided if proper foot care is practiced.

If any of the following warning signals are noted they should be called to the doctor's attention immediately: a tingling or burning sensation in the feet; a feeling of coldness or numbness of the feet; cramps in the calves of the legs; a change in foot or toe color to white, deep red, or purple; and any swelling, soreness, cuts, bruises, frostbite, or fungus infection such as athlete's foot.

Dieting

The health and comfort of the diabetic patient depend upon the amount of insulin (or oral hypoglycemic agent) taken, the diet, and the amount of exercise. Ordinarily, the diet consists of the same foods that are found in the diet of a healthy person, except that less carbohydrate is consumed. The patient should adhere to a standard pattern of food distribution

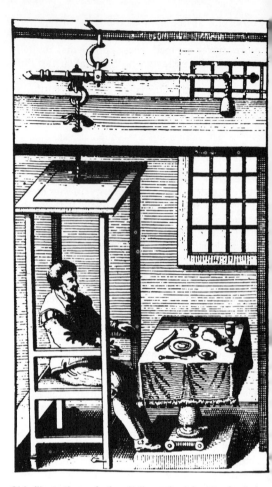

Old illustration of the Italian physiologist, Santorio (1561-1636), performing an experiment on the relation of weight to nutrition. *Bettmann Archive.*

from day to day. In other words, meals should be taken at regular intervals and should be of about the same amount from one day to another. Depending on an individual's activities, a greater quantity should be eaten at one meal than another. If the patient exercises a great deal, he may either increase the amount of carbohydrates in his diet or decrease the dosage of insulin. If he increases his insulin, he must abstain from overactivity or increase the intake of carbohydrates. However, these changes are to be decided only by the physician until such time as the patient has become thoroughly familiar with the individual manifestations of the disease within himself. Indeed, as the patient learns more about diabetes and his particular reactions to it, he will take over many of the decisions which at first were made by the physician. And he will be more healthy for it. As one authority has stated: "Conditions being equal, those who know the most can live the longest."

HOW URINE IS TESTED
FOR ACETONE AND SUGAR

The diabetic patient may be required to perform tests at home in order to assess the degree to which the disease is under control. These tests are generally performed upon a specimen of urine and are important supplements to the clinical laboratory tests that the physician performs upon a blood sample. They are simple to execute, and allow the patient to keep a closer check upon his condition at all times. Tests for sugar in the urine are routine, but in uncontrolled diabetes, tests for the presence of acetone should also be performed. Presence of the latter substance indicates that acidosis exists, and that immediate treatment should be obtained from a physician. A number of simple home testing kits are now available to the patient, and these carry with them complete instructions for their use. As with any chemical test, directions must be followed carefully in order for results to have significance. The following sequence of pictures shows the procedure employed in one common type of test for acetone and sugar, with typical results that may be obtained. Other tests are similar to the principle involved, but may give other endpoints.

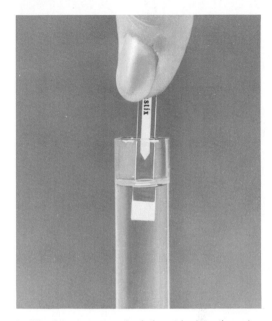

1. Dip the reagent end of the strip into the urine specimen for two seconds and remove. (As an alternate method, wet the reagent area of the strip for two seconds by passing it through a urine stream.)

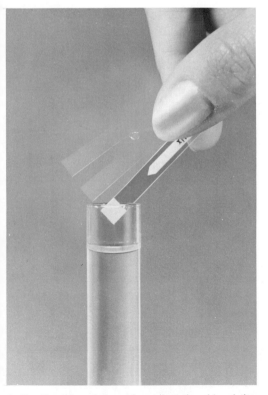

2. Tap the edge of the strip against the side of the urine container or sink to remove excess urine.

Photos courtesy of Ames Company

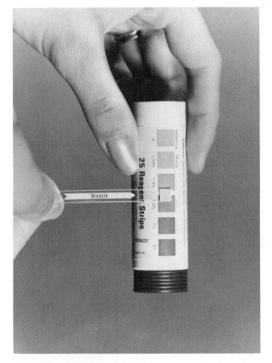

3. *Exactly 30 seconds* after removing from the urine, compare the reagent side of the strip to the closest matching color block. (The original color of the reagent area of the strip is light blue—disregard color changes that occur after 30 seconds.)

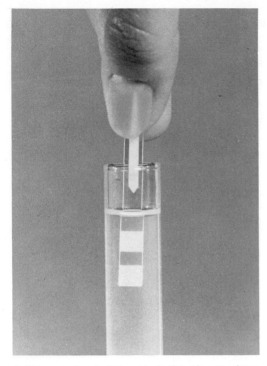

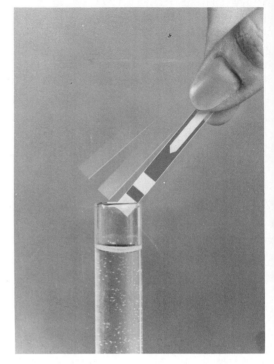

4. Dip reagent end of the strip in the urine specimen for two seconds and remove. (As an alternate method, wet reagent areas of the strip for two seconds by passing through a urine stream.)

5. Tap the edge of the strip against the side of the urine container or sink to remove excess urine.

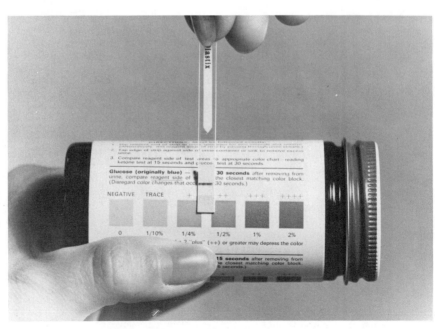

6. Compare the *reagent side* of the strip to appropriate color blocks.

HOW INSULIN IS MEASURED AND INJECTED

For the diabetic that must take insulin, there is no more important detail in his life than assuring that daily routine of insulin injection is cared for properly and without fail. Only a few decades ago the benefits of this drug were not available, and the patient had little hope for life. As the result of recent advances, the standardization of insulin and the improvement of its therapeutic value have made it practical for the diabetic to become accustomed to its routine use with little real inconvenience. Although most patients rapidly become acquainted with the necessity of developing a habit of taking their insulin, many soon cease to pay adequate attention to details of sanitary injection techniques and consequently suffer from the damaging effects of infection. Administration of insulin, like the administration of any other drug, may be a dangerous matter if not performed properly, so that careful attention must be given to details. Insulin is one of the very few therapeutic agents that is routinely administered by the patient to himself, and the diabetic must realize this fact and accept the responsibility that comes with it. The following sequence of photographs illustrates some of the major steps in the administration of insulin. Physicians may prescribe certain variations in the details for different patients, but it is important that in every case the diabetic patient follow carefully the precise directions that are given by the physician.

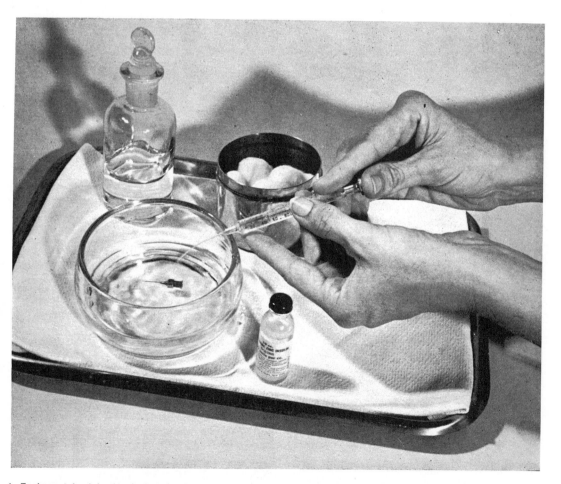

1. Equipment for injection includes a jar of 70 percent alcohol, alcohol-soaked cotton pledgets, and a hypodermic syringe and needle. Insulin should be stored on the bottom refrigerator shelf. Dishes, syringe, and needle must be boiled 20 minutes weekly. The cap of the insulin bottle, the syringe and needle are rinsed before each use, with alcohol.

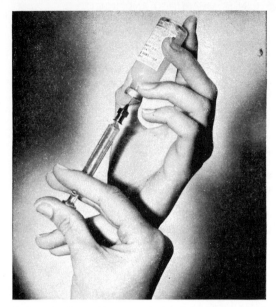

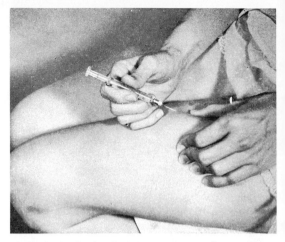

4. Each site for insulin injection should be located at least an inch from other recent sites, and the location sterilized with alcohol-soaked cotton.

2. In order to avoid vacuum in insulin bottle, air must replace insulin withdrawn. Syringe is therefore filled with air to equal amount of insulin to be withdrawn, needle injected through rubber cap of inverted bottle, and plunger of syringe forced in to drive air into bottle. Syringe, needle, and bottle must be held in a straight line to prevent bending needle; and rubber cap of bottle, needle and syringe must be kept sterile. If protamine zinc insulin is used, the bottle must be shaken before the insulin is withdrawn into the syringe.

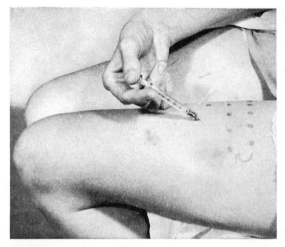

5. With needle and syringe at slight angle to skin, needle is pushed into skin with quick motion of wrist, and the plunger pushed all the way down.

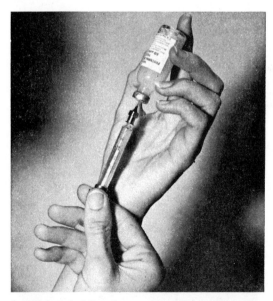

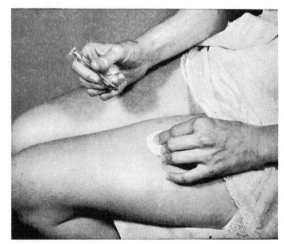

3. Withdrawal of the plunger of the hypodermic syringe now will result in filling of the syringe with the proper amount of insulin up to the indicated marking on the barrel. Any bubbles may be forced out by injecting part of insulin back into the bottle. The needle is now removed from the bottle and wrapped with alcohol-soaked cotton pledget, so that it may be kept sterile and laid down while the area for the injection is selected.

6. Needle is withdrawn from skin with one hand as skin is held down with alcohol-soaked cotton, assuring sterility. Equipment is then washed.

HOW THE DIABETIC SHOULD TAKE CARE OF HIS FEET

Proper foot hygiene is particularly important for the diabetic, since even the slightest damage to the skin may result in an infection that is intensified by the diabetes. The feet are particularly subject to minor injuries from poorly fitting shoes, improperly clipped toenails, and inadequate cleanliness. Blisters, bunions, corns, calluses, and hangnails must all receive prompt treatment in order to prevent infection, and the reasons for the occurrence of such disorders must be discovered so as to prevent recurrence. A thorough daily bathing of the feet is essential for the diabetic, and the care taken in this process will reward the patient in both comfort and freedom from many common foot disorders. The following sequence of photographs illustrates the major steps in this daily regimen of foot care. Each of the measures shown must be given careful attention in order to assure that the skin of the feet will remain healthy.

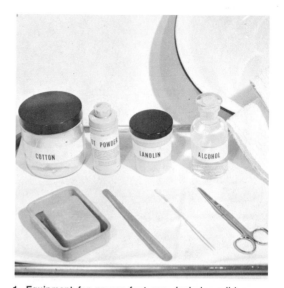

1. Equipment for proper foot care includes mild soap, an emery board, an orangewood stick, scissors, absorbent cotton, foot powder, lanolin, rubbing alcohol, a tub or basin, and soft type of washcloth and towel.

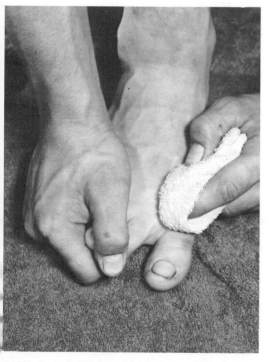

2. The feet should be washed gently with warm, but not hot, soapy water, care being taken not to break the skin between the toes. In drying the feet, the toes should be spread apart and very gently wiped dry.

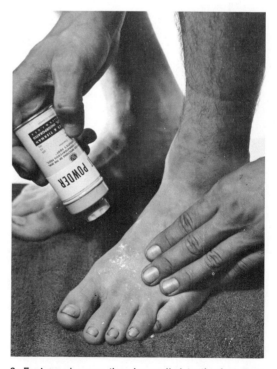

3. Foot powder may then be applied to the feet once they are thoroughly dried. Since the regions between the toes are particularly subject to chaffing and infection, they should receive a liberal amount of powder.

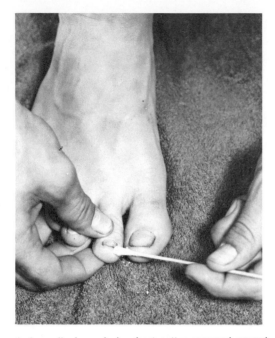

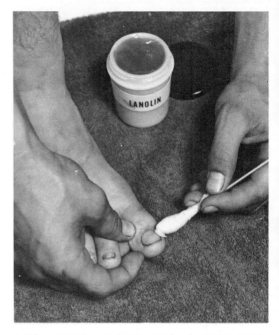

4. A small piece of absorbent cotton wrapped around the tip of an orangewood stick may then be used to clean the toenails. Toenails should be clipped straight across, rather than rounded, and even with tip of toe.

5. When toenails are brittle and break readily and irregularly, lanolin should be applied under the nail and around the cuticle by means of an orangewood stick to the tip of which has been wrapped a bit of cotton.

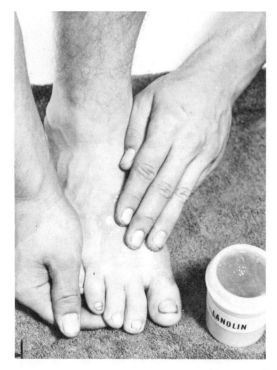

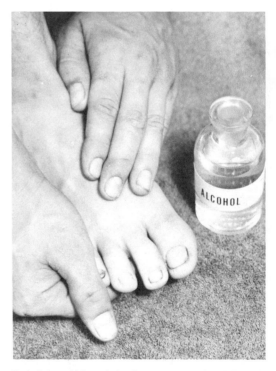

6. Dry and scaly feet also present a potential source of infection, so that they too should be rubbed each day with lanolin. Areas between toes should not receive lanolin, nor should feet be allowed to become tender.

7. A light rubbing of the feet once or twice daily with rubbing alcohol helps to overcome excess perspiration, but as with all other treatment, rubbing should not be vigorous enough to cause abrasions or roughened skin.

11 THE BRAIN AND NERVOUS SYSTEM

WHAT IT IS AND DOES

The nervous system is the governing agency of the body. It controls all muscular movements, whether voluntary or involuntary. It is responsible for all conscious, subconscious, and unconscious thoughts and regulates many vital processes such as circulation, respiration, digestion, and elimination.

Constantly sensitive to changes on the inside and outside of the body, the nervous system detects and differentiates all kinds of stimuli. Depending on the nature of the stimulus, this system may react immediately, may delay response, or may never react. For example, the pupil of the eye immediately narrows in a bright light; one may willfully hold a hot object to keep from breaking it; or one may see something he desires, but never seek to obtain it.

The nervous system is made up of two main divisions: (1) *the central nervous system*, composed of the brain and spinal cord; and (2) *the peripheral nervous system*. The latter consists of twelve pairs of nerves arising from the brain (*cranial nerves*), 31 pairs of nerves coming from the *spinal cord*, and the nerves of the *autonomic nervous system* which supply the internal organs and blood vessels.

The brain

The brain is the control station for nerve impulses. It is composed chiefly of nerve cells with their fibers interwoven in a complex relay system. In the average adult, it weighs approximately 45 ounces. At birth, it weighs only 11 to 13 ounces, but it increases in weight until about the twentieth year. After this, there is a steady loss of weight for the remainder of the person's life.

The brain is divided into four parts: (1) the *medulla oblongata*, continuous above with the midbrain and below with the spinal cord; (2) the *midbrain*, the part between the cerebrum and cerebellum; (3) the *cerebellum*; and (4) the *cerebrum*, composed of two large cerebral hemispheres. The medulla oblongata is about three fourths of an inch to one inch in length. Externally, it looks like an expanded part of the spinal cord. Internally, however, its structure is quite complex and consists of nerve tracts passing into the brain. From some of the nuclei come fibers that eventually emerge to form the VIIIth, IXth, Xth, XIth, and XIIth cranial nerves. Cell centers in this area also are concerned with swallowing, vomiting, breathing, speech, digestion, metabolism, and the beating of the heart. In the medulla oblongata, the large bundles of fibers, which originated in the two halves of the cerebrum and which transmit the impulses of voluntary movement, cross to the opposite sides. Thus, movement in the *right* arm, for example, is controlled by the centers in the left *half* of the cerebrum.

Lying above the medulla oblongata and continuous with it is the *pons*. It is made up of massive bundles of fibers that start in the cerebrum and sweep backward to the cerebellum. This connection makes possible many skilled acts that require co-ordination of sight, hearing, muscular movement, and various other sensations. The playing of a musical instrument is an example of such an act. The pons contains a space called the *fourth ventricle*. In the floor of this ventricle is the nucleus of the VIth cranial nerve. This nerve, which has the longest course inside the skull of all the cranial nerves, is concerned with turning the eyeball outward.

The *cerebellum,* the second largest part of the brain, is back of the pons. It lies in the back of the skull. It is made up of many narrow, leaflike folds arranged into two large masses, and of a middle portion. Rich in cells, it has many complex connections with the brain above it and with the spinal cord below. The chief function of the cerebellum is to co-ordinate more or less complex movements into special acts. This may be movement in different parts of the same limb; combined action of the limbs; combined action of the head and limbs; or combined action of the head, limbs, and body. For example, picking up a pencil, writing with it, and laying it down again requires smooth interaction of many muscle groups. The cerebellum correlates the actions of the various groups. To do this, range, direction, rate, and force of movement must be synchronized and maintained with the movement of the eye. Disease in the cerebellum does not cause paralysis. It does produce disturbance of muscular co-ordination. Tremors, staggering gait, and excessive relaxation of the muscles result from disease in this part of the brain, as well as disturbances in the above-mentioned components of muscular activity.

The midbrain is a small area between the pons and the cerebrum. It is an important relay station for the sensory impulses. It also governs some muscle activity of a reflex nature. Many of the involuntary acts of the eye, such as narrowing of the pupil in bright light, originate here. The IIIrd, IVth, and Vth cranial nerves originate from cell collections in this area of the brain.

Just above the midbrain is the *hypothalamus,* an important group of nuclei. Beneath it, the two large nerves from the eyes meet, and part of their fibers cross to the opposite sides. Other cells of this region are concerned with such vital functions as regulation of body temperature, metabolism, and heart rate. Sexual development, sleep, and the body's use of fat and water are influenced by this region in the brain. The relationship of the hypothalamus and the nervous system to the endocrine system is discussed in Chapter 10, "The Endocrine System." The *thalamus,* which is found next to this group of cells, contains another group of nuclei which integrate sensations of many sorts. Also, it is the site of a crude form of consciousness and plays a role in the production of emotion. When this

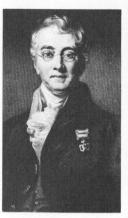

BELL, Charles (1774-1842) Scottish physician. Perpetuated his name in *Bell's law* which states that anterior spinal roots are motor, while the posterior roots are sensory. *Bell's nerve* is the exterior respiratory nerve, and *Bell's palsy* involves the facial nerve. He also observed that the trigeminal nerve was both motor and sensory. An internationally known anatomist and neurologist, Bell artistically illustrated his many published studies.

part of the brain is diseased, spontaneous laughter or crying may occur. The crude emotional responses that arise are further elaborated and controlled by the *cerebral cortex.*

Above these nuclei are two *cerebral hemispheres* which represent 70 percent of the entire nervous system. This is the area of the nervous system in which all the sensory experiences are mixed and blended. Specific sensory impulses thus become associated with many others and expand the experience and consciousness. The individual's capacity for many and varied activities, memory, emotions, and ideas is dependent on the action of this part of the nervous system.

The surfaces of the hemispheres are marked by large, rounded folds and deep grooves. Partly on the axis of the main grooves and partly on imaginary lines, the cerebrum is divided into four lobes: *frontal, parietal, temporal,* and *occipital.* Each lobe has special functions, but these functions are only partially understood.

The occipital lobes at the back of the skull are the site where visual impressions are made. Color, size, form, movement, and distance are evaluated in this portion of the brain, leading to the identification of a particular object. Also, the differences between similar objects are discerned. For example, two objects high in the air can be recognized as a bird and an airplane on the basis of past experience. Injury to this area may cause blindness.

The temporal lobes receive the fibers concerned with hearing, speech, balance, and smell. Diseases related to these lobes cause loss of smell, or they may be responsible for imaginary smells.

The parietal lobes are concerned with taste sensations and some other sensations such as the ability to judge weight, shape, and textures. By the action of this area, one is able to tell what various objects are by feeling, rather than by seeing them.

The frontal lobes are concerned with some of the most complex abilities of the mind. Reason, emotions, and judgment have their site here. In addition, there are a group of large cells in the posterior region of the frontal lobes which are involved with complicated voluntary movements. For instance, the speech center is located here. It is found to predominate on the left side in right-handed individuals and vice versa. However, if the speech function is lost because of injury to only one side of the brain, it can sometimes be re-acquired by re-education. The area responsible for these complex voluntary movements is called the *motor cortex*. The muscles of the body are controlled by various areas of the motor cortex. Irritation of the cells in these zones will cause spasms of the muscles they supply. Destruction of the cells will produce complete loss of voluntary movement of the muscles. Another function of the cells of the motor cortex is to keep the muscles in balance between relaxation and contraction. If this region of the brain is seriously damaged or destroyed, this inhibiting power is lost; consequently, the muscles become contracted and stiff (*spastic paralysis*).

The frontal lobes have many connections with the thalamus as well as with the other lobes of the brain. In the frontal lobes, feelings or emotions are added to the other associations. The combination of feeling and knowing determines most voluntary action of the body. A baby, seeing a piece of candy for the first time, may or may not reach for it. But the baby who has enjoyed candy tries hard to get a piece of it, when he sees it. Thinking, reasoning, judgment, and imagination result as the sensory and emotional associations become more complex. Disease in the frontal lobes of the cerebrum causes personality changes, errors in judgment and insight, and poor emotional control.

Twelve pairs of nerves arise from the brain itself. The Ist is associated with the sense of smell; the IInd with sight; the IIIrd and IVth with the eye muscles which move the eyeball or the muscles of the pupil; and the Vth carries sensations from the head and mouth and causes the muscles of the jaw to move. The VIth is concerned with the movement of the eye to the side. The VIIth carries impulses to all the muscles of the face. The VIIIth conducts impulses having to do with hearing and with balance; the IXth transmits taste sensations from the posterior third of the tongue, and other sensations from the throat and mucous membranes; it also aids in swallowing. The Xth is an exceedingly long nerve that extends down the neck and into the chest and abdomen; it is concerned with swallowing and talking; its action also slows the rate of the heart and regulates the movement of the stomach. It is a large part of the parasympathetic system in the upper part of the body, including the esophagus, stomach, intestines, liver, bronchi, lungs, heart, and blood vessels. The XIth supplies some of the muscles that turn the head and some of those in the neck. The XIIth is responsible for the movement of the tongue.

The spinal cord

The nerve tracts passing to and from the brain are contained in the spinal cord, which is continuous with the lower part of the brain. It is about 18 inches long and is rounded in shape. It is larger in the regions which give rise to the nerves to the arms and legs, since these parts have many complex functions thus requiring a large nerve supply. From the neck to the lowest part of the vertebral column, 31 pairs of nerves emerge from the spinal cord. Each nerve is attached to the cord by two roots. Because the spinal cord is not as long as the vertebral column, the roots of the nerves must gradually increase in length before they can emerge from between the vertebrae. These longer nerve roots collect in a mass that fills the lower end of the vertebral canal. The structure resembles a horse's tail and is called the *cauda equina*.

A cross section of the spinal cord reveals a gray figure, roughly shaped like an "H," imposed on a white background. The nerve cells make up the gray matter, while the nerve bundles form the white matter. Bundles with specific functions occupy specific areas of the spinal cord. Therefore, injury to the cord will result in certain abnormal reactions which will be evident on neurological examination. The abnormal findings will suggest where the diseased part is located.

Impulses which arise in the brain and are concerned with voluntary muscular movements are received by specific cells in the spinal cord. They relay these impulses to the nerves which control the various muscles. These cells have connections with other cells in the nervous system that act together to bring about *reflex activity*. Reflexes control the position of the head so that it automatically assumes the normal position. Withdrawal or *flexion* reflexes pull limbs away from painful or disagreeable stimuli. *Extensor* reflexes straighten out the limbs and work with the flexor reflexes. Bladder and bowel actions result from reflex action over which there is some voluntary control; in injury to the spinal cord, the tracts allowing voluntary control may be interrupted, so that the action is then reflex in origin.

The cells on the front and anterior side of the spinal cord connect with cells in the cerebellum to control the direction and precision of normal muscular movement. From still another part of the brain, connecting fibers come to these cells to bring about certain automatic, associated muscular movements—for example, the swinging of the arms as one walks. Another function of these cells is the maintenance of the proper amount of constant contraction or *tone*

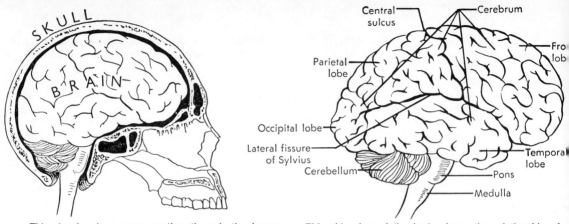

This drawing is a cross section through the human head which shows the relationship of the brain to the cranium. The picture shows how well the brain is protected from injury by bone.

This side view of the brain shows the relationship of its important structures to each other. The cerebrum, where thinking takes place, is much larger in humans than in the lower animals.

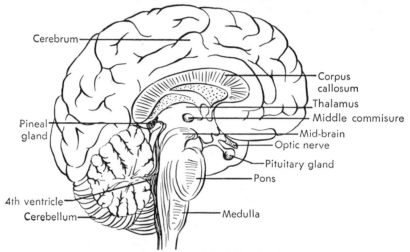

Drawing of a sagittal section of the brain showing some important internal structures, which are not visible from the surface. The function of the pineal gland is not well understood.

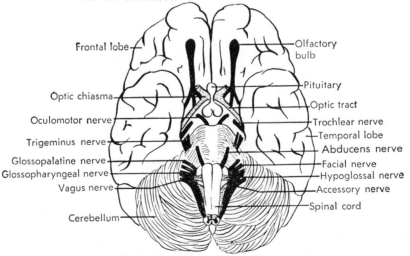

Illustration of the brain as seen from below, showing the cranial nerves in their relation to the structures of the brain. The cranial nerves are a part of the peripheral nervous system.

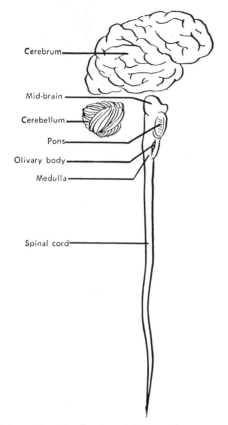

Cerebrum

Mid-brain

Cerebellum

Pons

Olivary body

Medulla

Spinal cord

This is a schematic drawing of the central nervous system which consists of all of the brain, together with the spinal cord. This is the most important division of the human nervous system.

of the muscles. If the muscles are too contracted, they move too slowly and rigidly. If they are too relaxed, too much stimulation is needed to make them respond.

The cells along the side of the cord send out fibers that unite with others to form the *sympathetic chain*. These cells are concerned with the action of involuntary muscles in the intestines, arteries, and other internal structures. Various glands receive fibers from these cells.

Cells on the back or posterior side of the spinal cord receive the sensations of touch, pain, vibration, temperature, pressure, and position. They then transmit these various sensations to other cells in the brain.

From this, it can be seen that impulses of many sorts travel down the paths in the spinal cord while others enter it and travel upward to the brain. Still others enter and travel only part of the way up and set off the spinal reflexes.

The peripheral nerves

As stated before, the peripheral nervous system is composed of the cranial nerves, already

described; the spinal nerves; and the autonomic nervous system. The autonomic system supplies nerves to most of the "automatic" organs of the body—the glands, heart, blood vessels, and involuntary muscles in the internal organs.

The autonomic system consists of its network of nerves and a series of nerve-cell collections called *ganglia*. Some of these ganglia are connected to the spinal cord by means of fibers, which arise in its gray matter and pass out over the roots of the spinal nerves. These vertebral ganglia lie on each side of the spinal cord and send out meshworks of fibers to the organs of the abdomen and pelvis. Other ganglia arise within the brain and supply such structures as the tear and salivary glands and the pupils of the eye. They also send out fibers in some of the cranial nerves. One important and familiar ganglion is the *solar plexus*. The dramatic symptoms of being struck here result from the momentary effects on the heart, arteries, and lungs.

One part of the autonomic nervous system prepares the person for "fight" or "flight." This part is responsible for a shift in circulating blood to skeletal and heart muscles, increasing heart and lung functions, dilating the pupils of the eyes, and moistening the skin with perspiration.

The other division of this system is concerned with conserving and restoring bodily resources. Thus, it protects the eyes by causing the pupils to constrict in bright light, and prevents the heart from overexerting itself. All the digestive processes are promoted by this part.

It can be seen that these two divisions counterbalance each other. Together, they are responsible for the physical reactions and sensations that accompany the emotions. The language is rich in expressions which recognize these physical accompaniments of emotion—"a sinking feeling in the stomach," "white with anger," etc. These many reactions of the body to emo-

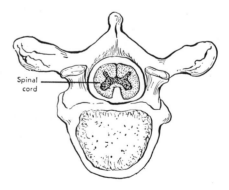

Spinal cord

THORACIC VERTEBRA

This is a cross-sectional drawing of one of the vertebrae and spinal cord. The vertebrae interlock with each other to form the backbone. The spinal cord is composed of nerve cells and bundles.

tional states enrich life, but they also become symptoms of emotional disturbances. Thus, suppressed resentment may easily cause overactivity of the muscles and glands of the stomach. The pain produced is not imaginary because of its emotional origin. If these physical reactions persist long enough, actual changes may occur in the affected organs.

Microscopic anatomy

The operation of the central nervous system depends on two substances: the *gray matter* (nerve cells), and the *white matter* (the nerve fibers given off by the cells). The function of the gray matter is the generating and dispatching of nerve impulses. The function of the white matter is the conduction of these impulses to and from the cells in the gray matter. Other cells in the nervous system have no nervous function, but instead are concerned with the support and nourishment of nerve cells.

Nerve tissue itself consists of cells giving off threadlike processes (*axons*) some of which are extremely long. The axons connect with other cells in the brain or spinal cord. These cells constantly generate, receive, or store up energy. Unlike most body tissues, nerve cells are never replaced once they are actually destroyed. If the cells are destroyed, their axons degenerate.

Some cells concerned with generating or receiving similar impulses may be collected into definite groups called nuclei. The axons from these cells unite and form bundles of nerves which then transmit the impulses. The nerve cells are not collected into nuclei in the cerebral hemispheres, but form a uniform layer (*cortex*) of gray matter over the surfaces.

A series of highly specialized organs called *receptors* detect changes in and about the body. They rapidly transmit this information to definite stations within the nervous system. This is called *sensory* activity. Receptors, called exteroceptors, gather information from a distance—seeing, hearing, and smelling. Interoceptors detect things in contact with the body—pain, touch, and temperature. And proprioceptors pick up information from within the body, giving a sense of bodily position. Fibers from the receptor organs pass into the spinal cord as a part of the nerve. Within the cord, they unite to form ascending tracts which connect with other spinal cells or enter the brain. Fibers from some special receptors, such as the eye, form nerves which enter the brain directly.

It is thought that when a sensory impression reaches the brain, it stimulates a nerve cell which, in turn, stimulates another cell. A third cell is then stimulated and so on, until a circle has been completed, and the last cell restimulates the first one. The circuit continues to *fire* or *reverberate*, thus retaining the impression which

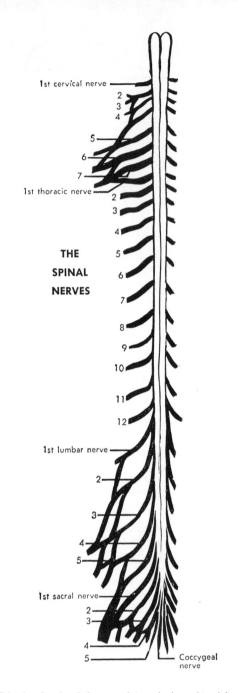

1st cervical nerve — 2 3 4
5
6
7
1st thoracic nerve — 2
3
4

THE

SPINAL 5

NERVES 6

7

8

9

10

11

12

1st lumbar nerve —

2

3

4

5

1st sacral nerve —

2

3

4

5 — Coccygeal nerve

This drawing is of the complete spinal cord and its 31 pairs of nerves. For clarity, the vertebrae are not shown. The nerves are named according to the region of the body they are opposite.

set it off. It is believed that these reverberating circuits hold the impressions so that they can be recalled later or compared with other impressions. It is further thought that a cell may participate in more than one circuit, thus accounting for various associations of sensory and muscular activity.

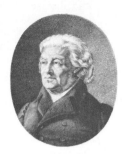

SOEMMERING, Samuel T. (1755-1830) German anatomist. Defined and classified the cranial nerves (1778). With remarkable skill at illustration, he produced fine drawings of his anatomical investigations, and with him descriptive anatomy is said to have reached its greatest height. Other body structures, organs, and areas bear his name, including the yellow spot on the retina of the eye.

In many ways, the nervous system resembles a vast electrical network, the brain acting as the chief control panel for the ascending and descending tracts. The nerve cells may be likened to tubes or batteries, while the nerve fibers resemble connecting wires. Impulses received and sent over the nerves are thought to be electrical in nature.

Electrical activity does occur in the brain itself and can be recorded with the proper instrument (*electroencephalograph*). Some of the electrical impulses from various lobes of the brain are detected by means of wires applied to the scalp. The impulses are recorded in waves. These assume a certain form—the rate, height, and length varying in different parts of the cerebrum. Age and the degree of consciousness also produce normal variations in the pattern. This test gives valuable information about such abnormal conditions as tumor, epilepsy, infections, and hemorrhages.

The central nervous system is well protected by the rigid *skull* and the flexible backbone (*vertebral* or *spinal column*). The skull consists of a dome of thin, porous, but strong, bones. The bones of the forehead contain the sinuses of the nose. The floor of the skull is composed of somewhat thinner bone and contains more sinuses that connect with the nasal passages. The deeper structures of the ear are embedded in the bones forming the base of the skull. The floor of the skull consists of three irregular depressions (*fossae*) that form three descending levels. The fossa in the back of the skull is the largest and deepest. The cranial nerves arise from different parts of the brain and emerge through various bony canals and openings of the skull.

Inside this hard shell, three separate tissues provide additional coverings for the brain and spinal cord. The outermost, *dura mater*, consists of layers of dense, fibrous material. The outer layer of the dura adheres tightly to the bones of the skull. The inner covers the brain and spinal cord, forming a tough, saclike structure. Within the skull itself, the dura is folded into partitions which separate and support the various parts of the brain. One such fold is called the *falx cerebri*; it divides the cerebral hemispheres into right and left halves. Another fold, the *tentorium*, separates the back fossa from the vault of the skull; it provides a horizontal support for the back part of the brain and separates that part from the cerebellum. Between the layers of the dura are large blood vessels called *venous sinuses* which collect blood from the brain and return it to the heart.

The middle of the three covering tissues is a delicate membrane called the *arachnoid* (which means cobweb-like), a layer that encloses the brain and the spinal cord in a loose-fitting sack. The space below this layer is the *subarachnoid space*.

The third covering is a thin, delicate sheet that follows closely all the irregular surfaces and fissures of the brain and spinal cord. This is called the *pia mater* and is next to the nerve tissue itself.

Between the arachnoid and the pia mater circulates the *cerebrospinal fluid*, which acts as a shock absorber for the central nervous system. Also, it probably helps in nourishing the nerve tissue itself. This clear, watery-looking fluid—formed within certain cavities (*ventricles*) of the brain—flows out from small openings into the brain and spinal cord before it is absorbed back into the blood stream. When the flow or absorption of the fluid is impaired, it accumulates in large quantities. The head enlarges and "waterhead" (*hydrocephalus*) results.

The spinal fluid is affected by various disorders and is easily drawn off to be examined for diagnostic purposes. Its pressure can be measured; it is above normal in some conditions involving brain tumors, brain hemorrhages, and certain infections. The presence of red blood cells signifies hemorrhage somewhere in the central nervous system. White blood cells are increased when there is infection or other inflammatory disease of the central nervous system; the number and type of the white blood cells in the spinal fluid offer clues to the identification of these processes. Changes in protein content, sugar, salt, and other chemicals of the fluid may help in the diagnosis of certain conditions. Other tests reveal specific diseases.

Lesions of the brain may be studied by *encephalography*. This x-ray procedure involves removal of spinal fluid by lumbar puncture and injection of air (pneumoencephalography). The air thus fills the cavities in the skull so they can be visualized in x-rays. A distortion of the cavities would suggest a possible brain tumor, blood clot, etc. An alternate method is to inject the air directly into the cavities (ventricles) in the brain. In this case, small holes are placed in the skull and the air injected following ventricular puncture (ventriculography).

DISORDERS OF THE BRAIN AND NERVOUS SYSTEM: POLIOMYELITIS

Poliomyelitis, or infantile paralysis, is an acute, infectious viral disease of the nervous system, in which the inflammation attacks the anterior part of the spinal cord. This disease is particularly feared because it may result in paralysis of any part of the body and leave the victim crippled for life, although this happens in a minority of cases.

There are four major types of poliomyelitis, and only one, the paralytic type, is actually associated with disabling paralysis. The abortive, nonparalytic and encephalitic types account for more than half of the cases diagnosed during epidemic periods. It is believed by some that many mild cases are unrecognized as poliomyelitis due to their resemblance to colds or intestinal disorders. The victims of these cases may recover without knowing that they have had poliomyelitis. Even such mild experiences with the disease offer future immunity to the virus.

Paralytic poliomyelitis may occur in several forms, depending upon the extent of viral involvement and the area of the central nervous system which is affected. *Spinal* poliomyelitis involves the muscles of the extremities or trunk, and is the form most frequently encountered. *Bulbar* poliomyelitis involves the cranial nerves arising from the brain stem, and the vital centers of circulation or respiration are affected. *Bulbo-spinal* poliomyelitis is usually severe and is associated with respiratory impairment and with paralysis involving both the spinal cord and brain stem. Ten to 25 percent of paralytic cases seen during an epidemic are of the bulbar or bulbo-spinal type.

Infantile paralysis has been a problem to man since the early beginnings of civilization. An Egyptian skeleton, dating back to 3700 B.C., shows bone malformations which indicate that the individual had been afflicted with polio during childhood. It was not until 1907 that polio was confirmed to be an infectious disease by Otto Ivar Wickman, a German physician. The United States had several mild epidemics early in its colonial history, but the disease was virtually unknown to the general public until 1916. During that year, New York City was ravaged by the most telling epidemic of polio on record. About 9000 children contracted the disease, and 2000 of these died.

Until recently, there were no means of preventing the disease. The Salk vaccine, introduced by Jonas Salk in 1953, was the first successfully applied antipoliovirus immunization. The Sabin live, attenuated oral vaccine was licensed for use in 1961–1962, and is now generally used. Since the advent of these two vaccines, epidemic outbreaks of the disease have been dramatically reduced.

The summer months, usually beginning in June, are the "polio season," or the time in which infantile paralysis is most prevalent. There is an increase of cases in July and August, a decrease in October, and by November the disease practically disappears for the winter. Any illness of the respiratory tract or intestinal disorder should be treated with rest and observed closely during these months, and persons acutely ill should be avoided as a precautionary measure. But complete avoidance of crowds during the polio season is no longer necessary by immunized persons.

Symptoms

Poliomyelitis is caused by a specific virus, which is an infectious agent too small to be seen with an ordinary compound microscope. In early stages of the disease the symptoms are so slight or so akin to symptoms of other, milder ailments that they often go unnoticed. For the first three or four days, the child may complain only of a headache and stomach upset, which causes vomiting. He may have fever up to 104°, a sore throat, and loose bowels. Often the child will appear drowsy, irritable, and listless, and will cry frequently for no apparent reason. If the diagnosis is made while these are the only symptoms, the chances of saving the child's life and preventing paralysis are good.

The next symptoms, however, are those of general weakness and paralysis. At first, there may be a stiffness of the back or resistance to movement of the neck. These symptoms can progress until one or more parts of the body are completely paralyzed.

In many cases, the paralysis may not occur or be so slight that the child will recover without the parents ever realizing that he had poliomyelitis. When this happens, the child may resume playing and then suffer a severe attack in a few days. Thus, it is imperative that the disease be

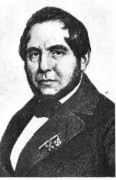

HEINE, Jacob von (1800-1879) German orthopedist. Most remembered as the man who first described the spinal paralysis found usually in infants and young children, and commonly known today as poliomyelitis or simply, "polio." The famous orthopedic institution at Cannstatt was founded by Heine, whose wise use of physiotherapy and surgery made it a model of its kind throughout the world.

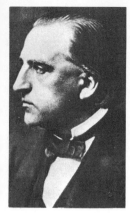

CHARCOT, Jean Martin (1825-1893) French neurologist and clinician. Creator of the greatest modern neurological clinic, at La Salpetriere, Paris. Universally regarded as one of the finest neurologists, he exerted a formative influence on Freud, who studied with him. He is author of many early descriptions of nervous disorders, and increased our knowledge of diseases of muscles and the nervous system, many of which bear his name. *Bettmann Archive.*

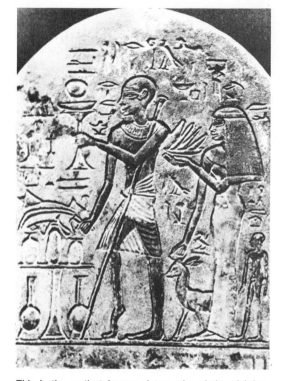

This is the earliest known picture of a victim of infantile paralysis. It appears on an Egyptian stele ca. 1400 B.C., and shows the priest Ruma with an atrophied right leg. *Bettmann Archive.*

diagnosed even in its mildest forms; and if the diagnosis is poliomyelitis, the child must stay in bed for a week to ten days following even the slightest attack.

It is a good rule to consult a physician whenever a child shows any symptoms of fever and vomiting during the summer months. The physician can probably tell if the child has poliomyelitis by physical examination, but he may have to examine a sample of the spinal fluid. Early diagnosis and proper care—i.e., during the first three days—can usually prevent or decrease the effects of the severe form of the disease.

Treatment

Infantile paralysis can be controlled through immunization by vaccine. Three oral doses of the Sabin vaccine are necessary before immunity is achieved. The first may be given at the age of six weeks or later. The second is given four to six weeks after the first, and the third is given approximately a year following the second dose. Another dose is desirable three to four years later, in order to insure a continuing high level of resistance to the virus. Although infantile paralysis is rarely seen in infants under one year of age, and is again rare although more severe among persons over 40, there is no "safe" age and all persons should be immunized.

Other than rest and comfort, there is no means of altering the course of poliomyelitis if the disease has developed. Treatment measures are directed toward preventing extension of the disease to other neuromuscular units of the body. Absolute bed rest and expert nursing care are essential for the patient. The application of moist, hot packs over the affected arms, legs and back is the best method for the relief of pain and prevention of muscle spasms, which, if not prevented, may cause deformity of the limbs.

When the acute stage is past, the physician will examine the child's muscles to determine which have been weakened and which have lost

their power of movement entirely. If the doctor believes the child is ready, treatment is begun to re-establish the use of as many muscles as possible. Surgical correction of some defects may be necessary before the muscles can undergo re-education. If the child is ready, the physician will probably prescribe a set of exercises. However, only the doctor can say when the child is ready or what exercises are needed. If the child walks too soon, is allowed to stand in deformed positions, or practices the wrong exercises, he may lessen the chances of overcoming his handicap.

After the physician has selected the exercises, the mother should be taught these exercises by a qualified physical therapist and begin a daily schedule, helping the patient to perform them. It is preferable to place the exercise period in the morning when the muscles are less tired; but in any case, the exercises should be done every day.

The mother begins by telling the child what movement he is to do, and the child attempts to do it. Then the child relaxes, and the mother puts the arm or leg back in the starting position. She should not help the patient in making a movement until he has done as much for himself as he can; then, the remainder of the movement is finished for him while he still endeavors to complete it.

When a movement can be performed ten times correctly without help, some resistance can be applied by the mother to make the exercise more difficult. This resistance should not be so great as to stop the movement or to make it jerky.

Although fatigue is to be avoided, the child should not be allowed to turn or twist his body to aid the movements. This only substitutes the use of nonparalyzed muscles for those that are weak.

As the exercises progress, the mother should concentrate on movements which are hardest for the child to do. Otherwise, there may be overdevelopment of stronger muscles at the expense of the weaker. If the legs are too weak, the child will have to wear splints, corsets, jackets, or braces for the first few months.

Prevention

The oral poliovirus vaccine has been established as safe and effective and has largely supplanted the injected vaccine because of its ease of administration and ability to induce immunity rapidly in young children. The oral vaccine consists of three separate types of inoculum; each represents a different strain of poliovirus. For infants, this course of vaccination is usually started in the first year of life and is integrated with other immunization procedures.

The poliomyelitis virus has been recovered from secretions of the nose and throat and from the feces of poliomyelitis patients; therefore, it is thought that the disease can be spread by means of coughing and sneezing. All persons should be immunized by poliovirus vaccine to prevent infection.

Direct contact of poliomyelitis patients should be avoided. In addition to actively infected persons, healthy persons may unknowingly be carriers of the virus and thus be sources of infection. Flies and other insects can carry the virus.

Other than vaccination, the best means of preventing infection are general cleanliness, good sanitation, rest and proper eating habits, and isolation from carriers of the disease.

All diseases of the respiratory tract and intestinal irregularities should be closely observed during the summer months, particularly if they occur in persons who have not been immunized. During epidemic periods, children should avoid fatigue and over-exertion, and should not mingle in large crowds where viruses could be spread.

It has been noted that tonsil operations or tooth extractions weaken a child's resistence to the disease. Therefore, it is best to postpone any such procedures during the summer months, when the disease is prevalent, until the child has been immunized—unless, of course, the child's health would be impaired by postponement.

Those interested in obtaining more information on poliomyelitis may contact The National Foundation at 800 Second Avenue, New York, New York.

REHABILITATION OF THE POLIOMYELITIS PATIENT

Rehabilitation of poliomyelitis patients combines use of physical medicine with psychological and vocational adjustment in an attempt to achieve maximal function and prepare the patient physically, mentally, socially, and vocationally for fullest possible life compatible with his abilities. After some degree of muscular coordination has been well established, a detailed program of muscle training is begun. If the affected part is used in the normal manner as far as possible, the various coordinating muscles and neurons will begin to interact with each other in new patterns to produce the rhythmic motion which has been lost. A great variety of equipment and techniques have been devised for all stages of muscle weakness. Psychologically, the

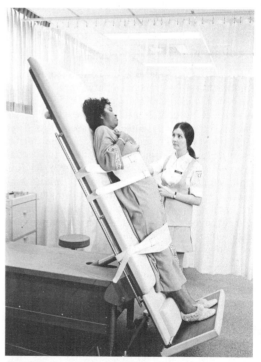

Rehabilitation of the cancer patient is similar to the rehabilitation of the poliomyelitis patient and the programs use similar equipment. The tilt table allows this formerly bedridden cancer patient's cardiovascular system to readjust to the upright position. *Courtesy The Rehabilitation Annex of The University of Texas M. D. Anderson Hospital, Houston, Texas.*

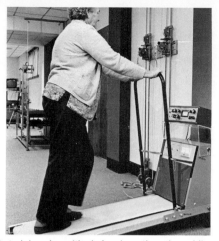

Gait training is critical for long-time immobile patients. This treadmill has a continuous range of speeds and several monitoring devices.

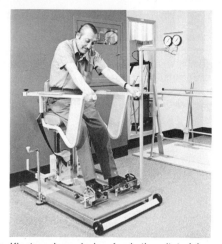

The Kinetron is a device for both gait training and development of muscular strength and coordination which adjusts to patient pressure.

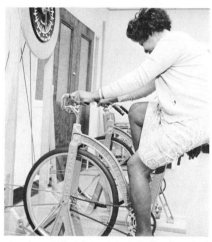

The classic gait training and strengthening device is the stationary bicycle. A simple coupled gauge provides ready monitoring.

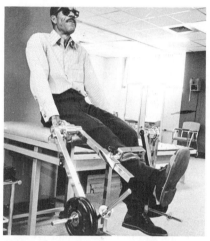

The N-K table is a device used to strengthen the legs of the patient. The load can be continuously varied by adding weights.

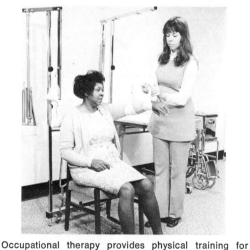

Occupational therapy provides physical training for the upper extremities. This Deltoid Aide is a simple arm exercise device.

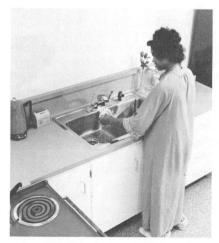

Here also, patients relearn normal household tasks in which they may have lost their normal coordination and confidence, as in the kitchen.

Courtesy The Rehabilitation Annex of The University of Texas M. D. Anderson Hospital, Houston, Texas.

effect of muscle training is important. Once the patient begins working, he no longer lies in bed passively waiting for help. Such persistent activity results in increased muscle strength, shortening of hospitalization, improved morale, and a speeding-up of the tedious recovery process.

DISORDERS OF THE BRAIN AND NERVOUS SYSTEM: LOCKJAW

Lockjaw (*tetanus*) is an acute disease of the nervous system caused by poisons from wounds infected with tetanus bacteria (*Clostridium tetani*). These organisms are found in dust, rust, sewage, and soil, and particularly in the feces of domesticated animals.

Tetanus bacteria thrive only in the absence of air. Entering through breaks in the skin, they establish themselves in dirty wounds such as result from accidents with automobiles and farm implements, fireworks, knife and nail punctures, or any penetrating wound regardless of how trivial it may seem. Any area of tissue destruction provides an ideal environment for the bacillus to produce its powerful poison.

Symptoms

The incubation period is variable, so from two to 50 days may elapse after contact with the germ before symptoms appear. The first signs may be stiffness in the neck and jaw, often preceded by chills, fever, and stiffness of the muscles near the wound. The patient may be restless, apprehensive, and yawn frequently. Soon the jaw muscles contract so strongly that the mouth cannot be opened (lockjaw), and pain follows any attempt to force the jaws apart. The rigidity spreads to the other muscles of the face, neck, and back. The eyebrows are raised, and the corners of the mouth turn up in a perpetual grin. Difficulty in swallowing sets in. In later stages violent, intensely painful muscular spasms intermittently involve the entire body, being set off by slight stimulations, such as air currents, noise, or light. These spasms last a variable period of time and may be sufficiently severe to cause fractures of the spine. Usually, the longer the period before symptoms appear and the longer the survival after the onset, the better is the outlook for the patient. If the disease is fatal, death usually results from paralysis of vital centers in the brain, starvation, heart failure, or asphyxiation. There is no permanent damage to patients who survive and no immunity is acquired by recovery.

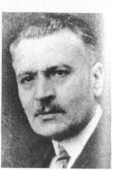

CARLE, Antonio (1854-1927) Italian surgeon. Noted for his valuable studies on the surgery of the brain. His work on the thyroid gland, and on the gastrointestinal and biliary tracts is also famous. But even more important for medicine than this was the profound effect that his school at Turin, guided by his eminent pupils, had on the general progress of Italian surgery. In 1884 he and Rattone demonstrated the transmissibility of tetanus.

The tetanus bacillus produces a poison, or *toxin*, which has a special affinity for nerve tissues; the main effect of the poison is thought to be on the nerve endings in the muscles. It is probable that the blood carries the poison from the infected area to distant muscle-nerve junctions, which become affected.

Prevention

Lockjaw is entirely preventable by vaccination, but a surprisingly large number of the American population is not vaccinated with preventive tetanus toxoid. In 1965 and 1966, 535 cases of tetanus with 363 deaths were reported in the United States. The need for immunization against tetanus applies to everyone.

The routine immunization schedule for children, known to reduce chances of contracting tetanus to essentially zero, is as follows: three DTP (diphtheria, tetanus, pertussis) injections are given at least one month apart in infancy. About a year later a fourth, reinforcing DTP injection is given. A fifth or "booster" injection is given upon entering school, whether it is nursery school, kindergarten, or first grade. Subsequent routine tetanus boosters should be given at about ten-year intervals. If validated by reliable records, this schedule of immunization eliminates the need for special tetanus boosters when a child enters camps, schools, or colleges. With a documented history of immunization, emergency tetanus boosters at the time of accident should not be given, to minimize toxoid reactions.

Tetanus immunization for infants and the elderly is extremely important; for with these two groups, the recent mortality rates are high. After the basic five-dosage pediatric schedule, single booster doses should be given every ten years regardless of age. Pregnant women and presurgical patients should have their immunization history clarified, for they have a greater chance of infection.

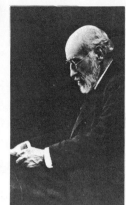

RAMÓN Y CAJAL, S. (1852-1934) Spanish neurologist. Received with Golgi in 1906 the Nobel prize for physiology and medicine for his work on the microscopic anatomy of the nervous system. Using their own original stains, which revealed the most intimate details of nerve and brain tissues, Cajal and his Spanish school of neurologists discovered many cell types. His *Histology of the Nervous System*, published in 1909, is a medical classic.

In cases where immunization is questionable and a wound is prone to tetanus, the physician may decide to administer hyperimmune human globulin.

Treatment

Once tetanus develops, early hospitalization is essential. Antitoxin in large amounts must be given. It cannot act, however, on toxin already fixed to nerve tissue. Therefore, dramatic relief of symptoms on administration of the antitoxin should not be expected. It can neutralize only the poison that is being produced and which has not yet been absorbed. Sedatives may prevent or lighten the spasms. Treatment may require prompt and drastic measures, especially if several hours have elapsed after the injury to the tissues. Immunization, as has been suggested, is always a good precaution. Some investigators have reported a decrease in mortality rate by the use of penicillin and of curare, a drug which relaxes the muscles.

DISORDERS OF THE BRAIN AND NERVOUS SYSTEM: SLEEPING SICKNESS

Disease processes of the brain which give rise to persistent drowsiness, stupor, or coma are often called "sleeping sickness." This group contains two separate types of diseases—one a disease of the brain tissue (*encephalitis*), and the other a disease caused by infection with a parasite called a *trypanosome* (African sleeping sickness).

Encephalitis is a disease which is the result of an inflammatory process in the brain, and can be caused by a number of agents, some known and some unknown. In all cases, there are pinpoint hemorrhages scattered through the brain, loss of nerve cells, and some degree of inflammation of the brain covering (*meningitis*), as well as of the brain itself. Symptoms may vary greatly, depending on which parts of the brain are most involved.

Encephalitis can occur in the course of any disease in which the brain is affected, such as syphilis or meningitis. Sometimes the disease may be a variant of poliomyelitis. Encephalitis may follow or occur during the course of infectious diseases, such as measles or whooping cough, or following vaccination for smallpox or rabies. Frequently, encephalitis occurs as a complication of influenza. Intoxication by various chemicals may cause the condition; certain viruses cause specific forms of primary encephalitis.

The onset of encephalitis is usually acute, but the condition may become subacute or chronic. As a rule, there is a fever which may be mild or high. Mental symptoms—irritability, insomnia, or coma—are almost always present, as are disturbances of the eye. Muscle activity is abnormal, varying from paralysis to overactivity.

In the forms of encephalitis caused by viruses, the symptoms and course of the disease may vary greatly in different patients. It may be a brief illness, so mild that the patient does not go to bed. Or it may be a grave illness with high fever lasting several weeks. Stupor and weakness of eye muscles are the most notable symptoms in some patients, while violent delirium, insomnia, and involuntary muscle activity are seen in others. Muscular rigidity and rhythmical tremor are seen, as in paralysis. There may be a rapid fatal termination, or the illness may be chronic. Treatment is largely directed toward making the patient comfortable. Permanent brain damage sometimes results.

The forms of encephalitis which occur during the course of acute infectious diseases usually begin with high fever, vomiting, headache, and rigidity of the neck and back. The patient becomes drowsy or even comatose. Difficulty in swallowing and speaking is often present, as is paralysis and relaxation of bladder and bowel muscles. The course to recovery or fatality may be rapid, or the patient may remain comatose for weeks. There is no specific treatment.

Parkinsonism, or Parkinson's syndrome, is a frequent result of epidemic encephalitis and has been related to the 1915–1926 epidemic of encephalitis. This condition consists of rigidity of the muscles, rhythmical tremor especially marked in the thumb and forefinger, impairment of arm movements, and a "poker face." Excessive yawning and coughing and breathing disorders may be experienced. Brief periods of deep depression, concern over physical health, irritability, forgetfulness, or even psychoses may occur. The condition may be steadily progressive, it may become arrested at any stage, or in some cases it may regress.

In some forms of viral encephalitis, domestic animals, birds, and small reptiles are the natural reservoirs of the virus, and the virus is transmitted by mosquito. The mosquito, after biting the carrier animal, transmits the virus to man. Control of mosquito proliferation is the only known means of preventing outbreaks of viral encephalitis. Encephalitis has occurred on epidemic scale in St. Louis, Missouri; Australia; Japan; and Central Europe. Recent sporadic outbreaks have appeared in Great Britain and various parts of the United States. No satisfactory vaccine has been developed to immunize human beings.

African sleeping sickness

Sleeping sickness (*African trypanosomiasis*) can be caused by either of two related parasites, *Trypanosoma gambiense* or *Trypanosoma rhodesiense*. The parasite is transmitted to man by the bite of infected tsetse flies. Usually occurring in tropical regions, the disease is characterized by fever, weakness, weight loss, and lethargy which may resemble a coma. There may be tremors of the tongue and fingers, headache, hysteria, delusions, and finally constant sleep. When the disease has advanced to the sleeping stage, recovery is rare. Sleeping sickness can be prevented by providing protection from the bite of tsetse flies in those areas where the fly is prevalent.

DISORDERS OF THE BRAIN AND NERVOUS SYSTEM: MENINGITIS

Meningitis is not a single specific disease but any inflammation of the membranes covering the brain, especially the *pia* and the *arachnoid*. The cerebrospinal fluid circulating over the brain and spinal cord has little sterilizing power; consequently, infection spreads rapidly through the entire subarachnoid space, usually producing pus.

Meningitis may follow head injuries and infections, especially those involving the eyes, ears, nose, or sinuses. It may be a complication of such systemic diseases as tuberculosis, whooping cough, pneumonia, influenza, scarlet fever, syphilis, and many others; in these cases, the organisms reach the brain by way of the blood

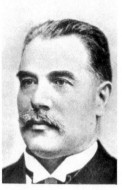

WEICHSELBAUM, Anton (1845-1920) Austrian pathologist. Known for his discovery of the *Micrococcus meningitidis* (1887). This organism, which is also called *Weichselbaum's coccus,* was found in the spinal fluid of persons who were afflicted with cerebrospinal meningitis, which affects the membranes of the brain and spinal cord. Weichselbaum, in investigating this fact, proved that this micro-organism was the cause of epidemic cerebrospinal meningitis.

stream. In some cases, meningeal involvement occurs before the primary disease produces its symptoms.

Whatever the cause, early symptoms of an acute meningitis are similar. Headache is one of the most striking. Usually intense, it may involve the entire head or be localized near a point of infection. Rapidly rising fever, ushered in by chills or a rigor, appears, and the patient is often irritable and drowsy. Stiffness of the neck is another early and reliable sign of meningitis. The patient holds his neck as still as possible; any attempt to bend it forward provokes great pain.

The later course of the disorder depends partially on the cause. In epidemic meningitis, the patient may be dead or recovering within a few days, while tuberculous meningitis persists for months. The nerves arising from the base of the brain may be affected so that deafness, weakness of the muscles of the eyes and face, or other signs of nerve paralysis appear. These effects may be permanent, but they usually disappear. Many patients recover fully and completely; but mental retardation, convulsions, and disturbances in behavior or thinking remain in a few cases. "Waterhead" (*hydrocephalus*) may result in some patients.

The sulfonamides and antibiotic drugs are used in treatment of patients with this condition. Blood transfusions, oxygen, and other measures may be required for the general support of the patient. While the outlook is still poor for patients with some types of meningitis, the new drugs have had a dramatic effect on many others. Tuberculous meningitis, which used to be invariably fatal, is one of the types that responds to early and prompt treatment with antibiotics. Although meningitis remains a serious disorder, its killing and crippling power has been greatly reduced.

DISORDERS OF THE BRAIN AND NERVOUS SYSTEM: RABIES

Rabies is a virus-produced disease which causes swift destruction of the nerve cells in the hindbrain. Although it is usually carried to man by dogs, other animals also spread the infection. In Mexico, the vampire bat is often infected. After a person is bitten and infected, the disease usually requires from four to eight weeks to develop; but it may lie dormant for as long as a year. In most cases, the incubation period is shortest when there are deep bites on the neck, head and face.

Soreness and numbness around the bite are the first symptoms. The patient may be irritable and anxious and complain of headaches and inability to sleep. Soon, mild muscle spasms make the throat feel full, and the voice becomes hoarse; swallowing and breathing are difficult. The anxiety mounts to terror, and the patient is extremely restless. Water is craved, but the mere sight of it sends the throat muscles into such painful spasms that it is dreaded; hence the name *hydrophobia*, or "fear of water," has been suggested. Later, convulsions rack the entire body; the behavior is wild; and the patient is delirious. In a day or so, the patient lapses limply into a quiet state that progresses into unconsciousness and death. The disease lasts two to four days and is always fatal.

The only treatment is to lighten the spasms and convulsions with medication or general sedatives. Food and water are given by a stomach tube passed through the nose.

While rabies always ends fatally once it develops, it can be prevented. When a person has been bitten by any animal, the wound should be washed thoroughly with soap and water, as this is known to destroy the rabies virus.

A healthy-looking animal which bites should

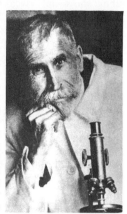

ROUX, Pierre Paul Emile (1853-1933) French bacteriologist. Working with Pasteur, Chamberland, and Yersin, Roux pioneered in the discovery of the causes of infectious disease, and the development of serum therapy. He proved the existence of diphtheria toxin in 1888 with Yersin. With Pasteur and Chamberland he first used a weakened bacteria culture in the treatment of disease, and demonstrated the presence of rabies virus in the blood. In the year 1898 he developed an antitetanic serum.

not be killed. It should be penned up alone and carefully watched for at least twelve days for any symptoms of rabies. If any develop, vaccination of the patient should start at once. The doctor injects vaccine under the skin daily for 14 days. If there are many bites on the head and shoulders, antirabies vaccine is given because the virus may reach the central nervous system before the injected antibody is adequate in amount.

The physician also gives tetanus antitoxin and penicillin to control other possible infections. Small children who have been around a rabid dog should undergo the treatment even when no break in the skin is seen, because the dog's saliva may have entered the mouth or eyes. It is the latent period between the bite and the development of the disease that allows for the period of treatment. If the animal stays healthy, there is little possibility that it is infected. The rabid dog is at first excited and restless, then snaps at or bites anything nearby. Occasionally,

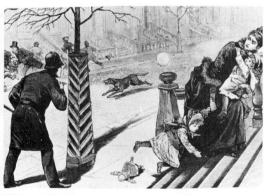

This old woodcut depicts a London policeman shooting a rabid dog. *Courtesy Bettmann Archive.*

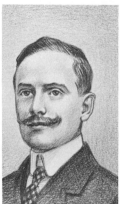

NEGRI, Adelchi (1876-1912) Italian physician. Negri is most famous for his discovery of microscopic round or oval bodies seen in the protoplasm and sometimes nerve processes of animals dead of rabies. These bodies are called *Negri bodies* and are considered conclusive proof of rabies. When a dog or other animal is suspected of having rabies, the animal's brain is examined for the Negri bodies. Rabid dogs should never be killed by shooting through the head, because the brain may be so destroyed that an accurate diagnosis is difficult.

they show only weakness which begins in the hindquarters and extends to the front legs and jaw. Death occurs in a few days. The value of vaccination against rabies was demonstrated by Pasteur, who on July 6, 1885, innoculated a boy, Joseph Meister, who had been bitten by a mad dog.

Until the early 1960s, rabies vaccine was made much as Pasteur made it—basically an extract from the brain of virus-injected rabbits. Reaction to the vaccine was often severe. A new vaccine made in fertilized duck eggs is much less likely to cause ill effects. A pre-exposure vaccine is also being developed for those who run special risks, such as veterinarians and persons going into countries where rabies is endemic.

In the United States, death from rabies has become rare. Dogs, however, should still be immunized yearly against rabies virus. Wild animals, especially foxes and skunks, are carriers of the virus.

DISORDERS OF THE BRAIN AND NERVOUS SYSTEM: EPILEPSY

From two to five per 1000 of the population are thought to have some form of convulsive disorder. About 75 percent of the cases start before the patients are 20 years of age, with the largest number starting in the first five years of life. Strong emotional reactions may bring on seizures. The flickering light of a faulty television tube has been known to trigger convulsions in children. Many of the childhood diseases which produce high fever may be accompanied by convulsions. This does not mean that the child in whom this occurs is an epileptic, nor does it predispose to convulsions later in life. The factors which may later precipitate the attacks usually are ones that change the physiological state of the body—such as puberty, menstruation, and pregnancy.

The exact mechanism which produces convulsions is not well understood. It is known that the normal patterns of electrical activity of the brain are disrupted. Many investigators believe that the "convulsive capacity"—that is, the ease or difficulty with which a convulsion is set off—plays an important role in all seizures. For reasons still poorly understood, brain tissue is sensitive to chemical changes, and responds with electrical discharges that result in convulsions. Thus, slight changes in the water or acid-base balance, alterations in the oxygen supply, or changes in concentration of certain chemicals in the blood will provoke seizures in predisposed persons but not in persons with less "convulsive capacity." Head injuries, high fever, tumors or scars in the brain substance, disturbances in blood supply, or damage to nerve tissue may be responsible for the physical and chemical changes.

Epilepsy is characterized by a sudden, brief disturbance in brain function, causing loss or change of consciousness if the disturbance is widespread. When it is localized, consciousness may not be impaired. In either case, there may be muscle contraction, abnormal sensations, or unusual mental experience.

The public is poorly informed about epilepsy. Many people consider it a great stigma; they think it occurs only in the mentally retarded or that it leads inevitably to loss of mentality. Since epilepsy is not a disease, but rather a group of symptoms, many investigators in the field feel the term "convulsive states" should be substituted for epilepsy. Epilepsy is divided into two groups. If there is no known organic injury to the brain before the first seizure, the condition is called *idiopathic epilepsy*; if such damage exists, it is known as *symptomatic epilepsy*.

Types of seizures

Whether the convulsions are idiopathic or symptomatic, they assume several different forms or combinations of forms. In *grand mal* epilepsy, the patient may feel unusually good or bad for a day or so prior to the attack. This vague state warns the patient of an impending attack. It is peculiar to the individual and identical in different attacks. There may be queer sensations in some part of the body. Flashes of light or color may be seen, strange sounds may be heard, and pleasant or disturbing emotions may be experienced. The face becomes pale, and the eyes dilate. Consciousness is swiftly lost, often with a wild, harsh cry. Breathing stops; the legs and body stiffen; and the patient falls to the ground, the elbows bent at rigid right angles. During this part of the spasm, which lasts from ten to thirty seconds, the bladder or bowel, or both, may empty. The face becomes blue as the features contort, and the patient seems about to die when the spasm breaks. Rhythmic muscular contractions, at first small and rapid, begin and then become slower and more powerful. Gasps for breath come through heavy froth, often blood-stained from a bitten tongue or cheek. The contractions become less and less frequent. This phase usually lasts two or three minutes but may persist longer. At the end, the patient may sleep heavily for several hours or rouse with aimless, thrashing movements, dazed and forgetful and unable to understand what is said to him. There is often a severe headache for several hours. Occasionally, the patient may have one convulsion after another without regaining consciousness. This dangerous state is called *status epilepticus* and demands immediate attention by the physi-

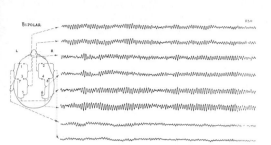

Electroencephalogram from a normal adult, showing the low amplitude of the tracings that are obtained from electrodes variously placed on the head. *Photography by F. W. Schmidt.*

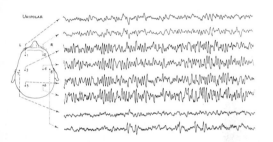

Electroencephalogram taken from a 4-year-old child suffering from a convulsive disorder, showing high amplitude waves, in marked contrast to those of the normal. *Photography, F. W. Schmidt.*

cian, since it can result in death from exhaustion.

In *petit mal* attacks, the mildest form of epilepsy, the loss of consciousness is fleeting and variable—from one to 40 or 50 times a day. It may be so short that it goes unnoticed. The head may nod momentarily, the flow of speech may halt a second or two and then may be normally resumed; or perhaps only a vacant stare marks the attack. Sometimes there are one or two contractions of the arms or flickering of the eyelids.

Psychomotor epilepsy may follow grand or petit mal seizures or occur independently. These attacks last from a few minutes to a day or so. There is no loss of consciousness, but the patient may remember nothing of the episode on recovery. The behavior is confused and unusual. There may be uncontrollable emotional outbursts which may be violently destructive, or the patient may be dazed and apathetic. There is also evidence that some psychomotor cases may be the result of subtle injury to the brain at the time of birth.

Focal seizures (*Jacksonian epilepsy*) assume two forms. There may be unusual sensations or uncontrolled movements remaining localized to one part of the body, while consciousness is undisturbed. Thus, the head and eyes may turn ir-

resistibly to one side despite the patient's awareness. In the other form, the movements or sensations which begin in one part of the body spread upward in a slow, orderly fashion, or they may cross to the other side. This form may develop into a typical grand mal attack with loss of consciousness. Many convulsive seizures resulting from brain injury are of the Jacksonian type.

Care of the patient

During a seizure, the family should take care of the patient rather than calling the doctor. Petit mal seizures are too short to require special attention. Patients in a psychomotor attack should be restrained as little as possible. A grand mal convulsion, once started, cannot be stopped, but is self-limited. Tight collars and belts should be loosened. A folded handkerchief or a gauze-padded tongue depressor can often be inserted between the back teeth to prevent biting the tongue. This should not be put between the front teeth, as they may be loosened by the powerful jaw movements. The patient should be turned on his side to allow saliva and vomitus to drain out.

The treatment of a patient with convulsive seizures depends on the cause. In idiopathic epilepsy, three fourths of all patients can be relieved of at least three fourths of all their seizures; and in certain cases, control is even better than this. The patient has most of the responsibility of controlling the attacks, because good control depends on his complete and consistent co-operation. He should avoid fatigue, irregular eating and sleeping, unusual excitement, and alcohol. Fasting or a special diet high in fat and low in carbohydrate, and moderate restriction of water, are sometimes helpful in regulating the abnormal electrical activity of the brain. He should take his prescribed medicines regularly, and he and his family must understand several things about the medication prescribed. Finding

GOWERS, William R. (1845-1915) English neurologist. In 1888 Gowers and Horsley successfully removed a spinal cord tumor for the first time in medical history. He was interested in the anatomy of the nervous system, and the pathological conditions which affect it. In 1881, he described epilepsy and in 1902, he described a form of progressive muscular atrophy, now called the *distal myopathy of Gowers*. He also invented a hemoglobinometer which is still being used.

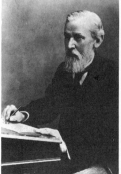

the proper drug or combination of drugs and adjusting the dosage is a highly individualized matter. They must be prepared for persistent trials until there is effective control. Many falsely believe that the medicine is "dope" or habit-forming; under proper supervision, the medication is harmless even when taken over a period of years. There is now a whole battery of drugs available which, either alone or in combination, can effectively control the convulsions.

In mixed seizures, two or even three medications may be needed for prevention. Phenobarbital is one of the oldest and most effective anticonvulsants, but produces drowsiness when given in large amounts. Dilantin suppresses grand mal convulsions and can be taken in larger doses than Phenobarbital without causing lethargy. When these drugs fail to control grand mal seizures, Mesantoin alone or in combination with them may give the desired control. Phenobarbital and Dilantin make petit mal worse, so Tridione is used in this type. In addition to these representative drugs, there are others which in recent years have been found effective. None of these drugs must ever be administered except under the physician's supervision. Further, some of these medications have various harmful side effects that must be watched for by the patient. Unexplained skin rash in patients on anticonvulsant drugs is a warning to consult the physician. Under no circumstances should the patient take it upon himself to lower the dosage or stop the medication, as this may cause a return of his convulsive seizures. He should have an adequate supply of medicine at all times; indeed, it is wise to carry a 24-hour supply on the person. Once good control is established, the medicine is taken indefinitely. When there have been no convulsions for a long time, the medicine may be gradually reduced over a two- or three-year period and stopped if no attacks occur. Treatment must be resumed if there is a seizure. When the attacks are numerous and severe, or when the treatment is started years after the convulsions have begun, it may be impossible to discontinue medication. The electroencephalograph is of great diagnostic value. This instrument records the electrical activity of the brain by means of electrodes pasted or otherwise attached to various points on the head. By this means, the source and nature of the trouble in the brain can often by identified. The "EEG," as it is called, may also serve as a guide in the choice of drug or other treatment. New EEG techniques utilizing FM transmitters should enable physicians to learn more about the exact mechanism which produces convulsions.

Patients may be treated by neurosurgical measures if a focal abnormality of the brain is the cause of seizures. Surgical treatment is indicated by the character of the lesion. For example, the less violent form of epilepsy, psychomotor, is not relieved by drugs in about 50 percent of the cases. Surgical treatment is sometimes effective. The location and extent of surgical removal are determined by the seizure pattern, electroencephalogram and air studies.

Both the patient and his family should look upon the epileptic as a normal individual, not a chronic invalid or some sort of social outcast. The family must guard against rejecting or overprotecting him by placing too many restrictions on his activities or by excusing him from his just responsibilities. The child should attend regular schools and associate freely with his usual playmates, so that he will not feel "different." He should be encouraged to play games and indulge in sports appropriate to his age. Any patient whose convulsions are not well-controlled should avoid dangerous situations. It is not true that mental deterioration is the fate of most epileptics. A recent effort toward job rehabilitation provides workshops where epileptics can gain confidence and skill in various industrial tasks. After training, many epileptics can be placed successfully in private industry.

Two epileptics, or even two normal persons, with a high incidence of convulsions in each of their families, should not be encouraged to have children. It is generally safe for well-controlled epileptics to have children if the mate and his family are free of the disorder. Most epileptics lead happy, useful, and normal lives.

DISORDERS OF THE BRAIN AND AND NERVOUS SYSTEM: CEREBRAL PALSY

Cerebral palsy denotes a group of disorders in which the patient has little or no control over his muscular motions. It is caused by damage in one of the three main areas of the brain that regulate muscular activity. All movements that are planned and controllable start in the part of the brain known as the *motor cortex*. Damage here results in stiffness of the muscles (*spastic paralysis*). A group of nerve cells in the brain (*basal ganglia*) normally restrain certain types of muscle activity, so that injury in this area allows unplanned movements to occur. There are two kinds of involuntary movements. There are slow, squirming, twisting movements that spread from the smaller joints to the larger ones without pattern (*athetosis*); these are more common in the arms than in the face and legs. The other type of involuntary movement is a tremor. Tremors are characterized by rhythmic motions which may vary from slight shaking to violent jerking. The *cerebellar* area of the brain controls muscle coordination as well as balance; if this area is involved, the *ataxic* type of cerebral palsy is seen in which there is clumsiness and lack of balance.

Cerebral palsy has many causes. Before birth the brain may not develop as well as it should. Antagonistic blood factors between the mother and child is another influence, as is injury or disease of the mother during pregnancy. At birth, difficulty in delivery may damage the brain. A premature baby's soft bones do not protect the brain as well as those of a full-term baby, thus allowing harmful pressures on the brain. After birth, bleeding into the brain may destroy cells. Difficulty in breathing at the time of birth may prevent sufficient oxygen from getting into the blood; therefore, the nerve cells, which are easily destroyed by lack of oxygen, may suffer. Infection and injury after birth may harm a control area and produce the symptoms.

After birth, the baby with cerebral palsy may look and act like any normal infant. However, blueness, twitching, or convulsions should make one suspicious that damage has been done. Because a normal baby's nervous system is incompletely developed at birth, the physician often cannot make a definite diagnosis until the second six months of life. When the baby is closely watched by the parents, signs may be seen as early as the first two or three months. Perhaps the baby does not move much, or the legs seem unusually stiff. Failure to follow the normal rate of babyhood accomplishments is important. Thus a child who cannot grasp an object at three months, or turn over at five months, or sit alone at seven months, may be showing the first signs of cerebral palsy.

Later, the diagnosis is somewhat easier to make, as the child's symptoms will probably be like some of those described below. The spastic type is most common (66 percent). The child's stiff, tense muscles do not remain quiet and relaxed when not in use, as normal muscles do. They tighten up even more as the child tries to move or if he is excited or frightened. Muscles often work in pairs—one relaxing or stretching so the other can contract. In the spastic child, these muscles contract at the same time so that neither muscle can move. The posture of spastic children is characteristic; the legs turn in, bending at the hips and knees, and the heels are off the ground. The arms are bent at the elbows and wrists, while the fingers are clenched. This constant contraction may cause the muscles to shorten permanently in the position described. The child has great trouble speaking and swallowing. He is shy, prefers to be alone, and is generally afraid. In the athetoid child (19 percent), unwanted motions begin when the child starts a planned motion. In reaching for a ball, for example, the arm may wave about so that the hand never comes near its goal. This aimless activity affects the muscles of the throat, face, and tongue and seriously hampers speech and swallowing. This child's personality is in marked contrast to the spastic's. He is fearless, lovable, and patient.

The ataxic form makes up 8 percent of the total. These clumsy-looking children have a sense of balance and try to keep from falling, but they find it difficult to walk on a narrow base. Muscle co-ordination is lost, and they have great trouble with skillful acts such as writing and throwing a ball. Speech and swallowing are fairly normal.

When the entire brain suffers, rigidity (4 percent) results and is often associated with severe mental deficiency. The body is rigidly arched backward, and the head is thrown back. The victims relax some in sleep.

In the tremor type (2 percent), the child has control of his muscles until he starts to do something or becomes excited. Then the vibrations get worse and interfere with the use of his hands. In severe cases, the movements are present even when the child is quiet and at rest.

A limp child that slumps or collapses like a rag may have brain damage just in front of the motor area. Unlike the other palsied children, he is extremely weak and will not try to start voluntary movement.

In addition to muscular incapacity, some children show other defects. Sometimes, the child lacks a sense of line direction, so that he cannot copy words or geometric forms such as squares or triangles. He seems unable to store mental images which can be used as patterns for later motions. Writing and arithmetic are apt to be difficult because the child needs mental pictures of words and numbers. Children with this additional defect are difficult to train because of their inability to recall the desired movements. Sometimes sight and hearing also are impaired.

Some palsied children drool saliva because they cannot swallow it. They may only grunt instead of speaking. Thus, they look mentally deficient even if they have superior intellect. They are unable to learn many things by experience, especially those having to do with muscle activity. The responses they do make are slow. Mental deficiency is seen with all types of cerebral palsy and may be mild or severe, but only one third of affected children are below the acceptable educational levels. Ataxic or spastic children are a little more apt to be deficient mentally.

Treatment is slow, long, and constant—a fact which parents should face before beginning, so that the child will not feel their impatience or disappointment. The parents also should understand that the aim of the treatment is *not* to restore to normalcy but to make the child useful to himself and society, and therefore happier.

Of all the defects to be overcome, those of speech and swallowing are most urgent. A child who can talk is not lonely and isolated from people. He may be left alone with safety which is impossible with a mute child. Arm and hand function are the next most valuable, because with these functions he will not be dependent on another person to feed, dress, and care for him. With arm function, a wheel chair can be operated. Leg movements are of least importance, but they should be developed if at all possible.

Many measures are used in helping these children. Braces will guide athetotic movement, support weak muscles, and keep muscles from permanent shortening. Surgery is helpful at times. When only a few muscles are spastic, cutting some of the nerves which carry movement impulses to these muscles may give highly satisfactory results. Muscles or ligaments that are permanently shortened may be freed or lengthened surgically. In a few cases, after careful study, the doctor may recommend operations on the brain and spinal cord. Some drugs are being used to relax muscle spasm and relieve tremors.

Muscle training is the most valuable way of treating these children, and a way in which intelligent, co-operative parents can be immensely helpful to their crippled children. This training is done by a physiotherapist, but many of their routines can be learned by parents and repeated at home. Relaxation is the first phase of training. The child learns how relaxed muscles feel, then he learns to relax them himself and to let them stay that way. When relaxation is mastered, passive motion is started. The trainer carries out motions of the child's muscles with no help from the child. This teaches correct movements, timing, and rhythm. Then, the child assists in some of the movements. When these are done correctly, he is ready to put two or more motion patterns together to form a skill. This skill is an everyday act which must be mastered—eating and dressing are examples.

Routine manipulations must be taught these children with the aid of many devices. Specially-made skis and canes with wide, weighted bottoms help them walk. Playing with a ball, simple woodwork, sewing, and knitting train them in many hand and arm movements. Forks and spoons with large specially-angled handles make eating easier.

It is essential that the child learn to speak. On this, to a considerable extent, depends his happiness, as well as much of his social and intellectual development. Work done before a mirror shows him how to mimic lip and tongue movements. If the parents cannot be unemotional when dealing with speech difficulties, they probably should leave this phase to persons with better control.

The child should find a sympathetic, encouraging environment in which he is accepted by others and given opportunity for relationships with others. In a friendly way, he should be encouraged to do what he can for himself, but he also should be able to accept the necessary help without shame and self-consciousness. The chances for improvement depend not only on the child's ability, but on his willingness to follow instructions. Such a willingness depends upon the persons around him. An attitude of optimism and genuine belief in the child's worth will do much to sustain him in his difficult struggle to participate in life.

DISORDERS OF THE BRAIN AND NERVOUS SYSTEM: STROKES AND PARALYSIS

High blood pressure with strokes as a leading cause of death has received much attention in the past decade. About 200,000 persons die each year from strokes, the most common injury to the brain. In stroke or "apoplexy," the flow of blood to a part of the brain is suddenly cut off. This, in turn, causes injury to all the structures connected with that part.

Parts of the brain may fail to be adequately supplied with blood because of: hemorrhage from rupture of a blood vessel; the formation of a clot within a blood vessel (*thrombosis*); spasm of an artery; or the occlusion of a blood vessel by a small particle, usually a blood clot, floating in the blood stream (an *embolus*). Most cases of hemorrhage and thrombosis occur in vessels previously damaged by thickening of the walls of the arteries (*arteriosclerosis*), although some hemorrhages in young people result from faulty development of the arteries causing a weak spot which may dilate (*aneurysm*) and rupture. An embolus in the blood vessels of the brain is usually associated with heart disease, but it may occur in other diseases. Disturbances in the blood supply to the brain may be determined by arteriography, an x-ray film of the brain following intra-arterial injection of radiopaque solution. Regardless of the cause of the stroke, that area of the brain through which pass the nerve fibers controlling voluntary motion or sensations of pain, temperature, touch, vision, etc., may be damaged.

When apoplexy is caused by hemorrhage, the individual may experience headache, dizziness, ringing in the ears, numbness, and nausea for several days or for only a few minutes before the attack. Sudden severe headache and unconsciousness may occur after such exertion as straining for a bowel movement, coughing, vomiting, or heavy eating. The patient complains of headache and topples over, with his head thrown back. Breathing is difficult and sounds like snoring. The cheeks puff out when the air is expelled; saliva drools. The half-closed eyes with wide black pupils stare from the extremely red face. The temperature is often below normal; the pulse is strong but slow. At first the paralyzed limbs may be limp. The bowels and bladder are controlled poorly or not at all. The spinal fluid, if examined, may reveal an increase in pressure and contain blood, when the blood has leaked into cavities or onto the surface of the brain. In severe cases, the coma deepens and the patient dies in a few hours or days. Some gradually regain consciousness and get over the attack. If so, for many days the patient will have severe headache, a stiff neck and back pains, and attempts to raise the outstretched hand will cause pain. In general, the longer the coma lasts after the first 24 hours, the poorer the chances are for complete recovery. With fatal hemorrhage, death may occur in a few minutes or the patient may live two or three days.

Thrombosis is by far the most frequent cause of stroke, although stroke caused by thrombosis is less dramatic and severe. Unlike hemorrhage, it is apt to occur after periods of inactivity. The patient often awakens in the morning to find that an arm, leg, or perhaps an entire side is useless, or that he can speak little or not at all. The patient may lose consciousness entirely or may gradually lapse into coma; the other signs, as described for hemorrhage, occur. Strokes from this cause have a better outlook for recovery, although there is usually some permanent disability.

When embolism produces apoplexy, the onset is even more sudden than in hemorrhage, and there is no warning. The symptoms resemble those caused by thrombosis. If the embolus has reached a vital area of the brain, death follows in a few hours. This is a frequent cause of stroke in young adults, especially those who have had a history of rheumatic fever. It is a rare cause of apoplexy, however.

In spasm of an artery, the sudden dizziness, paralysis, numbness, or visual disturbances disappear in a few hours, leaving few or no signs.

In treating these cases, the physician needs a history of the illness so that he will know what type of vascular damage he is dealing with. Even after the diagnosis of apoplexy is made, it is occasionally impossible to tell which mechanism caused it. Some vascular obstructions may be diagnosed accurately by angiography. Treatment is varied in accordance with the cause of the stroke. Surgical treatment is often effective in clearing arterial obstruction or repairing a rupture if the operation can be performed within the first 24 hours after the stroke. Surgical methods include removal of the diseased section; removal of clotting material; patching the artery with plastic material to increase its diameter; making a detour of plastic tubing to bypass the blocked part of the artery. Drugs may be given to reduce the swelling in the brain, to prevent further clotting, or to support the heart. Antibiotics are often given to prevent pneumonia, especially if the coma persists.

The patient crippled by a stroke can often be amazingly rehabilitated. His capacity for rehabilitation may depend on which side of the brain has been damaged and how severely, and his own motivation to relearn. In right-handed persons, the left side of the brain is usually dominant, almost always controlling language skills and movements of the body. In severe cases, the patient may be left speechless and helpless. Retraining through repetitive exercises can result in some improvement. Slight damage to the nondominant side of the brain may blunt the patient's sensory awareness and spatial judgment, which can be retrained. Rehabilitation must be begun early if it is to succeed. Footboards and sandbags should be used from the beginning to keep the legs and arms in good position. As soon as the acute phase of the illness is over, the active procedures start. A soft rope tied to the foot of the bed to form a "U" helps the patient pull himself into a sitting position. Muscular tone of the affected side is aided if the patient holds the paralyzed hand to the rope with the good one as he pulls up. This simple maneuver aids muscle strength, tone, and a sense of balance, thus saving the patient many hours of practice later. Exercises with an overhead pulley also aid blood vessel and muscular tone and shorten the period of rehabilitation. Later, the patient learns to sit on the side of the bed and next to stand. Much later he can stand between two kitchen chairs, using them to support himself as he attempts walking. Braces are used often to support the foot and leg in good positions. With help, the patient can learn to take care of most of his personal needs.

When speech is impaired, correction should start early. If a trained speech therapist is not available, a high school speech teacher may help the patient, or a member of the family may be instructed in what to do. The family must understand that the patient has not necessarily lost his intelligence, even though he may mutter unintelligibly.

Function may return rapidly, and there may be some increase in function for twelve months. Limb function may always be incomplete, particularly when there was complete paralysis of the entire extremity at the beginning.

Most of the retraining procedures are quite simple. Yet, with consistent use of them, the majority of these patients can be taught self-care. Some may even return to part- or full-time work.

Paralysis produced by cord injury

Paralysis caused by injury to the spinal cord differs from that produced by apoplexy. The spinal cord may be damaged by infectious diseases, tumors, or direct injury. Diving into shallow water, automobile accidents, and airplane crashes account for many injuries of the cord. Hard falls in the sitting position are likely to injure the lower part of the cord, while head-first falls that bend the neck frequently damage the upper part. Blasts from high explosives may cause small areas of damage throughout the entire length of the cord. A broken vertebra may crush the part of the cord directly below it. In any case, the symptoms that result will depend on what section of the cord is involved—upper, middle, or lower—and how far across the cord the injury extends; when the damage is high on the cord, more structures below the injury are rendered useless. Since it is known at what level of the cord the nerves to various muscles arise, the physician can locate the level of the cord injury by determining which muscles are paralyzed.

When there is severe injury to the cord high in the neck, the patient usually dies quickly. If he survives, both arms and legs are paralyzed (*quadriplegia*). Lower in the neck, a few muscles of the upper arm may be spared while the forearm and hand may be paralyzed as well as the legs. If damage is below this level, the legs only are paralyzed (*paraplegia*).

Three stages are seen following sudden injury to the spinal cord. The first is *spinal shock*. The patient experiences severe pain and sudden paralysis of all the muscles below the site of injury. Even involuntary or reflex movements are gone, and the muscles are flaccid. All sensations in the paralyzed parts are lost; but just above the level of the injury, there is spontaneous pain or increased sensitivity to pain, or there may be a tight, girdle-like sensation around the body. The blood pressure falls. The bladder and anal muscles go into spasm, so that urine and feces cannot be passed. The duration of this stage depends on the extent of the injury. If these symptoms clear up shortly, it is likely that there was only a concussion of the cord. When the injury extends across the width of the cord, this period lasts about three weeks. If the patient survives, the second phase sets in and is known as *paraplegia in flexion* or paralysis of the legs in a bent position. In some cases, however, extension paraplegia may occur instead, in which case there is an extension reaction to stimuli, in contradistinction to flexion. During this stage, which takes from two weeks to seven months to develop, reflex activity returns. The automatic acts that protect by withdrawing—for example, jerking back from something hot—are the strongest and first to return. If the sole of the foot is stroked lightly, the whole leg may draw up, although the patient is unable to move the limb voluntarily. Reflex spasms of the limbs are so easily produced that the light weight of bed clothes or even air currents may cause sudden, violent contraction of the legs. Often a *mass reflex* response occurs when the skin of the thigh or genital region is lightly brushed. The limbs withdraw, perspiration bursts out over them, and the bladder and the bowel empty automatically. Also in the second stage, muscles lose their former relaxation and become spastic; unless special precautions are taken, the limbs will become permanently fixed in bent positions. Because the sulfonamides and antibiotics control infection, the death rate for spinal cord injuries has been lowered. As a result, patients may live indefinitely in the second stage.

Bed sores and infections usually appear in the final stage, during which the reflex centers in the spinal cord may fail. The withdrawal responses are harder to produce, and mass reflex response may not occur. The paralyzed muscles waste away. The automatic action of the bladder and bowel is lost, so that the patient cannot pass urine or feces or dribbles both all the time. Death comes in a short time after these vital actions disappear.

Damage to only one side of the spinal cord results in symptoms that are quite different from those just described. Voluntary motion is lost only on one side of the body—the same side as the cord injury—and the muscles are spastic rather than relaxed and flexed. On this same side, only part of the sensations are lost—those that detect vibration and position—while sensations of pain and heat are unimpaired. On the side of the body opposite the cord injury, sensitivity to pain and heat is lost; the other senses are unaffected and muscle power on this side is normal. This type of injury is the result of accidents, such as knife wounds, and diseases which cause destructive pressure on one side of the cord.

In the early phase, the physician may be able to do much to help, but later little can be done to alter the damage done to the spinal cord itself, and from that standpoint treatment is still unsatisfactory. However, much can be done to help the patient function in spite of his handicaps. When the spine has been injured, the patient should be moved gently in a flat and prone position. The physician will manage the shock and other severe injuries first and then decide whether operation is necessary. If the vertebrae are dislocated or fractured so as to press on or continue to cut into the cord, operation may be required immediately. The physician will not operate if it is evident that the cord is completely divided, as this is useless. It may be necessary to operate much later if new bone formation puts pressure on the cord or if there is persistent pain from scar formation around the nerve roots. Casts are used to straighten the spine, thus relieving pressure on the cord. Traction on the lower extremities and braces may stretch and straighten the back.

Good nursing care is the greatest need of most paraplegic patients. The patient's weight must be distributed as evenly as possible in the bed, because those parts which bear the weight for long may ulcerate. Air mattresses are best, and sponge rubber mattresses are next best. Rubber rings, quilted pads, and rough material should not be used; the bed must be as smooth as possible at all times. The areas that need special watching are the heel, the bony prominences of the ankles and hips, and the skin over the lower back. Turning the patient every two hours with the patient on a Stryker frame will allow better circulation and will prevent prolonged pressure on any one region. Wrapping the heels in thick layers of cotton will protect them during the vigorous withdrawal responses. Injury to the cord leads to poor circulation in the skin, so that the skin may tear or bruise easily. Proper skin care consists of careful washing with water, usage of cold cream, and dusting with powder. The skin should be dried as often as it gets damp. If the patient is wet, ulcers invariably develop; this is another reason for giving continuous and careful attention to bladder and bowel function. Hot water bottles and heating pads should be avoided, since the patient is insensitive to pain, and heat is poorly conducted by the body, so that burns may develop.

In the stage of spinal shock, the bladder is particularly likely to overflow. The physician can handle this in several ways. He may insert, through the urethra, a catheter connected with bottles of solution to wash out and drain the bladder periodically. The bowel is easily controlled by enemas.

The patient can be kept in better general condition if he has a diet rich in protein. Bed exercises for the impaired part of the body preserve strength and the appetite. Passive motion and correct bed posture prevent paralyzed limbs from "freezing" in poor position.

Persistent pain is experienced by a number of these patients, and is often hard to control. If it is severe, surgery may be required for relief. It has been noted, however, that with good nutrition, occupational therapy, and recreation, the pain decreases. Frustration and irritability seem to play a role in causing the pain. Sexual function may be normal or absent.

As the stage of spinal shock wears off and the next stage begins, the appetite improves. The muscles which had wasted away gradually begin to lose their limpness and become stiffer and regain some of their size. If ulcers have developed, they begin to heal, and the large ones may be closed with skin grafts. The bladder may develop automatic action at this stage. If the bladder remains stretched and relaxed, the physician must decide whether to make a permanent abdominal opening or to use other surgical procedures to allow free-flow of the urine. If automatic action is established, fixed amounts of fluid should be taken according to a schedule. Exercise now is more important than ever and is directed toward teaching the patient to get in and out of his bed and wheel chair and to develop new movements and strength in the remaining useful muscles. The spastic muscles can be helped by passive motion, stretching, and warm baths. Vigorous exercise of the unaffected muscles reduces the spasticity of the paralyzed muscles. It is noted that the best influence over this spasticity is persistent activity and a good emotional adjustment. The patient can be measured for braces and begin learning to ambulate with the aid of crutches, as soon as any fractures have healed.

A depressive reaction usually follows a spinal cord injury, and the way the patient handles this period depends largely on his personality pattern prior to the injury. The adjustment is better when the patient understands his future in terms that are neither over-optimistic nor over-pessimistic. Dependence on others for assistance often leads to a childlike emotional attitude. All phases of rehabilitation are smoother when the patient is attempting to regain security through his own efforts rather than looking to others.

To promote self-reliance, early attempts should be made to ascertain the vocational interests of the patient. If he can no longer carry on his previous occupation, a psychologist may help determine the patient's mental capacities as well as his interests and aptitudes. If the patient has no special plans or interests, many may be suggested and tried tentatively. Occupational therapy not only helps improve the muscle co-ordination, but also develops work habits. Many vocations are open to paralyzed patients. A number attend college and high school. Manual arts, such as television and radio repair, printing, etc., are popular. Art is popular, and even quadriplegic patients can paint with the aid of special devices. The choice of work should take into consideration the shorter working day required by the patient; and it should be in a field of limited competition in order that employment be assured.

The family must be prepared to accept the paraplegic patient for what he is and to make a home for him that takes his physical needs into account. The patient who has learned to care for his daily needs, to live with pain that cannot be further eased surgically, to ambulate with crutches, to drive a car or use public transportation, and to partially or completely support himself is considered a fully rehabilitated patient.

REHABILITATION OF THE PARALYZED PATIENT

Even when the spinal cord of a paralyzed patient has been severely damaged, if he is willing to work, usually he can be taught to walk on his "dead" legs, or to use his partially paralyzed arms. The rehabilitation of a patient to the extent that he can walk across a street requires long hours of tedious work and patience on the part of those entrusted with the training. In addition to the physical training, the patient must be helped to achieve emotional adjustment. Further, he must be reassured that he can become almost completely independent physically, and he should be helped to become economically independent. Of the 2,600 para- and quadriplegic veterans of World War II, the majority have been trained to walk and have left V. A. Hospitals for jobs or further education. The pictures on this and the following pages were taken at the Veterans Administration Hospital in Houston, Texas.

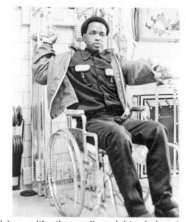

Exercising with the wall weights helps to develop muscle coordination and strength. This single exercise involves the use of the hands, wrists, arms, and muscles of the shoulder and chest in preparation for locomotion.

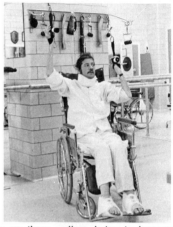

Practice on these pulleys helps to increase range of shoulder and arm movement. After many hours of hard work, the patient who at first could move his arm only a limited distance, is able to move the pulleys freely.

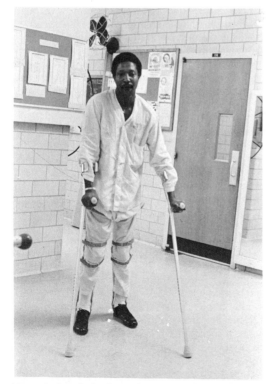

Many devices help the patient learn to walk unaided and drive a specially built car. Such patients often return to their old jobs, or train for new ones. Many occupations are open to them.

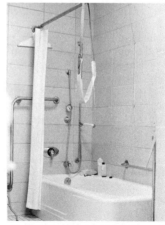

Devices such as bars and handrails are easy and inexpensive to install in the home of the paralyzed patient. This frees the patient from a life of invalidism, and enables him to care for many of his personal needs.

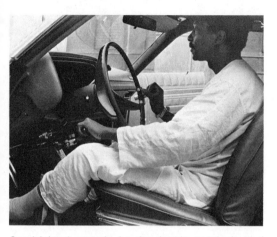

Special hand controls for the throttle and brake and a wheel nob enable the paraplegic patient to drive a car, thus giving him the independence he desires.

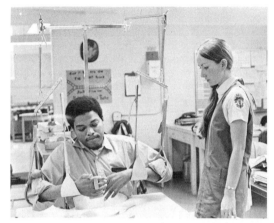

Loss of ability to lift the arm is compensated by sling supports which do this for the patient, enabling him to use his hands.

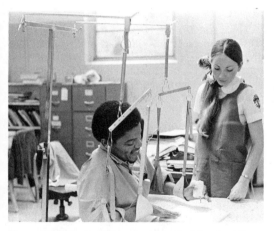

Since all lifting motions are performed by the slings, the patient is enabled to continue using his fingers and hands. This preserves strength of unimpaired muscles.

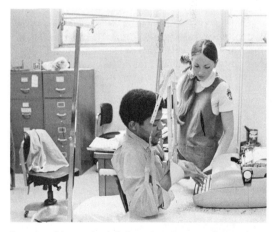

A motor driven wheelchair and various special devices in his home and office enabled this patient to learn several new skills before he returned to his old clerical job.

Photos on this and preceding page by Walter J. Pagel.

DISORDERS OF THE BRAIN AND NERVOUS SYSTEM: ST. VITUS' DANCE

Sydenham's chorea—or "St. Vitus' dance"—is associated with rheumatic fever. Rarely seen in adults, children between the ages of seven and 14 have it most frequently. Girls have it twice as often as boys. It is most common in the spring.

Involvement of parts of the brain that control and regulate muscular movements causes the choreal symptoms. The attack comes on gradually with fever, loss of appetite, and sometimes vomiting. The patient has trouble writing, or he drops objects because the muscles cannot sustain normal movements. Difficulty in walking and climbing stairs is noted, because the legs are affected early when the jerky movements first start. The affected child is often punished for making impudent faces. Later, all or part of the body contorts with quick, uncontrolled, spasmodic jerks that are worse in excitement or attempted movement. The child may control them for a few minutes, but they soon burst out again. Sleep usually stops the activity except in severe cases. Movements may be so wild and strong that restraints are needed to keep the child from hurting himself. The emotions are as variable as the motions. The child changes from laughter to tears easily, is fretful, and hard to control. Speech may be disturbed to such a degree that the person is not understood. General health is below par, and the appetite is capricious. The patient tires easily and sleeps poorly. Fever is absent in the uncomplicated case, and if present, indicates that rheumatic fever is active.

Ordinarily the attack ends spontaneously in six to ten weeks; rarely, it may last three to four months. The following spring the child often has another attack, and attacks may continue to recur annually for four or five years.

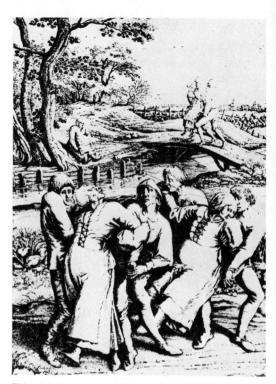

This picture, from a painting by Brueghel, shows people afflicted by St. Vitus' dance. This disease is now known as chorea, and is most often seen in children under fourteen. *Bettmann Archive.*

Treatment

The child should be kept in bed. Emotional tension will be less if there are no visitors. The physician will decide on the basis of laboratory tests and physical examination how long the child should remain in bed. A generous, attractive diet aids the patient to regain his health. Massage, prolonged warm baths, and various drugs help control the spasms. Sometimes the doctor will recommend "fever treatments." By artificial means, the body temperature is raised to approximately 104°–105° Fahrenheit and is kept there four to five hours. This is repeated two or three times a week.

Although the disease recurs, the single attack invariably regresses. The danger to the heart, in those cases where the rheumatic fever is also actively involving this organ, is to be most feared. Chorea should be recognized as an active phase of the generalized disease of rheumatic fever; there is brain disease because of the symptoms of rheumatic fever. The condition therefore cannot be considered harmless.

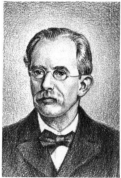

RECKLINGHAUSEN, Friedrich D. von (1833-1910) German pathologist. Distinguished in his field and famous for his pathological descriptions, especially for one explaining neurofibromatosis, often called *von Recklinghausen's disease*. He also recognized and described new varieties of tumors. Minute lymph channels of connective tissue, as well as a particular form of osteitis, bear his name for his early account of them.

DISORDERS OF THE BRAIN AND NERVOUS SYSTEM: NERVE DEGENERATION

Injury to a nerve results in degeneration of that nerve, the extent of which depends on the type and severity of the injury. If the injury is a mechanical one, such as cutting, the degeneration occurs simultaneously throughout the nerve below the site of injury and also for a short distance above this site. All injuries to nerves, whether by trauma, infection, or other systemic disease are called *neuritis;* the nerves degenerate in varying degrees throughout their courses. Nerves may regenerate if the cells from which they arise are intact. A regenerating nerve grows about 1/16 inch per day.

Spinal nerves carry both sensory and motor fibers; therefore, injury will result in disturbances in these functions. The severity of disturbance depends on the severity of injury. Pain is the most frequent symptom of neuritis. The intensity varies, but the pain is apt to be sharp, burning or boring; it will follow the course of the nerve or nerves affected. If the nerve is completely severed, pain is absent; it may be severe in mild degeneration. Disagreeable sensations, such as numbness or tingling, may also be experienced. The nerve is often tender and swollen. The muscles are flabby and may waste away; they may be slightly weak or completely paralyzed. The deep reflexes are lost. The skin may become thin, shiny, and cold. It may thicken, scale off, or show disturbed sweating and increased or decreased growth of hair.

Causes

Nerve degeneration has both local and general causes. Local causes of nerve degeneration are usually mechanical and affect a single nerve or a group of nerves that lie close together. Some local causes of this condition are cutting, stretching, tearing, pressure, and tumors. General causes usually affect more than one nerve. Some of the causes are intoxications from chemicals, infectious diseases, and deficiency states.

Diagnosis of the nerve degeneration itself is not difficult, but determination of the cause may be. Treatment is directed toward the underlying cause. Contractures are avoided by proper positioning and support of the limbs. Pain is controlled with aspirin or, in severe cases, with narcotics. It is imperative to avoid injury to the affected part.

DISORDERS OF THE BRAIN AND NERVOUS SYSTEM: NEURALGIA AND NEURITIS

Neuralgia may be defined as paroxysmal pain in an area, not associated with any demonstrable pathological change, and of undefined cause. Neuritis, in contrast, refers to pain or disability resulting from lesions of a nerve, even though the lesions may not always be readily demonstrable. Neuralgia is a symptom of some disorder, and not a specific disease, as is neuritis.

Neuralgia

There are two general types of neuralgia. The *typical* neuralgias manifest pain along the path of a definite sensory nerve distribution. They are further characterized by repeated attacks of short duration, frequently initiated by contact with some specific area or "trigger zone." The typical neuralgias are designated by the area affected, the chief being *trigeminal, glossopharyngeal,* and *geniculate neuralgias. Atypical* neuralgias do not manifest pain that follows a definite nerve area. There is no "trigger zone," and the pain may last for periods of several days, weeks, or months. *Atypical facial*

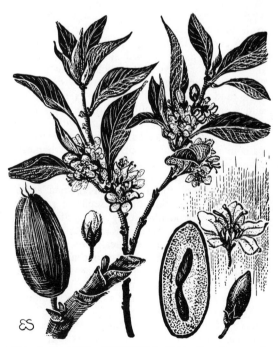

The coca plant. *Erythroxylon coca,* the leaves of which contain cocaine and other alkaloids. Cocaine paralyzes the peripheral ends of sensory nerves.

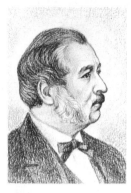

PANCOAST, Joseph (1805-1882) American surgeon. In the year 1859, he performed the first successful surgical operation on a patient who was suffering with an exstrophy of the bladder and an accompanying epispadias. He devised a surgical procedure which is now named after him. In this operation one of the branches of a facial nerve is divided in order to relieve the pain occurring in patients suffering from such disorders as facial neuralgia.

neuralgia is a common type that may be characterized by diffuse pain in the eyes, behind the nose, at the side and back of the head, and sometimes even in the shoulders. It has been suggested that such neuralgias may be closely related to the pain of migraine headache. Treatment of patients with the condition is variable, depending on the patient's symptoms. There is no specific cure.

Trigeminal neuralgia (Tic Douloureux) is the most common form of neuralgia. It may affect one or all of the three branches of the trigeminal nerve. A trigger point in the gums, near a tooth, or on the side of the tongue frequently starts the pain. These points may be so sensitive that shaving or washing the face or teeth are neglected lest a bout of pain be set off. The pain may radiate over the upper, middle, or lower part of the face. Variable but violent, it is described as sharp and shooting, as though hot needles or knives were sticking into the patient. The face twists in spasms of pain, and tears and saliva flow. In a few seconds, the attack stops. The condition may clear up spontaneously, but it is apt to return with shorter intervals between attacks. Dilantin relieves the pain in a large number of patients, carbamazepine gives relatively long-lasting relief to about 75 percent of patients, and inhalation of trichlorethylene several times daily has helped some. If these fail, injection of the separate roots of the nerve with alcohol may give relief which lasts for months or years. In some cases, it may be necessary to have a surgical resection of the *gasserian ganglion root*. This operation which formerly was regarded as dangerous, has been perfected so that it is now safe.

Glossopharyngeal neuralgia is quite similar to the trigeminal variety, excepting that the pain radiates from the area of the tonsils, pharynx, and ear zones. Tonsils act as the trigger zone, and swallowing typically brings on the attack. Division of the glossopharyngeal nerve is curative for this type of neuralgia. *Geniculate neuralgia*

is a less common form in which the pain is in the external auditory canal; the trigger zone is in the external ear. Section of the nerve is again the only successful remedy.

Neuritis

Neuritis may be of an almost limitless number of kinds, depending upon which nerves are affected. Neuritis of the sciatic nerve or *sciatica* is one common form which occurs predominantly in men past middle age. Arthritis, infection, malignant disease of the vertebrae, and rupture of an intervertebral disk are among the common causes. The pain usually occurs in only one leg and is constant, reaching its greatest intensity in a few days, remaining for weeks or months, and then gradually disappearing. The treatment of sciatica patients depends upon the underlying cause of the condition.

Other common forms of neuritis that result in pain or disability may result whenever the circulation or normal function of a nerve is impaired. The young bridegroom who sleeps with his bride's head across his arm all night and awakens to find that he has lost control over the arm or a portion of it is suffering from a common case of "honeymoon" neuritis. "Saturday night" neuritis occurs when the drinker sits on the end of a park bench with its back under his arm, and falls asleep in this position, causing a paralysis due to injury to a whole plexus of nerves below the arm. Pain or loss of movement of a leg due to sitting cross-legged for some time is another type. The weight of the fat of obese people causes nerve injury in some cases. The sensation that occurs when the foot "goes to sleep" results from a diminished flow of blood to the nerve involved. Most of these types of neuritis are of a temporary nature, and disappear spontaneously after a period of time, depending on the extent of the injury. In more severe cases, a variety of special measures are available to alleviate pain and to restore the injured nerve.

BABINSKI, Joseph Francois F. (1857-1932) French neurologist. Noted for Babinski's sign, a reflex of the great toe upon stimulation of the sole, and a sympton found to be peculiar to organic hemiplegics. His contributions to knowledge of cerebellar disorders, such as asynergia, a condition effecting incoordinate muscular action, are abundant. Illuminating studies on hysteria, and descriptions of several nervous syndromes are also credited to him.

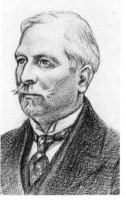

DISORDERS OF THE BRAIN AND NERVOUS SYSTEM: HEADACHE

Headache is always a symptom and never a disease. It is among the most common symptoms of disorder of not only the nervous system, but other parts of the body as well. Thus, discovery of the primary cause of a headache may be a difficult task. The severity of the pain is not always proportional to the gravity of the cause. Some of the most violent headaches arise from relatively minor bodily changes, while fatal disease of the brain may produce only mild pain.

Patients who consult a physician about headaches will be asked for certain basic information. The diagnosis may be facilitated if accurate answers can be given. The physician will want to know if he is dealing with a single acute headache, recurrent acute headaches, or chronic headaches. Events occurring before the headache—such as emotional stress, exertion, and eating, etc.—may give clues as to the cause of the trouble. The time of day the headache occurs and the exact type and location of pain are also important. Anything that accompanies the headache—for example, nausea, flashes of light, ringing in the ears—should also be reported. Any factors that relieve or intensify the pain are important. The way the attack begins and ends, whether slowly or abruptly, may be significant.

Pain-sensitive structures

Head pain arises from certain structures inside the skull. The large veins *(venous sinuses)* and their tributaries that drain the surface of the brain are sensitive to pain, as are the arteries. The brain substance itself is not sensitive to pain, but the coverings of the brain are. Most of the structures on the surface of the skull are pain-sensitive, particularly the arteries, and may give rise to headaches. The sinuses, teeth, ears, and muscles may be so affected that pain from them is at first local, but later covers a wider area.

Mechanisms of headache

Although headache is certainly one of the oldest symptoms known, only recently have the mechanisms by which the pain is produced been learned. Eight of these mechanisms of pain have been discovered and examined in some detail. They are: (1) dilation of the cranial arteries; (2) pulling or traction upon pain-sensitive intracranial structures; (3) traction on and dilatation of intracranial blood vessels; (4) inflammation of structures within the skull; (5)

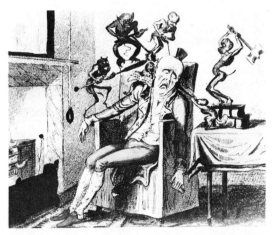

This engraving by George Cruikshank, an English humorist and illustrator of the 19th century, fancifully depicts the torments undergone by the sufferer of a headache. *Bettmann Archive.*

contraction of skeletal muscles over the head and neck; (6) spread of pain from stimulation elsewhere within the head; (7) pain from allergic reaction; and (8) mentally-produced, *psychogenic,* pain. The vast majority of headaches which eventually drive the patient to seek medical aid are caused either by dilatation of the cranial arteries or contraction of the muscles of the head and neck or by combinations of these two mechanisms. These headaches stem from conditions in the body that are usually easy to correct.

Headaches caused by dilatation of the cranial arteries *(vascular headaches)* account for the headaches associated with general infections, migraine headaches, or those resulting from taking certain drugs. This mechanism is responsible for hunger and "hangover" headaches, as well as for those which come on when people "don't get their morning coffee." The headaches of suddenly increased blood pressure belong in this group, as do those which follow convulsive seizures or head injury. These headaches usually have a throbbing quality, but this may be absent if the headache is prolonged.

In general, the treatment of persons with vascular headaches must be directed at the underlying cause. Inhalations of high concentrations of oxygen are especially helpful to persons who have headaches which are caused by lack of oxygen or with headaches resulting from "hangover" or a convulsive seizure. Headaches caused by traction or pressure on intracranial structures are associated with expanding intracranial masses. Brain tumors, abscesses, and hematomas are examples. The pain may be produced by primary pressure of the mass on a pain-sensitive structure, or it may arise secondarily from gen-

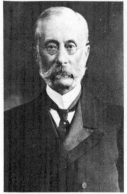

FERRIER, David (1843-1928) Scottish neurologist in England. Internationally famous for his studies on the localization of the various functions of the brain, which established the foundations of our knowledge in this area. Along with his other investigations in neuropathology, these studies first made possible operative surgery for brain tumors. He is generally considered to be one of the greatest experimental physiologists of his time.

eral displacement of the intracranial structures. These headaches are aggravated by coughing or straining. They are not relieved by drugs which constrict the arteries.

The headache associated with brain tumor may be intermittent and mild to moderate in severity. Usually, the headache does not interfere with sleep.

The headache produced by a hematoma is dull, steady, and felt throughout the head. The pain from brain abscess is similar to that of tumor. However, the abscess must be large enough to cause traction before pain is felt.

In healthy people, a sudden vigorous jolt or twist of the head may cause a slight headache. This results from traction on the pain-sensitive structures. It also accounts for the increased pain on sudden movement in vascular headaches. The management of headaches which arise by this mechanism of pain depends on the underlying condition. Aspirin and related compounds ordinarily relieve the pain, but stronger drugs may become necessary.

Headaches caused by traction upon and dilatation of the intracranial vessels is typified by the headache which frequently follows lumbar spinal puncture. At times, despite precautions, there may be slow leakage of the spinal fluid through the hole made by the needle. This results in headaches which are ordinarily mild, but which may become quite severe. Once the headache develops, bed rest is about all that is needed; the condition heals spontaneously.

Headaches caused by inflammation of cranial structures are experienced if the patient has any infection within the skull, such as meningitis or encephalitis. Such a headache also occurs as a result of the inflammation that follows brain hemorrhages. This type of headache arises from inflammation involving the pain-sensitive structures within the head. Headaches resulting from this mechanism may be intense and require narcotics.

A headache may occur secondary to pain arising elsewhere in the head and outlast the original pain. This is typified by the headaches associated with sinusitis. Certain diseases of the eye, or eye strain resulting from long use, or excessive attempts at accommodation in eyes that need glasses also cause this sort of headache. Infections which involve muscles, especially rheumatic fever, cause this type of head pain. Arthritis of the upper part of the neck or tumors in this area produce headache also.

Headaches also may be caused by sustained contraction of the muscles of the head and neck. The contraction may result from local muscle or nerve injury. Muscle contraction sometimes is associated with emotional tension.

Headaches produced by muscle contraction are located frequently over the back and lower part of the head and upper part of the neck. The pain is a steady, deep ache often associated with a feeling of pulling or tightness. The headache may be aggravated by movements of the head. The muscles themselves may be tender and tight. Massage of the muscles and heat applications often relieve the pain.

Headaches caused by allergy often go unrecognized, for they are not distinguished from other types by location and duration of pain. The most common allergens are pollens, house dust, animal dander, and foods such as chocolate, nuts, milk, and fish. Desensitizing injections and diet restrictions have proven helpful in preventing allergy-related headache.

Headache caused by emotional mechanisms is not well-understood. This type of headache is often bizarre. The patient may experience a wide variety of unusual sensations. While it may be described by the patient as being terribly intense, it ordinarily is of moderate severity and usually does not respond to the medications which relieve other forms of headache. In many cases, the treatment of patients with headaches of this type is primarily psychiatric.

GOLGI, Camillo (1844-1926) Italian neurologist. Golgi identified the nerve cells in the posterior horn of the spinal cord. The cells are called *Golgi's cells*. Many advances in microscopic anatomy have resulted from new staining methods. Under the microscope, nearly all body tissues are transparent, and all will not stain with the same dyes. To bring out one portion of a cell for study without overstaining the rest of the cell requires much research and good technique. Golgi developed staining techniques for studying nerve cells.

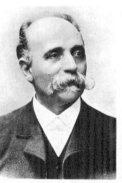

THE SPINAL NERVES

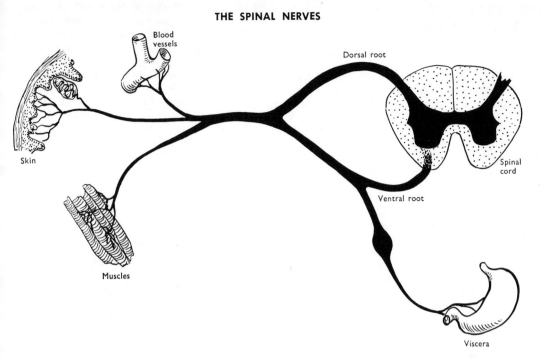

A typical spinal nerve. The spinal nerves play an important role in the involuntary activity of the body. They also carry impulses to and from the brain, and thus may be involved in many different types of disorders.

SEGMENTAL INNERVATION
OF THE SKIN

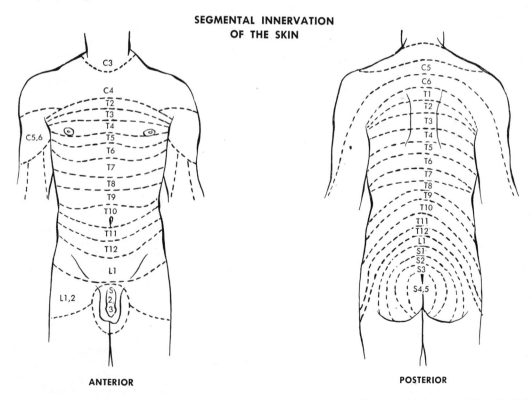

ANTERIOR   POSTERIOR

Anterior and posterior innervation of the skin. The spinal nerve which is distributed to each segment is indicated by its initial letter and number. Pain in one area may result from nerve injury farther along. Cervical, thoracic, lumbar and sacral nerves are designated by the capital letters C, T, L and S, respectively.

DISORDERS OF THE BRAIN AND NERVOUS SYSTEM: MIGRAINE HEADACHE

Migraine headaches, often called "sick headaches" or "recurrent headaches," have plagued mankind since earliest times. Mention of them is found in the literature of antiquity; Aretaeus of Cappadocia (second century) observed these headaches in his patients and wrote the first medical description of them. Migraine has been called one of the most common complaints of civilized people, and it is thought that from two to eight million persons in the United States suffer from these headaches. However, less than half of all migraine victims consult their physicians, so that there are no reliable data as to the numbers of sufferers.

The onset of migraine headaches usually occurs between ages 12 to 25; but they can begin at any age. Rural people and manual laborers are not as likely to be affected as urban dwellers and persons who perform mental work. The typical victim is a highly intelligent person, who is ambitious, hard driving, and meticulous.

The outstanding features of migraine headache that differentiate it from other types of headache are that one side of the head is affected; the attacks recur periodically; and it is probably hereditary. In the majority of cases, the headaches occur about once every two weeks. In women, they may be associated with the menstrual period. However, the attacks in some persons do not show this regularity, and they may even be separated by months or years.

A migraine headache may last from a few hours to more than a week. In any individual, the characteristic pain, accompanying symptoms, and time length are usually the same for each attack. In fact, the average sufferer can generally predict exactly what he will experience during any given episode of migraine.

Symptoms

As in any type of headache, the predominant symptom of migraine is pain. Most often, the pain is intense and of a sharp and boring character. It begins in the temple, eyeball, or forehead, and soon spreads from the initial spot to include either the left or right half of the head. Sometimes, however, pain will involve all of the face and neck, and even the arms.

In many migraine patients, the headache is preceded by disturbances of vision, which can occur in the form of complete blindness, dullness of vision, blinding flashes of light, sensitivity to light or sound, or dizziness. As the attack begins, the patient may notice a blind spot; that is, if he looks at a printed sentence, he will not

be able to see several of the words. This spot, in rare instances, increases in size until vision in one field is completely gone. The patient may regain the ability to see in the later stages of the attack, but he may still be troubled with dazzling black and white flashes of light.

During the attack, the victim's face usually appears pale and sallow, and his skin may be sweaty and clammy. His arms and legs will feel cold to him, even though he might have a fever. Nausea and violent vomiting often mark the climax of the attack.

After the attack has run its course, if there has been no vomiting, the patient usually feels relaxed and relieved. In fact, he may be filled with energy and tend to be overactive, although a dull headache may persist for a day or so.

Warnings of approaching attack (aura)

A large number of migraine sufferers report that their attacks seem to occur in relation to periods of "let-down" or exhilaration. Many have noted that their headaches will begin on weekends, the first days of a holiday, or on days of planned social engagements or travel. Often, on the night before onset of a migraine attack, the victim will be in especially high spirits. He may be unwilling to go to bed and have an unusually increased appetite. However, the next morning he may arise with a very depressed or melancholic attitude. As the day begins, he becomes restless, irritable, and confused. There may be an inability to concentrate on routine tasks or to make decisions. Just before the attack begins, relatives or associates of the patient may note a tendency to absent-mindedness which victims attribute to a sense of unreality. Warning that the headache is almost upon them may come with a visual disturbance, a tingling sensation in the hands and arms, or with ringing or other noises in the ears. Many persons have noticed either immediately before or during an attack of headache that finger rings are difficult to remove. Then the pain begins.

Numerous investigations have been made into the cause of migraine headaches, and many theories have been offered. Most authorities are agreed that distention of the cranial arteries in the scalp is the immediate cause. However, numerous and varied factors are responsible for this distension, some of which are known and some unknown. The personality traits of migraine patients—exacting, hard driving, etc.— are like those of persons having high blood pressure. It has been noted that about 50 percent of the children of migraine patients also suffer from migraine. This evidence is strong enough to suggest some hereditary influence. However, the possible inheritance of migraine has not been proven.

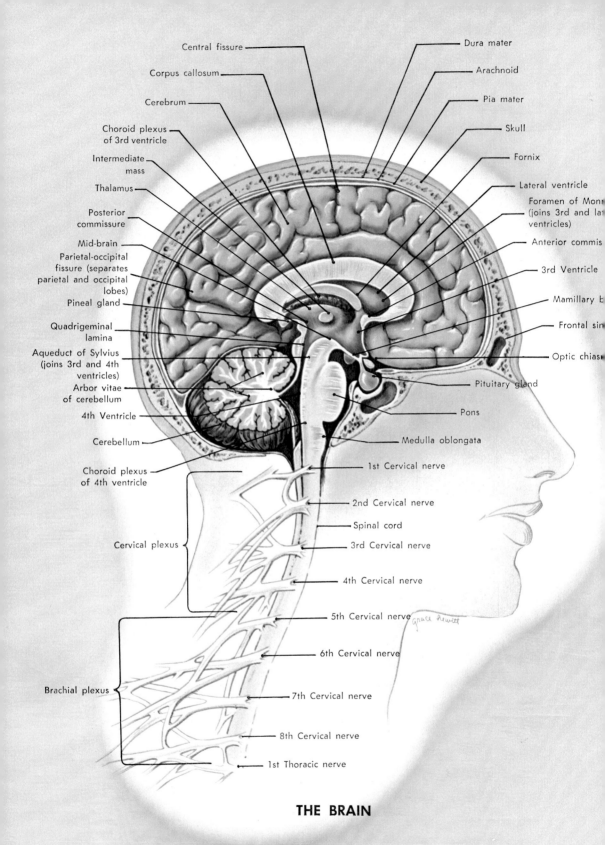

Central fissure

Corpus callosum

Cerebrum

Choroid plexus
of 3rd ventricle

Intermediate
mass

Thalamus

Posterior
commissure

Mid-brain

Parietal-occipital
fissure (separates
parietal and occipital
lobes)

Pineal gland

Quadrigeminal
lamina

Aqueduct of Sylvius
(joins 3rd and 4th
ventricles)

Arbor vitae
of cerebellum

4th Ventricle

Cerebellum

Choroid plexus
of 4th ventricle

Cervical plexus

Brachial plexus

Dura mater

Arachnoid

Pia mater

Skull

Fornix

Lateral ventricle

Foramen of Monro
(joins 3rd and lat
ventricles)

Anterior commis

3rd Ventricle

Mamillary b

Frontal sin

Optic chias

Pituitary gland

Pons

Medulla oblongata

1st Cervical nerve

2nd Cervical nerve

Spinal cord

3rd Cervical nerve

4th Cervical nerve

5th Cervical nerve

6th Cervical nerve

7th Cervical nerve

8th Cervical nerve

1st Thoracic nerve

Grace Hewitt

THE BRAIN

Some investigators believe that migraine headaches occur as the result of allergy, probably to certain protein-containing foods. Chocolate has been an offender, according to some patients. Thus, migraine in some may be akin to asthma. In other patients, however, the headaches are thought to occur because of eyestrain; and in others, certain factors of imbalance in the endocrine system might be responsible.

Care during the attack

Whatever the cause, the method of treatment is essentially the same in all persons. The victim should be left alone as much as possible in a quiet and darkened room. Patients are extremely sensitive to light and odors. An ice bag on the head and hot water bottle at the feet may offer some relief from pain. The intensity of the pain is sometimes reduced if the patient sits upright rather than lies down. The physician may advise the administration of a medicine called *ergotamine tartrate,* which has been found to terminate the headache in many instances *if given at the beginning of an attack*. This medicine has shown more promise than any other form of medical treatment. Another method is to allow the patient to inhale 100 percent oxygen; this may terminate or alleviate the pain.

While it is good procedure for the patient to take aspirin or other mild sedatives, *he should never take strong drugs for a migraine attack*. It is too easy for migraine sufferers to develop a drug habit, which is worse than the migraine. Furthermore, the drugs may not be absorbed during the attack; thus, the dangerous symptoms of overdosage by powerful drugs may become manifest when the patient begins to recover from a bout with migraine.

Actually, the best way for a patient with an attack of migraine to be treated is to prevent the attack. This is not always possible. However, the victim should certainly attempt to find the cause of his attacks by co-operating with his physician, and then try to eliminate that cause. If it can be found that certain foods are responsible, then these foods should be excluded from the patient's diet. It is quite possible that co-operation between patient and physician can lead to the cause and best treatment of this disorder.

Avoidance of fatigue, late hours, strain, and worry tend to reduce the frequency or severity of the migraine attacks. In most persons, physical or mental tension is often the immediate cause of the onset of an attack.

When no organic cause can be found, the migraine patient will do well to regulate some of his life habits. He must particularly avoid *excesses* of eating, drinking, playing, and working in order to keep from becoming mentally or physically fatigued. This is not to say that he should not get any open air exercise, because a regular routine of appropriate physical activities may be the solution to the prevention of migraine in many persons. He simply should not overdo it.

Most probably, migraine attacks will eventually cease spontaneously. Women who suffer attacks of migraine usually do not have any episodes during pregnancy; and the attacks may disappear entirely after the change of life. The disease may disappear in men and women at all ages, but most frequently the attacks cease at around 50 years of age, when the elasticity of the blood vessels has diminished, so that the dilatation mentioned as involved in the etiology of migraine has decreased.

DISORDERS OF THE BRAIN AND NERVOUS SYSTEM: BRAIN TUMOR

A brain tumor is an abnormal new growth of tissue in the brain. Brain tumors which originate within the brain seldom spread to adjacent or distant structures within the body. All such tumors inside the skull are potentially fatal by reason of their confinement within the closed cavity of the skull and their consequent encroachment upon the vital volume of the brain substance. A malignant brain tumor is, of course, difficult to remove. With modern brain surgery a benign tumor can be completely removed in many cases. When this is possible, the outlook for recovery is quite good. Early diagnosis facilitates the possibility of surgical removal.

Unfortunately, the signs and symptoms of brain tumor are quite variable and depend upon the portion of the brain that is compressed or disturbed by the expanding new growth. Headache is only occasionally the first, and not the most frequent symptom. Headache is usually

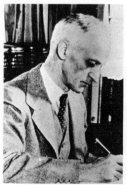

CUSHING, Harvey W. (1869-1939) American surgeon. Among the greatest surgeons of his time. His brain operations, especiallly for tumors, are famous, and his operative mortality was phenomenally low. In all of his work he combined an exhaustive study of the pathology, physiology and clinical observations involved with a brilliant surgical technique. He won the Pulitzer Prize for his fine biography of William Osler.

Illustration: Anatomy of the Brain . . . Grace Hewitt

of the intense, bursting type which may be localized in one particular section of the cranial cavity, but which is most often generalized. Headache is often accompanied by nausea and vomiting and is particularly significant if the vomiting is spontaneous and unaccompanied by preceding nausea.

Other early symptoms of brain tumor are various types of visual disturbance, including poor vision, blurring of vision, and double vision. Very often, the visual difficulty takes the form of what is called *hemianopsia* or inability to see with either eye to the right or to the left.

Following these symptoms, perhaps the next in frequency are those of in-co-ordination, weakness, and paralysis which may affect one arm, one leg or one half of the body, depending upon the location of the expanding growth. These symptoms are variable sometimes from week to week and sometimes from day to day.

Contrary to popular belief, personality or mental changes are the exception and not the rule in cases of brain tumor. When they occur, the patient may seem mentally dull, have lapses of memory, or lose all initiative.

Brain tumors occur in any location of the brain within the cranial cavity and also occur at any age including very early childhood. At various ages, tumors are more likely to occur in certain localities of the brain. In childhood, the tumors tend to occupy the hindbrain, resulting in early disturbances of co-ordination, stiff neck, severe headache and severe visual disturbance. Such children frequently cock the head to one side and sit and move in a rather rigid attitude.

In recent years, important advances have been made in the diagnosis of tumors and other disorders of the brain by the technique of *arteriography*. In this technique the blood vessels are injected with an opaque contrast medium, as close to the suspected lesion as is feasible. Radiograms are then made of the area to detect the flow of the contrast medium through and around the suspected lesion. Various types of tumors and other disorders are thereby differentiated. Likewise, the technique of *radiotopography* has enabled a much more accurate diagnosis of brain tumors, as well as tumors of other areas. By this method, a radioisotope is injected into the area under study and a scintillation camera or scintiscanner measures the distribution of the isotope in and around the suspected lesion.

Any combination of neurologic symptoms may result from brain tumor; there may be loss of smell, loss of sight, loss of hearing, loss of taste, or there may be distortion of any of these senses such as seeing flashes of light to one side or the other of the visual field, smelling odors which are not actually existent, or hearing non-existent noises.

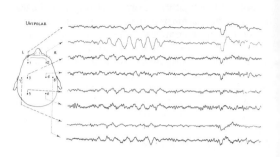

This electroencephalogram shows the abnormally slow wave action (second recording) of the right frontal lobe of a patient with a tumor in this area. *Photography, F. W. Schmidt.*

One of the most frequent disturbances incident to new intracranial growths is disturbance of the speech mechanism. This may take several forms, varying from the situation in which the patient is unable to make himself intelligently understood to others, to the opposite situation, in which the patient is unable to comprehend the speech of others. These disturbances are called aphasia. The various weaknesses or palsies accruing from brain tumor may vary from small losses of co-ordination to absolute paralysis of one or more extremities. Such in-co-ordination often results in staggering gait, swaying from side to side in standing and altogether grotesque locomotion.

One of the most prominent initial symptoms of brain tumor is the onset of convulsive disorders, or what is commonly called fits. This is such a commonplace occurence that there is a rule of thumb that convulsion occurring for the first time after the age of thirty years should be regarded as caused by a brain tumor until proved otherwise.

If any of the above symptoms are noticed, the patient should see his physician immediately. If brain tumors are correctly diagnosed early, there are very good chances for survival and rehabilitation. Approximately 70 percent of the patients whose tumors are completely removed by surgery can resume useful and comfortable living with little loss of original function.

New surgical techniques offer some hope for patients with especially difficult brain tumors. When extensive tumor pervades one side of the brain, hemispherectomy (removal of one half of the brain) may be undertaken. Though rare, this operation has also been used in other kinds of disease severely affecting one hemisphere of the brain, when the only alternative is death. If one side is removed, the other side may take over some of the higher brain functions. This is especially true for children, if the damaged half is removed before left- and right-handedness and speech have developed.

Aside from tumors which originate in the brain, tumors arising in various parts of the body may spread *(metastasize)* to the brain by way of the blood or lymph streams. Primary tumors of the lung are the most frequent to metastasize to the brain; breast tumors and gastrointestinal tumors somewhat less frequently spread to the brain, as do melanotic, thyroid and tumors of other areas.

DISORDERS OF THE BRAIN AND NERVOUS SYSTEM: SPINAL CORD TUMORS

A tumor of the spinal cord is an abnormal new growth of tissue in or about the spinal cord. The growth may originate in the spinal cord, or it may be an extension from a distant growth elsewhere in the body, or from adjacent structures. However, the symptoms are identical, so far as those referable to the spinal cord are concerned, because the symptoms result from compression of the spinal cord.

The most characteristic symptom of a spinal cord tumor is pain, usually located in the neck and shoulders, chest, abdomen, pelvis, or the extremities. This pain may trouble the patient constantly or intermittently. However, it usually occurs when the patient is at rest, and it is relieved by exercise. Often the patient will be awakened by pain from four to six hours after retiring; the pain may become so severe that the victim is compelled to walk the floor or to sleep in a sitting position. In most cases, the pain will be aggravated by laughing, coughing, sneezing, or lifting. The symptoms of a spinal cord tumor vary greatly, depending upon the structures involved or compressed.

Later in the course of the disease, the patient will become generally weak, and he may experience a feeling of numbness. His sensitivity to touch and heat may be diminished. At this time, there may begin a progressive loss of bladder function and control. The bowel control may be similarly affected.

After the disease has reached an advanced stage, the patient will become paralyzed in one or more areas of the body. These paralyzed areas will be located below the site of the tumor in the cord. By this time, bladder and anal control will be completely lost.

When the physician diagnoses a tumor of the spinal cord, he will probably recommend surgical removal of the growth. Eighty percent of spinal cord tumors are benign and removable. Intraspinal operations now can be performed with a minimum of danger. In those cases in which the diagnosis is made early, all functions are restored in many of the patients following surgery; and a cure often is possible to achieve, depending on the nature of the tumor. Consequently, recovery in a great many cases depends upon early diagnosis and adequate treatment.

OTHER DISORDERS OF THE BRAIN AND NERVOUS SYSTEM

Myasthenia gravis is a disease characterized by excessive fatigability of the muscles after mild or moderate exertion. The muscles about the head and neck are most seriously involved. Thus, toward the end of a meal, the jaw muscles may be so tired that further chewing is impossible. After a few minutes of rest, there is enough strength to start again, but the fatigue returns rapidly. Difficulty in swallowing or keeping the eyes open may be noted. Death may result from fatigue of the heart or respiratory muscles. Treatment has greatly improved within recent years. Mestinon, Mytelase, or Prostigmin may be used, but the dose must be carefully regulated for each individual by the physician.

Degenerative diseases of the nervous system include many disorders whose cause is unknown. Hereditary factors are obvious in certain diseases of the nervous system; in these disorders, the specific disease may not be inherited, but rather a general inherent weakness of the nervous system. Important examples of hereditary diseases of the nervous system are: *amaurotic idiocy, Huntington's chorea, familial periodic paralysis, hereditary spastic paralysis, progressive muscular dystrophy, Friedreich's and Marie's ataxia, hereditary tremor, progressive lenticular degeneration, feeble mindedness*, and certain psychoses.

A nonhereditary degenerative disease of the nervous system is *syringomyelia*. It is characterized by cysts, usually located in the central part of the spinal cord or in the lower part of the brain. It usually starts when the patient is 20 to 30 years of age. Ability to feel pain, heat, and cold are lost, although sensitivity to touch and pressure are preserved. Muscle weakness and wasting occur.

The rare Sturge-Weber syndrome is marked by a localized atrophy and calcification of the cerebral cortex and a large port-wine stain on the face and neck at birth. Such stains often have no medical significance, but with this disease the coloration is caused by excessive blood vessels in the skin, scalp, and brain surface. After a few weeks or months, the child develops disabling convulsions and seizures. Drug control of seizures requires increasingly heavy dosage. Hemispherectomy (removal of half of the brain) performed in infancy has been used successfully in a few instances of the disease.

Multiple sclerosis usually develops early in adult life in people who are otherwise healthy. It is characterized by periods of remission, followed by periods of recurrence in which the symptoms reappear. The illness may extend over a period of years. It ultimately becomes completely disabling for most people.

In recent years, researchers have speculated that multiple sclerosis may be classed among diseases which result from "autoimmunity," a condition in which the body becomes allergic to part of itself. Some form of antibody circulating in the blood attacks nerve cell junctions and destroys the protective sheathing of nerve fibers. There is destruction of the white matter of the nervous system, in the spinal cord as well as in the brain. This occurs in tiny spots which are scattered throughout the nervous system. The symptoms are diverse and fluctuating. This disorder is difficult to diagnose, particularly at the beginning of the illness.

Often multiple sclerosis starts with temporary mistiness of vision which may not be accompanied by pain and which usually does not amount to blindness. This may be so mild as to pass almost unnoticed by the patient or may not be severe enough to make him seek medical aid. The patient may experience double vision (*diplopia*), a tingling or burning sensation of the skin (*paresthesia*), in-coordination, weakness, tremors, an oscillatory movement of the eyeballs (*nystagmus*), or stammering. Often the speech becomes monotonous or slurred. Eventually, the muscles of the legs become stiff or spastic and go into spasms. At times, mental symptoms develop, in which case there is deterioration of the intellect. There may be depression or an overelated state. By far the most common mental symptom is that of extreme well-being, so that the patient is characteristically optimistic and feels well despite the severe symptoms. He frequently smiles or giggles with no provocation. It is often difficult to make the diagnosis of multiple sclerosis since it resembles many other disorders of the nervous system. At the present time, there is no useful treatment known. During the acute attacks, the patient should be encouraged to remain in bed.

Parkinson's disease, also known as shaking palsy, is a disease of later life, usually appearing when the patient is 50 or 60 years old. In 1960, there were 34,000 reported cases of Parkinson's disease in the United States. Since that time, the number of cases has been declining. It is speculated that eventually the disease will cease to be a major medical problem. The disease has been related to the encephalitis lethargica epidemic of 1915 to 1926. This virus disappeared in 1931. In persons infected at that time, the virus is thought to have damaged or lain dormant in the part of the brain that controls muscular movements. Only one victim of Parkinson's disease born since 1931 has been reported by one group of investigators. Slow-acting viruses such as that thought to cause Parkinson's disease may be related to other diseases of the nervous and muscular systems.

Parkinson's disease is progressive in severity, beginning so mildly that the patient may be unaware of any disability until others notice the characteristic symptoms of a rhythmic tremor of muscles, a gradual slowing of voluntary movements and masklike expression of the face. Later, a peculiar, slightly hunched posture and hurried, unbalanced gait develop.

Until recently, the condition was considered to be incurable, but the development of neurosurgical techniques have benefitted many cases. By one technique, cryothalamotomy, a permanent lesion is produced in the substantia nigra region of the brain. This lesion is created by reducing the temperature to $-60°$ C for three minutes at the site of damaged cells. Since the early 1960s, an amino acid, levodopa (levodihydroxyphenylalanine), has been under investigation for relieving the symptoms of parkinsonism. Numerous investigators have now confirmed that this drug is effective in relieving the rigidity, tremor, mental depression, and other symptoms of the disease. There are adverse side effects, however, to the use of this drug; it should never be taken except under a physician's direction.

Disease of the nervous system may also be a complication of certain other general disorders. An example is *pernicious anemia* in which there is a secondary degeneration of the spinal cord, particularly in the tracts on the sides, or the pathways from the motor cortex to the spinal cord. This condition produces spastic paralysis in the legs and involves the centers that control the action of the bladder and bowel.

BIOCHEMICAL DISORDERS OF THE BRAIN

Certain enzyme abnormalities may result in brain damage from biochemical imbalance. The lack of the enzyme essential to the metabolism of phenylalanine, contained in most protein foods, causes phenylpyruvic acid to accumulate and inflict permanent brain damage. This is an inherited disorder, present in about 4 persons in 100,000; among mental defectives, the incidence is 500 per 100,000. If the defect is detected promptly at birth, the infant can be placed on a special diet and escape almost all brain damage. The PKU test, as it is called, has become a routine part of neonatal examinations.

Mongolism is associated with the presence of an extra chromosome and varying degrees of brain damage. A metabolic abnormality is also involved. The system produces too much of the enzyme that breaks down tryptophan, an essential component of protein involved in brain function. These are only two examples of the effects of biochemical alterations on brain tissue. There are others, some of which are related to inherited genetic defects; they are discussed elsewhere.

HEAD INJURIES

By the year 1969, 1,690,000 persons had been killed as a result of automobile accidents in the United States. Head injuries accounted for many of these deaths and large numbers of the permanently crippled.

Head injuries may be classified according to the structure involved. The scalp alone may be injured, or the skull may be fractured. Within the skull, either the coverings of the brain and/or the brain itself may be damaged. Any of these injuries may be present alone or in any combination.

The scalp may merely be cut, or great areas of it may be torn away. A cut scalp, which bleeds freely, often gives the impression of severe injury when only slight damage has been done. If the laceration causes no disfigurement and if there is no infection, scalp injuries alone are of relatively little importance.

Skull fractures

Most persons are unduly alarmed when the diagnosis of skull fracture is made. Actually, uncomplicated skull fractures without brain damage seldom cause death or disability. Skull fractures are of two types: closed (*simple*) and open (*compound*). Either may be complicated further in various ways. Simple fractures vary from a small fracture line to extensive cracking of the bones throughout the skull. Simple uncomplicated fractures require no specific treatment other than good nursing care and bed rest. A simple skull fracture in a child ordinarily requires four or five months to heal; in adults, adequate healing may take a year or longer.

Simple fractures of the skull are complicated if one of the pieces of bone is depressed so that it presses on the brain. Other complications arise when the fracture occurs across a major artery or vein or involves one of the cranial nerves. In a depressed fracture, the shape and volume of the inside of the skull may be so altered that an operation is needed to restore the contour. Bone fragments that are markedly depressed must be elevated to prevent irritating the brain, and possibly causing the patient to have convulsive seizures. If the depression results in little or no pressure on the brain, it is usually left alone. In many fractures involving the cranial nerves, little can be done because the nerve usually is irreparably damaged at the moment of injury. Fractures across a major artery have to be managed surgically.

Compound fractures of the skull are generally more serious than simple fractures, because the brain is exposed, and bacteria may enter, causing infection. In the dome of the skull, the bones may cut through the scalp. In fractures of the floor of the skull, the break may occur through the mucous membranes of the nose, the sinuses, the orbit of the eye, or the middle ear. If there is clear fluid running from the nose or ears with no visible evidence of injury, or if there is blood running from the mouth, nose, or ears, one should suspect such a fracture. Compound fractures in any location of the skull predispose the patient to meningitis unless proper measures are taken. This threat has been greatly reduced by the use of sulfonamides and the antibiotics. These drugs are ordinarily given at once to any patient who has had a compound fracture of the skull. Compound fractures may be complicated still further by depressed fragments or fracture lines extending through major vessels.

Brain injury

Within the skull, either the brain or its covering (*dura*) may be damaged. Injury to the dura causes bleeding which may, in turn, injure the brain tissue. When bleeding is on the under surface of the dura, it is called a *subdural hematoma*; if bleeding is above the dura, it is called an *extradural hematoma*. Extradural hematomas almost always occur in the region of the temple. Patients with these hematomas have a characteristic course of symptoms. An individual receives a blow on the head, which may or may not cause temporary loss of consciousness. Soon he begins to complain of headache, which becomes increasingly severe during the next two or three hours. Nausea and vomiting are often experienced. The patient may become a little drowsy. There may be speech difficulties or weakness in various parts of the body. If the drowsiness continues, the patient becomes stuporous and finally goes into a deep coma. Blood collects in the area of the wound. Since the skull is rigid and nonexpansile, the collecting blood can only depress the brain tissue. If this lasts for only a short time, there may be no permanent damage. If it lasts for a long period, there usually is permanent damage to the brain tissue. The only treatment is prompt operation. Once the diagnosis of extradural clot is suspected, there should be immediate surgical exploration. This is a

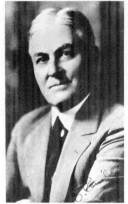

CRILE, George W. (1864-1943) American surgeon. Developed a technique of reducing operative shock by controlling post-operative nervous activity, through block anesthesia of nerve trunks. This proposal stimulated further study on the control of shock. Crile's experimental studies on shock, as well as his ingenious but difficult method of direct blood transfusion from donor to recipient, are well known. He was especially interested in the surgery of goiters.

rather simple procedure; two small holes are bored into the skull, and the clot is located. Then a larger hole is made; the clot is sucked out; and the bleeding artery is tied off. When treated promptly, there is an excellent chance the patient will recover.

Subdural hematomas usually develop over a period of days or weeks. Chronic subdural hematomas are much more common than formerly suspected. They often follow minor head injuries and usually occur in infants and persons over forty years of age. The bleeding is slow, and often fluid from the surrounding tissue is drawn into the clot. This results in a slowly enlarging mass which allows the brain tissue some adjustment to the increased pressure. The symptoms which appear after weeks and months are usually similar to those of brain tumor. Headache is present in most cases; drowsiness is another conspicuous sign. Both of these symptoms may fluctuate from day to day in the same patient. Dizziness often accompanies these symptoms, and vomiting may also occur. Older patients usually are confused; personality changes are so insidious and vague that the family cannot state just what is wrong, but only that the patient is "different." There may be weakness or complete paralysis of various parts of the body. Diagnosis of this condition is sometimes difficult, and made only through an exploratory operation. This may be a simple procedure like that already described for extradural hematomas or may be more extensive. Recovery is good in many of these cases, particularly if the underlying brain tissue is healthy.

Injuries to the brain are extraordinarily varied in their effect. For example, the trauma of a bullet entering the brain may cause life to cease almost immediately; or the tearing and depriving brain tissue of blood and oxygen can make the difference between functional living and vegetable-like existence. In rare instances, a bullet entering the skull has been known to miss vital areas and leave the victim with little more than a severe headache. Brain injury may occur without damage to other structures of the head. It usually is subdivided into the following classes: *concussion*, *contusion*, and *laceration*. Concussion is a jarring of the brain which usually results in a transitory period of unconsciousness. It is one of the commonest and mildest forms of brain injury. Recovery is almost always complete. Contusion is a bruising injury to the brain. The patient's symptoms are a combination of two effects; nonfunction of some nerve centers and overactivity of others which are normally inhibited by higher control centers. Disturbance of consciousness is a sign of generalized disturbance in the brain, whatever the cause. This may be a mild, transient change or profound and prolonged coma. A boxer's "k.o." is an example of concussion. Many fighters have no lasting effects while others become "punch-drunk" and portray unusual symptoms; this condition is discussed later.

Recovery from complete loss of consciousness is attained by certain stages. The entire process may require only a few minutes; however, any of the phases may be prolonged for hours or days. In severe injury, paralysis of major brain functions, even of respiration, may occur. The latter returns quickly in nonfatal cases. Death occurs rapidly if artificial respiration is not applied in those instances when return of respiration is delayed. Deep coma is marked by flaccid paralysis and even loss of involuntary motion. As coma lightens, the patient passes into stupor, and reflex activity returns. He responds automatically to forceful commands but is unaware of his surroundings. The next phase, excitement or *delirium*, is marked by extreme restlessness and confusion, and often the patient is violent. He gradually becomes quiet but remains extremely confused mentally. In the next stage, *automatism*, the patient answers questions and performs simple tasks in a fairly orderly but automatic way. The highest functions—judgment and insight—are the last to return.

Laceration of the brain results in actual tearing or destruction of the brain tissue itself.

DANDY, Walter Edward (1886-1946) American surgeon. Aided in the development of neurosurgery, which had its beginnings toward the end of the nineteenth century. He introduced ventriculography, a diagnostic procedure using radiographs of air-injected ventricles of the brain, to localize tumors. His work on hydrocephalus, as well as certain neurologic procedures including operations for ruptured intervertebral disk, became well known.

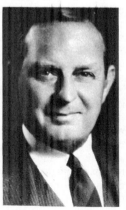

Swelling of the brain occurs and probably accounts for at least part of the widespread changes that follow. Slowing of the blood flow results in poor oxygen supply, which further increases the damage.

On recovery of consciousness, there may be loss of memory (*amnesia*) for the accident itself. Often this amnesia includes events that occurred before the accident (*retrograde amnesia*) and a variable period of time after the accident (*posttraumatic amnesia*). The presence of retrograde amnesia is evidence of the severity or extensiveness of the brain injury. The duration of posttraumatic amnesia varies, because the patient often has isolated memories of events before the complete return of memory.

Care of the patient

An unconscious person should be handled as little as possible. He should be placed on his side; his lower jaw and tongue must be kept forward to prevent blockade of his air passage. Care must be taken that vomitus is not breathed in. Bleeding from the scalp may be stopped temporarily by pressure bandages. If the patient is in a state of shock—cold, clammy skin and rapid, feeble pulse—he should be kept warm, but not hot, until the physician can take other measures. In profound coma, a nasal tube for feeding is used. Skillful nursing care, sedation, adequate fluid intake, and maintenance of an airway are mandatory. Establishment of a tracheotomy may be necessary for aspiration of excess mucus, to provide an avenue for unobstructed breathing. A humid room with a temperature of 65° to 70° F may assist breathing. Two days of bed rest is the minimum.

In slight injury with incomplete or brief loss of consciousness, complete recovery within 24 hours is usual. In moderate head injuries in which unconsciousness lasts up to two or three hours, the patient passes through the various recovery stages, already described, within a few hours or over a period of several weeks. Recovery may be arrested at any of these stages for various lengths of time. In severe injuries where unconsciousness lasts three hours or longer, the mortality rates are higher. As a rule, if after severe injury, the patient arouses sufficiently to answer questions, he is fairly certain to recover from the initial generalized brain injury; but he is still liable to such complications as meningitis and hemorrhage. Personality and intellectual impairment may occur. In general, the older the patient, the slower and less certain is the improvement, and full restoration is doubtful in patients over 60 years old. Children tolerate head injury with fewer aftereffects than adults. Some, however, show behavior disorders. In general, the duration of post-traumatic amnesia is the best single criterion for prognosis; the longer

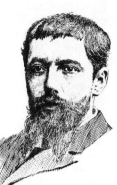

DEJERINE, Joseph Jules (1849-1917) French neurologist. Considered one of the greatest European neurologists of his time. He is famous for many studies on tabes, muscular atrophy, interstitial neuritis, spinal radiculitis, the spinal arthropathies, the optic thalamus syndrome, and other related syndromes caused by lesions in the pons and medulla. His treatise on the anatomy of the central nervous system was a most important study.

it lasts, the poorer the outlook. Improvement may continue slowly for twelve to 18 months.

Complications

Infections, such as brain abscess or meningitis, may complicate head injury. Abscesses may develop from improperly managed scalp wounds. These become infected, and this process may penetrate the skull to the dura. Ordinarily, this tough membrane prevents the infection from passing into the brain, but it may fail occasionally. Most brain abscesses result from compound fractures or from penetrating wounds, both of which introduce bacteria into the brain. The injured brain provides an ideal place for the growth of bacteria. If the organisms are *virulent*, meningo-encephalitis may develop rapidly and cause death before the abscess can form. If they are less virulent, a brain abscess develops. This may begin acutely within a day or so after injury with such symptoms as headaches and fever. Chronic abscesses may begin months after the injury, but most develop within a few days or weeks. The onset of headaches, listlessness, and vomiting is slower than in the patient with acute abscess.

Posttraumatic meningitis results from infection at the time of injury and usually follows compound fractures or penetrating wounds. Its onset is abrupt, and the usual signs of meningitis are present.

Convulsive seizures

Convulsive seizures of any type may occur at any time after brain injury. The occurrence of seizures immediately following the injury does not necessarily mean that the patient will continue to have them, nor does their absence during the acute phase guarantee against them in the future. At any rate, they may develop months or years after the original injury. They are more apt to occur in those injuries which produce penetration of the dura and brain damage. Retention of a foreign body of any sort leads to a higher incidence of convulsions. Laceration of the brain and small intracerebral hemorrhages also result in tissue changes which may cause convulsions. The best treatment is preventive. Clean removal of all injured brain tissue at the time of original operation allows minimum formation of scar tissue, thus minimizing the chance of later seizures.

The condition known as "punch drunk" is seen in people who have had repeated head injuries—professional football players and particularly boxers. The condition is thought to result from small hemorrhages throughout the brain which the patient receives as a result of blows on the head. The changes begin gradually with the loss of dexterity, which the patient may claim is as good as ever. Lack of attention, concentration, and memory follow. Impediments of speech and glazed, staring eyes make this too-talkative and too-social person look partially drunk, hence the term "punch drunk." Tremor of the hands, unsteadiness of gait, and failing vision and hearing develop in severe cases. Headache, dizziness, and roaring in the ears may be present. The victim is unable to engage in even simple intellectual activities and is without insight regarding his disability.

Unlike the "punch drunk," the person with *postconcussion syndrome* complains of greater incapacity, of which he gives little outward sign.

Authorities differ as to its cause. Some believe that it is caused by organic damage to the brain while others think it is the result of psychologic factors. This condition is not related to the severity of the injury. Headache, which is quite variable in character, is the most common complaint. It is usually located near the site of injury. It may be caused by mental or physical effort, light, or noise, or may occur spontaneously. Rest and quiet usually give relief. The patient may suffer from intolerance to cold, easy fatigability, and insomnia. Some memory impairment and confusion in thinking may be noted; in the more severe cases, the patient may have an emotional outburst, particularly of rage. Treatment usually consists of the administration of mild sedatives and psychotherapy.

In cases of severe brain injury, occasional patients have permanent mental changes. In general, these are characterized by slowness or inability to grasp new ideas of time and place, and poor perception. The memory is poor, and there is a tendency to fill in gaps with stories which are not told with the intent of lying. This type of mental reaction is often noted in patients during the acute phases of their head injury, but the eventual outlook in uncomplicated cases is good. Alcoholism or arteriosclerosis make this prognosis poorer. Mental deficiency following head injury in childhood, contrary to the common idea, is rare.

12 THE TEETH

WHAT THEY ARE AND DO

Teeth are the pearls of the body. They are not only highly ornamental, but extremely useful as well. Their chief function is to grind food from large to small pieces so that it may be swallowed and digested. They are also used for working, aiding expression, making love, forming words during speech, music making, and in many other ways. They are an important part of the body, as they contribute much to the individual's sense of well-being. Their loss is associated with the fear of old age and death. Some women have never let their husbands see them without their artificial teeth. The young person confronted with an early loss of teeth undergoes a major psychologic readjustment. This is especially true in young women. Men often feel that they lose some of their masculinity with the loss of their teeth. Decayed teeth and diseased gums serve as pathways for germs to enter the body. Sound teeth contribute to good health, both physiologically and psychologically.

Anatomy

Each tooth is composed largely of mineral salts. Calcium and phosphorus are the most prominent, while magnesium, fluorine, and others are found in small quantities. These inorganic salts are embedded in an organic matrix of fine tissue fibrils to form the hard portions of the tooth. That portion of the tooth that protrudes into the mouth is called the *clinical crown* and it is covered by the hardest substance found in the human body, *enamel.* The root surface of the tooth, hidden from view beneath the gum, is composed of a bonelike tissue called *cementum.* The remaining bulk of the tooth is made up of *dentin.* Dentin has much the same composition as bone, but has a different structure microscopically. Within a chamber in the center of the dentin and extending through a canal down to the apex of the root is the *dental pulp.* The pulp is a soft tissue containing nerves, lymphatics, and blood vessels supplying the tooth.

The enamel is made of epithelial cells, or cells that line the external tissue and are not supplied by the blood vessels. Dentin, cementum, and pulp arise from vascular connective tissue. Enamel is derived from the same source as hair and nails. This point is important because when the tooth erupts into the mouth, the enamel loses contact with blood-rich tissue and can only gain nutrients from the saliva. When enamel is damaged by disease or accident, it cannot repair itself. Drugs and vitamins taken after eruption of the tooth cannot reach the enamel through the circulatory system. However, certain drugs taken by children can affect their permanent teeth before they erupt. This situation complicates the management of tooth decay, for decay originates on the surface of the enamel, or in a fissure of the enamel.

Dentin, unlike bone, does not serve as a storehouse for inorganic salts that may be drawn upon in time of need. Once calcium and other minerals have been laid down in dentin, they remain there permanently, except during the period of resorption of the roots of the primary tooth, when shedding, and in certain cases of

	Tooth	Calcification Begins	Eruption	Root Completed
PRIMARY DENTITION Upper and Lower	Central incisor	4 mos. in utero	6—8 mos.	1½ yrs.
	Lateral incisor	4½ mos. in utero	7—9 mos.	1½—2 yrs.
	Cuspid	5 mos. in utero	16—18 mos.	3¼ yrs.
	First molar	5 mos. in utero	12—14 mos.	2¼—2½ yrs.
	Second molar	6 mos. in utero	20—24 mos.	3 yrs.
PERMANENT DENTITION Upper	Central incisor	3—4 mos.	7—8 yrs.	10 yrs.
	Lateral incisor	10—12 mos.	8—9 yrs.	11 yrs.
	Cuspid	4—5 mos.	11—12 yrs.	13—15 yrs.
	First bicuspid	1½—1¾ yrs.	10—11 yrs.	12—13 yrs.
	Second bicuspid	2—2¼ yrs.	10—12 yrs.	12—14 yrs.
	First molar	at birth	6—7 yrs.	9—10 yrs.
	Second molar	2½—3 yrs.	12—13 yrs.	14—16 yrs.
	Third molar	7—9 yrs.	17—21 yrs.	18—25 yrs.
PERMANENT DENTITION Lower	Central incisor	3—4 mos.	6—7 yrs.	9 yrs.
	Lateral incisor	3—4 mos.	7—8 yrs.	10 yrs.
	Cuspid	4—5 mos.	9—10 yrs.	12—14 yrs.
	First bicuspid	1¾—2 yrs.	10—12 yrs.	12—13 yrs.
	Second bicuspid	2¼—2½ yrs.	11—12 yrs.	13—14 yrs.
	First molar	at birth	6—7 yrs.	9—10 yrs.
	Second molar	2½—3 yrs.	11—13 yrs.	14—15 yrs.
	Third molar	8—10 yrs.	17—21 yrs.	18—25 yrs.

localized disturbances of unknown cause. A diseased dentin also has no means of repair.

The dental pulp lies within a chamber in the center of the tooth. On the periphery of the pulp are many special cells that have small tubules extending through the width of the dentin to the enamel. When decay touches the dentin, these peripheral cells act to protect the pulp. They deposit a "wall" of calcium salts in the dentin between the decay and the pulp chamber. Although this makes the dentin harder and requires more time for decay to break it down, it does not stop or repair the damage done. It does serve a useful purpose in healthy teeth by forming a hard barrier to the wear or abrasion that takes place gradually when gritty substances are chewed and as the teeth wear down with age. Additional calcified tissue also forms on the wall of the pulp chamber. This is called secondary dentin. Nodular calcifications within this pulp tissue often occur. They are called pulp stones and have little significance, although some think they are responsible for certain types of toothache.

The dentinal tubules may transmit sensation to the pulp. Since each dentinal fibril is connected to a cell on the periphery of the dentinal pulp, it is reasoned that any stimulus to the fibril will result in a stimulus to the pulpal tissue. When a "wall" of calcium salts (sclerotic dentin) is deposited in the dentin to resist advancing decay, the dentin will no longer conduct pain sensations. Some investigators believe that, in addition to the tubular content of dentin, there are actual nerve endings embedded within the dentinal matrix which are responsible for its sensitivity.

Enamel, harder than dentin, has no sensitivity. Dentin is exquisitely sensitive in some places while in other areas it will transmit no sensation. Neither of the tissues, because of the manner in which they are formed, has ability to repair damage once the tooth has erupted into the mouth.

The root of the tooth is covered by *cementum*. This tissue closely resembles bone in structure. In that part nearest the crown of the tooth, the cementum is thin and contains no cells. This fact accounts for the ease with which the cementum may be worn away by abrasive dentifrices once the gum recedes from the neck of the tooth.

Since that portion of the cementum and dentin beneath the gum is nourished by the blood stream, it is possible for these tissues to repair themselves when injured. Fracture of a tooth root may heal, as does fracture of any bone. Tearing of cementum from the tooth root may also heal and frequently does. Failure of root fracture to heal is usually the result of the arrangement of the dentinal pulp within the root of the tooth. The pulp is dependent upon its blood supply from those vessels that enter through several tiny openings at the apex of the root. It is possible for this pulpal tissue to die following fracture for lack of oxygen and other nutrients. If circulation is maintained, there is a better chance of healing.

The membrane that holds the tooth within the jawbone socket is known as the *periodontal mem-*

brane. It is composed of many strong connective tissue fibers embedded on one side within the cementum and on the other within the bony wall of the tooth socket, the *alveolus*. These fibers form a basketwork in which the tooth is suspended. Each tooth has its own set of fibers. Their structure and arrangement is such that great pressure in the direction of the bony socket may be exerted on the teeth without undue discomfort being suffered. Relatively little pulling, or twisting force applied gradually, intermittently, and in certain directions, will eventually allow easy removal of the tooth. This knowledge allows the dentist to extract teeth gently and without undue traumatic effect upon the supporting bone. It also should suggest the harmfulness of certain acquired habits such as tapping the teeth with a pencil or other hard object and forcing wire or rubber bands about the teeth. Any gentle force applied over a period of time steadily or intermittently will result in tooth movement, and in damage to the periodontal membrane and *alveolar bone*. The same effect can be produced by excessive masticatory force on individual teeth in malocclusion.

The alveolar bone supports the tooth and anchors it to the jaw. Unlike the dentin and enamel, it serves as a storehouse for calcific salts that are drawn upon by the rest of the body in time of need. It continually undergoes change. It must give way in advance of erupting teeth to allow for their emergence into the oral cavity. It must then be rebuilt in order to support the teeth as they erupt.

Teeth located side by side in the jaw and suspended independently of each other usually shift slowly toward the midline as they wear at their proximal areas of contact. This loss of tooth substance is compensated by a removal of the alveolar bone on the front side and a new deposition on the posterior side; thus the tooth migrates forward through the bone. Alveolar bone is readily affected by any disease that interferes with calcium metabolism.

The *gums* are the soft tissues that cover the alveolar bone and are continuous with the mucous membranes of the mouth, lips, and cheeks. Their blood supply comes from the vessels of the jaws and face. They respond to injury as do other mucous membranes of the body. A weak place in the anatomical arrangement of these tissues is the line of junction of the gum margin around the neck of the teeth. During eruption, the tooth moves through the gum until it emerges into the mouth. As it comes through, the tooth loses its intact epithelial covering.

The *gingival tissues* adapt closely to the necks of the teeth and form a working seal due to the strength of the connective tissue fibers in the edge of the gum. Covering epithelium lines the tooth sides of the gingiva for a short dis-

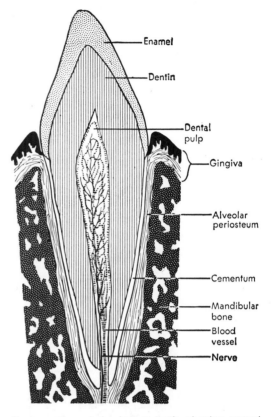

Cross section of the human tooth, showing enamel, dentin, and cementum which make up its mineral structure; and the living tissue pulp.

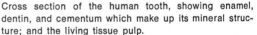

tance. As the mucous membranes secrete, tooth and gum are covered by mucoid substances that keep the surface slippery. These slimy secretions aid passage of foods during chewing and swallowing and help keep the mouth clean as they flow slowly from the tissues over the teeth and through the mouth into the throat.

Eruption

There are usually two sets of natural teeth. The first are called the baby teeth, or milk teeth, and are relatively small in size. The scientific name is *primary* or *deciduous teeth*. There are 20 teeth in the first set. Each tooth has a name that designates its position in the jaws and tells something of its form and function. The front tooth nearest the center of the mouth in the upper jaw is called an upper central incisor. It is shaped like a chisel and is used to incise food and other things. The tooth in the same relative position in the lower jaw is called the lower central incisor. As one goes back into the mouth of the child, one finds next the lateral incisor, then

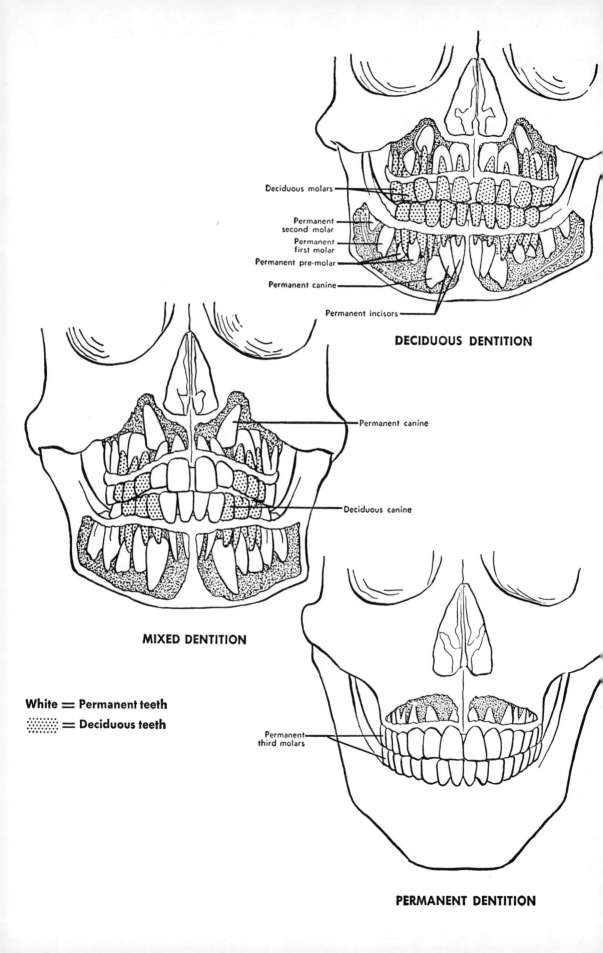

Deciduous molars

Permanent second molar

Permanent first molar

Permanent pre-molar

Permanent canine

Permanent incisors

DECIDUOUS DENTITION

Permanent canine

Deciduous canine

MIXED DENTITION

White = Permanent teeth

:::::: = Deciduous teeth

Permanent third molars

PERMANENT DENTITION

the cuspid or eye tooth, then the first and the second molars. The arrangement is the same in the upper and lower jaws and on the right and left sides.

The cuspids are strong sharp-pointed teeth, well-fitted for tearing food, while the molars are principally used for grinding. When the molars first appear in the mouth, their chewing surface has several cone-shaped eminences known as cusps. The deciduous first molars have four cusps. The deciduous second molars have either four or five cusps. All the teeth in the primary dentition are usually erupted and functioning by the time the child is about two years of age.

The second set of teeth is called the permanent or adult set. These are 32 teeth in an adult, 20 of which gradually replace the primary dentition, starting at about the age of seven and finishing at about 18 or later. In addition to the permanent central incisors, lateral incisors, and cuspids, there are first and second bicuspids which take the position of the first and second deciduous molars as they are shed. The bicuspids have two cusps, and are used for tearing and grinding. There are usually three molars in the permanent set; they are the first, second, and third molars. The third molar is the last tooth to erupt and is commonly called the wisdom tooth. The lower first permanent molar usually has five cusps; the others have four. This pattern may vary in the upper first molars which occasionally have five cusps also and in the third molars which frequently have more or less than four cusps. All incisor teeth have one root; bicuspids, one or two; and molars, two or more.

Since teeth begin to form in the embryo, long before birth, they are affected during their early development period by the health of the mother. Any severe metabolic upset of the mother can deform the teeth of the child, since they depend for their healthy growth on nutrients supplied by the mother's blood stream. Consequently, a correct diet with abundant vitamins and minerals is indicated. As calcium and phosphorus are the chief minerals concerned in the development of the teeth, these should be supplied by natural foods such as pure fresh milk, cheese, eggs, meat, green vegetables, and fresh fruits. If there is any indication of inability to assimilate enough vitamins and minerals, proprietary preparations may be advised as a dietary supplement.

A marked disturbance of the mother's health must be experienced before changes are seen in the teeth that form and calcify prior to birth. There seems to be a natural protective mechanism that takes necessary tooth ingredients from the mother's body and even from other parts of the baby in order to obtain a supply for the teeth.

The usual sequence in which the baby's teeth erupt is: central incisor, lateral incisor, first molar, cuspid, second molar. Lower teeth usu-ally erupt a month or so ahead of the upper ones. (See chart on p. 418 for usual age of occurrence.) It is essential for the health, happiness, and comfort of the child to maintain these primary teeth in their correct positions and free from dental disease. The necessity for professional dental supervision during this early and important growth period cannot be overemphasized. Brushing the teeth with a small, soft pure bristle brush should begin as soon as the incisors appear. At the age of three, the child should visit the dentist whether any dental service is needed or not. Prevention of dental diseases begins in early childhood.

Around the age of six, a permanent first molar erupts behind the last deciduous molar. It should serve the child for the rest of his life, for unlike the deciduous teeth, it has no successor. Of all the permanent teeth, this is one of the most important to maintain in position and is the most frequently lost. Its loss is primarily the result of neglect on the part of the child and disinterest on the part of the parents.

As the primary and permanent teeth erupt into the mouth, they assume positions that allow for an intermeshing of the cusps and incising edges of the lowers with those of the uppers. This arrangement is called *occlusion* and provides an efficient grinding apparatus during chewing, as the jaw moves up and down and sideways, as well as slightly forward and backward. Should this arrangement be disturbed during development of the child, he is said to have malocclusion; and the function of his teeth is impaired.

It is quite natural to think of the teeth individually. They should be thought of, however, as units in a chewing (*masticating*) machine. After the incisors have cut off a piece of food, the tongue passes it back to the broad-surfaced molar and bicuspid teeth for grinding. From the tip of each cusp a ridge with a pointed crest extends down to the central portion of the surface.

As the lower jaw moves, in chewing, from one side across to the other, the lower teeth are dragged, under pressure, across the upper teeth. When the teeth are properly placed in both jaws, the cusp ridges of lower teeth glide downward across the ridges of upper teeth; each cooperating upper and lower ridge serves as a pair of shears. Ideally, many pairs of "shears" operate simultaneously on both sides of the mouth, with two results: the food is effectively ground and prepared for digestion, and the force of chewing is equitably distributed to the posterior (bicuspid and molar) teeth. This equitable distribution of force, rather than excessive force on a few teeth and none on others, is important in maintaining the health of the bone through the years and in avoiding pyorrhea. Mastication is the first step in metabolism, the digestion, and utilization of food.

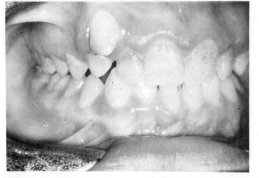

This picture illustrates a case of Class I malocclusion in a 12-year-old child. The permanent cuspid is abnormally placed.

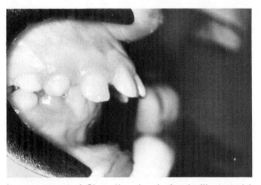

A severe case of Class II malocclusion is illustrated in this picture. This child's lower teeth bite into his palate.

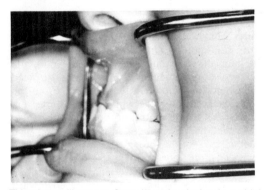

This picture illustrates Class III malocclusion in a child 4 years of age. The lower teeth protrude beyond the uppers.

Malocclusion

Irregularities in position and relation of teeth and arches may be found in both deciduous and permanent dentitions. Such disturbances fall in the general classifications of malocclusion and have led to the development of a specialty of dentistry known as *orthodontics*, which is concerned with the correction of such abnormalities. There are many causes of irregularity of teeth, dental arches, and jaws. One of these is heredity. Many authorities think the role played by heredity is small in comparison to acquired causes that have been shown to produce certain types of malocclusions. Another is mouth breathing, caused by blocked nasal passages, enlarged adenoids, severe allergies, or asthma. Acquired causes include early loss of deciduous or permanent teeth, prolonged retention of primary teeth, habits such as thumb or finger sucking, lip-biting, tongue thrusting, sleeping or leaning on one's hand and other practices which bring undue pressure on the upper teeth or jaws. These malocclusions frequently result in facial disfigurement, as well as greatly reducing chewing ability and contributing to subsequent gum disease.

It is important to correct malocclusion because the malposition of the jaws and teeth prevents correct chewing of food, which affects the general health and causes tooth decay. Irregular tooth position allows retention of food between the teeth causing bacterial growth. This in turn creates decay and gum disease, or *pyorrhea*. The disfiguring effects of malocclusion are usually of great psychological importance to the adolescent child.

Malocclusions are usually separated into three major classes according to the manner in which the teeth of the lower jaw (*mandible*) meet the teeth of the upper jaw (*maxilla*) when the patient bites or chews.

In the first class, there is a fairly normal position of the mandible in relation to the maxilla, resulting usually in a nice profile except where abnormal pressure habits, such as thumb-sucking, cause protruding upper front teeth. The malocclusion or disfigurement is caused by individual teeth or groups of teeth not being in correct position and functioning properly. Examples of this might be teeth in the maxilla or mandible that are widely spaced, rotated, crowded, overlapped or unerupted. Ocassionally, in contrast to protruding upper front teeth, these teeth erupt toward the tongue to such an extent that when the child bites, the upper teeth are locked inside the lower teeth. Children with these conditions should be placed under dental supervision as soon as the condition is noticed. Often, treatment is instituted early, while the teeth are still erupting; this eliminates a longer treatment later.

In the second class of malocclusion, the mandible and teeth are in a more backward position in relation to the maxilla. Patients of this group, in profile view, appear to have a deficient chin. The upper teeth may protrude so far forward that when the patient chews, the lower front teeth bite into the gum covering the palate. The lips are kept apart and in many instances the lower lip rests between the upper and lower teeth. The upper lip is frequently short. It is difficult for the child to bring his lips together

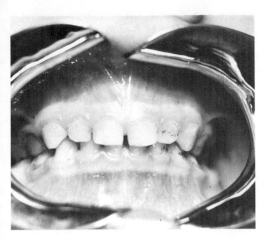

Normal occlusion of the deciduous teeth, in a child 3 years old, is illustrated here. Upper teeth extend beyond the lowers.

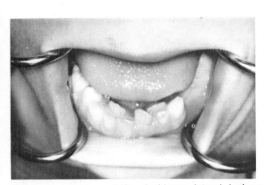

Prolonged retention of the deciduous lateral incisors forced the eruption of permanent teeth toward the tongue.

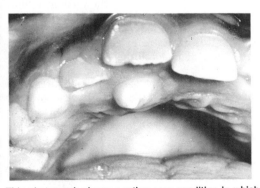

This photograph shows a rather rare condition in which an extra tooth erupts in the palate. The child is 9 years of age.

without straining. These children are usually mouth breathers and the palate is high, arched, and narrow. Thumb sucking and mouth breathing over an unduly long period of time are considered major causes of this disfiguring condition. Other patients in this group, however, possess such a muscular lip that the front teeth are not allowed to protrude but rather are forced to lean back toward the tongue, causing these upper teeth to almost cover the lower teeth when the mouth is closed. This is called a deep overbite. In these cases the palate is usually of good width and the patient breathes normally instead of through his mouth. The lower teeth may still bite into the palate, however, as described before. Failure of development of the lower jaw creates an appearance similar to those just mentioned and ofttimes underdevelopment of the mandible and malrelation of the mandibular teeth to the maxillary teeth exist together, causing quite a facial disfigurement.

In the third class, the mandibular bone and teeth are protruded in relationship to the upper arch and teeth. This class is just the opposite from the second class. When the individual closes his mouth, the lower teeth are located on the outside of the upper teeth. This holds true not only for the front teeth, but the back teeth as well. The profile of the face of a child with this type of malocclusion gives the appearance that the child is belligerent, angry, or pouting. The lower lip is forced out of position by the teeth, so that it overlaps the upper lip. The mandibular arch is usually oversized, while the maxillary arch is normal or undersized. The teeth in the upper arch may be crowded or bunched together, or may have fairly good alignment. Overgrowth of the lower jaw gives the same type of appearance but is associated with *acromegaly*, which is caused by dysfunction of the pituitary gland. (See Chapter 10, "The Endocrine System: *The pituitary*.")

The time required for orthodontic corrective treatment of patients with the second and third class malocclusion is usually longer than for those with the first class, but this does not always hold true. In many instances, the orthodontist will recommend that permanent teeth be removed from either the maxillary or mandibular arch, or both, to facilitate treatment and produce a more stable result. The length of time necessary for treatment of malocclusion is dependent upon its severity, the body response to treatment, and the cooperation of the patient in following the prescribed instructions. Children are often requested to wear elastic ligatures between the upper and lower teeth. Sometimes a head gear is made for the patient which helps to control the forces placed on the teeth.

When a patient with malocclusion is first seen, the orthodontist will make a thorough examina-

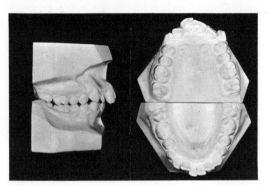

This photograph shows a side and occlusal view of models before orthodontic treatment was initiated.

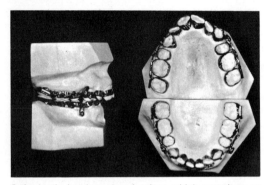

Orthodontic bands and arch wires, which constitute an orthodontic appliance. Treatment is about half completed.

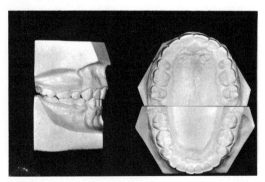

This photograph shows a side and an occlusal view of models after orthodontic treatment has been completed.

tion, including a complete mouth x-ray; he will compile the patient's medical and dental history; make plaster models of the teeth and gums; and possibly he will take face and tooth measurements which will be of value in analyzing the individual's condition. With these diagnostic aids, the orthodontist is then able to arrive at a treatment plan for the patient.

After an interview with the patient and the parent, in which all the conditions of the case and probable results have been discussed and understood, the treatment is started. Bands made of precious metals or stainless steel are made to fit many or all the teeth in the arch, and having been adapted, are cemented to the teeth with dental cement. This takes a great deal of time and patience on the part of both the patient and the orthodontist. Small, springy wires are fashioned and attached to these bands on the teeth. Slight force is exerted by these springy wires upon the teeth which have to be moved. Treatment must be gradual, since the force exerted is designed to change the bone surrounding the teeth, allowing the teeth to be moved through this changed bone and then permitting deposition of new bone around the tooth root in the new position.

Visits to the orthodontist must be made by the patients at intervals of two or three weeks after the plate is placed in the mouth. During the treatment, which lasts from twelve to 24 months, it is absolutely necessary that the patient maintain the highest possible degree of oral cleanliness. After the teeth have been moved to correct positions, the bands are removed from the teeth and the teeth cleaned of any remaining cement. A small acrylic plate known as a Hawley retainer is then fashioned to hold the teeth in the new positions. This retainer is worn for as long as a year or more, being removed by the patient only for eating and for cleaning the teeth.

Orthodontic treatment is not painful, although the patient may feel some discomfort for a day or two after an adjustment has been made. Many times it is not feasible to correct a malocclusion entirely during a specific period. Frequently, in the younger age groups the treatment is interrupted, bands are removed, and the child is allowed to develop and grow before the second phase of the treatment is started. The correct age at which to begin treatment must be determined by the orthodontist through careful mouth examination and study of the patient's history. It is advisable to place a child who has any degree of malocclusion under dental supervision as early as possible. The family dentist will refer the patient to an orthodontist if the condition warrants orthodontic consultation or treatment. Although children's teeth are the easiest to correct, adults can also benefit from orthodontics. Damage caused by malocclusion can be severe in an older person and can cause bone disease and loss of teeth. If at all possible, inconspicuous braces are used on adults.

In most cases, correction of malocclusion is accomplished completely by the orthodontist. Severe misplacement of the jaw, however, may require surgical correction. This can be performed best on adults who have stopped growing. In some cases, either the upper or the lower jaw can be reconstructed from inside the mouth, leaving no disfiguring scars. This is an advancement over older surgical methods which entered the jaw from outside the neck and ran the risk of damaging nerves and leaving scars.

The best treatment for malocclusion is prevention. Prevention is obtained when the deciduous dentition is maintained in a healthy state and when premature loss of teeth is avoided. Habits predisposing to tooth irregularity, such as finger sucking, should be interrupted as soon as possible. Little can be done, of course, about hereditary influences.

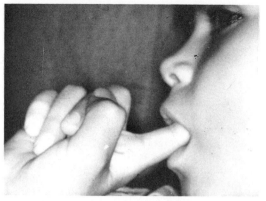
Finger sucking habit in a child, age 9.

Systemic disturbances

In rare instances there is a total or partial lack of deciduous or permanent teeth. In some cases, the condition is hereditary. It is often associated with other disturbances, such as dryness of the skin, partial baldness, and fingernail deficiency. Complete absence of teeth is referred to as *anodontia;* and partial anodontia signifies a partial lack. The cause of these conditions is not known. Some investigators believe it to be associated with endocrine disturbances, but little scientific evidence has been presented to support this view.

Supernumerary or extra teeth are rather common in both the deciduous and the permanent set. Such teeth may or may not resemble those found in the natural dentition. The cause of the condition is unknown. In some persons, the presence of these teeth goes undetected throughout life. Later in life, when artificial dentures are constructed, extra teeth may erupt, causing the patient to think another set of teeth is making its appearance. When these teeth closely resemble their neighbors and erupt into a functional position, they may go unnoticed until seen by the dentist. Some cases of fourth functional molars are reported, being fairly common in the American Indian.

Variations in time of eruption and slight variations in position are not unusual and should give little concern. Extreme divergence in eruption time may be associated with systemic disturbances. *Rickets* is well known as a cause of delayed eruption. Cretinism is also associated with a delay in the appearance of the teeth. Administration of thyroid hormone may be helpful in such cases.

The premature eruption of teeth has little significance except in the psychological sense. Many individuals believe that a baby born with teeth is apt to develop an undesirable personality; other persons consider this condition a good omen. The general custom of removing

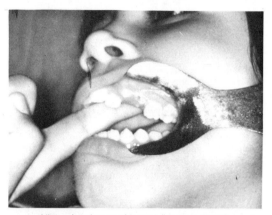
View showing position of finger in mouth.

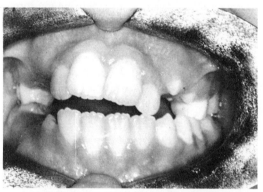
Malocclusion caused by finger sucking.

these teeth shortly following birth should be discouraged unless x-ray pictures are made to determine whether they are extra teeth or a part of the normal complement. If they are a part of the normal dentition, the mother should be encouraged to retain them in spite of some discomfort during breast feeding. In many countries it is the custom to breast feed babies long after all deciduous teeth are in place. This custom does not harm the mother or child.

Deciduous teeth sometimes are retained beyond normal shedding time. If the retention time is unduly prolonged, an x-ray examination should be made to determine whether permanent teeth are present. Delayed shedding of teeth, when the adult dentition is present, may be associated with rickets, cretinism, or a hereditary factor.

The two types of teeth that cause most anxiety during the eruptive process are the permanent cuspids and the third molars. The cuspid often emerges high on the outer surface of the gum and seems to protrude abnormally. This situation often disturbs parents; but if sufficient space is available for the tooth, it will assume correct position in a relatively short time. If space is not available for this tooth, as may occur when primary teeth are neglected, special orthodontic treatment may be indicated.

Third molars, or wisdom teeth, often fail to erupt properly. Partially or fully impacted third molars may cause crowding and subsequent malocclusion. If these molars, which grow slowly, erupt out of correct position and not in functional occlusion, disease of the surrounding gum may be started and the patient may suffer much discomfort. These circumstances have led to the loss of many third molars that might have been preserved as useful members of the masticatory mechanism. As these teeth may play a useful role following the loss of others, every effort should be made to preserve them as long as there is indication that they may be in a functional position following complete eruption.

Mottling, pitting, and discoloration of the enamel are disturbances caused during the formation of the teeth. Lack of complete calcification is known as *hypocalcification*. Lack of complete form is called *hypoplasia*. Rickets is one disorder that disfigures the appearance of the teeth. The hypoplasia that accompanies rickets results in stunted teeth, pitting of the enamel surface, and hypocalcification of that part of the tooth which is developing at the time of the disease.

White, mottled spots, and hypoplastic pits are also formed on individual teeth as the result of infection, trauma, or any localized disorder of the tooth-forming organ. This is in contrast to a disease state which affects all teeth forming at the time. Single lesions of the enamel seldom give trouble unless they serve as retentive areas for food debris which predispose to tooth decay.

Mottled enamel may be very disfiguring, since the white, opaque, hypocalcified areas eventually acquire a brown stain. These stains may be removed by treatment with drugs, or the tooth crown may be replaced. Mottling can also be caused by an excess of fluorine in water or food. A small amount of fluorine, in the form of sodium fluoride at one part per million parts of water, protects against tooth decay and does not produce disfigurement. A very great amount

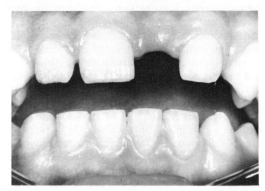

This child lost a front tooth in an accident. The space is gradually closing because of lack of a replacement.

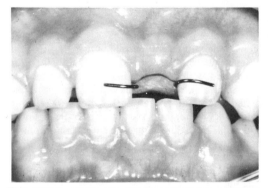

This picture shows the simple orthodontic appliance used to push the teeth apart and thereby regain the lost space.

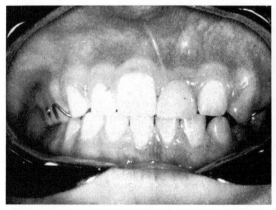

The temporary replacement shown here may be worn until the child is old enough for a permanent replacement.

of fluorine must be ingested before ill effects are seen.

Tetracycline antibiotics, administered for respiratory illnesses, can cause a peculiar yellowing of the teeth in young children and in babies whose mothers received the drug while pregnant. The discoloration usually covers only the primary teeth, and does not stain the permanent teeth. However, if the dosage is heavy or prolonged, damage can be done to the permanent anterior teeth of children, stunting the teeth's growth as well as discoloring them.

It is important that teeth function correctly, for the food should be mixed thoroughly with saliva during mastication. Digestion actually begins in the mouth. The saliva contains an enzyme, *ptyalin*, that acts upon starch and starts its breakdown. Thorough chewing of food is also of physiologic value, for the chewing motion and salivary secretion stimulate gastric secretion. Food, finely divided, is more readily acted upon and the minerals and vitamins more easily extracted.

DISORDERS OF THE TEETH: DENTAL CARIES

Dental caries or tooth decay is a microbial disease that attacks almost every individual. It begins early in life. Some children lose all their baby teeth by the time they are four years of age as a result of rampant tooth decay. This disease process attacks the hard tissues of the teeth, resulting in their decalcification and eventual destruction through loss of both organic and inorganic elements. The cause is not fully known.

Plaque formation

Dental caries is a process in which bacteria adhere to the tooth surface, especially in pits and other harbored areas, to form plaques. Plaque is made up of microbes that are able to attach to the teeth's surface because the bacteria secrete a sticky slime called *zooglea* (living glue). Plaque is also known as the microcosm, or "little world." The microcosm keeps out substances that might harm the bacteria. Water, mouthwash, and saliva have little ability to penetrate the sticky mass, but sugar and fermentable carbohydrates penetrate easily. These foods are sources of energy for the caries bacteria.

These bacteria with their enzymes are capable of acting on fermentable foods to form acids. When sugar or carbohydrates contact the plaque, acids are produced in one-half to one and a half minutes. They increase in concentration up to one-half hour or more. The acidity at the end of 30 minutes may be sufficient to dissolve enamel.

When acid concentration is sufficient to react with the inorganic salts of the tooth, there is partial decalcification of tooth substance. This produces a porous, opaque, white spot within the enamel substance. The process of acid formation and decalcification continues until all fermentable food is used and the acids are neutralized by saliva and minerals of the tooth substance. Decalcification stops when the acids are neutralized until more fermentable substance is brought into the plaque; then the cycle is repeated. Through food stains, the white, opaque, porous enamel may become light or dark brown. Organic material of the tooth is said to be destroyed by *proteolytic* bacteria normally present in the plaque.

Any condition that leads to the formation of a bacterial film upon the tooth's surface will predispose to dental caries if acid-producing bacteria are present. Such conditions are irregularity of tooth position, poor mouth hygiene, developmental defects (the hypoplastic pits that occur in a small percentage of individuals who have had severe rickets), excessive consumption of highly refined foodstuffs (white flour and sugar), between-meal eating, and the bedtime snack. When one eats at frequent intervals throughout the day, the cycle of acid production is reinitiated with each new ingestion of suitable food.

If it is not removed, plaque will flourish for weeks, months, or years to produce acid and demineralize the teeth whenever fermentable carbohydrates are eaten. Most people who appear to be resistant to dental caries can be shown to have very low intake of carbohydrates. Often these apparently resistant individuals become susceptible when they eat carbohydrates frequently. Those microbes dependent on carbohydrates then begin to grow and crowd out nonacid-producing bacteria. The microbes that produce acid are *acidogenic*. Those that can live in an acid medium are *acidophylic* organisms.

Any condition that diminishes salivary flow, thereby contributing to poor natural cleansing of the teeth and a diminished quantity of saliva in the mouth, will elevate the incidence of carious lesions. This has been observed frequently by the rapid production of decay in patients who have received radium or deep x-ray therapy for mouth cancer.

Treatment

The first sign of dental decay is a white spot in the enamel. The white spot occurs because some of the mineral has been removed by the acid and the light is refracted differently than off the sound enamel. As demineralization proceeds, an actual hole or *cavity* is produced. When a cavity forms, the area becomes more difficult to clean and the microbes flourish.

The most successful means of stopping a carious lesion is the use of *fillings* (restorations). These fillings, made of amalgams, cast gold inlays, and gold foil have served for years as effective agents for repair. When the diseased portion of the tooth is completely removed and the remaining tooth substance cleaned and prepared to receive a filling, the caries will usually be arrested.

Basically, the treatment of tooth decay consists of thorough removal of diseased tooth substance and a restoration of its anatomy. The aim of this is to restore the tooth's ability to chew food, and to seal the tooth as permanently as possible against further invasion by bacteria. Since some metal restorations are subject to shrinkage and expansion while others depend upon cement, which in time disintegrates in the mouth, this is an operation for which meticulous care is needed.

The remaining portion of the tooth that has not been restored is still susceptible to attacks by the disease. Recurrent caries near a filling may appear in the tooth. Mouth x-ray films taken at regular intervals are necessary for early diagnosis of tooth decay. It is especially important to have all decay eliminated as soon as it is detected.

If a cavity is not filled when it is small, decay progresses through the enamel and dentin of the tooth until the dental pulp is reached. At this time the patient experiences excruciating pain; there is no relief until the pulp dies or is removed, or the tooth is extracted. As the bacteria enter the pulpal tissue, they may be confined there or may enter the blood stream and invade other organs of the body. When they are localized within the pulp chamber, the condition is called a pulp abscess. Part of the pulp may be dead or necrotic while the remainder is still alive. This leads to intermittent toothache that may be hard to localize and is seldom relieved completely until the dentist is consulted. Treatment may consist of removal of the pulp and filling the pulp chamber and root canal, or removal of the tooth. (For other restorations, see p. 433.)

Should the infection proceed further along the canal into the root, with eventual death of all the pulp, an abscess or dead tissue may form around the apex of the root with the jawbone. This abscess, or *granuloma,* may cause the patient little trouble, or it may serve as a focus from which bacteria and their toxins are spread to other organs in the body. These germs are thought to be responsible for kidney or heart diseases. Some authorities believe they may also play a role in rheumatic disease. This source of dissemination of bacteria from one lesion to other parts of the body is called the focus of infection.

Whether for the purpose of preventing focal infection or preserving the teeth for mastication, the importance of minimizing tooth decay by preventive measures and arresting it by corrective measures cannot be overemphasized.

Prevention of tooth decay

There are three basic steps to prevent tooth decay: diet control, effective hygiene, and fluoridation.

The aim of dietary regulation for the improvement of dental health is to limit those foods which are high in starches and sugars. These foods may replace more valuable ones, and by their local action in the mouth, stimulate the growth of organisms associated with dental caries. A physician or dentist should be consulted before any dietary change is made. It is emphasized that dietary regulation is not "diet," but rather a way of eating which is probably different from the accustomed one. The foods to be limited are those containing large quantities of sugar and sometimes starch which tend to cause acid formation on tooth surfaces. Some foods, such as crackers or cookies, are objectionable because they lodge between and on the teeth and furnish material for acid formation for several hours. While ideally, from the standpoint of dental health, such foods might be completely eliminated from the diet, such a measure would be impractical for most persons,

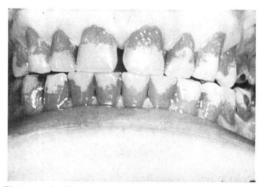

Photograph illustrating poor job of brushing teeth. Mercurochrome has been added to show plaque.

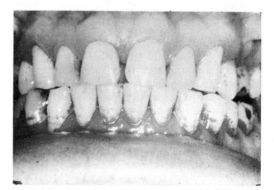

Good job of brushing teeth. The mercurochrome reveals that little plaque has been left on teeth.
Courtesy, Dr. S. S. Arnim, The University of Texas Dental Branch.

so that intelligent regulation of their amounts seems more desirable. The value of a piece of raw fruit or vegetable, such as celery, carrot, or apple, taken at the end of the meal is stressed. This stimulates salivary flow, partly cleanses tooth surfaces, and dislodges foods left in the mouth.

The following foods are desirable dietary materials, and from the point of view of controlling caries, should comprise the major part of the daily diet:

1 pint, preferably more, of milk—whole, skim, or buttermilk.
1 egg.
Vegetables, especially leafy greens and yellow ones. A raw one daily.
Potato—preferably cooked in the skin.
Butter or substitutes—enriched margarine.
Cream, cheese, other fats.
Meats, poultry, fish, liver.
Fresh fruits, or unsweetened fruit juices, fresh or canned without sugar.

By limiting the following foods in the diet, dental health will be improved, particularly when carious activity is severe:

Bread: limit to one or two slices per meal.
Biscuits: limit to one a day.
Cereals: limit to one serving a day—preferably cooked.
Hot Breads: limit to one piece.

The following list of items includes those that are thought to be the most effective in promoting dental caries, and should therefore be regulated most carefully, if it is impractical to omit them:

Sugars, syrups, molasses, jams, jellies, preserves, honey, candy, soft drinks, sundaes, ice cream, sherbet, milk shakes, sodas, cookies, crackers, cakes, pastries.
Fruits, canned or prepared with sugar.
Salad dressings containing sugar or starch.
Sweet pickles, ketchup, chili sauce.
Chewing gum.

Dental health may be promoted by substituting oranges, apples, and other fresh fruits or vegetables for the in-between snack that too often consists of candy, sweet carbonated beverages, cake, coffee with sugar and cream, and other similar acidogenic foods. Natural cheeses are recommended for in-between meals for children. Many of the "process" cheeses contain added sugar. Natural cheese contains minerals and vitamins as well as needed calories. Should all mothers feed their children vegetables, fruits, cheese, milk, nuts, and other similar items, instead of more refined substitutes, there would be a marked improvement in mouth health.

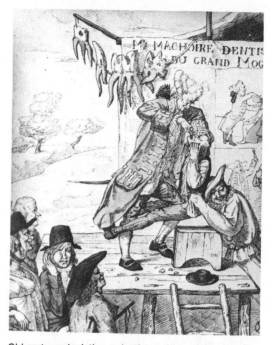

Old cartoon depicting a dentist at the work of extracting teeth "without effort." *Armed Forces Medical Library, Washington, D.C.*

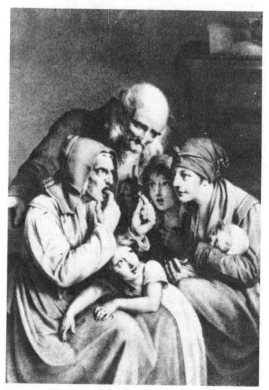

The Last Tooth. An early 19th Century lithograph by Boilly.

Dental hygiene

Another effective method of preventing tooth decay involves good *mouth hygiene*. In the past, this technique has been relatively ineffective because little was known about caries. First, the significance of the attachment of the dental plaque to the tooth in relatively thick, large masses was not realized. For hygiene to be effective, the bacterial plaque must be removed from the tooth before it has had an opportunity to develop a size and thickness capable of producing sufficient acid to dissolve the tooth. By removing plaque material from the tooth surface at least once a day, it is possible to eliminate one of the chief items in the production of more caries.

We are told by dentists, parents, teachers, radio, and television advertising that we should brush our teeth to avoid decay. We are also told to limit the carbohydrates in our diet to prevent dental caries. Yet, when we seem to practice these teachings, why do we continue to get cavities in our teeth? It is because even though people brush their teeth, it is rare to find a person who *really* cleans the microcosms from the surface of his teeth. Brushing but not really cleaning is a common practice.

It is also rare to find a person who uses or has been taught to use dental floss. A toothbrush will not reach those in-between surfaces of the teeth. This means that approximately one half of the teeth surfaces are not cleaned. It is in these uncleaned proximal surfaces of the teeth where cavities develop and where peridontal disease starts. These ideas are not new. The following was written by Dr. Levi S. Parmly, a New Orleans dentist, in 1819:

> "Young persons should be urged to keep their teeth very clean, and the daily use of a toothbrush, with water only, will in most cases be quite sufficient. In addition to the use of the brush, great advantages may be derived from the employment of waxed floss silk. In this way the impurities that cannot be reached with a brush are removed from between the teeth, and which, when permitted to remain, cause their decay. If it were possible to keep the teeth thoroughly and constantly clean, they would never decay."

Dr. Parmly did not know, writing a century and a half ago, that the impurities he spoke about were bacterial by-products, but he did know that this material which was not removed caused decay of the teeth.

To prevent dental disease, you should first visit your dentist. He can provide you with proper dental aids to help clean your teeth and teach you how to use them effectively.

How to brush: The toothbrush should have soft, rounded-end bristles, which are small in diameter so that plaque can be removed next to the gum that surrounds the tooth. The bristles should be directed *toward* the gum and tooth margin and moved slowly so that the bristle ends gently work between the tooth and gum. Hard, jagged bristles may harm the gums. Toddlers and very young children should be taught the brushing habit. A soft infant toothbrush and a careful rotary movement are all that are needed.

How to use floss: Unwaxed dental floss is used to clean the proximal surfaces between the teeth. Unwaxed floss is preferred because waxed floss may leave a waxey residue on the tooth, thus preventing fluoride to come in contact with the tooth. Also, waxed flosses are usually large in diameter and do not pass as easily under the gum margin as the smaller floss. The floss is gently passed between the teeth and underneath the edge of the gum. It is then held firmly against the tooth and passed toward the biting edge. Whether brushing or flossing, none of the procedures should cause pain.

How to use water sprays: Water sprays are used to irrigate the teeth and gums. They are beneficial aids that help remove loose food particles, bacteria, and bacterial irritants from the base of the teeth, braces, and bridges. Sprays flush out those particles loosened with the brush and floss. They should never be used with a forceful stream of water for it may damage the tissues. The water spray does *not* take the place of the brush or dental floss since sprays cannot remove the microcosm attached to the tooth surface.

Test of effective cleaning: After the teeth have been brushed, flossed, and sprayed, a "disclosing wafer" should be dissolved in the mouth. These wafers have a red stain that only colors the unremoved plaque. The clean tooth surface will not stain red. Remember that the microcosm is transparent and cannot be located unless it is stained. When stained, the microcosm can be seen and removed. By using the disclosing wafer, you can soon learn where the hard-to-clean areas are.

A second means of preventing dental caries with mouth hygiene is by removal of food before it has time to serve as a raw material for acid formation. This could be done by altering the order in which we consume foods, so that high carbohydrate foods are eaten before the proteinaceous and fatty ones. It is believed that such an order of eating would tend to eliminate most of the highly refined flour residue from about the teeth. Although many mothers may object, a child will suffer less from sweet desserts if he is allowed to eat them *before* his regular course. This is because the sugar does not remain long in the mouth since it is washed down by other foods. Thorough rinsing with water following eating is also helpful. (For further discussion of the diet, see Chapter 21, "Nutrition.")

Another specific recommendation to help clean the mouth following eating is the use of a small piece of paraffin wax as a substitute for sugar-sweetened chewing gum. Children love to chew. Ordinary paraffin, used to seal jams and jellies in home canning, is a good chewing cleanser. It tends to crumble if taken directly into the mouth when the weather is cold, but if held in the palm of the hand for a few moments until it becomes warm, it has a gumlike consistency. When chewed immediately after eating, it aids in cleansing the teeth and in stimulating salivary flow. This dilutes and washes away food residues from the tooth surfaces. Ammoniated, sugar-free chewing gums may be used for the same purpose.

Recommendations on mouth hygiene may be summarized by saying one should wash the teeth with brush and water immediately after eating sweet foods or foods made with white flour. At least once a day, carefully floss the in-between surfaces of the teeth (*approximal surfaces*).

Fluoridation

Dentists have learned, through many years of research, that when fluoride is added to drinking water, the teeth are stronger and more resistant to decay. Fluorine, in the form of sodium fluoride, may occur naturally in drinking water, but as a rule is present in inadequate amounts. More than 3000 communities in the United States now add fluoride to their drinking water in amounts of one part sodium fluoride to one million parts water. The amount varies slightly according to the average temperature of an area. In hotter climates, people drink more water so that the concentration of fluoride must be weaker. People in cold climates must have slightly stronger concentrations to compensate for the small amounts of water they drink. It has been conclusively demonstrated that the addition of the proper amount of sodium fluoride to drinking water reduces caries by as much as two-thirds. It is particularly useful during childhood and adolescence. Fluoridation also appears to prevent malocclusion due to decay of the back teeth. Those children who drink fluoridated water have fewer decays of their permanent molars, which determine the structure of the mouth.

In addition to drinking-water fluorides, teeth may also be painted by the dentist or dental hygienist with a fluoride solution. The teeth are first thoroughly cleaned of bacterial plaques, then blocked from the salivary flow by using cotton rolls; the fluoride solution is then daubed

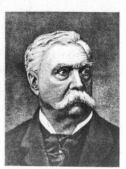

KINGSLEY, Norman W. (1829-1913) American dentist. Credited by many as being the founder of modern orthodontics, a branch of dentistry dealing with the repair of irregularities of the teeth. One of Kingsley's important contributions to dental orthopedics was a metallic splint with a plaster-bound headpiece, which was designed for the support of fractures of the maxilla. From Dr. H. Prinz: *Dental Chronology*, Copyright by Lea and Febiger, Inc., 1945.

on the teeth, where it is allowed to remain undisturbed for approximately five minutes. When teeth are so painted with fluoride solution, the enamel becomes slightly more resistant to acid action.

Fluorine substances have been incorporated in toothpastes and toothpowders as decay preventatives for adults as well as children. Stannous fluoride has been shown to be useful for this purpose by several clinical studies on relatively large numbers of people. The exact mechanism of the action is not completely understood. Significant reduction (as high as 90 percent) in the numbers of new cavities occurring in the teeth brushed with stannous fluoride has been reported by large studies conducted by the U.S. Army and Navy. While fluoride in drinking water mainly benefits children, fluoride applied directly to the teeth helps adults.

As knowledge concerning the mechanisms of dental caries becomes more comprehensive and exact, better methods for prevention of this disease will develop.

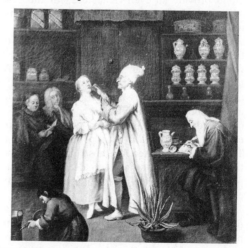

Reproduction of the old painting, The Tooth Extractor, by Longhi, showing the appearance of a dentist's office as it was several centuries ago.

DISORDERS OF THE GUMS: PYORRHEA

Even if a person is in that extremely small group of individuals that are caries immune, he still may not be free from dental disease and eventual loss of teeth. Pyorrhea is a serious disease of the gums that destroys the soft tissue and bones which support the teeth, causing the teeth to loosen, the gums to abscess, and the jawbone to waste away.

Pyorrhea is known by many names. *Periodontoclasia* is destruction of the tissues around the teeth. *Periodontitis* is inflammation of the tissues surrounding the teeth. Pyorrhea caused by systemic disease such as tuberculosis, diabetes, or endocrine imbalance is called *periodontosis*. The term *chronic marginal gingivitis* is used to describe the inflammation caused by debris and bacteria lodged at the margin of the gums.

Periodontal disease (*perio*—surrounding; *dontal*—tooth) is thought to be a disease of older people. But it is important to know that it often starts in children when the teeth erupt and may continue through several years until the teeth are lost.

Periodontal disease begins at the edge of the gum, an area that is often missed when teeth are cleaned. The microcosm produces toxic products that irritate the tissues, causing swelling and redness. These noxious products are absorbed by the gum, and in time the underlying connective tissue fibers are destroyed. This leaves the gum tissues weak. A space is formed between the edge of the gum and the tooth that is called a *periodontal pocket*. The pockets provide an ideal place for bacteria to grow and produce more destructive products which continue to destroy soft tissue and bone. Serum and blood provide an even richer diet for the germs at the gingival margin. This process continues until the teeth are lost.

The microbes that cause pyorrhea act differently than those that produce dental caries. Caries bacteria need an outside carbohydrate food source. But pyorrhea-causing agents live off nutrients in the tissue and are not dependent on the food we eat. Therefore, if we never ate carbohydrates, we probably would not have cavities, but we *could* have periodontal disease. This is demonstrated in those countries where there is little to eat and no dental care. Such people have few cavities, but periodontal disease is everywhere.

No specific organism causes pyorrhea. Many different kinds are found in the periodontal pocket, such as streptococci, actinomyces, leptotricia, staphylococci, spirochetes, and many others.

Danger: tartar

If plaque is not removed from the teeth, it soon serves as a matrix in which mineral salts of calcium and phosphorus are deposited forming a hard, cement-like, rough material called tartar *(calculus)*. Calculus can cause pyorrhea. It firmly affixes the injurious mass of bacteria to the tooth surface at the edge of the gum and also acts as a mechanical irritant. Each time that the gum is pushed against the hard rough mass during chewing or brushing, it abrades the soft tissue and bleeding results. Blood furnishes nourishment for the pyorrhea bacteria and the process continues.

As the periodontal membrane loses its attachment, the epithelial covering of the gum grows down along the root. The calculus is now found within the pocket between gum and root as well as at the gum margin. The patient may experience no symptoms as the teeth are slowly detached from the supporting bone by this disease.

Other factors that predispose to pyorrhea are, in general, any that injure the gum, such as early loss of teeth with resulting malocclusion, drifting, food impaction, excessive forces on individual teeth during chewing, grinding of teeth during sleep, and ill-fitting restorations. More important than all of these is the failure of the patient to remove the debris from the neck of the tooth at the gum margin at least once every day.

Treatment

Treatment for pyorrhea is effective if started early enough. With extensive bone loss and tooth drifting, however, there is little that can be done to keep the teeth in the mouth. It is often advisable to remove all teeth so affected before trying to save the remainder.

Those with adequate bony support are treated by the dentist with root *curettage*. This term means the removal of the tarter deposits from the roots with curettes designed to reach between the gum and the tooth. Once the debris is removed, the patient must keep the area clean by brushing, flossing, and rinsing at least once a day.

Treatment requires many appointments and much time. The dentist must gently search out deposits, curette them from the root surface, and wait several days to see whether small pieces still lie hidden beneath the gum, and if the signs of inflammation, redness, swelling, and pus formation still persist. In those areas where curettage is ineffective, the gum is removed to eliminate the pocket in which the organisms thrive.

Pyorrhea is easier to prevent than to cure.

Persons cannot prevent the formation of tartar at the necks of their teeth. With the best home care, it soon makes its appearance following eruption of the tooth. Effective prevention is the result of good teamwork between patient and dentist.

DISORDERS OF THE GUMS: VINCENT'S INFECTION

There is another dental disease which affects the gums and causes much distress. It is acute in character, appearing suddenly for no apparent reason. The common name is Vincent's infection, but it is also called ulceromembranous stomatitis, trench mouth, and acute necrotizing gingivitis. This disease is a painful inflammation of the margins of the gums which rapidly involves the deeper tissues. On occasion it may penetrate all the way to the underlying alveolar bone. As the condition progresses, a slough forms between the teeth and the ulcerated gum in that area. This entire gum tissue (interdental papilla) is soon destroyed. The ulcer and sloughing spread to the gum margin on the sides of the teeth and may involve the cheeks, lips, throat, and tongue.

Accompanying this ulceration, necrosis, and sloughing of tissue, there is a distinctive and peculiarly offensive odor. One can almost diagnose the disease from this characteristic odor. Bleeding is also a common and constant symptom. The slightest touch to the affected gum will lead to free and ready bleeding. Affected persons may experience a sense of deep depression, some fever, very painful gums, an increase in salivary flow, and possibly a metallic taste in the mouth.

A contributing cause of Vincent's disease is thought to be a lowered resistance on the part of the patient and an unhygienic local oral condition. There is not one specific organism responsible for the infection, but a complex of spirochetes, bacteroides, fusiforms, and diphtheroids. The predisposing factors include a general lack of mouth cleanliness; slow, difficult eruption of teeth with irritated gum flaps; ill-fitting dental restorations such as bridges, partial dentures, overhanging edges of fillings; and all systemic disturbances that lower resistance to disease.

Treatment

The condition may be eliminated easily within two or three weeks unless it has progressed so far that much tissue has been damaged. Therapy includes thorough cleaning and treatment by the dentist and careful hygienic measures by the patient at home. All the debris must be removed from the teeth by rinsing, brushing, and flossing gently. Deposits of calculus and other hard irritants must be removed by the dentist. Rinsing with one and one-half percent hydrogen peroxide aids in the treatment.

RESTORATIONS

Following the loss of one or more teeth as a result of caries or periodontal disease, the intelligent individual has them replaced with suitable restorations. These artificial teeth may be fixed to others in the mouth or they may be removable. A fixed restoration is usually called a *bridge*. It should be cleaned as carefully as the teeth to which it is fastened, for accumulation of food and bacteria upon its surfaces will lead to gum disease and decay of adjoining teeth. The cleaning is done with dental floss and a toothbrush. On occasion it is found necessary to thread the floss underneath the bridge in order to clean the restoration correctly.

Investigators in dental research are attempting new methods to replace lost teeth. Transplants of whole tooth and root are sometimes possible within the same mouth. Plastic implants are being tried to see if tissue will form around the base of the artificial tooth to hold it. These implants are put in place seconds after a tooth is pulled.

Restoration of the partial loss of one or more teeth is possible through *capping*. The damaged enamel is removed and a plastic or cement cap is fitted around the remaining stump.

If more than one tooth is lost, they are replaced by a removable restoration called a partial denture. Partial dentures may be fixed or removable. They are a necessary adjunct to the later years, for they make it possible to masticate food satisfactorily at a time when chewing food thoroughly has special significance. There is a tendency, on the part of people lacking several teeth, to eat only those foods that are soft and easily swallowed. This habit leads to nutritional disorders, to diet selections that promote digestive disturbances, and to the fostering of chronic disease.

When complete artificial dentures finally replace all the natural teeth, these problems become more acute. One is rarely able to masticate food with the same ease or dexterity with a "set of false teeth" as he could with those that nature provided. There are some exceptions to this statement. Certainly, complete dentures fill a great need for the toothless, since it is only through their use that food may be satisfactorily consumed. Dentures need frequent adjustment to compensate for the shrinkage of the gums and alveolar bone as time passes and occasionally they need refitting. The gum ridges, like the eyes and feet, change with time and use.

A well-fitting denture will cause no sore spots on the gums. It will remain relatively stable in the mouth during chewing and talking. It should be cleaned following eating and before retiring by washing thoroughly with water and a soft brush. Should it have a sharp edge or rough bumps, these should be rounded and polished by the dentist, for they can irritate the gums. Dentures aid in maintaining good health, and are a valuable safeguard against deficiency diseases in the aged.

13 THE DIGESTIVE SYSTEM

WHAT IT IS AND DOES

The digestive system is the group of organs that receive and absorb food into the body and eliminate the unabsorbed residue. Food may be of many types with widely different physical characteristics. It may be wet, dry, solid, or liquid, and consists of various chemical components. Before food can be used by the body, it must be acted upon both mechanically and chemically to convert it into forms which can be readily absorbed. The process of performing these mechanical and chemical changes is called *digestion.*

The simplest kind of digestive system, found in the lower animals, consists of a straight tube passing through the body from the anterior opening, or mouth, to the posterior opening, or anus. The human digestive system is of that general pattern, for it is a continuous tube with specialized parts. The successive parts of this tube are the *mouth, pharynx, esophagus, stomach, small intestine, large intestine,* and *anus.*

The linings of the intricate, convoluted tube comprising the digestive system perform mechanical and chemical actions on the food. They are equipped to absorb products of digestion and transmit them to adjacent blood and lymph vessels. The circulatory system, in turn, carries the food products to the near and distant body cells.

Several glandular organs open into the digestive tube. Some, the *salivary glands,* open into the mouth. Others, the *liver* and *pancreas,* open into the small intestine. Still others, *mucous glands,* provide lubrication for the passage of food and waste materials throughout the digestive tract.

The mouth

The mouth is bounded externally by the lips and cheeks, and is roofed by the *palate.* Within it lie the teeth and the greater part of the tongue. The space between the cheeks and teeth is called the vestibule. Normally, the cavity or the vestibule is obliterated by the lips and cheeks pressing against the teeth. A pair of the larger salivary glands, the *parotid glands,* open into the vestibule, one on each side.

The mouth cavity proper begins at the teeth or gums and is separated from the nasal cavity by the palate. The front two thirds of the palate are hard and bony; the back third is soft and muscular, and continues backwards into the pharynx. The soft palate is hinged on the hard palate, and it can be raised to meet the posterior wall of the pharynx; it does this every time food is swallowed, thus preventing the food from being pushed up behind the nose. In the middle of the back part of the palate is the *uvula,* a conical projection which points down to the tongue. This small organ operates the "gag reflex," which prevents over-large pieces of food from being swallowed. On either side of the soft palate in triangular recesses are the *tonsils,* which are masses of lymphoid tissue.

The muscular *tongue* lies in the floor of the mouth and curves backward to form part of the front wall of the pharynx. The movements of the tongue help in the chewing of food and in

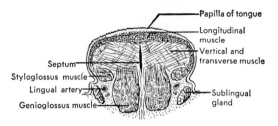

CROSS SECTION OF THE HUMAN TONGUE

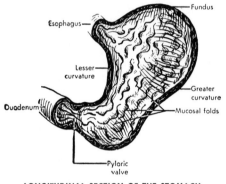

LONGITUDINAL SECTION OF THE STOMACH

PAROTID

SUBLINGUAL

SUBMAXILLARY

THE SALIVARY GLANDS

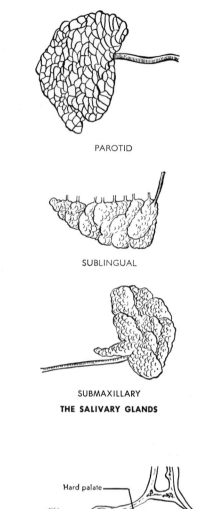

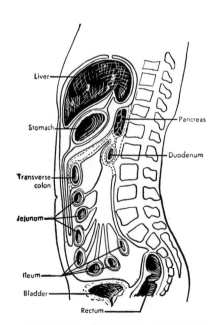

CROSS SECTION THROUGH THE HUMAN TRUNK

CROSS SECTION THROUGH PART OF THE HEAD

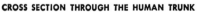

Details of the Digestive System

swallowing. Free tongue movement is essential for articulate speech. On the surface of the tongue are specialized organs for tasting (the taste buds), as well as multishaped projections (*papillae*) of the covering membrane. The caps of these papillae are constantly being shed and renewed. A diminished or excessive rate of shedding or renewal, together with the presence of various organisms (*bacteria*), are responsible for the altered appearance of the tongue that can be seen in certain diseases. However, the surface of the tongue does *not* reflect changes occurring on the lining membrane of the stomach.

Salivary glands

A clear watery fluid (*saliva*) is secreted into the mouth from three paired glands: the *parotid, submaxillary,* and *sublingual glands.* There are also numerous small salivary glands of the cheek and tongue. Saliva moistens the mouth, enables the food to be rolled into a plastic mass, and lubricates the food. It also enables a person to taste solid food, for the taste buds on the tongue are only stimulated by dissolved substances.

Saliva cleanses the mouth and prevents growth of bacteria by removing food particles which may act as culture media. Salivary secretion is decreased in fevers and the mouth soon becomes foul-tasting and must be cleansed by artificial means. Saliva also contains a ferment or enzyme, *ptyalin,* which slowly breaks down starch into the less complex, absorbable sugar, *maltose.*

The largest salivary gland is the parotid, which lies on the side of the face below and in front of the ear. The salivary secretions of the gland reach the mouth through a duct which runs inward through the fat of the cheek and opens on the inner surface of the cheek at the levels of the crown of the second molar tooth.

The saliva secreted by the parotid is thin and watery; secretion from the sublingual gland is thick and viscid, although the sublingual is the smallest of the main salivary glands. It rests immediately below the mucous membrane of the floor of the mouth, beneath the tongue. Its ducts open into the floor of the mouth through small conical elevations (*papillae*), which can be seen by the naked eye.

The submaxillary gland can produce either thick or thin saliva. It can be felt against the inside edge of the lower jaw. A long duct, about two inches in length, carries the saliva from the submaxillary gland to the floor of the mouth.

The secretion of the salivary glands is under control of the nervous system. Usually, secretion of the body's glands may be stimulated either by nerve impulses or by hormones, the nervous type of stimulation occurring when secretion is needed quickly. When rapid response is not essential, hormone stimulation is employed. A rapid response is obviously necessary for salivary glands, because food remains such a short time in the mouth; consequently, only nervous mechanisms stimulate their secretion.

Food, or even inedible material placed in the mouth causes a secretion of saliva within two or three seconds by stimulating nerve endings. This reflex is called an *unconditioned* or inherent reflex. The type of saliva secreted—either watery or viscous—depends on the type of substance initiating the reflex. A dry biscuit produces a thin watery saliva, while a piece of meat causes a highly viscous saliva which lubricates the meat and enables it to be swallowed easily.

When saliva is produced as a result of stimulation of nerves not in the mouth—for instance, from the smell or sight of food—then the reflex is said to be *conditioned.* A conditioned reflex is one in which training and experience are the basis of the reflex process.

The pharynx and esophagus

The pharynx is the vertical passage beginning behind the nose and mouth and extending from the base of the skull above to the esophagus below. The pharynx is equipped with three semicircular muscles located one under the other which enable the pharynx to squeeze food down toward the esophagus.

One of the most muscular parts of the digestive system is the esophagus. It is a flattened tube passing through the lower part of the neck, the whole length of the chest, and joining the stomach just below the diaphragm. The esophagus is ten to twelve inches in length in the adult. Normally, the entrance into the stomach is kept closed by a muscular contraction in the lower inch or so of the esophagus, which opens as a piece of food approaches, but prevents reflux of acid from the stomach to the esophagus.

The stomach

The stomach is a receptacle in which food accumulates. Some of the earlier processes of digestion take place here, namely, the conversion of food into a viscous fluid. The normal stomach is J-shaped, with a bulge above and to the left of the junction with the esophagus. The shape varies according to whether the person is standing, sitting, or lying down; and according to whether the stomach is full or empty. The stomach lies in the upper left portion of the abdomen, its long axis being nearly horizontal. The inner curved edge of the stomach is called the *lesser curvature,* and the outer, longer curved edge is the *greater curvature.*

The stomach narrows to join the small intestine forming a canal (the *pyloric canal*), which has a thick muscular valve (the *pyloric sphincter*). This sphincter remains closed so long as the food in the stomach is solid. The pyloric sphincter relaxes only when the gastric contents have been changed into a semifluid state. If only liquids are taken into the stomach, the pylorus opens and the fluid passes into the small intestine almost immediately. Usually it takes from three to four and one-half hours before the stomach completely empties a meal into the small intestine.

Minute glands in the stomach manufacture hydrochloric acid and certain ferments which break down portions of the food into simpler substances. The muscular coats of the stomach grind and mix the food with the stomach secretions. The physical grinding and crushing is of great importance to normal digestion.

The bowels

Intestines, the portions of the digestive system from the stomach to the anus, are divided into two main parts, the *small intestine* and the *large intestine*. The small intestine begins at the pyloric sphincter and lies in the abdomen in coiled loops; it is 20 to 22 feet long. Thus, the small intestine occupies the greater portion of the abdominal cavity. It gradually diminishes in size as it extends downward, having a diameter of about two inches where it joins the stomach, and about an inch where it joins the large intestine. The first portion of the small bowel is called the *duodenum*, which is about eight to ten inches in length. The duodenum differs from the remainder of the small bowel in that it is fixed to the posterior abdominal wall. The ducts of the liver and pancreas open into the duode-

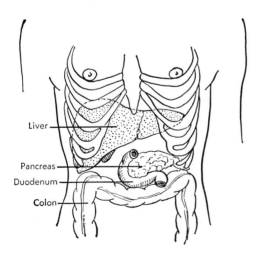

Part of the liver may lie within the ribs, although it is separated from the chest cavity by the diaphragm. The pancreas and duodenum are lower.

num. The remaining small intestine is divided into the *jejunum* and the *ileum,* the upper eight feet being regarded as jejunum and the lower twelve feet as ileum. The coils of the small intestine are able to move about freely in the abdominal cavity, being connected to the posterior abdominal wall by a fan-shaped sheet of tissue (the *mesentery),* which measures about 20 feet at its free edge and only five or seven inches at the attachment to the abdomen. The blood vessels, lymph vessels, and nerves serving the intestine lie between the layers of this sheet of tissue.

Digestion proceeds to its completion in the small intestine. By means of excretions of pancreatic juice from the pancreas and *bile* from the liver, together with juices secreted by the intestine itself, the splitting of proteins and digestion of carbohydrates and fats are accomplished. These secretions are alkaline in comparison to the acid secretion in the stomach.

The piece of food *(bolus)* travels along the small intestine in a series of rushes; the bowel contracts just behind the bolus and relaxes in front of it. This contraction and relaxation occurs in a series of alternating wavelike motions along the small intestine for a variable distance. In addition to this *peristaltic* movement, which conveys the food through the intestine, there are also regular constricting movements of the intestine. These occur at a rate of 20 to 30 a minute, kneading the food thoroughly and insuring that the digestive juices are well mixed with it. These latter movements do not propel the food onward through the bowel; they merely exert a churning action.

The small intestine opens obliquely into the large intestine. A valve (*ileocecal valve*) is located at the junction. This valve permits the passage of the contents of the small intestine into the large intestine, at intervals. It also prevents the return of material into the ileum.

The large intestine begins on the right side of the abdomen just above the rim of the pelvis, and is about five feet long. Arranged in an inverted horseshoe shape around the small intestine and about three inches in diameter at its commencement, the large intestine gradually narrows to the anus.

The large intestine is divided, for purposes of description, into the following parts: the *cecum* and *vermiform appendix*, the *ascending colon, right flexure* of the colon, *transverse colon, left flexure, descending colon, sigmoid colon, rectum,* and *anal canal.* That portion of the large bowel which hangs below the opening of the ileocecal valve is called the cecum; it is a blind sac to which is attached a wormlike tube, the vermiform appendix. The appendix is usually about three inches long, but may be as long as nine inches or shorter than one inch. As an adult

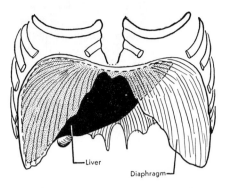

The location of the human liver. It is beneath and in close approximation to the diaphragm.

gets older, the lumen of the appendix gradually gets narrower.

The nearly fluid contents of the ileum pass through the ileocecal valve and collect in the cecum. Slowly the contents are forced up into the ascending colon. Movement through the large intestine is slow and takes place in periodic rushes, like the peristaltic rushes of the small bowel. This movement, which is actually a series of peristaltic waves, occurs only at long intervals—probably about every eight hours. It may occur immediately after the entry of food into the stomach (the *gastrocolic reflex*). Also, the desire to have a bowel movement, so commonly experienced after breakfast, is the result of this reflex. Mental disturbances may generate the reflex, for some people desire to defecate if they get nervous and upset.

In order to reach the outside of the body, it is necessary for the large bowel to penetrate the floor of the pelvis. At this juncture, the large bowel is enclosed by two muscles, the internal and external *sphincters,* which compress the sides of the tube and reduce its cavity to a narrow passage. That part of the large intestine immediately preceding the muscles is termed the *rectum.* The terminal portion of the passage, from the rectum to the external opening or *anus,* is called the *anal canal.* The sphincters remain closed most of the time, but are opened when the person defecates. These muscles are voluntary muscles.

The waste material of digestion deposited in the rectum is known as *feces* or *fecal* matter. Most of the time the rectum is empty. Then, when the colon becomes full, the fecal matter passes into the rectum. The desire to defecate is a reflex initiated by pressure on the walls of the rectum by the feces.

Absorption of food is effected almost entirely in the small intestine, and the waste material that passes into the large intestine consists of nonabsorbable matter and inorganic salts mixed with water. The large intestine secretes some ma-terial and absorbs water, so that the amount of material finally excreted is only about one third of the weight of material entering. Most of the absorption of fluid takes place in the cecum and ascending colon, with smaller amounts being absorbed as the material progresses through the ascending, transverse, and descending colon and the rectum.

The solid matter finally excreted is feces. The fat, protein, and carbohydrate of the food is nearly all absorbed, and only the cellulose framework of vegetables and fruits remains unabsorbed. The color and odor of the feces are caused by the action of bacteria, which inhabit the large bowel, and by the pigments present in bile. During starvation, feces continue to be formed from bile, which is emptied into the digestive tract from the liver, and from bacteria and other secretions from the bowel itself.

The anatomy of the gut

The structure of all the parts of the long tube forming the digestive tract, the *alimentary canal,* generally conforms to the same plan. From the inner surface of the tube outward there are four layers of tissue—*mucous, submucous, muscular,* and *serous.* Each layer has a specialized function.

The mucous coat contains numerous tiny glands which secrete digestive juices.

The submucous coat consists of loosely arranged but strong and elastic tissue, which enables the other tissue layers to slide freely over one another. The submucous coat also furnishes a bed in which the blood vessels and nerves form branches before entering the mucous coat. Masses of lymphoid tissue are scattered throughout the mucous and submucous coats of the small intestine, especially in the jejunum and ileum. These aggregations are known as *Peyer's patches* and are from one to three inches long and about one inch wide. They are connected by lymph vessels which drain away milky-looking, fatty fluid *(chyle)* from the intestine during digestion.

The muscular coat of the alimentary canal is in two layers (three in the stomach). The muscle fibers of the inner layer are arranged in a circular pattern around the canal, while those of the outer layer are arranged longitudinally. There is an inner oblique layer of muscle between these coats in the stomach. The muscle layers are responsible for the churning and peristaltic movements.

The serous layer of the tube is formed of a tough membrane *(peritoneum)* and comprises a complete or partial covering in different parts of the tract. The peritoneum has two separate layers forming a closed sac. One of the layers covers the wall of the abdominal cavity *(parietal* peritoneum), and the other covers the organs of the abdomen *(visceral* peritoneum).

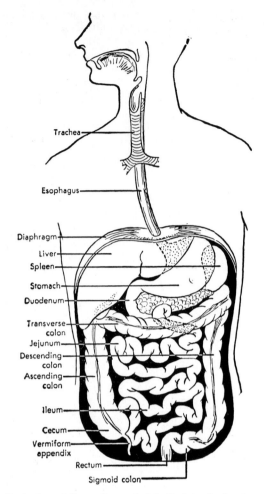

Illustration of the entire gastrointestinal tract, showing the relative positions of the various parts of this long tube and the organs connected to it.

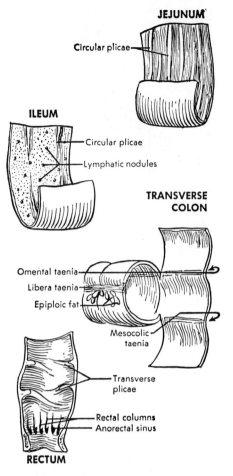

These drawings show the appearance of the inner and outer walls of segments of the gastrointestinal tract and their distinctive folds or plicae.

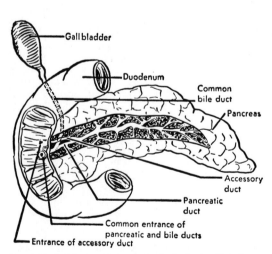

Drawing showing arrangement of ducts leading from the pancreas and gallbladder, through which bile and pancreatic juices flow into duodenum.

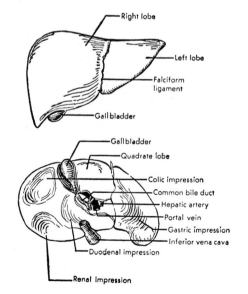

Detailed drawing of the human liver with its parts labeled. Depressions in its surface allow it to fit snugly among the other organs of the abdomen.

DETAILS OF THE DIGESTIVE SYSTEM

A Modern Operating Room and Its Staff

● THIS OUTLINE DRAWING shows the most important details in the composition of a modern surgical operating room. On the succeeding two pages there is a full color photograph of this same scene, the details of which may be identified by the numbers shown on the outline drawing. *(1)* is the head surgeon at the operating table, across from his first assistant, *(2)* and beside his second assistant, *(3)*. *(4)* is the instrument nurse; *(5)*, the anesthetist; and *(6)* a nurse who moves about the room as needed. Patient is on the operating table, *(7)*. *(8)* is the instrument table on which all required instruments are arranged in an orderly fashion so that they may be rapidly passed by the instrument nurse to the surgeon. *(9)* is the anesthetic machine which provides the controls by which the anesthesia may be accurately adjusted. *(10)* is a suture table, and *(11)* a large operating light that gives good illumination to the field of the operation. The arrangement of the personnel permits them to operate as a team with speed and proficiency and eliminates every possibility of lost time and motion. The well trained surgical team can therefore perform a complex major operation in a relatively short period of time with a minimum of danger to the patient. *Photograph by Courtesy of Hermann Hospital, Houston, Texas. R. A. Kolvoord, photographer.*

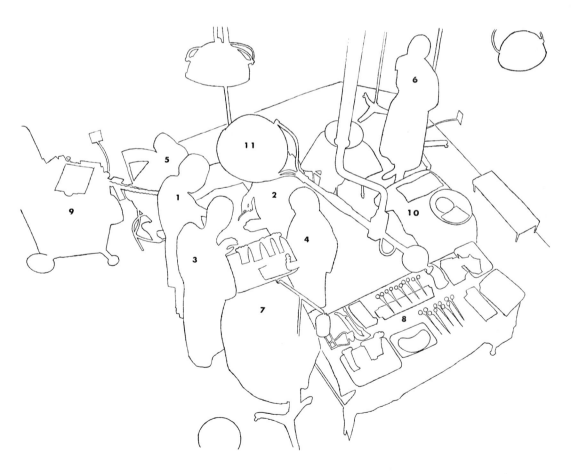

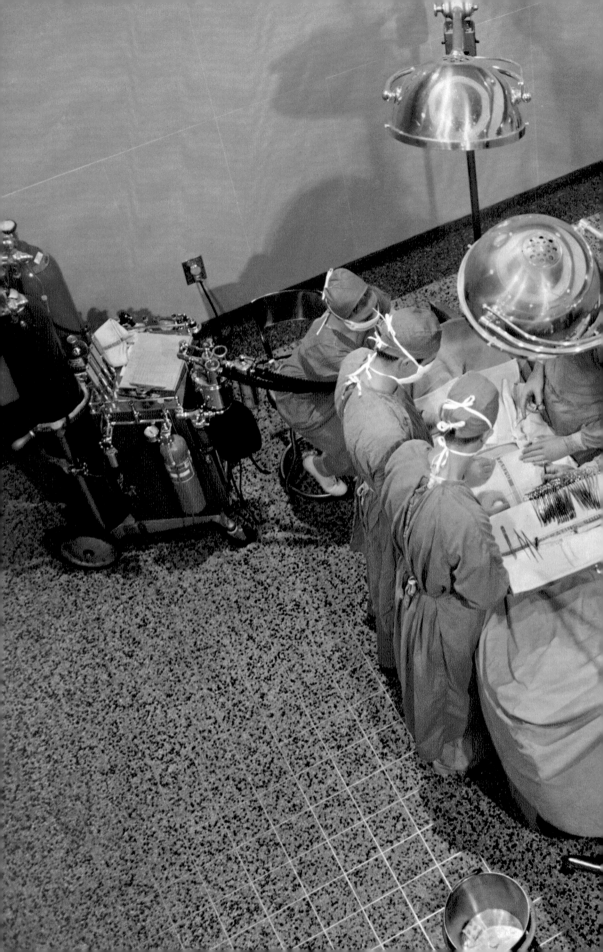

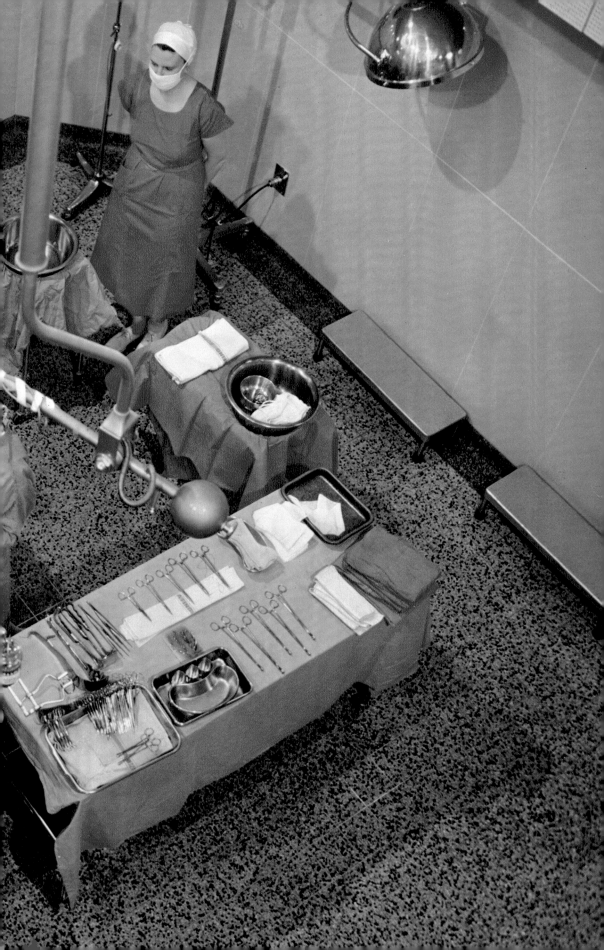

X-ray is a Valuable Aid in Diagnosis and Treatment

● THE DISCOVERY OF THE X-RAY by Roentgen in 1895 heralded the advent of a new era in medicine, for the first time making it possible for the physician to see the outline of areas on the inside of the body. Subsequent developments in radiology have made the use of x-rays in diagnosis and therapy one of the most skilled specialities of medicine. Early workers, unaware of the effects of large doses of radiation on tissues, often became martyrs to their field. More recently, however, these effects of radiation have been put to use in the treatment of patients suffering from a variety of infectious diseases and from cancer. The accompanying photographs show some of the details of the routine activities of the radiology department of a hospital. *Courtesy Hermann Hospital, Houston. Photography by Bob Sallee.*

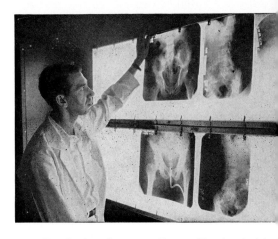

Examination of an x-ray film provides the physician with information regarding the internal body structure.

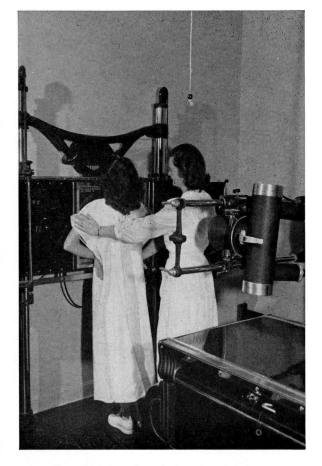

For a chest x-ray, the patient stands against the x-ray machine with her head and arms in the position shown.

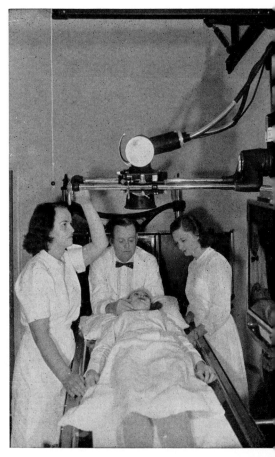

X-ray machine in use. Source of radiation is above patient. Machine can be raised or lowered as needed.

The peritoneal cavity

The cavity lined by the peritoneum is known as the *peritoneal cavity*. The intestines and other abdominal organs do not lie within the peritoneal cavity. They are covered over by peritoneum and thus are external to it. The peritoneal cavity, then, is empty. The peritoneum produces sufficient moisture to lubricate its surface; therefore, the stomach and intestines are free to move with little friction. Infections of the peritoneum *(peritonitis)* caused many postoperative deaths before the introduction of modern drugs.

The peritoneum also forms the external covering of the mesentery, the sheet of tissue which binds the intestines to the posterior abdominal wall and provides their blood, nerve, and lymph supply.

The liver

The liver is a large glandular organ, weighing nearly four pounds, which occupies the upper portion of the abdominal cavity, mainly on the right side immediately underneath the diaphragm. It produces a yellowish-green or brown fluid of bitter taste called *bile,* which is conveyed from the liver by two ducts (the *hepatic ducts).* The ducts unite to form a common bile duct, which eventually opens into the duodenum. Connected with the bile duct is a pear-shaped sac, the *gallbladder,* which serves as a reservoir for the bile.

The chief components of bile are *bile salts* and *bile pigments.* Bile is strongly alkaline in reaction and thus neutralizes the acid coming into the duodenum from the stomach. The bile not only performs important functions in the process of digestion, but also serves as a vehicle for the excretion of waste products from the body.

Bile salts help in the breakdown of fat in the intestines and in fat absorption through the intestinal wall. The bile salts are injected into the digestive canal at the duodenum. They are not excreted, but are almost totally absorbed through the walls of the intestine, to be used over and over again. Bile pigments are derived from the hemoglobin of broken-down red blood cells and are excreted with the feces. When the pigments appear in excessive amounts in the blood, the mucous membranes and conjunctiva of the eye become stained a pale yellow, and the patient is said to be *jaundiced.*

Bile is continually secreted by the liver and stored in the gallbladder. Here the bile is concentrated by the absorption of water through the walls of the gallbladder. It is released from the gallbladder into the intestine when food passes through the pyloric valve from the stomach into the small intestine. *Gallstones* are formed of constituents of the bile which have settled out of solution. The stones vary in size, color, and structure according to the materials composing them.

Besides producing the bile, the liver is the site of many other important biochemical reactions and has been compared to a chemical factory. Proteins are synthesized by this organ. Iron and copper are stored there; the body's surplus of sugar is kept in the liver; *fibrinogen,* the material necessary for the clotting of blood, is made there; vitamin A is formed there; poisonous substances are detoxified and by a similar process many hormones are neutralized when no longer needed.

The pancreas

The pancreas is a long, soft, yellowish-grey gland which lies transversely on the posterior abdominal wall, its right end enclosed by the curve of the duodenum and its left end touching the spleen. It lies for the most part behind the stomach. The pancreas is about six inches long, and weighs about three ounces. The gland secretes a clear, watery, alkaline fluid (the *pancreatic juice),* which passes to the duodenum through the *pancreatic duct.* Pancreatic juice is one of the chief chemical agents in digestion, for it contains enzymes that break down starch into sugar, fats into glycerine and fatty acids, and proteins into peptones and amino acids. In addition to the pancreatic juice which is excreted into the duodenum, the pancreas also secretes directly into the blood stream the antidiabetic hormone, *insulin.* This aspect of pancreatic function is further discussed in Chapter 10, "The Endocrine System: *The Pancreas."* A sufficient quantity of food can be digested by the intestine to maintain life for an indefinite period, without the presence of pancreatic juice. However, death occurs if the pancreas is completely destroyed or removed surgically, unless insulin is supplied artificially. Thus, patients who must have the pancreas removed are able to live only so long as they receive injections of insulin.

WILLIS, Thomas (1621-1675) English anatomist and physician. Presented the first, though crude, demonstration of the chemical nature of diabetes mellitus by describing the sweetness of the urine, from which he isolated a crystalline mass similar to grape sugar. His *Cerebri Anatome* (1664) was the best account of the nervous system then in existence. The spinal accessory nerve and the arterial "circle of Willis" have both been named after him.

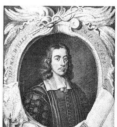

Pancreatic juice flows into the intestine when acid material comes into contact with the duodenal mucosa. A hormone, *secretin,* is liberated from the mucous coat of the duodenum by any acid substance coming in contact with it. This hormone enters the blood stream and is conveyed to the pancreas in a few seconds. There it stimulates the glandular cells to produce pancreatic juice. There is also nervous control of pancreatic secretion, so that even the thought of food may stimulate its secretion.

The act of swallowing

When food is taken into the mouth, it is chewed until much of it is finely divided, and then swallowed. It is thoroughly mixed with saliva while being chewed, and the ferment, ptyalin, begins to break down the starch into sugar. The act of swallowing consists of three parts; first the food, pounded into a soft ball, is placed on the back of the tongue and then the tongue is quickly pressed against the hard palate, projecting the bolus into the pharynx. This is the only voluntary part of swallowing; all the other muscular movements concerned in moving the food into the stomach are reflexes and not under the control of the will.

There are three possible pathways for food when it enters the pharynx—it can go forward and upward into the nose, forward and downward into the trachea and lungs, or downward into the esophagus. The tongue pushed against the palate prevents food from coming back into the mouth. The soft palate rises and meets the posterior pharyngeal wall, thus blocking entry of food into the nose. Food is prevented from going into the lungs because the larynx is raised and the vocal cords closed during swallowing, and the epiglottis at the base of the tongue projects backward over the larynx. This movement has the effect of opening the upper end of the esophagus; so the bolus takes the path of least resistance and enters the gullet. Once in the esophagus, the food quickly travels down into the stomach, being moved by a wave of contraction preceded by an area of relaxation *(peristaltic wave).* The whole process of swallowing takes about six or seven seconds.

The chemical process of digestion

The stomach expands to contain the meal, and churns it into a semifluid consistency. The gastric juice secreted by the glands in the stomach wall is acid in nature, because the acid-secreting cells *(oxyntic cells)* of the stomach produce a weak solution of *hydrochloric acid.* The acid is necessary to provide the optimum conditions for the protein-splitting enzyme *(pepsin)* to work, and it destroys many kinds of bacteria clinging to the food. Pepsin is also secreted by specialized cells *(zymogenic cells)* in the mucous coat of the stomach. The acid gastric juice is produced continuously, even during sleep. However, it is produced more abundantly when food is placed in the mouth. Food is better digested when it is agreeably flavored and pleasant to look at. If food *looks* unattractive, there may well be a decrease in the secretion of gastric juice. In fact, there is evidence that the activity of the stomach is regulated by a hormone released from the brain and carried to the stomach via the blood stream.

In the stomach, then, much of the protein is reduced to simpler soluble substances by hydrochloric acid and pepsin. The fat and starch are macerated and suspended in solution. Simple sugars taken with the food pass readily into solution. The semifluid mass in the stomach passes through the pyloric valve into the small intestine, there to undergo further processes of digestion.

When the partially digested food passes into the duodenum from the stomach, the mere contact of the material with the intestinal wall sets off a reflex which stimulates secretion of intestinal juice, pancreatic juice, and bile. Besides the nervous reflex controlling the secretion of intestinal juice, there is probably also a hormonal control.

Intestinal juice *(succus entericus)* is derived from the innumerable glands scattered diffusely over the mucous lining of the small intestine. This juice is alkaline in reaction, and neutralizes the acid secretions carried over from the stomach. Its alkalinity is caused by the presence of *sodium carbonate* and *sodium bicarbonate.* The intestinal juice also contains ferments to break down the various sugars—cane sugar, milk sugar, and malt sugar—a small amount of starch ferment, and some fat ferment. It also contains a substance necessary to activate pancreatic juice, which in turn contains powerful ferments of protein, fat, and carbohydrate. The pancreatic juice breaks down the raw food substances into simpler materials; and the intestinal juice breaks down the products of pancreatic digestion still further into more readily absorbable substances.

The intestinal juice is alkaline in reaction and the various ferments act efficiently only in an alkaline medium; their digestive power is destroyed in the presence of acid material.

Bacteria, which are normally present in the intestines, play an important role in digestion. Their constant chemical activities aid in breaking down large food molecules into smaller chemicals suitable for absorption into the body. They also produce certain chemicals, especially vitamins, which are required by the body, but may not be supplied in sufficient quantity by the average diet. Bacteria become established in the intestines shortly after birth. In the adult, approximately 50 percent of the stool is bacteria.

The absorption of food occurs almost exclusively in the small intestine. The intestine is the first line of defense against any injurious substances entering the body through the digestive tract. Water, glucose, and other materials are absorbed in negligible quantities through the stomach wall. Alcohol, however, is absorbed in the stomach. Consequently, intoxication occurs quickly when the stomach is empty.

The absorbing units in the small intestine are small, finger-like processes (villi) which occur in the mucous coat. Each villus contains a tiny blood vessel and a lymph vessel. Because the mucous coat of the intestine is arranged in folds, the total absorbing area is about 90 square feet.

Amino acids, which are the products of the digestion of proteins, and glucose are absorbed into the blood stream through the capillary loops of the villi. Fat is mainly absorbed by the lymph vessels.

No chemical process of digestion occurs in the large intestine, and only water and glucose and certain salts (electrolytes) can diffuse through its wall. The secretion of the large intestine is mucus, which lubricates the feces in their passage to the exterior. The complete passage of food through the digestive tract usually takes 24 to 48 hours.

Bacteria are present in great numbers in both the small and large intestine. Normally the bacteria of the former are quite different from those of the latter, and they feed on carbohydrate-producing organic acids, such as are found in vinegar. So long as adequate amounts of carbohydrate are taken in the food, the acid-producing organisms flourish and prevent the entry of bacteria from the large bowel. In young children, however, the acid-producing bacteria may diminish in numbers, and then bacteria from the large intestine invade the small bowel, causing vomiting and diarrhea.

The intestines are insensitive to such stimuli as would readily cause pain in the skin or superficial tissues. Yet pain is a common symptom of disease of the digestive tract. It is generally believed, although definite proof is still lacking,

that pain of this type arises from two conditions. Excessive contraction of the bowel, which causes distention of itself or a neighboring organ, causes pain. Pain also occurs if the bowel becomes obstructed by a hernia, twisted on itself (volvulus), or blocked by a mass of feces or by a growth. If the contraction is not powerful, then nausea only may be experienced.

Hunger is the result of the peristaltic contractions occurring in an empty stomach. This sensation originates in the stomach, because it may occur when the intestines are filled with unabsorbed food. Hunger and appetite are not synonymous. Appetite is the complex craving for food which is developed by past enjoyment of savory food and probably is related to the state of elasticity of the stomach wall.

Thirst is a sensation probably caused by the drying of the walls of the pharynx. As long as the water content of the body is satisfactory, the salivary glands keep the pharynx moist. If the water content falls, the secretion of the salivary glands is depressed, and the consequent drying of the mucous membrane of the pharynx produces the typical sensation of thirst.

DISORDERS OF THE MOUTH

The mouth is the first segment of the digestive tract and is also in close relation to the respiratory system. Its development is influenced by hereditary and constitutional factors. The mouth contains an important organ of speech, the tongue. Further, the mouth prepares food for swallowing by grinding the food between the teeth and moistening it with the saliva.

Nutrition, metabolism, and endocrine imbalance affect the mouth, and by virtue of its position, it is one of the areas of the body most vulnerable to disease-producing organisms. While some diseases do arise in and are confined to the mouth, oral disorders often are manifestations of generalized disease. Specific diseases of the teeth and gums are discussed in detail in Chapter 12, "The Teeth."

Generalized disease of the mouth

Acute inflammation of the lining membrane of the mouth may interfere seriously with the normal intake of food, particularly in children. Any generalized and simple form of inflammation is referred to as *catarrhal stomatitis.* In children the condition may be associated with measles, scarlet fever, smallpox, chicken pox, or other infectious diseases, while in adults it is usually found in conjunction with poor oral hygiene. The excessive use of tobacco is often a

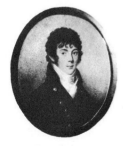

YOUNG, John Richardson (1782-1804) American physician. Contributed notably to the physiology of digestion while still a student at the University of Pennsylvania. In his graduating thesis from that school, entitled *An Experimental Inquiry Into Principles of Nutrition and the Digestive Processes,* Young demonstrated that gastric digestion was due to the solvent action of the gastric juice.

contributing factor. The membrane of the mouth becomes reddened, and there is increased secretion of saliva from the salivary glands. Although the condition causes discomfort, it is not often painful. The condition subsides fairly rapidly when proper dental hygiene is instituted. During the acute phase the physician may prescribe a mild alkaline mouthwash.

Painful *ulcers* in the mouth may occur singly or in groups and may recur for years. This condition is known as *aphthous stomatitis,* and is thought to be precipitated when certain forms of bacteria in the mouth multiply until they reach a critical level, particularly in association with a vitamin deficiency or a latent neurogenic viral infection. Cure is difficult, but the pain can be lessened by a bland antibiotic mouthwash and strict attention to mouth hygiene.

When a painful superficial ulcer covered with a whitish-gray membrane occurs in the mouth, it may result from infection by the organisms of *diphtheria* or *Vincent's angina*. Vincent's angina is a painful ulceromembranous disease of the tonsils and pharynx, commonly referred to as trench mouth. Diphtheria is a generalized disease, and the patient with a diphtheritic patch in the mouth will have severe generalized symptoms, while the patient suffering from Vincent's angina usually will have symptoms of sore mouth, swelling of lymphatic nodes, soft ulcers, and fever.

Blisters forming on one side of the mouth, which break down to form painful ulcers and which never cross the midline, are most likely a form of "shingles" (*herpes zoster*). These lesions usually heal spontaneously in a few days but may remain painful for weeks.

Whitish patches, which begin as small white spots that run together to form large uneven areas, may be caused by a yeast-like organism. The condition is a form of stomatitis commonly known as *thrush*. It occurs most commonly in undernourished children, but may occur in adults whose resistance has been undermined by a chronic disease. The patient is easily cured by the frequent use of a mouthwash containing sodium bicarbonate, and a proper diet.

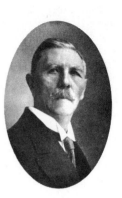

REHN, Ludwig (1849-1930) German surgeon. Performed, in 1880, the first thyroidectomy for exophthalmic goiter, a condition in which the thyroid gland becomes enlarged and the eyeballs protrude from the eyesockets. In addition, he made important contributions to surgery of the heart and the circulatory system, and made a number of important observations on certain forms of malignant tumors. Notable also is his operation for rectal prolapse.

Another form of stomatitis caused by yeast or fungus can occur as a fairly common complication of antibiotic treatment given for a separate disorder. The small sores flourish in the lining of the mouth and on surfaces of the tongue. The normal bacterial inhabitants of the mouth that usually kill such fungi have been destroyed.

Ill-fitting dentures, dentures that are not cleaned properly, or the chewing of tobacco may cause the mucous glands on the palate to enlarge and appear as small inflamed elevations with a central pore. This condition will subside when such irritants are removed.

White areas of membrane which cannot be peeled away from the underlying tissues sometimes occur, paticularly in response to the irritation of smoking. This condition must be carefully watched by a physician, because it may lead to cancer. The term given to this condition is *leukoplakia*.

Three stages of syphilis may cause lesions in the mouth. In the primary stage of the disease, a painless hardened ulcer (*chancre*) may be formed. In the secondary stage, white mucous patches in the mouth and warty masses near the angle of the mouth are often seen. In the tertiary stage a painless punched-out ulcer may occur. The tertiary form also causes the degeneration of the mucous membrane of the mouth, leading to the formation of leukoplakia.

Tuberculous ulcers may form in the mouth from infected sputum. These are painful, multiple ulcerations. The antibiotic drug, *streptomycin*, is effective in healing the ulcers, although they are likely to reappear unless the underlying tuberculous disease is adequately controlled.

Fungi may invade the mouth and cause chronic swellings which produce a discharge. *Actinomycosis* is such a condition and occurs most frequently after a dental extraction. A hard inflamed mass appears on the jaw, and this forms sinuses which discharge to the surface of the cheek. Penicillin, the sulfonamides, and exci-

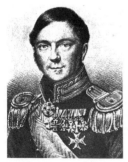

GRAEFE, Carl Ferdinand von (1787-1840) German surgeon. He was prominent among the German group which pioneered in the growth of modern surgery through a better organization of clinics and increased emphasis on fundamental principles. He is referred to as the "Father of Modern Plastic Surgery," for his original work in rhinoplasty.

sion have been effective in treating patients with this disease.

The tongue

The tongue is normally pinkish-white in color, and has three kinds of projections (*papillae*) on the upper surface. At the junction of the mouth and pharynx, there are eight to twelve large, rounded papillae (*circumvallate papillae*), lying across the tongue in the shape of an inverted V. Most of the taste buds occur on the sides of these papillae. Over the entire upper surface, but more numerous near the tip and lateral margins, are mushroom-shaped papillae, while hairlike or *filiform* papillae occur over the entire upper surface of the tongue. These papillae, with enmeshed food particles and bacteria, form the coating of the tongue. Changes in the coating are the result of shredding or regeneration of the papillae and the growth of bacteria. A fold of membrane joins the under surface of the tip of the tongue to the floor of the mouth and is called the *frenum*.

Sometimes the frenum is abnormally short and results in "tongue-tied" speech, but this is a rather infrequent developmental anomaly. It was formerly thought to occur commonly, and to be associated in some way with mental deficiency, so that unnecessary efforts were made to cut the "tongue-tie" of many normal children. Actually, the operation for "tongue-tie" needs to be performed only about once in three thousand newborn babies.

Changes in the tongue's coating

The appearance of the tongue was once thought to reflect the changes occurring in the gastric mucosa, but this is not necessarily true, although a few conditions which cause degeneration (*atrophy*) of the tongue also cause atrophy of the gastric lining.

If the coating or mucous membrane of the tongue is thin, and the tongue is pale and atrophied, some form of blood deficiency (*anemia*) may be present. Incorrect diet can also cause atrophy of the tongue coating, and when the diet is brought up to normal standards and perhaps supplemented with vitamin B, the atrophy is stopped. *Pernicious anemia* will cause atrophy of the tongue coating, which will not progress when the anemia is corrected. The chronic alcoholic develops a thin tongue coating in contrast with the occasional drinker who wakes up the "morning after" with the sensation of having a furred tongue.

A heavily coated tongue is not necessarily indicative of constipation or any other digestive upset, but is simply caused by stoppage of the normal cleansing mechanisms—that is the flow of saliva and the movements of speech and mastication. During fever, the tongue may be coated because the patient is taking a liquid diet; because the amount of saliva formed is less, resulting from the general dehydration of the body; or because the normal attention to oral hygiene is likely to be suspended.

Burning, painful tongue

Some people complain of a burning or painful sensation in the tongue, which is severe enough to keep them awake at night. While a few of the sufferers show other changes in the tongue which seem to indicate that vitamin deficiency, anemia, lack of iron, or allergy to cosmetics is the cause, the majority of patients show no tongue changes which might account for their pain. In this latter group are women who have passed the menopause and are worried about the possibility of developing cancer. Psychotherapy is the best treatment after a thorough search has been made to rule out any possible organic lesion.

Diseases of the salivary glands

The saliva secreted by the salivary glands is essential for comfort and good health, and in the rare instances where salivary glands fail to develop, there has been early and extensive dental decay. Saliva not only cleanses the mouth mechanically, but contains substances which inhibit the growth of bacteria.

An excessive amount of saliva may be secreted by the stimulating effects of drugs containing metals such as bismuth and mercury, or by the acquisition of dental plates.

Decreased salivary flow is called *xerostomia*. This is not a specific disease, but rather a symptom that may arise from a number of causes. Fear or anxiety will cause a temporary cessation of salivary flow, as will a fever or drugs such as *atropine*. Atropine is frequently given shortly before surgical operations, and so the dry-mouthed feeling that the patient experiences just before the operation is understandable. Lack of saliva may cause the mouth to become rough and dry, and in chronic cases, painful cracks and fissures may develop which bleed easily. Chewing or swallowing food may become impossible without first coating the mouth with paraffin oil.

A common cause of decreased flow of saliva is the formation of a stone in the duct leading from the gland to the mouth, with resulting obstruction of the duct. The obstruction causes a back pressure of saliva and swelling. Since the salivary glands are contained in firm capsules, any appreciable swelling causes pain. This pain has the peculiarity of occurring merely at the thought or sight of food and is more pronounced after eating. Obstruction of the salivary gland predisposes to infection of the gland. Calculi (stones) lying within the duct of a salivary gland can often be seen on an x-ray film, and they can usually be surgically removed easily.

Infection of the parotid gland (*parotitis*) sometimes occurs after surgical operations, particularly operations on some part of the digestive tract. Poor care of the teeth and mouth predisposes to infection, which may be painful. Penicillin is effective in the treatment of patients with parotitis.

The most common disease of the salivary glands is *mumps*, a highly infectious, painful virus disease. The disease is most common in children between the ages of four and 14. In adults, the disease is more serious because of complications such as inflammation of the testes or ovaries, pancreas, and brain. There is no specific treatment, but the disease quickly subsides in children. It may last for a month in an adult. This disease is discussed in detail in Chapter 2, "The Child."

Enlargement of all the salivary glands is known as *Mikulicz's disease*. It may also be caused by such diseases as leukemia, Hodgkin's disease, or syphilis.

Sometimes a portion of one of the sublingual salivary glands becomes enlarged and appears as a soft, bluish, painless mass in the floor of the mouth. This swelling is called a *ranula*. It is a saclike, cystic growth and can be easily removed surgically.

Tumors of the mouth

Tumors may be benign or malignant, and many benign tumors occur in the mouth. Because the malignant tumors of the mouth are almost invariably fatal unless treatment is early, any swelling or ulcer in the mouth should be reported immediately to the physician, who can make a correct diagnosis by removing a portion of the growth for examination under the microscope or by oral cytology smears.

Cancer of the lower lip is a comparatively common disease in older men who work outdoors without benefit of a protective hat. At first, the cancer looks like a small sun blister and seems quite innocuous. However, the ulceration fails to heal and increases gradually in size. Sometimes cancer of the lip takes the form of a small, hard, button-like tumor, often surmounted by a hard scale; this growth increases steadily in size for a time before it finally ulcerates.

Cancer of the lip can be eradicated in the early stages by treatment with radium, x-rays or surgical removal. The lesion is far more dangerous than it looks, because microscopic pieces may become detached and enter the lymph stream. They are then carried to a lymph node in the neck, and there they may grow as rapidly as the primary growth on the lip. Even at this stage, a cure often can be affected by removing all the lymph nodes on one side of the neck. If the cancer originally developed near the center of the lip, then there is a good possibility that cancer may spread to both sides of the neck. If the cancer is unchecked, it may eventually cause the death of the patient. However, if treatment is given early, the patient's chances for cure are good.

In contrast to the frequency of the occurrence of cancer on the lower lip, the upper lip is rarely affected by this disease. Cancer of the upper lip usually spreads more slowly and generally does not spread to the lymph nodes until very late.

Cancer of the tongue is more aggressive than cancer of the lip. Since this muscular organ is constantly in motion, small bits of the cancer are more likely to break off and be carried to the lymph nodes. The disease usually appears first as a small lump on the tongue. *Leukoplakia*, a disease characterized by thick, white patches on the membrane of the cheeks, gums, and tongue, is considered a precursor of mouth cancer. The frequency of leukoplakia and cancer of the lip and mouth is much greater in smokers than nonsmokers. The hazard is particularly high for pipe smokers. The use of alcohol is also strongly implicated in the development of cancer of the mouth.

Cancer may also occur on the inside of the cheeks or on the hard palate and may seem, in the early stages, to be merely a small harmless lump. Because pain usually accompanies only advanced cancer, a person with an early cancer may delay in showing it to a physician. It is in this early stage, however, that chances of curing the patient are the greatest.

Patients with cancer of the tongue or the lining of the cheeks are treated usually by surgical, x-ray, or radium therapy or by a combination of surgical and radiation therapy. The planning of such treatment is highly specialized. Sufficient radiation must be given to destroy the cancer without severely damaging adjacent nomal tissues, which are essential for the proper healing of the affected area. Too little radiation will fail to cure the patient. The lymph nodes in the neck on one or both sides may require surgical removal, especially if they have become involved with the malignant disease.

The chance of curing the patient who has cancer of the tongue, after spread to the lymph nodes has occurred, is decreased; obviously the longer the patient delays in seeking treatment, the more likely it is that cancer cells will have spread to other parts of the body.

The salivary glands, too, are sometimes the sites of cancer. Usually a hard painless lump forms in the gland, and this may remain dormant for many years. If the patient is not treated, however, the lump eventually enters a phase of rapid growth and spreads to the lymph nodes and eventually to the lungs. Therefore, any lump, no matter how long it has been present and how innocent it may seem, should be investigated by a physician. It may not be cancer; but if it is, prompt treatment may result in the eradication of the disease.

Cancer of the mouth occurs more often in unclean mouths and those containing broken teeth with sharp edges, or poorly fitted dentures. The periodic mouth examination, when thoroughly performed, offers an excellent opportunity for the education of the public in proper oral care, and for the timely detection of precancerous and early cancerous lesions. The elimination of sharp teeth, overhanging margins or fillings, poorly fitted dentures and bridgework, infections, or other sources of chronic irritation is an important factor in the prevention of mouth disease, probably even cancer.

Harelip and cleft palate

Harelip is the term given to a fissure through the upper lip which exists at birth and is caused by a failure of two adjacent parts of the face to unite properly at an early stage of development in the womb. The cleft may extend only through the flesh of the lip and cause but slight deformity. Sometimes the cleft may extend further back into the upper jaw, the floor of the nose, and even into the palate. The resultant large deformity of the nose and mouth will interfere with sucking and later with speech if not surgically corrected. The term "harelip" is not correctly descriptive since a hare's lip is cleft in a Y-shaped manner in the center of the lip. Harelip can never occur centrally in the human baby's upper lip because there is no fusion of processes in the midline. A harelip may be associated with other deformities such as a club foot or imperfectly united spine. The condition may have a familial origin. Usually, a harelip occurs on one side of the lip. However, double harelip does occur and is usually more serious than the unilateral type, because the jaw and palate are also frequently cleft. Sometimes, although the lip is not actually fissured, there can be seen a thin red scar on one or both sides of the center of the lip, which is the union of adjacent facial processes.

There is no scientific evidence to support the common misconception that external factors during pregnancy influence the development of deformities in any way.

A simple harelip involving only the substance of the lip does not interfere seriously with the baby's feeding. Nevertheless, it should be corrected surgically when the child is about three

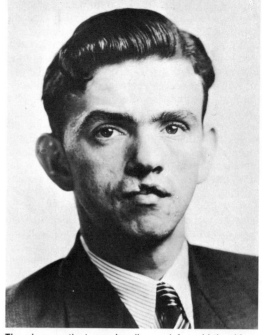

The above patient was handicapped from birth with a facial disfigurement (harelip) and speech impairment because of a cleft palate. Satisfactory employment was difficult to locate, so that at twenty years of age he was employed in an unskilled trade at a very low salary.

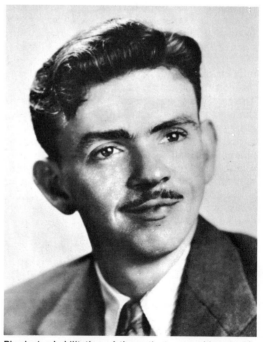

Physical rehabilitation of the patient was achieved with the result portrayed above. There was a great uplift in his morale, and his earning capacity rose. *Courtesy Federal Security Agency, Office of Vocational Rehabilitation, Washington.*

months old. When the operation is skillfully performed, feeding can proceed normally and the cosmetic effects are gratifying.

In rare cases, a cleft in the upper lip will occur vertically through the cheek, just outside the nostril, into the lower eyelid, or if there is not an actual cleft, there may be a thin scar. Such a deformity is referred to as an *oblique facial cleft*. Sometimes the cleft is at the corner of the mouth and extends horizontally into the cheek producing an abnormally large mouth opening. Small accessory ears are an additional anomaly often present in infants with this abnormally large mouth. The treatment is usually surgical.

Just as fusion of adjoining parts of the lip may be incomplete, so fusion may occasionally progress to a greater extent than usual, resulting in an abnormally small mouth. Often this deformity is associated with defective development of the lower jaw. If the opening of the mouth is extremely narrowed, the corner of the mouth can be slit transversely on each side and more normal looking lips fashioned by skillful surgery.

Cleft palate is a defect of the roof of the mouth existing at birth, the cleft being on the midline and allowing direct communication between the nose and the mouth. The mildest forms of cleft palate involve only the *uvula*, the conical mass of tissue which hangs down toward the tongue from the back of the soft palate. The cleft may produce a double uvula. However, the soft palate or both the hard and soft palates may be cleft. In extreme cases, the cleft may extend forward through the jaw and lip on one or both sides of the midline. The effect of cleft palate on the infant is serious. Sucking is impossible, and milk taken into the mouth tends to escape through the nostrils instead of being swallowed. These children must be carefully spoon-fed with the head extended backward. As the child grows older, speech is indistinct and may be impossible to understand. All the sounds requiring a certain amount of air pressure within the mouth for correct pronunciation such as *b, d, p, t, g,* and *f* are difficult for the afflicted child to utter. Moreover,

the membrane lining the nose is exposed to more air than is normal; this leads to excessive drying of the membrane, loss of secretion from the mucous glands, and diminution of the blood supply. The senses of taste and smell are much less acute than normal, partly because of the unhealthy state of the mucous membrane and also because the food cannot be pressed down onto the taste buds on the surface of the tongue.

Operation for repair of cleft palate is essential. Successful surgical repair provides a roof to the mouth, thus preventing the food from regurgitating through the nose; allows the soft palate to be pressed against the posterior wall of the pharynx in swallowing and speaking; and eradicates the obvious external deformity. The operation is usually carried out before the child has learned to speak, between one year and 18 months of age. At this age, the child is better able to withstand the operation, and enough time has not elapsed to allow bad speech habits to have been formed. In patients with severe deformity, the operation may be done at an earlier age.

If the cleft penetrates completely through the soft and hard palate and through the upper jaw, the operation should be performed as early as possible. A complete soft palate is fashioned from the deformed tissues, and the cleft in the hard palate also is closed. When surgical procedures cannot completely close the fissure, a modified denture is made to cover the cleft. This may be fastened to the teeth, arched to fit the curve of the mouth, and extended into the pharynx to allow the person to speak and control food. The dentist usually co-operates with the surgeon and speech therapist in the fashioning of this special plate, which is called an *obturator*.

After operation for repair of cleft palate, it is essential that the child be trained to speak clearly by a speech therapist. The child may not be aware of the faulty enunciation which is so obvious to those around him. Although the operation may be completely successful, he may continue to speak indistinctly if he is not thor-

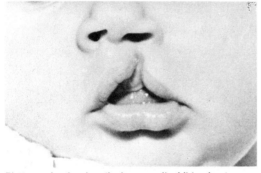

Photograph of a harelip in a small child prior to corrective treatment. Harelip should be corrected surgically when the child is about three months old.

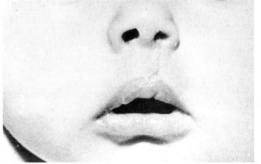

Following surgical correction, little indication of the harelip defect remains. *F. W. Schmidt, Photography Dept., Univ. of Texas Medical Branch.*

oughly trained in the correct enunciation of sounds.

Diseases of the throat

Cancer of the tonsils is not common. There are two main types, and both are very treacherous because the disease spreads beyond the tonsils to nearby lymph nodes at an early period in the disease. As with all other forms of cancer, early diagnosis and treatment by either surgical or x-ray therapy are essential. No known medicine, paint, or spray can effect a cure of the disease. The prospect of cure, if the patient is treated at an early stage, is much better than is generally thought.

Clergymen, politicians, and public speakers may suffer from a chronic inflammation of the larynx because of the continual exertion that is imposed upon it. The mucous membrane becomes thick and red, the throat dry and irritated, and the voice becomes husky. Excessive smoking and drinking can bring about the same result. Usually a period of complete rest with abstinence from smoking, alcohol, and condiments will cure a chronic laryngeal inflammation.

A bone from food caught in the throat may open a pathway for infection, forming an abscess in the back of the throat. Nasal infections in children may also cause an abscess to form in this site. A chronic abscess can occur here also as a result of spinal tubercular infection. Whether acute or chronic, this abscess in the back of the throat forms a tense swelling. If it is not relieved surgically, it may burst into the throat or erupt sideways, penetrating the skin of the neck.

Either small sacs or herniations of the mucous membrane on the back part of the pharynx can cause *dysphagia*, or difficulty and pain in swallowing. The hernias or diverticula are usually found in older people, and once developed, cause severe symptoms of gagging and regurgitation. The diverticula are formed because of pressure within the digestive tract caused by a pulsion disorder, or a malfunction of the swallowing motion. Immediate surgical relief can be given by a physician after x-ray diagnosis.

Complaints of a burning feeling in the throat, a sensation of fullness, or a lump in the throat are sometimes made by people in whom no disease or lump in the throat can be found. These symptoms may be produced by anxiety, and most often occur in young adults who are experiencing economic or emotional difficulties.

Cancer of the throat commonly occurs in the recesses which lie on either side of the back of the larynx. Unless the growth actually invades the larynx, there is no huskiness or change in voice. The first symptom is usually the feeling of a lump in the throat, or there may be actual visible swelling in the neck.

Treatment involves the use of surgery or x-rays or both. The increasing sophistication of x-ray techniques has made it possible to administer sufficient quantities of radiation to these tumors without causing excessive damage to the patient.

For a detailed discussion of the *tonsils* and *adenoids*, and associated diseases, see Chapter 2, "The Child: *Tonsils and Adenoids*." Sore throat and disorders of the larynx are discussed in Chapter 5, "The Respiratory System."

DISORDERS OF THE ESOPHAGUS

The esophagus is the passage from the throat to the stomach. There are two main symptoms of diseases of the esophagus, pain and difficulty in swallowing. Congenital abnormalities, inflammation, ulcers, spasm, tumors, varices, rupture, foreign bodies, and diverticula are the principal pathologic conditions of the esophagus.

Many developmental anomalies occur in the esophagus. The esophagus, for example, may not connect with the stomach but may end blindly or connect directly with the trachea. Surgery offers a chance of survival to infants with such a defect.

The opening through the diaphragm for the esophagus may be unusually large, allowing a portion of the stomach to bulge through (*diaphragmatic hernia*); this is the so-called upside down stomach. Gastritis often develops in this displaced portion of the stomach. This unusually large opening may be present at birth, and it may not become evident until adult life.

Severe injury may, of course, tear the muscle fibers of the diaphragm apart, forming a *traumatic diaphragmatic hernia*. Not only the stomach, but also portions of small and large bowel may pass through the opening and may cause intestinal obstruction. Surgical repair is usually advised. However, if a physician decides that the opening is small, he may recommend a regulated diet and administer antacids to alleviate the symptoms caused by the hernia.

Inflammation of the esophagus (esophagitis) is characterized by pain, burning beneath the *sternum* (breastbone), difficulty in swallowing and an increase in the secretion of mucus in the pharynx and mouth. Vomiting may occur in conjunction with extreme thirst. Treatment requires a bland liquid diet, or at most strained solid foods. Alcohol and tobacco should be avoided.

Hiatus hernia or hernia of the esophagus is similar to inflammation in its symptoms and initial treatment. Esophageal hernia is more common in overweight persons. Clothing which constricts the abdominal region should not be worn, and bending and lifting should be avoided. If the hernia increases in size or leads to complications, surgical treatment may be necessary. Occasionally, hiatal hernia and esophagitis caused by regurgitation of acid from the stomach occur together. Correction of the hernia is necessary to heal the inflammation. A bland diet and avoiding use of alcohol and tobacco promote healing.

Esophageal ulcers are similar in symptoms and treatment to peptic ulcers, discussed later in this chapter, under "Disorders of the Stomach."

Spasm of the esophagus, or *cardiospasm*, may be painless and presents usually the symptom of difficulty in swallowing, but it may cause such severe substernal pain that it could be mistaken for angina pectoris. However, the physician will be able to detect the true cause of the discomfort and bring about its relief.

Cancer may occur in the esophagus, usually in the lower or midportion of the tube. The annual incidence of this disease is 7.9 per 100,000 persons. The symptoms, which are caused by the cancer's obstructing the free passage of food into the stomach, include difficulty in swallowing, a sensation of food sticking in the chest, loss of appetite, and loss of weight. Cures of this type of cancer have resulted from surgical removal of the esophagus and by x-rays generated at extremely high voltages. A special form of x-ray therapy for patients with this type of cancer was developed in Denmark and is now practiced in many countries throughout the world. The patient sits upright on a revolving stool in the path of the x-ray beam. The stool is slowly rotated within the beam of x-rays. By this method, the tumor will receive the maximum possible amount of radiation from points of entrance all around the body. Thus, no normal tissues at a point of entrance will receive too large a dose of the powerful rays. If the disease is detected in an early stage, as many as 25 percent of the patients may survive.

Rupture of the esophagus is a rare occurrence, usually caused by sudden, violent vomiting. In a diseased esophagus, the effort to force food down sometimes causes a rupture which may even extend into the respiratory tract. Foreign bodies which become lodged in the esophagus must be located and promptly removed by the doctor.

Bulges or pockets in the esophageal wall (*diverticula*) occur in the upper, middle, or lower sections of tube. Those occurring in the upper section may retain food particles thereby causing difficulty in swallowing and regurgitation. If there is danger of constriction, they may be relieved by surgical removal. Serious congenital abnormalities, such as incomplete esophagus, are not compatible with life, causing death within a few hours or days after birth. The other eso-

phageal abnormalities are either accommodated without treatment or by surgical repair.

Ulceration of the esophagus may occur, particularly in people with abnormally short gullets or hiatal hernias, because regurgitation of stomach acids takes place easily. Symptoms and treatment are the same as for esophagitis associated with hiatal hernia.

An acute burn of the esophagus from the drinking of caustic liquids accidentally or suicidally may produce ulcers, perforations, or delayed stricture. Lye solutions should never be put in containers that can be mistaken for food and should never be left within reach of a child. Cleaning fluids also should be kept out of a child's reach.

DISORDERS OF THE STOMACH

Indigestion is a vague term given to any upset of the digestive processes. Indigestion may be caused by spasm of the esophagus; failure of the opening between the esophagus and stomach to relax properly; inflammation of the stomach wall; peptic ulcer; cancer of the stomach; gallbladder disease; intestinal disorders; or emotional upset.

"Heartburn" is an intense burning sensation under the breastbone. It is a symptom of esophageal spasm and occurs frequently in the early months of pregnancy and in overactive individuals who are usually tired at mealtimes. Excessive smoking is also a causative factor. The pain may be caused by a regurgitation of acid from the stomach into the esophagus, or by a spasm of the muscular coat of the esophagus at its lower end. Usually heartburn can be relieved by the adoption of regular habits, putting aside worry at mealtimes, and cutting down on the number of cigarettes smoked during the day.

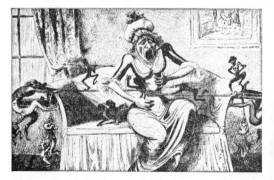

Engraving by the English illustrator Cruikshank of his impression of the symptoms of colic, a common term for digestive upsets. *Bettmann Archive.*

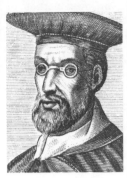

CAPIVACCIO, Girolamo (d. 1589) Italian surgeon. Gave the first description of a gastric ulcer which was thought to have changed from a benign to a malignant lesion; it was named after him, the ulcer of Capivaccius. The discovery was not fully appreciated until the present century. Today, the ulcer patient is watched carefully so that if he develops a cancer at the site of the ulcer, it may be removed in an early, curable stage.

While heartburn usually occurs without the presence of actual organic disease, occasionally it may occur as a result of gallbladder disease, nutritional disease of the nervous system, pressure on the esophagus from disease of the respiratory system or even cardiac disturbance. Therefore, the physician may order x-ray studies of these organs.

Difficulty in swallowing, vomiting, and pain in the pit of the stomach (*epigastric pain*) may result from *cardiospasm* (spasm of the sphincter muscle which joins the esophagus to the stomach). Usually this form of indigestion occurs in young, overactive, neurotic people, and the fundamental cause is unknown. The esophagus becomes dilated above the constricted area, and the vomiting occurs once the esophagus is filled with food. The condition is usually relieved by the avoidance of bulky, irritating, or extremely cold foods, and alcohol, provided that the underlying emotional difficulties are recognized and resolved.

Although persistent indigestion is usually caused by disease of the esophagus, stomach, or gallbladder, in many instances distress or discomfort follows a meal because of nervousness or anxiety. Nervousness and anxiety may cause an increase in the movements of the stomach; fear and emotional strain may inhibit them. Food taken when one is anxious, agitated, or fatigued may be followed by heartburn, belching, vague discomfort, and other symptoms of indigestion. This inhibition may cause reversal of the normal stomach movements. There is a definite relationship of emotional factors to gastric symptoms. Normal, healthy emotions facilitate the efficient working of the digestive system, while emotional disturbances can lead to a breakdown of the process of digestion.

In certain forms of heart attacks, the symptoms may closely resemble those of acute indigestion. Confusion of these two diseases can be fatal to the patient; consequently, when symptoms of acute indigestion occur, the physician should be summoned to evaluate the condition.

Gastritis

Inflammation of the stomach wall is termed gastritis and is the most frequent form of stomach upset. Gastritis may be acute or chronic; the acute form is often caused by food poisoning. Acute inflammation may occur from the eating of spoiled food. Further, there are many instances in which an inflammation develops as a result of too much food, even though the food is neither spoiled nor poisonous.

The person developing acute gastritis first loses his appetite and feels a sense of pressure and fullness in the pit of his stomach, which is not relieved by belching. Nausea develops, often accompanied by headache and a slight rise in temperature. Copious vomiting may then take place, and this is followed by a sense of relief. However, the patient feels completely fatigued.

In the great majority of instances, healing takes place quickly if the patient remains on the diet prescribed by his physician for a week or more. The use of drugs is unnecessary. Diarrhea frequently accompanies acute gastritis and may require a special diet.

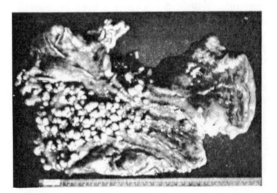

Photograph of the inner surface of a human stomach containing polyps. This condition is known as *multiple polyposis* or *polyposis ventriculi.*

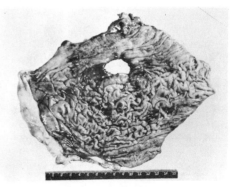

Photograph of the inner surface of a stomach which has been perforated by an ulcer. *Courtesy of the surgical staff, Memorial Hospital, Houston.*

Corrosive substances which have been swallowed either by mistake or with suicidal intent cause an acute gastritis with severe cramping pain and collapse. There is always the danger that the lye or acid may perforate the stomach wall and cause acute peritonitis. The fate of the patient depends on quick, effective treatment by a physician. The first step is usually that of washing out the stomach thoroughly by means of a stomach tube and neutralizing the poison by counteractive substances. Milk or limewater is used as the neutralizing agent if the poison was an acid, or vinegar if it was an alkali. Surgical treatment will be necessary if the stomach perforates or if tough scars develop in the esophagus and stomach as an after-effect of the poisoning.

Peptic ulcer

The gastric juice manufactured by the stomach contains hydrochloric acid, mucus, and a ferment, *pepsin*, which breaks down protein in the food into simpler substances. Sometimes the mechanism for secreting gastric acids does not shut off after all the food has been consumed, and the pepsin-hydrochloric acid mixture goes to work on the digestive tract itself. Thus, a *peptic ulcer* occurs in the walls of the stomach or the duodenum which are the regions bathed by the gastric juices. Peptic ulcers may also occur in the esophagus as a result of the backflow of juices. The vagus nerve is believed to be largely responsible for the continuous overproduction of gastric acids. It receives stimulation from the sight and odor of food, and from the emotions. The vagus nerve is sometimes overactive at night when there is no food in the stomach. The juices go directly through the pylorus into the duodenum. This causes destruction of the mucous membrane of the intestine and can result in a duodenal ulcer. Also implicated are the regulatory mechanisms of the stomach wall. The antrum, or lower portion of the stomach, contains a hormone to halt the production of acid when gastric juices begin to fill the antrum. Ulcers can be produced by a malfunction of this regulatory mechanism.

People with a low concentration of hydrochloric acid in their gastric juices rarely develop peptic ulcer. Most ulcer patients have a higher concentration of gastric acids, although the quantity of juices secreted may be lower. Thus food may take longer to digest and the corrosive acids may remain too long in the stomach.

Smoking may aggravate ulcer formation or delay the healing of an ulcer which has already formed. It has been found in animal experiments that coarse food also will retard the healing of an ulcer by subjecting the stomach wall to minor trauma. A tense, ambitious, hard-driving person is more likely to develop a peptic ulcer than the calm phlegmatic type. Indeed, a healing ulcer may become reactivated as a result of worry or an emotional shock. However, the disease may occur in any type of person at any age, so that a person with ulcer symptoms should consult his physician.

Peptic ulcer is relatively common. About ten to twelve percent of all Europeans and Americans suffer from the condition at some time in their lives. The condition occurs about four times more frequently in men than in women, and it may occur at any age, although it is rare under the age of ten. The frequency of peptic ulcers occurring in patients with blood type O may point to a genetic factor in ulcer incidence. Duodenal ulcer occurs about ten to twelve times as frequently as ulcer of the stomach. Usually only a single ulcer is formed in the duodenum but there may be multiple stomach ulcers.

Peptic ulcers usually occur in definite sites which are bathed freely in gastric juices. Stomach ulcers usually occur on the upper, lesser curvature. Ulceration occurring on the lower,

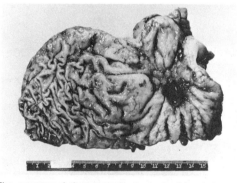

The mucosa of the stomach shown in this photograph is interrupted by a large ulcer, probably resulting from the presence of lymphosarcoma.

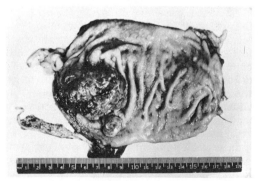

Photograph showing appearance of gastric mucosa of a patient with gastric carcinoma. Size of cancer may be judged from the centimeter scale.

greater curvature must be regarded as possibly cancerous.

The size of peptic ulcers varies from a quarter of an inch to several inches in diameter. The ulcer may be deep or shallow, depending on the length of time it has existed. Peptic ulcers may invade gradually deeper and deeper into the stomach or duodenal wall until a large blood vessel is penetrated, causing massive hemorrhage; or the wall may be completely perforated. Thus, it is important that treatment be given as early as possible in the course of the disease.

Peptic ulcer is a chronic disease, and most patients complain of symptoms over a period of five to eight years before seeking medical advice. However, some patients are brought into the hospital emergency room with an acute perforated ulcer, although they have never suffered from any recognizable symptoms.

Pain is the outstanding symptom of peptic ulcer. The reason for this pain has long been a subject for study, because the gastrointestinal wall is insensitive. The pain is apparently related to the contact of acid with the base of the ulcer, because the pain is relieved by emptying the stomach, or neutralizing the acid. Continued neutralization of the gastric juice, results in complete relief of the pain.

The periodicity of pain is striking; pain seems to be more prevalent in the spring and fall of the year. The pain may last for only a few days or weeks at a time, but it usually persists for two or three months. Then there may be a remission, which may last for even longer or shorter periods. As the disease progresses, the painful episodes become longer and the intervals of remission shorter. Fatigue, worry, and acute infections occurring in a period of remission may cause an abrupt recurrence of pain in many patients.

Usually the pain is burning in character. It may be felt in the pit of the stomach, in an area perhaps no more than an inch and a half to two inches in diameter, which can be pointed out exactly by the patient.

The symptoms of duodenal and stomach ulcer are similar, the chief difference being in the time of onset of pain. The pain resulting from a duodenal lesion may appear as late as three to four hours after a meal. Pain occurring 30 to 60 minutes after eating is most frequently caused by a stomach ulcer. The pain of peptic ulcer of the stomach or duodenum is almost invariably relieved by eating. Symptoms are rarely present in the morning since the flow of gastric juice generally is reduced until food is eaten. After breakfast there may be some pain which may be relieved by milk or an alkaline drink. Pain usually follows after lunch and dinner, the time of occurrence depending upon the type of lesion. Ulcer pain may occur at night, usually between midnight and two a.m. It is thought that an acutely inflamed lesion and high acidity are the combination necessary to provoke nocturnal pain.

Nausea is not a common symptom of peptic ulcer, although nausea and vomiting may occur if the ulcer has become chronic and has scarred the stomach to such a degree that normal emptying is no longer possible. Vomiting without nausea may occur if the pain is severe.

Constipation is a common complaint of peptic ulcer patients. Often, the constipation is regarded as the cause of the pain, with the result that the patient may take laxatives habitually. The resultant bowel upset may be severe.

Loss of appetite is an unusual symptom of peptic ulcer, and loss of weight sometimes occurs. Some patients gain weight as a result of learning that eating continuously relieves pain.

Often patients with ulcer are anemic, because the continued loss of blood from the ulcer will deplete the store of hemoglobin in the body. Ulcer incidence is also high in patients with rheumatoid arthritis.

Diagnosis: The physician diagnoses peptic ulcer with the aid of x-rays. The ulcer can be seen on the x-ray screen in 95 percent of cases when it occurs in the stomach, and in about 70 percent of cases when it occurs in the duodenum. The patient first drinks a suspension of barium sulfate, which is visible on the x-ray plate and shows the outlines of digestive tract as it passes through. Examination by the *gastroscope* is of value in confirming the diagnosis and in locating stomach ulcers not seen by x-ray examination. The gastroscope is an ingenious system of mirrors and lenses combined in a long tube which is flexible in its lower half. This instrument enables the physician to look into the stomach. The instrument is inserted through the mouth, down the esophagus and along the posterior wall of the stomach. A rubber bulb pumps air into the stomach, distending it and allowing the walls to be inspected. A small electric bulb in the tip of the instrument supplies the illumination, and a system of lenses allows the operator to see what lies in front of the gastroscope. Although the lower half of the instrument is flexible, the system of lenses is arranged in such a fashion that no matter how the flexible portion is bent, the view obtained through the instrument is always clear. Examination by the gastroscope is not a painful procedure nor is hospitalization necessary. The instrument is swallowed just as if it were a stomach tube, and once the examination is over, the patient can return to work immediately if he wishes.

Modification of the gastroscope has led to development of the fiberscope, a similar but completely flexible instrument. This flexibility makes passage easier and more comfortable to the patient. In addition light transmission is sufficient to provide color photographs without additional

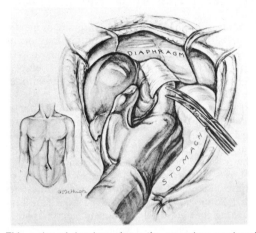

This series of drawings shows the procedure employed in the Dragstedt operation for benign peptic ulcer. A high left-of-center incision has been made in the abdomen, as shown in the small sketch.

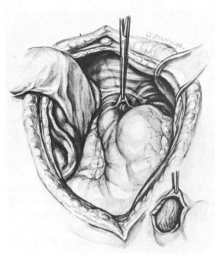

In the above illustration, the liver is being held to one side, the peritoneum over the esophagus at the margin of the diaphragm is divided, and a small opening has been made in the diaphragm.

illumination. With the introduction of the Japanese gastrocamera gastric photography has found greater utilization. The gastrocamera consists of a small camera placed in the tip of a completely flexible tube. The combined technique of roentgenologic and gastrocamera examination may have improved diagnosis of more advanced malignancy.

Treatment: When a patient is proved to have peptic ulcer, the physician will place him on a regimen of diet, rest, and avoidance of fear and worry. This regime must be thorough, prolonged, systematic, and constantly supervised if it is to succeed, because the symptoms of ulcer vanish long before the ulcer heals. The diet is one of soft nutritious foods, containing a high proportion of milk and cream. The usual schedule is about three ounces of equal parts of milk and cream to be taken hourly from 7 a.m. to 7 p.m., for the first few days. Orange juice is then added; and then rice pudding, poached eggs, custards, and omelets are gradually allowed. After about a month, the patient is usually able to begin taking three full meals a day, but all the food must be cooked soft and must be well chewed; highly seasoned foods are to be avoided. A rather high percentage of adults who cannot tolerate milk because of a common enzyme deficiency are put on a bland, but milk-free diet.

Antacid powders or pastes are given sometimes to insure neutralization of the acid present in the gastric juice. The efficiency of any particular powder or paste to neutralize hydrochloric acid in a test tube is no guarantee that it will act just as well when taken internally. Many factors are involved in neutralizing the stomach contents, of which the most important are the rate at which the stomach secretes acid

and the rate at which the stomach empties its contents. Antacids may actually increase gastric secretion, and it is difficult to neutralize the acid in a stomach which empties rapidly. Modified licorice compounds can give relief to patients with duodenal ulcers.

The stomach continues to secrete gastric juice during the night, and a drug such as *atropine* may be prescribed by the physician to be taken in the evening, so that the amount of gastric juice secreted during the night will be considerably diminished.

Rest and avoidance of emotional upset are quite important in the care of the ulcer patient. Complete bed rest in a hospital for two to four weeks is usually desirable. However, this is often impossible when the patient is the breadwinner of the family. Tranquilizing drugs may be given initially, but ultimately the patient must develop the habit of mental relaxation without the aid of drugs. If a peptic ulcer of the stomach does not heal immediately while under treatment, or if it recurs, it requires surgical exploration and biopsy to determine whether it is malignant. The mortality of removing the ulcer-bearing and ulcer-prone parts of the stomach today is less than the mortality of uncontrolled peptic ulcer.

Another technique for relief of ulcer pain is freezing all or part of the stomach with a cooling liquid and then rewarming the organ. This reduces secretion of hydrochloric acid for weeks or months, and lowers the flow of gastric juices to the duodenum. It is employed principally to relieve the pain of duodenal ulcers, and to prevent massive bleeding.

Complications of peptic ulcers: One of the most serious complications of peptic ulcer in the stomach or the duodenum is acute perforation

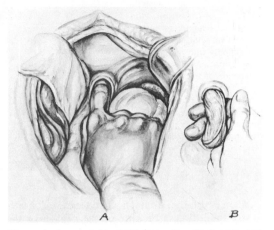

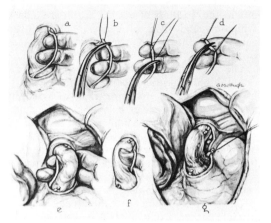

Finger is inserted in opening in the diaphragm and the esophagus is pulled down below the diaphragm to permit removal of the vagus nerve segment by the process shown in the next illustration.

Cutting of the vagus nerve frequently relieves peptic ulcer. Pictures courtesy *Lester R. Dragstedt, M.D., Copyright 1947, Annals of Surgery, by permission of J. B. Lippincott Co., Philadelphia.*

through the organ wall. Perforation occurs without warning; there may be no increase in severity or frequency of symptoms to herald the attack. Vigorous exercise, coughing, vomiting, and straining at stool may precipitate the perforation. Acute perforation rarely occurs in a patient undergoing adequate treatment.

Surgical methods: When the stomach or duodenal wall has been perforated, an operation is necessary to repair the tear by closing the perforation or by a definitive operation to prevent recurrence.

There are many surgical procedures for ulcers, depending on their severity and location. Subtotal gastrectomy removes 75 percent to 80 percent of the stomach and rejoins the duodenum to the remaining upper part. Hemigastrectomy removes 50 percent of the stomach and rejoins the remainder to the small intestine, by-passing the duodenum. In gastroenterostomy, the whole stomach is opened directly into the small bowel. Vagotomy, or severing the vagus nerve, usually accompanies these procedures to cut down the over-production of gastric acid. Vagotomy is also teamed with pyloroplasty, or widening the valve between the stomach and the duodenum. Vagotomy alone is sometimes used.

In addition to surgical repair, measures must be taken to offset the great amount of shock that occurs with the perforation. Unremitting care for a week after the operation will usually prevent such complications as generalized peritonitis, or intestinal obstruction.

Destruction of a large vessel in the wall of the stomach or duodenum, causing massive hemorrhage with vomiting of blood and the appearance of black tarry stools, is a more frequent complication of peptic ulcer than perforation. Probably one untreated person in four with pep-

tic ulcer has massive bleeding into his stomach at some time. Treatment is not usually surgical, but consists of complete bed rest, blood transfusion if necessary, and the consumption of small, frequent, bland meals. Under this regimen, the bleeding usually ceases and healing of the ulcer begins. Should bleeding continue, emergency surgical procedures may be necessary.

Obstruction of the passage of food may occur if the ulcer is of long duration, because of the contraction of the scar tissue in the base of the ulcer and stricture of the normal outlet. Persistent vomiting, or the vomiting of food eaten the previous day may occur. If this condition proves to be the result of organic constriction, only surgical intervention can bring relief. In some instances, the obstruction may be caused by swelling (*edema*) of the tissues and can be relieved by medical measures.

Cancer of the stomach

Cancer of the stomach causes approximately nine deaths for every 100,000 people in the United States each year. Japanese and Norwegians have an even higher percentage incidence of this disease.

Men past the age of 45 years are the most frequent victims of cancer of the stomach. However, women do develop the disease. While the actual cause of cancer in any site is unknown, a few unhealed peptic ulcers probably become malignant. It is thought that chronic gastritis is frequently associated with stomach cancer.

Because stomach cancer commences insidiously, any digestive upset occurring after middle age should be reported immediately to the doctor. Similarly, any person at any age with persistent abdominal discomfort should have a full and thorough examination. Loss of weight, loss of appetite, and loss of normal health are indeed symptoms and signs of cancer; but, unfortunately, they are often symptoms of advanced cancer.

The diagnosis of stomach cancer is made by examining the gastric juice (acid often absent), by investigating the stools for traces of blood, by x-ray and gastroscopic examinations of the stomach, by surgical exploration and biopsy and by microscopical examination of smears of material obtained by gastric lavage. The x-ray examination of the stomach is especially informative, as the exact location and approximate size of the cancer can be determined.

Three types of stomach cancer occur: an ulcerating cancer, a tumor growing in the cavity of the stomach, and a diffuse thickening of the stomach wall. Most cancers of the stomach have a high degree of malignancy and spread to nearby lymph nodes or distant areas early in the disease. The regional nodes are the most common sites of malignant spread (*metastasis*). Another node often involved is the node located just above the left collar bone (the *supraclavicular node*); sometimes a painless enlargement of this node is the first indication that the patient has cancer of the stomach. The liver, peritoneum, and lungs are also frequent sites of metastasis.

Cancer of the stomach is said to be in an *early* stage when it is still confined to the stomach; after spread to regional nodes or other areas has occurred, the disease is in a *late* stage.

There is only one curative treatment for patients with cancer of the stomach—early and complete removal of the lesion with a portion or even all of the stomach. The ability to cure a patient with cancer of the stomach by surgical therapy depends upon whether this operation is undertaken in an early or late stage. If performed early, surgical procedures can cure a large percentage of patients; however, when diagnosis is made after the disease has spread beyond the stomach, the cure rate falls considerably.

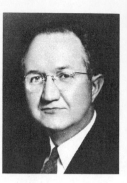

Cancer of the stomach is too often a hopelessly fatal disease because of the neglect of the patient to consult his physician for what may have seemed to be only trivial symptoms of indigestion. "He who treats himself has a fool for a patient" is an old saying that is tragically true in so many cases of digestive upset.

Benign stomach tumors include gastric *polyps*. These tumors often grow on stalks and usually do not cause pain unless they are long enough to be caught and pulled into the duodenum. Anemia may be a prominent symptom. These tumors are potentially malignant, and therefore should be removed surgically. Other benign stomach tumors produce symptoms only if the tumor bleeds, ulcerates, or causes obstruction. They, too, should be removed surgically.

Food poisoning

Food poisoning occurs as a result of eating food or drinking water that contains either bacteria or poisons produced by bacteria. Organisms capable of directly infecting a human are *Salmonella* and *Shigella*. Poisonous bacterial by-products are called *toxins*. By far the most prevalent toxin associated with food poisoning is that produced by the *Staphylococcus*. Less common is *Clostridium botulinum*.

Public health measures now control outbreaks of the more severe diseases caused by Salmonella (typhoid) and Shigella (bacillary dysentery). But food and waterborne outbreaks due to nontyphoid Salmonella have now emerged as a serious public health hazard. Nontyphoid Salmonella has found a home in poultry, eggs, livestock, and improperly built water supply systems. The organisms are also transmitted by flies and rats.

Living Salmonella organisms taken into the stomach cause a gastritis which may be mild, or severe enough to mimic typhoid fever. If the bacteria become established in the intestinal tract, they produce fever, nausea, vomiting, cramping, and diarrhea in various combinations and degrees over a period of days. These infections are always self-limited and require only symptomatic treatment. Meat, milk, and eggs are

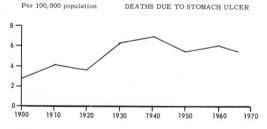

Per 100,000 population   DEATHS DUE TO STOMACH ULCER

Increase in the number of deaths resulting from ulcers in the stomach is partly due to the fact that more persons now live to the age at which ulcers occur. Also stomach ulcer is more easily recognized by modern diagnostic procedures used today.

disorders of the vermiform appendix

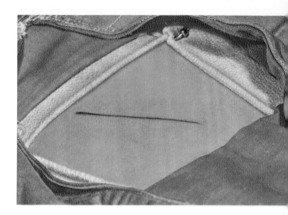

1

1. Prior to the appendectomy, the surgical field is prepared by washing the skin and painting it with an antiseptic. The prospective line of incision is then marked.

2. The scalpel used for the initial skin incision is discarded after the incision has been made. This is done to avoid carrying any outside contamination into the peritoneum.

3. The surgeon then makes an incision through the subcutaneous fat, thereby exposing the peritoneum. The other tissues are held aside by the use of surgical retractors.

4. An incision is next made in the peritoneum, and the appendix is located. It is then carefully manipulated into the surgical field in order to facilitate its removal.

5. The appendix is shown here prior to its removal. It is then separated from the intestine (cecum) in such a manner that none of the contents are allowed to seep out.

6. The hole in the intestine that results is now carefully sutured shut in such a manner as to insure that it will remain closed and that no postoperative leak can possibly occur.

7. With the appendectomy complete, the incision must be carefully repaired by suturing both the opening in the peritoneum and then the original wound in the skin.

8. Sutures used for closing the peritoneum are of catgut which will be absorbed by the body. The sutures used for closing the skin are of thin but quite strong black silk or synthetic material.

9. The wound that remains after an appendectomy is small and will heal rapidly, permitting the patient to be active in a day or so. Skin sutures are removed some days later.

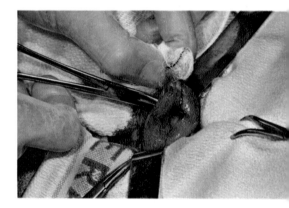

4

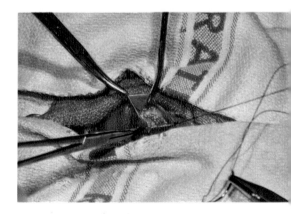

7

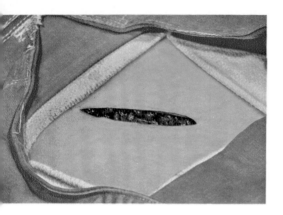

2

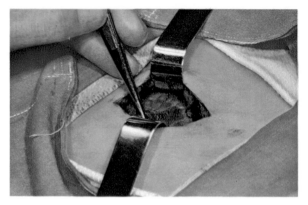

3

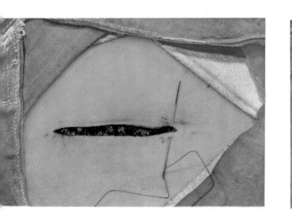

5

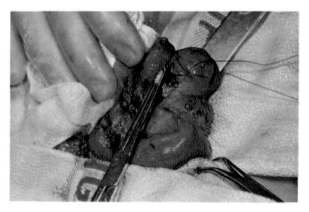

6

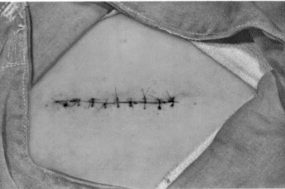

8

9

the most common foods carrying Salmonella. Sanitary measures can control the organism. Particular care should be taken to discard cracked eggs. Care should also be taken to separate utensils used for pet feeding, since pet foods may be contaminated. Pets, especially turtles, may be infected when purchased and children are often infected by handling them. If meat and eggs are properly cooked, water and milk supplies adequately purified, and fresh food properly cleansed, outbreaks of Salmonella poisoning should rarely occur.

A more unusual form, *Salmonella cubana,* has been found sometimes in a red food dye used in gum, candy, and cough syrups.

Food poisoning caused by toxin-producing Staphylococcus is by far the most common form encountered in the United States. The chemical toxins are produced by the bacteria when certain foods are prepared and allowed to remain unrefrigerated for an hour or more. The bacteria are introduced by food handlers who carry the organisms in their nose and throat. Sauces containing eggs or cream, salad dressing, mayonnaise, and custards are particularly favorable to Staphylococcus when left at ordinary room temperature. Neither the bacteria nor their toxins will alter the taste or appearance of the food. Symptoms of staphylococcal food poisoning occur within about three hours after eating infected food. In a typical instance, nausea, vomiting, abdominal cramps, prostration, and diarrhea occur. There is no specific drug treatment available, and the poisoned patient usually recovers with the aid of a fluid diet in 12 to 24 hours. Since staphylococci are present everywhere, it is almost impossible to prevent their access to food. It has been found, however, that the staphylococci cannot manufacture their toxin in a cold environment. Therefore, the best control is adequate refrigeration of all perishable food. When this not possible, only freshly prepared foods should be eaten, especially in warm weather.

Botulism is the term given to the gastritis

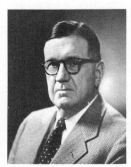

MILLER, Thomas Grier (1886-) American physician. Refined the methods of gastric analysis by inventing, with W. O. Abbott, a two-channel tube of small calibre, with which they worked out a technique for studying the secretory and motor functions of the small intestine in man. This same technique has been used to drain the intestine, and to diagnose and treat a number of disorders such as obstruction of the intestine. *Fabian Bachrach.*

caused by consuming the toxins of *Clostridium botulinum.* The condition is usually associated with the eating of improperly prepared home-canned foods. Botulism was named by physicians in Germany over two centuries ago. The term was derived from the Latin "Botulus," meaning "sausage," and the early outbreaks were caused by eating improperly cooked sausage. Besides nausea and vomiting, paralysis of the muscles may ensue, so that there is double vision because of derangement of the eye muscles, and difficulty in speaking and swallowing may occur. The diaphragm may be paralyzed, so that an iron lung is necessary to maintain life. The bacteria may or may not cause any detectable odor or taste in food; consequently, home-canned food cannot be assumed to be free of these organisms in the absence of odor. No home-canned food should be tasted—even in small samples—until it has been thoroughly cooked. Antitoxin serums are available and if given early enough, can neutralize the toxin. Even so, the disease has been fatal in approximately half of the people affected in the United States. Fortunately, with modern commercial canning procedures, this disease has become a rarity.

Fruit and vegetables should be washed as soon as possible after picking, before they are canned. Meat, fish, and poultry should be cooked in a pressure cooker for the prescribed length of time prior to canning. Any canned food not so treated should be boiled before eating. Boiling at 212° Fahrenheit for four hours destroys the bacillus itself, while the toxin is destroyed at 167° Fahrenheit in ten minutes. Canned food with a disagreeable odor or gas formation should never be tasted, but should have several spoonfuls of lye added to the can or jar, and then be destroyed.

Ptomaine poisoning is the term commonly applied to outbreaks of food poisoning. Ptomaines are substances formed in food when it putrefies. For a time, the theory was widely accepted that these substances were responsible for the symptoms in food poisoning. However, it is now known that the majority of "ptomaine food poisoning" outbreaks are caused by the toxins of the staphylococci. Many putrefied foods, in the absence of food poisoning germs, are without ill effect when eaten. Limburger cheese is a popular putrefied food and the Eskimo considers putrefied meat a delicacy.

Poisoning may be caused by the ingestion of substances, besides food infected with bacteria. The ice trays of some refrigerators are cadmium coated; and if acid foods are placed in them, sometimes enough cadmium is dissolved in the food to cause vomiting and diarrhea within 15 or 30 minutes after eating. If sodium fluoride, an insect poison, is eaten, abdominal pain, vomiting, and diarrhea occur, sometimes accompanied by paralysis of eye and facial muscles.

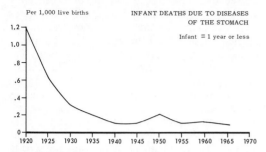

This chart depicts the decrease in infant deaths resulting from diseases of the stomach during the period 1920-1966, within the United States.

Otherwise edible mussels may at times contain a poisonous substance produced by infection with the protozoa *Gonyaulax catenella.* Outbreaks of Gonyaulax poisoning occur during the "red tides," when the ocean becomes so overgrown with the tiny red organism that it actually appears red. Infectious hepatitis can be carried by clams and oysters grown near sewage outlets. Although not a true food poison, the infection is a serious threat. The virus is also found in drinking water contaminated by sewage.

Mushrooms often cause food poisoning. There are 70 to 80 known poisonous varieties. The most poisonous type is *Amanita phalloides,* which contains a poison, *amanitotoxin,* that causes the death of many tissues of the body. Usually mushroom poisoning develops 6 to 16 hours after eating.

When food poisoning has occurred, the physician makes every effort to recognize the type of poisoning, so that proper treatment can be instituted and further cases may be prevented. It is fortunate that, in most instances, the diarrhea and vomiting which accompany the disease eliminate poison not already absorbed. The illness is usually short, and recovery proceeds uneventfully, if the patient adheres to the diet

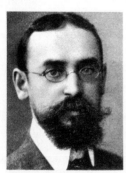

PFANNENSTIEL, Hermann Johann (1862-1909) German gynecologist. Described in 1900 an incision for entering the abdominal cavity. The major virtue of this particular operation consists in the fact that it is designed to avoid visible scarring of the abdomen. To accomplish this, Pfannenstiel employed a long, horizontal incision curving over the *mons pubis.* Thus the scar is so located that it is rendered virtually unnoticeable by the pubic hair.

prescribed. When vomiting and diarrhea are persistent, however, hospitalization may be required.

Food poisoning often affects American tourists in foreign countries. The native population may be immune, even act as carriers for the causative organism. For this reason, drinking water of unknown quality should be boiled or otherwise purified. Food should be thoroughly cooked; only those vegetables and fruits which can be peeled and then washed should be eaten raw. Certain sulfonamide drugs may be taken as a preventive measure, at the physician's discretion.

Bezoars

Bezoars are stone-like balls which form in the stomach or intestinal tract. Most often they are found in nervous young girls who have a habit of biting their hair. A concretion forms around the swallowed hair particles. Bezoars can also be formed from eating a quantity of persimmons, a fruit containing highly sticky resin. Symptoms include abdominal pain, loss of appetite for solid foods and increased appetite for liquids, inability to eat much at one time, vomiting, bowel upset, foul breath, anemia, and exhaustion. Treatment is usually surgical and is simple removal of the foreign body.

Congenital abnormalities of the stomach

The most important congenital abnormality of the stomach is an enlargement of the muscle forming the pyloric valve between the stomach and the small intestine with resultant narrowing and obstruction of the passage of food from the stomach.

Infants about two or three weeks old are the usual victims, although the condition may occur at any time between the age of ten days and four months. A similar condition is sometimes found in adults; but it is doubtful if the condition existed since birth, and there is usually some other gastric disorder associated with the diseased valve, such as gastritis or gastric ulcer.

Babies with a malformed pyloric valve usually show no symptoms in the first few days of life, but then they begin to vomit, lose weight quickly, and fail to excrete the usual amount of urine because of the loss of fluid from the stomach. The vomiting is of a particular type—it is effortless and projectile. Sometimes a hard lump, the size of a marble, can be felt through the abdominal wall to the right of the midline just below the ribs.

The treatment of a child with this anomaly is surgical division of the malformed muscle.

Sometimes there is pyloric obstruction without overgrowth of the pyloric muscle. It is thought that, in these cases, there has been a failure of the newly developed nervous system to co-ordinate properly, with the result that the pyloric valve remains in continuous spasm. No lump can be felt in the abdomen in these cases, and operation is usually not needed. A sedative just before feeding time usually causes the pylorus to relax, and then the food passes through the stomach normally.

Sometimes, a child may be born with an "upside-down" stomach (diaphragmatic hernia), but this is a rare event. This abnormality usually causes annoying dyspeptic symptoms and bowel dysfunction. Surgical intervention should be employed to correct the defect in most instances. This condition is discussed further under "Disorders of the Esophagus."

DISORDERS OF THE SMALL INTESTINE

The length of the small intestine, approximately 20 feet, is arbitrarily divided into three parts for descriptive purposes. The first inches which are relatively fixed to the posterior abdominal wall are called the *duodenum*. Below the duodenum is the *jejunum,* which comprises the upper two-fifths, and the *ileum* which comprises the remaining three fifths of the small bowel. The major part of the processes of digestion and absorption takes place in the small intestine.

Ulcer: The most frequent pathologic condition of the duodenum is *peptic ulcer.* True peptic ulceration of the duodenum is more frequent than that of the stomach. The symptoms of duodenal ulcer differ from those of stomach ulcer only in that in cases of duodenal ulcer there is usually a longer time interval between eating and the development of pain. The medical treatment is the same in both cases, and has been previously described in the section on stomach ulcer. Surgical procedures for duodenal ulcer as well as the new technique of freezing are also discussed under stomach ulcers.

Acute inflammation: Because the small intestine plays such an important part in the functioning of the body, all but the most trivial disorders in this area are accompanied by general bodily upset. *Acute inflammation* of the intestine results in poor absorption of its fluid contents; consequently, the body has to utilize whatever water is already present. Water is removed from the blood, and the skin becomes dry, the tongue coated, and less urine is excreted by the kidneys. There is a consequent building up of toxic substances in the blood stream. The normal movements of the intestine are interrupted, with resulting distention of the abdomen.

If disease of the small intestine becomes chronic, loss of appetite, lassitude, weakness, and anemia may result. Chronic inflammation may produce a progressive incomplete obstruction from scar tissue formation. Also there is a condition of unknown cause called *Crohn's disease* or *regional ileitis* that may cause severe scarring and inflammation of the small bowel with chronic obstruction and fistula formation. Surgical intervention is the only known remedy.

Pain, nausea, vomiting, audible intestinal rumblings, diarrhea, or constipation are the symptoms which characterize most disorders of the small intestine. Intestinal pain is of two kinds—one being caused by acute inflammation, which gives rise to pain in a specific area; the other being caused by obstruction of the bowel, which causes a diffuse pain.

Vomiting may occur whenever the stomach or intestines are irritated, either from inflammatory or mechanical disturbances. Rumblings are caused whenever intestinal action moves a mixture of fluid and gas (usually swallowed air) quickly. Diarrhea results when the excess mobility spreads to the large bowel; constipation occurs when intestinal movements cease or an actual obstruction to the passage of materials exists.

Intestinal obstruction: Complete or intermittent blockage of the small intestine may be caused by the presence of adhesions between adjacent portions of bowel or between the bowel and the abdominal wall; by the presence of a hernia; by the formation of an *intussusception* (invagination of the bowel); by a twisting of the bowel (*volvulus*); by swallowed foreign bodies; by tumors; or by other constricting lesions of inflammatory nature.

The chief symptoms of intestinal obstruction are pain and vomiting. Distention appears when the obstruction has become established. The pain is intermittent and cramplike and occurs in episodes lasting one to three minutes. Abdominal tenderness does not occur early.

Cancer: Cancer of the small bowel is rare, but may occur anywhere along the length of the bowel. In some cases, the tumor arises in association with the appendix. X-ray therapy is of little benefit, and surgery is the treatment of choice. As in the case of most cancers throughout the body, the chances of cure are greatly enhanced if treatment is administered early in the course of the disease.

Meckel's diverticulum: A congenital abnormality of the small intestine which is a remnant of the simple intestinal tract of the fetus that empties through the umbilicus and usually closes at birth is known as Meckel's diverticulum. If it does not close completely, a blind alley, or pouch, forms about 20 inches from the ileocecal valve, the point where the small intestine meets the large intestine. The other end of the duct may be attached to the abdominal wall at the umbilicus, or may adhere to any part of the abdominal wall. It then acts as a band or adhesion and may cause intestinal obstruction. Acid-producing cells may occur in its wall. Eventually the accumulation of acid may cause ulceration and hemorrhage, or the duct may become acutely inflamed and produce symptoms of acute appendicitis. Treatment necessitates surgical removal of the duct. Malabsorption of food in the small intestine may cause some skin disorders such as rosaria and generalized acne. A gluten-free diet will help to clear the skin.

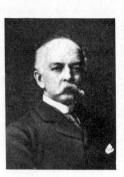

McBURNEY, Charles (1845-1913) American surgeon. Acquired fame as an authority on appendectomy, largely through improved surgical techniques and diagnostic discoveries related to the operation and the disorder. His gridiron incision for appendectomy obviated the need for cutting the abdominal muscles; instead it simply separated them. The tender pressure point on the abdomen, known as *McBurney's point*, is important in diagnosing appendicitis.

DISORDERS OF THE VERMIFORM APPENDIX

The appendix is a small blind tube attached to the cecum, at the beginning of the large intestine. *Appendicitis* is an inflammation of the appendix. The infection may be acute and lead to perforation of the appendix, or it may subside spontaneously. There may be mild recurrent attacks. Adhesions, stricture or kinking of the appendix, or obliteration of the appendiceal canal may occur as a result of infection, causing "chronic" appendicitis. The restraints placed on the proper exercise of bowel function in modern civilized communities may account for the great frequency of appendicitis. The disease is rare among nomadic tribes.

The lumen of the appendix is narrow, and the intestinal contents which pass into it contain large numbers of bacteria. Frequently when the appendix becomes blocked by particles of fecal matter, foreign bodies (such as seeds), or intestinal parasites, the circulation of blood through the appendix becomes impeded, with resulting perforation and development of localized abscess or diffuse *peritonitis* (infection of the peritoneum).

The accompanying picture series shows the details of an *appendectomy* (removal of the appendix.) (Between 456-457)

Pain, tenderness, and spasm in the right side of the abdomen are the typical symptoms of appendicitis. Other symptoms vary with the extent of the disease and the individual reaction of the patient. Nausea and vomiting are common but not invariable symptoms. There is usually slight fever, but the temperature may not become elevated for some hours after the onset of pain.

Pain may first be felt in the pit of the stomach, becoming localized subsequently in the right side of the abdomen. However, the development of the typical right-sided pain depends on the position of the appendix. If the appendix has folded beneath the cecum (termed *retrocecal*

appendix) pain may occur in the back; if it hangs down into the pelvis there may be no localized pain, the pain being diffused over the abdomen or in the pit of the stomach. When the appendix lies immediately beneath the abdominal wall, pain, spasm, and tenderness are localized in the lower right side of the abdomen. Thus, there are two types of pain in appendicitis. First, there is the pain caused by obstruction of the appendix; second, spasm and tenderness occur in localized areas when the infection reaches the overlying peritoneum.

Sudden disappearance of pain in the course of an attack of appendicitis does not mean that the infection has subsided, because recovery is a gradual process. On the contrary, it indicates an even more acute process and need of a surgical operation, because sudden cessation of pain is

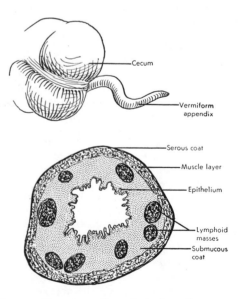

The vermiform appendix projects from the cecum as shown in this drawing. Cross-sectional drawing above shows the layers that compose its wall.

usually caused by rupture of the appendix. If operation is not performed, the abdomen will become intensely painful, with accompanying rigidity. The formation of an abscess usually results in pain, tenderness, and rigidity becoming more localized.

Crying, vomiting, and the refusal of food may be the first symptoms of appendicitis in children. Because such symptoms commonly occur from dietary indiscretions, parents may administer a laxative before consulting a physician, with the result that perforation of the appendix may be precipitated. A laxative or enema must not be given in the presence of abdominal pain without a physician's advice.

Many conditions may produce symptoms similar to those of acute appendicitis, particularly in female patients. Rupture of a cyst in the right ovary, rupture of a tubal pregnancy occurring in the right tube, or even an acute infection of the tube may produce right-sided pain, nausea, and vomiting. In both sexes and especially in children, pneumonia in the right lower lobe of the lung may irritate the diaphragm and cause spasm and tenderness of the whole right side of the abdomen. Stones and infection in the right urinary tract may also cause this type of pain. The physician can usually differentiate these conditions by various diagnostic procedures.

There is only one treatment for a patient with acute appendicitis: immediate operation as soon as the diagnosis is made. To refuse or delay operation is to invite inevitable complications and even death. Even if the patient has experienced several mild attacks of appendicitis and made an uneventful recovery from each, operation is still imperative, because a more serious infection may occur at any time.

Removal of the appendix is a simple procedure. The development of modern surgical and anesthetic techniques has reduced the mortality to a negligible figure. Even when peritonitis has occurred, the use of antibiotics has enabled the surgeon to save all but the most critical cases.

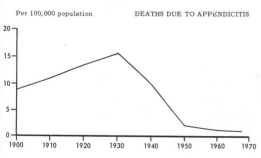

Per 100,000 population   DEATHS DUE TO APPENDICITIS

Deaths due to appendicitis, usually because of infection, have greatly decreased in the United States through the use of new antibacterial agents.

The earlier the operation is performed in the course of the disease, the more certain is the survival of the patient. Moreover, early therapy may prevent complications which demand a protracted convalescence.

DISORDERS OF THE LARGE INTESTINE

The large bowel usually exceeds five feet in length and includes the *cecum* (with the *appendix),* and the *ascending, transverse, descending,* and *sigmoid colon.* The functions of the large intestine are principally the absorption of water and salts from the material delivered into it by the small bowel, and the formation of feces, which, after concentration and storage, are excreted through the anus.

Distention

Distention or dilation of the colon is one of the most common affections of this part of the digestive tract. The distention may be caused by an accumulation of gas, an obstruction from mechanical causes, or nervous tension resulting in inhibition of the bowel's normal movement or spasm of the anal sphincter.

Gaseous distention may occur through the influence of the emotions, which upset the normal rhythmic movement of the colon. The distress caused, while uncomfortable, is not usually severe. The more severe types of distention occur as a complication of peritonitis or infectious diseases, such as pneumonia, or following abdominal operations. The distention of the bowel may be so great that breathing is hindered by pressure of the inflated bowel on the diaphragm.

Lesions that may obstruct the large bowel include: bands and adhesions; hernias; strictures caused by old scars of inflammatory processes; torsion of the loop of bowel; and tumors, including cancer. Bands, strictures, and adhesions may occur as the result of old inflammatory lesions. Although it is usually the small bowel that becomes caught in a hernia, the large bowel also may slip into such an opening.

Torsion, or twisting, of the loop of bowel around itself occurs when an unusually large loop of bowel with a long mesenteric attachment hangs freely in the abdominal cavity. When the loop of bowel becomes twisted upon itself, the blood supply is impaired. In cases in which the distention of the loop is extreme, it may be seen outlined through the intact abdominal wall. The sigmoid colon is the most common site of torsion of the large bowel.

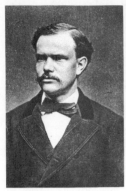

FITZ, Reginald Heber (1843-1913) American physician. Demonstrated the clinical symptoms of the inflamed vermiform appendix in 1886, and is claimed to have first used the term, "appendicitis" to designate the condition. He showed moreover that the old "inflammation of the bowel," or perityphlitis, was usually a peritonitis following appendiceal rupture. His studies on acute pancreatitis were valuable contributions to knowledge of the disease.

The treatment of patients with intestinal distention consists of application of heat to the abdomen in the milder cases, and limitation of food to fluids such as weak tea, soup, and soft eggs. A tube inserted into the rectum may facilitate the passage of gas.

In more severe cases, nothing is given by mouth. In order to remove the gas, the physician may pass a tube through the mouth, the stomach, and small bowel, down to the distended intestine. Distention secondary to complete obstruction usually requires immediate surgical intervention to remove the obstruction or uncoil and remove the twisted loop of gut.

Sometimes an extreme degree of chronic distention of the large bowel (*megacolon*) occurs in children, when there is a defect of nerve cells in the bowel wall (*Hirschsprung's disease*). This is usually present from birth or manifests itself early in life. The child is usually stunted, and the abdomen is enormous. Days or weeks may pass without a bowel movement. The condition is probably caused by a disorder of the nerves controlling the stimulation and inhibition of the intestinal muscles.

Since many serious complications can occur, treatment is best begun immediately upon diagnosis in the newborn. At this time an opening or colostomy is formed to the outside from the zone between the normal and affected colon. Later, often when the child is about two years old, a second surgical resection may then be performed for permanent correction.

Irritable bowel habits

An irritable colon is a frequent cause of abdominal distress. Such terms as "unhappy," "unstable," and "spastic" colon, and "hypertonic constipation" are used to describe this disorder. It is sometimes referred to as nervous indigestion, gastric neurosis, and intestinal neurosis. The condition is characterized by an abnormal irritability of the bowel with resultant abdominal distress and alteration of function. If there is no

organic disease present, bowel irritability may be related to some excessively irritating substance such as laxative foods, cathartics, or enemas.

Emotional upsets may be responsible for irritable bowel habits. The symptoms are often associated with psychoneuroses; symptoms develop in sensitive persons in the event of insoluble personal problems. Chronic anxiety states are a common result of such conflicts. The symptoms of functional bowel distress range from fullness and discomfort after eating or drinking to severe, cramplike abdominal pains. The pain is usually more noticeable in the lower abdomen. Ordinarily, defecation or the expulsion of flatus affords temporary relief of the symptoms. Nausea is a frequent symptom, and some individuals are not able to eat a meal of moderate proportions without experiencing an unpleasant sensation of fullness and distention. Belching, rumbling, gurgling in the abdomen, and excessive flatus are additional symptoms.

Many persons have the idea that they are constipated, when actually they are not. As a result, they form the habit of taking laxatives and enemas which cause irritable bowel symptoms. The concept that defecation should occur after a meal or that copious evacuations are necessary is unfounded, but many individuals are obsessed with notions that their bowels do not move frequently enough. In fact, many such persons subscribe to the following erroneous ideas: that the retention of waste matter in the body beyond one day is detrimental to health; that if the bowels fail to move for one day they must do something about it; that a large mushy stool or series of stools is normal and beneficial; that the colon is a sewer to be emptied as often and as thoroughly as possible; that the resting period of the bowel which follows purging is a sign of constipation and can only be cured by more

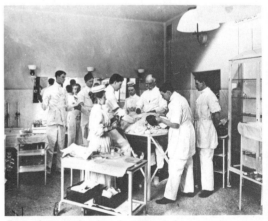

Rare photograph taken in 1901 of the operating room of Dr. Charles McBurney, who introduced new methods into diagnosis and surgery of appendicitis. Dr. McBurney is operating. *Bettmann Archive.*

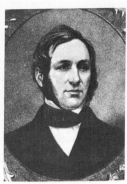

purging; and that many common symptoms, such as headache, fatigability, and vertigo, are best treated by cathartics and enemas.

A weakening of normal bowel function and the development of increasing instability in bowel habits always follow the habitual administration of laxative agents. The incidence of hemorrhoids is much greater in cathartic users than in other persons.

Headaches, fatigue, and countless other manifestations accompanying bowel distress usually have a "nervous" or "emotional" basis. A sense of weakness, sweating exhaustion, or even fainting preceding or following a bowel movement is often described by affected persons. This phenomenon resembles mild shock in particularly unstable persons.

Usually the physician's diagnosis of irritable bowel is made on the basis of the person's history of cathartic or enema habit, dietary indiscretion, emotional strain, generalized or lower abdominal distress, abnormality of the bowel habit, and tenderness along the course of the colon. A person having these symptoms may have some organic disease. This must be decided by the physician because these same symptoms could be indicative of a number of more serious conditions. Evidence of cancer of the colon can be ruled out by negative findings by x-ray examination, proctoscopy, and stool examination; however, an exploratory operation must be performed in some instances to make certain of the diagnosis. Diverticulitis and ulcerative colitis may be detected by x-ray and proctoscopic examinations. Cancer of the stomach and cancer of the pancreas may also precipitate abdominal distress. Persons with gallbladder disease may present symptoms of bowel distress.

However, most cases of irritable bowel are not the result of organic disease. As an initial step in treatment, the patient must relieve his mind of anxiety concerning any other organic disease. He should become adapted to obtaining satisfactory bowel movements without the use of laxatives or cathartics. Ordinarily, there is no

danger in waiting several days or even a week for feces to come down into the rectum.

Some persons are unable to evacuate the bowel normally because of a loss of the normal defecatory reflex. Glycerin suppositories used at regular intervals are often helpful in reestablishing the reflex; these should be used only on the advice of a physician. In patients with irritable colon, rest is of great value; but in patients with lax abdominal muscles, exercise is recommended. The amount of rest needed depends on the severity of the symptoms. When pain is severe, complete bed rest is desirable. For the average patient, long hours of sleep at night and perhaps a nap or rest period in the afternoon are adequate. The application of heat to the abdomen in the form of hot towels, an electric pad, or a hot water bottle is advisable.

The main effort should be directed toward restoration of the normal bowel function. The dietary management of bowel disturbance is based upon the varying laxative effects of different foods. Anything which stimulates peristalsis may produce spasm and disordered function in a sensitive intestine; therefore, diet must be adjusted to the sensitivity or irritability of the bowel. All foods stimulate intestinal activity and thus are laxative to a degree. There are no really constipating foods, but there are marked differences in the effects of different foods. Dietary irritants of the bowel include orange juice, bran, and coffee. The best way to manage bowel distress is to maintain a diet in which coarse, irritating, or laxative foods are avoided. Usually with this method, it is possible to establish normal bowel function within a few days and to relieve the distress, but the diet should be continued for a few weeks before returning to the normal full menu. Many persons must maintain diet restrictions permanently, if they are to live comfortably.

There is no reason for pain and distress to persist when the bowel function becomes normal. If pain does continue, then the associa-

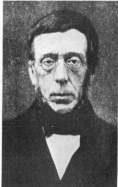

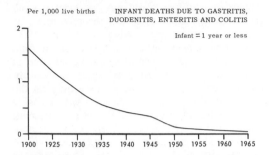

Per 1,000 live births   INFANT DEATHS DUE TO GASTRITIS, DUODENITIS, ENTERITIS AND COLITIS

Infant = 1 year or less

The number of infant deaths due to enteritis, gastritis, duodenitis and colitis has dropped over recent decades to its present low value. Better sanitation is partly responsible for decline.

tion with some other organic disease must be considered, or involvement of some emotional factor.

Tobacco is a well-recognized intestinal stimulant, poorly tolerated by some persons. Its use should be omitted when necessary, although in the majority of persons, bowel function may be regulated and bowel distress relieved regardless of tobacco usage.

The following is a list of foods and their effect in the dietary management of irritable bowel symptoms:

I. Foods causing little irritation and hence best tolerated in acute disturbances:

Water, weak tea, rice or barley gruel, meat broth, Cream of Wheat, oven-toasted bread, Zwieback or toasted soda crackers with butter, soft-cooked eggs, boiled milk, custard, plain gelatin.

II. Foods more substantial but relatively bland and easily digestible:

Cereals with milk or cream: refined rice, Rice Krispies, Puffed Rice, cornflakes, Puffed Wheat, oatmeal (well-cooked), macaroni, noodles, spaghetti, vermicelli.

Soups: consomme, strained chicken broth, strained vegetable soup, strained cream of rice soup, strained cream of potato soup, strained cream of mushroom soup.

Cheese: cream cheese, American cheese, Edam cheese, Swiss cheese, cottage cheese.

Fish: salmon, tuna, whitefish.

Fowl: chicken, turkey, squab.

Meats: broiled, boiled, roasted, or baked beef, veal, lamb, ham, liver.

Potatoes: baked, mashed, or au gratin.

Breads: white bread, toast, croutons, whole-wheat breads, bread sticks, milk toast, hot biscuits of white flour, hot rolls.

Milk products: milk, eggnog, butter, cream, cocoa.

Other beverages: tea, coffee, Sanka, Postum (laxative to some persons).

Desserts: vanilla custard, floating island, rice custard, caramel custard, angel food cake, cream puffs, eclairs, ice box cake, bread pudding, ice cream, snow pudding, chocolate, tapioca pudding, cornstarch pudding, Spanish cream, plain cake, lady fingers, sponge cake, Boston cream pie, custard, plain jello, Bavarian cream, cottage pudding.

Pies: lemon cream, banana cream, cocoanut cream.

III. Cooked vegetables, more laxative chiefly because of greater residue:

A. Moderately irritating: asparagus, string beans, carrots, beats, spinach, sweet potatoes, peas.

B. More irritating: artichokes, parsnips, onions, cabbage, cauliflower, broccoli, squash, corn, rutabaga, eggplant, green peppers, turnips, kohlrabi, navy beans, lima beans.

IV. Cooked fruit, more laxative because of chemical irritants: prunes, peaches, apricots, rhubarb, tomatoes, pears, pineapples, plums, fruit pies, grapes, figs, cherries, applesauce, baked apples, berries of all kinds.

V. Raw vegetables, more laxative: Lettuce, celery, watercress, endive, tomatoes, radishes, onions, cabbage, cucumbers.

VI. Raw fruits, more laxative: Bananas (least laxative), oranges (juice, sections, whole), grapefruit (juice, sections, whole), apples, melons, pineapples, avocados, grapes, plums, apricots, berries, pears, peaches, cherries.

Diarrhea

The term *diarrhea* means the passage of watery, unformed stools, but without the presence of blood and pus. When blood and pus are present in the stool, the term "dysentery" is used. This is generally due to a specific infection. Diarrhea may be either acute or *chronic,* and is present in so many disorders that a thorough investigation of the whole body by a physician is necessary in order to establish the correct diagnosis and treatment.

Attacks of *acute diarrhea* last only from one

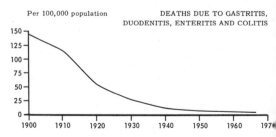

Per 100,000 population   DEATHS DUE TO GASTRITIS, DUODENITIS, ENTERITIS AND COLITIS

The importance of these diseases as a cause of death in the United States has become negligible, due to improved sanitation and methods of treatment.

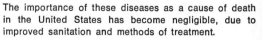

to three days, and are characterized by the passage of watery stools—sometimes three or four and sometimes 15 to 20 in a day—distressing and ineffectual straining at stool, abdominal cramps, and often nausea and vomiting.

The stools may be light brown, gray, or green in color. They usually have a foul odor and are often flecked with mucus. The vomiting and abdominal cramps usually subside after the first day. There may be mild fever during the attack, the temperature usually not rising more than a degree or two. There are present, however, varying degrees of collapse and prostration, and occasionally these are severe.

Until the physician arrives, the patient should be kept in bed; rest is of great importance in treatment. Hot water bottles or heating pads applied to the abdomen are comforting. Calomel and castor oil are omitted, as are enemas and irrigations, because the irritating substance causing the attack is swept out of the bowels by the diarrhea. If a purge is given, a complete cessation of bowel movements for one or two days frequently results, retarding the return of normal bowel function.

When the nausea and vomiting have subsided, such liquids as hot water, weak tea, broth, or barley gruel usually will be allowed. Later, boiled rice, toast, custard, and soft-cooked eggs will be given when the patient's desire for food has returned.

The cause of many cases of simple acute diarrhea is not always discovered. Infections, poor sanitation, poisoning, and nonspecific infections are contributing factors in various instances. If, however, acute diarrhea occurs frequently and without apparent cause, the influence of nervous and emotional factors should be investigated. Some people have diarrhea on a day before they are to make a public speech. A tendency to nervous diarrhea is thought by some investigators to be inherited, and has actually been observed in experimental breeding in rats.

Chronic diarrhea, uncomplicated by specific organic disease, has become recognized as an important symptom of emotional disorder. The constant expectation of frequent, large bowel movements may become the individual's major concern, and can even result in inability to carry on daily work.

Episodes of diarrhea may often be identified with dietary indiscretions; more often they may be traced to emotional tension. An understanding by the patient of the relation between his symptoms and his worries may lead to the relief of chronic diarrhea. This might require that the patient keep some sort of a daily record of his symptoms and his emotional crises.

While the cause of many attacks of diarrhea may not be discovered, all cases of acute diarrhea must be regarded with suspicion by the physician. Diarrhea may be the first indication of poisoning by arsenic, mercury, silver salts, and other inorganic poisons. Addison's disease, thyrotoxicosis, chronic nephritis, and cirrhosis of the liver may cause diarrhea. Benign or malignant tumors of the stomach, pancreas, or intestine may cause diarrhea. Increased production of the hormone, *adrenalin,* by the adrenal glands during times of stress or fright may so alter the muscle tone of the gut that diarrhea results.

Management of diarrhea, when a specific cause has been determined and corrected, requires a thorough study of any accompanying emotional disturbance. Often diarrhea can be controlled by the elimination of fat from the diet, or of other foods such as strawberries, shellfish, and eggs, to which the individual may have become sensitive. Diet control alone, however, is not always sufficient to effect a cure of diarrhea. Rather, dietary control must be related to and based upon the particular condition that causes the diarrhea in the individual.

Constipation

A person is said to be constipated when the feces become unduly hard and dry and some difficulty is experienced in the act of defecation. Although the term *constipation* is often applied when daily evacuation does not take place, this is not truly constipation, as there may be a good physiological reason for the bowel to rest. Also, some individuals in the best of health defecate only, one, two, or three times a week. In true constipation, the ease and sense of completeness of evacuation of the rectum and lower part of the colon is lacking.

Constipation is more common among women than men. Habitual constipation occurs in young adults and becomes established in their twenties. Although practically half the population will give a history of constipation at some time, x-ray studies have shown that true constipation is not as frequent as imagined.

Many factors may be responsible for, or contribute toward, the production of constipation. Apart from obvious gross mechanical obstruction—caused by tumor, adhesive bands, or stric-

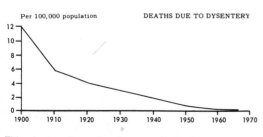

Per 100,000 population   DEATHS DUE TO DYSENTERY

This chart portrays the decrease in deaths per 100,000 population in the United States due to dysentery, during the period between 1900 and 1968.

tures—constipation may be caused by habit, diet, or the state of the muscles of the bowel.

The act of defecation can be readily inhibited by an effort of the will, and a habit of refusing to respond to the urge to defecate is a common cause of constipation. The sensation of a full rectum usually occurs regularly at some definite time each day, and refusal to respond causes the desire to defecate to pass. The rectum becomes accustomed to the increased fecal bulk and there is retention of feces in the distal colon and rectum. This leads to excessive absorption of fluid; hence, the feces becomes dry, hard, and less easily expelled.

As a result of continued overloading, the bowel musculature becomes sluggish in its action, and thinning and lack of tone may result. Properly regulated habits, rather than purgatives, are more likely to correct this type of constipation.

The diet may be responsible for constipation when it contains too little of undigestible residue, or roughage, which normally stimulates intestinal activity, or when the diet is not fluid enough. The times at which meals are taken are also important, because regular meals stimulate regular emptying of the large bowel.

Senility, obesity, lesions of the central nervous system, and generalized disease may rob intestinal muscles of their normal reactivity so that the propulsive mechanism of the bowel may not function efficiently. A diet low in calcium, potassium, or vitamin B, also may cause this condition.

A segment of the large bowel may be the site of muscular spasm and cause only spasmodic contractions which have little value in moving the feces onward. Such a contracted bowel may be felt through the abdominal wall as a thick cord. This type of spasm may be caused by disease of the gallbladder, duodenum, or appendix, or it may be the result of overwork, worry, or shock.

Certain individuals are born with abnormally long colons and this condition may be accompanied by constipation. Passage of material is naturally slower through a greater length of bowel and there is more opportunity for fluid absorption. Individuals with this congenital abnormality may have the desire to defecate only once or twice a week. Distention of the elongated bowel occurs, and pressure on other parts of the bowel, bladder, or blood vessels results. Heartburn, fullness, or belching may accompany constipation.

Hemorrhoids or fissures of the anus may aggravate constipation because of the pain that occurs with every bowel action. Since the hemorrhoids or the fissures may have been initially caused by constipation, a vicious cycle may be set up which is relieved only with cure of the anal lesion.

Constipation is usually relieved by adequate amounts of laxative foods in the diet. Foods which stimulate bowel action are fats, fruits, vegetables, and coarse cereals. Fruits contain a high proportion of undigestible cellulose, as well as sugars, acids, and salts which have a chemically stimulating effect on the bowel. Undigested fat supplies a mild lubrication to the feces, while partially digested fats are mildly irritating and activate the bowels.

Patients with stubborn cases of constipation should consult their physicians, as each case will need individualized treatment. Proper diet, adequate fluids, routine habits, and the use of brewer's yeast, mineral oil, suppositories of glycerin or wetting agents, and enemas are some of the means available to them for re-establishing the defecatory reflex.

Ulcerative colitis

Ulcers may form in the colon as the result of invasion by bacteria or parasites, but the cause of the most common form of *ulcerative colitis* usually cannot be determined. Certain deficiencies and personality disorders may have some influence in causing the disease.

The symptoms of ulcerative colitis may vary from the painless passage of blood with each stool to dysentery and fever, with death resulting from exhaustion, perforation of the colon, and generalized peritonitis. The less severe cases recover completely. Frequently, periods of remission alternate with periods of relapse. Occasionally, the disease becomes chronic, with the passage of several bloody stools daily, but without causing severe disability. In these patients, the colon becomes a scarred tube, thickened with ulcerations throughout its length. At this stage, complications are frequent, and nutritional deficiencies, intestinal obstruction, perforations and malignant disease may occur. Ulcerative colitis is sometimes found in children. Surgical intervention is usually required to prevent perforation of the bowel and physical retardation. Emotional disturbances do not appear to be a factor in this childhood ulcer.

The treatment of patients with ulcerative colitis is persevering medical supervision, providing for rest in bed, diet control, sedatives, blood transfusions when necessary, and control of infections. Cortisone, ACTH, nonabsorbable sulfonamides, and new antibacterial agents have proved of value in some cases. Occasionally, surgical removal of the colon becomes necessary when the disease proves resistant to medical treatment or complications develop. If emotional factors are thought to have any role in causing the disease, the patient probably should receive psychotherapy.

Diverticula

Small pouches or pockets (*diverticula*) often occur in the walls of the large intestines in older persons, and are most frequently found in the descending and sigmoid colon. They are formed by a spreading of the muscular coat of the bowel wall at the point of passage of a blood vessel, which causes the inner lining of the bowel to protrude through the wall as a blind pocket. Infection of these diverticula (*diverticulitis*) occurs in a small percentage of cases; usually, the diverticula cause no untoward symptoms. When diverticulitis occurs, however, the infection may be chronic, mild, or severe. An abscess may be formed with resultant localized peritonitis, and even perforation may result. The bowel may develop spasm, or obstruction may develop as a result of the inflammation. The symptoms of diverticulitis are cramplike pains in the lower abdomen with tenderness and perhaps spasm of the muscles of the abdominal wall in the left quadrant, very similar to the right-sided pain experienced by the patient with appendicitis.

Treatment of mild cases consists of rest in bed with heat applied to the abdomen, supplemented by dietary and medicinal control of the bowels, chemotherapy, and intestinal antiseptics. If the abscess causes obstruction or perforation, surgical side-tracking or removal of the affected portion of the colon may be required.

Tumor

Both benign and malignant tumors occur in the large intestine. Indeed, nearly half of all tumors of the digestive tract occur in this region. Benign *polyps* of glandular or fatty tissue occur frequently in persons past middle age, and chronic infection of the bowel may play a part in formation of these small, pendulous tumors. Polyps may or may not be cancers, and usually cause no symptoms unless they become ulcerated and bleed, or encroach on the lumen of the bowel, and cause obstruction. In such instances, the polyps cause the same reaction as foreign bodies, causing contractions of the bowel. As a result, a segment of the bowel may become pushed into an adjacent segment, a process known as *intussusception.*

Sometimes a diffuse area of multiple polyps is discovered in the large bowel of an adolescent. In many such cases, the polyps probably have been present since birth, perhaps as an inherited defect. Cramping pains in the lower abdomen, diarrhea, hemorrhage from the bowel, and the passage of mucus are frequent symptoms. The treatment of patients with benign tumors is surgical excision of the area, because there is danger that one or several of the polyps eventually will become malignant.

Malignant tumors of the large bowel are among the most frequent cancers occurring in the body. The right and left sides of the colon have different functions; the right side absorbs fluids and salts; the left side stores feces. Cancer occurring in the right half of the bowel usually spreads up the bowel wall; cancer of the left side tends to encircle the bowel. Cancers of the right side disturb function, but seldom cause obstruction; however, obstruction is a common feature of left-sided growths. Surgical removal is the only method of treatment for patients with cancers of the large bowel, and few locations in the body respond with such good results. It is imperative, however, that these lesions be diagnosed and that adequate surgical resection be done while the growth is still confined to the colon.

Intestinal parasites

Lower forms of animal life may invade and live in the digestive tract of man. At times they produce acute distress such as the passage of bloody stools mixed with mucus, or a chronic draining of vitality. At other times the parasite may live with its host without producing symptoms; in such cases the infected individual serves as the reservoir of infestation for those around him. The effect produced depends upon the number and virulence of the parasites and the natural resistance of the host to the toxins of the organism.

Intestinal parasites may be single-celled organisms (*protozoa*) or multicellular (*metazoa*). The most important single-celled parasite is

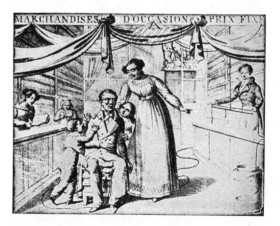

Old French lithograph carrying a humorous suggestion that especially long tapeworms might be sold to stores as wrapping cord. *Bettmann Archive.*

called *Endamoeba histolytica*. It causes amebic dysentery and amebic colitis. The multicellular organisms may be flat worms, such as flukes and tapeworms, or round worms, such as pinworms.

Protozoan parasites: It has been estimated that from 1.5 to ten percent of the population of the United States are infested with *Endamoeba histolytica*. The organisms are taken into the body in contaminated food and drink, and naturally the chance of contracting amebic dysentery or amebic colitis is greatest in districts having poor sanitary conditions. The disease is more frequent in hot than in cold or temperate climates. Although the number of people infested tends to be fairly constant in any one locality, sudden epidemics do occur from time to time. The most shocking epidemic on record occurred in a hotel in Chicago in 1933 when there were 1,050 cases and 70 deaths. The cause of the outbreak was found to be a plumbing defect through which sewage seeped into the water system. Modern sewage methods avoid such catastrophies. The sewage of the average city is either disposed of several miles from the water supplies or is completely decontaminated and used in industry and agriculture. For further details, see Chapter 25, "Sanitation."

The amebae are able to exist in an encysted form which has much greater resistance to external conditions than have the mobile forms. The cysts may survive in cool damp places for as long as three months, while the mobile forms die quickly outside the body. The organism enters the body as a cyst, and the tough shell around the cyst passes through the stomach and upper portion of the small bowel and dissolves in the lower portion of the small bowel, thus liberating a mobile organism. This organism passes into the large bowel and the appendix, makes a breach in the lining membrane, and then burrows into the soft submucous tissues, forming a "button-hole" ulcer. There the organisms divide and multiply, with some of them being propelled into the lumen of the large bowel. Here they are rapidly reconverted into the cystic form. When they reach the exterior with the feces, they have a good chance of surviving long enough to be picked up in the food of another host and there continue the life cycle.

The ulcers formed by the amebae may be small and discrete, or they may spread and merge with resultant sloughing of the intestinal lining and hemorrhage. The symptoms may be mild—some constipation, nausea, decline in appetite, gas, and abdominal cramps. Sometimes there may be no symptoms other than a feeling of fatigue and depression. Diarrhea usually occurs only after excesses of eating or drinking.

When the organisms spread throughout the wall of the bowel, however, diarrhea results and becomes severe, with up to 15 bloody stools in 24 hours; there is great weakness and prostration, vomiting, and right-sided abdominal pain. There is little or no fever. Recovery takes place slowly and the disease may become chronic, with occasional increased severity of the diarrhea and anemia interspersed with the passage of frequent stools. The organisms may find their way to the liver and lungs, and form abscesses there if the disease is not cured.

Amebic dysentery, as the disease is popularly known, is diagnosed by examining the stools under the microscope and identifying the amebae. Dysentery may be difficult to control and treatment must be frequently repeated. One method of treatment consists of giving iodine-containing compounds for eight to ten days after an initial dose of castor oil, with a diet of milk and milk foods until the acute phase of the disease has passed. Emetine hydrochloride, carbarsone and terramycin are usually prescribed in treatment. If organisms have found their way to the liver or lungs, chloroquine is the drug of choice.

Since the cysts of amebae may be present on fruit or vegetables, be carried by flies or cockroaches, or have infested the water in unsanitary areas, travelers would do well to avoid any water which has not been boiled, to avoid raw fruits and vegetables, except those which can be peeled at the table, and to guard against flies in these areas. Especially should these precautions be taken when traveling in countries where human manure is used. Endamoeba histolytica is further discussed in Chapter 4, "Disease Producing Organisms."

Another protozoan parasite, *Balantidium coli*, occasionally infests the digestive tract. This parasite occurs wherever its natural host, the pig, is found, and it causes an infection similar to that caused by Endamoeba histolytica. It is similar in appearance to Endamoeba, but has numerous rows of short thread-like processes (*cilia*), which serve as a means of propulsion, like the banks of oars in a Roman galley. The disease is usually milder than the amebic infection, but severe diarrhea may occur. Because this organism is present in the feces of practically every pig, pig feces should never be used as fertilizer, and pigs should not be allowed near any wells or springs which serve as a drinking supply for man. *Escherichia coli*, an intestinal bacterium, can cause diarrhea in infants. It is often transmitted by household pets.

Metazoan parasites: Metazoan parasites are multicellular organisms, in contrast to the single-celled protozoa. Several hundred are known to infest man, but only a few are important. Most important as intestinal parasites are certain of the roundworms and flatworms. The roundworms include *Ancylostoma duodenale* and *Necator americanus*, both of which are hookworms; *Trichinella spiralis*, which causes *trichinosis*; *Ascaris*, the largest of the roundworms;

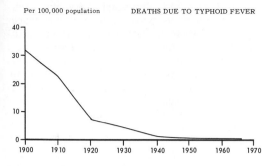

Per 100,000 population   DEATHS DUE TO TYPHOID FEVER

Immunization and other improved sanitation procedures have virtually eliminated typhoid fever as a cause of death within the United States.

and *Enterobius vermicularis*, the pinworm. The flatworms include the tapeworms and the flukes. These forms are discussed in Chapter 4, "Disease Producing Organisms: *Animal Parasites*." Aside from these species, mention might be made of the whipworms (*Trichuris trichiura*) which may infest the cecum and appendix of children. In severe infestations almost the whole bowel will be involved. In mild infestations, with few worms, there may be no symptoms. Occasionally children are very sensitive to the infestation, and loss of appetite, sleeplessness, and nervousness with convulsions may result.

The worms can be removed from the digestive system by certain drugs. Prevention of the disease can be obtained by careful personal hygiene and avoidance of contaminating food with infested soil.

Strongyloidiasis is caused by a delicate threadworm (*Strongyloides stercoralis*), which thrives in a hot, moist climate. The male threadworm is superficially attached to the wall of the upper bowel, but the female becomes embedded in the wall and lays eggs which hatch there. The hatched larvae enter the lumen of the bowel and are passed to the exterior with the feces. Their distribution is similar to that of the hookworm.

Infestation of the human host occurs when the larvae penetrate the skin from infested ground, gain entrance to the blood, and travel to the blood vessels of the digestive tract after traversing the lungs. Pain in the pit of the stomach and dull headache are common, and the sufferer tends to undergo periods of despondency. If the parasite becomes trapped in the lungs, there may be paroxysmal cough, with blood-tinged sputum.

Although *strongyloidiasis* may be cured by the administration of certain drugs, it is almost certain to recur if preventive measures are not taken. Prevention of the disease may be accomplished by avoiding walking barefoot on infested ground, and the proper disposal of infested feces.

Typhoid fever

With the advent of modern sanitary practices, particularly with reference to the control of food and water-borne diseases, some of the world's most devastating diseases have been virtually eradicated. Particularly is this true of typhoid fever and cholera; in communities that have adequate sanitation, these diseases are seldom observed. In more backward regions, however, they still exact a heavy toll of life.

At the turn of the century typhoid fever was responsible for an untold number of deaths. Occasional cases still occur, either sporadically in small groups, or singly.

Typhoid fever is caused by the bacillus *Salmonella typhosa*. It differs from other Salmonella organisms, such as those responsible for certain food poisonings. The organism is contained in the products of excretion. The bacilli can exist after leaving the body, but they do not multiply. Infected persons occasionally continue to excrete bacilli in the stools for years after they have recovered from the disease, and the perpetuation of typhoid fever is aided by these healthy carriers. Sewage contamination of water or shellfish, or direct contamination of uncooked foods by the soiled hands of a carrier cause many outbreaks of typhoid fever. Flies also may carry the organism from feces to food.

The organisms enter the body through the mouth. By invading the lymphoid tissue in some part of the digestive tract, usually the small intestine, they are carried to lymph nodes in the abdomen. Here they multiply and enter the blood stream. They usually are found in heaviest concentration in the biliary tract. They are also found in the lymph nodes, spleen, lungs, bone marrow, and liver. One attack of typhoid fever usually makes the infected person immune for life.

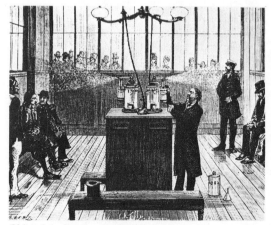

Old print showing a disinfection chamber at Lyons, France, for travelers coming from the cholera areas of Toulon and Marseilles. *Bettmann Archive.*

The onset of typhoid fever is rather gradual, causing the person to feel generally ill and feverish. Headache accompanied by a nonproductive cough may be the first notable symptom. The fever may be higher each day, reaching 102° to 105° Fahrenheit by about the third week. Chills and sweats usually are present, as well as periods of delirium. Loss of appetite, nausea, nosebleed, vomiting, and constipation are also frequent symptoms. A blank, staring expression is a common manifestation. Diarrhea may be present and several watery, grayish, or greenish stools may be passed each day. The fever finally reaches a high level, where it remains for a week or two; then it begins to subside. In about 30 days, if the patient survives, a normal temperature is reached. A rash ("rose spots") appears during the second and third week and is seldom generalized. Often less than a dozen spots can be seen at a time, principally on the trunk, upper abdomen, and lower chest. At the height of the illness, abdominal swelling and generalized abdominal tenderness are present. All the effects subside as the fever diminishes, and by the time the temperature has returned to normal the other symptoms also have usually disappeared. It is a most devastating disease, but not hopeless with modern methods of therapy. Treatment with *chloramphenicol* has proved effective. The nursing care is extremely important in obtaining recovery.

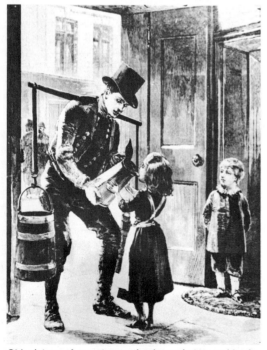

Old picture of a water carrier in a cholera epidemic, an unwitting spreader of cholera through unsanitary drinking vessels. *Bettmann Archive.*

One of the most important preventive measures in controlling typhoid—other than proper sanitary handling of water and sewage in a community—is to eliminate the handling of food by persons who might be carriers; and all persons in their households should be immunized. Chloramphenicol, used in treating the disease, is not effective against the carrier state. In some instances penicillin will clear up the condition, but often surgical removal of the gallbladder is necessary to reduce the chances of transmission of the disease by a carrier.

Vaccination for typhoid fever is both practical and effective. Except with unusual exposure, immunity is reasonably sure for twelve months and generally lasts for a number of years. However, strict sanitation measures should not be relaxed.

Cholera

This is an acute infectious disease, caused by the ingestion of food or drink contaminated by feces which contain the organism, *Vibrio comma.* The digestive tract is the principal site of infection. In the United States, cholera is no longer a serious problem, even though it occurs more or less constantly (is *endemic*) in many parts of the world. In the United States, deaths from cholera are extremely rare. The effects of extreme dehydration in cholera cause the features to become gaunt and pinched and the eyes to appear sunken. The skin becomes bluish and in some places, such as on the fingers, it becomes shriveled. Cholera strikes its victim suddenly and the speed with which the symptoms attain overwhelming proportions is amazing. Voluminous, watery stools passed with great frequency, copious vomiting, and severe prostration are characteristic. Almost nothing that is taken by mouth can be retained, and great thirst is experienced by the patient, as the loss of fluid increases. There may be generalized and painful muscular cramps.

Procedures of strict isolation should be followed for both patients and proved carriers. Clothing, bedding, and eating utensils should be disinfected. As in typhoid fever, stools, vomitus, and urine should be thoroughly disinfected. Prompt replacement of water loss is essential. Failure to recognize this or delay in action may result in fatality. To prevent and control cholera, it is essential that isolation measures be enforced. Strict control of the water supply, food, food handling, and flies is necessary. If the water supply is not subject to general control, drinking water should be boiled and chlorinated. Raw foods should not be eaten in choleraic areas and all food should be protected from flies. Vaccination provides only partial immunity.

DISORDERS OF THE RECTUM AND ANUS

The rectum and anal canal combined are about six to eight inches in length and form the terminal portion of the digestive tract. Foreign bodies are particularly likely to become lodged in the rectum, whether they are swallowed or introduced through the anus, because powerful sphincter muscles are present to close the lower part of the anal canal. The presence of a foreign body in the rectum will cause constipation or diarrhea, the passage of mucus and blood, muscular straining and pain. When the rectum is not ruptured, the surgeon exerts every effort to remove the object through the anus, because the risk of infection is greater if the abdomen has to be opened.

Cancer of the rectum

The rectum is a common site of cancer of the gastrointestinal tract. More men than women develop cancer of the rectum, and the disease usually occurs after middle age.

As in the case of most cancer, the cause of cancer of the rectum is unknown. Polyps may occur in the rectum, just as elsewhere in the large bowel, and may predispose the patient to the development of cancer. Constipation is not considered a factor.

The most frequent symptoms of rectal cancer are bleeding, irregular bowel actions, frequent urge to defecate, and pain. It is common for patients with these symptoms to delay for a long time in seeking medical advice. The success of treatment is jeopardized by such delay, because the cancer may have spread through the wall of the intestine, involved other organs, or spread to neighboring and distant lymph nodes.

The blood which appears is generally bright red, and may be mixed with the stool or simply form streaks in it. Change of bowel habit may

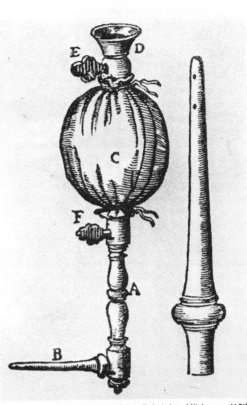

Enema apparatus designed by Fabricius Hildanus (16th century) showing the water bag and anal insertion tip. *Copyright 1944, CIBA SYMPOSIA.*

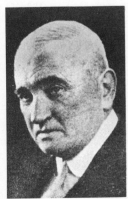

MILES, William Ernest (1869-1947) English surgeon. Miles contributed a method of performing an abdominoperineal excision for cancer of the rectum and lower portion of the colon. Introduced in 1907, it has become the method of choice throughout the world. This complete and radical removal offers the best chance for cure without recurrence. Miles also investigated the ways in which rectal cancer spreads, and its control by surgery.

be slight, but is usually persistent. Diarrhea may vary from mild irritation of the bowel to the passage of eight to ten stools daily. Constipation caused by rectal cancer may be masked by the taking of purgatives. Pain is not present in all cases; in fact, it usually develops only when the cancer has become advanced and is causing partial obstruction to the passage of feces or when it occurs next to and involves the dentate margin of the anal canal. Loss of weight or strength does not occur until late in the course of the disease. Cancer of the rectum can easily be diagnosed by the physician. Examination of the rectum with the gloved finger may suffice to establish diagnosis, or the physician may use a special instrument (*proctoscope*) which permits the interior of the rectum to be observed.

Treatment is surgical excision of the rectum and anal canal, an artificial anus (*colostomy*) being established in the abdominal wall. Less drastic operations in which the anus and anal sphincter are preserved are yielding encouraging results.

The prospect of an abdominal anus may seem repugnant. However, when it is realized that such an anus allows a normal, comfortable, useful, and profitable existence, the abhorrence of

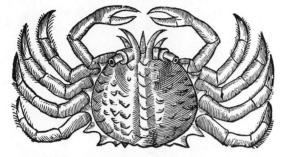

One of the earliest uses of the illustration of the crab to symbolize cancer. This picture appeared in a text-book of surgery, published in 1634. *Courtesy of Universiteits-Bibliotheek, Amsterdam.*

the procedure can be overcome. A part of the secret of comfortable living with a colostomy is the careful management of diet and the empty-ing of the colon. This should be done at regular intervals. After irrigation, the area is cleansed and covered with vaseline, aluminum paste, or a plastic or silicon spray, and a gauze pad. Various types of bags may be attached with special water-proof adhesives. Evacuation of the bowel once or twice daily can be achieved by eating a suitable diet. Usually a constipating type of diet is required during the first six months after the operation. After that, the diet can be broad-ened somewhat, but foods which irritate the colon should always be avoided.

A colostomy is, in reality, an artificial fistula. Other such artificial fistulae may be surgically constructed for relief of obstruction or for other reasons. They are called by a prefix representing the area involved plus the ending "ostomy" (Greek for "opening"). Examples are gastros-tomy, jejunostomy, ileostomy, etc.

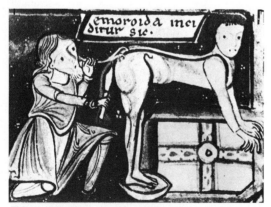

This painting from an eleventh century manuscript por-trays methods then used for treatment of patients with hemorrhoids. *Bettmann Archive.*

Cancer of the anus

Anal cancer is rare in comparison with can-cer of the rectum and usually arises in the skin surrounding the anal opening or in the anal canal itself. In many instances in which the can-cer is confined to the skin, it may be possible to treat the lesion with radium needles implanted under it or by x-ray therapy or a simple oper-ation. If the cancer has begun to spread, then radical surgical measures are usually necessary. Invasion of the rectum by an anal growth usually infers longstanding neglect of the tumor. The negligence of patients in seeking medical at-tention for such an obvious tumor is lamentable. Recognition of anal cancer while it is still in an early stage of development, followed by proper treatment by the physician, may save the patient from an extensive operation, and may even save his life.

Imperforate anus

Failure of the anus to develop, resulting in the rectum ending blindly in the pelvis or connecting with the bladder or vagina, occurs once in every 5,000 births. The occlusion is known as *imper-forate anus* and may vary from a thin diaphragm to occlusion of the entire anal canal and rectum. The problem may be solved by a simple pro-cedure or it may require an extensive corrective operation.

Anal fissures, abscesses, and fistulae

Infection of the anus is the cause of anal *fis-sure*, hemorrhoids, *abscess*, and *fistula*, and is usually the result of invasion of the numerous tiny glands or crypts, which abound in the tis-sues adjacent to the anus. If the infection is not checked, either by the natural resistance of the body or by treatment, the infection may spread into the surrounding tissues.

An anal fissure is an ulcer of the anal canal. It appears as a crack in the skin usually at the anal margin. The ulcer is increased by the act of defecation. The pain may last for a few min-utes or several hours.

Although relief from the pain of an anal fis-sure may be obtained from hot baths and anes-thetic ointments, the cure for the persistent condition is the alleviation of the infection and excision of the ulcer by surgical operation.

If the infection spreads through the wall of the anus, an abscess may occur in the tissues around the anus, and this may burst through the skin around the anus or back into the rectum. In either case, the abscess cavity has two openings—the original site of entry of the in-fection and the point where it bursts through.

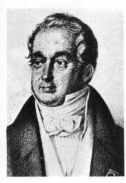

DUPUYTREN, Guillaume (1777-1835), French surgeon. In 1828, he devised an operation using his instrument, the enterotome, for making an artificial anus. Considered to be one of the greatest of the early vascular surgeons, Dupuytren ligated the external iliac artery and the subclavian artery during the early part of the 19th century. He was also an orthopedic surgeon.

PHYSICK, Philip Syng (1768-1837) American surgeon. First American physician to use the stomach pump, which he introduced into America in 1805. Another important contribution relating to the alimentary canal was his development of an operation by which an artificial anus (1826) was constructed. Often called the "Father of American Surgery," he pioneered the use of absorbable animal ligatures.

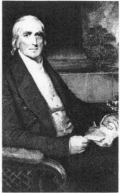

Fistula is the term by which such a condition is designated.

The symptoms of an acute abscess—redness, local heat, swelling, and tenderness—usually cause the patient to seek medical aid. However, when the abscess bursts, the tension and pain are relieved, and the visit to the physician is sometimes erroneously postponed. A chronic discharging fistula is formed. Both the gland in which the infection originated and the infected tract must be removed once the infection is under control.

Hemorrhoids

Hemorrhoids, or "piles," are tender, painful, bluish, localized swellings which appear at the anal margin, frequently after abnormal function of the bowel or strenuous work. They are varicose veins infected by material from the anus. The veins may become filled with blood clots (thrombosed) which cause pain, bleeding, and protrusion. Hemorrhoids are classified as external (covered with skin and outside the sphincter muscle) or internal (covered with mucous membrane and protruding through the sphincter). Infection of the overlying skin or mucous membrane may occur and there may be sloughing of the area. The anal sphincter may be constricted.

The palliative treatment of a patient with acute hemorrhoids is usually the application of cold wet packs, avoidance of heavy labor, and correction of constipation. Chronic hemorrhoids may be relieved by injection therapy. Rubber bands are sometimes used to tie up internal hemorrhoids. These procedures, however, may only postpone curative measures. When hemorrhoids are large and of long duration, surgical removal will have to be undertaken for permanent relief.

Anal pruritus

Itching, smarting, or burning of the anal region (*anal pruritus*) may be caused by hemorrhoids or by infection. There are many people, however, who suffer from these symptoms without a demonstrable cause. Usually, they are young to middle-aged, tense, and nervous individuals. The itching may vary in intensity, but it is usually worse at night or whenever the individual is laboring under nervous tension. Sleep may be disrupted, and often the sufferers will scratch themselves until they have drawn blood. Anal pruritus is more common in men than in women.

The treatment of a patient with anal pruritus usually is unsatisfactory. Where an underlying disease such as eczema, diabetes mellitus, allergy, psoriasis, or hemorrhoids has been discovered, correction of the condition may help. However, where the pruritus is aggravated by emotional factors, cure is difficult. The patient may require the combined services of a surgeon, dermatologist, and psychiatrist. The use of x-ray therapy may give temporary relief, but such treatment is usually avoided because repeated courses of x-ray therapy may damage the anal skin.

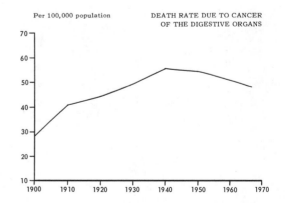

This graph shows the increase in the death rate in the United States from cancer of the digestive organs during the period from 1900 to 1966.

IRRIGATION OF A COLOSTOMY

Cancer of the rectum frequently necessitates surgical resection of the rectum and the creation of a permanent artificial anus in the anterior abdominal wall (colostomy). One of the major problems that colostomy patients face is the psychological effect of loss of control over bowel movements, and the difficulties that this presents to normal social activities. Regular irrigation of the bowel at suitable intervals provides a solution to these problems and eventually makes it possible for the patient to return to a normal life. Pictures copyrighted 1952, The Medical Arts Publishing Foundation.

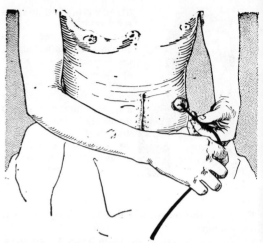

1. Insertion of a catheter and irrigation should be as simple for the patient as the giving of an enema, once the patient has been trained.

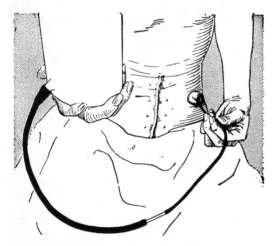

2. After the tube is inserted a few inches into the stoma, the bucket containing the water is lifted up to start the flow of water into the bowel.

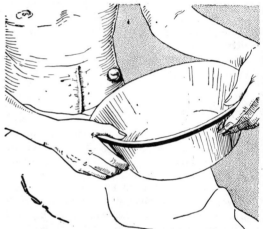

3. When the prescribed amount of water has entered the bowel, the tube is removed and discharge is caught in pan held against abdomen.

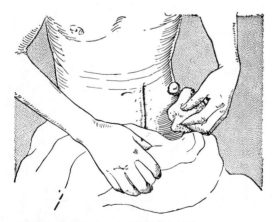

4. After drainage from the bowel, the patient should cleanse the area around the stoma with a gauze pad soaked in weak antiseptic solution.

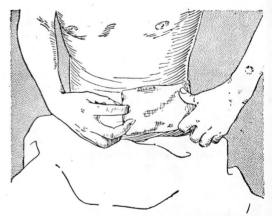

5. A gauze pad rather than a bag is preferred for protection against spillage because pad is disposable, easily replaced, and allows more freedom.

DISORDERS OF THE LIVER

The liver is the largest gland in the body and is absolutely essential to life. It stores the products of digestion and transforms the foodstuffs into complex tissue elements, while it also breaks down complex substances into simpler ones for the production of energy. In addition, to list only a few of its other functions, the liver detoxifies certain poisons, forms and secretes bile, and partly regulates the volume of blood in the body.

Sugar (*glucose*) taken into the body as food is brought to the liver and stored there as *glycogen*; then, during a period when no food is being taken into the body, the liver sets free part of its store of glycogen, converts it back to glucose, and releases the glucose into the blood stream, where it is taken up by the muscles and used as fuel for energy. As a rule, the liver contains enough glycogen to supply a normal amount of energy during a 12-to-24 hour fast, depending on the amount of physical exertion that is undertaken.

When the muscles perform work and use up the glucose, lactic acid is produced and enters the blood stream. The lactic acid is then taken to the liver where it is converted into glycogen, stored, and eventually returns as glucose to the muscles.

There are, of course, sugars other than glucose in food, and normally they are taken to the liver, converted into glycogen and released as glucose whenever necessary. *Galactose* is such a sugar. If the liver is diseased, then galactose may not be converted into glycogen and will enter the blood stream unchanged, to be excreted by the kidneys as waste. The finding of galactose in the urine may, therefore, be an indication of liver disease.

The liver can also make glucose from the proteins of meat, milk, and vegetables; and so it plays a most important part in maintaining the amount of sugar in the blood at its proper level.

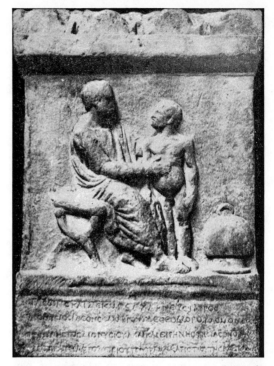

This photograph of an Athens tombstone shows the Greek physician Jason feeling the liver of a patient as a diagnostic measure. *Bettmann Archive.*

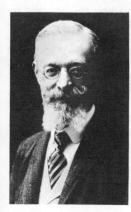

BANTI, G. (1852-1925) Italian physician. Remembered for his splendid description in 1882 of the splenomegaly which bears his name. This disease of undetermined origin is often referred to as a syndrome, evidenced by a complex of symptoms, including an enlargement of the spleen, anemia, leukopenia, hemorrhage, and cirrhosis of the liver. He explained the nature of leukemia, typhoid septicemia, and pneumococcic infection.

Diabetic patients have practically no stores of glycogen in their livers, for the glycogen-storing function is damaged by the lack of pancreatic hormone.

Fat is stored in the liver, and alcohol speeds up the deposition of fat. Prolonged consumption of alcohol and an inadequate diet may cause an excessive deposition of fat in the liver and an overgrowth of fibrous tissue, which may permanently damage liver function.

The liver manufactures vitamin A from the yellow pigment (*carotene*) of vegetables and milk and stores vitamin D and the vitamin B complex. It also manufactures the *fibrinogen* of the blood, which is essential for normal clotting, as well as other blood proteins, bile salts, bile pigments, and numerous other products. Certain cells of the liver act as scavengers, removing bacteria and foreign proteins from the blood. Poisonous substances are either neutralized by chemical combination, stored, or excreted into the bowels by the liver. The liver contains a store of fluid which can be drawn upon to maintain the normal volume of blood in the vessels.

Liver disorders may be studied by testing the function of the liver. Some tests consist of injecting certain substances into the blood and later testing the blood to determine how efficiently the substance was removed from the blood by the liver. For example, a normal liver

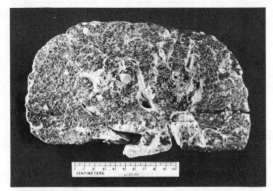

This photograph shows a surgical specimen of a diseased human liver. The blotchy areas that can be seen are pathological manifestations of portal cirrhosis, a chronic, progressive liver disease.

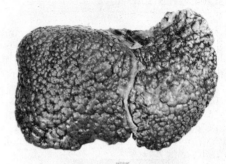

Surgical specimen of liver of a patient who suffered from Laennec's cirrhosis. This disease, formerly thought to be caused by alcoholism, is now known to result from nutritional disturbances.

will remove certain dyes from the blood within a certain length of time. If a patient has a cirrhotic liver, one of these dyes may remain in the blood beyond the expected time period, indicating that the liver is probably not functioning properly. Other tests define liver function according to the presence or absence of particular chemicals in the feces or urine. Still other liver function tests involve testing the blood serum for qualitative or quantitative changes in liver-produced serum proteins.

Jaundice

When an excess of bile pigment is released into the blood, a yellowish staining of the skin and mucous membranes results, which is referred to as jaundice. It is a symptom rather than a disease. Jaundice may be caused by the production of bile pigment in excess of the amount which the liver can excrete, or it may result from liver damage, the liver then being unable to excrete a normal amount of bile pigment. The pigment is derived from hemoglobin of broken-down red blood cells. Normally, most bile pigment is excreted by the liver into the intestines and then is absorbed from the intestines back to the liver, so that little pigment is present in the blood.

The three main causes of jaundice are excessive destruction of red cells, infection or poisoning of liver cells, or obstruction of the bile passages through which the pigment is normally excreted into the intestine from the liver. The last condition is the most common cause of jaundice. The obstruction may occur from gallstones, tumors or parasites within the ducts, or from compression of the ducts by a tumor of the pancreas. Frequently, a combination of causes exists.

The first evidence of jaundice is a yellow staining of the white of the eye. This is usually followed by staining of the skin of the entire body. The tint of the skin may range from a pale yellow to a deep olive green, and often an irritable itching accompanies the jaundice. In obstructive jaundice, the stools become clay-colored because of the absence of bile pigment from the intestines. The urine may range in color from light yellow to brownish-green because of the presence of the pigment in excessive amounts. The liver enlarges, and if the obstruction to the passage of bile is not removed, its function gradually fails. The treatment of a patient with obstructive jaundice entails an operation to remove the cause of the obstruction.

Jaundice may be caused by damage to the liver's cells by viruses, bacteria, parasites, and chemicals such as carbon tetrachloride, phosphorus, and coal tar derivatives. Virus infection resulting in jaundice has become relatively common. There are two viruses which may cause the condition. *Infectious hepatitis* (camp jaundice) is transmitted through the feces and thus occurs under conditions of poor sanitation. The disease begins with fever, loss of appetite, lassitude and headache, followed by jaundice. *Serum hepatitis* exhibits similar symptoms, but may result in a longer illness; in addition, serum hepatitis is thought to have a higher death rate. As the name implies, this virus is transmitted through contact with the serum or blood of a person who has, or has had, the disease. Anyone donating blood for medical use is always asked, "Have you ever been jaundiced?" An honest answer is extremely important, since a donor who has once been jaundiced may actually have had serum hepatitis and may pass it on to an already dangerously ill patient.

Jaundice caused by chemical poisoning may occur as the result of absorption of the toxic agents by mouth, by inhalation, or through the

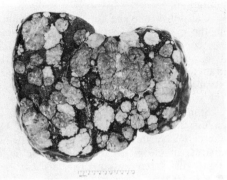

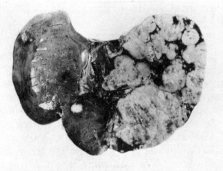

This surgical specimen is a human liver which has been widely invaded by a primary cancer. It is not usually possible to cure a patient unless diagnosis is made before such an advanced stage.

Cancer metastases in the liver, from the stomach. *Copyright 1950, Medical Radiography and Photography. Courtesy R. B. Schnick and W. F. Sullivan, Veterans Administration Hospital, McKinney.*

skin. A large dose of the chemical may be absorbed quickly, or small amounts may be absorbed over a long period of time. In either case, the treatment consists of removal of the patient from all possible exposure to the poison, rest in bed, and a regulated diet. In severe cases, the intravenous injection of glucose and whole blood may be required. Fatiguing exertion must be avoided for as long as six months after the poisoning to avoid taxing the liver's depleted stores of glycogen.

Excessive destruction of the red cells is an uncommon cause of jaundice. Sometimes the red cells of the patient are abnormal and break down easily because of structural defects. In other cases, the destruction is caused by septicemia or the transfusion of an incompatible type of blood. Newborn infants are frequently slightly jaundiced after birth, but this seems to be normal. The newborn infant possesses many more red cells than are needed for life outside the womb, and it is thought that the jaundice results from destruction of these extra cells. The most severe form of jaundice in infants is caused by erythroblastosis fetalis. (See Chapter 6: "Blood and Blood Forming Organs.")

Weil's disease, caused by spirochetal infection, also produces jaundice along with chills, fever, muscle pain, and nephritis. Treatment consists of supportive measures and chemotherapeutic drugs. (See Chapter 24, "Tropical Diseases.")

Cirrhosis

The term cirrhosis was used by Laennec, the famous French physician, more than a century ago to describe a condition of the liver in which the organ was of a yellow color (from *kirrhos,* tawny). The chief feature of the condition is an increase in fibrous tissue which usually causes contraction (*atrophy*) of the liver and impairment of its function. Classification of the types of cirrhosis is difficult, because the causes are multiple and in many instances obscure. There are two general categories of the disease, portal cirrhosis and biliary cirrhosis. The mechanism of the gradual destruction of liver tissue and replacement by fibrous tissue is not known. A variety of toxins, bacteria, and metabolic conditions undoubtedly are contributory factors. Biliary cirrhosis is caused by obstruction of the bile passages or by infection. There may be a remarkable freedom from symptoms of liver insufficiency even when the organ is damaged extensively. The main symptoms are those of obstruction. In portal obstruction there is congestion of the entire blood supply which causes distention of the veins at the lower end of the esophagus (*esophageal varices*) and the cardiac end of the stomach. These vessels may rupture and internal hemorrhage may result, leading to the vomiting of large quantities of blood. Another complication of portal cirrhosis is the collection of fluid (*ascites*) in the abdominal cavity. Biliary cirrhosis is characterized by severe jaundice, but there is usually no ascites.

Cancer of the liver

Cancer of the liver is rare in the white race. However, liver cancer is relatively common among Japanese, Chinese, Malays, and the Bantu natives of South Africa. It is thought that the difference in diet between the majority of the white and colored races may be a factor in the variant incidence of the disease. Secondary growths of cancer in the liver from cancer in other sites of the body are common; however, about 30 percent of all patients dying with cancer have liver involvement.

DISORDERS OF THE GALLBLADDER

The formation of gallstones in the gallbladder or bile ducts is the most common source of symptoms referable to this part of the digestive system. Gallstones are composed of constituents of the bile which slowly solidify out of solution, and the most common constituents are *cholesterol* and bile salts and pigments. They vary considerably in size and color and are frequently multiple. Several factors enter into the formation of stones. Infection or injury of the wall of the gallbladder or bile duct is thought to be the main cause while disturbances in cholesterol concentration and a slowing of the biliary flow along the bile ducts are both contributing factors. The stones can sometimes be seen by means of x-ray photographs.

Symptoms of gallstones usually occur after the age of 40, although they are frequently encountered in younger women who have had one or two pregnancies. While it is probable that gallstones produce symptoms within a few months of their formation, many gallstones are discovered by physicians, without having produced symptoms.

One method of diagnosing gallstones involves the use of a radiopaque dye, *tetraiodophenolphthalein*. Drs. Evarts Graham and Warren Cole developed the technique by which this dye is used. They noted that the substance concentrated in the mucosa of the gallbladder; consequently they hoped to visualize the bladder on x-ray films taken after injection or ingestion of the substance. Much to their surprise, only the normal gallbladders could be visualized in this manner; the abnormal or diseased bladders failed to concentrate the dye. Therefore, the test was given to determine the functioning of the gallbladder: if the organ could be visualized it was functioning normally; if it could not be visualized on the x-ray film, an operation was indicated. A new compound, Telepaque, is now used for this test, chiefly because it causes less unpleasant side-effects.

Women are affected by gallstones more commonly than men, probably because of pregnancy, obesity, and sedentary habits. Overeating probably plays an important part in their formation. The relatively rare occurrence of gallstones among Oriental people suggests that the type of diet may be of considerable importance in their formation. Although there is no conclusive evidence to link gallstones to diet, gallstones in animals have been produced by feeding them fatty foods and bile acid products and it is known to occur in certain aboriginal races whose diet is very restricted or where sanitation is at a minimum.

Gallstones may be found in the gallbladder, in the *cystic duct* (between the gallbladder and the common bile duct), in the ducts within the liver, in the *common bile duct*, or at the entrance of this duct into the duodenum. The symptoms vary in relation to the position of the stone.

Stones in the gallbladder do not cause pain unless they obstruct and cause cramps. Usually there is a vague sensation of fullness and dull distress in the pit of the stomach or under the right ribs, after eating. The distress is often more apparent after eating pork, cabbage, or fried foods as they cause the gallbladder to contract. The pain caused by gallstones may sometimes be confused with that of peptic ulcer. Whereas the pain of the latter is regularly relieved by eating food or drinking milk, the pain of gallstones is not so influenced.

Gallstones in the cystic duct cause an accumulation of fluid in the gallbladder which may on occasion amount to several ounces. This fluid forms a favorable medium for bacteria and the great danger of stones in this portion is that the gallbladder will become infected. If the wall becomes infected, an abscess may form and break through the wall of the organ, causing peritonitis.

Stones cause colicky pain as they pass into and along the common duct. Frequently, the stone will become lodged in the duct, forming a ball valve which results in jaundice of fluctuating intensity. In these cases, infection frequently occurs in the distended duct and liver above the stone.

Sometimes the stone is passed down the length of the bile duct and into the intestine, to be eventually passed in the feces. Frequently, however, the stone becomes lodged at the entrance of the duct into the duodenum. In this position, gallstones cause an intense chronic jaundice and the itching produced is usually severe. The colicky pain which accompanies the passage of the stone along the duct is variable in intensity from one of the most severe to which the body is subjected, to being completely absent after the stone has become lodged at the entrance of the intestine.

The attacks of pain caused by movement of the gallstone within the bile passages (*biliary colic*) usually commence several hours after eating a heavy meal; hence, pain usually occurs during the night. These attacks are caused by spasm or stretching of the walls of the bile duct. They usually are so severe that they cause the patient to roll and groan with each spasm. Usually the pain is felt underneath the right ribs and radiates around to the back beneath the right shoulder blade. It may last for several hours.

Vomiting usually occurs during the attack and brings some relief. A few hours after the attack, the urine becomes dark from the presence of bile pigments, and the stools become light in color one to three days later.

A stone passing down the ureter from the kidney to the bladder will also cause colicky pain, but the pain begins in the back and shoots down and around to the front of the abdomen, down into the sex organs, and often into the inner surface of the thigh; the urine is bloody. Colicky pain caused by intestinal obstruction is more generalized over the abdomen and more severe below the level of the navel.

Mild attacks of gallstone colic may often be relieved by bed rest and hot packs placed on the abdomen. A severe attack, however, will require the attention of a physician and the injection of pain-relieving drugs. The further treatment after the pain has been alleviated depends on the general condition of the patient.

Usually removal of the gallbladder is advised, as attacks of colic are likely to recur, and infection may complicate the disease, causing rupture of the gallbladder. The operation removes the diseased gallbladder and the stones. If the gallbladder is not removed, it may burst into the abdominal cavity, causing peritonitis, or it will continue to form stones. If the gallbladder does not rupture, the infection may spread from the bile ducts to the pancreatic duct, causing acute or chronic infection of the pancreas (*pancreatitis*).

If operation is not possible, and this is rare indeed, the physician will attempt to prevent further attacks by placing the patient on a strict diet in which fat and greasy foods, pork, spicy foods, and alcohol are avoided. Such medical treatment, however, cannot replace surgical resection as a cure for gallstones.

Although infection of the gallbladder is usually associated with the presence of gallstones, it occasionally occurs without the presence of stones, particularly as a complication of typhoid fever. Such infections are believed to arise from organisms gaining direct entrance to the gallbladder through the bile duct from the duodenum. Also, the microbes may be carried there from some focus of infection in the body, by the blood.

In an acute infection of the gallbladder, the patient is prostrated, and there is pain and tenderness in the right upper abdomen. The pain becomes generalized over the whole abdomen if perforation of the gallbladder occurs. Nausea and vomiting are common, and the fever which accompanies the infection may reach 104° Fahrenheit. Jaundice occurring during the attack is usually indicative of the presence of stones in the common bile duct but may occur in the absence of stones if the infection spreads to the liver. Attacks of gallbladder infection usually subside quickly, but they may be recurrent and in time become chronic.

The treatment of acute infections of the gallbladder is the administration of one of the antibiotic drugs, such as penicillin or aureomycin, and omission of all food, although the patient may be allowed to suck ice. The decision must be made by the surgeon as to whether to operate immediately to remove the gallbladder or to wait and perform the operation when the acute attack has subsided. Operation is usually imperative if the infection does not subside in one to three days.

Sometimes the bile ducts fail to develop a lumen and are represented by solid cords of tissue. Persistent and deepening jaundice after the first few weeks of life usually results, together with gradual enlargement and hardening of the liver. Life may be prolonged for as much as twelve months without treatment, but then the condition usually terminates fatally. Plastic repair of the defect is sometimes possible.

Cancer of the gallbladder

Cancer of the gallbladder is uncommon and is usually associated with gallstones. This constitutes another reason why surgical rather than medical treatment is usually advised when gallstones are discovered. The tumor usually grows through the wall of the gallbladder and invades the liver. The patient then loses weight and strength rapidly. The only hope of cure is surgical removal of the growth at an early stage. Unfortunately, this is seldom possible because the patient usually presents himself for treatment at an advanced stage of the disease. Women develop the disease about five times more frequently than men, perhaps because gallstones are so much more common in that sex.

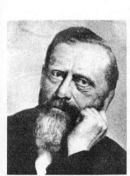

GRUBER, Max von (1853-1927) German bacteriologist. Discovered with Durham in 1896 that certain bacteria clump together (agglutination) when placed in the presence of serum from a person who is immune to the disease to which the bacteria give rise. The immunity may be caused either by prior infection or may be produced by inoculation. The reaction was first utilized in the Widal test for typhoid fever, but has proved of value in the diagnosis of cholera and cerebrospinal meningitis.

DISORDERS OF THE PANCREAS

There are three principal parts of the pancreas: the head, which is connected to the duodenum via the pancreatic duct; the body, which produces enzymes and insulin; and the tail, which touches the spleen. The pancreatic duct and the bile ducts share a common entrance to the intestine. Consequently, infection of the pancreas is commonly associated with disease of the bile ducts, while jaundice frequently results from swelling of the pancreas from infection or cancer. The long axis of the pancreas lies behind the stomach and duodenum and chronic peptic ulcers may penetrate its substance.

Infection of the pancreas

Acute infection of the pancreas may result from invasion of the gland by bacteria. It also may follow the retention of the powerful digestive ferments in the gland when there is an obstruction of the pancreatic duct. Another cause of pancreatic infection is the rupture of a blood vessel within the substance of the gland. In any case, it is the escape of pancreatic ferments into the gland with subsequent digestion, hemorrhage, and even death of the affected tissues that causes the violent symptoms of the disease.

The disease usually begins suddenly with excruciating pain in the upper abdomen which frequently radiates to the back. The pain is usually constant, in contrast to the colicky pain of gallstones. Vomiting may be severe, particularly if the attack occurs after a heavy meal or excessive drinking. The patient becomes pale and develops shock.

Chemical block of the sympathetic nerves leading to the pancreas is used in treating acute pancreatitis. Blockage of the nerves usually relieves the pain. Drugs also are used to control the pain, and nothing is allowed to be swallowed. The necessary fluid and salt are given intravenously. Some form of therapy may be necessary to combat the shock state. Improvement in the patient's condition usually follows,

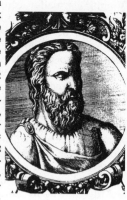

ARETAEUS of Cappadocia (ca. 2nd century A.D.) Greek physician. First to describe diabetes, centuries before such a complex thing as the endocrine system was known to exist. From his two most important works on the causes, symptoms, and treatment of chronic diseases, Aretaeus emerges as a physician cast in the Hippocratic mould. These writings reflect the emphasis on direct observation, on bedside study, and on the desire to be useful to men. *Bettmann Archive.*

and the patient is kept in bed. His progress is carefully followed, sometimes for several weeks, to see whether an abscess forms in the gland. If an abscess forms, surgical drainage is performed. If the patient's condition fails to improve, intravenous fluid is given; and, especially if jaundice develops, immediate operation to drain the gallbladder and bile ducts is imperative. Use of antibiotic drugs has somewhat improved the treatment of patients with this condition.

Recovery from an acute infection of the pancreas may be complete. However, a diffuse infiltration of the organ by fibrous tissue may result and slowly choke the cells producing the digestive enzymes and damage the insulin-producing cells. Such a condition is termed *chronic pancreatitis.* The patient with this disease passes foul, bulky, greasy stools because of the upset of fat digestion. He may develop diabetes. The physician is able to give such a patient considerable relief by administering capsules of pancreatic extract to correct the digestive processes and sufficient insulin to control the diabetes. Often the pain may be relieved by cutting the splanchnic nerves.

Cancer of the pancreas

Middle-aged or elderly men are the most common sufferers from cancer of the pancreas; the disease is only one-third as frequent in women. When the tumor originates in the head of the gland and blocks the bile duct, a steadily increasing jaundice appears, and increasing itching of the skin develops. When the cancer begins in the body of the organ, pain is the most common symptom. The pain is usually constant and of a deep, penetrating character that radiates through to the back, between the shoulder blades. If the cancer occurs in the tail of the gland, there may be no symptoms until the growth has spread to the liver, with resulting loss of weight and general impairment of bodily

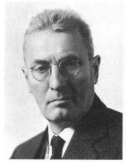

CARLSON, Dr. Anton Julius (1875-1956) American physiologist. Aided in the formulation of correct concepts of the physiology of the alimentary tract, principally with his analysis of the hunger sensation. Long a professor of physiology at the University of Chicago, Carlson was respected for his genius as a teacher and for his many famous pupils.

function. The only treatment possible is the removal of the whole gland, a surgical procedure which is possible today because of the means available for controlling shock and the availability of substances which can substitute for the secretions of the gland.

Sometimes agglomerations of glandular tissue occur in the pancreas which simulate cancer. These are called *islet cell tumors*. These tumors may not be malignant, and if not they do not spread through the gland or invade other structures. Because of the possibility of their becoming malignant, however, these tumors are always removed. Sometimes this mass of glandular tissue secretes so much insulin that weakness and faintness occur. The patient may even lapse into coma, because of the extent to which the blood is depleted of its sugar. Surgical removal results in the disappearance of symptoms. In recent years, cases have been reported in which islet cell tumors are associated with peptic ulcerations of the jejunum.

Diabetes

The most common affliction involving the pancreas is *diabetes mellitus*. This disease is discussed in detail in Chapter 10, "The Endocrine System."

OTHER DISORDERS OF THE DIGESTIVE SYSTEM

Poor circulation of the blood may cause several types of digestive upset. Chronic heart failure will lead to blood being dammed up in the liver with resultant increase in its size. As a result of this congestion of the liver, the abdominal cavity may become filled with fluid *(ascites)*. This fluid at times may enormously distend the abdomen. The fluid may be drained by a needle passed through the abdominal wall, or the kidneys may be forced to eliminate the fluid by the administration of compounds of mercury *(diuretics)*.

Ascites is also common in patients with tuberculous infection of the peritoneum and in those with cancer which has spread through the peritoneal cavity. Tubercular ascites will disappear with eradication of the disease; ascites caused by cancer usually indicates that cure is no longer possible. Until recently, the only treatment that could be given was to drain the fluid with a tube as often as the abdomen became distended; this was needed as frequently as every week. Now, drugs and radioactive metals are used to halt the formation of fluid, although they do not cure the patient with cancer.

Lung disorders may affect the digestive tracts of some patients. Those with obstructive pulmonary disease have a high incidence of ulcers, probably because of diminished tissue resistance.

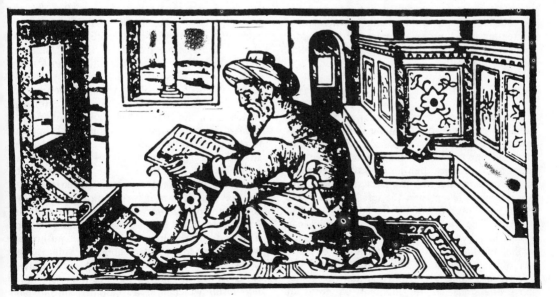

Avenzoar, the twelfth century Arabian physician in Spain, studied both gastric carcinoma and carcinoma of the esophagus. *Bettmann Archive.*

14 THE URINARY SYSTEM

WHAT IT IS AND DOES

The general function of the urinary system is to cleanse the blood by filtering out waste substances and excreting them as urine. The normal urinary system of a human being is made up of two kidneys, two ureters, the bladder, and the urethra. Urine is produced in the kidneys and passed by wavelike muscular contractions down the tubelike ureters to the bladder, which serves for temporary storage. At intervals the bladder opens, usually voluntarily, and urine is expelled through the urethra.

Kidneys

The kidneys are two bean-shaped organs located on each side of the spine and in approximately the middle of the back. They are about four and one-half inches long, two inches wide, and a fraction more than an inch thick. Because of a crowding effect of the liver, the right kidney is slightly lower than the left. Normally the upper parts of the kidneys lie beneath the last two ribs. The very top portion of each kidney is attached by strong fibers to the diaphragm, so that the kidneys rise and fall about one-half inch during breathing. The lower ends of the kidneys are generally from one to two inches above the crest of the hipbone. In front of the right kidney lie portions of the liver and of the gastrointestinal tract. In front of the left kidney are parts of the stomach, spleen, pancreas, loops of the small intestine, and parts of the colon. The *adrenal glands* appear as caplike bodies on the upper end of the kidneys.

The kidneys lie behind and outside of the lining membrane *(peritoneum)* of the abdominal cavity. Thus, it is possible to operate on the kidney without opening the peritoneum with the ensuing risk of its becoming infected *(peritonitis)*. In fact, the relations of the entire urinary tract are such that the great majority of operations are performed outside of the peritoneum.

The kidney is surrounded by a thin capsule of supporting tissue and by a layer of fat. This fat layer, in turn, is enclosed in a thin sheath of connective tissue. From the outer surface of this sheath, fibers connect with the walls of the niche in which the kidney lies and with the peritoneum in front of the kidney.

At the concave medial portion of each kidney is a depression known as the *hilus*, through which pass the artery and vein supplying the kidney. However, the major portion of the hilus is occupied by the *renal pelvis*, a small funnel-shaped reservoir which collects urine from the kidney and transmits it to the ureter to which the renal pelvis is connected. Within the hilus the pelvis divides into two or more cuplike divisions known as *major calyces*, and these in turn form a total of four to twelve *minor calyces*. The ends of the minor calyces are pushed inward by one to three projections of kidney tissue known as *renal papillae*. Each papilla contains from twelve to 80 minute openings *(foramina papillaria)* which are the ends of the *papillary ducts* through which urine passes into the pelvis.

The specialized tissue of the kidney proper is composed of an external *cortex* and an internal *medulla*. The medulla is formed into some eight to 18 cone-shaped segments called *renal pyramids*. When the kidney is sectioned, the pyra-

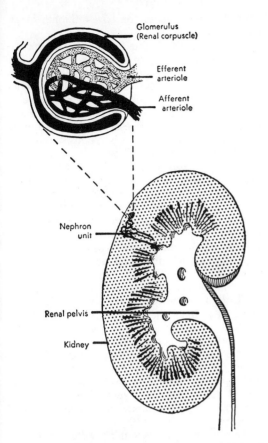

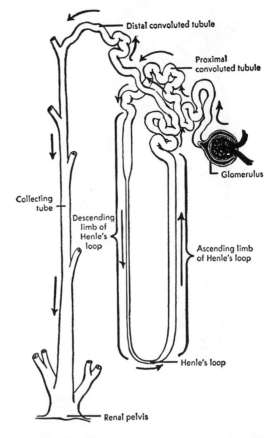

Cross-section diagram of kidney, showing position of glomerulus and nephron unit in the outer layers. Renal pelvis and center of kidney serve as a collecting system for urine formed in nephron units. Arterioles carry blood to and from glomerulus.

An enlarged illustration of a nephron unit. In each kidney over a million such nephron units filter fluids from the blood and convert these filtrate fluids into urine in the tubules. The collecting tubes then transport the urine into renal pelvis.

mids have a somewhat glistening appearance and contain delicate radial lines or striations. These striations mark the course of kidney tubules which empty into the calyces of the pelvis through the renal papillae mentioned above. The papillae are thus formed by the apices of the renal pyramids.

The cortex proper forms the outer layer of approximately one-half inch of the kidney tissue between the *capsule* and the bases of the renal pyramids. Cortex tissue also dips between the pyramids to form the *renal columns* which extend to the cavity *(sinus)* of the kidney.

From the standpoint of both what it is and what it does, the basic unit of the kidney is made up of the so-called corpuscle and its associated small tubes. A kidney corpuscle consists of a filtering unit *(glomerulus)* and its surrounding envelope (capsule). The capsule is formed by the end of a filtrate-collecting tube being pushed inward, much as one might push the wall of a tennis ball inward with the finger. A very small artery enters the space formed by

the process just described and divides into a mass of smaller vessels *(capillaries)* which are rolled together. This mass of capillaries is the filtering unit. The capillaries then reunite to form a small, outgoing blood vessel.

Extending from the double-walled capsule around each glomerulus is a small tube *(tubule)* which becomes highly contorted and rolled together to form the nearby convoluted tubule. It then becomes a straight tubule of small diameter called the descending portion *(limb)* of a loop known as Henle's loop. This part of the loop extends down into the inner part *(medulla)* of the kidney and then reverses direction to form the ascending part of the loop. The ascending limb emerges from the medulla and becomes the more distant convoluted tubule. By means of a connecting tube the convoluted tubule empties into a collecting tube. Thus the unit which began with the glomerulus is completed.

The unit beginning with a glomerulus and ending in a collecting tube is sometimes referred to as a *nephron*. It has been estimated

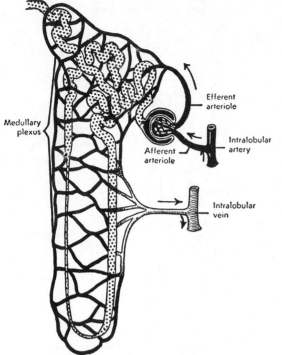

Medullary plexus

Efferent arteriole

Intralobular artery

Afferent arteriole

Intralobular vein

The flow of blood to and from the nephron unit. Afferent arterioles carry the blood from the intralobular arteries to the glomerulus. Efferent arterioles then carry the blood to a network of capillaries surrounding the tubules and the medullary plexus; it then passes into the intralobular veins.

that there are at least a million of these units in each kidney. The collecting tubules themselves finally unite with other collecting tubules to form larger channels known as papillary ducts. These ducts empty into the collecting funnel (pelvis) of the kidney through the foramina papillaria of the renal papillae.

The function of the kidneys is to aid in removal of waste products from the blood stream. By far the best blood supply of any organ in the body is provided the kidney. In fact, it has been estimated that one fifth of the output of the heart, or over a quart of blood per minute, passes through the kidneys. In the capillaries of the glomeruli the blood is under sufficient pressure to cause part of the fluid portion (plasma) of the blood to filter through the capillary walls into the glomerular capsule. It has been estimated that 16 percent of the blood plasma passing through the kidneys is filtered through the glomeruli. The total filtrate is about 100 to 175 quarts per day. It is thought that this filtrate contains all the substances found in blood plasma except proteins and certain fatty materials. These latter materials are retained because the pores in the capillary walls of the glomeruli

are only approximately one five-millionth of an inch in diameter.

The glomerular filtrate has a volume approximately 100 times that of the urine excreted. The chief function of the uriniferous tubules is to reabsorb water and other substances. Normally all of the glucose is reabsorbed, as well as some of the minerals and building blocks of protein (amino acids). Selective resorption in the tubules aids in maintaining in the blood stream the proper concentration of water, salt, etc. For example, in cases of limited intake or excessive loss of water because of sweating, diarrhea, or vomiting, more water is resorbed from the filtrate, and the urine is more concentrated than normal. Conversely, in cases of excessive intake of water, resorption is decreased, and the urine may be much more dilute than usual. The concentration of salt and substances regulating the degree of alkalinity of the blood are controlled in a similar manner.

Most of the nitrogenous waste products are excreted through the kidneys, principally in the form of urea. This substance normally is present in urine in a concentration about 70 times greater than its concentration in blood. The capacity of the kidney to remove urea from the blood serves as a criterion of kidney function in the "urea clearance" test. Creatinine is another type of nitrogenous waste substance, and is excreted partly by the tubules.

The ureters are two thick-walled, muscular tubes which serve to conduct urine from the kidney pelvis to the bladder. They are approximately one foot in length and have an average caliber of about one-fifth inch. Like the kidneys, the ureters are located behind the peritoneum, or lining membrane, of the abdominal cavity. In order to reach the bladder, the ureters curve toward the midline. In men, the ureters in this region lie close to the seminal vesicle and are crossed by the vas deferens. In women, the ureters pass close to the mouth of the uterus and the upper part of the vagina, a fact of considerable importance in surgical procedures involving these organs. (For further discussion of the reproductive organs, see Chapter 15, "The Reproductive System.")

The ureters enter the bladder at its lower and back portion. The entrance is generally at such an oblique angle that the ureters traverse the wall of the bladder for almost an inch. The openings are small slits which may have a valve-like action. Furthermore, muscle fibers of the ureter appear to exert a clamplike (sphincter) effect. Urine does not pass into the bladder in a steady stream, but rather in small spurts every ten to 30 seconds. This is caused by waves of muscular contractions (peristalsis) passing downward along the ureters. When the bladder is distended, pressure of the urine tends to close off the portion of the ureter traversing the bladder. Nevertheless, urine at such times may escape and flow backward toward the kidneys.

Bladder

The urinary bladder is a muscular reservoir which serves for temporary storage of urine received from the ureters and discharged at intervals through the urethra. It is somewhat Y-shaped when empty and spherical when distended. The capacity without overdistention is about one pint. When empty, the uppermost part of the bladder is approximately at the level of the union of the two pubic bones (*pubic symphysis*). The upper surface is covered by peritoneum, while the lower portion is supported by the floor of the bony pelvis. In front, the space between the pubic bones and bladder is filled with loose fatty tissue. At the junction of front and upper portions of the bladder a strong fibrous cord connects the bladder with the navel.

In men, the lower back portion of the bladder is in contact with the two seminal vesicles and the vas deferens running from the testes to the seminal vesicles. Part of the posterior border of the bladder is also in contact with the rectum, which lies just behind it. Bands of connective tissue from the bladder to the rectum help keep the former in proper position. Beneath the posterior portion of the lower surface of the bladder is the prostate gland, through which the *urethra* passes. Ligaments from the prostate to the walls of the pelvis also help support the bladder.

In women, the posterior lower part of the bladder is in contact with the neck (*cervix*) of the womb (*uterus*) and the upper part of the front wall of the vagina. The bladder is attached to these structures by connective tissue. The triangular area between this opening and the opening of the two ureters is known as the *trigone*.

Urethra

The urethra is a canal extending from the bladder to the external opening (*meatus*) of the urinary tract. In both sexes the urethra serves for the elimination of stored urine from the bladder, and in men it also functions as the passage of secretions of the reproductive organs. The urethra in men averages about eight inches in length and is divided into three parts. The prostatic portion is about one inch in length and extends downward from the bladder through the prostate gland. In its central part the prostatic urethra is enlarged to form a bulge into which open the ducts of the prostate, the ejaculatory ducts, and the prostatic utricle. The middle or membranous part of the urethra is approximately one-half inch in length and passes

through the muscular urogenital diaphragm. The remainder of the urethra is called the cavernous, or spongy, portion because it is surrounded by the cavernous portion of the underside of the penis. Along the entire urethra, but most numerous in the spongy portion, are located mucous glands. Though the clear mucus secreted is thought to have a genital function, it may also serve as a means of lubrication to prevent the urethra from becoming dry between urinations. The slitlike opening of the urethra at the tip of the penis is the urethral meatus.

In women, the urethra is from one to two inches in length and extends downward and forward to open just in front of the vaginal opening. The urethra is normally about one third of an inch in diameter and is surrounded by the urethral glands. The function of the female urethra is wholly urinary. The *para-urethral glands,* or *Skene's glands,* open into the urethra just within the external opening.

Urination, or micturition, is the act of excreting urine. As the bladder fills, the *internal sphincter* muscles at the upper portion of the urethra automatically contract to keep the bladder outlet closed. As the individual becomes conscious of the filling, the desire to urinate causes a voluntary closure of the *external sphincter* muscle (located just beneath the prostate in men, and in approximately the same position in women) by a reflex stimulation. As the urge increases, the muscles of the perineal region (the area between the anus and the genitals) become contracted somewhat.

Voiding is a complex function, generally controlled at will. Contraction of the bladder muscle (detrusor) forcibly widens the bladder outlet. In addition, the voluntary relaxation of the muscles in the pelvic floor aids in the dropping and funneling of the bladder outlet and thus helps to widen the bladder outlet.

Thus waste material is removed from the blood by the kidneys, sent as urine down the ureters to the bladder for temporary storage, and then passed through the urethra to the outside.

DISORDERS OF THE KIDNEY

There are many different types of kidney abnormalities. Complete absence of both kidneys occurs in some stillborn infants, in connection with other defects. More commonly, only one kidney is present, and persons with such a defect may lead entirely normal lives. The so-called double kidney is observed with relative frequency; although in reality this is one kidney proper with two collecting funnels (kidney pelves) and partial or complete duplication of the ureters.

When one kidney is small and has limited function, the opposite kidney is likely to become enlarged. Fusion of the kidneys may occur to give various abnormalities in form, such as an L-shaped kidney, a cake-shaped kidney, a shield-shaded kidney, or the so-called horseshoe kidney. The last type occurs in approximately one out of 500 to 1000 persons.

One or both kidneys may be in an abnormal position, often located in the pelvic region. This condition is called ectopy. In crossed ectopy both kidneys may be on the same side of the body with one above the other. This condition, present at birth, is to be distinguished from so-called "floating kidney" (ptosis). In this uncommon condition the kidney is movable; pain, obstruction of urinary flow, and infection may occasionally occur. "Floating kidney" occurs more frequently in women than in men. Although pregnancies may have something to do with this, in years past tight lacing of corsets also was blamed for the condition. The position of a floating kidney may be fixed by an operation known as nephropexy. Many such kidneys cause no symptoms and require no correction.

Kidney stones

The occurrence of stones in the urinary tract is one of the most important problems of urology (that special branch of medicine dealing with the urinary tract in both sexes and with the reproductive organs in men). The way in which stones form is not known, but either organic or inorganic material may serve as a central core on which the stone grows. Recently, evidence has been presented that, in some cases, bacteria may form the core. Further, it is thought that diet and consumption of highly mineralized water (hard water) can contribute to the formation of stones. There may also be a climatic factor. Regions where large numbers of people have kidney stones are called "stone belts." These include hot, dry, areas such as southern Florida and California, south China, Egypt, and south-central Russia. The dry heat may cause concentration of urine, thus producing stones. Stones also are more probable in the presence of hyperexcretion of calcium, i.e., in persons with a parathyroid tumor.

However, the greatest percentage of stones appears to be caused by a metabolic abnormality that increases the concentration of crystalloids in urine. These stones consist mainly of inorganic materials or salts. The chief constituent of kidney stones is calcium. The composition of stones depends to a large extent on whether the urine is acid, alkaline, or neither (neutral). Salts of uric acid are common in stones formed in acid urine; salts of oxalic acid (oxalates) in neutral urine; and salts of phosphoric acid (phosphates) in alkaline urine. Stones formed from cystine (an amino acid used as a protein building block in the body) may be dissolved when the physician administers drugs which make the urine alkaline.

Kidney stones may be single or multiple. They may be uniform in structure or be in concentric layers. They often possess sharp points or edges which produce considerable damage to the funnel-shaped collecting tube (kidney pelvis) and cause blood to appear in the urine (hematuria). The stones may completely fill the collecting tube, reaching a large size. Such stones often follow the contour of the kidney pelvis and are called stag-horn calculi. Stones in the kidney may block the ureteral entrance at times, thus causing obstruction of urinary flow and dilation of the kidney pelvis with urine (see later discussion of obstruction). Resulting damage causes a blood protein, albumin, to appear in the urine. Infection may also occur, in which case pus may be found in the urine.

Kidney-stone colic usually occurs when the stone passes from the kidney pelvis down the ureter to be expelled into the bladder. While it is in the ureter, the stone may cut the mucous membranes of the walls of the ureter and cause excruciating pain and bleeding. The pain may come on suddenly or gradually, and usually runs from the midportion of the back down into the corresponding thigh (and testicle in men). Such pain, occurring distant from the area involved, is known as referred pain, and is felt because nerves serving other body areas lie close to the nerves which go to the kidney. Consequently, sensations of pain are observed in areas distant from the kidney, as though the pain had actually arisen in the distant area. Other manifestations of kidney-stone colic are nausea, vomiting, blood in the urine, and even collapse. In the majority of cases, the stone is passed spontaneously; its passage is greatly aided by fluids and drugs that relieve spasm and control pain.

Fortunately, many kidney stones and other stones of the urinary tract are opaque to x-rays and can therefore be seen on the K.U.B. x-ray picture (of kidneys, ureters, and bladder). At times "silent" kidney stones which have failed to cause symptoms are discovered by x-ray examination. However, stones composed entirely of uric acid or its salts are not visible on x-ray film.

Most patients with kidney stones that are too large to pass are treated surgically. After operation, the patient is required to drink an abundance of water or to follow a diet that will change either the acidity of alkalinity of his urine, to aid in prevention of new stones. If the kidney is badly damaged, it may be necessary to remove it totally (nephrectomy).

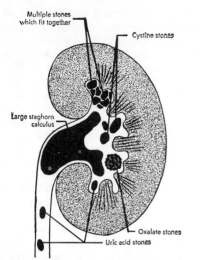

Cross-sectional diagram of a human kidney illustrating the various categories of kidney stones (calculi) and where they occur. Oxalate and phosphate stones are commonest. The latter type occur frequently in the presence of a kidney infection.

Effect of obstruction

Various conditions in the kidney and its pelvis may obstruct the flow of urine. Examples are: abnormalities of development, stone, or tumor. However, obstruction anywhere in the urinary tract produces similar changes in the kidney. The kidney pelvis, or collecting portion of the kidney, becomes dilated with urine under a certain amount of back pressure. This condition is known as *hydronephrosis*. Since the kidney continues to secrete urine, the pressure increases; because of this pressure on the blood vessels, the blood supply to the kidney is lowered. If continued long enough, the kidney substance completely degenerates and becomes functionless. This condition is termed *hydronephrotic atrophy* (degeneration and shrinkage of the kidney caused by retained urine). Infection often occurs as a complication.

Patients with hydronephrotic atrophy may have no characteristic symptoms, though pain is generally present and tenderness may occur. Blood and pus may be present in the urine, and urination may occur with greater frequency than usual. The condition may be readily diagnosed by a procedure in which a solution of a substance opaque to x-rays—such as a salt of iodine —is injected into the kidney pelvis through a hollow flexible tube known as a *catheter*. This tube is introduced through another hollow metal instrument called a *cystoscope*, which is first guided from the outside of the body through the urethra and into the bladder. A solution of the iodide compound may also be injected intravenously and allowed to pass through the urinary tract, thus making it opaque to x-rays. After the kidney pelvis has been made opaque in one

of these manners, an x-ray picture (pyelogram) is taken.

The treatment of patients with hydronephrosis involves removal of the cause of obstruction by surgical or other means. If the patient has an associated infection, he is treated with appropriate drugs. The kidney may have to be removed if the kidney destruction is far advanced. In this and other such conditions an estimate of damage is made by the *renal function tests,* one of which measures the ability of the kidney to excrete a dye injected into the veins. The rate at which the dye is excreted is measured with a catheter extending into the kidney pelvis, as described above. The catheter is sometimes left in place in the kidney to determine whether the injured kidney can improve its function within a few days. The ability of a damaged kidney to repair itself depends on the relief of the obstruction and the extent of damage.

Infections of the kidney (nephritis)

The term *nephritis* means inflammation of the kidney. The term includes inflammations produced by the toxins of disease-producing agents and the presence of other substances in the blood, such as bacteria. There is a higher incidence of nephritis among children than adults, although children recover more quickly and completely.

Bacteria probably cannot pass through the filtering apparatus (*glomeruli*) of the normal kidney. But in case of kidney damage caused by obstruction or a stone, the organisms gain a foothold. If only the kidney pelvis is involved, the infection is called *pyelitis;* but if both pelvis and kidney proper are involved, the condition is known as *pyelonephritis*, which is the most common type of kidney infection. Shrinkage of the kidney substance occurs in *atrophic pyelonephritis*. At times, accumulated pus causes obstruction and degeneration of kidney tissue, and this condition is known as *pyonephrosis*.

Except in occasional cases in which the infection is localized in the outer layer (*cortex*) of the kidney, pus and bacteria are present in the urine of most patients with pyelonephritis. Generally, there is a burning sensation felt on urination, and urination occurs more frequently than usual. The white blood cell count is usually high,

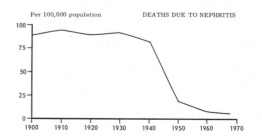

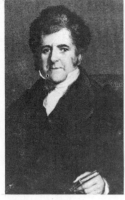

BRIGHT, Richard (1789-1858) English physician and clinician. It was in 1827 that he published his universally famous description of those disorders of the human kidney that have since then been known as *Bright's disease*. He also pointed out the difference between the edemas having a renal and a cardiac origin. He described pancreatic jaundice and many other associated varieties of degeneration of the tissues of the liver.

and fever may run up to 106° Fahrenheit. Tenderness in the loin is often noted. Treatment depends largely on the particular type of bacteria present. This fact is determined by examination of urine, which in most cases is obtained by use of a catheter passed into the bladder. Identification of the infecting organism and its probable response to prospective drugs requires the services of a competent bacteriologist.

Tuberculosis of the kidney may occur with or without active tuberculosis elsewhere in the body. In most cases, the germ responsible is thought to reach the kidneys by way of the blood stream. Frequency of urination and a burning sensation may occur, but the sudden appearance of blood in the urine may be the first symptom. The urine is often cloudy with pus. Although tuberculosis can completely destroy a kidney, various drugs have brought new hope to persons suffering from this condition.

Noninfectious diseases

The term *Bright's disease* has been used loosely to refer to several types of kidney disease associated with the presence of abnormally large amounts of fluid in the intercellular spaces of the body *(edema)* and the presence of protein in the urine *(albuminuria)*. In this group of diseases, the kidney is *affected*, but not *infected*. There might be a bacterial infection in the nose, throat, or some other region of the body, but the kidney itself is not invaded. In the main, there are three kinds of Bright's disease: degenerative, hemorrhagic, and sclerotic.

The degenerative type, nephrosis, is characterized by death *(necrosis)* of the outer layers of cells in the tubules of the kidney. This condition can be brought on by such factors as a long course of high fever and mercury poisoning. Albumin and dead cells in the urine are the chief indications.

The second type of Bright's disease, the hemorrhagic type, is probably caused by poisons formed by a bacterial infection elsewhere in the body. It may occur as a complication of such diseases as scarlet fever, diphtheria, pneumonia, and typhoid fever. Blood and albumin may be present in the urine, and the patient has swelling of various parts of the body *(edema)*. The function of the kidneys may be reduced and chills, fever, and vomiting may occur. The hemorrhagic type of Bright's disease is essentially an inflammation of the capillary blood vessels in the filtering units *(glomeruli)* of the kidney, and is often called *glomerulonephritis*.

The third type of Bright's disease is characterized by a hardening *(sclerosis)* of the tiny arteries *(arterioles)* of the kidney and is known as *arteriolar nephrosclerosis*. The disease is primarily of the blood vessels, and high blood pressure *(hypertension)* usually is present. As the walls of the arterioles become hardened and thickened, many of these vessels may cease to carry blood. The kidney substance then shrinks in such areas, and the kidney appears finely granular. Although this disease is generally slow in progress, it may be acute and rapidly fatal when kidney function is lost.

Various other types of noninfectious kidney diseases are known. The "uremic poisoning" of pregnancy is associated with accumulation of waste products in the blood, and degeneration of kidney tissue. Swelling may be noted in parts of the body, and albumin may be present in the urine. In severe cases, convulsions and unconsciousness may occur. There may be complete absence of urine *(anuria)*.

Physiological albuminuria

Albuminuria refers to the presence in the urine of protein from the blood. Although this condition usually indicates damage of some sort to the filtration apparatus of the kidney, it may occur at times in apparently healthy individuals. Strenuous exercise, cold baths, intense mental strain, and other common events may bring on a harmless type generally called "physiological

EDEBOHLS, George Michael (1853-1908) American surgeon. He is most celebrated for his numerous contributions to the knowledge of procedures for surgery of the kidney. He attempted to operate for hydronephrosis, and later performed nephropexy. In 1899 he performed the first operation designed to bring about the relief of Bright's disease by the removal of the renal capsule. The procedure subsequently has been given the name *Edebohls' operation*.

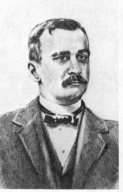

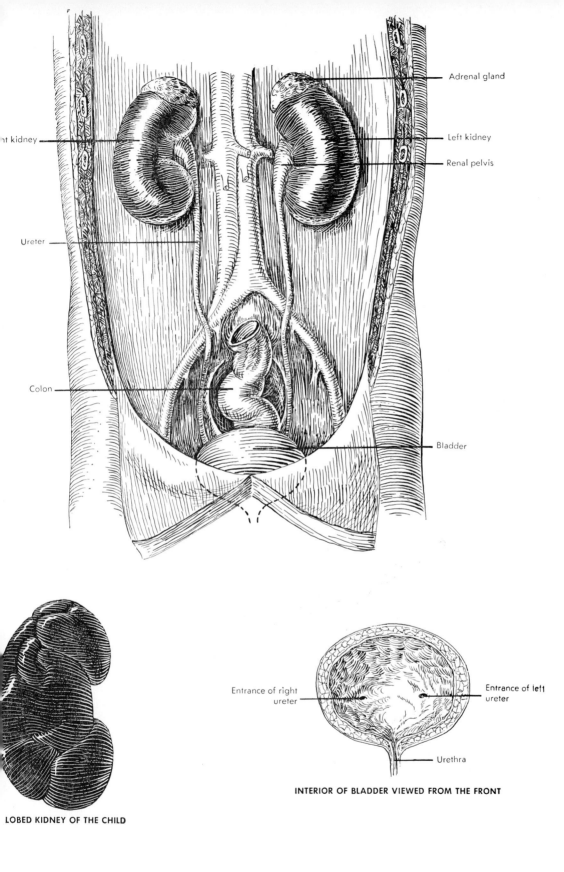

Adrenal gland

Left kidney

Renal pelvis

...ht kidney

Ureter

Colon

Bladder

LOBED KIDNEY OF THE CHILD

Entrance of right ureter

Entrance of left ureter

Urethra

INTERIOR OF BLADDER VIEWED FROM THE FRONT

THE URINARY SYSTEM OF THE MALE

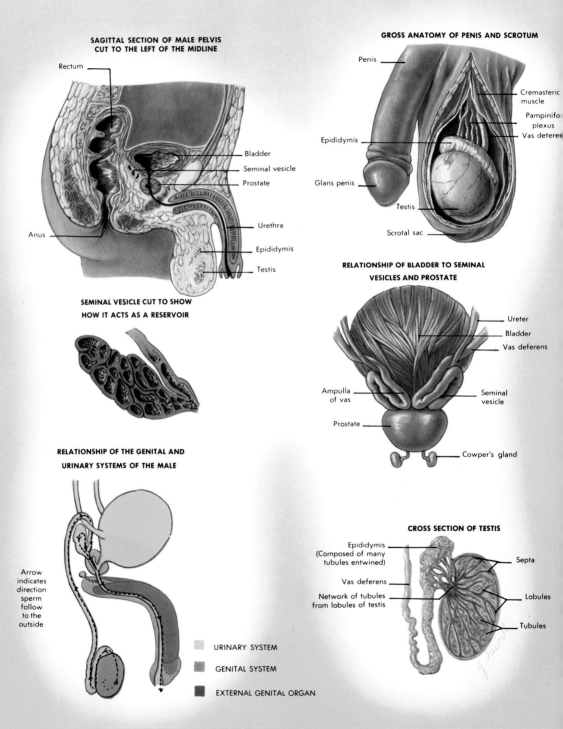

SAGITTAL SECTION OF MALE PELVIS
CUT TO THE LEFT OF THE MIDLINE

Rectum

Bladder
Seminal vesicle
Prostate

Urethra

Anus

Epididymis

Testis

GROSS ANATOMY OF PENIS AND SCROTUM

Penis

Cremasteric
muscle
Pampinifo
plexus
Vas deteren

Epididymis

Glans penis

Testis

Scrotal sac

SEMINAL VESICLE CUT TO SHOW
HOW IT ACTS AS A RESERVOIR

RELATIONSHIP OF BLADDER TO SEMINAL
VESICLES AND PROSTATE

Ureter
Bladder
Vas deferens

Ampulla
of vas

Seminal
vesicle

Prostate

Cowper's gland

RELATIONSHIP OF THE GENITAL AND
URINARY SYSTEMS OF THE MALE

Arrow
indicates
direction
sperm
follow
to the
outside

URINARY SYSTEM

GENITAL SYSTEM

EXTERNAL GENITAL ORGAN

CROSS SECTION OF TESTIS

Epididymis
(Composed of many
tubules entwined)

Septa

Vas deferens

Network of tubules
from lobules of testis

Lobules

Tubules

THE MALE GENITAL SYSTEM

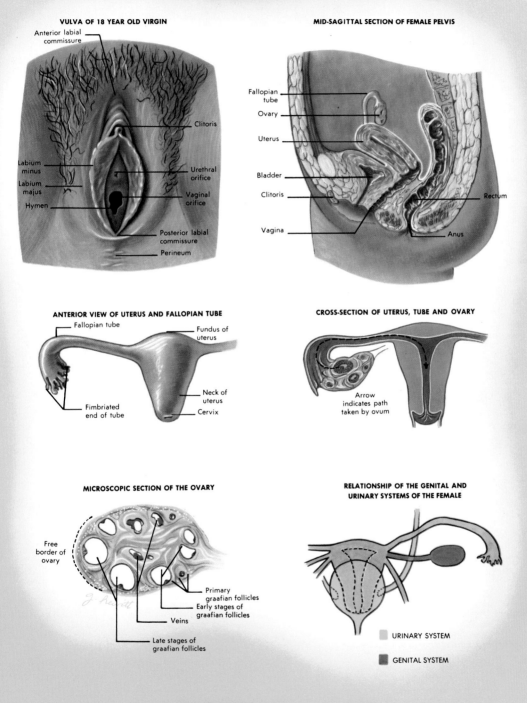

VULVA OF 18 YEAR OLD VIRGIN

Anterior labial commissure

Clitoris

Labium minus

Labium majus

Urethral orifice

Vaginal orifice

Hymen

Posterior labial commissure

Perineum

MID-SAGITTAL SECTION OF FEMALE PELVIS

Fallopian tube

Ovary

Uterus

Bladder

Clitoris

Vagina

Rectum

Anus

ANTERIOR VIEW OF UTERUS AND FALLOPIAN TUBE

Fallopian tube

Fundus of uterus

Neck of uterus

Cervix

Fimbriated end of tube

CROSS-SECTION OF UTERUS, TUBE AND OVARY

Arrow indicates path taken by ovum

MICROSCOPIC SECTION OF THE OVARY

Free border of ovary

Primary graafian follicles

Early stages of graafian follicles

Veins

Late stages of graafian follicles

RELATIONSHIP OF THE GENITAL AND URINARY SYSTEMS OF THE FEMALE

URINARY SYSTEM

GENITAL SYSTEM

THE FEMALE GENITAL SYSTEM

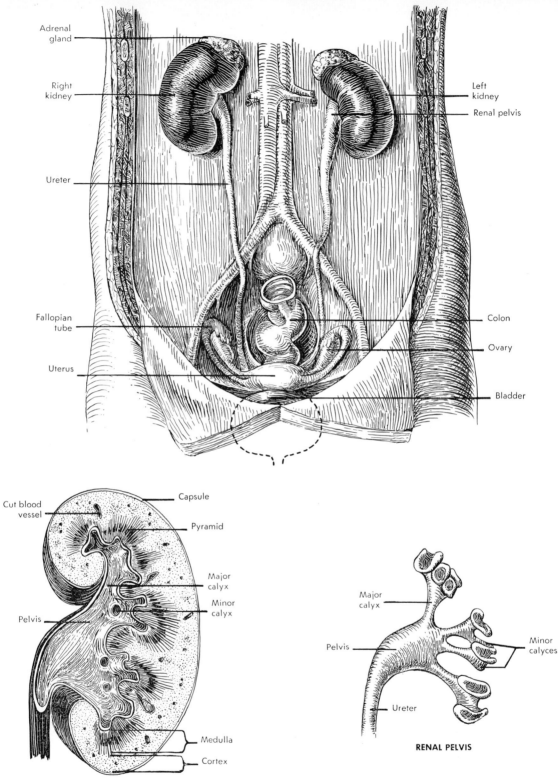

Adrenal gland

Right kidney

Ureter

Fallopian tube

Uterus

Left kidney

Renal pelvis

Colon

Ovary

Bladder

Cut blood vessel

Capsule

Pyramid

Major calyx

Minor calyx

Pelvis

Medulla

Cortex

CUT SECTION OF KIDNEY AND RENAL PELVIS

Major calyx

Pelvis

Minor calyces

Ureter

RENAL PELVIS

URINARY SYSTEM OF THE FEMALE IN RELATION TO THE REPRODUCTIVE SYSTEM

albuminuria." In some individuals, the albumin appears in urine excreted during the day, but is absent in urine formed during sleep. This condition is believed to be related to the shape of the spine; when the individual stands up, the vein of the left kidney may be pressed upon at the point where it passes the spine. The back pressure on the return blood from the kidney probably results in albumin escaping into the urine.

Cysts

Cysts are sacs containing a fluid-like material. Their cause is uncertain. Simple cysts may be removed surgically.

Polycystic disease is a condition in which the kidney is filled with numerous cysts. Both kidneys usually are involved, and the disease probably is present at birth. The condition may be hereditary, so that persons with polycystic disease are advised to consider this before having children.

Tumors

Tumors of the kidney that do not spread to other parts of the body are known as benign. They may occur in either the kidney substance or its pelvis. Blood in the urine is the most common symptom, although pain may also be present. X-ray study is of value in diagnosis, and treatment consists of surgical removal where necessary.

Malignant tumors or cancers of the kidney are much more serious, since they may spread *(metastasize)* to other parts of the body. In children, the most common type of cancer of the

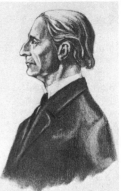

LUDWIG, Karl Friedrich Wilhelm (1816-1895) German physiologist. He developed the present theory of urine formation as a filtration of the blood followed by resorption of water in the tubules. He also showed that secretory glands were more than simple filters. He developed the kymograph and applied it to the study of the human circulation and respiration. He carried out investigations on the composition of the gases in blood.

kidney is the *Wilms' tumor*. This type of tumor frequently grows to great size and causes the abdomen to protrude. It is seen most often in children under six. The physician may be able to feel with his fingers the abdominal mass caused by the tumor, before blood in the urine or pain appears. At times weakness and vomiting are present. The current method for treating patients with Wilms' tumor is threefold: drugs to shrink the large, vascular growth, surgical resection to remove it, and irradiation to halt any cells that may have escaped while handling it. This method has improved long-range chances for many children considered hopeless. It is essential, however, that the tumor be recognized while it is still in the early stage of development. If the patient is not given treatment, this tumor is invariably fatal.

The problem of early diagnosis is likewise of great importance in other types of cancer of the kidney. Usually the first symptom of all types is blood in the urine *(hematuria)*. Pain is apt to occur later. At the first sign of blood in the urine, a physician should always be consulted. This is advisable even if the blood appears in the urine for a few days only, since blood may appear and disappear at intervals when cancer is present. Many advances have been made in the surgical treatment of patients with cancer of the kidney, but success depends to a large extent on early diagnosis.

Unlike many other internal organs, the kidney daily sends its product to the outside. Consequently, abnormalities of the kidney frequently give warning via the urine. Any urinary condition varying from normal deserves the physician's attention.

The artificial kidney

When extreme kidney damage impairs the system's ability to cleanse the blood, the patient can be helped by a mechanical device to filter out the waste material. This process is called *dialysis*. There is an increasing array of these

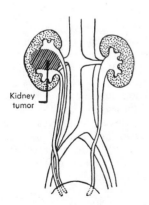

Kidney tumor

Illustration of a tumor in a kidney which also happens to have a congenital double ureter. There are a number of types of renal tumor and they may be either benign or malignant. They may affect the renal pelvis or various portions of the kidney proper, and smaller ones may not be detected for many years. Understanding of these structures from a medical standpoint has greatly improved since the first kidney removal in 1861.

life-saving machines, sometimes termed artificial kidneys, for use in hospitals and homes.

First, a small plastic tube is implanted in the arm or leg to connect a vein with an artery. Two or three times a week, the tube is opened to be hooked up to the dialysis machine. The arterial blood flows into the machine and passes through an intricate plastic filter that centrifuges out the waste material. The blood then flows back into the venous system.

Each session with the dialysis machine takes many hours. These expensive and often inaccessible machines have been increasingly simplified to help patients who are not near large medical centers or who cannot afford the cost of hospital dialysis. One simpler machine uses gravity to pump the blood through its filter. A small, portable filter has been developed to make home dialysis more practical. Often, dialysis machines are used until a donated kidney becomes available for transplantation.

Kidney transplantation

Transplantation of internal organs has made rapid progress in recent years. Kidney transplants are now the most successful and numerous of attempts to replace organs in man. There are several sources for organ replacement. *Homografts* are transplants between unrelated members of the same species. *Heterografts* are transplants between members of different species. *Isografts* are grafts between two genetically close members of the same family. Transplantation among identical twins has had the greatest rate of acceptance. This is because the body more readily accepts tissue it recognizes as its own, but rejects "foreign" tissue. This phenomenon is known as the *immune reaction*, and is a major hazard to transplantation of blood-supplied organs.

Immunity is an active biochemical response by *antibodies* (defenders) to *antigens* (invaders). The body has its own antigens which it does not normally challenge. But if strange antigens enter, antibodies are produced by the lymphatic system, causing severe inflammation and death to the transplanted tissue. The immune reaction does not affect corneal transplants, since that tissue does not receive antibodies from the lymph glands via the blood.

Transplant donors are typed by the kind of antigens carried by their blood cells. If they match, or nearly match, the recipient's serotype, the transplant has a better chance of acceptance by the host. Immunosuppressive drugs and radiotherapy increase the chances for successful transplants from nonrelated donors and from siblings who are not twins by halting production of antibodies.

Most transplanted kidneys are from live donors. Cadaver transplants are also used when donated by a dying patient and his family. Because of the scarcity of available donors, transplants from baboons and chimpanzees have been attempted as a substitute until a human kidney can be found. Animal transplants have been the least accepted, and the longest survival rate of a heterograft is nine months. In the future, organ banks may be feasible, where donor kidneys can be frozen or kept alive in animals until needed by a patient.

Transplantation of internal organs became possible with the development of surgical techniques for joining blood vessels (*anastomosis*). Chemotherapy, radiology, and precision operating room equipment have been quickly developed to meet the demands of transplantation procedures. Indeed, transplantation techniques are so successful that women who have only one kidney, whether donor or receiver, can bear and deliver children.

DISORDERS OF THE URETER

The *ureter* is the tube through which urine passes from the kidney to the bladder. It often is affected by diseases of the urinary tract above or below the ureter itself.

Abnormalities of development

Duplication of the ureter on one or both sides is a fairly common abnormality. The entire ureter, or a portion of it, may be double, and it is fairly common for two ureters from a so-called double kidney (see section on the kidney) to unite before entering the bladder. Such a union forms what is known as the "Y-shaped ureter."

Kinks in the ureters may be present at birth. They generally occur after birth, however, as a result of lengthening of the ureter secondary to obstruction of the urinary flow. Narrow places (*strictures*) in the canal of the ureter, as well as enlargement of the canal, have been observed at birth. The latter condition results in a gigantic ureter known as *megalo-ureter*. It may be caused by a failure of normal development of muscle tone in the ureter of the unborn child.

Defects in development may cause the ureters to open into the rectum or the female urethra. Abnormal openings into the reproductive tract have also been observed. The ureter may open into the prostate, seminal vesicles, vas deferens, or ejaculatory ducts. Ureteral openings into the vagina, uterus, and fallopian tubes have likewise been found (see Chapter 15 for discussion of these structures). Abnormal openings of the ureters may be corrected surgically. If untreated, however, these conditions may lead to infection or an inability to retain urine.

In rare cases, at birth the part of the ureter entering the bladder may be dilated or ballooned. This condition is known as a *ureterocele* or *ureterovesical cyst*. In women, the ureter may protrude through the bladder and appear at the external opening of the urethra. Ureterovesical cysts can generally be removed surgically or by burning with an electric current (*fulguration*).

Obstruction

Obstruction of the ureter itself, or any part of the urinary tract below the ureter, may result in dilation. This often causes the ureter to grow abnormally and become kinked. Infection is common in such cases.

Infections

In most cases, infection of the ureter occurs by upward extension of a bladder infection or downward spread of an infection in the funnel-shaped collecting tube (*pelvis*) of the kidney. Strictures in the ureteral canal may occur, especially in patients with tuberculosis.

Stones

Stones weighing as much as one third of a pound have been found in the ureter. Diagnosis is usually performed by x-ray techniques. A great many ureteral stones can be removed by special instruments without resorting to an operation. (For passing catheter tubes, see section on the kidney.)

Tumors

Tumors of the ureter are rare. Usually the symptoms produced resemble those of tumors of the kidney. Benign (nonspreading) tumors often may be removed by local resection, but malignant tumors (cancers) require removal of both ureter and kidney. As in kidney cancer, early diagnosis is extremely important. A physician should be consulted if blood appears in the urine, as this is the most frequent symptom.

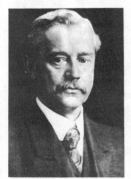

KELLY, Howard Atwood (1858-1943), American surgeon. He was famous for the many novel procedures and devices that he introduced into surgical methods for the urinary system. Although he was a specialist in women's diseases, he was the first clinician to insert a rubber tube (catheter) through the male urethra, across the bladder and thence on up into the narrow ureter.

DISORDERS OF THE BLADDER

Since the bladder occupies a position between the kidneys and the urethra, it is often called the middle portion of the urinary tract. Most abnormal conditions of the bladder are associated with, or the result of, conditions affecting the upper or lower portions of the tract.

Abnormalities of development

Rare abnormalities of the bladder may be listed as complete absence, double bladder, or the more or less incomplete division of the bladder by *septa*, such as the hourglass bladder. Outpocketings (*diverticula*) of the bladder are relatively common, and may be present at birth or develop as the result of increased pressure caused by obstruction to the normal flow of urine.

In the condition known as *exstrophy*, the front wall of the bladder and the abdominal wall covering the organ are absent. The back (*posterior*) wall of the bladder protrudes and the ureters excrete urine to the outside of the body continuously. Exstrophy has been corrected surgically with some success.

Hernia

The tissues which hold the bladder in place may become weakened and allow the bladder to bulge into various abnormal positions. If the bladder protrudes into the vagina, the condition is known as *cystocele*. It is often secondary to childbirth, and is due to relaxation of perineal support. It can be repaired surgically.

Fistulae

Abnormal channels allowing the passage of urine from the bladder into other hollow organs, or directly to the outside of the body through the skin, are known as *fistulae*. Fistulae are of many types. In *vesico-intestinal fistula*, a communication exists between the bladder and some part of the intestine. In the more common *vesico-vaginal fistula*, the channel lies between the bladder and vagina. Although other causes exist, vesico-vaginal fistula may result from childbirth. In such women, urine leaks almost constantly from the bladder into the vagina. Treatment for patients with fistulae consists usually of closing the abnormal opening surgically.

Inflammations

Inflammation of the bladder is known as *cystitis*. Although inflammation of the kidneys and ureters may frequently accompany cystitis, usually there is no clinical evidence of upper urinary tract involvement. When the upper urinary tract is involved, the patient usually has fever. Cystitis is most commonly caused by one of the bacillary group of bacteria. Many of these bacteria are motile, and ascend into the bladder on the mucous membrane of the urethra. Consequently, the urethra may also become inflamed, resulting in *urethritis*. Urethritis and cystitis cause an increased frequency of urination, an increased urgency to urinate, as well as pain on urination. When cystitis is caused by *Staphylococcus* or other cocci, it is usually the descending type of infection. This type of infection begins in the kidney and descends into the bladder via the urinary tract. The ascending type of infection is far more common.

In suspected cystitis, examination of the urine is done first; often, this is all that is necessary to diagnose the disorder. If diagnosis is uncertain, an examination of the bladder and urethra may be made with a *cystoscope*, an optical instrument used for inspecting the inside of the bladder. By such an examination (*cystoscopy*), the physician is able to determine the extent and general type of the inflammation. If the cystitis is caused by infection, a bacteriologist or pathologist identifies the specific organism or organisms responsible; with this information, a decision can be reached as to what antibiotics

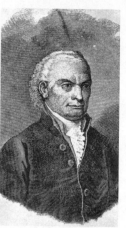

COTUGNO, Domenico (1736-1822) Italian anatomist and scientist. The first person to establish experimentally the abnormal presence of albumin in the urine. Cotugno described the *nasopalatine nerve*, which carries sensations from the mucosa of the nose and mouth to the brain. He was the first person to describe the cerebrospinal fluid and was also a pioneer in the prophylaxis of tuberculosis. Cotugno was the originator of the term *sciatica*, to designate pain along the sciatic nerve.

or other drugs are most apt to be effective. Although treatment with appropriate drugs is of great value, other types of treatment may be necessary to prevent relapses. This is particularly true of so-called *trigonitis*, which is an inflammation of the triangular part of the bladder at the corners of which the ureters and urethra open. In this condition the back portion of the urethra usually is involved also.

Bilharziasis is an inflammation of the bladder caused by a flatworm, *Schistosoma haematobium*. It is also known as *schistosomiasis*. This disease is rare in the United States, but its growing incidence in the East, Middle East, and parts of Africa and South America has made it a major world health problem. The larvae live in fresh-water snails in marshy areas, rice paddies, and lakes. When they develop into swimming, forktailed embryos known as *cercariae*, they leave the host snail and penetrate the skin of human beings who may be walking in the water or swimming. They quickly enter the blood stream and go into the bladder and liver where they may live for years, producing eggs. These eggs may be excreted and enter the water supply system through inadequate sewage treatment.

Symptoms of schistosomiasis are infection, anemia, stunting of growth, intestinal bleeding, and extreme debilitation. With the cystoscope, flat reddened areas with opaque, yellow raised spots are seen on the bladder. Diagnosis is often made by finding eggs in the urine. There are three principal strains of schistosomae in humans. Treatment is difficult. Large-scale attempts are being made to eradicate snails. Drugs, particularly antimony preparations, are effective for some patients. To treat patients with resistant strains, a mechanical filter is surgically placed in the saphenous vein of the thigh to catch and remove the eggs from the blood. If the organisms are present in the bladder for a number of years, cancer may result.

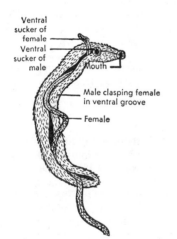

Enlarged drawing of an adult male and female *Schistosoma haematobium*, the flatworms which are the causative agents of a severe bladder inflammation. The adult stage worms are from one quarter to one inch in length. At various stages in their life history these worms live in the lungs, the liver and the bladder. The female will lay her eggs in the finer venules of the mucosa of the bladder. Afterward she lives with the male in the illustrated manner. Eggs are passed in the urine, after which the young hatch. They must then infect a snail, before they can continue to develop into later stages and infect human beings.

Ventral sucker of female
Ventral sucker of male
Mouth
Male clasping female in ventral groove
Female

Stones

Stones (calculi) in the bladder are generally associated with faulty elimination of urine from the bladder. This is often caused by some type of bladder outlet obstruction, e.g. an enlarged prostate. Stones also quickly form if a catheter has to be left in the bladder for long periods. Stones may be single or multiple and are usually associated with infection.

Most stones may be diagnosed by x-ray examination or cystoscopy. Symptoms include pain and blood in the urine, especially at the end of urination. Furthermore, the urinary stream may stop suddenly if a stone in the bladder suddenly closes off the opening of the urethra.

Patients with bladder stones often are treated by a procedure known as *litholapaxy*. An instrument called a *lithotrite* is inserted into the bladder, and the stone is grasped between the jaws of this instrument and crushed. In some cases, the bladder must be opened for removal of the stone.

Tumors

Both nonspreading (benign) tumors and spreading tumors (cancers) of the bladder occur. The bladder is the most common site of cancer in the urinary tract (this does not include the prostate). Bladder cancer is about twice as common in men as in women, and usually occurs after age 50.

The outstanding symptom of cancer of the bladder is blood in the urine, without pain, and it is probably the first symptom in most cases. Other conditions may cause blood in the urine. However, this symptom is a serious one in any case, and its cause must be determined. Blood may not occur in sufficient amounts to give a

bright red color to the urine, but instead may result in pink or smoky-colored urine. Blood may appear and then as suddenly disappear.

Blood in the urine always calls for a complete urological investigation, including a cystoscopic examination in order to exclude cancer. Cancer of the bladder is diagnosed through the use of the cystoscope; through this instrument a small piece of the suspected growth can be taken for microscopic examination by a pathologist, in order to determine the diagnosis. If cancer is present, surgery is required in most cases. However, radium or x-rays may be used.

DISORDERS OF THE URETHRA

The *urethra* is the tube leading from the bladder to the exterior of the body and constitutes the lower part of the urinary tract. Disorders here may produce severe damage to the upper portions of the tract, particularly if the escape of urine is partially or completely prevented. Infections of the urethra may spread upward to the bladder, ureters, and kidneys.

Abnormalities of the urethra which are present at birth are more common in men than in women. In rare cases, the entire urethra may be absent in an unborn child. Unless an opening of the bladder is established, the bladder becomes distended with urine, and the kidneys are destroyed by back pressure. An abnormal opening (fistula) of the bladder into the rectum may occur. In other instances, there may not be a channel throughout the normal course of the urethra. This condition is known as *imperforation,* and its consequences are similar to those of complete absence of the urethra. More common than either of these abnormalities is a narrowing (*stricture*) of the urethra.

Valves present at birth in the back portion of the urethra also may cause obstruction in the flow of urine. The resulting back pressure may lead to greatly dilated ureters and dilated kidneys (*hydronephrosis*). The patient commonly has urinary difficulties throughout life, such as a small stream of urine, dribbling, and a frequent urge to urinate. Some patients with this disorder are unable to retain urine (*incontinence*), or it may be one of the causes of bedwetting (*enuresis*). Kidney function may be reduced, and symptoms of *uremic poisoning* may appear. Frequently, infection ensues. Surgical removal of the valves, or their division with an electric current, is readily accomplished by a physician, and provides the patient with relief. The success of this treatment, however, depends largely on an early diagnosis.

Abnormalities of the urethra are similar in both sexes except for defects involving the ex-

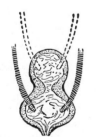

This illustration is of an hourglass bladder with ureters entering into the bottom chamber. The dotted lines show how the ureters may also enter into the upper portion of the bladder in a more normal fashion. Only twenty-two cases of this rare condition have ever been reported since its first discovery in 1848. The hourglass bladder is said to have a relatively normal capacity for storage of urine.

ternal opening of the urethra, the *meatus*. Abnormal development in this area is considered in the following section on the meatus.

Although the great majority of inflamed urethras are caused by bacterial infections, chemical irritation also can be responsible. For example, strong chemicals used in self-treatment of gonorrhea may produce inflammation. If the urine is too acid or too alkaline, inflammation may occur, and a burning sensation may be felt on urination.

The most common inflammation of the urethra is sometimes called "nonspecific urethritis" and may be caused by chronic, nongonorrheal inflammation of the prostate gland. Inflammations of the urethra are the most common urinary tract disorders in women. Gonorrhea and certain nonvenereal diseases which produce infections of the urethra are discussed in detail in Chapter 15.

Symptoms of any urethral inflammation generally include a frequent urge to urinate, and a burning sensation when urination actually occurs. In men, "stripping" the penis causes a drop of cloudy fluid to appear at its opening (*meatus*). The urine contains pus, and at times blood cells. In any particular case of urethral inflammation, a bacteriological examination is required for positive identification of the offending microorganism and for determination of the probable value of drugs. With this aid, the physician is nearly always able to effect a rapid cure by administration of one or more of the antibiotics or sulfonamide drugs.

Stricture

An abnormal narrowing of the urethral canal is known as *stricture*. A complete closing off of the urethra may occur in severe cases. Strictures are more common in men than in women, and the majority involve the back (*posterior*) part of the anterior urethra. They may be present at birth, or they may be acquired through infection or injury.

Strictures present at birth already have been mentioned. Functional disorders of urination may be caused by irritation from hemorrhoids, or by anxiety as to a coming event, such as making a public speech. Local applications of heat may induce relaxation of the muscle concerned and result in urination. In some cases, the physician must prescribe drugs, or he may empty the bladder by introducing a hollow flexible tube (*catheter*) through the urethra. Acquired strictures of the urethra are most frequently caused by gonorrhea, but may be the result of other types of inflammation, injuries or instrumentation.

Strictures cause difficulty in urination, and in some cases may be the cause of a urethral discharge or bleeding. The desire to urinate may be more frequent than usual, and dribbling may occur after urination. If the stricture is of severe degree and of long duration, the resulting stoppage of the flow of urine may cause the urethra back of the stricture to become dilated and to form pouches. Increased pressure from dammed-up urine can also cause the bladder, ureters, and kidneys to become dilated and infected. A frequent and annoying condition of narrowing of the urethra occurs in many women during the menopause and can become a true stricture.

When symptoms suggest stricture of the urethra, definite diagnosis is made by the passing of probelike instruments known as bougies into the urethra. A solution which is opaque to x-rays may be injected and an x-ray picture of the urethra then taken to demonstrate whether strictures are present. Such a picture is known as a *urethrogram*. Stricture may be treated surgically or by dilating the urethra with bougies. The surgical procedure may be accomplished internally with a special instrument called a urethrotome, or externally by removing the area of stricture.

Stones and tumors

Most frequently stones (*calculi*) in the urethra are formed elsewhere in the urinary tract and lodge in the urethra. Although the cause is not always clear, stones often are associated with outpockets (*diverticula*) of the urethra, especially in women. Single stones are most common. Obstruction of the flow of urine may result from stones in the urethra.

Urethral stones sometimes may be passed by pinching the opening of the urethra during urination. The pinching causes the urethra to swell with dammed-up urine which may float the stone and result in its passage in the spurt of urine which follows. Stones may also be removed with forceps, or crushed with a special instrument inserted into the urethra. Stones firmly lodged (*impacted*) may require surgical removal. All stones may cause injury and bleeding.

Tumors of the anterior urethra are uncommon. Benign inflammatory *polyps* occur most often in the posterior urethra; their symptoms include frequency of desire to urinate, difficulty in urination, and a discharge from the urethra. Hemorrhage is not common. Apparently they are secondary to a prostatic disorder; they are not associated with loss of sexual vigor or potency. The usual treatment for benign tumors is destruction by electric current (*fulguration*).

Malignant tumors (cancers) of the urethra are rare. When they occur, the symptoms are similar to those of stricture. Patients with cancer of the urethra are usually treated by radiotherapy and sometimes surgically.

DISORDERS OF THE MEATUS

The *meatus*, or external opening of the urethra, is the end or outlet of the urinary tract. Through the meatus the urine, produced by the kidneys and stored temporarily in the bladder, is expelled from the body. In males, the meatus is located on the head (*glans*) of the penis; in females, the meatus is in the vestibule which is the space between the inner lips of the vulva.

Abnormalities in development

The meatus may be narrowed at birth. If narrowing is sufficiently pronounced, the passage of urine is retarded, with resulting damage to the remainder of the urinary tract. These changes, caused by the pressure of dammed-up urine, have been described in previous sections. Narrowing of the meatus generally produces an abnormally small stream of urine. Treatment consists in widening the opening by an operation known as meatotomy.

The meatus may be double, with partial or complete duplication of the urethra. The extra opening may be on the head of the penis, or on the undersurface of the penis back of the glans.

More common than two openings in the urethra is the urethra in which the single meatus is abnormal in position. Such abnormal openings are present at birth. If the abnormal meatus is on the upper surface of the penis, the condition is known as *epispadias*. The opening may be on the upper surface of the head of the penis, or on the shaft. In the latter case, the roof of the urethra is missing, and the meatus is a wide, open slit or trough. Complete epispadias occurs with *exstrophy* of the bladder, in which the bladder is protruded through the abdominal wall. The penis may be small, flattened, and held

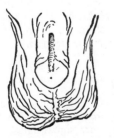

One type of epispadias is illustrated here. In this type the meatus is seen as an open trough along the top of the penis. An even more extreme form may occur in which the urethra is open along the entire length of the shaft. Another variety occurs when the meatus is located at the base of the penis. Although displacements of the meatus are commoner among males, extreme upper displacement is found in women.

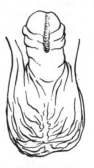

Hypospadias, shown in a typical form in the drawing, is a relatively common congenital defect in which the meatus lies on the underside of the penis. This condition is about 150 times more common than epispadias. Hypospadias is in many cases accompanied by a bending down and backward of the shaft of the penis. Other deformities of the foreskin and glans may be present.

against the pubic region by a band of supporting tissue. There is complete loss of the ability to retain urine (*incontinence*). In these rare cases, a conduit is formed surgically to divert the urine through the ileum.

Much more common than epispadias is the opposite condition, *hypospadias*, in which the meatus is on the underside of the penis. The opening may be on the glans of the penis, the shaft of the penis, at the junction of the penis with the scrotum, or at the junction of the scrotum with the *perineum* (region between the scrotum and the anus). In the last two types, normal sexual intercourse may be difficult or impossible. Most cases of hypospadias can be corrected by reconstructive surgical operations upon the penis and urethra.

Epispadias in women is more infrequent than in men. The *clitoris* (see Chapter 15) may be split, and the front wall of the urethra may be absent to varying degrees. The splitting process may involve the bones of the pubis and result in exstrophy of the bladder.

Tumor

Both benign (nonspreading) tumors and malignant tumors (cancers) of the meatus occur. The most frequent tumor of the female urethra is the *caruncle*. This benign tumor resembles a raspberry and bleeds easily. Caruncles may be extremely tender to the touch and urination may be quite painful. Women with these tumors may find sexual intercourse unbearable. The patient frequently is extremely nervous and of low morale. Such tumors may be destroyed by burning with an electric current (*fulguration*), removed surgically, or may be managed by a combination of both methods. Prolapse of the urethra, which consists of the protrusion of redundant mucous membrane through the urethral meatus, is often confused with caruncle. The mass is not so sensitive as a caruncle.

Cancer at the meatus is rare; in women, it usually involves the vulva. (For a detailed discussion of vulvar cancer, see Chapter 15.)

DISTURBANCES OF URINATION

Urination at frequent intervals is one of the most common symptoms of disorders of the urinary tract. Frequency may be caused by an increased production of urine, as in diabetes or inflammation of the kidney (*nephritis*). Local irritations arising from infections, strictures, prostatic obstructions, stones, tumors, or from a too acid or alkaline condition of the urine, also may cause frequency. Frequency may be a result of various nervous disorders, ranging from dread of an approaching event to diseases in the brain or spinal cord.

Difficulties in the act of urination

Difficulty of urination most commonly is caused by an obstruction of some type. Narrowing of the urethra usually results in a small, forked stream or a stream shaped like a corkscrew. Enlargement of the prostate often causes delay in beginning urination, though this condition may also result from diseases of the nerves involved in urination. Dribbling of urine at the beginning of the act is characteristic of retention of urine in the bladder. In certain nervous disseases, there may be abnormal dribbling at the end of urination. Stones in the bladder may cause an intermittent stream of urine.

Pain

Pain during urination (*dysuria*) most often is a burning sensation and usually is caused by inflammation in the bladder or urethra. In cases of inflammation of the back portion of the urethra, burning occurs chiefly at the start of urination; in cases of inflammation of the bladder, burning is present throughout urination. Persons with ulcerated bladder or bladder stones usually experience pain at the end of urination.

Abnormalities in urinary output

An abnormally large output of urine is known as *polyuria*. If the increased excretion or frequency occurs mainly or entirely at night, the symptom is called *nocturia*. Polyuria naturally follows unusually high fluid intake, but also occurs in diabetes, certain kidney conditions, and nervous disorders.

An abnormally low urine output is known as *oliguria*, and a complete absence of urine is called *anuria*. These symptoms often are caused by obstruction at some point in the urinary tract, or by a decrease in production of urine. Excretion of urine is curtailed when the body is in a state of dehydration (from diarrhea, vomiting, etc.), when there is insufficient functioning of the kidneys, and when there is spasm of certain blood vessels. Although oliguria and anuria are symptoms which ordinarily disappear when the underlying abnormality is corrected, they are of sufficient seriousness to require emergency treatment. Correction of fluid intake may be all that is necessary, along with drugs designed to relax muscles and promote excretion of urine. However, the condition may be of a very serious nature and should be appropriately evaluated.

Incontinence

Inability to control the emptying of the bladder is known as *incontinence*. This condition may be partial or complete. Temporary loss of control may accompany excitement or fright. Irritation of the neck of the bladder or inflammations of the back portion of the urethra may cause involuntary dribbling of urine. In *paradoxical* or *passive* incontinence, the bladder fills but cannot be emptied normally either because of an enlarged prostate, or diseases of nerve centers in the brain or spinal cord, or injury to local nerve centers. A constant dribbling from the overfilled bladder results. Benign and malignant prostatism is discussed in Chapter 15, "The Reproductive System." Diseases of or injury to the spinal cord may produce the so-called *neurogenic bladder*. The bladder fills normally, but cannot be emptied at will. However, if the skin of the leg or the penis is pinched, the bladder may empty itself automatically as the result of a nerve reflex action. In *true incontinence*, there is a constant, uncontrollable dribbling of urine. True incontinence may be caused by abnormalities present at birth, false passages (*fistulae*) for excretion of urine, or injury or disease of nerves. Treatment is primarily surgical.

Bed-wetting

Most children achieve bladder control by day and night by the time they are three or four years old. Boys are somewhat slower than girls to do so. If, after he has reached this age, a child continues to wet his bed at night, he is probably suffering from some emotional rather than physical disturbance. There are cases where the child's symptoms or a test of the urine (*urinalysis*) may suggest an organic cause. But by far the great majority of children have nothing physically wrong. However, a careful search must be made to determine if there is an abnormality present; and when a pathological condition exists it is essential that it be corrected at an early date, in order to preserve kidney function. When benign urinary obstruction is relieved in children, they are cured if kidney function has not been destroyed and dilatation of the urinary tract has not occurred.

Bed-wetting is one of the most common indications of emotional unrest in children, and is considered so significant a psychological problem that it is discussed in most manuals of child psychiatry. The technical term for the disorder is *enuresis*. Physicians have discovered that bedwetting frequently begins in a child who had formerly remained dry at night, following some mental conflict which upsets the child. The child may have developed feelings of insecurity because of harsh treatment, the absence of his parents, or the arrival of a new baby who threatens his position in the family sphere. A searching effort should be made to discover a possible source of emotional tension. With the help of their physician, parents can examine the situation existing in the home, to ascertain whether friction, coercion, or pressure has prevailed to undermine the self-confidence of the child. If parents make too much fuss over the wet bed, the child can be kept in a state of dread and nervousness, which makes control increasingly difficult for him to attain. Nagging, scolding, or threatening does more harm than good. Above all, parents should avoid suggesting to the child that there is anything shameful or dirty about such lapses. This not only contributes to the child's feelings of insecurity, but may also lead to mistaken ideas connected with the sexual function. Since a child cannot distinguish between the organs of sex and excretion, he may retain the idea in later years that everything connected with sex is dirty. This attitude has been responsible for many an unhappy marriage.

Although the reason for bed-wetting lies in his troubled mind, it must be remembered that the child *does not wet his bed deliberately*. Therefore, it should not be attacked as a disciplinary problem. Cutting down on the fluids allowed at night, particularly those containing caffeine, has been suggested and is a logical measure, provided it does not form the basis for an argument. If it does, argument may be even more conducive to bed-wetting than the fluids would be.

Parents of the child who wets his bed can be of the greatest help by creating an atmosphere of affection and security around the child, and by maintaining a casual attitude to his difficulty. When his emotional tensions finally become dispelled, he may then be able to achieve complete bladder control.

15 THE REPRODUCTIVE SYSTEM

WHAT IT IS AND DOES

From the standpoint of the species, the most important function of the body is the ability to reproduce life. Among the higher animals the function of reproduction is dependent on the union of cells—one from the male and one from the female. Not only must the male reproductive cells (*spermatozoa*) and female reproductive cells (*ova* or *eggs*) unite, but the minute fragment of life thus produced must be nurtured within a protective environment until the new organism is able to survive apart from that environment.

Male reproductive system

The male reproductive system is comprised of the genital glands also known as the *testes*, held in a pouch of skin outside the body (the *scrotum*). The secretion of the testes is conveyed to the *urethra* (the tube which leads from the bladder to the exterior) by two ducts (*vasa deferentia*). Two receptacles (*seminal vesicles*) open into these ducts; and an external introductive organ (the *penis*) conveys the male reproductive cells or *spermatozoa*, from the male body and into the body of the female. Other accessory sex organs (the *epididymis* and the *prostate*) share in providing the necessary fluids for making up the *seminal plasma*, which is a viscous liquid containing the sperm cells.

The sperm cells are sensitive to change but can survive outside the body for a short time if the environment is suitable. The seminal plasma furnishes the ideal environment for the sperm cells. Like most biological fluids, the seminal fluid is made up of a large proportion of water, in which are dissolved proteins, sugars, mineral salts, and many other substances. The seminal plasma constitutes the bulk of the ejaculate.

A mature spermatozoon consists of the *sperm cell*, which is composed of a head and a tail. The sperm cells propel themselves by a flailing action of the tail portion. When the sperm cells have attained maturity, in the testes, they move partly by their own propulsion to the seminal vesicles, where they are stored until ready to be discharged. The discharge of the sperm cells with the contents of the seminal vesicles is preceded by a discharge of prostatic fluid, mixed with the seminal plasma, to form the *semen*. The amount of semen discharged in one ejaculation varies and depends largely upon the frequency of ejaculation.

The *testes:* Production of sperm cells takes place in the *testes*. The testes are two oval-shaped organs located outside the abdominal cavity below the penis, and held by a pouch called the *scrotum*. In addition to the reproductive function, the testes produce male sex hormones which are secreted into the blood stream. In this respect the testes are endocrine glands; they determine the degree of sexuality developed by an individual. Rarely, an individual is born with both testicles and ovaries; this is *true hermaphroditism*. These and other abnormal conditions are discussed in detail in Chapter 10, "The Endocrine System."

Before a boy is born, the testes are present within the abdominal cavity where they have been formed, and descend gradually until, by the time of birth, they make their exit through a passage called the *inguinal canal* and have become localized in the scrotum.

For the testes to function effectively, they must be at a lower temperature than that of the abdomen. When the temperature increases, the testes do not produce mature spermatozoa. Because they are located within the scrotum outside the abdominal cavity, the testes are kept at a temperature a few degrees lower than that of the body. When the outside temperature is lowered, the spermatic cord that is attached to the testes and the scrotum draws upward, keeping the testes close to the body and allowing them to be warmed by the body's heat. When the outside temperature is raised, the testes are lowered away from the body by the scrotum and spermatic cord. This is possible because the scrotum and the spermatic cord are endowed with a degree of elasticity, and the testes possess free movement within the scrotum.

The surface of the testes is covered by a layer of fibrous tissue called the *tunica vaginalis*. The internal structure of the testes is divided into sections separated by thin membranes. Within each section are long, thin, tubelike strands, called the *seminiferous tubules*. It is within these tubules that the spermatozoa are produced. In the spaces or "interstices" that exist between the tubules are the *interstitial* cells. These are not directly concerned with the reproductive function, but produce the male hormone, which is an important factor in the development of the accessory sex organs.

In the cells that make up the seminiferous tubules, the spermatozoa are produced. If a section of the testes is observed with a powerful microscope, a number of circular structures representing cross sections of the tubules can be seen. Within the circular structures are seen the spermatozoa at different stages of development. Toward the center of the tubules are seen the mature spermatozoa with complete heads and tails.

The *epididymis:* During the maturing process, the spermatozoa pass into multiple small tubes (*vasa efferentia*) which lead to the *epididymis*. The epididymis is a long, coiled tube in which the touring spermatozoa are stored for a few days to gain further maturity. The epididymis establishes contact with a long, thin duct (*ductus* or *vas deferens*). Upward in its course toward the abdomen, the vas deferens is joined by the testicular arteries, veins, lymphatics, and nerves to form a thick tube, the *spermatic cord*. The spermatic cord, containing the vas and other vessels, passes into the abdomen through the inguinal canal, and descends by the side of the urinary bladder to the prostate, through which it passes to reach the urethra. It is there joined by the small duct of the *seminal vesicles*. For each testis, there is one spermatic cord, one vas deferens, and one seminal vesicle.

The *seminal vesicles:* The seminal vesicles are two pouches located between the bladder and the rectum, although not connected to either. The lower ends of the two seminal vesicles unite to form two short ducts that serve to carry the spermatic fluid to the large duct in the penis (the *urethra*) and outside the body. These are the *ejaculatory ducts,* which are two small ducts that penetrate the prostate. From this point both the semen and the urine share the same passage, the remaining portion of the urethra. The relationship between the seminal vesicle, the prostate, and the urethra manifests itself when one of these organs becomes infected; the infection spreads quickly from one to the other if it is not arrested in its early stages. Moreover, prostatic infections may spread to the urinary system, affecting the bladder.

The *prostate:* The *prostate* is an organ located at the base of the bladder; it completely surrounds the portion of the urethra that leads from the bladder. The prostate is an accessory organ of reproduction, containing numerous glands that produce the *prostatic fluid,* an important component of the *semen*. The secretion is produced at a low but constant rate, and is poured into the urethra in small amounts; small quantities escape into the urine. Sexual stimulation accelerates the production of prostatic fluid; during ejaculation the prostatic fluid is delivered in larger quantities and is mixed with the seminal plasma to form the *semen*. In addition to serving as a housing and transporting vehicle for the sperm, the prostatic fluid appears to be necessary to maintain viable spermatozoa in the vagina, possibly by protecting the sperm from the acid condition of the vagina.

The function of the prostate is essentially reproductive; it is not known to produce hormones or any substance that the body may need otherwise. The product of prostatic activity—the prostatic fluid—does not enter into the blood stream, but is always excreted outside the body, except under disease conditions. Normally, prostatic fluid is clear and slightly opalescent. It contains a few cells, bacteria, and crystals from substances that accumulate in this organ.

The spermatozoa, produced in the testis, are thus seen to progress through a complicated network of organs to reach the outside of the body. It is generally thought that in ejaculation the several components of the genital tract discharge their contents in orderly sequence. The *bulbo-urethral glands* in the penis discharge first, their secretion serving to lubricate the urethra. The prostatic secretion with its neutralizing action is added next, and finally the seminal vesicles project their bulky secretion.

A single ejaculation may contain over a quarter of a billion spermatozoa. If fertilization does not occur, all of these cells die; if fertilization does occur, only one spermatozoon will survive; it will fertilize the egg. Occasionally, two ova may be produced within a short period of time and two spermatozoa will fertilize them, producing *fraternal* twins. *Identical* twins develop from a single ovum. Fraternal twins may be of different sexes, but identical twins are of the same sex and look alike.

The sperm cells which swim in the semen are microscopic. Their propulsion is brought about by movements of their tails. When sperm are deposited in the vagina during sexual intercourse, they move gradually upward toward the womb. The fatality rate of the sperm is high, but the chances of one's arriving alive in the womb are usually good. The life span of a sperm cell is not known precisely, but it is believed that the sperm has the ability to penetrate and fertilize an ovum for only about 48 hours. The energy necessary for maintenance and propulsion of spermatozoa is derived mostly from the various types of nourishment present in the seminal plasma.

The *penis:* The *penis* is the male organ of copulation and urination. In sexual intercourse it serves to convey the semen into the vagina of the female.

The shape of the penis varies greatly depending on whether it is flaccid or erect. In the flaccid state, the penis is a cylindrical organ, but when erect, it assumes a triangular shape in cross section. The penis consists of three cylindrical masses of erectile tissue held together by fibrous tissue and covered by skin. Two of the cylindrical bodies lie side by side, and the third one which holds the urethra is located underneath the other two. The lower cylinder ends in a cone-shaped body (the *glans*), which constitutes the free end of the penis; in the center of the glans is the opening of the urethra. The skin that covers the penis is thin and has no hairs except near the root of the organ, but possesses numerous glands that produce secretion.

The glans of the penis is covered by a circular fold of skin called the *prepuce.* In many instances the prepuce, or foreskin, may cover the entire glans, obstructing the passage of urine. Under these conditions the secretion of the skin glands accumulates, creating a constant source of irritation and infection. Therefore, surgical removal of the foreskin *(circumcision)* may be desirable as a prophylactic measure, and is usually performed shortly after birth. Circumcision is a simple operation and consists of cutting away the excess foreskin so that the glans is free. The operation was performed in ancient Egypt before it was introduced among the Hebrews. Today, it is still practiced among the Jews and Mohammedans as a religious rite.

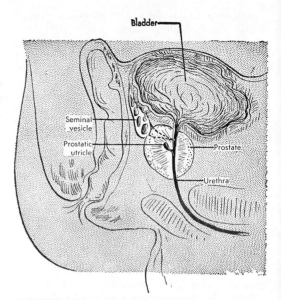

POSITION OF PROSTATE AND SEMINAL VESICLE

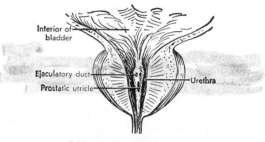

DETAIL OF PROSTATE

Detailed drawings showing, above, the position of the prostate and seminal vesicle, and below, some details of a cross section of the prostate gland.

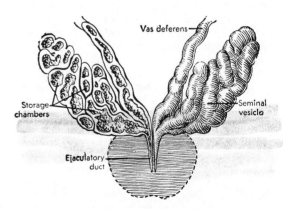

DETAIL OF SEMINAL VESICLE

Detailed drawing of the seminal vesicles and the vas deferens, with organs on the left cut away to show the details of the small storage chambers.

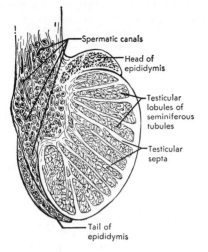

Detailed cross-sectional drawing of a human testis, showing the location of the epididymis, the spermatic canals, the seminiferous tubules, and septa.

However, it is practiced also as a hygienic measure by peoples native to all continents. Whatever the reason for this ancient practice, the result is certainly beneficial.

The mechanism of erection: Erection is necessary for normal transmission of semen into the body of the female. Sexual stimulus, either mental or physical, sets off a series of reactions that culminate in erection. The sexual stimulus received by the nervous system causes a flow of blood from the arteries that lead to the penis, and within the penis, to the many vessels and cavities of the erectile tissue to occur at a faster rate than the blood flows *from* the penis via the veins. The penis becomes engorged with blood, thus becoming firm and erect. The penis returns to its original flaccid state when the process is reversed after erection.

Female reproductive system

The female reproductive system is composed of a pair of *ovaries*, two *Fallopian tubes*, the womb *(uterus)*, the *vagina*, and the *vulva* or external genitalia. In the latter are included the *labia majora, labia minora, clitoris*, and *vestibule* —a space within which are openings of the *vagina, urethra*, and the *vestibular glands*. The ovaries represent the counterpart of the male testes, since they are the organs which produce the egg cells *(ova)*.

The two ovaries establish contact with the uterus by means of the two Fallopian tubes, which convey the egg cells from the ovaries to the womb. The womb, or uterus, is a muscular organ with great capacity for expansion. The inside of the womb is hollow and the walls are covered by a mucous membrane known as the endometrium. Here, the fertilized ovum develops into a baby.

The hollow portion of the female reproductive system constitutes a continuous structure, so that the ovaries, tubes, and womb may be regarded as a unit. The uterus forms the center of this unit, and is located in the pelvic cavity between the urinary bladder and the rectum, and the tubes form a passageway to the ovaries which are located on each side of the uterus.

The female reproductive system does not produce a fluid corresponding to the male seminal fluid. Under the influence of sexual stimulation, however, the walls of the vagina secrete fluids which serve as lubricants that facilitate intercourse.

The egg cells or ova are periodically produced in the ovaries at intervals of approximately four weeks. At the end of each four-week period, one egg reaches maturity and passes into one of the Fallopian tubes. The egg descends gradually and remains viable for a short while. Following intercourse, the sperm cells swim toward the tubes, in one of which fertilization may take place. Since neither the male nor the female reproductive cells live long, successful fertilization can occur only during a short period of time each month. This period of maximum fertility in women can be ascertained by various means, which will be discussed in detail in a following section of this chapter.

If the egg is fertilized by the sperm, the fertilized ovum enters the uterus and becomes attached to the uterine wall where the child develops. Ordinarily, only one egg is produced each month although more than one egg may be produced and in some cases may lead to multiple birth. If pregnancy occurs, usually no eggs are produced until after the child is born or pregnancy is interrupted.

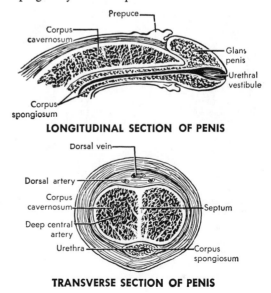

LONGITUDINAL SECTION OF PENIS

TRANSVERSE SECTION OF PENIS

The *ovaries:* The *ovaries* are the organs in which the egg cells (ova) are produced, and also the organs in which the female sex hormones are manufactured. The other organs of the female reproductive system are commonly called the accessory organs of reproduction. The relationship and the influence of sex hormones upon the accessory sex organs as well as on other parts of the body are discussed at length in Chapter 10, "The Endocrine System."

The female reproductive system normally has two ovaries. The ovary is an organ roughly the size and shape of an unshelled almond. The surface of the ovary is almost white and smooth in the child, but becomes irregular and pitted in the adult; the senile ovary is fibrous and wrinkled. The ovaries are located on each side of the womb and are each intimately related to the distal opening of the tubes, which serve to convey the egg from its ovary into the womb. The ovaries, Fallopian tubes, and womb are

anatomically so related that they function as a single organ. They are held together by a strong sheet of tissue called the *broad ligament.*

The Fallopian tubes, or *oviducts,* pierce the walls of the womb, forming a continuous channel from the interior of the womb to the ovary. The opening at the intersection of the womb and Fallopian tube is so small that a bristle would enter with difficulty. However, it is sufficiently large to allow the passage of the egg that comes from the ovary. The egg is not endowed with self-propulsion like the male sperm cells; thus it needs to be propelled from the tubes into the womb. The inner walls of the tube are made up of tissue that has many hairlike processes which sweep the egg into the womb.

When the egg has matured in the ovary, it is freed from the ovary and passes into the tube; from the funnel-shaped end of the tube that is in contact with the ovary extend a series of fingerlike processes (the *fimbriae*), toward the ovary; these aid in securing the egg after it has been freed from the surface of the ovary. Fertilization of the egg, if it occurs, usually takes place in the inner portion of the tube. The fertilized egg is carried toward the womb and eventually becomes lodged in the mucous membrane covering the inner surface of the womb.

Development of the egg (ovum): The maturing of the egg is a continuous process regulated by the endocrine system. This process can be understood better by visualizing the microscopic structure of the ovary.

Within the organ, there is a layer of cells called the *germinal epithelium.* Here, the potential egg begins its existence and continues to develop gradually until a *primary follicle* is formed around it, which is a clump of cells isolated from the main layer. The central cell of the clump is the egg, the remaining cells forming a ring around the egg. During a lifetime each ovary forms between 200,000 and 400,000 follicles. Of all these potential eggs, only a few develop into mature eggs; most of them degenerate at the follicle stage or at a more advanced stage of development. Those follicles that do not degenerate increase in size; meanwhile, the egg cell itself enlarges until the original size is doubled. The one-ring layer of cells around the egg then multiplies and forms several layers. Fluid begins to accumulate in little pools which merge and form larger ones until one large pool is formed with the egg inside of it.

Other changes occur in the areas adjacent to the follicle. As the follicle matures, it moves toward the surface of the ovary; when the maturation process is complete, the follicle protrudes from the surface of the ovary. At this time ovulation occurs. The follicle bursts and the egg, with its fluid, is expelled from the surface of the ovary, leaving a cavity. Consequently, the

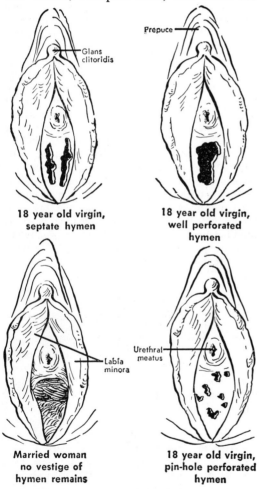

18 year old virgin, septate hymen

Prepuce

Glans clitoridis

18 year old virgin, well perforated hymen

Married woman no vestige of hymen remains

Labia minora

18 year old virgin, pin-hole perforated hymen

Urethral meatus

Appearance of various types of hymens. The hymen of an 18-year-old virgin may be perforated, septate or have pin-hole perforations, as in the first three drawings. A married woman usually has no trace of a hymen, as in the fourth drawing.

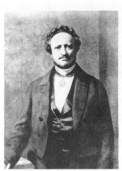

MÜLLER, Johannes (1801-1858) German anatomist and physiologist. In Müller's study of the developing human embryo, he discovered a pair of tubes or ducts, which have been named *Müllerian ducts*. These ducts appear early in the development of the fetus. In the female these primitive structures evolve into the oviducts, uterus and vagina. In the male they atrophy and leave vestigial appendages.

adult woman who has ovulated many times possesses ovaries that have a pitted appearance.

The *uterus:* The *uterus,* commonly known as the womb, is a pear-shaped organ the size of a small fist; it is located in the pelvic cavity of the female. The uterus is the organ that receives the fertilized egg from the Fallopian tube, provides the necessary nourishment and protection of the fetus during the various stages of pregnancy, and expels the developed child by the action of its muscular walls. The walls of the uterus are elastic, allowing for distention during pregnancy and return to the original thickness after childbirth.

The cavity of the womb is lined with a mucous membrane called the *endometrium.* The endometrium is not of the same thickness and consistency all the time, but varies considerably during the menstrual cycle. During menstruation, the endometrium disintegrates and is expelled with the menstrual blood, but a new endometrial lining begins to form immediately following each menstruation.

The womb possesses two parts called the "body" *(fundus)* and the "neck" *(cervix).* The cervix is below the fundus and connects with the vagina at a right angle. The position of the womb is not always the same. In general, the long axis of the womb extends from front to back and slightly downward. The neck of the womb is then pointed toward the rectum and meets the vagina at a right angle. The urinary bladder lies in front and the rectum in the back of the womb.

The cervix, or neck of the womb, is an important organ that has numerous functions in the reproductive system. During pregnancy, the cervix protects the fetus, and during childbirth it distends to permit passage of the child. The cervix may be the origin of a variety of disorders and the site of numerous infections.

The *vagina:* The *vagina* is the female organ of copulation. During sexual intercourse, the vagina receives the male organ (penis) and is the depository for the sperm cells.

The vagina is made up of muscular tissue

which possesses a considerable degree of elasticity; this permits distention without tearing when the child passes from the womb to the exterior of the body. The vagina is located between the urinary bladder and the rectum, although it is not directly connected to either. The vagina serves as a passageway between the opening of the vulva and the opening of the cervix.

In the adult woman, the size of the vagina varies, but the average length is approximately three inches. When the woman is in a standing position, the direction of the vagina is backward and upward, forming almost a right angle with the long axis of the uterus. The outer opening of the vagina is surrounded by a mucous membrane called the *hymen.* In the virgin woman, the hymen covers a considerable area of the vaginal opening; in rare instances it may cover it entirely *(imperforate hymen)* causing retention of the menstrual flow. The hymen varies considerably in shape but in general is semicircular. Because of the highly active life led by young girls of today, such as horseback riding, skiing, volleyball, etc., an intact hymen is not common even among virginal girls. If the hymen is intact at the incident of first intercourse, it is usually ruptured at that time, although not always; sometimes it does not tear, but merely stretches. Consequently, absence of a hymen or a ruptured hymen should never be construed to mean that a woman is not a virgin.

The lining of the vagina secretes a fluid that is acid in nature and serves as a cleanser and lubricant. In an acid environment only certain types of bacteria can live, most of which are harmless and even helpful. The vaginal lining is smooth only in women that have borne children or after the menopause in childless women. In the young virgin, the lining forms a series of folds.

The *vulva:* *Vulva* is the collective name applied to the external female organs of reproduction and includes the *mons pubis, labia majora, labia minora, clitoris, vestibular bulbs, vestibule, Bartholin's glands, Skene's glands,* and *hymen.* The *urethra,* which is part of the urinary system, is often regarded as a structure of the vulva.

The *mons pubis* is located on top of the pubic bone just above the genital organs. The mons pubis is a pad of fatty tissue covering the underlying bone. It forms an inverted triangular area which is covered with hair in the adult woman. The sides of the triangular area are delimited by the groins. From the top of the triangle, the mons pubis bends gradually downward and backward, dividing in the center to form two distinct sides that eventually, toward the perineum, become indistinguishable from the labia majora. The mons pubis contains many erogenous nerve endings which, when stimulated, add to the woman's excitement.

Labia majora means "major lips," and as the

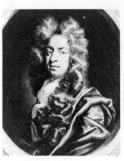

COWPER, William (1666-1709) English surgeon. Cowper is well known for his famous description in 1697 of the bulbourethral glands which are situated just behind and to each side of the urethra. These small bodies are called *Cowper's* glands. His descriptions of many other parts of the anatomy and also of various circulatory disturbances such as aortic insufficiency, assure Cowper of an important place in medical history.

name indicates they are two large "lips" or folds of tissue located around the vaginal opening. When the woman is in the erect position, the labia majora conceal most of the other external organs of reproduction. Extending downward they gradually decrease in thickness until they disappear into the region of the *perineum.* The perineum is the area between the vulva and the anus. When the labia majora are pulled aside, the remainder of the female external organs of reproduction become visible.

Within the labia majora lie the *labia minora,* which means "minor lips." As the name implies, they are two "lips" or folds of skin which form an angle. The area bounded by this angle is called the vestibule, and within this area is located the opening of the vagina. The labia minora have also been referred to as the "sex skin" because of the abundance of erogeneous nerve endings found in this tissue. When properly stimulated during sexual excitement, the "minor lips" thicken two to three times their normal size.

The *clitoris,* which is located at the apex of the triangular area delimited by the labia minora, is a relatively small organ made up of erectile tissue. Erectile tissue is tissue that becomes firm and engorged with blood in response to stimulation. The clitoris in the female and the penis in the male are somewhat similar in structure and response. The clitoris is covered by a fold of skin, which is known as the prepuce; the tip of the clitoris is called the glans.

The openings of the urethra and the vagina are located in the vestibule. The urethral opening and openings of the *Skene's glands* lie just below the clitoris, and below these lie the opening of the vagina. Skene's glands secrete an alkaline substance which reduces the acidity of the vagina. In the lower portion of the vestibule are located two small glands which secrete into the vagina. These glands, called *Bartholin's glands,* are not normally conspicuous but become prominent when they are inflamed and infected. Bartholin's glands produce a drop or so of mu-

cous secretion which previously was thought to serve as a lubricant during sexual intercourse. Secretion produced by these glands is insufficient, however, to actually serve such a function. As previously indicated, such lubricant actually is produced by the lining of the vagina.

Menopause

When, at puberty, a girl enters into young womanhood with its concurrent physical changes, it is largely the increased quantities of estrogen produced by her ovaries that are responsible for the change. Throughout her reproductive life, the ovaries continue to produce quantities of estrogen and another hormone, progesterone, which, in most women, are sufficient to maintain good physical and reproductive health. By about the age of 50, however, the ovaries have withered and are no longer able to produce estrogen in quantity. Either rapidly or gradually, the amount of estrogen produced by the individual declines to very little. This is the period of menopause.

If untreated, a woman ages much more quickly than a man of similar years. She may experience hot flushes, tension, irritability, and profuse sweating. When her estrogen is gone, a woman undergoes a loss of physical attractiveness. There are marked skin changes, disfiguring fat deposits appear, the breasts begin to atrophy, and the external genitals begin to regress. An irritated or inadequate vagina may make intercourse difficult. The bones become brittle and easily broken, and a woman is more susceptible to heart disease and often feels tired, ill, and depressed. As an elderly woman, she would be stiff, frail, bent, wrinkled, and apathetic. She might have skin cancers, osteoporosis (excessively brittle bones), irritating vaginal discharges, and cracked and bleeding vulvar tissues.

These are some of the symptoms which can

GRAAF, Reinier de (1641-1673) Dutch anatomist. Graaf was particularly interested in the anatomy of the genital organs and digestion. He is best known for his discovery of the *Graafian follicles,* which are small globular transparent vesicles in mammalian ovaries. Each follicle contains one ovum (egg). The menstrual cycle is initiated by the discharge of an egg from a follicle. Another contribution of Graaf included methods of preserving anatomical specimens by injection with solidifying substances.

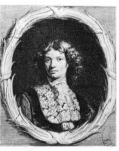

happen to a woman as her ovaries cease to produce the hormones estrogen and progesterone. Naturally, all symptoms do not happen to every woman, and some women experience virtually none.

There is now a treatment known as estrogen replacement therapy which can eliminate the ravages of menopause. This treatment is simply administration to the woman, in a dosage determined for her by her physician, of an amount of synthetic estrogen which will act to keep her body youthful. The results are the same whether the woman is started on the treatment during menopause, before her own supply of estrogen is completely gone, or years afterward. Even women who are 20 years past menopause can have most of their symptoms reversed.

The plan of administration of estrogen is similar to that for the birth control pills. For about 20 days, beginning on the fifth day after the beginning of the menstrual cycle, a pill containing estrogen is taken. The last eight to twelve pills contain progesterone as well as estrogen. This schedule delivers these two hormones to the body in just the same cycle in which the ovaries produced these hormones. When medication is discontinued after 20 days, menstruation follows, just as it does in women with functioning ovaries when hormone levels drop at the end of a cycle.

This rhythmic administration of hormones in the same pattern that the body formerly followed results in periodic "planned bleedings" or menstruation. For the woman who is still close to menopause, the physician usually elects to schedule the bleedings on the same 28-day cycle that her menstrual periods have always followed. However, for the woman whose ovaries definitely no longer produce hormones, it is effective and more convenient to use a 40- or 50-day cycle. Thus, a woman can experience only six or seven planned bleedings, or menstrual periods, yearly.

Many women are confused by the continuance of menstruation, believing that this indicates they are still capable of becoming pregnant. Once the ovaries have withered, however, there is no possibility of pregnancy, no matter what medication is taken. The continuing menstrual bleeding is simply a response to the administration of hormones. Further, postmenopausal women menstruate with almost no discomfort whatever, even women who previously experienced menstrual pain.

Almost always when a woman undergoes "artificial" menopause through an operation which removes her ovaries, hormonal replacement is prescribed. In cases of hysterectomy, when the uterus is also removed, the woman will no longer menstruate. However, some hormonal replacement is generally maintained to control the other symptoms which result from lack of estrogen.

The treatment should be continued to the end of a woman's life. Should she ever stop taking the hormones, the symptoms and signs of menopause will again become evident.

Often, many people associate the word estrogen with cancer. The reason for this is that, more than 35 years ago, in an early study of hormones and cancer, it was found that cancerous growths resulted when large quantities of certain chemicals (among them a few with estrogenic properties) were administered to certain mice (a strain which was inbred to have a high incidence of cancer spontaneously). There is no proof, however, that estrogen can cause cancer in human beings. Even in monkeys, the animal most like man, enormous doses of estrogen fail to produce any cancerlike changes.

Further, there is some evidence that the administration of estrogen may exert a protective effect against cancer. It is now believed that menstruation has a cancer-protective effect, because any tiny, beginning nests of abnormal cells in the endometrium (the lining of the uterus) are automatically washed away in the cyclic bleeding. Heretofore, 92 percent of cases of endometrial cancer have occurred after the menopause, when estrogen levels were radically reduced. It may be that the planned bleeding brought about by the relatively new hormone replacement therapy will exert the same cancer-protective effect, by washing away foci of abnormal cells.

DISORDERS OF THE TESTES

Infections of the testes are usually spread from adjacent areas; or systemic infections such as typhoid fever, undulant fever, or mumps may affect the testes. Mumps, particularly in the adult male, sometimes localizes in the testes, producing swelling and fever. A severe case of mumps in the adult may be followed by atrophic change in the testicle, and sterility may result. In prepubetal children, however, these serious consequences do not occur.

Descent of testes

Normally, the testes descend from inside the abdomen into the scrotum by the time of birth, but sometimes the descent is interrupted in one of the various stages. In a small percentage of cases, the testes remain in the abdomen after birth—a condition known as *cryptorchism*. In this position the testes do not function, because the temperature of the body is too high for the production of spermatozoa. Undescended testes may provoke a series of complications in addition to that of sterility. Undescended testicles appear to be somewhat more vulnerable to malignant growth than do normal ones. Incomplete development of both testes can induce changes in the secondary sexual characteristics of the individual. These changes are apparent in the external genital organs, which remain infantile, and in the absence of hair on the face, chest, and limbs. Treatment of such patients consists of administration of hormones, and, in some instances, surgical correction. Normal descent of the testes is influenced by hormones from the pituitary gland, and if it has not occurred by the time of puberty, it probably will not occur at all. Surgical measures are carried out only after careful evaluation of all factors, particularly the age of the subject. The condition should be corrected as early as possible to prevent damage to the cells which produce spermatozoa.

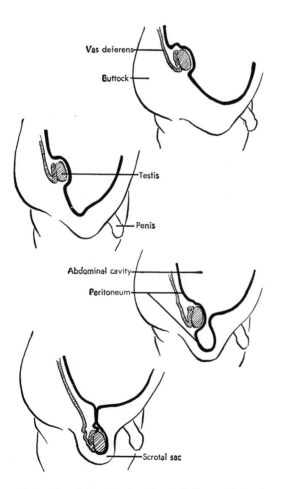

The series of drawings from top to bottom portrays the normal sequence of changes by which the testes descend from the abdomen into the scrotum.

Even when the testicular descent is not completely arrested, there may be an incomplete closure of the muscular floor of the viscera at this point. *Hernia* is frequently associated with the condition. Another possible complication is the development of *hydrocele,* in which an accumulation of fluid seeps through from the abdominal cavity into the spaces of the scrotum, forming a tight and sometimes painful swelling. Hydrocele may also be caused by infection or injury to the testes.

Cancer of testes

The most serious disorder of the testes is cancer; fortunately it is not common. The incidence of cancer of the testicle is estimated to be only two per 100,000 of the male population in a year. When cancer attacks the testes, its existence may first be noted by enlargement of one testis. Pain is regarded as a late symptom. Often, before pain appears, cancer will have spread to the lymph nodes above the collar bone and will appear as a lump in the neck region before any other symptoms are noted. When it has spread this far, cure is unlikely, but surgical and hormonal therapy may lessen discomfort and pain.

DISORDERS OF THE PROSTATE

Men over the age of 50 often become afflicted with conditions that render urination difficult. Among these conditions, enlargement of the prostate gland is the most common. The causes of prostatic enlargement (prostatic *hypertrophy)* are not known. However, it is known that about 30 percent of men over 50 years of age develop this condition, which in some cases leads to urinary obstruction. As a result of the enlargement, pressure is exerted against the upper portion of the urethra and often upon the bladder. As the size increases, the patient becomes unable to empty the bladder completely.

The first symptom of prostatic enlargement appears as a frequent desire to urinate, particularly at night. The quantity of urine voided is then less than normal and urination itself is begun with considerable effort. As the condition progresses, urination becomes more difficult, and accumulation of urine in the bladder causes inflammation, discomfort, and loss of vitality. At this stage, catheterization, or removal of the urine by means of a rubber tube may become necessary. This must be done by experienced professional persons, as it is a dangerous procedure in unskilled hands. The condition eventually causes a chronic infection of the entire urinary tract, and a series of complications ensue. In this event, hospitalization and surgery become necessary. The surgical operation removes all the obstructing tissues and clears the urinary passages.

Acute prostatitis

Prostatic enlargement is a disease that progresses gradually. As previously stated, it is a disease of men over the age of 50. In younger men, the prostate is more often affected by acute infections *(acute prostatitis);* in some instances, the infection may be chronic. Acute prostatitis may result from a number of causes, such as a stone in the prostate, a narrow urethra, or spread of infections from other sites of the body, or an extension from an infected urethra.

In acute prostatitis there is a feeling of urgency of urination, accompanied by a feeling of fullness in the rectum; chills and fever are common; urination is difficult and painful; and the patient cannot sit comfortably for any length of time. The patient may achieve comfort after the application of heat, and urination is frequently made easier when the patient takes a hot sitz bath.

The form of treatment varies, depending on the type of infection. In general, bed rest is required; reduction of fluids and a bland diet without condiments are prescribed. Sexual excitement and the use of alcohol aggravate the condition. The infection is arrested by the use of antibiotics or sulfonamides, depending on the nature of the infection.

Chronic prostatitis

Acute prostatitis is a common disease that affects both the young and the old. *Chronic prostatitis* is less common and results from persistent infection of the prostate. The disease is of long duration and requires long periods of treatment. The symptoms of chronic prostatitis are somewhat different from those of the acute form. The patient suffers pain about the groin, the back, the penis, and throughout the pelvic region. There is a discharge from the urethra most of the time, particularly in the morning. The disease is difficult to cure but seldom has serious consequences.

Examination of the prostate

Examination of prostatic fluid is important in the diagnosis of prostatic diseases, and is done routinely by the physician. Prostatic fluid is drawn from the patient by massage. The patient stands on the floor and, bending over, rests his elbows on a table. The doctor introduces his gloved and lubricated index finger into the anus and locates the prostate through the anterior wall of the rectum. To massage the prostate, the

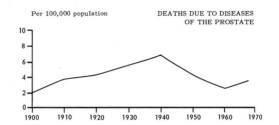

Increase in deaths due to prostate disorders, during the first half of this century, was partially due to the fact that more individuals lived to the age when these disorders appear. The present decline in the death rate is thought to be associated with the development of more efficacious antibiotics and other drugs.

index finger strokes the surface of the gland several times. The prostatic fluid is then expelled from the penis and is placed on a slide for microscopic examination. The massage also serves other purposes besides diagnosis; it is part of the treatment in many prostatic conditions. The forcible expulsion of fluid from the prostate clears away large quantities of bacteria when the organ is infected. Prostatic massage is also performed to relieve congestion of the prostate when infection and enlargement cause difficulty in urination.

The doctor also can ascertain by feeling with his finger the approximate size of the organ, the texture, the presence of tumors, and other qualities that are of importance in diagnosis. Thus, cancer of the prostate, discussed in more detail later, can often be detected at an early stage. The texture of the prostate discloses the state of this organ; if soft and tender, the chances are that the prostate is inflamed as a result of infection.

The examination of the prostate is not limited to manual examination. Often it is necessary to observe this organ in detail. An examination is made using an instrument called a *cystoscope;* this is a hollow tube in which there is an optical system and a source of light. The patient is anesthetized and the tube is introduced into the urethra until the end reaches the part to be examined. The doctor obtains a clear view of the prostatic urethra and the urinary bladder. The instrument is used also for surgery that can be performed through the urethra. Delicate instruments can be introduced through the cystoscope to perform the various operations. Most of these instruments function electrically, burning rather than cutting the tissues, and causing little bleeding.

The doctor obtains much information regarding the state of the prostate by examination of the urine. Three urine specimens are obtained in glass containers. The first glass contains the first portion of urine, whereas the second and third glasses contain the urine that passes after the urinary passages have been cleansed. When the first urine specimen is cloudy but the others are clear, it usually means that the urethra is infected. When all specimens are cloudy, the infection may have spread to the upper portions of the urinary system. Shreds may indicate prostatic infection.

Cancer of the prostate

The most serious prostatic disorder is cancer of the prostate, a disease that occurs in about 20 percent of all cases of prostatic enlargement. Like most types of cancer, prostatic cancer must be detected early to be cured. Often, cancer of the prostate cannot be detected readily because the symptoms may appear only after the condition has become advanced and perhaps has spread to other parts of the body. In late stages, prostatic cancer may spread to the bones, where growth of the malignant cells continues at a rapid rate. When the bones have become involved there is no hope of curing the patient. However, much can be done by the physician in relief of pain, extension of life, and prevention of invalidism. Regular medical examinations, particularly in men over 50, are the best means of detecting early cancer in this organ.

Optimism increases as new means of treating patients with prostatic cancer are discovered. Undue optimism sometimes leads to a misunderstanding of the new form of treatment, and the word "cure" is too readily applied. Thus, the treatment of patients with prostatic cancer by means of female sex hormones is directed to control rather than cure. It has brought comfort to many patients and has served as an aid to surgical treatment. The female sex hormone and compounds that have similar properties act upon the normal prostate and accessory sex organs of the male, causing them to become smaller. Castration (surgical removal of the testes) brings about a similar effect, because removal of the testes also removes the source of male sex hormone. This basic principle has been translated into a new form of treatment, and most patients with prostatic cancer find relief of symptoms almost immediately after castration. The administration of female sex hormones brings about the same relief, but its action is slower. After either castration or female sex hormone treatment, the prostate and the tumor decrease in size, sometimes to the extent that urinary obstruction is relieved. The pain in the bones, that characterizes advanced cancer of the prostate, may be reduced or totally eliminated after this form of treatment in some patients. Life may be extended many useful years.

Radical surgical treatment is preferred for patients with prostatic cancer when the disease has

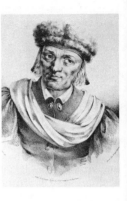

LEONICENUS, Nicolaus (1428-1524) Italian physician. Leonicenus was the author of one of the earliest descriptions of syphilis. He recognized that the disease caused internal damage as well as disfiguring lesions of the skin. He also was aware of the infectious nature of syphilis, but did not seem to realize that it was contracted primarily through sexual contact. He insisted that the disease was of great antiquity, and was known to Hippocrates. At that time syphilis had not yet acquired its present name.

not spread, but not all patients are able to undergo this type of treatment. A combination of treatments often proves effective.

DISORDERS OF THE SEMINAL VESICLES

The seminal vesicles, which are the two pouches containing the seminal fluid and spermatozoa, are frequently affected by prostatic infections since these organs are anatomically continuous. Usually the seminal vesicles are examined at the same time the prostate is examined. The entire length of the seminal vesicles cannot be reached by the examining finger, but when they are inflamed, they are distended and can be felt. As in prostatic examinations, the doctor ascertains the size, contour, and texture of the seminal vesicles. He also notes whether one or both sides are affected.

Acute infections

Acute infections (acute vesiculitis) spread to these structures from the urethra. When the vesicles become infected, the patient suffers pain and tenderness above the groin; he feels desire to urinate frequently, and has frequent and painful erections, especially at night. When the doctor examines the patient, the vesicles may be felt through the rectum; they may be swollen, distended, and tender. The patient must remain in bed, take hot sitz baths, and apply hot compresses to the perineum. The infection is arrested with sulfonamides and antibiotics. With the advent of these drugs, serious infections are becoming relatively rare.

Other disorders

The diseases just mentioned are the more common conditions associated with the prostate and seminal vesicles. There are other diseases that occur less frequently, either from direct causes or as complications arising from other diseases. Tuberculosis, for example, may attack any part of the genital system, but usually attacks the testes and the seminal vesicles; the prostate is rarely affected by this disease. Prostatic *abscesses* sometimes follow acute prostatitis. The abscess can be drained by manipulation by the physician; also, drainage may occur spontaneously.

Infections of the accessory sex organs are no longer highly painful diseases of long duration. With the sulfonamides and antibiotics most infections usually can be arrested in a short time.

DISORDERS OF THE OVARIES AND FALLOPIAN TUBES

The ovary is susceptible to a variety of disturbances. Disorders of ovulation, painful or irregular menstruation, and other conditions related to the female sexual cycle result in most instances from improper function of the endocrine system. These conditions are discussed in detail in Chapter 10, "The Endocrine System."

Tumors of the ovaries

The diseases not related to the endocrine system that affect the ovaries comprise a large number, of which tumor formation is the most important. Tumor does not necessarily imply cancer, and actually most ovarian tumors are *not* cancers. There are a number of tumors that grow in the ovary, which vary in size, shape, consistency, and many other characteristics. They can grow to enormous proportions without causing symptoms. Others may rupture abruptly without having presented any symptoms; in such instances, prompt surgical intervention may become necessary. Fibroma of the ovary and other fibrous type tumors are identified by the symptoms of fluid in the abdomen and chest. These tumors are usually benign, and the distressing symptoms are relieved by removal of the tumor.

Most ovarian tumors develop without presenting symptoms, except those that produce hormones. Eventually, pain is caused by the tumor pressing against neighboring organs, tension of the tumor mass, rupture, or infection.

When a positive diagnosis of tumor has been made, surgical exploration becomes necessary in almost every case. Abdominal exploration is

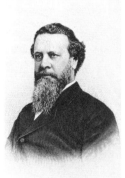

THOMAS, Theodore Gaillard (1832-1902), American physician. Thomas was the author of a textbook on diseases of women which was published in 1868, and was considered to be one of the outstanding books of the day on that topic. He devised a vaginal speculum, a device which exposes the interior of the vagina for examination, which he described in his book. He is credited with performing the first vaginal ovariotomy (removal of an ovary through the vagina), in the year 1870.

necessary to secure a complete diagnosis and to remove the tumor. All ovarian tumors may be dangerous if not removed, because it is almost impossible to decide which will develop into a cancer and which will not.

By the time a tumor is noticed by the patient, it is often too late to effect a cure if the condition is a cancerous one. The extensive growth of tumors of the ovary can be prevented only by early discovery and removal. Therefore, periodical pelvic examinations are extremely important in the early detection of cancer. Also, a pelvic examination is of great importance for early detection of cancer of the cervix. When cancer is detected at an early stage of development, treatment is possible and most often successful.

Infection and tumors of the Fallopian tubes

Infections of the Fallopian tubes frequently cause permanent sterility. The Fallopian tubes are attacked most often by the organisms caus-

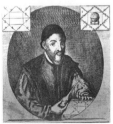

FALLOPIUS, Gabriel (1523-1562) An Italian anatomist who described the ovaries (the egg-bearing organs in the female), and the oviducts which are the tubes that connect the ovaries with the uterus. The oviducts are now called *Fallopian tubes* in his honor. Fallopius also gave the present name to the vagina and the placenta. The placenta is the structure which supplies the unborn child with food and oxygen. He made a detailed study of the ear and was the first to describe the semicircular canals. *Bettmann Archive.*

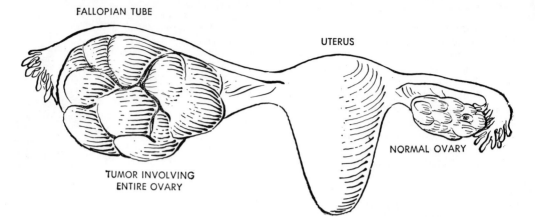

FALLOPIAN TUBE

UTERUS

NORMAL OVARY

TUMOR INVOLVING
ENTIRE OVARY

Drawing showing the relationship of the Fallopian tube to the ovary and uterus as well as a tumor involving the entire right ovary. Left ovary is normal, for comparison.

ing gonorrhea, infections produced during childbirth, tuberculosis, and a variety of systemic infections. These infections may be either acute or chronic, and in some instances they may involve the entire reproductive system.

Tumors may develop in the Fallopian tube, usually as a secondary growth which originated in some other organ of the body. The growth of a tumor in the Fallopian tube manifests itself by pain caused by tension exerted by the tumor. This symptom may be followed by a discharge from the vagina, which is usually watery and bloody. Menstrual irregularities may occur. Tumors of the Fallopian tubes are relatively rare, and the obscure symptomatology often makes their diagnosis quite difficult.

Tubal pregnancy

The Fallopian tube is at times the site of an abnormal type of pregnancy, called *tubal* pregnancy. In these cases, the embryo fails to descend into the womb and develops instead in the Fallopian tube. As the fertilized egg grows within the tube, the tension increases, and the tube may rupture, causing death of the fetus. Once existence of tubal pregnancy has been established, surgical intervention to remove the tube and the embryo is usually necessary. Often there may be no symptoms of tubal pregnancy prior to rupture. This condition endangers the patient because hemorrhage is imminent in nearly every case. Tubal pregnancies are probably caused by some abnormality of the tube that interferes with the normal progress of the fertilized egg through the tube. Tubal pregnancy is not the only form of abnormal pregnancy that takes place outside the womb, but it is perhaps the most common abnormal type. Other types of abnormal pregnancy include abdominal and ovarian pregnancies.

DISORDERS OF THE UTERUS

The uterus is held in place by the floor of the pelvis and a series of tough bands of tissue called ligaments. Thus, the womb is not rigidly fixed in one position, but is movable. Abnormal displacements may occur when the position of the womb changes beyond certain limits. The uterus can turn backward causing *retrodisplacement*. The condition has several causes, but the most common cause is childbirth. During labor there is often considerable stretching of the supports that keep the womb in place. To avoid displacement, the physician instructs the mother to lie on her abdomen or side during convalescence. The degree of displacement varies, depending on how much stretching has occurred. When displacement does occur, secondary symptoms may arise. The patient may feel uncomfortable, have a backache, and often suffer bladder and rectal distress. In most instances, retrodisplacement of the uterus causes no concern or symptoms. Once the condition has been discovered, the physician institutes treatment dependent on the degree of displacement and on the severity of the symptoms. In general, treatment consists in bringing the uterus to a normal position by manual manipulation and maintaining it in a normal position by some mechanical support. Mechanical supports vary in design and shape. These supports are called *pessaries;* they consist of a flexible ring made of rubber or plastic. The shape of the ring is adjusted by the physician to avoid discomfort for the patient. The object of the pessary is to push the neck of the womb backward; by so doing, the body of the womb moves forward. The ring is placed around the neck of the womb, leaving the passage unobstructed. After the pessary has been fitted properly, the doctor instructs the patient

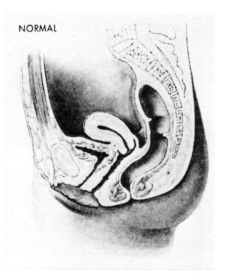

NORMAL

to return periodically to observe and follow up the treatment, and to return immediately if there is pain or if the pessary moves away from the fitted position. The patient is instructed to take frequent vaginal douches. Under certain conditions, retrodisplacement of the uterus may necessitate surgical operation to restore the normal position of the womb. Types of retrodisplacement of the womb are illustrated on this and the next page.

At childbirth, the stretching of the uterine supports may cause both retrodisplacement and *prolapse* of the uterus. In the latter condition the womb falls from the normal position and the cervix pushes far into the vagina. Severe pro-

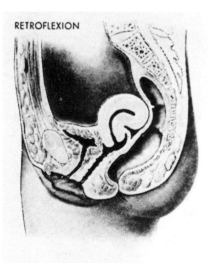

RETROFLEXION

lapse can cause the womb to push the cervix through the vagina. Complications ensue, usually associated with ulcerations of the cervix as a result of irritation produced by continuous contact with the clothing of the patient. The pressure exerted by the prolapsed womb upon the urinary bladder causes *incontinence,* or inability to retain urine. Frequently, incontinence is the complaint that induces the patient to consult the physician.

Like other displacements, prolapse is corrected with pessaries and by surgical means. Pessaries are not of the same shape as those used for retrodisplacement. Some are shaped like doughnuts and are inserted edgewise into the vagina, then moved to a position that fits the cervix like a collar. Other pessaries are similarly shaped but have small handles that aid in removing them. Still others have longer handles and are supported by abdominal belts. Curative measures for a prolapsed womb are surgical. The restoration of the normal position of the womb does not necessarily involve loss of reproductive function.

Endometriosis

The lining of the womb, as previously mentioned, is a remarkable structure that grows and disintegrates about every four weeks. The mechanisms that regulate this cycle are controlled mostly by hormones produced in the ovaries. The lining, or *endometrium,* sometimes behaves abnormally and grows not only on the walls of the womb but within the walls, or on adjacent pelvic organs, causing a condition known as *endometriosis.* The patient with this condition may suffer irregularities in the menstrual cycle. Menstruation is often painful and copious.

In endometriosis, the endometrium will grow outside the uterus and has been found in nearly all the surrounding organs and even in organs remote from the organs of reproduction. In other sites of the body the displaced lining of the womb continues to undergo the same periodic changes which take place within the womb. When ovarian hormones act upon the endometrium, stimulation takes place, and the menstrual phases are discernible.

The manner in which bits of lining are transported from the womb and lodge in other parts of the body is not clear. Apparently they can be transported by way of the Fallopian tubes, the blood, and the lymph. Also, it is thought that endometrial tissue may be spread by rupture of a cyst or as a result of surgery.

Endometriosis of this type *(external endometriosis)* may necessitate surgical treatment. The results obtained from surgical treatment of patients with endometriosis are satisfactory in the majority of cases.

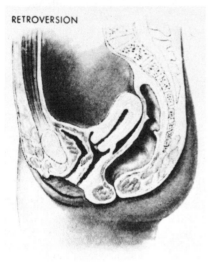

RETROVERSION

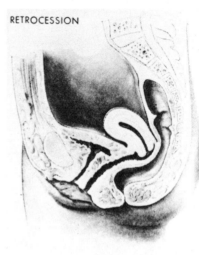

RETROCESSION

Tumors of the uterus

The uterus is one of the most frequent sites of tumor formation, being second only to the breast. Tumors develop in nearly any part of this organ. The body of the uterus (fundus) also can be the site of infections, irritations, and other diseases. Tumors of the fundus are of many types, but most common are fibroids (*leiomyomata*) of the uterus which develop from muscle tissue. Fibroids of the uterus usually occur as multiple growths in the walls of the womb. The patient may have a group of small fibroids for many years and suffer no ill effects. However, the size of the tumors varies, sometimes reaching large proportions. As a result of the growth of the tumor, pressure may be exerted upon adjacent organs, thereby causing

complications. The urinary bladder may be displaced as a result of the tumor, and there may be difficulty in urination. Other symptoms caused by fibroids of the womb are pain, excessive menstrual flow, and sterility.

Treatment of patients who have fibroids varies according to the type and size of the tumors. If the tumors are small and cause no symptoms, usually no treatment is deemed necessary. Others that may endanger the health of the patient usually are removed surgically. There are many other forms of tumors that can grow in the fundus and that can arise from any of its component tissues. In their early stages of development, many of these growths can be treated successfully either surgically or radiologically. Some, such as choriocarcinoma, respond to chemotherapy.

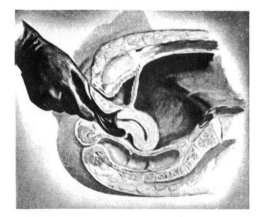

This illustration portrays the manner in which the corrective pessary may be inserted into the vagina to modify uterine position. *Sharp & Dohme Seminar.*

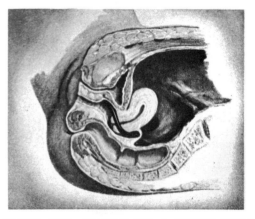

Diagram which illustrates how a correctly inserted pessary helps to maintain the uterus in its forward abdominal position. *Sharp & Dohme Seminar.*

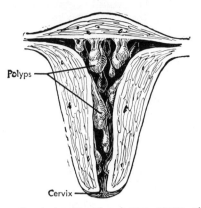

Cross-sectional drawing of a human uterus, showing the appearance presented by numerous polyps growing on the inner mucosal wall of the uterus.

Both benign and malignant tumors occur in the cervix. Tumors may appear at first as harmless growths, but a transformation may occur, and the benign growth becomes a cancer. The cervix is one of the most frequent sites of cancer. Fortunately, the chances of early detection of cervical cancer are favorable. The importance of detecting cancer at an early stage cannot be overestimated, since early detection and proper treatment are necessary to prevent spread of the growth. Periodic pelvic examination is the best means of detecting cancer of the cervix and other genital organs.

Therapeutic means have been improved greatly and cervical cancer is cured frequently by modern means of treatment.

When cancer develops in the cervix it is at first confined to this organ, but, depending on the type of growth, spreads at different rates to the adjacent organs. In the early stages of the disease, there are no specific symptoms except perhaps irregular bleeding and discharge, which are also symptoms elicited by numerous conditions of the reproductive system. Consequently, the patient may delay the visit to the doctor until she is sure that the bleeding will not disappear. After such delay, the cancer may have advanced beyond hope of cure. Any unusual bleeding or discharge, other irregularities in the menstrual cycle, periods in which there is profuse bleeding, and the recurrence of a period after several months without periods should be recognized as danger signals, and prompt medical consultation should be sought.

Some patients with cervical cancer may have no symptoms, not even appreciable bleeding. The disease may not be diagnosed in the earliest stages. Usually an apparently healthy individual will not consult a physician when there is no discomfort, pain, bleeding, or other complaint. Hence, the problem of early detection of cervical cancer can be solved only when *all* adult women undergo periodic examinations, regardless of the state of their health. When this is done, many lives will be saved.

An examination of the cervix by the doctor is a simple procedure. Although early cervical cancer may present a perfectly normal appearance and there may be no symptoms, there is a test which can detect the unsuspected cancer, permitting treatment at a time when the opportunity for cure is very good. This procedure, the "Pap" test, is a cytologic examination and was developed chiefly by the late Dr. George N. Papanicolaou. The test involves the microscopic examination of cells collected from the vagina. These are cells shed from the uterus into the vagina as part of the normal life process.

A vaginal specimen can be obtained from a woman of any age. The quick and painless procedure is performed in the doctor's office, a clinic, or a hospital. The specimen, which consists of a bit of mucus scraped from the cervix, is placed on a glass slide and sent to a laboratory to be studied through a microscope to determine whether cells in the specimen appear to be abnormal.

If microscopic examination of the smear reveals any abnormal cells, bits of tissue are taken from the cervix for further microscopic study. This process of removing and examining tissue from a living body is known as a biopsy. It is the only method of diagnosing cancer.

The biopsy study may show that the abnormal cells are not cancerous, but are indicative of a benign tumor or other abnormal condition. However, biopsy also may show that the abnormal cells come from surface areas of the cervix that have been eroded by injury or infection. Such a condition, in the presence of persistent secondary infection, may fail to heal and thereby serve as a contributing cause in the develop-

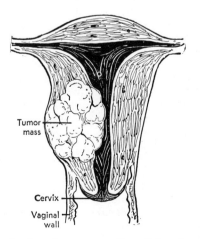

This drawing of a cross section of the uterus shows the appearance of one type of uterine tumor that is occasionally found in the muscular layers.

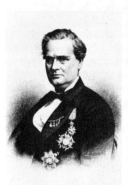

SIMS, James Marion (1813-1883) American surgeon. Sims made many important contributions to the field of gynecology. He invented the duckbill vaginal speculum, called the *Sims' speculum*, which is still in general use today, and devised the *Sims' position* for gynecological examinations. In 1858 he developed a successful operation for closing vesicovaginal fistula (an abnormal opening betwen the vagina and the bladder). In 1861 he introduced a procedure for amputation or removal of the uterine cervix.

ment of cancer. Treatment of the infection and primary abnormality is an essential preventive measure.

Cervical cancer rarely appears in women under the age of 20. It sometimes occurs before 30, but is most common in women around 45 years of age. Cancer of the body of the uterus usually affects women at the time of or after menopause. Every woman going through menopause should be under the observation and care of a physician. She should have periodic checkups, which include a "Pap" smear and pelvic and breast examinations. In recent years, large numbers of women have been screened for cervical cancer, by microscopic examination of the vaginal fluids. Although formerly the method was regarded as too time-consuming and laborious to be used on a large scale, investigators have refined the methods to the extent that now these methods are being widely used in discovering cancer. In one study, in Memphis, Tennessee, 108,000 women were examined; 393 intraepithelial cancers were discovered, of which 353, or 90 percent, had not been suspected. Also, 373 invasive cancers were found, of which 112, or 30 percent, were unsuspected.

When cancer is still confined to a small area, immediate treatment can be successful. There are only two effective forms of treatment for patients with cancer of the uterus: surgery and radiation. Too frequently, unscrupulous charlatans make claims to possess some miraculous cure. Such claims are false, and such "cures" only cause delay in proper treatment and decrease the chance for recovery.

In a surgical operation for cervical cancer, the entire womb, the ovaries, the Fallopian tubes, and the pelvic lymph nodes usually are removed. Hence, no chances are taken that bits of cancerous tissue may be left that could spread to other parts of the body.

There are two principal ways of using radiation to treat patients with uterine cancer: (1)

radiation may be beamed to the cancerous tissue from a source outside the body, such as an x-ray or cobalt therapy machine, or (2) a radioactive material, such as radium, can be placed within the cancerous growth. Often radium is enclosed in a capsule which is inserted through the vagina and uterine cavity to the cancer site. No matter what type of radiation is used for therapy, however, the objective is always to deliver a dose powerful enough to destroy the cancer, but not so great as to damage normal tissues seriously. Fortunately, most cells of the uterus are more sensitive to x-irradiation than are the normal cells.

The treatment that exists is good and if the disease is local, many patients can be cured. Consequently, the disease must be diagnosed early, while it is still confined to a local area. The disease usually will be diagnosed early if the patient will have periodic pelvic examinations, conducted by her physician.

Other disorders of the uterus

Tumors of the womb represent only a fraction of all diseases that may affect this organ. Infectious diseases are common in the uterus, even though they often do not originate in the womb, but in some adjacent organ. Tuberculosis, which usually begins in the lung, may spread to the organs of reproduction, affecting the uterus or any other area of the reproductive system. The symptoms are similar to those produced by ir-

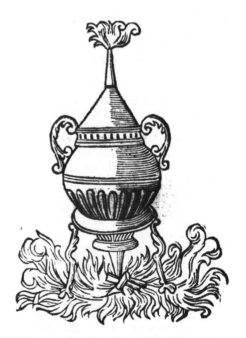

Old Italian woodcut showing a kettle filled with water, the steam from which was used in combatting womb inflammations. *Bettmann Archive.*

ritation of the endometrium. Formerly, the only recourse was surgery, but now certain drugs are recognized as useful in genital tuberculosis.

DISORDERS OF THE VAGINA AND VULVA

Vaginal infections are caused by a large number of disease-producing organisms. Gonorrhea may produce vaginal discharge at any stage of the disease, particularly in the acute form. Certain parasites live in the vagina and other organs of the genitourinary tract, where they often cause infection when the environment is favorable.

Trichomonas vaginalis, a parasitic protozoan, may infect the vagina, producing a foul-smelling, frothy, irritative discharge. *Moniliasis,* a fungus infection caused by *Candida albicans,* may affect the vaginal wall causing a white discharge and white patches.

Nonspecific infections, caused by a number of bacteria, may be present in the vagina. These infections are characterized by an increased production of vaginal secretions. When these infections are severe, the vagina becomes inflamed and swollen, and sometimes the irritation extends to the external genital organs.

Treatment of vaginal infections depends upon the type of organism causing the condition. Local applications of chemicals in the form of tablets, jellies, solutions, etc., are the usual treatment. Bacterial infections can usually be controlled by administration of one of the antibiotic drugs.

Tumors occur in the vagina but they are relatively uncommon. The most common type of tumor is called "inclusion cyst," which in most instances is not serious. Although cancer occurs rarely in this area, any abnormal growth or lump in the vagina should be examined by a physician.

In extremely rare cases, there may be congenital absence of the vagina. The condition is not readily recognized because the external organs are usually present, including the vaginal opening. Penetration is possible only to a minor degree, and the patient may be unaware of the condition until a medical examination is performed. When the vagina is absent, the condition may be corrected by plastic surgery. The operation consists mainly in dissecting the space between the rectum and bladder, then forming a lining with a tube formed from skin, a section of the intestine, or other structures.

There are some instances in which sexual intercourse is a painful experience or even is impossible for the woman. Pain during sexual intercourse is an abnormal condition and requires medical attention. Pain may result from a variety of causes. Among them, abrasions of the genital organs are common immediately after marriage. The condition is mild and usually disappears after a short period of postponement of sexual intercourse. More serious is the pain caused by excessive sensitivity of the vagina, as in the condition known as *vaginismus.* This malfunction is frequently psychological and characterized by spasmodic contractions of the vaginal orifice, thus creating a physical obstacle to sexual intercourse.

Disorders of the vulva

Among the most common diseases that attack the external genital organs are infectious diseases. Organisms that produce gonorrhea and other venereal diseases find a suitable environment in these organs where they grow and invade neighboring structures. These diseases are discussed in the section on "Venereal Diseases."

Inflammation of the vulva is called *vulvitis,* and may be caused by a number of factors. Since the external portion of the vulva is covered by skin, many conditions which affect the skin of other parts of the body—e.g., eczema, ringworm, erysipelas, contact dermatitis, etc.—may affect the vulva. Acute vulvitis occurs in children and obese women as a result of constant irritation. Vulvitis occurring in diabetic patients is caused by the increased sugar content of the urine which produces irritation and provides a favorable environment for the growth of yeasts and fungi. Vulvitis often produces considerable itching and reddening of the external genital organs. The irritation often is spread from the vulva to the folds of the thigh and causes burning of the skin.

Many disease-producing organisms invade the vulva and cause inflammation. Certain protozoa *(Trichomonas vaginalis)* may infect the vulva, especially if the infection is present in the vagina. *Moniliasis* may affect the vulva as well as the vagina. Bacteria, most often streptococci, may invade the vulva and cause an infection. In most instances, the infections can be cured by administration of sulfonamide drugs and antibiotics.

Pruritus vulvae means itching of the vulva. This condition may result from a number of factors such as uncleanliness, leukorrhea, or a reflex from disease in the uterus, or ovaries. Pelvic abnormalities, tumors, the menopause, diabetes, or even emotional disturbances can give rise to pruritus vulvae. The treatment depends entirely upon the cause. It is important in all instances to prevent scratching of the affected area. The physician usually will prescribe some medication that relieves the itching, at least temporarily.

Leukoplakia means "white plaque" and refers to areas of thickening of the skin. It usually occurs in the area of the clitoris, the labia, and perineum. Itching often is associated with leukoplakia. The cause of this condition is not known; however, it can usually be eliminated by proper medication.

Both benign and malignant tumors occur in the vulva; however, cancer of the vulva is rarely found in young women; it occurs most often in women past the menopause. The average age of patients with cancer of the vulva is approximately 60 years. Patients with cancer of the vulva are usually treated surgically. The chances of effecting a cure depend upon whether the disease is diagnosed in an early or late stage.

IRREGULAR BLEEDING AND DISCHARGE

Normal menstruation is always periodic; therefore, any irregularity in interval, type, or amount of bleeding is a sign of abnormality. Medical investigation of any irregularity should not be delayed, because the sole chance of curative treatment of the serious causes of irregular bleeding—cancer, for instance—depends upon early diagnosis.

During adolescence, menstrual periods may be irregular during the first year and should not cause alarm; hormonal function in the ovaries has just begun, and it may be several months before the menstrual cycle becomes stabilized. Following this initial fluctuation in ovarian activity, regular periods become established. This cycle recurs throughout the normal menstrual life, unless pregnancy intervenes.

Hormone imbalance is discussed in Chapter 10, "The Endocrine System." Certain disturbances in the endocrine system causes profuse, prolonged, irregular uterine bleeding. This type of hormone imbalance may first occur after termination of pregnancy.

Benign tumors of the uterus may produce irregular bloody discharge. The most common of such lesions is an ulceration of the cervix, which may bleed on contact. This type of bleeding must always be considered serious until the exact nature of the causative lesion is determined by the physician. Other growths on the cervix or lining of the uterus, such as small pear-shaped masses (polyps), cause bleeding because of their abundant blood supply. Infections of the lining or wall of the uterus (endometritis) that sometimes occur after childbirth or abortions, cause irregular uterine bleeding. Adequate medical treatment will stop the irregular bleeding.

Tumors of the uterine muscle, commonly referred to as fibroids, sometimes cause irregular bleeding, because of their size or location in the uterine wall. Many ovarian tumors, because of their increased hormone production, modify the lining of the womb, and thus cause bleeding.

Another type of bleeding between menstrual periods may occur at the time of ovulation. At the exact time the egg cell is extruded from the ovary, the patient may experience some pain in the lower abdomen lasting for three to six hours, together with a small amount of bloody vaginal discharge. This is a phenomenon recognizable by its timing; namely, that it occurs only at the midcycle interval (in women who menstruate every 28 days) and usually lasts only a few hours to one day.

The most serious cause of irregular bleeding from the female genital tract is cancer. The cervix is by far the most frequent site of cancer in the female reproductive organs. Persons between 40 and 50 years of age, the so-called "menopausal age," are most likely to develop cervical cancer. However, no age group is immune. Bleeding following intercourse or douches should never be ignored, because such bleeding may originate from a soft cancerous lesion of the cervix. Spotting of blood, watery malodorous discharge, or obvious bleeding in the woman past the menopause must always be considered a sign of malignant growth until proved otherwise. This age group is far more likely to report bleeding to their physician, as they have previously stopped menstrual bleeding. Many of these women, however, are likely to attribute intermittent bleeding to the "change of life," and neglect to consult a physician. Such neglect forfeits the chances of early recognition and treatment if cancer is the cause of the bleeding. Periodic pelvic examinations at intervals of not longer than six months are recommended for every woman over 30 years of age.

Bleeding irregularities are not the only symptoms of disease in the reproductive tract. Leukorrhea, commonly referred to as "discharge," often indicates an abnormality. "Discharge" from the vagina occurs frequently and may be insignificant or serious, depending upon the underlying cause. The mucus-producing glands present in the vagina and cervix normally secrete a small amount of whitish material for moistening the tissues. Sometimes there is an exaggeration of the normal amount. Minor inflammation of the genital lining, congestion, and other conditions may produce a discharge. Activity of the mucous glands is increased by sexual stimulation and by premenstrual hormone effects. The mucous secretion thus produced varies in quantity, but is colorless, odorless, and nonirritating.

Thus, leukorrhea is a symptom of a variety of conditions, many of which are of little clinical significance. However, it may also be a warning signal of a more dangerous condition. Inflammation of the Fallopian tubes resulting from gonorrhea, tuberculosis, or other infection, may cause leukorrhea. Cancer of the uterus may be accompanied by a similar discharge.

Since there are numerous causes of leukorrhea, any discharge that is abnormal in quantity, color, or odor should be reported to the physician.

It should also be recognized that psychological causes also produce a large percentage of menstrual difficulties. Studies have shown that menstrual cramps are virtually unheard of among certain South Pacific Island women, and that in modern cultures such as our own most women who suffer from premenstrual tension and difficult menstruation have a background of parental discord and sex education from a mother who presented it in a deprecating manner.

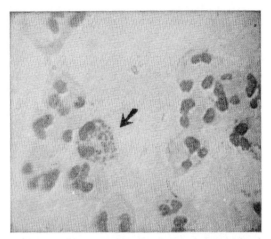

Photograph showing gonococci inside the pus cell as indicated by arrow. This causative agent of gonorrhea is the bacterium *Neisseria gonorrhoeae.*

VENEREAL DISEASES

The venereal diseases are gonorrhea, syphilis, chancroid, lymphogranuloma venereum, and granuloma inguinale.

Gonorrhea

Gonorrhea is a contagious, pus-producing (*pyogenic*) inflammation of the genital mucous membranes, caused by a microorganism, *Neis-* *seria gonorrhoeae*, commonly called the *gonococcus*. It is the most common of all venereal diseases and is worldwide in distribution.

Gonorrhea is transmitted in adults by sexual intercourse. Gonorrheal *vulvovaginitis* in young girls, however, is an epidemic form of gonorrheal infection which is transmitted by nonsexual contacts, such as towels, toys, etc. Adults who have been apparently cured may still be infectious. Gonorrheal infection of women is thought to be the most frequent cause of disease of the female reproductive organs. Gonorrheal infection can occur from contact with contaminated articles; such instances, however, are rare in adults, since gonococci die quickly at a temperature lower than that of the body or in the absence of moisture. The time from exposure to development of symptoms (*incubation period*) of gonorrhea is generally three to ten days, but may be longer.

Symptoms and types of infection

In the male, gonorrheal infections usually begin in the anterior urethra, causing severe inflammation. Because of this inflamed condition, urination causes an intense burning sensation. A large amount of pus is produced for a period of two to three months, if the patient is not treated. If not successfully controlled in the early stages, gonorrhea may produce a chronic infection which can last for years.

Complications in men include inflammations of the prostate (*prostatitis*), epididymis (*epididymitis*), and testis (*orchitis*). Epididymitis may produce sterility by sealing off the tubes which carry sperm from the testes.

In the female, the external genitalia usually become infected first. If the infection is not con-

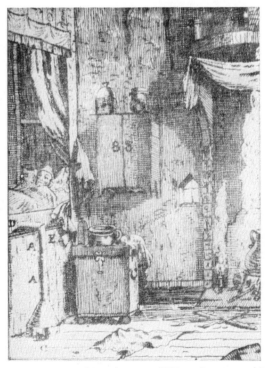

This engraving from the year 1688 portrays an old method for the treatment of syphilis patients with a high temperature bed. *Bettmann Archive.*

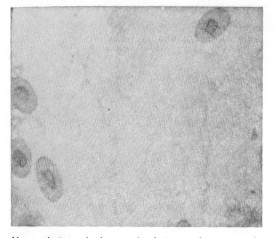

Above photograph shows spirochetes as they appear in a blood smear. The spirochete which causes syphilis is known as *Treponema pallidum*. Spirochetes are identified by their corkscrew shape.

trolled, it may spread to the other reproductive organs. Complications in women include inflammation of the Fallopian tubes (*salpingitis*) and of the ovaries (*ovaritis*). Pyosalpingitis (pus tubes) is a frequent cause of sterility in women, since the Fallopian tubes may become sealed off.

Other complications occurring in both sexes are inflammation of the bladder (*cystitis*), rectum (*proctitis*), mouth (*stomatitis*), joints (*arthritis*), kidneys (*nephritis*), bones (*osteomyelitis*), heart valves (*endocarditis*), membranes covering the brain and spinal cord (*meningitis*), and lining of the body cavity (*peritonitis*). Blood poisoning (*septicemia*) may also occur.

Gonorrheal infection of the eyes (*ophthalmitis*) may occur in adults, but most frequently occurs in newborn infants who are infected in passage through the birth canal. At one time, nearly one third of all blindness in children was the result of such infection; however, this type infection has been almost completely eradicated by physicians treating all newborn babies with preventative medication.

Treatment

It is imperative that a physician supervise any treatment of patients with venereal disease. This is particularly true in the use of penicillin for gonorrhea, for two reasons. First, the patient may appear to be cured and yet be capable of transmitting the disease. Second, penicillin may cure gonorrhea but only "mask" an unsuspected case of syphilis, which is also present at the same time. Syphilis cannot be cured except by larger doses of the drug. This is particularly important, because penicillin may suppress the early and more easily recognized stage of syphilis, but the

disease may nevertheless develop at a later time and in a later stage, with more serious consequences. For this reason, physicians sometimes use one of the sulfonamide drugs in cases of gonorrhea where the presence of syphilis is also suspected, since the drug does not "mask" developing syphilis. Other drugs, such as terramycin and aureomycin, have also been used successfully in the treatment of patients with gonorrhea. However, it must be emphasized that no single drug is effective in all cases of gonorrhea.

Prevention

Prevention of the spread of gonorrhea is a matter of public health concern. There is a need for effective public health education. Such an educative program must emphasize the need for prompt treatment to those who contract gonorrhea. It will also alert young people who do not have gonorrhea to the possibility of infection. The use of prophylactic devices and thorough cleansing of exposed parts with soap and water are of great value in the prevention of gonorrhea, although such measures are not thought to be entirely effective against syphilis.

Physicians are required by law to use penicillin or a dilute solution of silver nitrate in the eyes of newborn infants to prevent gonorrheal infection and possible resultant blindness.

Syphilis

Syphilis is a contagious venereal disease which can infect any of the body tissues. Until recently the disease was sometimes called lues, since the word syphilis was considered taboo. The term "hard chancre" has been used to distinguish the skin lesion of the primary stage of syphilis from "soft chancre," or chancroid (caused by another type of bacteria), while the synonym "great pox" was used to distinguish the skin eruption of the secondary stage from "smallpox."

The origin of syphilis is not known. It is debated whether Christopher Columbus and his crew brought it to the new world from Europe

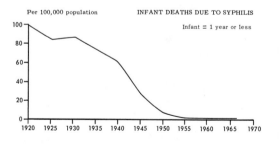

This chart shows the pronounced decrease which occurred in the death rate due to syphilis among infants in the United States between 1920 and 1966.

or whether they contracted the disease from the women of the new world and took it with them to Europe. It is known, however, from studies of bones of American Indians that syphilis existed in America at least 500 years before Columbus made his first voyage. It is furthermore known that some of Columbus' crew accompanied Charles VIII of France in the invasion of Italy in 1494. A terrible epidemic of syphilis began in Italy at this time and spread over all of Europe as the troops returned.

Today syphilis is worldwide in its distribution. Although the disease is perhaps not as severe as in the days of Columbus, or even during World War II, it is still one of the major scourges of mankind. The United States Public Health Service has estimated that half a million new cases occur each year in the United States alone. In World War II positive blood tests were obtained in 4.5 percent of men examined by Selective Service Boards. The incidence in Negroes in this group was slightly over 25 percent. It has been estimated that between one and two percent of the children of the United States are born with syphilis.

Cause and transmission

Syphilis is caused by a corkscrew-shaped microorganism (*spirochete*) known as *Treponema pallidum*. At least 99.9 percent of all cases of syphilis in adults are acquired by sexual means, such as kissing and sexual intercourse. Although treatment generally seems to render an infected person incapable of transmitting the disease, there is some evidence that persons apparently cured may still infect others.

Syphilis is the only one of the venereal diseases that may be acquired congenitally with passage of the causative organism from the mother to the unborn child. Syphilitic infection may cause abortion or stillbirth. Surviving infants have advanced, generalized (*tertiary*) syphilis at birth. Even third generation syphilis has been reported.

Within a few hours after exposure, the syphilis spirochete penetrates the skin or mucous membrane and enters the blood stream and tissues. However, symptoms appear only after ten to 90 days—averaging about three weeks. Then, the "hard chancre" of the primary stage of the disease may appear. The chancre ordinarily is found on the genitals or in the mouth, but may occur elsewhere. In occasional cases no chancre develops. Chancre fluid is extremely infectious.

Even though no treatment is given, chancres generally disappear in ten to 40 days; then two to six months later, the secondary stage appears. Small raised red areas (*syphilids*) may be found on the skin, or small *mucous patches* in the mouth or on the reproductive organs. Lymph nodes over the body usually become enlarged.

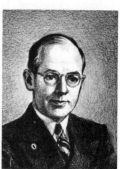

KAHN, Reuben Leon (1887-) American bacteriologist. He introduced a flocculation test for syphilis (1923-1928) which is now used in conjunction with the Wassermann complement-fixation reaction. Neither of these tests is infallible, both showing on occasion false positive or negative reactions. When they are used together, however, the chances of a correct interpretation are greatly improved. The Kahn test has fewer steps than the Wassermann and is thought by many to be more accurate.

Generally, the lesions of secondary syphilis heal spontaneously in three to twelve weeks, but may recur later.

Symptoms of tertiary syphilis may develop soon after the secondary symptoms have disappeared, or may be delayed for many years. Ulcer-like draining sores appear on the skin; hard nodules (*gumma*) occur in the tissue under the skin or in the internal organs. The heart and blood vessels are frequently damaged, and lungs may also be affected.

Syphilis of the central nervous system (*neurosyphilis*) can occur in the secondary stage, but usually accompanies late tertiary infection. Involvement of the spinal cord may cause loss of co-ordination of the limbs, and infection of the brain may cause "softening" (*general paresis*) with deterioration of mental faculties and paralysis of limbs. It has been estimated that ten to 15 percent of the inmates of institutions for the insane are victims of neurosyphilis.

Treatment

Treatment of syphilis with mercury ointment dates back at least to the sixteenth century. In a quest for a "magic bullet" to cure syphilis, Dr. Paul Ehrlich in 1912 tested over 600 compounds, one of which was the famous drug, *arsphenamine*. Other arsenic-containing drugs, such as mapharsen and bismuth compounds have been widely used in treating syphilitic patients. In recent years, penicillin has largely replaced these drugs, and other antibiotics such as aureomycin, chloromycetin, and terramycin have also been used. It is extremely important that all treatment be prescribed and supervised by a physician. Inadequate treatment may cause syphilis to remain dormant for years and finally reappear in the late stages when a complete cure is more difficult. Improper treatment may cause severe reactions, which may even be fatal.

Prevention and control

Today this disease is not under proper control. There is no method of immunization against syphilis; avoidance of exposure to infected persons is of paramount importance. If exposure does occur, prophylactic measures should be instituted as promptly as possible.

During World War II, the armed forces of the United States developed a rigorous control program for venereal disease, consisting of intensive indoctrination of all personnel. Prophylactic stations were set up at all bases and complete instructions for the correct administration of chemical prophylaxis were disseminated. In many areas clinics were available, staffed with trained attendants to give medication. In addition to the chemical prophylaxis, mechanical prophylactics were issued to the men in service. As a result of the widespread educational campaign and the strict enforcement of prophylactic measures, venereal disease was kept to a minimum.

The prevention and control of syphilis is largely an educational problem. Doctor Thomas Parran, for many years Surgeon General of the United States, has summarized the task as one of (1) finding cases, (2) prompt treatment, (3) examination of all contacts, (4) prevention of birth of syphilitic babies by compulsory blood tests before marriage and early in each pregnancy, and (5) public education.

Largely because of the efforts of Doctor Parran and the Public Health Service, much progress has been made in the control of syphilis in this country. The adult death rate in 1958 had dropped to less than one-eighth that reported for 1920. However, between 1958 and 1961, the reported cases of infectious syphilis in the United States increased by 75 percent. In the late 1960s, public apathy to this major problem was somewhat overcome and the medical sciences again began to gain on the disease.

An estimated 60,000 babies are born with

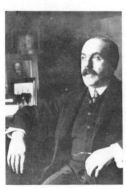

WASSERMANN, August von (1866-1925) German bacteriologist. He is known internationally for the specific blood reaction test (complement-fixation test) for the diagnosis of syphilis, which he developed in 1906 along with Carl Bruck and Albert Neisser. He was at one time director of the department of experimental therapy at the Koch Institute for Infectious Diseases. Later he was director of the department of experimental therapy in the Kaiser Wilhelm Institute. *Bettmann Archive.*

congenital syphilis each year in this country. This figure is tragically high since congenital syphilis can be prevented by treatment of the pregnant woman, even though the treatment may not be sufficient to cure the disease in the mother.

Chancroid

Chancroid is often called "soft chancre" to distinguish this initial soft sore from the "hard chancre" of syphilis. Chancroid occurs throughout the world and has been estimated to make up ten percent of all venereal infections. Chancroid is usually transmitted by sexual contact, but it is thought that infection may occasionally occur indirectly from soiled dressings or towels. The causative organism is the bacillus, *Hemophilus ducreyi.*

Four to ten days after exposure to chancroid, a small lesion appears on or near the genital organs. This sore soon becomes an ulcer with irregular edges and is surrounded by a reddened and swollen area. More than one soft chancre may occur. The infection frequently spreads to the lymph nodes of the groin, causing swellings known as buboes.

The best method of prevention of chancroid is refraining from sexual relations with infected persons. Thorough cleansing of exposed areas with soap and warm water is thought to be of more value than specific methods of prevention recommended for other venereal diseases. For treatment of patients with chancroid, physicians have successfully employed sulfonamides. Streptomycin also has been found useful.

Lymphogranuloma venereum

Lymphogranuloma venereum is a virus-produced disease affecting the lymph organs in the genital areas. This disease was described by Nicolas and Favre of Paris, France, in 1913 and is still known in France as "La maladie de Nicolas et de Favre." It is found all over the world, and there is some evidence that the number of cases is increasing. In the United States, the disease is particularly prevalent in the South, especially among Negroes.

Lymphogranuloma venereum is usually transmitted by sexual intercourse. However, the virus causing this disease *may* enter the body by way of the mouth or the eye. After an incubation period of seven to twelve days, a small hardened area (*papule*) appears, usually on the penis in men. After the local sore heals, men are generally considered no longer capable of transmitting the disease, but women may infect subsequent sexual partners for years. In the early phases of the disease, fever, inflammation of the joints, skin rashes, and even infection of the brain and its covering membrane may be present.

From the local lesion, the disease spreads to the lymph nodes, especially those in the groin. The swelling produced in the lymph nodes may reach the size of a walnut. These swollen areas have been called buboes but they seldom break open and drain pus. If not treated they may remain for months. In women, the vulva may become enromously enlarged, a condition known as *elephantiasis*. Narrowing (*stricture*) of the rectum may also occur and necessitate surgical correction for its relief.

Lymphogranuloma venereum is the only venereal disease known to be caused by a virus. Although this virus can be cultivated in developing fertile chicken eggs, the usual methods of diagnosis do not involve direct observation of the virus. Clinical symptoms are suggestive, but a skin test is generally used for confirmation. A small amount of heated virus is injected into the skin by the physician. If the patient has lymphogranuloma venereum, a hard inflamed area develops in 24 to 48 hours. The skin test, known as the *Frei test*, will apparently be positive throughout life, even after the disease is cured. One attack of this disease is thought to render one immune for life.

Unlike most virus diseases, lymphogranuloma venereum has been successfully controlled with sulfonamides or penicillin. Excellent results have also been obtained with other drugs, such as terramycin and aureomycin.

Granuloma inguinale

Granuloma inguinale is a disease characterized by deep ulcerations of the skin of the genitals and believed to be caused by the microorganism, *Donovania granulomatosis,* sometimes referred to as Donovan body. Although this disease is generally regarded as venereal, there is no absolute proof that it is transmitted from one person to another by sexual contact. In fact, the husband or wife of a person with granuloma inguinale usually does not have the disease. However, it is possible that natural resistance to the disease is so high that only relatively few of those exposed are affected. Granuloma inguinale is associated with uncleanliness. It has been estimated that there are 5000 to 10,000 cases in the United States.

After exposure, one to four weeks elapse before the disease is noticeable. Swelling, usually in the groin, appears first. The swollen area then ruptures to form an ulcer. New ulcers continue to appear as the old ones heal, and the disease may cover the reproductive organs, buttocks, and lower abdomen. Such extensive lesions develop a foul odor. Persons with granuloma inguinale appear to develop little immunity, and the disease may be present for many years.

Fuadin and other antimony compounds were first used, but in recent years streptomycin has been found more effective than older methods

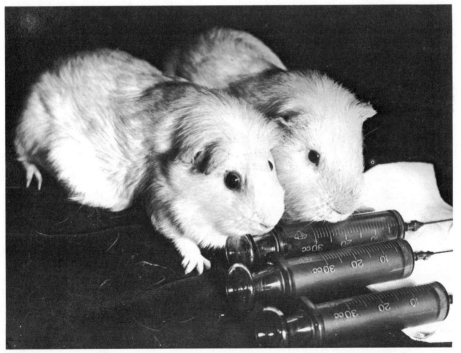

Blood from guinea pigs contains one of the important constituents of the Wassermann test for syphilis. Other essential elements are derived from sheep blood and rabbits. In obtaining blood from guinea pigs, the animals are bled from the heart with a syringe and needle. Operations of this type are performed with animals under ether. Animals recover quickly and may be used often. *Medical Research Bulletin. Jay A. Smith photo.*

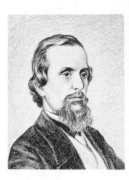

HUTCHINSON, Jonathan (1828-1913), English surgeon. Described the three signs of congenital syphilis, now called *Hutchinson's signs*. They are notched teeth, interstitial keratitis (chronic inflammation of the cornea), and eighth nerve deafness (deafness caused by a lesion of the 8th cranial nerve). When these three signs are found in children, they are considered to be diagnostic of congenital syphilis. He also described *summer prurigo*.

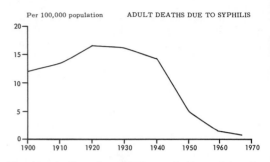

The introduction of antibiotics probably explains the decline in deaths due to syphilis since 1940.

in the treatment of patients with this disease. Excellent results have also been obtained with terramycin. By use of these drugs, definite progress has been reported toward eliminating this disease.

SEX AND MARRIAGE

Marriage may be defined either as the ceremony or act by which a legal relationship of husband and wife is formed, or as a physical, legal, and moral union between man and woman for the establishment of a family. Most primitive unions were more or less casual alliances between the male and the female. As the culture advanced in complexity, the period of helplessness of the children became longer, and the need for parental care became greater. Much of the responsibility for the care of the children fell upon the woman, for her dependent condition during pregnancy rendered her unfit for more strenuous activities. Hence, the role of each parent became defined. The father provided food and shelter, and the mother prepared the food and cared for the young. Thus, the family was established. In its biological aspect, the origin of marriage is to be found in the family, rather than the origin of the family in marriage.

Forms of family and marriage

The individual functions of the man and woman within the family vary among different cultures. There have been many instances in which the family unit centered around the mother and children, with the father occupying a position of little social significance or prestige. Such matriarchal societies, in which the mother is the dominant figure, have consistently failed to endure through the years. By far the most prevalent type of family is the patriarchal, or father-dominated family. Today in America, however, mother-domination of society is constantly increasing.

The term "forms of marriage" is used to indicate the *numeric* variation, the definition depending upon the number of consorts united to each other. There is no conclusive evidence that the varieties of marriage correspond to stages of social evolution. Rather, the forms of marriage are regarded as the product of each particular culture, being determined by the type of community, and its economic, social, and political organization.

Polyandry is the form of marriage in which several men are legally married to one woman. It is the rarest type of marriage. It occurs chiefly in regions in southern India and central Asia, and in a few African and Eskimo tribes. The rarity of this form of marriage may be caused in part by the possessive attitude of men toward women, but polyandry is usually the result of scarcity of women. In Tibet, there exists a fraternal type of polyandry in which several brothers live in the same household and share a common wife. Children born of these marriages are usually regarded as the legal descendants of the eldest brother. However, in some societies, the children may be allotted individually to the brother upon whom the mother chooses to bestow the honor of social paternity.

Polygyny is the form of marriage in which several wives are legally united to one man. All of the offspring are regarded as legal descendants of the husband. Polygyny has probably existed at one time or another in every culture. The reasons for the existence of polygyny are largely economic and political. Multiple wives may increase a man's wealth and his social importance and authority. The maintenance of separate households for each wife is more common than keeping all the wives under one roof. In the Western world, polygyny was practiced legally and accepted by both church and state as recently as the seventeenth century. Where polygyny still exists, it is not usually practiced throughout the entire community, as this would require an enormous surplus of females. Rather,

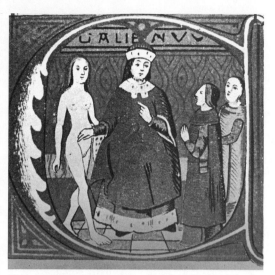

This medieval picture shows Galen, who lived in the second century, lecturing to a group of students on the topic of gynecology. *Bettmann Archive.*

it is largely confined to members of the wealthy and ruling classes, who can afford the luxury of more than one wife. Many wives are an economical asset, since they can care for the children and keep the household without the need of many servants. Another contributory reason for polygyny among some societies is the high valuation placed on children. This seems to have been the chief reason for polygyny in the history of the Hebrew patriarchs. In some cultures, polygyny has received the explicit sanction of religion, as in Mohammedanism and Mormonism. With the advance of higher civilizations, however, polygyny as a rule gives way to monogamy.

Monogamy is the form of marriage in which one man is married to one woman. This form of marriage exists in most communities, largely because of biological necessity, since under normal conditions the numbers of males and females in most populations are relatively equal. Also, economic conditions usually make it impossible for a man to support more than one wife and her offspring.

The marriage ceremony: Among all peoples, uncivilized as well as civilized, legal marriage is usually accompanied by some form of ceremony that expresses group sanction and social acceptance of the union. The ceremony is usually of a religious or magical character, although it may be a purely social ceremony in some cultures. Among primitive societies, group desires, hopes, and fears became closely associated with the various deities. The classical figures idealizing the image of womanhood and femininity have assumed various forms which are remarkably similar in different cultures. To all cultures there is the primal nude figure: Aphrodite to the Greeks, Venus to the Romans, and Eve to the Jews and Christians. Many cultures developed ideal types to symbolize the subordinate functions of woman. The Greeks revered Pallas Athene, protectress of the hearth and household crafts, and the Romans cherished Diana, protectress of the hunt and of chastity. The various deities were invoked as part of the marriage ceremony and were believed to protect the home and community against evil. Mythology and folklore the world over are rich in the varied and highly ritualistic ceremonies of early marriage.

Exogamy and endogamy: Almost universal among the various cultures, even among strictly "clannish" societies, has been the requirement that marriage take place between persons who are not near kin. The custom of forbidding marriage within the clan is known as *exogamy* as opposed to *endogamy*, or marriage within the clan. This incest taboo has existed over many years, as indicated by the early Greek plays concerning Oedipus and Electra, which reveal an ancient abhorrence of incest. Within the few cultures that have practiced family intermarriage, endogamy is generally justified on the grounds that such marriages take place among the ruling classes, who supposedly are immune by royal prerogative from the physical effects of incest.

Marriage by capture and purchase: Among warlike tribes, marriage by capture was often common. However, capture of wives rarely took place outside the tribe. Since the beginning of recorded history, marriage by capture was only ceremonious as practiced among the ancient people. The presence of the best man at modern weddings may owe its origin to its ancient counterpart—the chief abettor of the bridegroom in the act of capture. Further, some authorities hold that today's wedding ring has evolved from a shackle put around the feet of the captive wife.

Marriage by capture was slowly transformed into the practice of marriage by purchase. This stage occurred particularly in early barbarism, with the development of slavery and the concept of the wife as property. The evolution of altruism which goes hand in hand with human progress brought about consideration of the female as an individual, not as an article of property. Thus, with the advance of civilization, the practice of purchasing wives was gradually abandoned. The bride price was reversed in its operation and became the dowry, a token of respect and kindness toward the woman. The practice of bestowing a dowry on the bride is still prevalent in some modern societies.

The effect of Christianity on marriage: The early Aryan peoples of Europe regarded marriage primarily as a religious bond, since the family life was based on ancestor worship. The early Aryan view of marriage later gave way to

TABLE OF THE LEGAL REQUIREMENTS FOR MARRIAGE IN THE UNITED STATES

State	With Consent/ *Without Consent* Men	Women	Physical and Blood Tests	Wait for License/ *Wait After License*
Alabama[7]	17, *21*	14, *18*	2, 4	None, *None*
Alaska	18, *21*	16, *18*	2, 4	3 days. *None*
Arizona	18, *21*	16, *18*	2, 4	48 hours, *None*
Arkansas	18, *21*	16, *18*	1	3 days, *None*
California	18, *21*	16, *18*	2	None, *None*
Colorado	16, *21*	16, *18*	2, 4	None, *None*
Connecticut	16, *21*	16, *21*	2, 4	4 days, *None*
Delaware	18, *21*	16, *18*	1, 3	None[8]
District of Columbia	18, *21*	16, *18*	2	4 days, *None*
Florida	18, *21*	16, *21*	2, 4	3 days, *None*
Georgia	18, *19*	16, *18*	2, 4	None,[7] *None*
Hawaii	18, *20*	16, *20*	1, 3	3 days, *None*
Idaho	18, *21*	16, *18*	2, 4	None,[7] *None*
Illinois[6]	18, *21*	16, *18*	2, 4	None, *None*
Indiana	18, *21*	16, *18*	1, 3	3 days, *None*
Iowa	18, *21*	16, *18*	1, 3	3 days, *None*
Kansas	18, *21*	18, *18*	2, 4	3 days, *None*
Kentucky	18, *18*	16, *18*	1, 3	3 days, *None*
Louisiana[6]	18, *21*	16, *21*	1[9] 3	None, *72 hours*
Maine	16, *21*	16, *18*	2, 4	5 days, *None*
Maryland	18, *21*	16, *18*	5	48 hours, *None*
Massachusetts	18, *21*	16, *18*	2, 4	3 days, *None*
Michigan	18, *18*	16, *18*	1, 3	3 days, *None*
Minnesota	18, *21*	16, *18*	5	5 days, *None*
Mississippi[7]	17, *21*	15, *18*	1	3 days, *None*
Missouri	15, *21*	15, *18*	2	3 days, *None*
Montana	18, *21*	16, *18*	2, 4	5 days, *None*
Nebraska	18, *21*	16, *21*	2, 4	None, *None*
Nevada	18, *21*	16, *18*	5	None, *None*
New Hampshire[6]	14, *20*	13, *18*	2, 4	5 days, *None*
New Jersey	18, *21*	16, *18*	2, 4	72 hours, *None*
New Mexico	18, *21*	16, *18*	1, 3	3 days, *None*
New York	16, *21*	14, *18*	1, 3	None, *24 hours*
North Carolina	16, *18*	16, *18*	2, 3	None, *None*
North Dakota[6]	18, *21*	15, *18*	1, 3	None, *None*
Ohio[6]	18, *21*	16, *21*	2, 4	5 days, *None*
Oklahoma[7]	18, *21*	15, *18*	1, 3	None, *None*
Oregon	18, *21*	15, *18*	1, 4	7 days, *None*
Pennsylvania	16, *21*	16, *21*	1, 3	3 days, *None*
Rhode Island[7]	18, *21*	16, *21*	1, 3	None,[6] *None*[8]
South Carolina	16, *18*	14, *18*	5	24 hours, *None*
South Dakota	18, *21*	16, *18*	1, 3	None, *None*
Tennessee[7]	16, *21*	16, *21*	2, 4	3 days, *None*
Texas	16, *21*	14, *18*	2	None,[7] *None*
Utah	16, *21*	14, *18*	2, 4	None, *None*
Vermont[6]	18, *21*	14, *18*	2, 4	None, *5 days*
Virginia	18, *21*	16, *21*	2, 4	None, *None*
Washington	17, *21*	17, *18*	5[10]	3 days, *None*
West Virginia	18, *21*	16, *21*	1, 3	3 days, *None*
Wisconsin	18, *21*	16, *18*	2, 4	5 days, *None*
Wyoming	18, *21*	16, *21*	2, 4	None, *None*

1. Blood test required. Must be administered within state.
2. Blood test required. May be administered out-of-state.
3. Physical test required. Must be administered within state.
4. Physical test required. May be administered out-of-state.
5. No premarital tests required.
(Where out-of-state tests are acceptable, they should comply with the laws of the state in which they are to be used, and the applicant should also determine whether these tests must be on forms supplied by the state in which they are to be used and whether certification is required.)
6. Special laws apply to nonresidents.
7. Special laws apply to those under 21 years.
8. 24 hours if one or both parties are residents; 96 hours if both parties are nonresidents.
9. Blood test at option of physician.
10. Male must make affidavit that he is not afflicted with any contagious venereal disease.
Note: The District of Columbia, Delaware, and Maryland require that the marriage be performed by an ordained officer of a church.

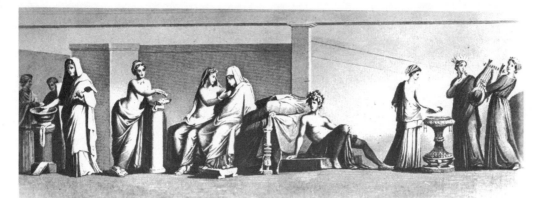

Picture from a famous old Roman wall painting known as the *Aldobrandini Marriage*, showing a group of goddesses supervising and counselling the bride on her conduct during the first night of marriage. *Bettmann Archive.*

the Roman concept of marriage as a private contract, to be formed and dissolved by the man and woman of their own accord. The Christian church sought to restore the concept of marriage as a religious bond, which was finally realized by making marriage one of the sacraments of the church. Even the church, however, was forced to recognize that consent and legal contract were essential means of entering the marriage relation. In early Christian Rome, manners and morals so lacked restraint that the Roman Catholic Church adopted many rules which departed from the original purpose of suppressing sexual gratification, but were by necessity included in the basis of the sexual code. It is obvious that the *social* purpose of this regard for chastity was to safeguard the sanctity and entity of monogamic patriarchal marriage.

Protestant reformers revived the idea that marriage was a civil relation, to be created and broken only by civil authority, rather than a religious bond or sacrament. In an effort to overrule this view, the Roman Catholic Council of Trent in 1563 declared that a valid marriage could be created only by the Church and annulled by the Church. This still remains the Roman Catholic view of marriage. The concept of marriage as a private and civil contract has been revived in many modern nations among many elements of their populations.

Genetic aspects of marriage

People marry for personal reasons and not for the conscious betterment of the species. In many instances, the maximum welfare of the individual may well be the maximum welfare of the group also. While the existence of the family perpetuates the species, it may also improve the species biologically. The branch of science known as *eugenics* pertains to the biological improvement of the inherent qualities of the human organism by application of knowledge of the laws of genetics.

A great amount of positive evidence regarding inheritable traits now exists. Both healthy and unhealthy traits are inheritable. It would appear sensible, therefore, for intelligent persons to give thought to how the genetic stock might be improved through legislation that would prevent the procreation of unhealthy individuals. Many states have laws that permit sterilization of inmates of mental institutions who have low grade mentality. But since democratic countries maintain respect for individual rights and differences, only voluntary eugenics is possible as a positive measure. However, a majority of states do require premarital blood tests. Although such laws may prevent transmission of venereal disease to the marriage partner and to the children, they fall far short of improving the biological structure of the species by an effective genetic approach.

The family physician can be of help in evaluating the desirable genetic traits of two people contemplating marriage. From the family history of both parties, the physician may be able to tell whether two people have genetic traits which will result either in healthy children or in the transmission of latent disorders, of which the persons themselves may be unaware.

The sexual drive and how it affects marriage

It is paradoxical that even though sex is the biological foundation of marriage, many adults are misguided, reticent, prudish, or even ignorant of many important and rather obvious factors concerning sex. Popular understanding of the reproductive function is permeated by superstition and false ideas. One of the common mis-

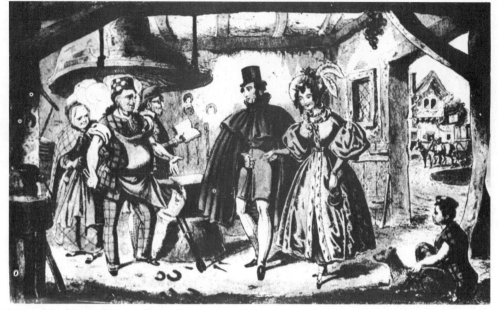

Old picture of the famous forge at Gretna Green, where the young couples were married before the anvil to insure the forging of a strong marital union. *Bettmann Archive.*

conceptions among young boys, for instance, is fear of sexual depletion, that they might "use up" their potency. Many men also subscribe to the common misconception that the intact hymen is an infallible sign of virginity. Among young women, the attitude toward sex may be strongly affected by the feeling that sex is not "nice," or that it is a burden inflicted upon the woman by the aggressive, voracious male. Such women perform their "marital duty" perfunctorily, perhaps even feeling superior because they receive no satisfaction from their sex life; they consider sex as a one-sided affair, without understanding that their marriage relationship is incomplete, and that the deficiency is their own. Many women, because they fail to obtain sexual gratification early in marriage, consider themselves hopelessly "frigid." To avoid such mistaken ideas, an understanding of both the psychological and physiological aspects of sex is helpful.

In both sexes, the period of life known as *puberty* is marked by the development and manifestation of the sexual drive. At puberty, the young male becomes conscious of a desire to gratify his sexual impulse, with masturbation as the earliest manifestation. Masturbation may be practiced by both sexes and is considered a more or less normal phase in the sexual development of the individual.

The sexual impulse varies greatly from one individual to another. In general, the capacity for sexual intercourse is at the highest between the ages of 20 and 40 in the male, although there is a gradual decline in sexual outlet frequency from the teens. However, marital coitus among older men occurs considerably more frequent than is commonly believed. About three fourths of all men between the ages of 65 and 69 experience satisfactory coitus as do about 60 percent of the men between the ages of 70 and 74.

In the sexually mature male, the accumulation of the semen in the organs which store the semen results in physical pressure. This physical tension occurs spontaneously, but may also occur as the result of mental images and desires. In the sexually abstinent male, involuntary seminal loss may take place during sleep, usually associated with erotic dreams. Erection and ejaculation during sleep is a motor reflex, responding to the need to relieve physical tension, although the erotic nature of sex dreams has either a causal or resultant relationship with the physical tension. This need is separate from the emotional urge to attain sexual gratification, which often occurs when there is no backlog of seminal pressure. Repression of the sexual impulse is physically possible in the male, but it is difficult unless the mind and body are kept vigorously at work.

The sexual impulse in young women is far less dependent upon the craving for relief of sexual tension. The anatomical difference between the sexes explains this difference to some extent. Erection and nocturnal emissions disclose to the

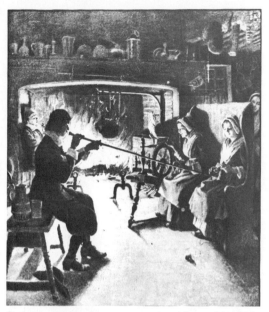

During colonial days a young couple could obtain privacy in their conversations only by talking through a *whispering rod. Bettmann Archive.*

young man the functional significance of his reproductive organs. But in the young woman, the copulative and reproductive purposes of her genital organs do not become immediately obvious. In most women, the sexual impulse remains dormant for a much longer time than in the male, being awakened to full activity, culminating in orgasm, only after repeated sexual intercourse. Much more time is needed in overcoming the sexual taboos women have had forced upon them than the fewer ones and less severe ones endured by men, also attributing to the delay in full sexual awakening of women.

The physiological mechanism of the orgasm for both man and woman has been carefully described recently in rather exacting details in the writings of Masters and Johnson, researchers in the field of human sexual behavior. It is known that the heart rate is substantially increased at orgasm, and that the blood pressure rises sharply. The experience of orgasm involves the crossing of a sensory-psychical threshold of overwhelmingly intense impressions, an extremely complex reaction which involves the sympathetic-spinal reflexes as well as the cerebral cortex. The definition of orgasm—as a summation of sexual excitement rising in crescendo until a summit of enjoyment is reached, followed by a feeling of physical and emotional relaxation and relief— only partially describes this mechanism. In the normal male, ejaculation of semen occurs simultaneously with the subjective pleasurable sensation of the orgasm. There is, of course, no ejaculation that accompanies the woman's orgasm

although in some instances vaginal muscle contractions at the time of orgasm may force a few drops of lubricating fluids from the vagina and mistakenly lead one to believe that a woman, too, may ejaculate.

Few women experience orgasm in the first few times they have intercourse. Consequently, a newly married woman may think that she is frigid. This "false frigidity" is the result of inexperience and lack of adjustment between the two partners. The temporary frigidity is common and should not be a permanent barrier to sexual gratification. In many instances, however, sexual experience for the woman may never amount to more than that of mild enjoyment and the satisfaction of giving pleasure to the sexual partner. This lack of complete gratification may or may not arouse any sense of loss or deficiency; but if it does, neurotic symptoms may become manifest. Thousands of women never attain sexual gratification, but still become pregnant, give birth to children, and may even regard themselves as happy wives. However, when the male partner is emotionally demonstrative and skilled in erotic technique, the woman of average sensibilities who has regular sexual intercourse should sooner or later begin to experience orgasm. Throughout life, however, sexual gratification of the woman will depend largely upon the degree of physical and mental accord with the husband. Both husbands and wives should realize that while many women are not able to reach orgasm by sexual intercourse, especially during the early months of marriage, they can be made to respond fully sexually by other means of stimulation, either manually, orally, or mechanically. Once the woman is able to reach orgasm via other methods, the anxiety, fear, or guilt that interfere with her responding in sexual intercourse will often disappear and she will then be able to respond orgasmically during coitus. Far more women than most people realize actually prefer to reach orgasm by methods other than sexual intercourse and it is the responsibility of both husband and wife to see to it that the spouse is given as complete satisfaction as possible in each sexual experience.

There is another difference in the sexual life between the male and the female. The sexual impulse in the female is frequently associated with the urge to reproduce; she experiences the longing for a child, a longing to experience maternity. This urge is much less pronounced in the male. In men, the urge to reproduce may sometimes reflect a longing to have a child by some special love object. However, the male motives to reproduce have become largely modified by such factors as family descent, monetary considerations, social convenience, or even personal vanity. Thus, in the modern man, the urge to reproduce becomes a lesser component of the sexual drive.

Mental and physical factors affecting sex

The physical and mental factors affecting sex continually interact and influence one another in the attainment of health and happiness in marriage. These factors differ with individuals and with the passage of time. In the beginning of marriage, the first intercourse poses problems. The woman who has never experienced sexual intercourse may offer both physical and mental resistance. Physically, the hymen may have to be broken. The hymen has often been considered an infallible symbol of virginity, but many women fail to bleed on first intercourse, for any of several causes. As explained earlier, the hymen is elastic and may distend upon penetration; and even upon penetration and rupture of the membrane, little blood may be lost. Also the hymen may have become ruptured by other physical means. The absence of an intact hymen cannot be regarded as a sign of previous intercourse, any more than the presence of the intact hymen proves virginity. *Defloration*, or rupture of the hymen, causes some discomfort to the majority of women. If, in rare cases, the pain is unendurable, the hymen must be ruptured by surgical means.

In addition to this physical resistance, because of outmoded notions taught women in a Victorian culture, the inexperienced woman usually feels some degree of fear, no matter how intense her emotional feeling for her mate, nor how complete her theoretical knowledge. It is difficult for women to achieve complete sexual gratification during the first intercourse for these reasons.

The beginning of marriage is an apprenticeship for both partners. Sexual adjustment must be *learned*, and the exercise of sexual technique must be adapted to the individual needs and preferences of each couple. This should be achieved slowly, in order to avoid severe demands during the first phases of adjustment. The complicated and advanced erotic techniques may well be left until at least a successful degree of sexual adaptation is attained.

The thought of pregnancy influences the sexual relations of most people. When the couple desire children, continued failure to conceive may change their feelings about coitus. Also, and more frequently the case, when the couple do not desire children and cannot liberate their minds from the fear of pregnancy, sexual intercourse may not realize all its potentialities. Fear of pregnancy can so inhibit the bodily reactions that marriages may be deeply affected. In persons whose religious restrictions do not prohibit the use of contraceptives, these devices may be helpful in relieving this fear. Contraception can also be of value in preventing pregnancies from occurring too close together, or when the woman should not bear children for medical reasons.

When a woman reaches sexual maturity, her

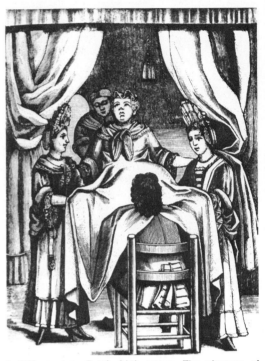

A 17th century Dutch birth scene. The absence of adequate medical knowledge made childbearing a very hazardous procedure. *Bettmann Archive.*

desire for intercourse should become at least equal to that of her husband. Indeed, the healthy, erotically mature woman may have a greater sexual vigor than the average man. A decided discrepancy between the sexual drive of the man and the woman may result in either chronic nervousness in the woman, or chronic sexual overstrain and fatigue in the husband. Actually, though many women never realize it, the female is probably more richly endowed to enjoy sex than is the male. The female body has many more easily stimulated, or erogenous, skin areas than the male. Orgasm, when achieved by the woman, is longer in duration than that of the man, and there can be a deeper involvement of the entire being in the sex act itself. The sexual awakening in a woman may reach its fullest power in the later years, and may even become intensified after the menopause. As the woman reaches the height of her ability to obtain sexual gratification, often increased by release from the fear of pregnancy, the man may be experiencing a decline in sexual potency. An understanding of this difference in sexual drive in men and women may help in the maintenance of sexual harmony in the later years of marriage.

Sexual activity in marriage

Men are not born with intuitive knowledge of sex and its technique, and all too often the man

Percent

PHYSICAL DEVELOPMENTS IN ADOLESCENCE

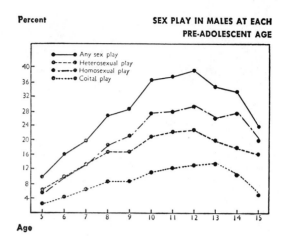

Age

This chart portrays the percent of American males undergoing the indicated changes in physical development at the various ages during adolescence.

Percent

SEX PLAY IN MALES AT EACH PRE-ADOLESCENT AGE

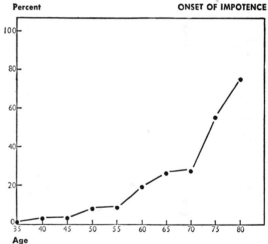

Age

This chart depicts the percent of pre-adolescent males who have engaged in various forms of sex play indicated at ages from five to fifteen years.

Frequency per week

DECREASE OF MARITAL INTERCOURSE

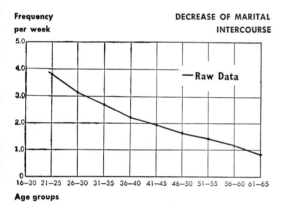

Age groups

Chart showing the progressive decrease with age of the average frequency of marital sexual intercourse by white male Americans in the United States. *SEXUAL BEHAVIOR IN THE HUMAN MALE by A. C. Kinsey, W. B. Pomeroy and C. E. Martin. Copyright 1948 by W. B. Saunders Company, Philadelphia, Pennsylvania.*

Percent

ONSET OF IMPOTENCE

Age

Chart showing the age of onset of impotence. The increasing percent of the total male population which is impotent at each age level is indicated.

feels that satisfaction for himself is sufficient to insure gratification for his partner. Some men do not even know that a woman's sexual sensation develops and culminates to a slower rhythm than their own. Also, there are many men who do not know that sexual pleasure comprises a great vista of total experience, which includes many kinds of activity, all within the bound of "normality." With no variety of stimulation or modification of sensory perception, the monotony of perfunctory sexual activity can imperil the most sound marriage. Actually, sex can be an art, a skill that can be acquired through learning and experience. If the natural faculty is not improved, the sexual activity after a time may suffer a decline in sensory and emotional gratification. The term "sexual activity" includes the

full and varied range of contact and function that result in sexual consummation, or coitus.

The sex act need not be restricted to immediate coitus, but rather should develop over such a period of time that will allow for the slower rhythm of the woman's sexual sensation to attain a sufficient degree of excitation to evoke emotional as well as physical responses. In order to reach this desirable goal, the complete sexual act includes progressive phases of activity: a preliminary phase, a period of bodily stimulation, the actual sexual union or orgasmic response, and the concluding phase, or aftermath.

The preliminary phase is actually an anticipation of the sex act that heightens the enjoyment

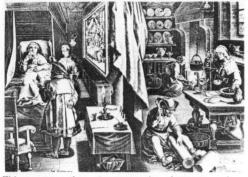

This seventeenth century engraving shows a number of persons engaged in the preparation of aids for treatment of syphilis. *Bettmann Archive.*

of sexual intercourse. Usually, the most effective stimulus during this preliminary phase is conversation, for in this early stage, the mind is more stirred than the body. This phase is marked by activity reminiscent of courtship—of approach and retreat, aggression and defense. If this preliminary stage of mental stimulation is adroitly performed, it will arouse in the mature man and woman a physical desire for mutual bodily contact.

The stimulation of the body is graduated in intensity, erotic sensibility increasing as the genital area is approached. The lightest touch can be the most effective touch. If the stimuli of the preceding phase have aroused the desired degree of excitement, the female genital organs will become expanded by an increased blood supply and the internal tissue will moisten the vagina with its lubricating secretions. Until this response is evident, intercourse generally should not be attempted.

If the woman is inexperienced—and it takes time for the development of a strongly sexual temperament—the importance of the bodily

stimulus before intercourse appears obvious. Thus, additional excitation may be necessary if the woman is to attain excitement equal to that of the man. The normally potent man has other limited means of equalizing matters. He can, as far as possible, deliberately suppress his consciousness of local stimuli; and he can learn, to a degree, to control or postpone the reflex of ejaculation, but this is difficult. With experience and practice, the woman can learn to accelerate or prolong her reactions in accord with those of her partner.

The accumulation of excitement necessary to attain orgasm is reached through rhythmic motion until the intensity of feeling reaches a peak. The stimulation of the woman during coitus is twofold, being both clitoral, for physiological pleasure, and vaginal for psychological pleasure. To attain this twofold stimulation, the man must know something of the anatomy of the female organs.

The sexual desire and pleasure of each partner greatly enhance the other. Because this is so, it has often been considered that ideally the act of sexual intercourse should terminate in simultaneous orgasms for the partners. There are circumstances that more often than not cause simultaneous orgasms to distract from rather than add to the pleasures of both, although, of course, if a couple find that they actually prefer to have simultaneous orgasms then they should strive for that goal. In such planning, the following should be considered. To give the fullest pleasure to one's sexual partner one must devote full attention to that partner at all times during the sexual act, most especially at the time of the orgasm. If one is caught up in his own orgasmic response, he cannot give full attention to his partner and if he concentrates on his own needs or tries to divide his attention, he fails both. Furthermore, men are ordinarily capable of only one orgasm during any one sexual experience while almost all women are capable of multiple

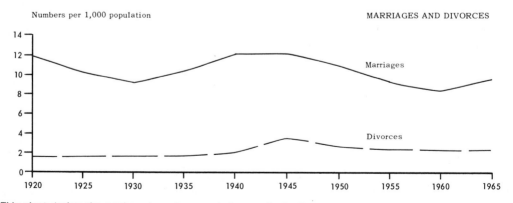

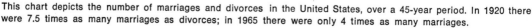

This chart depicts the number of marriages and divorces in the United States, over a 45-year period. In 1920 there were 7.5 times as many marriages as divorces; in 1965 there were only 4 times as many marriages.

orgasms and about one half of the women experience two or more orgasms during a sexual encounter. Thus, if the man has his orgasm at the same time as the woman has hers he may deprive her of the additional orgasms she may require if she is to be fully satisfied sexually. Most men not only lose the ability to continue the act of sexual intercourse after their orgasms but they also readily—for a while, at least—lose interest in any aspect of sex. And lastly, a physiological difference between men and women at the time of the orgasmic response should be considered. At the time of orgasm, the man's tendency is to plunge his penis as deeply as possible into the vagina and hold it there, to be followed perhaps by one or two deep, deliberate thrusts. The woman's tendency is to have the same stroking, plunging movements that led to the peak of her excitement to be continued during the orgasmic response. The incompatibility of these two movement patterns is easily recognized and the usual response for the couple is for them both to concentrate on the woman's pleasure until she is fully and completely satisfied and then both direct their attention to pleasing the man.

After the sexual experience, pleasurable feelings of relaxation and relief remain. This descending degree of pleasure forms the emotional basis for the concluding phase of sexual union. This last phase results in a release from the tension of mind and body. The sudden relaxation immediately after such intense demands on nerves and muscles necessarily results in a feeling of marked relaxation. When intercourse is carried out matter-of-factly, this relaxation is not so complete, because the tension was lower and the ebb of feeling more abrupt. Even though both partners are strongly inclined to sleep, the slower ebb of sexual feeling in the woman creates a need for emotional assurance from her mate that for him, too, the enjoyment endures. This emotional assurance may well be gratifying to both partners, but the emotional need is usu-

ally much more pronounced in the woman. A word, a touch, or an embrace will in most instances suffice for the emotional confirmation needed to prove that the total experience of sexual union was indeed mutual.

Position and action during coitus: During the act of sexual intercourse, there are many variations in the position and action of both partners. There is a certain amount of misunderstanding regarding this topic, as well as misconception as to what may be regarded as "normal." Sexual technique is of great practical importance as regards sexual pleasure itself, the prevention of physical disorder or injury, and the control of conception. With regard to conception, any position which facilitates orgasm in the man and retains the seminal fluid within the vagina also promotes the probability of conception. Any position which results in the ebbing of the semen away from the interior of the vagina diminishes chances of conception.

It is often assumed that there is only one "normal" position, that of the woman's lying on her back with the man above and facing her. The "normal" position is that which the couple finds mutually inoffensive and personally satisfactory.

The actual duration of intercourse varies widely among individuals and depends on the physical and emotional make-up of each person, although it generally takes the average man only from two to four minutes of sexual intercourse to have an orgasm while it takes the average woman about fourteen minutes. The frequency of intercourse varies from more than once a day to once a year, with an average of three times a week among the younger couples. Normal frequency cannot be determined, because there is a "normal" for each individual. The only criteria are physical exhaustion and fatigue. Hence, any frequency is regarded as normal as long as fatigue and discomfort do not result.

Among the erroneous ideas concerning sex is that the sexual act should always be initiated by the man. Opinions vary with individuals, but

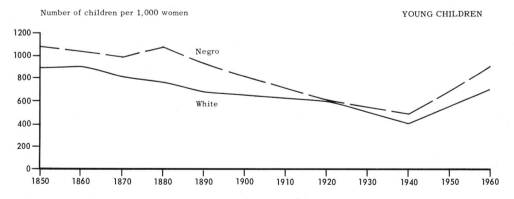

This chart shows the number of white children and Negro children under five years old, for every 1,000 women in the United States, aged 20-44 years old, during the period between the years 1850 and 1960.

it is not uncommon for the man to want and to enjoy having the sex act initiated by the woman rather than by himself. To expect the woman to be solely an inactive member in conjugation would be to inflict on her an unwarranted degree of submissiveness and passivity.

Sterility

Sterility or infertility is the term meaning inability to produce offspring. Often the term is confused with sexual impotence in the male, which is an entirely different condition associated with the inability to perform the sexual union. Sexual potency does not necessarily imply that the man is fertile, because sterility in man usually is the result of some defect in the number or the structure of the sperm cells. Until recently, male sterility was underestimated, and no attempts were made to ascertain the condition of the male in childless unions. A better understanding of human reproduction has led to more accurate diagnosis of sterility, and today the man, as well as the woman, undergoes careful examination before the final diagnosis is made.

It is not unusual that infertile unions result from a lack of understanding of the sexual cycle in women. The average woman is fertile only during a short period of each month, namely, during the time when the egg cell is in the Fallopian tube and still viable. The high peak of fertility, then, occurs approximately twelve to 16 days after the beginning of the last menstrual period in a woman with a 28-day menstrual cycle. In any event, the period of ovulation may be difficult to predict with certainty, since the menstrual cycle may vary in length, as well as in time of ovulation, among individuals. However, it is possible for the woman to ascertain with a fair degree of accuracy the time of maximum fertility. This is done by recording her body temperature every morning (rectal temperature is thought to be a more accurate method than oral recording). To maintain such a chart accurately, fairly even habits must be maintained, as a few drinks the night before, overstrain, fatigue, and many other factors will cause the temperature to vary. Ordinarily, the temperature of the body is constant from day to day if a constant regime of daily habits is maintained, and at the time of ovulation there is a sharp but transient rise in body temperature. At this time the egg has been ejected from the ovary and descends gradually into the Fallopian tube; this represents the time of maximum fertility.

The egg is viable for only one or two days at the most and soon loses its fertility. The change in body temperature is helpful in determining the best time of the month to attain impregnation. Similarly, the spermatozoa are viable in the

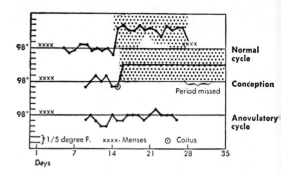

Top chart shows temperature elevation from ovulation to menstruation in normal menstrual cycle. The second chart shows continued elevation which permits an easy diagnosis of probable pregnancy. Bottom chart is a case where no temperature rise indicates no ovulation. *From WHAT'S NEW, Copyright 1946, Abbott Laboratories, North Chicago, Illinois.*

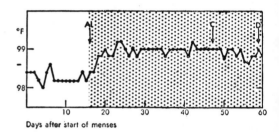

Pregnancy diagnosed by continued elevation of waking temperature. Artificial insemination (AI) was followed by a negative (C) and then positive (D) pregnancy test. *From WHAT'S NEW, Copyright 1946, Abbott Laboratories, North Chicago, Illinois.*

genital tract for only a short period of time, perhaps no more than two days. Thus, any union that precedes or follows the time of ovulation by more than two days will probably be unsuccessful.

Theoretically, the normal woman *can* conceive at any time during the month. However, in order to ascertain the most *fertile* period, she can construct a graph, plotting days on the horizontal scale and the temperature on the vertical. After she has plotted her daily temperatures for three or four months, she will be able to predict within fairly accurate limits when ovulation occurs. Until conception occurs, it may be desirable to confine sexual union to those periods of the month when the woman is most fertile. Recent research findings have shown that if a woman is to ovulate a second time during a monthly cycle or is to ovulate at a time other than at the expected 14th day of the cycle, the ovulation is most likely to occur during the peak of sexual excitement, even though that peak might be during the menstrual flow.

Fertility is a relative manifestation that varies greatly from one individual to another. In many instances, the male may prove infertile with one woman but not with another. Similarly, the woman may be fertile, depending on the male. As a result of this difference, fertility must be regarded as a reflection of the reproductive capacity of the couple and not of the individual.

Apart from these considerations, infertility in women may be caused by a variety of conditions. Pelvic diseases and infections may be conducive to infertility. Since the discovery of antibiotic drugs, however, most infections can usually be controlled effectively, thus preventing permanent damage.

In addition to infections, the organs of reproduction in the female are susceptible to other types of disease that may lead to sterility. Inflammation of the genital organs is often responsible for the production of mucus that is considered toxic, or poisonous to spermatozoa. In addition to this toxicity, the mucus constitutes a mechanical obstacle in the passage of the male germ cells into the uterus. The orifice of the cervix may become obstructed by mucus.

In the absence of inflammation or mechanical obstruction of the genital passage, infertility may be ascribed to endocrine disturbances. The endocrine system plays an important role in the sexual cycle of the female, and any disturbance of the endocrine balance may lead to abnormalities in reproductive function. Endocrine disturbances may affect reproduction at any one of the various stages from the maturation of the egg to implantation in the womb. The egg matures in the ovaries as a result of stimulus by hormones produced by the pituitary gland and by the ovaries. At various stages, the improper functioning of the endocrine system may lead to sterility by affecting the maturation of the egg, or by rendering it infertile after it has matured. Even if the egg has been fertilized, the endocrine system still exerts control over the growth of the lining of the uterus and either facilitates or inhibits implantation of the fertilized egg. Many conditions of endocrine imbalance may be modified by proper hormone therapy prescribed by the physician.

Infertility can also result from malformations of the organs of reproduction which are present at birth. An undeveloped uterus can cause infertility, and in some patients the uterus may be absent at birth, in which case conception is impossible.

An important factor in infertility, although not too well understood, is diet. Nutritional deficiencies may elicit conditions that affect the entire organism, and thus also affect the reproductive system. The infertile patient undergoing treatment is advised by the physician to eat well, but moderately, and to supplement meals with vitamin preparations. Vitamin E, which is present in large amounts in wheat germ, is usually recommended as an important supplement. The weight of the patient is also important. An overweight condition is generally as unhealthy as being underweight; both overweight and underweight may be controlled by an adequate diet.

In barren unions there is always the possibility that the man may be sterile. Examination of both husband and wife is necessary to determine which partner is sterile. The husband is given a physical examination and a specimen of semen is analyzed. A male may be sexually potent and may produce an adequate volume of ejaculate, but may nevertheless be sterile. In-

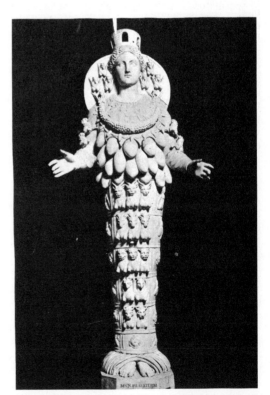

Photograph of a statue of Diana of Ephesus who was known as the Goddess of Fertility. All things were nurtured from her breasts. *Bettmann Archive.*

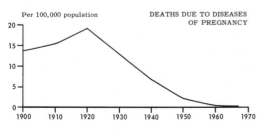

Per 100,000 population   DEATHS DUE TO DISEASES OF PREGNANCY

Recent years have seen. a dramatic decrease, in the United States, in deaths due. to disorders of pregnancy, as shown by this chart covering 1900-1966.

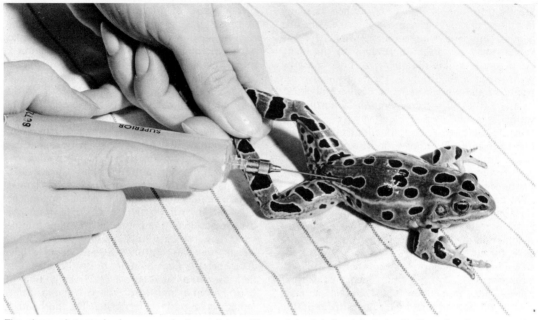

The above photograph shows a male leopard frog (*Rana pipiens*) being injected with the urine from a woman suspected of being pregnant. Within about 12 hours after injection, the urine of the frog is inspected for sperm. If sperm are present in the frog's urine, the test is positive for pregnancy. *Courtesy Hermann Hospital, Houston.*

fertility in this case may be the result of absence of spermatozoa in the ejaculate or the presence of an insufficient number of germ cells. In order for the sperm to be fertile, several conditions must be fulfilled. The number of cells is only one condition. Below a certain quantity, the sperm may be malformed or not sufficiently active to produce conception. The volume of the ejaculate is also important. There are variations in volume not only among different individuals but in the same individual. The volume of ejaculate is usually larger after a period of sexual abstinence.

The semen may be inadequate to produce conception if there are a large number of abnormal cells in proportion to normal ones. The average sperm cell is composed of a head and a relatively long thin tail. The movements of the tail are whiplike and serve as a means of propulsion. The head constitutes the major portion of the cell and also contains the germ plasm. Examination of semen often reveals abnormal cell forms, such as a double-headed cell, a split tail, or a shortened tail. The proportion of abnormal forms to normal spermatozoa in the semen constitutes an important factor in sterility.

Microscopic examination of the semen reveals the form and the motility of the cells. Spermatozoa are capable of swimming long distances and at relatively high speeds. The propulsion of the cells can be estimated when observed under the microscope. Motility becomes an important factor when the cells are in the vagina, where

they swim toward the uterus. Only those cells endowed with good capacity for self-propulsion can bring about fertilization.

The only decisive proof of fertility in the male is, of course, the production of offspring. However, semen examination is of great diagnostic value.

When consultation with a physician becomes necessary to determine the cause of sterility, a frank discussion is necessary in order to facilitate the diagnosis. To conceal pertinent facts defeats the purpose, because an incomplete history may be misleading to the physician.

The treatment depends upon the underlying cause which the physician must determine by examination and observation. In some cases, the cause of sterility is readily apparent, in others obscure. Supposedly sterile couples have produced offspring sometimes after many years of barren marriage. In other instances of apparent sterility of several years duration, conception has been successful after the couple have received advice from the physician to promote impregnation during the fertile period of the month by ascertaining the time of ovulation. The fertile period varies greatly, depending on the length of the menstrual cycle. Ordinarily, the days immediately before menstruation are regarded as relatively nonfertile periods of the month and intercourse at this time has a smaller chance of resulting in conception.

In instances in which the male produces healthy spermatozoa that fail to reach the uterus

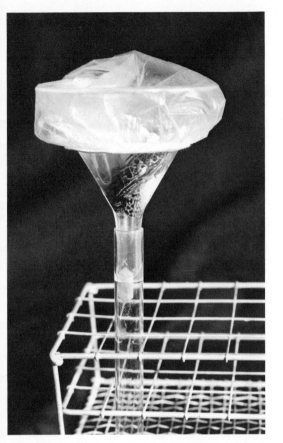

This picture shows the frog imprisoned in a funnel which is attached to a test tube. The urine of the frog is collected in the bottom of the test tube.

as a result of some abnormality in the female, *artificial insemination* may be employed. This is a highly specialized medical procedure in which conception has been attained on many occasions. The offspring are healthy and normal in all respects, just as often as in the more usual method of conception. Sperm from a donor may be used if the husband's sperm is absent or inadequate.

Birth control

There are instances in which pregnancy may constitute a serious threat to the woman's health. Contraceptive measures or sterilization may be recommended in such conditions. Contraceptive measures prevent pregnancy by creating a mechanical barrier that prevents spermatozoa from entering the uterus, or by creating an unfavorable chemical medium in which the sperm cannot survive and fertilize the ovum.

Many women, usually for religious reasons, cannot use chemical or mechanical measures to prevent conception. These women may use what is called the rhythm method of contraception. This method is based on the normal cyclic changes in the reproductive organs which result in periods of fertility and infertility. During the fertile periods, intercourse is avoided. The basal body temperature (temperature during absolute rest) is a fairly accurate indicator of the fertile period. The woman can prepare a daily temperature curve by taking her temperature orally immediately upon awakening each morning and recording it promptly. The typical temperature graph will highlight the fertile period. A physician can instruct the woman further and inform her where to obtain suitable graph paper and basal thermometers for easy reading.

The most common type of mechanical barrier is the rubber diaphragm which is inserted into the vagina to completely occlude the orifice of the cervix, thus obstructing the migration of spermatozoa upward into the Fallopian tubes. Before the diaphragm is inserted, a specified amount of one of the chemical agents should be deposited on its inner surface. A diaphragm should be obtained from a physician, who will fit it to the individual woman.

Another means of mechanical obstruction to conception is the condom. This rubber device surrounds the penis and contains the sperm after ejaculation, thus preventing the sperm from coming into contact with the cervix and possibly proceeding to fertilize the ovum.

Chemical or spermicidal contraceptives consist of jellies or creams which provide partial obstruction and in addition contain nontoxic chemical agents that immobilize sperm at relatively low concentrations. Creams and jellies are inserted high into the vagina with an applicator provided in the package. Capsules or suppositories are placed in the vagina about 15 minutes before coitus to allow sufficient time for them to melt, spread, and release their active ingredients. Regardless of the measure employed, douches should not be taken within eight hours after intercourse.

A relatively new means for preventing conception is the intrauterine device (IUD), small plastic or stainless steel devices which come in a variety of shapes. When placed in the uterus by a physician, the IUD is a very effective method of birth control. Although the reason for its effectiveness is not clear, some physicians believe that the presence of the device in the uterus so increases the speed of passage that the ovum cannot become implanted on the uterine wall. The intrauterine device is effective as soon as it is fitted. When further pregnancies are desired, it is removed and fertility is restored.

The contraceptive method which has probably received more widespread publicity than any other is "the pill." The oral contraceptive, when taken as directed for approximately three fourths of each menstrual cycle, is virtually 100 per cent effective against pregnancy.

The oral contraceptives work by suppressing ovulation. They are administered as follows: Beginning on the fifth day after the beginning of the menstrual cycle, one pill is taken each day for 20 or 21 days (depending on the brand taken). The pills are then stopped to allow menstruation to occur. On the fifth day after the menstrual flow begins, the cycle of pills begins anew.

There are two types of oral contraceptives. In the first type, all of the pills contain a combination of estrogen and a particular steroid. In the second type, called the sequential type, the first 14 or 16 pills contain estrogen alone; the pills taken for the remainder of the cycle contain estrogen plus a progestin. The use of the estrogen alone at first and then in combination with a progestin is believed to be a more physiological approach and to more closely simulate the cyclic secretion of these steriods by the ovaries.

The pills containing estrogen and progestogen combined appear to have an advantage over the sequential group in that they also create a barrier to the sperm by creating a "hostile" cervical mucus. In addition, the endometrium resists implantation of the fertilized egg. Thus, if a woman forgets one of the combined preparations for one day, pregnancy would not occur because of the persistent cervical and endometrial deterrents. However, skipping the sequential pill for one day may result in pregnancy.

There are also a few other situations in which the pill may not be effective. When shifting from the combined to the sequential drugs or when first starting the sequential drugs, mechanical contraception should also be practiced for the first month to prevent pregnancy. Also, pregnancy is possible during the first eight days of the *first* cycle during which the combined drugs are taken.

Occasionally, undesirable side effects may occur when a woman first takes the oral contraceptive. These include nausea and vomiting, increase in breast tenderness and engorgement, accentuation of acne, fluid retention, weight gain, increased vaginal discharge, and breakthrough bleeding. These symptoms usually disappear within the first three cycles. If not, they should be reported to the physician. If at the end of the first cycle the menses do not occur when expected, medication should be resumed on the seventh day after termination of the previous 20-day course.

Generally, women suffering from thrombophlebitis, carcinoma of the breast or genital tract, hepatic disease, cardiac dysfunction, or renal disease should not use oral contraceptives. Some interesting therapeutic benefits said to result from use of these compounds include im-

proved texture of the skin in patients with acne and the elimination of dysmenorrhea (painful menstruation).

Impotence

The sexual adaptation upon which a successful conjugal life depends can be impaired by both physical and emotional aberrations. Among the most frequent disorders affecting marriage are impotence in the male and frigidity in the female.

Impotence is characterized by incomplete erection of the penis. Temporary impotence is common following the completion of intercourse. Failure to maintain erection of the penis throughout intercourse may be regarded as *emotional* impotence. The man finds that erection is normal until the actual time of insertion; then erection is lost, and intercourse becomes impossible.

Rapid response and brief intercourse on the part of the man do not indicate impotence. On occasion, as a result of prolonged continence or excessive excitation, orgasm may be attained immediately after penetration of the penis, or actually even before penetration. This is not an unusual reaction and may well be a manifestation of a sexually potent male. However, when this condition persists and premature ejaculation becomes a regular pattern, there is the possibility of illness or at least a problem. In this event, the man should seek medical advice to attempt to correct the condition.

The age of the man is, of course, an important factor in impotence. Some men past the age of 55 begin to lose erotic interest and capacity for erection. However, the variations are great; many men remain sexually active until advanced years. Actually, there is little reason for a man's sexual ability to decrease any more rapidly or to a greater degree than the other physical capabilities. When such is the case, emotional factors may well be the cause of the loss.

In instances where surgical removal of the

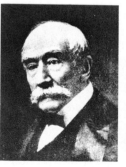

EMMET, Thomas Addis (1828-1919) American gynecologic surgeon. Emmett made early investigations into the causes of sterility in women. He developed a method of vaginal cystotomy (an incision of the bladder through the vagina to afford complete drainage of the bladder). He also devised an operation to repair lacerations of the cervix which occur in childbirth. The latter operation was useful in avoiding complications from subsequent pregnancies and labor.

gonads becomes necessary, impotence is often thought to be an inevitable consequence. This is not true, because removal of the testicles after puberty does not end the capacity for erection and does not necessarily diminish sexual desire.

Frigidity

True frigidity may be the result of *dyspareunia*, which signifies difficult or painful sexual intercourse. This condition usually involves spasm of the muscles surrounding the vagina (vaginismus) and may be caused simply by a lack of adequate lubrication.

Pseudo, or false, frigidity may have many causes. In many instances, the woman's early training and ethical background prohibit the understanding and enjoyment of the sex act. Early impressions that sex is "nasty and shameful" or that pregnancy is an ordeal just short of martyrdom are naturally prohibitive. So also can a noticeable lack of affection between the woman's parents affect the woman's own attitude toward marriage and, therefore, her capacity for response. The husband, too, can hinder her response, by persistent premature ejaculation, by remaining clumsy, by clinging to unsavory personal habits, and by sheer ignorance of sexual technique, and by a selfish lack of concern for the wife's needs.

Fear of pregnancy can deeply affect the woman's response to sexual activity. Frigidity may occur soon after a baby is born, especially if the labor was difficult and prolonged, or if the husband insists on having sexual intercourse before the woman has healed properly.

Women who have too much self-love, especially when they marry men who are attracted by their immaturity and "little girl" attitudes, find sexual gratification difficult. Such women unconsciously seek paternal love, for they have never reached emotional maturity.

The problem of conflicting desires—even transitory ones in which the woman feels only a normal, passing sexual attraction towards men other than her husband—may engender feelings of guilt which render her frigid. Misunderstandings, quarreling, and poor health may also cause frigidity. Some women have strong unacknowledged homosexual impulses and cannot fully respond to men, since sex becomes more or less a competition, if not wholly repugnant. In women with masculine temperaments and in whom there are no impulses toward career or other creative activity, sublimation of the masculine tendencies may be replaced by aggression. They replace feminine gratification in favor of the masculinity they unconsciously imitate.

Hypo and hypersexuality

A disproportionate desire for sexual activity may exist which renders an individual either "undersexed" or "oversexed." Usually, these conditions result from emotional factors. Because of emotional disturbances, the so-called

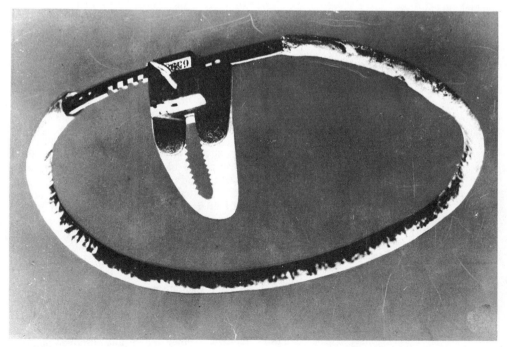

In the middle ages the *chastity belt* was sometimes employed to protect the woman's virtue. *Bettmann Archive.*

"undersexed" individual becomes inhibited concerning genital activity, so that the desire for sexual activity is diminished. Conversely, the "oversexed" individual suffers from mental upsets that result in heightened sexual energy. In this opposite extreme, the "oversexed" persons seek to express through genital activity the sexuality they strive to satisfy. Obviously, in many instances, the disturbances of sexuality are not sufficiently pronounced to have more than a superficial and unrecognized effect on the sexual life of the individual. Consequently, many persons suffering from a lack of sexual capacity or an exaggerated capacity are never consciously aware of being exceptional. Thus, the line of division between "normal," "oversexed," and "undersexed" is not a clear-cut boundary. However, psychological disturbances may result in pathological degrees of sexual activity.

Nymphomania

A complete inability to attain sexual gratification in women sometimes results in the pathological condition known as *nymphomania*. This is expressed in an insatiable desire for sexual orgasm. In some instances, unrecognized homosexual tendencies may result in the unconscious effort of the woman to "prove" her femininity by excessive sexual activity. With others, nymphomania may be the result of frigidity, or of only occasional experience of orgasm. Most often, however, nymphomania appears to be a result of marked feelings of insecurity or inadequacy which the woman attempts to resolve— but unsuccessfully—by excessive sexual acts. The fact that intercourse excites, but does not satisfy, creates the desire for renewed and increased attempts. Since the underlying cause of this disorder is thought to be primarily emotional, psychotherapy is probably the only treatment that can bring appreciable help in correcting the condition.

Satyriasis

The pathological condition in the male which corresponds to nymphomania in the female is *satyriasis,* or "Don Juanism." Among the underlying causes may be latent homosexual tendencies. The unconsciously homosexual male is attracted to women, but receives little or no satisfaction from his relations with them. Therefore, he continues to seek gratification by increased sexual activity. Or he may be attempting to prove his masculinity to himself and the world. The "Don Juan" usually is emotionally immature; he is little interested in the individual woman, but only in his conquests, and he constantly seeks new ones. The person so affected may give the impression of being "oversexed," when more accurately he is "undersexed"; that is, he lacks the ability to achieve complete sexual gratification. The person suffering from satyriasis is usually one who doubts his masculinity and questions that he is a worthwhile person.

Homosexuality

Sexual behavior may be studied in terms of both the aim, i.e., the type of activity desired, and the object, or person toward whom the desires are directed. The term homosexual refers only to the *object.* Therefore, by definition, any kind of sexual activity of any type whatsoever with a person of the *same sex* is homosexual. Conversely, sexual activity of whatever sort with a person of the opposite sex is *not* homosexual, even though it may or may not be considered "normal."

Human beings have organically bisexual dispositions. In the well-balanced individual, the various components are united to form a harmonious whole. Normally, the feminine components predominate in the female and the male components predominate in the male. Puberty is the period of sexual decision. During preadolescence and early adolescence in the female, these bisexual tendencies may become homosexual tendencies as the result of various emotional factors, such as fear of the opposite sex, identification with the father, and others. In the male, homosexuality may be caused by the same factors, only the process of identification is reversed.

This inclination to direct the sexual impulse toward persons of the same sex may be predominant but unrecognized by the individual. Many women, unaware of latent homosexual tendencies, may marry and discover that sexual relations are unsatisfactory or even untenable.

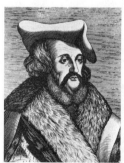

FRACASTORO, Girolamo (1483-1553) Italian pathologist and author of a famous medical poem which included all the knowledge of syphilis at that time. He is credited with giving the disease its name. He recognized the origin of the disease and suggested mercury compounds as treatment. He made many contributions to the knowledge of infectious diseases, and suggested a germ theory of infection. He gave the first accurate account of typhus and is called the founder of scientific epidemiology.

The complementary qualities of male and female are most fully realized in normal heterosexuality. This need for completion of one individual by another of the opposite sex is the basic emotional factor in sex in all major cultures. The sexual act combines the two incomplete parts to form the complete whole.

It is of interest to know that the average homosexual, whether male or female, cannot be identified as homosexual by physical appearance. Only 15 percent of males have physical characteristics that will correctly identify them as homosexual and only 5 percent of the female homosexuals (lesbians) can be so identified.

Sex hygiene

Sexual function, like any other bodily function, may become faulty through poor living habits that result in impaired physical and mental health. Sex hygiene is often taken to mean prevention of venereal disease, but actually the laws of health pertaining to sex include all the rules that promote general bodily and mental well being.

Many physical factors affect the sexual efficiency and vigor of both partners. Sexual activity is regarded as healthy and normal so long as extreme fatigue and discomfort do not result. The ill effects of sexual abuse are magnified when accompanied by other excesses, such as an overindulgence in alcohol. Alcohol taken in small quantities may give the impression of being a sexual stimulant. In large quantities, it inhibits the genital functions while at the same time it removes inhibitions, which may allow freer sexual indulgence. Habitual overindulgence in alcohol is deleterious to the sexual functions. The acute manifestations may occur in the form of physical debilitation and generalized bodily tension.

Chronic irritation of the sexual organs should not be ignored, but should be regarded as a possible symptom of disease. Acute genital in-

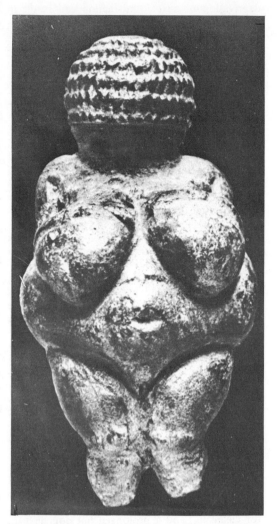

Photograph of a stone age idol, the *Venus of Willendorf*, believed to be the oldest statue of a human figure in existence. *Bettmann Archive.*

Similarly, a homosexual male may marry, beget children, and never realize that he is actually homosexually inclined. This situation may result in intense suffering from the conflict between the homosexual desires and the quasi-sexual attraction that still exists for his wife. The emotional factors are complex and numerous. Sometimes psychiatric help can engender normal heterosexuality, but this is not always successful. Correction or prevention of homosexuality is a complex problem and one for which medical science has only a partial answer.

Masculinity and femininity are fundamental qualities, expressed by how completely the man or woman accepts or rejects the respective sexual function. Masculinity and femininity are not direct opposites, for there are both male and female components in every normal personality.

CZERNY, Vincenz (1842-1916), German surgeon. He is best known for being the first to remove completely the uterus through the vagina (vaginal hysterectomy). This method avoids cutting the abdominal wall. He performed this operation in 1879. Czerny introduced the method of removing uterine fibroids (connective tissue tumors) through the vagina. His name is associated with several other operations such as the radical repair of an inguinal hernia.

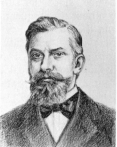

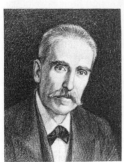

WAGNER von JAUREGG, Julius (1857-1940) A German physician who developed a nonspecific treatment of late syphilis now called fever therapy or the *Wagner von Jauregg treatment*. The method involves artificially raising the patient's body temperature. Von Jauregg did this by infecting the patient with malaria. In the treatment of neurosyphilis and paralytic dementia by this method, he got good results. For his work he received the Nobel prize in 1927.

flammation, as a rule, will preclude sexual intercourse, because pain may result. However, if coitus is attempted, the experience of any persistent or acute physical pain during intercourse indicates the need for medical attention. Normal coitus should not be painful, and if such pain persists, some pathological condition may be present.

There are many superstitions and taboos associated with menstruation, particularly with regard to intercourse. No physical harm is incurred by sexual intercourse during menstruation, and the woman's desire for intercourse may actually be heightened during the menstrual period.

The problem of intercourse during pregnancy is much more involved than during menstruation. Coitus is not considered harmful during the early months of a normal uneventful pregnancy except possibly during the days corresponding to the monthly bleeding phase of the menstrual cycle. Intercourse should not be attempted during the last six weeks before delivery, or at any time during pregnancy if it is followed by bleeding. However, each individual should be guided by the advice of her attending physician. Pregnancy influences sexual desire in diverse ways, according to the temperament, the constitution, and the stage of gestation. The pregnant woman may desire coitus and achieve satisfaction during pregnancy to an increased degree, since the subconscious "pregnophobia" is absent. Consequently, if the woman is healthy and the uterus shows no tendency to premature function, if necessary care is exercised, and if careful cleanliness is observed, the risk in coitus is slight. In the event of discomfort during intercourse, or the appearance of an infection of the female organs, the practice should be discontinued. According to some authorities, vaginal douching should be omitted during pregnancy, unless specifically advised by the physician.

Sexual activity has a healthy influence on both mind and body, and in many people continued deprivation of sexual satisfaction can result in mental and emotional conflicts that lead to neurotic behavior and unhappiness.

A rational means of preserving marital sympathy and interest is to maintain that no form of sexual activity be employed that is not mutually enjoyable to both the man and the woman.

Personal cleanliness influences both the emotional and bodily functions of sex. In addition to the general attention to physical cleanliness, frequent and adequate cleansing of the genital organs is of paramount importance to prevent irritation by removing glandular secretions and decaying organic material. Especially to avoid inflammation, the man should employ regular and thorough cleansing of the glans. Circumcision, or surgical removal of the foreskin, facilitates cleanliness and is an effective prophylactic against the accumulation of glandular secretion as well as possible infection.

Feminine hygiene is particularly important, because the folds and interstices of the interval genitalia are somewhat inaccessible, and the glandular secretions are adhesive. The majority of women have fixed ideas concerning the necessity for routine vaginal douches. Some authorities maintain that, in the absence of definite disease, there is no necessity for routine douching and that it decreases the natural secretions of the vagina. However, many women find regular douching indispensible for bodily cleanliness. A properly prepared and administered douche without irritating chemicals is harmless and almost universally used as a personal health measure. In order to avoid contamination and infection, douches should never be administered under pressure. Two types of douches are usually recommended: a warm douche solution for cleansing, and a prolonged hot douche with ordinary tap water to provide heat to the pelvic organs. The douche solution should usually be slightly acidic to promote the natural acidity of the vagina. The douche should be taken lying down with the knees drawn up and the hips raised slightly. No dogmatic rules can be given regarding the type or solution needed, as the physician alone can best prescribe the most desirable technique for the individual. Although many women are reluctant to use a douche during menstruation, if warm water is used it is not harmful.

Many women use an alkaline douche before coitus in the hope of neutralizing the usual acid condition of the vagina and thus enhancing the possibility of impregnation. The acid environment of the vagina is threatening to the vitality and life of sperm and neutralizing the area by douching with an alkaline solution is thought to enable the woman to conceive, especially if the man has a low sperm count or if his sperm are subnormally active.

Sex knowledge, like all knowledge, should be

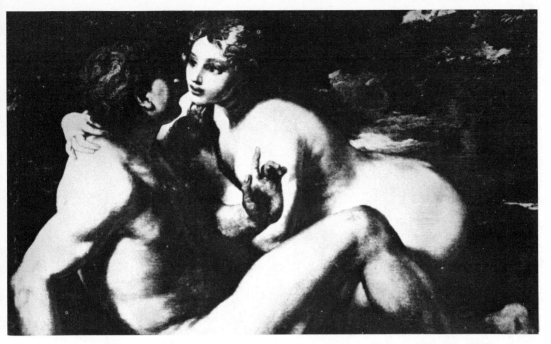

Adam and Eve, the biblical parents of man, as portrayed by Luca Giordano. *Bettmann Archive.*

acquired from an authoritative source. Information from books alone can often be misleading. In questions pertaining to personal bodily cleanliness, to possible malformations and dysfunctions, to the many reasons for lack of attainment of sexual adjustment, there is no better source than the physician.

The role of the physician as counselor in matters of marriage has become prominent in recent years and many people seek advice from their doctors before marriage. A premarital physical examination is now required by law in many states. This examination is desirable and should be complete. Special attention should be paid to the genital organs, which as a rule are not examined unless there is some specific complaint. A pelvic examination of the woman will reveal abnormalities that may be easily corrected

PAWLIK, Karel J. (1849-1914) Czechoslovakian surgeon and gynecologist. Pawlik described several anatomical landmarks of the female pelvis. *Pawlik's folds* are the anterior columns of the vagina which form the lateral boundaries of *Pawlik's triangle* and serve as landmarks in locating the opening of the ureters. In 1889 he performed a successful cystectomy (removal of the bladder). A grasping of the unborn child through the mother's abdomen to determine the child's location is called *Pawlik's grip*.

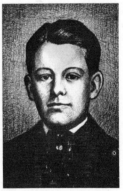

DÖDERLEIN, Albert Siegmund Gustav (1860-1941) German obstetrician. Döderlein is best known for his classic study of vaginal secretions in relation to puerperal fever. He demonstrated that an organism, now called *Döderlein's bacillus* and once thought to be of pathological importance, was actually a normal inhabitant of the vagina. Puerperal fever is now known to have no specific etiology. Several organisms are usually found.

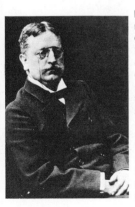

before marriage. The young couple, enlightened concerning the elements of sex physiology, will have a much better chance of achieving a happy marriage than the couple that must discover all the facets of marriage by experimentation. A frank discussion of the facts with the physician helps to dispel erroneous concepts which young people frequently obtain from unauthoritative sources. Moreover, the psychological effect of the premarital conference is of great value in the eradication of any stigma attached to sex. Such stigmata frequently exist in young people whose knowledge of sex and its relationship to marriage is based upon knowledge without understanding, or upon some unfortunate experi-

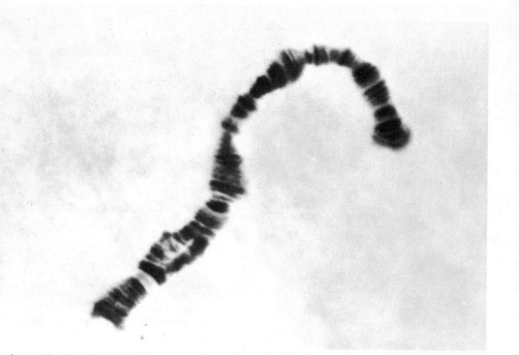

Photomicrograph of a single chromosome from the salivary gland of the small fly *Chironomus*, magnified several thousand times. Because of the large chromosomes, this animal has great value in experimental genetics.

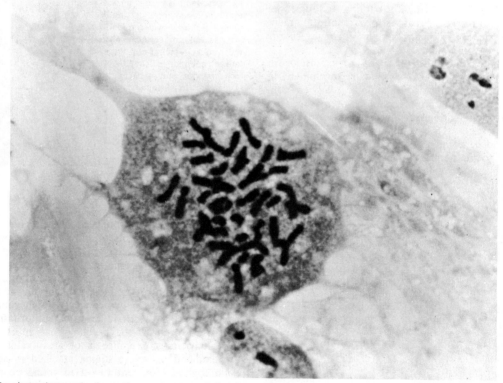

This photomicrograph shows the appearance of the chromosomes in one cell derived from a fetal human spleen as they appear at one stage in the life of the cell. Special staining techniques contribute to their visibility. *Courtesy of Dr. T. C. Hsu, The University of Texas M. D. Anderson Hospital and Tumor Institute.*

ence that they or persons close to them may have suffered. Proper psychological alignment to the true nature of this subject is most essential before the marriage occurs, in order to prevent the carrying-over of these deep-seated false impressions and the identification of them with the person's own married life. Although repeated visits to a physician, or perhaps to a psychiatrist, may be necessary in some cases, the ultimate value to the married couple will more than justify them.

16 THE BREAST

WHAT IT IS AND DOES

The breasts are modified skin glands, and are referred to as the *mammary glands*. They lie in the outermost layer of connective tissue, called the *fascia*. In men, the breasts remain undeveloped and without specific use. In women, however, they are active, functioning parts of the body throughout much of life. On a well-developed, well-nourished woman who has not borne a child, the breasts may extend from the second or third rib to the sixth or seventh rib, and from the outer border of the breastbone *(sternum)* to the folds of the armpit. A woman who has borne children normally has somewhat larger breasts.

The size and shape of the breasts in different individuals varies from round to conical. The consistency is usually firm and elastic, but varies a great deal, depending upon the presence and amount of fatty tissue. Rarely are the two breasts equal in size; the left is usually larger. Needless to say, there is a great divergence in breast sizes among individual women. The average breast in a woman who has not borne a child ranges from four to six inches in diameter and weighs between two and one half ounces to one half pound, or more. These figures depend to a great extent upon age, climatic conditions, race, and the general health of the individual woman.

The skin of the breasts is covered with tiny soft hairs associated with sebaceous glands and sweat glands like those found on the rest of the body. This skin is thin, and often superficial veins may be seen through it. The skin of the breast is elastic and flexible, despite the fact that it adheres to the fatty layer beneath it.

At the tip of each breast in both men and women is a projection called the nipple, surrounded by a pigmented area (the *areola*), which is about one and one half inches in diameter. The color varies considerably, depending upon the complexion of the woman. In childless women, it is usually reddish. The areola enlarges and the color deepens during pregnancy, becoming almost black in true brunettes. After the milk-producing period terminates, the color fades.

There are a number of superficial eminences erratically arranged on the surface of the areola. These are formed by large fat-producing (*sebaceous*) glands and undeveloped milk glands.

The *nipples* are not in the exact middle of the breasts, but slightly to the side. The skin is wrinkled and the same color as the areola. They are usually round or cone-shaped, and the tip contains the tiny depressions which are really the openings of the milk ducts. There are no hairs or sweat glands present, but many sebaceous glands are evident. The size of the nipple is usually directly proportionate to the size of the breast proper, but large nipples may be found on small breasts and vice versa.

In the deeper layers of the nipples, circular muscle fibers (as well as others) help to empty the breast of milk. When they contract, the nipple becomes harder, narrower, and more erect.

The breasts are composed primarily of a round, flattened mass of glandular tissue called

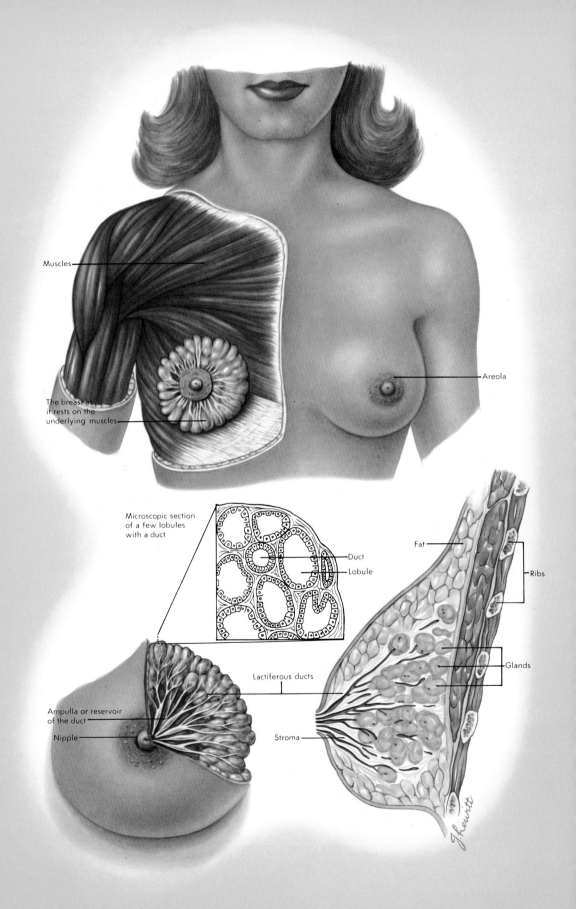

Muscles

The breast as
it rests on the
underlying muscles

Areola

Microscopic section
of a few lobules
with a duct

Duct

Lobule

Fat

Ribs

Glands

Lactiferous ducts

Ampulla or reservoir
of the duct

Nipple

Stroma

J Hewitt

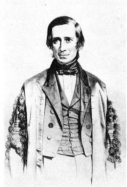

PAGET, James (1814-1899) English surgeon. Well known for his description in 1874 of carcinoma simplex, a condition now known as *Paget's disease of the nipple*. This affliction is now recognized as a breast carcinoma of ductal origin with metastases to the skin of the nipple, causing dermatitis. Osteitis deformans, a disease of the bone accompanied by deformity, is also frequently referred to as *Paget's disease,* in his honor.

the *corpus mammae*. This tissue is whitish or reddish-white in color and is thickest under the nipple and thinnest at the edges. The corpus mammae is a complicated structure consisting of 15 or 20 separate and distinct *lobes*, which are separated by varying amounts of fat. The lobes vary in size and shape but generally are pyramidal. They are arranged in a pattern which resembles a wagon wheel, with the nipple as the hub.

Each lobe contains a single milk duct (*lactiferous duct*) which opens into a tiny depression on the tip of the nipple. The ducts are side by side in the nipple and close to each other. At the base of the nipple (the part closest to the breast proper), they branch off in different directions. At this point they are large enough to be seen by the unaided eye. Underneath the areola, the ducts become even larger and form a reservoir (*ampulla*) called the *lactiferous sinus*, in which the secretions of the breast may accumulate for a short period of time. The ducts continue past this widening and gradually decrease in size, as they divide into smaller and smaller branches. They do not communicate with each other at any point on their course, although two or more may have the same opening in the nipple.

Each of the small branches of the ducts terminates in a tiny round or tubular sac-like structure, the *alveolus*. Several of these alveoli open into one portion of the duct and are held together with connective tissue, forming a lobule. The lobule is lined with specialized cells from which the milk is secreted. The small blood vessels (*capillaries*) which supply the area allow blood serum to escape from them. This serum is absorbed by the specialized cells, which assimilate certain materials from the serum. From these materials, milk is synthesized within the cells and then emptied into the lactiferous duct. The lobules whose ducts merge with one excretory duct constitute a lobe.

These various tissues—the lobes, lobules, and alveoli—are covered entirely by a thin, delicate membrane of connective tissue. The mammary gland in its entirety is sheathed in a fatty layer of tissue, the *adipose capsule*. This fat fills in the spaces or defects made by the lack of uniformity in the size and shape of the lobules, thereby giving the breast its smooth outline. The amount of fat determines the size of the breast. Much more of this fat is found in breasts of women who have borne many children than in those who are without children. During the milk-producing period following pregnancy and in thin, emaciated women, the lobules become more obvious as the fat is absorbed. Immediately under the nipple and the areola there is a dearth of adipose tissue. The nipple can be moved freely because of the loose connective tissue. For the same reason, the ducts and sinuses can expand more freely to allow the excretion of milk.

The connective tissues (*stroma*) form the foundation or framework of the breast. The layer directly beneath the breast (*ligaments of Cooper*) sends strands into the breast itself, thus causing the firm consistency of the organ. The deep layer of connective tissue sends strands in the opposite direction, directly into the covering of the chest muscles. The connection is a loose one, so that the breast moves freely over the chest wall.

The male breast until the age of puberty develops in the same manner as does the female breast. After this time the breast of a man grows slowly and is fully developed at approximately 20 years of age. The nipple is small in comparison to the female's, but both it and the areola are pigmented.

The first significant changes in the female breast usually occur when the girl is 11 to 13 years of age. The activities of the gland are apparently related to changes in the reproductive system. If no function of the ovaries has been established, the breasts remain underdeveloped. During puberty, the child's breasts become more prominent, and the projection of the nipple and areola form the tip. The breasts become elastic and firm in consistency. The areola begins to attain some coloring, and the skin becomes tense; sometimes mild pain may be felt as a result of this tenseness of the skin. The breast is usually somewhat cone-shaped. Between ages 14 and 16, a fat layer is deposited under the skin, softening the contour of the breast and making it more hemispherical in form. The greater part of the breast consists of this fatty layer and connective tissue. The milk glands are fully developed at this time, but only a small amount of glandular tissue has been formed; and this is found at the base and at the borders of the breast. After puberty, the amount of glandular tissue gradually increases, as well as the fat and connective tissue. Both before and after menstru-

Illustration: Anatomy of the Breast . . . Grace Hewitt

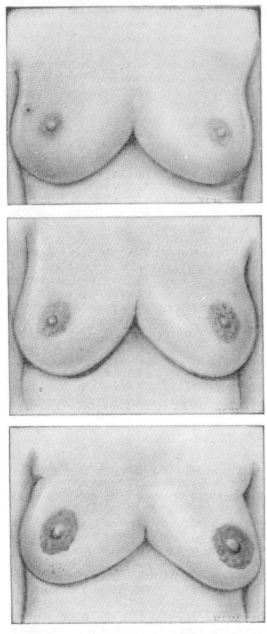

During the course of a normal pregnancy the breasts change in a characteristic fashion, as shown from top down, after two, six, and nine months. *Adapted from C. F. Geschickter, M.D., DISEASES OF THE BREAST 2nd Ed. Copyright, 1945. J. B. Lippincott Co., Philadelphia.*

ation, changes in the breast occur. Prior to the onset of a period, the gland is larger, more tense, and firm. Discomfort, pain, or tenderness may be present. Following the menstrual period, these symptoms usually disappear.

The adolescent girl should be taught what changes to expect in her person. Frightened or embarrassed by the physiology of adolescence, she may attempt to disguise or alter the appearance of her breasts by tight, ill-fitting brassieres or poor posture. Understanding and kindness are prerequisites for the adjustment and happiness of a young girl during this cycle. A series of pictures showing the development of the female breast from ages 8 to 14 may be found in Chapter 2.

Abnormal changes in the breasts peculiar to puberty may occur. A painful swelling and hardness of the breasts may develop, usually in both breasts, but often more intense in one than in the other. This condition, often called *puberty mastitis*, may last for several weeks and occurs because of the rapid development of breast tissue which usually occurs at this time of life. It arises rapidly and often begins first on one side. The areola darkens and the swelling assumes the form of a firm, tumorlike mass, varying in size from one to two inches. Sometimes a few drops of cloudy liquid may be squeezed out of the nipple. After several weeks, the breasts resume their normal shape and contour. Rarely, a true inflammation may be present.

Five to six weeks after pregnancy begins, the breasts begin to enlarge, and continue to increase rather rapidly in size until mid-pregnancy. The surface veins dilate; and if the breast has enlarged very much, bluish-white streaks may appear in the skin (*striae*). The nipple becomes larger, and the size of the areola increases. The pigmentation of the areola deepens. The sebaceous glands at the base of the nipple and on the areola become more obvious. The skin covering the nipple becomes thin and may be extremely sensitive.

Even though a milklike substance (*colostrum*) can be squeezed from the nipples about the fifth month of pregnancy, the real production of milk does not begin until three or four days after the baby is born. Following birth and before the milk secretion is apparent, the breasts become more distended and tender. They are hard and swollen, and tenderness is usually more severe in that part of the breast nearest the armpit.

Special attention must be paid to the nipples, particularly if the mother plans to nurse her child. All during pregnancy, any secretion which has caked on the nipple should be carefully and gently washed off. If tenderness is apparent, the physician usually will advise the patient to apply cold cream, cocoa butter, lanolin, or another emollient in order to increase the pliability of the breast.

If the nipples are inverted, the woman may make them protrude by gentle pressure with the fingers while applying cream or oil. It may be necessary to use a breast pump to evert the nipples.

For the first few days before true milk production begins, the physician usually will advise the mother to nurse the baby for only a few minutes at a time. Although the baby receives little nourishment, this trial period is important in accustoming the mother and the baby to each other. The sucking action of the child also helps to stimulate the secretion of milk. By the time the milk appears, usually on the third or fourth day, regular feedings can be initiated and the length of nursing time increased.

Milk production (*lactation*) is probably caused by hormonal influence. The ovarian hormones and the pituitary gland are thought to be the instigators of lactation. The actual secretion of milk is dependent upon a stimulus which arises in the anterior part of the pituitary gland. If this gland is removed from an animal which is in the milk-producing period, lactation ceases.

Although the breasts are developed sufficiently by the middle of pregnancy to permit lactation, the production of milk does not occur until after the baby is born and the placenta is delivered. Human milk is a bluish-white or slightly yellowish fluid with a characteristic odor and a rather sweetish taste. It is approximately seven parts water and one part solids. Human milk is an emulsion of fat, suspended in a solution of protein, carbohydrates, and inorganic salts; the yellow color comes from the emulsified fat. The composition of human milk may vary from day to day, and even hour to hour. The fat is subject to the greatest variations. The essential food elements—carbohydrates, fat, and protein—are present in sufficient amounts to make milk the most satisfactory food for the infant. Except for vitamins B and D, human milk also contains adequate vitamins and inorganic salts for the growing infant. Antibodies to infection are also found in breast milk. Indeed, breast-fed children seem to resist infection better than those who are formula-fed, and are less likely to have diarrhea, colic, diaper rash, and allergies. Furthermore, in addition to the benefits the infant receives from nursing, there is some evidence to indicate that women who nurse their children are less likely to develop malignant or benign diseases of the breast.

Certain drugs taken by the mother may pass into the milk, thus affecting the nursing child. Drugs which may be transmitted in this manner include iron, arsenic, lead, quinine, alcohol, and opium and its derivatives.

Nursing her child should never add extra strain to the woman's breast. She should not feel exhausted after the procedure. She should lie down comfortably, loosen any tight clothing, and hold the infant parallel to her own body. In this way, no additional strain is put on the breast, either by the baby or the weight of the breast itself.

If the mother does not wish to nurse the infant, or if her physician thinks it unwise for medical reasons, special care is taken to diminish the secretion of milk. The doctor often pre-

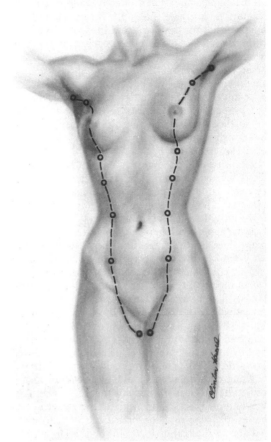

Additional nipples may appear anywhere along the lines shown. The condition is known as polymastia. Modified from an illustration by F. Netter, M.D., in *The Ciba Collection of Medical Illustrations.*

scribes medications to check the flow before it has begun. A breast binder may be applied, and the mother is cautioned to restrict the intake of fluids. Some women suffer no pain or discomfort during this process.

During the milk-producing period, a type of cyst called a *galactocele* may occur in rare cases. It is caused by obstruction of one of the larger mammary ducts and contains altered milk —butter, cheese, or soap-like contents. There are no symptoms of infection, such as pain and redness, although these symptoms may appear as the result of an old infection. As a rule, the physician waits until the baby is weaned before he removes the cyst.

The breast, following the change of life, becomes quite different in appearance. Although it may retain its size (because of added fat deposits), the amount of glandular tissue diminishes, and the fibrous tissue gradually becomes more dense. Changes in the size or shape, and any discharge from the nipple should be reported to the physician.

Through all stages of growth and development of the female breast, an effective and adequate support is desirable, not only for psychological purposes but for purely physical reasons. Women with pendulous breasts and pregnant or nursing women in particular benefit from proper support. The properly-fitted brassiere should gently support the breasts without tension or pressure over any area. The shoulder straps should be of the proper length and width. There should be complete conformation to nature's design, without rough seams to injure or irritate the nipples or breast tissue.

Occasionally an individual will have more than the normal number of breasts. This is known as *polymastia*, which means "many breasts." The condition appears about twice as frequently in men as in women. These extra breasts appear oftener on the left side of the body than on the right, and more such breasts are found below the normal breasts than above them. They are usually in line, along the so-called "mammary line." In the female, the extra breasts may become enlarged and painful during pregnancy, and some may even secrete milk. Most of these extra glands do not have a function and rarely develop fully. Another anomaly of the breast is absence of one or both breasts (*amastia*). This is an extremely rare condition.

Underdevelopment of the breasts (*hypomastia*) sometimes is seen in varying degrees. There is the "nipple" breast, in which the structure is barely palpable and the breast is small in comparison to the rest of the body build. The nipple itself may be infantile and undeveloped as may be the remainder of the breast. Sometimes the breast is adult size with the gland structure present, but the layer of fat is missing. It is thought that these conditions are caused by undersecretion of certain hormones, or by an aberration of their function.

DISORDERS OF THE BREAST: BENIGN CONDITIONS

Inflammation of the breast is called *mastitis*. The disease can have many causes and may occur in many different forms. It may occur following childbirth, while the mother is nursing her baby; or it may follow injury to the breast, or be associated with an infection. Acute mastitis developing after childbirth usually appears between the first and third weeks after delivery. More than one half of the cases of this form of mastitis occur in women who have just had their first child. The name given mastitis following childbirth is *acute puerperal mastitis*. It is often preceded by painful or cracked nipples. The patient complains of tenderness and pain in

the breast. A fever as high as 105° or 106° may be present. The lymph nodes of the armpit occasionally are enlarged. The skin over the affected area is hot, reddened, and tight. Sometimes a fluid exudes from the nipple. The symptoms may subside spontaneously; however, appropriate treatment should be instituted promptly. Massage is of no value, and is inadvisable. The mother cannot continue to nurse her baby, and the breast should be supported by a binder.

An abscess of the breast occurs most frequently within one month after childbirth. It is caused by infection entering through a "cracked nipple." The breast becomes tight and painful, and the patient develops fever which may become as high as 105°. The unfortunate consequences of a breast abscess are that the infant is deprived of breast milk, plus the fact that the new mother has a long period of discomfort and pain. Treatment is instituted as quickly as possible in order to avoid a prolonged convalescent period, as well as the possibility of the destruction of a large amount of breast tissue.

Mastitis following a breast injury of any kind is called *traumatic mastitis*. It usually clears up without complications, but occasionally an abscess forms. A lump of fatty tissue, or fat necrosis, sometimes appears in conjunction with mastitis as a result of the injury. Mastitis appears, though seldom, in newborn infants of both sexes.

Chronic mastitis sometimes follows acute mastitis, and usually involves both breasts. It can develop after a miscarriage or abortion. It can, however, occur in either males or females following injury to the breast tissue. Chronic mastitis sometimes appears in or even after the change of life (*menopause*). One form, *chronic interstitial mastitis*, appears most frequently in women with small breasts, and between the ages of 40 and 60. Usually, both breasts are involved. In these cases the breast often is tender and enlarged, and there may be a watery discharge from the nipple. The treatment depends upon the severity of the symptoms.

The term *chronic cystic mastitis* is somewhat misleading. Actually, the term is used to describe a group of abnormal but benign breast conditions: painful breasts (*mastodynia*), disorders caused by abnormal gland action (*adenosis*), and those caused by changes in the breast secretions (*cystic* diseases). Mastodynia occurs often in women with unusually large breasts, but also occurs prior to the menstrual period in women with small breasts. In both cases, the pain is more severe during the premenstrual period. Painful breasts are encountered more frequently in women in their middle thirties who have never had children, or have not given birth to a child for several years previously.

Adenosis is characterized by multiple nodules in the breast, and usually occurs in women between 35 and 44 years of age. Childless women with small breasts are more frequently subject to this disease.

Patients whose health is otherwise quite normal may develop cystic nodules in their breasts. They seldom have a history of discomfort or abnormalities connected with their menstrual periods or with childbirth. The cysts associated with the disease are occasionally discovered during pregnancy, but usually appear at or near the menopause. There may be only one cyst or several.

Treatment of patients with chronic cystic mastitis consists of surgical procedures or endocrine therapy. As the three types of this disease may be related to a later development of malignant conditions, careful diagnosis and continued observation of the patient's condition are necessary.

A *benign tumor* is an abnormal new growth of tissue that does not spread to other body areas. *Fibroadenoma* is the most common benign tumor of the breast found in young females. It is seen most frequently in women between the ages of 21 and 25 years. Such tumors grow rapidly during pregnancy. Occasionally they develop during or even after the menopause, and may occur in young girls before the onset of menstruation. Pain and discomfort are seldom present in these cases. Many of the patients discover a "lump" before other symptoms appear. Fibroadenomas, like all breast nodules, can be diagnosed with certainty only after surgical removal and microscopic examination.

The typical symptom of *intraductal papillary hyperplasia*, another benign tumor, is the discharge of blood or blood-tinged fluid from the nipple when the breast is compressed. Sometimes, however, the discharge from the nipple is watery and streaked with blood, or watery with no trace of blood. These growths occur most often in women between the ages of 35 and 55 years. Sometimes only one growth is present, but there may be many. A physician should be consulted on any discharge.

Hypertrophy

Abnormal enlargement of the breasts is called *hypertrophy*. This condition is less common in the United States than in the tropics. It may occur in males or females, and both breasts usually are enlarged, but generally are not painful. The four most common types of hypertrophy of the breasts are: (1) *infantile hypertrophy*, which occurs in girls before the age of puberty; (2) *gynecomastia*, which occurs in males, most often at the time of adolescence; (3) *virginal hypertrophy*, which occurs in young females during adolescence; and (4) *gravid hypertrophy*, which appears during pregnancy or lactation.

Infantile hypertrophy is seen in girls usually from one to five years of age. Accompanying the breast enlargement, there may be growth of pubic hair and onset of the menstrual period. Such premature sexual development is a symptom of disease of the ovary, adrenal gland, or midbrain, and is not a disease of the breast.

Gynecomastia of the male breast may involve one or both breasts. Two forms of the condition exist: enlargement associated with abnormal sexual development; and enlargement with no accompanying abnormal sexual development, which is by far the most common. Occasionally, tumors of the testicle may be associated with gynecomastia, and injury to the testicle has been followed by this disorder. Removal of the prostate gland occasionally results in enlargement of the breast in older males. Disturbances of the function of the endocrine glands also may be a causative agent in gynecomastia; the hormone balance may not be within normal limits, or a tumor of the adrenal gland may be present.

Virginal hypertrophy of the breast usually begins just before or at the beginning of a young girl's first menstruation. Usually both breasts are involved. Persistent growth may continue for as long as two years, but the enlargement usually is more rapid for a period of three to six months. There seldom are any related symptoms until the weight of the breasts causes discomfort. (In one case reported, the patient's breasts weighed 64 pounds.) Occasionally, plastic surgery may have to be performed.

Gravid hypertrophy of the breast occurs during pregnancy or lactation. The increase in size of the breasts usually is not noticed by the woman until the production of milk ceases.

Fat necrosis and skin eruption

Degeneration of fat within the breast (*fat necrosis*) occurs most frequently in the heavy, fat breast, and usually develops after injury. The symptoms are often mistaken for cancer of the breast. A painless, hard lump forms; the nipple is sometimes retracted; and the breast may be pulled out of shape. Surgical removal of the deteriorated area clears up the disorder.

Skin eruption frequently occurs on the breasts of nursing women. It may affect one or both breasts. The nipple and area surrounding the nipple (*areola*) become red and encrusted. The patient complains of burning and itching of this region. The disorder may be caused by "the itch" (*scabies*) or by the more serious *Paget's disease* of the nipple, a malignant disease of the skin arising from breast tumor. Severe eczema of the breast may develop following a minor injury to the skin of the breast. The attending physician will carefully determine the cause before beginning treatment.

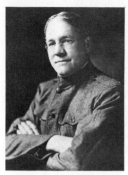

BLOODGOOD, Joseph Colt (1867-1935) American surgeon. Well known for his many contributions to knowledge of chronic mastitis, mammary carcinoma, and senile hypertrophy of the breast. He is also recognized for his description of the blue-domed type of mammary cyst. He devised an operation for the control of inguinal hernia by transplanting the rectus muscle. He also developed a theory to explain chronic mastitis.

Intertrigo

This is a common skin disorder of the breast, caused chiefly by friction; it appears underneath the fold of the pendulous breast, especially in patients who are not thorough in bathing. The affected area becomes red and itches. Patients with diabetes aften develop intertrigo, especially during the summer months. See also Chapter 8, "The Skin: *Skin Disorders—Dermatitis*."

Injuries to the breast

The location of the breasts makes them very liable to injury. A blow or injury to the breast may result in a bruised area or a localized collection of blood (*hematoma*); or a severe bruise may ultimately result in abscess formation. Bruises of the breast may result in a certain amount of bleeding from the nipple, which should be controlled before further treatment is given.

Lacerations of the breast are cared for in the same manner as cuts in any other part of the body. Sunburn of the breast is to be avoided since the reaction may be severe because of the thin skin and loose underlying tissue. There is no evidence that such injuries to the breast are related to the development of malignant disease.

Abnormal conditions of the nipple

Most abnormal conditions of the nipple occur in the pregnant or nursing woman, except for congenital abnormalities (which have already been described.) *Depressed nipples* are fairly common in the pregnant woman. Sometimes the nipple is only slightly erectile; or the nipple may be depressed below the level of the surrounding tissue. If possible, this condition should be rectified by *gentle* traction during the latter half of the pregnancy. Should the nipples fail to respond to this treatment, it may not be possible to breast feed the baby. In attempting to elevate the nipples, it is important for the infant to nurse. However, persistent attempts to have the baby

nurse when the nipple is quite depressed may result in infected breasts, and should be discouraged.

Cracked or fissured nipples develop usually during the first two weeks following delivery. The nipples become extremely tender and are more than ordinarily subject to infection. Careful cleaning and handling of the breasts before delivery can help to prevent this condition. If fissures develop, the baby should be permitted to nurse through a nipple shield; if the fissure does not heal with proper treatment, breast feeding should be discontinued. (For a discussion of the management of the breast during the period of lactation, see Chapter 1, "Life Begins: *The New Mother*".)

In *keratosis*, the "horny" outer layer of the skin thickens, and projections form around the milk ducts. The slightest provocation will result in a fissure formation. A lesion of this sort should be watched carefully, as it may prove to be an early stage of Paget's disease, a form of malignant disease, mentioned above.

Discharge from the nipple indicates an abnormality of the breast, either malignant or benign. The drainage may be milky, pus-like, watery, or watery but blood-tinged. The presence of any discharge should always call for an examination by a physician. In most cases, discharge is the result of a benign condition; nevertheless, it warrants professional attention.

DISORDERS OF THE BREAST: CANCER OF THE BREAST

Cancer of the breast is the most common malignant tumor in women. Almost one-fourth of all cancers in women are located in the breast, causing about 20 percent of all cancer deaths in females. Most of these deaths occur between the ages of 50 and 60, although the disease may

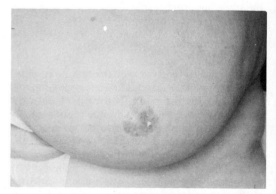

Eczematous lesion affecting the nipple. Copyright 1970 Year Book Medical Publishers, Inc., courtesy E. C. White, The University of Texas M. D. Anderson Hospital, Houston.

Per 100,000 white females   DEATHS FROM CANCER
OF THE BREAST

Chart showing death rates from cancer of the breast, among women of different age groups. Women between 75 and 79 are ten times more likely to have breast cancer than are those between 35 and 39. U.S. Dept. Health, Education, and Welfare, Public Health Service, National Office of Vital Statistics.

ating early in life and who have continued their cycles for more than 30 years, and those who have had no pregnancies, or only one or two.

Types of breast cancer

Breast cancer is classified in various ways. The microscopic appearance of the tissue and the site of origin provide the most commonly used classifications. Cancers originating in different sites, or having different microscopic appearances, may have quite different growth characteristics. They may be slow-growing or fast-growing and have a hard or soft texture. In general, a breast cancer appears initially as a small, *painless* lump in the breast—more frequently in the upper outer section of the breast. Should the growth be located near the surface of the breast, a "dimpling" of the skin overlying the tumor may be noticed. After the lesion has been present for

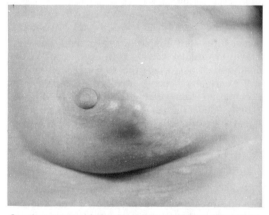

Small sarcoma of the breast in a 65-year-old patient. Copyright 1970 Year Book Medical Publishers, Inc., courtesy R. G. Martin, The University of Texas M. D. Anderson Hospital, Houston.

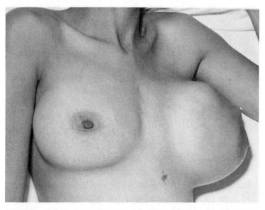

Typical, large breast sarcoma in a 37-year-old patient. Copyright 1970 Year Book Medical Publishers, Inc., courtesy R. G. Martin, The University of Texas M. D. Anderson Hospital, Houston.

actually develop years earlier. There are many population differences in cancer incidence around the world; for instance, women in the U.S. are five times more likely to die from cancer of the breast than are women in Japan. A small percentage of men also develop cancer of the breast.

Without treatment, about 20 percent of patients with breast cancer will live five years from the onset of symptoms. If the disease is diagnosed in its early stages, treatment will be more successful and may enable the patient to live a normal life span. Much can now be done to control pain for those whose cancers are unsuccessfully managed. Early detection is the primary weapon.

Cancer in the breast, like cancer elsewhere in the body, is an uncontrolled growth of cells. Little pieces of the growth may separate from the tumor and travel through the vessels of the lymphatic system to nearby lymph nodes, where the traveling cancer cells come to rest and form a secondary growth. It may also spread by way of the blood stream. These processes of spread throughout the body are called *metastases*.

The cause of breast cancer has not been established; an hereditary predisposition may exist. Studies conducted over the past several years have suggested the possibility that cancer of the breast may be associated with the improper functioning of glands which have to do with secondary sexual characteristics, pregnancy, and lactation. Although there are occasionally sharp changes in the breasts of women who are taking contraceptive pills, there is no evidence that the pill causes breast cancer.

In general, women considered to be in the high-risk group are: those with a family history of mammary cancer, those who began menstru-

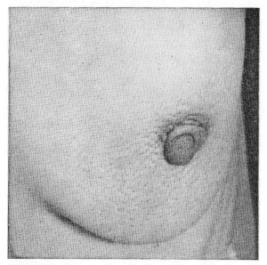

This photograph of a mature female breast with a retracted nipple shows clearly the characteristic "orange peel" skin associated with advanced cancer.

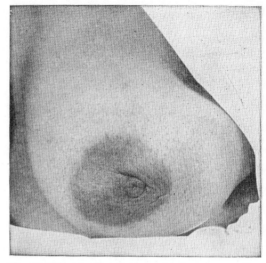

The severely retracted nipple on this breast, as well as the less distinct "orange peel" skin, results from cancerous involvement of underlying tissue.

some time, the nipple may become flat and drawn inward (*retraction*). In most cases, if the condition is neglected, the skin over the breast will eventually become involved, and pain may become an important feature of the disease. Finally, depending on the type of cancer, secondary growths may be discovered in the area of the armpit or elsewhere in the body.

Paget's disease of the nipple

Paget's disease of the nipple is a form of malignant disease of the nipple, a metastatic involvement secondary to an underlying tumor in the mammary gland. It usually affects only one breast and is characterized by eczematoid redness, cracks or ulceration, and tenderness of the nipple, from which there is frequently an abnormal discharge. The diseased area of the nipple will not heal. The associated breast cancer may antedate the nipple symptoms but is usually discovered one or two years after the disease of the nipple is first noticed. A persistent abnormality of the nipple must be regarded with suspicion.

Cancer of the male breast

Cancer of the male breast is relatively rare, comprising one percent of all cases of breast cancer. This disease usually occurs in men between the ages of 54 and 60. As in female breast cancer, the first symptom is usually a lump in the breast. However, the average victim is unaware that breast cancer occurs in men, so that he may delay longer in seeing a physician than would a woman with breast cancer. Later symp-

toms include ulceration of the skin over the breast and enlarged lymph nodes in the armpit; these signs usually indicate that the disease is far advanced. If performed early, surgical treatment may eradicate the growth. However, treatment falls short of success unless the patient sees his physician while his only symptom is a lump in the breast.

Pregnancy and breast cancer

Pregnancy has been found to affect the course of cancer of the breast. Cancer in a pregnant woman usually grows more rapidly than in a nonpregnant person. The chief danger of breast cancer among pregnant women lies in the fact that the victims associate the first symptoms of the cancer with their pregnancy (or lactation) and therefore may fail to consult their physician promptly.

Symptoms

Most of the deaths which occur as a result of cancer of the breast are among patients who visit their physician several months after the first symptoms have appeared. If all women would seek medical attention at the first appearance of any abnormality of the breast, the mortality rate from breast cancer would be greatly decreased. In general, the symptoms most patients describe are: (1) "a lump in the breast," which usually is discovered accidentally; (2) drainage from the nipple, frequently blood-tinged, and sometimes scant when first noticed; (3) pain, which is seldom present in the early stages of the disease, and indicates an advanced stage; (4) change in the size or shape of the breast, such as enlargement, shrinkage, or hardening; (5) "drawing-in" (retraction) of the nipple, which may be painless; (6) roughening or thickening of the skin to an "orange peel" appearance; and (7) swelling in the armpit region, which may be noticed by the patient as a "lump" or merely as a tender swelling of that area.

Means of diagnosis

When a patient with a suspicious symptom consults her physician, he will perform a complete physical examination with emphasis on the breasts. *Biopsy* is usually necessary for an accurate, definite diagnosis. Biopsy is the removal of a piece of the lump for study under the microscope, and is painlessly performed under anesthesia.

Getting a detailed view of the breast before taking a tissue sample has aided doctors in diagnosis and in pinpointing the area for biopsy. *Mammography* is the study of the breast by means of x-ray films. *Thermography* is the study of the breast by means of recording heat emitted by different types of tissue. Certain malignant tumors emit greater heat through the skin than normal or benign tissue. Mammography is also used to screen high-risk women before they show clinical symptoms, the most active stage of many cancers. Survival rates are highest if these elusive early cancers can be found.

Treatment

Breast cancer is under attack from an increasing array of methods. Surgical resection, x-ray

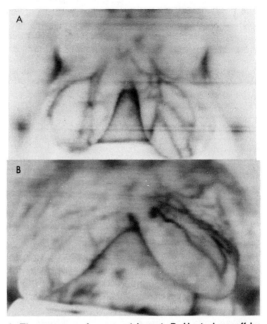

A, Thermogram of a normal breast. B, Heat given off by tumor in the left breast is a conspicuous addition to the regular thermal pattern. Copyright 1970 Year Book Medical Publishers, Inc., courtesy G. D. Dodd, The University of Texas M. D. Anderson Hospital Houston.

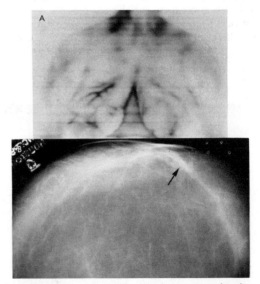

A, Small carcinoma of the right breast seen by thermography. B, Mammogram of the same tumor. Copyright 1970 Year Book Medical Publishers, Inc., courtesy G. D. Dodd, The University of Texas M. D. Anderson Hospital, Houston.

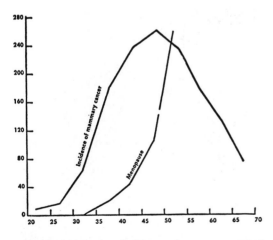

Chart showing the age incidence of mammary cancer and the age of menopause. Approximately 55 percent of women with mammary cancer have not passed the menopause; while 45 percent of them have. *Adopted from C. F. Geschickter, M.D., DISEASES OF THE BREAST, 2nd Ed., Copyright 1945 by J. B. Lippincott Co., Philadelphia, Pennsylvania.*

therapy (alone or in combination), and chemotherapy are accepted forms of treatment. When surgical resection is performed, it generally implies removal of the entire breast and adjacent

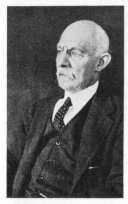

HALSTED, William Stewart (1852-1922) American surgeon. In 1882 he introduced an operation for the radical amputation of the breast as a means of combatting carcinoma. This procedure, along with several others in surgery, is known as Halsted's operation. He is said to have been the first to introduce use of sterile rubber gloves into surgical practice. Among his other contributions are regional block anesthesia, an operation for hernia, and a new type of hemostat.

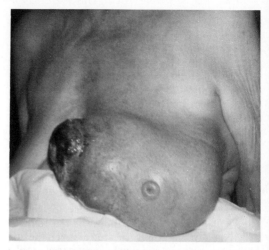

A large breast cancer that was removed by simple mastectomy. Copyright 1970 Year Book Medical Publishers, Inc., courtesy C. M. McBride, The University of Texas M. D. Anderson Hospital, Houston.

tissues, including the chest muscles and tissue in the armpit. A large number of patients require the radical operation, frequently followed by x-ray treatment. Reconstructive surgical procedures and new prosthetics allow women to achieve a completely normal appearance.

Many advances in equipment and technique have improved the use of radiotherapy in recent years. For patients with advanced breast cancer, radiotherapy alone may be used since the risk of recurrences on the chest wall and other nearby areas requires a wide-ranging weapon. Postoperative irradiation is given to halt any possible growth of the cancer cells in the surrounding areas by destroying them or imprisoning them in dense fibrous tissue. And to complement other methods, a variety of new drugs have

offered hope for increasing survival in patients with breast cancer.

Certain hormones including estrogens, androgens, progestational compounds, and corticosteroids can effectively alter the natural course of advanced breast cancer. In addition, alkylating agents, antimetabolites, and certain antibiotics and alkaloids have been established in the management of disseminated mammary cancer.

Most metastatic mammary carcinomas, although inoperable, respond to irradiation. Cutaneous metastases respond most favorably.

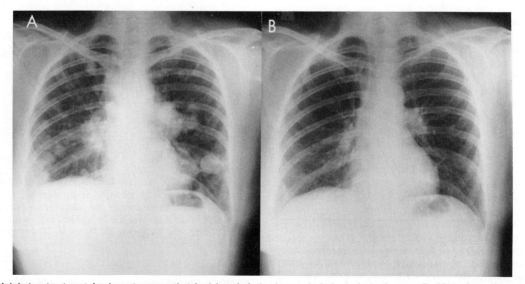

Melphalan treatment for breast cancer that had invaded the lungs. A, before chemotherapy. B, After chemotherapy. The tumor tissue, which appears as light areas in the lung region, is considerably reduced after treatment. Copyright 1970 Year Book Medical Publishers, Inc., courtesy Mary E. Sears, The University of Texas M. D. Anderson Hospital, Houston.

When metastasis to the vertebral column occurs, the patient often suffers severe pain, and the process may be accompanied by signs of compression of the spinal cord and severe neurologic disturbances. In metastases to the long bones pathologic fractures are sometimes the first symptoms which bring the patient under observation. The marked and often immediate relief of pain that follows irradiation of metastases to the vertebral column may be only temporary.

Today, the treatment of patients with cancer of the breast, as with all diseases, can be most successful, if the patient and physician work together as a team. The greatest enemy of cancer is an intelligent, observant, well-educated public. The medical profession has fought tirelessly to educate the public in regard to suspicious symptoms that might mean cancer, and the importance of reporting these symptoms quickly. Most *cancer is curable* if detected early enough. If everyone had a thorough physical examination every year, conducted by his own physician, there can be little doubt that many cancers would be detected in stages sufficiently early to make treatment successful. Women over 40 should have a physician examine their breasts at least every six to twelve months. A great aid to early diagnosis of breast cancer is the present trend toward self-examination of the female breast.

Reconstruction and rehabilitation

Reconstructive surgical procedures after injury, tumor removal, or simple mastectomy can often restore the appearance of the breast. Great care should be taken on the part of the patient to discuss the procedure with her own physician since there are many unacceptable and dangerous shortcuts. Performed by a properly trained surgeon, reconstruction of the breast can be done relatively safely. Some women even manage to nurse their children after insertion of an uplift device.

Materials *not* recommended are glass and paraffin. Other materials used with varying success to date are the body's own fat; sponges of rubber, plastic, silicone, and polyvinyl; and injections of liquid plastic gel. A method with few reported side effects consists of a silicone plastic bag backed on one side with a form of nylon mesh. A pocket is created between the breast tissue and the muscle of the chest wall. The device is inserted behind the breast tissue, with the mesh facing the chest. This allows the muscle to grow into the material and anchor the bag. The breast tissues come into contact only with the front of the impermeable nonreactive silicone plastic covering.

Any reconstructive method should leave the breast soft, should not shrink or move, should not bury or obscure the remaining breast tissue, and should not cause inflammation or disease. Also available are new prosthetic brassieres that can be fitted to give a normal appearance.

Self-examination of the breast

In the initial step of self-examination of the breast, the woman places herself squarely before a mirror, with her arms at her sides and posture erect. She carefully examines her breasts in the mirror for symmetry in size and shape, especially noting the contours of the breasts, any swelling or any dimpling of the skin, or change in shape, direction, or retraction of the nipple. After this portion of the examination, she raises her arms over her head and again studies her breasts in the mirror, looking for the same signs as before. In addition, she watches for any evidence of fixation of the breast tissue to the chest wall as she moves her arms and shoulders. The relative positions of the breasts on the chest wall are checked; if one has recently become larger or more shrunken than the other, her physician should be consulted.

To perform the second half of the examination, the woman reclines on her back on a bed. This position allows the breasts to spread over a greater area, and thins the breast tissue. Consequently, the structures within the breast will be more easily felt. In this position the breasts tend to spread apart and to hang slightly to the sides. A flat pillow or folded towel is placed under the shoulder on the same side as the breast she will first examine. This raises that side, distributing the weight of the breast tissue more evenly over the supporting chest wall.

The following picture series is reproduced by courtesy of The Cancer Bulletin, Copyright 1951.

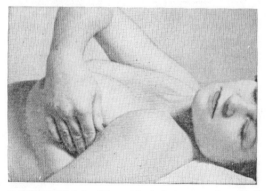

1. With padding in place under her shoulders and areas at the side, the woman begins the examination of her breasts by carefully feeling the tissues which extend into the armpit regions.

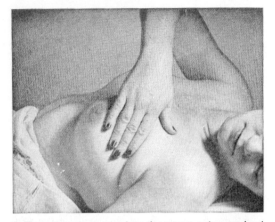

2. The woman now examines the upper, outer quadrant of her breast, making use of the flats of her fingers rather than their tips. She should give this area especially careful attention.

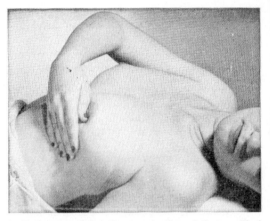

3. Having completed the examination of these critical areas, the woman now proceeds to the remainder of the outer half of her breast, feeling successively from margin to the nipple.

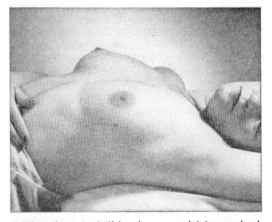

4. When the outer half has been completely examined, the woman raises her arm over head. This spreads and thins the underlying tissues for the remaining steps of the examination.

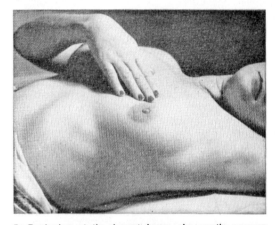

5. Beginning at the breast bone, she gently presses the tissue of the inner half of the breast against the chest wall, moving stepwise in this manner to the middle (areola) of the breast.

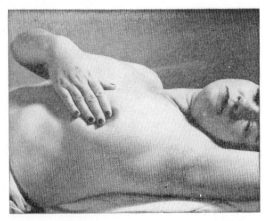

6. The woman then carefully palpates the nipple area and the underlying tissues. Still using the flats of fingers she notes normal structures and any previously unobserved lumps.

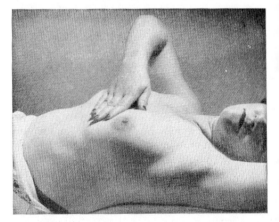

7. Examination is completed by feeling remainder of the inner half of the breast. The ridge of firm tissue along the lower margin of the breast is normal and no cause for alarm.

Most breast cancers can be cured if they are treated while the growth is still small and localized. However, if treatment is late, only a small percentage survive. As pointed out earlier, cancer of the breast seldom causes pain in the early stages, and often goes unsuspected until too late. Therefore, the only method at present of reducing the high mortality rate from this disease is the regular examination of the breasts of women who present *no* symptoms of cancer.

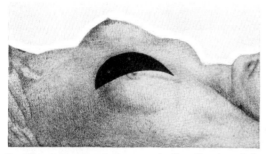

For the purposes of the examination the breast is divided into three areas. Less than 20 percent of cancers occur in inner half, shown here in black.

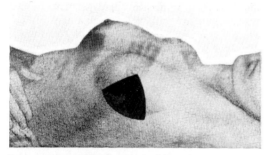

From seven to fifteen percent of breast cancers occur in the lower outer quadrant of the breast shown in black in this illustration of the breast.

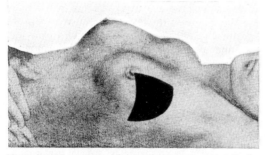

Many breast cancers, about 47 percent, occur in the upper outer quadrant, shown here in black. The 22 percent that remain occur in the nipple area.

Ideally, examinations should be performed monthly, in order that any new growth may be located in time to insure the most favorable outlook for cure. However, since a woman usually does not see her physician as often as this, it is more practical for her to learn to examine her own breasts. Self-examination is easy to learn and can be conveniently fitted into her normal routine. After a little practice, she will become familiar with the normal structures in her breasts and with their individual contours, and with alertness may be quick to note even a small new growth.

Among the abnormalities, aside from lumps, which she may find—and for which she should look—are dimpling or puckering of the skin of her breasts, any change in either nipple, any thickening which may be seen or felt, loss of mobility, or any pronounced lack of similarity in size, contour, or position of the two breasts (there is normally, however, a slight inequality in size). A discharge from the nipple demands investigation, even though it may not mean a cancer. Pain, swelling, and inflammation are usually indications of noncancerous conditions, but they are also symptoms of advanced cancer, and rarely may occur early. In general, the signs the woman seeks are not obvious signs.

The woman should set up a regular schedule for monthly breast self-examination. The ideal time is immediately following the end of her menstrual period. Temporary changes and tenderness occur normally in the breasts shortly before and may persist during menstruation. Therefore, an examination just before or during the period may be unsatisfactory. However, the menstrual period will serve as a reminder for the woman to inspect her breasts. After the menopause, or "change of life," monthly examinations should be continued, because breast cancer occurs more often between the ages of 40 and 70 than at earlier periods. A sleepless night of anxiety due to the suspected presence of an abnormal lump will be avoided if the examination is performed upon arising in the morning rather than at night.

After repeating breast self-examinations at regular intervals for a few months, the woman will become familiar with the feel of the normal structures within her breasts. Thus, she may be able to detect immediately any unusual lump as soon as it appears. She should be aware that not every lump in her breasts is a cancer. In fact, the majority will be some condition other than cancer. Nevertheless, when she detects a lump, she should consult her physician immediately. This course of action will certainly add to her peace of mind.

Self-examination of the breast is important, but should not be regarded as a substitute for periodic breast examinations by a physician.

17 THE EYE

WHAT IT IS AND DOES

The eye is one of the most important organs of the body. A large portion of all our information is acquired through vision; the remainder is provided by such senses as hearing, smelling, tasting, and touching.

The eye is frequently compared to an extremely delicate camera. Such a comparison is well advised, although most man-made cameras do not match the accuracy, the sensitivity, or the flexibility of the eye. Like a camera, the eye contains a lens which focuses light on a light-sensitive area, the *retina*, which is analogous to the film of a camera. The eye can "take" an unlimited number of pictures, some of which will be sorted out by the mind, stored in the memory, and recalled later. The normal eye takes all its "pictures" in color, at almost any distance.

The working parts of the eye are the lens which focuses the picture, the retina which receives it, and the *optic nerve* which transmits an impression of the picture to the brain. However, there are many other parts of the eye, most of which exist to protect this important organ from injury and disease.

Special tests have been designed to test the various working parts of the eye. The general examinations for aviators usually include tests for *visual acuity, depth perception* (the ability to estimate the space between two objects which are at different distances from the eye), *color vision, eye convergence,* and *motility*. These functions will be discussed later.

The eye is situated in a socket formed by the bones of the head, and thereby is protected from heavy blows. It rests on a soft pad of fatty tissue which further minimizes damage. The human eye is equipped with a *lid*, a thin flap of skin which can completely cover and protect the organ. The lashes and brows help to filter dust particles and microorganisms from the air, and help screen out perspiration. The *conjunctiva* is a membrane which covers the inner side of the lid and folds back onto the front of the eyeball. Near the upper and lateral folds of the conjunctiva, there are many small glands (*accessory lacrimal glands*) which secrete a watery solution, *tears*. The tears are spread over the surface of the conjunctiva to lubricate and protect it. The large tear gland is located just above the eye, toward the outside and under the bony structure above the socket. When the eye is irritated, this larger gland secretes large amounts of tears which wash away foreign particles in the eye. Some of the tears are removed from the eye through the *lacrimal duct* which opens into the inner part of the nose. The two openings to this duct can be seen on the inner corner of the eye, one on the margin of the lower lid and the other just above it on the upper lid. The eyeball itself is protected by its tough white outer layer, the *sclera*. The sclera is completely opaque, except in the transparent central region which is called the *cornea*. The conjunctiva and sclera protect the eye from dust, invading bacteria, and foreign bodies.

Besides protective devices, the eye contains many structures which improve the accuracy of the camera-like essentials. The *iris* controls the amount of light entering the eye. The iris is the doughnut-shaped colored structure in the eye. When light is bright, the hole (the pupil) in the iris becomes smaller; in dim light it may be quite large. In some persons absence of the iris (*aniridia*) is inherited. Although vision is impaired, it is not completely lost. Various corrective measures against hypersensitivity to light and refractive errors can be taken by the physician.

The anterior surface of the iris may be of different colors or shadings of color in different individuals, such as blue, brown, gray, or green, depending on the amount and distribution of pigment cells. The color of a person's eyes is determined largely by heredity.

The lens of the eye is a highly transparent, biconvex, nearly spherical body used to focus the rays of light upon the retina. It is located behind the iris. The *ciliary* body helps the eye to adapt to different circumstances. This is a circular structure, triangular on cross-section, lying immediately behind the iris, and containing the ciliary muscle. The ciliary body supports some 60 to 80 paired strands of suspensory fibers which are connected to the lens. At rest, these fibers are under tension and pull the lens into a flattened shape. When the ciliary muscle contracts, however, the ciliary body is pulled inward toward the lens; the result is that tension on the lens is relieved, and it assumes a more convex shape. This enables the eye to accommodate for near vision.

Within the eye are several chambers, the largest of which is located between the lens and the retina (which is described below). This chamber is filled with a gelatinous fluid (the *vitreous humor*) which is light-refractive. Between the lens and cornea is a smaller chamber which contains a weak salt solution, the *aqueous humor.*

The eyeball is connected to its socket by six muscles. The muscles are responsible for movements of the eyes within the sockets. One has a pulley-like action which permits rotation of the eyeball.

The eye muscles are also responsible for *convergence.* Convergence of the eyes is necessary so that each eye can present a similar picture to the brain. When an object is viewed at close range, the eyes may appear crossed or converged.

The retina

The retina is the light-sensitive area of the eye found on the inner surface at the back of the eyeball. Its sensitivity to light is brought about by the presence of many chemicals which become altered when the light strikes the retina. One of these chemicals, *rhodopsin* (*visual purple*), contains a large amount of vitamin A. If there is a deficiency of this vitamin, vision is im-paired. For this reason, people performing exacting visual tasks at night are often advised to eat a diet abundant in vitamin A, but it is doubtful that this has any beneficial effect in countries with a high standard of living.

The greatest concentration of nerve endings in the retina is found in a particular area called the *fovea*, which is located near the center of the retina. The nerve endings in this area are called *cones* and are responsible for direct vision and detection of both intensity and color of light. Scattered near the fovea and distributed in greater numbers elsewhere in the retina are other types of nerve endings called *rods*. These nerves have little ability to detect color, but are extremely sensitive to light. In daylight, in fact, they are almost unable to operate, but when the light is dimmed, their sensory ability returns (*dark adaptation*). The inability to see in dim light is called *night blindness*. About 30 minutes are required for dark adaptation to reach its maximum. Since only a few of the rods are located in the foveal region, one does not look directly at objects to view them in the dark; instead, the individual looks slightly to the side or just above or below the object.

There are a number of hereditary conditions which may cause an individual to be color-blind. In most instances, the cones of the fovea are operative but do not distinguish colors. The most common type of color blindness is termed "red-green" color blindness. The individual has defective recognition of reds and greens. Rarer types prevent differentiation of other pairs of colors. Total color blindness is the rarest type; the individual can distinguish only shadings of gray and black.

The inheritance of red-green color blindness usually follows a sex-linked pattern. Briefly, the disability appears more frequently in men than in women; although only one girl in 100 will be color-blind, the disability will appear in one out of every ten or twelve boys. The disorder will not appear in a color-blind man's son unless the boy's mother is either color-blind or is a carrier of the gene for color blindness. Consequently, the disorder only rarely is transmitted from father to son. More commonly, color blindness is transmitted from an affected man through his daughters (in whom the condition usually is not expressed) to about one half of his grandsons. (For additional details regarding the inheritance of physical characteristics, see Chapter 1, "Life Begins: *Heredity.*")

The types of color blindness other than red-green color blindness may be either inherited or acquired. In some instances, at least, total color blindness and pastel-shade blindness are thought to be inherited; the mode of inheritance is not known. Color blindness can be caused by disease or injury of the retina, the optic nerve, or the conduction paths of the eye to the brain.

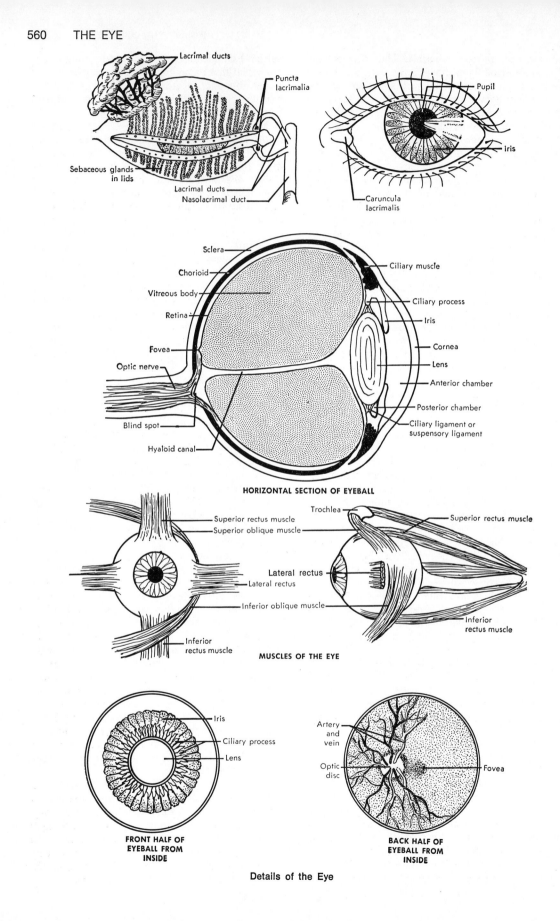

HORIZONTAL SECTION OF EYEBALL

MUSCLES OF THE EYE

**FRONT HALF OF
EYEBALL FROM
INSIDE**

**BACK HALF OF
EYEBALL FROM
INSIDE**

Details of the Eye

Corneal Transplantation

The eight illustrations below show important steps in the surgical process of grafting a new cornea into a human eye. There are believed to be thousands of persons in the United States who might be helped by such an operation, and yet they constitute only a small fraction of the blind, and only a portion of those who suffer from corneal opacity. This miracle of modern surgery is only practical in certain cases where the "window" to the eye has become opaque and the other working parts of the eye are in good functioning condition. When a large area of the cornea is opaque, when the opacity is too dense, or when there is accompanying pressure within the eyeball, the operation probably will not be successful. The operation can only be performed in places where eye surgeons trained in this technique are available, and where the facilites have been provided for obtaining the cornea to be transplanted. One of the major problems in this procedure is in obtaining suitable eyes. Individuals who are about to die, or who will have an eye surgically removed for some reason other than corneal opacity, may donate their eyes for this purpose. Previous ar-

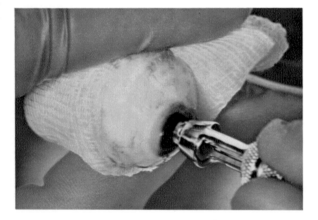

1. The corneal area to be used in the transplantation is removed from the eye of the donor with a *Paton Trephine*, after which it may be stored for up to two days.

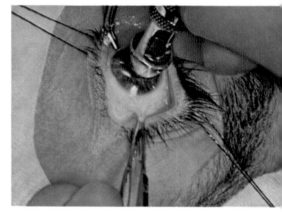

2. In the operation proper, the corneal area to be removed is outlined with a trephine to insure its proper removal. The lids are held back by means of sutures

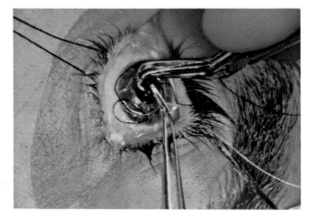

5. The old cornea may now be cut away from under these bridging sutures with an exceedingly delicate pair of special surgical scissors.

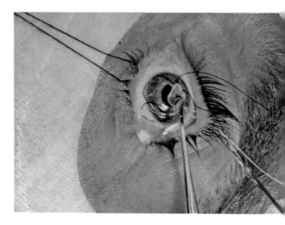

6. The surgeon cuts carefully along the stained area so that the aperture will exactly fit the new cornea, and so that no overlapping or unevenness can possibly result.

rangements must be made, and the eyes should not be offered in the donor's will, since they would be worthless by the time the will is probated. The eye must be sent immediately to a hospital where the cornea may be removed from it. This removal, as well as all subsequent surgical procedures, must be performed under aseptic conditions.

Five to eight days following operation the delicate bridging sutures may be removed from the eye, since the operation, if successful, will have resulted in a union of the transplanted cornea with the surrounding tissues. In most cases, the vision of the patient will have been improved appreciably, and it may even be restored to normal. A considerable stimulus to the success of this operation resulted from the establishment of the Eye Bank for Sight Restoration, Inc., which has been able te establish means by which suitable corneas may be made available and kept until needed. Cooperation in this work by the airlines, the American Red Cross, hospitals, and other agencies has been necessary in order to insure a supply of the needed corneas. These pictures have been reproduced from "What's New" by permission of the Abbott Laboratories, North Chicago, Illinois, by whom they are copyrighted (1947). Material in "What's New" was obtained through the permission and cooperation of the officers and medical staff of the Eye Bank for Sight Restoration, Inc., New York City, New York. The photography is by Sarra, Inc.

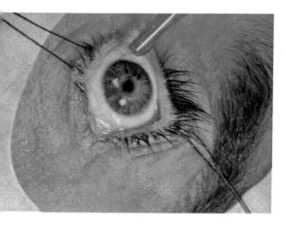

3. The dye *fluorescein* is now dropped into the eye to detail clearly to the surgeon the area to be removed, in order to insure that the new cornea will fit properly.

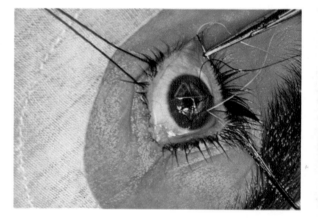

4. Bridging sutures are now placed into the patient's eye. These are to hold the new cornea in place after it is inserted into the orifice, in a later step in the operation.

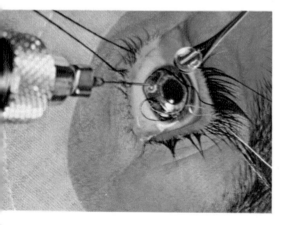

. The old cornea is discarded and a drop of sterile atropine is placed into the anterior chamber of the eye in order to prepare it better for the ensuing step.

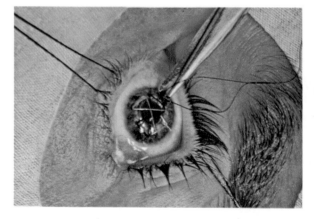

8. The new cornea is then inserted into place, the bridging sutures tightened, and excess threads removed. Operation takes about twenty minutes for its completion.

DISORDERS OF THE EYE: CONJUNCTIVA, EYELIDS, AND LACRIMAL GLANDS

The delicate membrane covering the visible surface of the eyeball (except for the cornea) is called the *conjunctiva*. This membrane also folds back onto the inner surfaces of the lid. Reddened or "bloodshot" eyes are caused by increased vascularity in the conjunctiva. However, the blood vessels of the conjunctiva are also readily apparent in the normal eye. The conjunctiva and eyelids are prone to infection and irritation more than many of the other eye structures because they are exposed to the atmosphere.

Conjunctiva

Conjunctivitis is the general term given to any inflammation or infection of the conjunctiva. This condition has innumerable causes and constitutes the most common eye disease of the Western Hemisphere. Most cases are caused by bacterial or viral infection. However, allergy, chemical irritation, and infection by fungus or parasites are sometimes responsible.

"Pink-eye" (*acute catarrhal conjunctivitis*) is a term rather loosely applied to inflammations of the conjunctiva in children, although adults are also susceptible. Pink-eye is sometimes associated with irritation from smoke, dust, wind, or intense light, as from electric arcs.

In the acute, highly contagious form of pink-eye, the eyes are red and watery at first. Then pus begins to accumulate. The eyelids may smart, burn, or itch, and become stuck together overnight by the discharge. General swelling and puffiness often surround the eyes.

Pink-eye usually represents an infection of the conjunctiva by pneumococci or staphylococci, but occasionally the Kochs-Weeks bacillus is responsible. Because the cornea can become involved in certain epidemic forms of this disease, medical attention should be sought whenever an eye is persistently or acutely inflamed. A physician's care is also important because occasionally what seem to be the symptoms of conjunctivitis actually mask more serious eye disease.

If pink-eye is diagnosed, scrupulous care must be exercised to avoid transmitting the disease to others (or to the opposite eye, if only one eye is affected). For this reason, isolation of the patient is usually advised. The hands must be washed thoroughly and frequently. Towels, washcloths, handkerchiefs, and pillowcases should be laundered daily. The eyes should be gently cleansed according to the physician's instructions, to keep them free of discharge. He may also prescribe antimicrobial preparations, alone or with steroid compounds, for the patient to apply to the eyes several times a day, to shorten the course of the disease. Protection from strong light may be required for the comfort of the patient. Promptly treated, conjunctivitis usually responds readily to therapy and causes no permanent eye damage.

Ophthalmia neonatorum is the term applied to any inflammation of the conjunctiva in newborn infants. The condition is acquired by contact with an infected birth canal during delivery of the infant. *Gonococcus* is usually the infecting organism, but other organisms are sometimes responsible. Most states now require the routine use of preventive measures in the delivery room. In most hospitals, two drops of a 1 percent silver nitrate solution are instilled into each of the infant's eyes at birth. Because even this weak solution sometimes causes a mild chemical conjunctivitis, many ophthalmologists now suggest that penicillin be substituted. Others favor the continued use of silver nitrate to avoid the possible emergence of penicillin-resistant strains of bacteria in hospital nurseries. The use of such preventive measures at birth has enormously reduced the incidence of eye damage and blindness resulting from ophthalmia neonatorum.

Trachoma, an eye disease which has an incidence approaching that of the common cold in some areas of the world, is a severe form of viral conjunctivitis. Because it occurs primarily under conditions of overcrowding and poor hygiene, it is rare in the United States. It occurs sporadically among certain of the American Indians. This condition is characterized by large, clear "granulations" underneath the eyelids. Without sulfonamide or other antibiotic treatment, trachoma eventually produces corneal damage and moderate to complete visual loss. Vaccines are being developed, and improved sanitation and modern drug therapy are lowering the world-wide incidence of trachoma.

Pinguecula is a yellowish nodule of tissue which appears gradually on the conjunctivas of both eyes in some persons. These nodules are usually located on the nasal side of the iris and are fairly common among persons over 35 years of age. The nodules consist of hyaline and elastic tissue. Generally no treatment is necessary.

Eyelids

Hordeolum (sty) is a common infection of one or more of the small glands of the eyelids, usually caused by staphylococci. Children are especially susceptible. A sty begins as a small reddened area on the margin of the lid. Pain is almost always present and is directly related to the amount of swelling. In severe cases, the entire eyelid is swollen. A few days after its appearance, the sty develops a yellow center, caused by the formation of pus, and usually erupts a few days later. A single sty may not require medical attention unless it is quite painful. Warm compresses are helpful. The physician may evacuate the sty and prescribe ointments to prevent further spread of infection. When a number of sties appear, or when they recur often, general health and diet should be evaluated.

Chalazion is a swelling or enlargement of one of the oil glands of the eyelid, caused by obstruction of its duct. Ordinarily the symptoms of chalazion are minimal, except that the individual feels or sees a slow-growing, round lump in the lid. The skin moves loosely over the swelling. Occasionally a chalazion disappears spontaneously or with the use of hot compresses. The physician may prescribe topical medication to alleviate the condition. If these measures fail, a simple surgical procedure is performed which removes the mass, leaving no visible scar.

Blepharitis is a relatively common condition in which the margins of both eyelids become red and inflamed. Blepharitis can be caused by bacterial infection or it may be an extension of seborrheic dermatitis (see page 260) involving the scalp, eyebrows, and at times the ears. The symptoms vary widely among individuals, from mild to severe. Blepharitis may produce only redness and slight crusting, or it may produce itching, burning, edema of the eyelids, falling out of lashes, lacrimation, and hypersensitivity to light *(photophobia)*. The lids often become stuck together overnight from the accumulation of dried secretions.

The physician usually prescribes ointments containing antibiotics if infection is present. Hot compresses are helpful in the acute stage. The lids should be kept free of scales and crusts with a damp cotton applicator. If the blepharitis is of the seborrheic type, the treatment is similar but additional attention is given to cleanliness of the scalp and eyebrows. Unless the seborrheic process is halted elsewhere, the blepharitis cannot be controlled. Frequently staphylococcic blepharitis occurs in association with seborrheic blepharitis.

Ptosis is a condition in which one or both upper eyelids droop. Ptosis is caused by failure of the levator muscles of the eyelid to operate properly. This abnormality may be congenital or acquired. Congenital ptosis, when severe, is treated by surgical alteration of the involved muscles. In acquired ptosis, the underlying cause of the muscle paralysis must be determined and dealt with.

Edema (swelling of the tissues with fluid) of the eyelids is usually the result of allergies to eyedrops, drugs, or cosmetics. Trichinosis—the disease caused by eating contaminated pork— can also produce eyelid edema, but other systemic symptoms are also present.

Lacrimal apparatus

The lacrimal glands produce tears for the lubrication and protection of the eye. The nasolacrimal duct is the passage which conveys excess tears from the lacrimal sac into the nasal cavity. When this duct becomes obstructed for some reason, infection of the tear-producing sac is likely. Infection of the lacrimal sac is called *dacryocystitis*.

Dacryocystitis appears most often in infants and in adults over 40 years of age. In acute cases, pain and fever may be present, with redness and edema around the visible portion of the infected eye. The secretions which cannot drain through the obstructed duct spill back out through the eye. Medical care should be sought to avoid such complications as infection of the cornea.

DISORDERS OF THE EYE: CORNEA

The cornea is the tough, transparent window which covers the iris and pupil. It protects the eye and acts as a "magnifying glass." If it becomes opaque, particularly in the center, vision is impaired, if not destroyed completely. Disease or injury of the cornea is almost always accompanied by severe eye pain. Hypersensitivity to light *(photophobia)* is another common warning signal of corneal disease.

Corneal ulcer

Corneal ulcer is, as it states, an ulcer of the cornea. It usually starts as a small, gray area of localized *necrosis* (tissue death). Corneal ulcer is considered a medical emergency because of its tendency to widen and deepen rapidly, until much of the cornea is destroyed. Causes of this condition include trauma (usually a foreign body in the eye), infection, and allergy. The most common infectious agent responsible for corneal ulcer is the herpes simplex virus. Characteristic symptoms are reddened eyes, discharge and lacrimation, pain, blurred vision, and photophobia, but individual symptoms vary considerably.

Immediate medical attention is imperative. Infections are treated with specific antibiotic therapy, and steroid compounds are often prescribed in addition to such supportive measures as hot compresses and eye patches.

Keratitis

Medical dictionaries list over 30 different types of *keratitis,* but all represent inflammation of the cornea caused by infection, trauma, or chemical irritation.

Interstitial keratitis is an inflammation of the deep layers of the cornea. It occurs most commonly among children afflicted with congenital syphilis, and appears between the ages of 5 and 15. The cornea becomes progressively grayish and opaque. Eventually both eyes are usually involved. If drug therapy fails, corneal transplantation may be considered in suitable cases.

Industrial keratitis takes many forms. Almost always, the source of inflammation is physical trauma or chemical irritation. Reaper's keratitis, for example, is produced when the cornea is wounded by the awn of some grain. Oystershucker's keratitis is caused by fragments of oyster shell which have entered the cornea. Workers in artificial silk manufacture are susceptible to still another type.

Keratopathy

Deterioration of the cornea with aging or in the presence of other eye disease may produce outgrowths of hyaline tissue on the back surface of the cornea. These transparent growths interfere with vision by scattering incident light. The condition is called *guttate keratopathy*. The cornea may also develop blisters on its front surface (*bullous keratopathy*) which interfere with vision and may be very painful.

Corneal Transplantation

In recent years, surgical techniques have been perfected for the replacement of all or part of a diseased human cornea by a corresponding segment of a clear human cornea obtained from another individual. Perfection of the methods of corneal transplantation has brought new hope to victims of corneal diseases. The patient has an excellent chance of regaining his vision through this procedure, provided his particular condition is one that can be corrected by the operation. One of the more common is the restoration of transparency to a cornea which has been scarred by injury or burn.

For the corneal transplant to be successful in restoring sight, the other parts of the eye must be in good condition. In addition, the eye must be free of infection. If there is an increased pressure from the fluids within the eye (*glaucoma*), the chances for success are decreased. In many cases, however, glaucoma will respond to treatment, thus permitting the surgeon to carry out the transplantation. In instances where the entire cornea has become opaque and blood vessels have established themselves in the corneal tissue, or in infants with opacity of the cornea, operation is less likely to succeed. The diverse conditions which can cause the cornea to lose its transparency require the careful evaluation of an ophthalmologist before transplantation is undertaken. The percentage of successful transplants is constantly increasing. However, it is highest in those conditions which do not require grafts extending all the way to the outer edges of the cornea.

Eye banks

Because of the difficulties of acquiring healthy corneas for transplantation when needed by patients with corneal diseases, *eye banks* have been set up. A person wishing to donate his eyes immediately after his death for the purpose of corneal transplantation should notify an eye bank, either personally or through his physician. He will be given a membership card to carry, and in the event of his sudden death, this will ensure that his wishes are carried out. In some states, permission to use the eyes of a recently deceased individual may be granted along with autopsy permission by the next of kin. Most hospitals also have simple release forms, which may be signed by the patient and his relatives during a period of hospitalization. Because this is not the most psychologically auspicious time for such a commitment, however, prior membership in an eye bank, while one is in good health, is preferable.

A donor should not will his eyes to the eye bank. This requires a probate of the will in court, with the result that so much time elapses that the eyes are no longer of medical value. Donor eyes must be removed shortly after death by sterile surgical technique and stored under certain prescribed conditions.

The ideal donor eye for a corneal transplantation comes from an adult 25 to 35 years of age who has just died of acute injury or disease. Eyes from donors of all ages are usable, as long as the corneas are healthy and clear. The entire eye is removed promptly on the death of the donor, after which it is carefully prepared and delivered to the eye bank. Here, the eye is tested for defects in the cornea and is preserved in completely sterile condition. The fresh cornea must then be used for transplantation within hours or days, unless special preparations are made for longer-term storage.

In recent years, a method has been devised by which donor corneas can be frozen for long periods of time without apparent damage of any kind to the corneal tissue. In transplantation operations using corneas frozen by this method, the results have been as good as those obtained by the use of fresh corneas. The new freezing process may greatly expand the scope of corneal surgical procedures, for it allows maximum utilization of donor eyes and removes the present limitations in scheduling transplantation operations for the recipients. The storage technique involves thorough preparation of re-

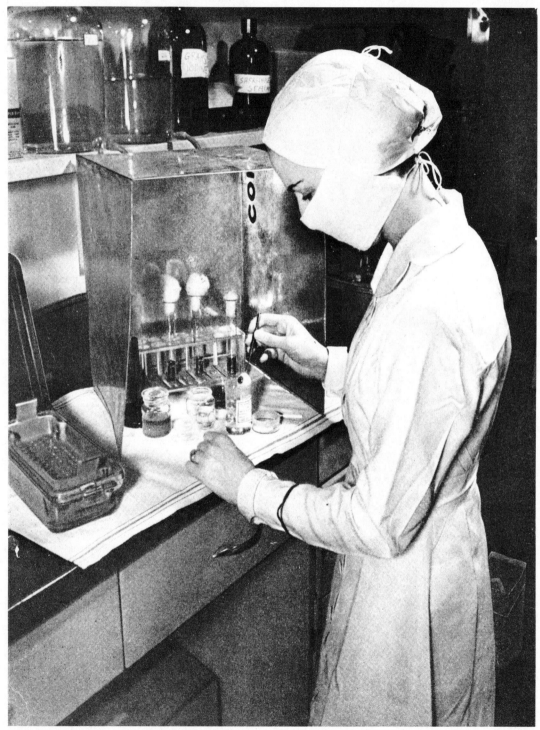

When the eye from a donor is received at the eye bank, it is promptly transferred through an antiseptic solution and then placed into a moist chamber for preservation. Each eye that is used is carefully checked for sterility.

cently removed donor eyes in several protective solutions, then freezing them in liquid nitrogen at −196° C. Other means of storing corneas for extended periods have been attempted (such as dehydration) but the consequent alterations in the corneal tissue have limited their usefulness.

Considerable research is being performed on the development of artificial corneas, but the work is still largely in the experimental stage. These artificial corneas, composed of such substances as clear silicone rubber and synthetic polymers, have been tried in a selected number of patients unable to benefit by conventional corneal transplantations. Many have been given useful vision for some time. One of the chief limitations of the artificial corneas developed to date is that the eye eventually rejects the foreign substance, which lacks the properties of living tissue.

DISORDERS OF THE EYE: LENS, IRIS, AND RETINA

Other diseases of the eye which the ophthalmologist encounters with some frequency involve the lens, the iris, and the retina. Cataract of the lens is perhaps the best known of these. The lens lies just behind the iris. The retina, which coats the inner surface of the eyeball, receives visual stimuli focused upon it by the lens, and transmits images to the brain via the optic nerve.

Lens

A *cataract* is a cloudy or opaque discoloration of the lens of the eye. It may not hamper vision noticeably, or it may cause almost complete blindness. The extent of visual loss depends upon the density of the cataract.

Senile cataract, by far the most common type, affects most persons over the age of 60 to some degree. However, clouding of the lens is usually so mild that most individuals are never bothered appreciably. Senile cataract, when present, generally involves both eyes. The characteristic gray or white appearance of the pupil which is ordinarily evident in advanced cataract may be difficult to detect in the aged because they tend to have small pupils.

There are numerous other causes for cataract formation. Cataracts may be congenital in origin, appearing at birth or during early life. They can result from physical injury or severe irritation of the eye. Less commonly, they may occur as a complication of some systemic disorder, such as diabetes, circulatory disease, or certain skin diseases. Some drugs can also produce cataract. The primary symptom is painless, progressive impairment of vision.

Whether a cataract should be removed depends mainly upon the extent of visual loss. When both eyes are involved, surgical procedure is sometimes performed on only one eye at a time, to avoid a long period of total blindness. Before operation, the eyes are thoroughly examined for other disorders. Complete medical tests are often performed to detect possible disease elsewhere in the body. Although most patients are apprehensive about eye operations, cataract removal by a competent eye surgeon carries little risk of failure. The history of cataract extraction dates back to antiquity. A basic surgical technique still widely used today was first developed in 1745.

A recent development in cataract extraction involves the use of an enzyme to dislocate the lens in its capsule. This method is of particular value in the young adult with a strong zonule.

Cryosurgery is coming into increasing use for cataract extraction. This recently perfected operative technique *(cryoextraction)* involves the use of surgical instruments cooled to subzero temperatures. The principle is this: A supercooled metal probe is inserted into the diseased lens, so that the tissue of the lens forms an iceball at the point of contact. Thus, the probe and the lens tissue adhere to one another. As the probe is withdrawn by the surgeon, the entire lens of the eye and its enclosing capsule share the forces of extraction with the probe. In effect, all are removed as a single entity. The advantage of cryoextraction is that removal of the entire lens is easier, and the capsule of the lens is less likely to tear—as it sometimes does in conventional methods.

Cataract extraction improves vision significantly in almost all patients who undergo surgery. After a suitable period of convalescence usually about six weeks, the eye can be fitted with a contact lens which performs much of the function previously served by the lens of the eye.

Iris

Aside from certain congenital malformations of the iris, *iritis* is the most common condition affecting this structure of the eye. Iritis is an acute or chronic inflammation of the iris, due to any of a variety of causes. When the ciliary body, which lies behind the iris, is also involved, the condition is called *iridocyclitis.*

In iritis, the iris looks muddy, dull, and swollen. Symptoms usually include throbbing eye pain, blurred vision, photophobia, and sometimes swelling of the upper lid. Prompt medical care is essential because of the danger of secondary glaucoma ending in blindness. The physician usually prescribes atropine drops to keep the pupil dilated and adrenocorticoid steroids to shorten the course of the disease. When the

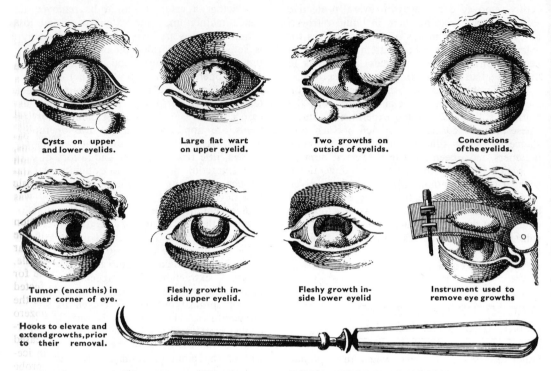

Cysts on upper and lower eyelids.

Large flat wart on upper eyelid.

Two growths on outside of eyelids.

Concretions of the eyelids.

Tumor (encanthis) in inner corner of eye.

Fleshy growth inside upper eyelid.

Fleshy growth inside lower eyelid

Instrument used to remove eye growths

Hooks to elevate and extend growths, prior to their removal.

EYE DISORDERS ILLUSTRATED BY AN EIGHTEENTH CENTURY SURGEON

Various eye disorders and surgical instruments, as illustrated in a monograph by Dr. Laurence Heister, published in 1745. This book, "A General System of Surgery," was one of the best illustrated surgical volumes of the time. *Courtesy Universiteits-Bibliotheek, Amsterdam.*

cause of the iritis can be determined, specific measures are directed at its removal.

Retina

The retina, which makes up most of the inner surface of the eyeball, actually consists of two loosely joined layers: the sensory layer, which receives visual stimuli, and below that, the pigment layer. The pigment layer is attached to the underlying choroid coat. When the sensory layer of the retina separates from the pigment layer, *retinal detachment* is said to occur. Retinal detachment may occur as a complication of some disease, it may result from injury to the eye, or its cause may be undetermined. Older persons with nearsighted eyes appear somewhat more susceptible to retinal detachment.

The detachment is partial at first, but without medical attention almost always becomes complete, resulting in total and permanent blindness in the affected eye. At first, the patient may "see" flashes of light. Then he may have the sensation of a curtain gradually moving across the eye. The field of vision becomes progressively cloudy, until vision is lost. The progressive nature of retinal detachment is due to the gradual seepage of fluid from the large vitreous cavity into the space between the two layers of the retina. As more fluid seeps through the original hole or tear in the retina, more of the sensory layer of the retina is separated from the pigment layer, until the detachment is complete.

Retinal detachment is usually treated by immobilization of the patient in bed and surgical closure of any breaks in the retina. Diathermy and cryosurgery are two commonly employed methods of reattaching the retina to the choroid coat. In either case, the principle applied by the surgeon is that the choroid coat and retina are irritated at the site of the break by heat or extreme cold so that an area of artificial inflammation is produced. A scar then forms which seals the break in the retina. Cryosurgery is considered superior to diathermy by many ophthalmologists. A supercooled probe (−70° C) causes a smaller area of damage and renders the operation less hazardous. In addition, the minimal scar formation in cryosurgery makes reoperation easier if it becomes necessary. Ultimately, cryosurgery may replace diathermy in the treatment for retinal detachment.

Experimental work with photocoagulation also shows promise in treatment for retinal detachment. By this method, an intense beam of light is projected through the pupil onto the tear, causing a reaction of the tissues, which then seals the hole. This may become an important

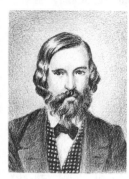

GRAEFE, Friedrich W. E. A. von (1828-1870) introduced iridectomy for treating glaucoma, iritis, and iridochoroiditis, and devised an operation for strabismus. Later diagnoses of ocular paralysis, sympathetic ophthalmia, and karatoconus were made easier and more accurate on the basis of his classic descriptions of their natures and symptoms. He is responsible for Graef's sign of exophthalmic goiter, and early noted the effect of cerebral disorders on vision.

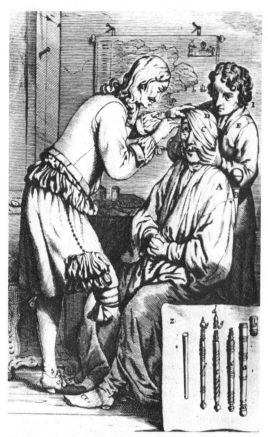

Eighteenth century engraving which portrays an operation for cataract, showing in the lower right corner the medical instruments which were employed during that period. *Bettmann Archive.*

medical application of the laser beam, which already has been employed by medical researchers for retinal detachment, with some success.

Retinitis is inflammation or edema of the retina which is often associated with inflammation of the choroid coat. Distortion and blurring of vision are common symptoms, along with a general sensation of eye discomfort. Prompt medical care is important in this as in other eye conditions, to avoid serious complications.

OTHER DISORDERS OF THE EYE

The eye is susceptible to other disorders not necessarily restricted to particular ocular structures. They may affect the eye as a whole or its muscular function. These widely disparate conditions are discussed below.

Glaucoma

Glaucoma is an increase of pressure within the eyeball. It is caused by an inability to eliminate, at an adequate rate, fluid produced by the ciliary body of the eye. As the pressure within the eye rises, the blood supply to the optic nerve is hampered and vision is reduced. Damage to the optic nerve is irreversible.

Glaucoma is a leading cause of blindness in persons over 40 years of age, tending to occur in members of the same family. In the United States alone, two million people are estimated to have glaucoma—and, of these, about half are undetected cases.

The disease has many causes, some of them unknown. In *acute glaucoma,* the increase of pressure in the eye occurs over a short period of time. The patient experiences extreme pain and blurring of vision. The eye looks red and the cornea steamy. Other symptoms include nausea, vomiting, and headache. Untreated acute

glaucoma can cause complete and permanent blindness within three to five days.

Chronic glaucoma, which may take years to develop, is many times more common. Few symptoms are present in the early stages of the disease. Gradual loss of peripheral vision over several years may be the only manifestation. Central visual fields are affected only late in the disease. When early symptoms are present, the patient often complains of vague disturbances such as seeing haloes around electric lights, finding increased difficulty seeing in the dark, or having mild headaches.

Glaucoma is most effectively treated when discovered early. For this reason, many ophthalmologists recommend that a complete physical examination of anyone over 40 include measurement of intraocular pressure. This is done with an instrument called a *tonometer.* The tonometer is a simple device with a footplate which rests gently on the cornea (after administration of a local anesthetic) and accurately gauges the pres-

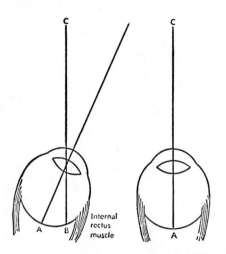

In "cross-eyes" the eye muscles do not properly align the eyes and cause object C to be focused at point B in the left eye rather than on the fovea A. Since different points are stimulated, abnormal vision results, although most cross-eyed persons suppress the image from the deviating eye.

sure within the eyeball. Early diagnosis of unsuspected cases by tonometry and adequate control measures thereafter usually preserve useful vision throughout life. Without treatment, or with late treatment, glaucoma is likely to cause blindness.

Glaucoma can often be controlled by medication. If this fails, a surgical procedure (iridectomy) is performed to relieve the pressure.

Strabismus

Normal *binocular vision* is the ability of each eye to look at the same point in distance. It is the result of balanced muscular co-ordination, allowing proper convergence of the eyes to take place. When one eye cannot achieve binocular vision with the other because it deviates inward ("cross-eyes"), outward ("wall-eyes"), upward, or downward, *strabismus* is said to be present. Strabismus may be caused by paralysis of one or more ocular muscles or by congenital imbalance of the muscles.

About one in 20 children is born with, or develops, strabismus of some degree. What frequently happens is that these children initially experience *diplopia* (double vision) but soon learn to suppress from conscious awareness the image from the deviating eye. Consequently, *amblyopia* ("lazy eye") prevents the vision from developing in the deviating eye. Because amblyopia due to strabismus occurs in such a high incidence, all preschool children should have a routine examination for visual acuity. Testing is particularly important because the degree of strabismus may be too minor to detect by looking at the child's eyes, but still it may be sufficient to cause amblyopia.

Amblyopia detected at the age of one year can often be cured by patching the strong eye for one week and forcing the "lazy" eye to work. By the age of six, a full year may be required to equalize the visual acuity of both eyes.

In treating children who have strabismus, the goal of the ophthalmologist is to achieve good vision in each eye, to co-ordinate the muscular activity of both eyes, and to "straighten" the eyes for cosmetic and psychological reasons. Strabismus may be treated with eye exercises, special glasses, or, if other methods fail, by surgical correction of the muscular imbalance. Operation usually involves shortening or lengthening one or more of the eye muscles. With present-day operative techniques, the child can generally leave the hospital within a day or two after operation and the eyes need not be covered.

The eye muscles, or the nerves which supply them, may also be affected by disorders which arise later in life. Double vision resulting from muscular imbalance frequently occurs after head injuries, stroke or other brain disease, tumor formation in an eye, and in diabetes. The occurrence of double vision should always be investigated by a physician to determine its cause. Correction of the condition varies from treatment for its cause by surgery, eye exercises, and proper glasses.

Exophthalmos

Exophthalmos is an abnormal protrusion of one or both eyes. It gives the individual a wide-eyed, staring expression. When both eyes are involved, thyroid disease is usually responsible. When only one eye is affected, some form of eye disease is more likely. Exophthalmos may be caused by injury, tumors, inflammation, edema, infection, or glaucoma. It is managed by attempting to remove the underlying problem.

Tumors

Tumors of the eye may be benign or malignant. They can involve outer or inner ocular structures. Although they occur seldom, they deserve special consideration because benign tumors can cause serious eye damage and malignant tumors are a threat to life.

Tumors of the eyelids closely resemble tumors of the skin elsewhere. However, they may interfere with vision and irritate the eyeball by friction or pressure. Tumors which arise within the eyeball may cause increased ocular pressure (glaucoma), bulging of the affected eye from its socket (*exophthalmos*), pain, defects in vision, and other symptoms. In the early stages of tumor growth, the patient may experience no symptoms at all. Thus, a benign or malignant tumor within the eyes is sometimes detected only on routine eye examination.

The two principal types of malignant tumors arising in the eye are *malignant melanoma* and *retinoblastoma*. Melanoma occurs almost exclusively in adults. It is found most often between the ages of 40 and 60 and involves only one eye. Melanoma generally arises in the choroid coat of the eye and is first noticed as a defect in the visual field. Eventually, retinal detachment takes place around the tumor.

Retinoblastoma is probably always a congenitally acquired cancer. It occurs in children under five years of age, usually in one eye but sometimes in both. Occasionally several children in the same family have the condition. It has been known to occur in the offspring of adults who were cured of retinoblastoma in childhood.

Primary malignant tumors are ordinarily treated by removal of the diseased eye, even though useful vision remains in the eye. This radical step is necessary because of the tendency of eye cancers to spread rapidly to other parts of the body. However, some malignant tumors are now amenable to other types of treatment. Benign tumors can be managed more conservatively, with attempts to preserve sight in the affected eye.

In rare cases, secondary tumors of the eye result from the spread of primary cancer elsewhere in the body. These metastatic eye tumors are most often associated with breast cancer. Treatment is directed first to control the primary tumor.

Secondary eye diseases

Degeneration of one or more of the structures of the eye may take place as an indirect result of other conditions. Vision may be impaired when the blood supply to the eye diminishes, as for example, in hardening of the arteries. High blood pressure sometimes causes hemorrhages in the retina, with consequent death of small areas of tissue. Multiple sclerosis, diabetes of long standing, brain tumors, meningitis, and other central nervous system diseases sometimes impair or destroy vision. Certain infectious diseases, such as syphilis, can cause blindness. Poisonous substances in the blood may also damage the tissues of the eye. Some of these are wood alcohol, carbon tetrachloride, arsenic, and quinine. Whenever eye damage is a secondary condition, treatment usually begins with attention to the primary cause.

In addition, degeneration of the various parts of the eye is a frequent concomitant of the aging process. The bright colors of the retina which are present in childhood begin to fade as age increases. The lens also undergoes changes, becoming rigid and less movable.

Eye injuries

Severe head injury may cause damage to almost any of the eye structures. Usually symptoms become apparent at once, but sometimes not for days or weeks. Any patient with moderate to severe contusions near the eyes should see an eye doctor to avoid the possibility of permanent damage.

Chemical burns are another common cause of eye damage. Whatever the chemical, the eyes should be washed immediately and thoroughly with large quantities of water. The face should be submerged in a container of tap water and the eyes opened and closed continuously. If a container is not available, the eyes should be opened and closed underneath a running tap.

Subconjunctival hemorrhage, or "red eye," may appear without any apparent cause. However, the accumulation of blood under the conjunctiva usually follows coughing or some exertion. The blood may change in color due to breakdown of blood pigments.

After any trauma to the eyelid area, ecchymosis, known as "black eye" may occur. Blood collects in the tissue, especially of the lower lid and remains for the duration of blood pigment breakdown. The discoloration lasts one to two weeks.

EYE FATIGUE, REFRACTORY DEFECTS, AND GLASSES

"Eyestrain" is a word which, for many years, has been used to signify abuse of the eyes by sustaining some kind of visual activity for too long (such as reading or watching television) or by working in poor illumination. Many ophthalmologists now consider the term "eyestrain" ambiguous from a medical standpoint, since the use of healthy eyes for long hours at almost any activity, even under poor lighting conditions, will not produce irreversible change in the eye. The primary penalties for overuse of the eyes are usually temporary fatigue, tension, or discomfort. Eye fatigue can be hazardous for other reasons, of course—such as increasing the chances of accidents.

Whenever discomfort regularly results from use of the eyes, some underlying condition should be suspected. Headaches, tension, or general eye discomfort associated with normal visual work are an indication that something is probably wrong, and medical attention should be sought. *Refractive error* (nearsightedness, farsightedness, and astigmatism), imbalance of the ocular muscles, or eye disease may be the cause. Reduced vision in one or both eyes also demands an eye examination, especially when the visual loss has been sudden or when glasses which have been obtained relatively recently become less effective.

Effect of lighting on eye fatigue

Proper lighting plays an important role in eye fatigue and work efficiency. Illuminating engineers have carried on extensive research over the years to determine the ideal lighting conditions for schools, homes, and business establishments. Good illumination improves individual performance and comfort, and decreases mistakes and accidents.

Glare of any kind quickly produces fatigue or discomfort in many individuals. High-quality sunglasses can be worn to reduce outdoor glare reflected from shiny or light surfaces such as snow, sand, and water. Indoor glare may result from the use of unshielded light bulbs or improperly placed light sources. This can be avoided by the use of indirect lighting, which casts a bright light upon the ceiling or walls so that the reflection is diffuse. Or, a number of shaded lamps may be placed around the room to create a diffuse light.

A single, strong source of light in a dark room is the least desirable type of illumination. When the work before a person is brightly lit and the background is dark, eye fatigue occurs more quickly. The diffusion of light surrounding the work area should almost equal the light reflected by the work itself. This reduces the constantly changing adaptation of the retina to varying intensities of light, as well as alterations in pupillary size.

The principles of proper illumination and guidelines for the purchase and placement of light fixtures are reviewed in a number of publications. A brochure on the fundamentals of good lighting and illumination requirements for various activities can be obtained at any local electric utility company.

Near- and farsightedness

Ideally, the lens of the eye receives light from the outside and bends it in such a way that an image is resolved upon a small point of the retina. In order to maintain focus on the retina, the lens must change its shape when objects are viewed from different distances. This process is called *accommodation.* For distant vision, the pupil becomes large, the lens becomes flattened, and the amount of *convergence,* or crossing of the eyes, is diminished. Reversal of these processes brings about accommodation for vision at close range.

An individual sees objects because light rays reflected from those objects pass through the cornea and lens of the eye and are brought to a focus upon the retina. The cornea has more than twice the focusing power of the lens. If the cornea-lens combination focuses the rays of light at a point in front of the retina, the person is nearsighted and cannot see distant objects clearly without glasses. If the light rays are focused at a point behind the retina, the person is farsighted. For farsighted persons, distance vision is less strained than near vision, but with normal accommodative power most of them can see both near and far objects clearly. The term "farsighted" is somewhat misleading, although it has become part of popular terminology.

These conditions may arise from structural variations of the eye itself or from disease. A newborn infant is almost always markedly farsighted; and this condition is increased constantly in intensity until about the sixth year. After that the farsightedness decreases until about the twentieth year, after which eyesight normally remains stable for some ten years more. However, many persons retain at least a slight degree of farsightedness. Rarely, farsightedness may be caused by tumor, inflammation of the eyeball, flatness of the cornea, or chemical changes of the fluids within the eyeball. Injury causing a backward displacement of the lens also leads to farsightedness. Absence of the lens causes extreme farsightedness.

Some persons who are farsighted may still be able to see at close range. However, they must exert a great deal of conscious effort to do so. The added effort of this voluntary accommodation for near vision is conducive to eyestrain and may cause the individual to tire rapidly.

Nearsightedness *(myopia)* is the condition in which the individual is able to see objects clearly when they are close to him, but his vision becomes blurred when he looks at distant objects. The condition often goes unrecognized by the

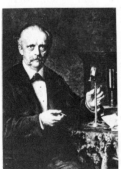

HELMHOLTZ, Hermann L. F. von (1821-1894) German physiologist and physicist. Inventor of the ophthalmoscope. This was a most brilliant gift to ophthalmology for it exposed the inner structure and activity of the living eye. Developer of Young's basic color vision theory, Helmholtz also measured nerve impulse velocity, and proved the muscular source of most animal heat. Acoustics, thermodynamics, and chemistry all received rich contributions from this fertile genius.

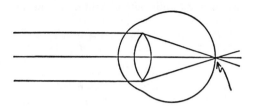

Normal eye. In a normal eye the light rays pass through the cornea and are caused, by the lens, to converge at the point at which the retina occurs.

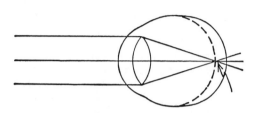

Nearsightedness results when light rays that come from a distance are focused on points which fall in front of the retina, along the broken line.

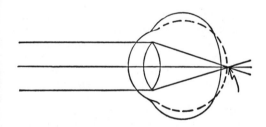

Farsightedness arises when the parallel light rays are made to converge at points beyond the retina, which fall along the indicated broken line.

individual, particularly if he has no need to see clearly at a distance. He apparently assumes that the fuzziness of the visual field is normal. Therefore, unsuspected myopia may be discovered only after routine medical examinations or in vision tests given to applicants for driving licenses.

Nearsightedness has long been known to occur with relatively great frequency among members of certain families; consequently, heredity is recognized as one of the possible causes of the disorder. The exact method of inheritance, however, is unknown. As a rule, the condition first develops during the early school years. By the age of 20, one person in four has developed myopia to some degree. Elderly persons may become myopic and able to read without glasses for the first time in years. This so-called "second sight" almost invariably signals the development of cataracts.

Close work, such as editorial, watch repairing, or bookkeeping work, probably does not lead to myopia. Many authorities believe, however, that myopia may cause the individual unconsciously to choose a profession or a hobby calling for close work.

Myopia is often the result of a slight lengthening of the eyeball and thinning of the fibrous wall. This may be caused by increased pressure of the liquids within the eyeball. Nearsightedness also may result from too great a curvature of the cornea or the lens, or by changes in the lens brought on by advancing age. Temporary myopia may occur because of injury or infection of the eye.

Presbyopea, a decrease in the ability of the eye to accommodate to various distances, is a normal concomitant of the aging process. It is common in persons over 40. Presbyopea also accompanies some disease processes. When accommodation becomes inadequate to focus the eyes at normal reading distances, special lenses such as bifocals or separate reading glasses are required.

Astigmatism

Astigmatism is a common optical defect, but in most cases it is so slight as to go completely unnoticed. It is manifested by a distortion of vision. Thus, in looking at an object, a straight line in the vicinity of the object may appear curved. When the eyes are moved, a motionless object may seem to move as it passes through the distorted area of the field of vision.

Astigmatism can be horizontal, vertical, or diagonal. In most cases, this distortion is so slight as to be detected only by careful examination by the eye specialist (ophthalmologist), and even then may require no correction whatever under normal circumstances. However, the astigmatism can be corrected by special lenses.

The cause of astigmatism usually is associated with the shape of the cornea, the clear part or "window" of the eye in front of the iris and pupil. Normally, the cornea can be pictured as a piece cut off of a round hollow ball or watch crystal. However, the cornea is not truly spherical. It may be slightly flattened horizontally or vertically. These irregularities are largely nullified by a compensating shape of the lens. When the lens fails to compensate properly, noticeable astigmatism results. In a few cases, therefore, astigmatism is caused by the lens rather than the cornea.

Examination for optical defects

When an individual realizes that he is suffering from optical defects, or when he suspects it because of eye fatigue, headaches, or other symptoms, the family physician or ophthalmologist can usually determine the cause of the difficulty.

For a thorough examination, the ophthalmologist may request that the patient undergo *dilation* of the pupils. This procedure is safely carried out by dropping into the eye a solution of certain drugs such as *homatropine, tropicamide,* or *cyclopentate.* These drugs relax the pupil and cause a dilation. In some cases, particularly if the patient is under 25 years of age, the drug should be used preceding the examination.

Dilation of the pupils results in the steady focusing of the eyes, usually at a point infinitely far away. For this reason near objects cannot be seen clearly, unless myopia is present. This impaired vision may last up to a day or two after the examination. In many cases dilation is not necessary.

The ophthalmologist employs a number of devices in examining the eyes. The *ophthalmoscope,* invented in 1851, revolutionized the science of ophthalmology. This small instrument, equipped with a light source, can be held in the hand of the physician. It allows him to examine the interior of the eye. Second in importance only to the ophthalmoscope is the *slit-lamp biomicroscope* combined with the *corneal microscope.* This instrument, too, is provided with a light source, and permits illumination and magnification of the cornea and lens. Many abnormalities can be visualized by the examiner which might otherwise be missed. The *tonometer* is a device for measuring the pressure within the eyeball and is used to diagnose glaucoma. The footplate of the tonometer rests gently on the cornea. A metal plunger in the center holds various small weights by which delicate pressure measurements are taken.

Glasses

The various optical defects usually can be corrected by the use of glasses prescribed by the ophthalmologist. It should be remembered, however, that glasses are corrective only in that they improve the individual's vision. They seldom affect the original cause of the defect or abolish it, unless there is a problem involving alignment of the eyes.

Glasses must be prescribed by the physician on the basis of his findings in the individual's eyes. By exact measuring, he is able to calculate the type of lens which will correct the defect. The patient must take the prescription to a specially trained dispensing *optician.* After receiving the glasses the patient should return to the physician in order that he may check them carefully. Minor errors such as improperly fitting frames may detract from the efficiency of the

glasses, add to difficulty of vision, and aggravate eyestrain.

Because the eyes themselves usually carry out certain processes designed to compensate for the visual defects, proper glasses may be uncomfortable at first and may seem to increase the eyestrain. This temporary discomfort should not cause the patient to discard the glasses. If they have been checked by the physician, such disturbances will clear, usually within a week or two. A patient who does not become accustomed to his glasses might well return to his physician to ascertain the exact cause of the failure.

After the patient has received the prescribed glasses, he must realize that he will have to return later for reexamination. Such a visit is necessary because the eyes are continually changing as a result of aging. In some conditions such as myopia of children, changes in the eye may occur rapidly, so that the patient must return frequently—sometimes as often as every three months.

Unfortunately, many people wait years before having their eyes reexamined. They are compelled to return only after it becomes apparent to them that the glasses are no longer able to give them good vision. Often, the need for a change of glasses will be manifested first, not by visual difficulty, but by eyestrain, headaches, pain in the region of the eyes, nausea, fatigue, etc.

Contact lenses are coming into increased use, especially since the development of the small *corneal lens* which covers only part of the cornea and requires no fluid for insertion. Contact lenses are usually worn for cosmetic reasons or for sports, where ordinary glasses might be broken. Although many individuals can wear these lenses with comfort for most of the day, learning to tolerate them requires considerable motivation. Furthermore, care must be exercised when the lenses are inserted and removed. As more and more individuals choose contact lenses over conventional glasses, ophthalmologists see an increasing number of complications resulting from improper insertion and removal, incorrect fitting, and overuse. Corneal abrasion is the most common of these. An individual who desires contact lenses should put himself in the care of a qualified ophthalmologist.

The necessity for *bifocal glasses* arises from the fact than man-made lenses are not adaptable to different distances, as is the normal lens of the eye. A person requiring a lens of one magnification to see at a distance, may not be able to see close work with the same glasses. In this way smaller lenses of a different appropriate magnification are used, usually at the lower level of the glasses. The individual then looks downward through the "second pair" of glasses when he desires to see clearly at close range. In this way, the extra pair of reading glasses is eliminated. *Trifocal lenses* are helpful in eliminating the blurred area between the point of focus of the distance glasses and the point of focus of the bifocal lens. They are useful in many occupations. Persons with extremely weak eyesight may require telescopic spectacles for distance vision and a very strong bifocal or other magnifying lens for near vision.

Glass Eyes

When for one reason or another it becomes necessary to remove an eyeball, restoration of a suitable cosmetic appearance is generally achieved with a glass or plastic prosthetic device. Although

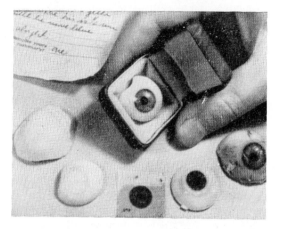

3. Stages in the manufacture include moulding of plastic to shape, sizing and fitting with disc. Coloring matches the natural eye when complete and includes veins.

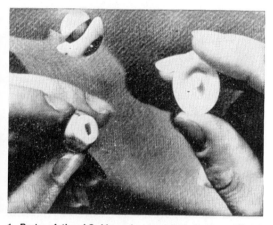

1. Parts of the AO Monoplex eye include an artificial eyeball and removable front shell which attaches with a peg. Eye muscles sutured to mesh provide mobility.

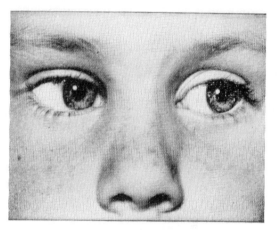

4. This child has been equipped with an artificial movable eye, but it is difficult to determine which one is the artificial replacement. It is the child's right eye.

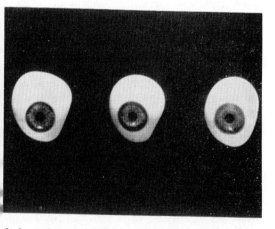

2. A number of standard shapes are provided so that a comfortable fit is obtainable, and so that the iris will normally be in its correct position, relative to the lids.

such replacements have been available for years, a number of mechanical limitations have always kept them from having the appearance of the natural eye. In recent times, great advances have been made in the improvement of eye replacements; at present, it is possible to obtain a "glass" eye that is practically indistinguishable from the natural one that was lost. Improvements include not only the artistry in preparation of the iris and sclera, but means for giving the eye mobility so that it follows its natural mate. This latter advance alone improves the modern product over older types which were difficult to maintain in anything resembling a natural position. At the present time a variety of models is available. Details of one type are shown here by courtesy of the American Optical Company.

Corneal Type Contact Lenses

The corneal type contact lens is a small, thin, smooth, nonirritating plastic lens only a little larger than the pupil of the eye—just about half the size of a dime. It is worn on the front surface of the eye—the cornea—and remains there by adhesion or capillary attraction. Their manufacture is a very precise process, and they must be ground far more exactly than regular glasses. Consequently, they can only be made by skilled specialists. Pictures by courtesy Obrig Laboratories, Inc.

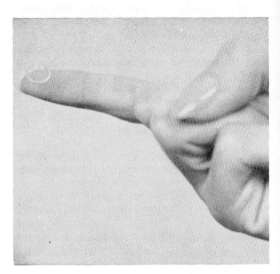

3. The completed lens.

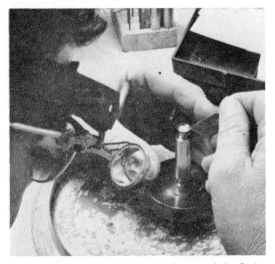

1. Polishing the front surface with pitch and tin oxide. *Photograph by Steinmetz, Sarasota, Florida.*

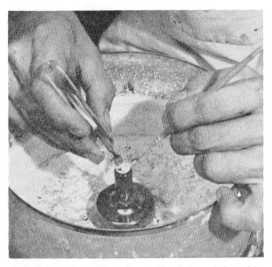

2. Reducing the size of the lens. *Photograph by Steinmetz, Sarasota, Florida.*

THE BLIND: THEIR CARE AND OPPORTUNITIES

Blindness may be caused by any of a number of conditions. Emotional upsets and hysteria may produce temporary blindness. Permanent blindness can be caused by pressure on the optic nerve by tumors, brain damage by skull fracture or loss of adequate blood supply, eye injuries, or certain of the eye diseases discussed previously in this chapter. The inability to see may be complete, although most blind persons are able to perceive at least some light. Depending on the cause, blindness may be permanent or temporary. Only a few years ago most blind persons were considered incurable, but the rapid advances made in medical science in recent decades have brought a more hopeful outlook to many blind persons. At the present time, many cases of blindness which involve the lens, cornea, and sometimes the retina, may be alleviated by surgical methods. Other forms of blindness due to damage to the retina, the optic nerve, or the central nervous system are usually more permanent.

In 1967, there were approximately 426,000 blind persons in the United States; 33,500 of these people became blind that year. Blindness affects all age groups, but most of those so afflicted are elderly, although about 60 percent of the blind are not sightless in the real sense of the word. In some states, a person is considered "industrially blind" when he has a visual acuity of less than 20/200 in his better eye, with properly fitted glasses. These figures mean that the person taking the test for visual acuity can only see at 20 feet what one with normal vision can see at 200 feet. Normal vision is 20/20 vision or better. The test itself consists in determining the size of print the person under observation can see at a fixed distance.

Some persons classified as blind can see clearly, but over only a small area. That is, their vision may be limited to an area approximately the size of that to be seen by looking through the barrel of a gun. Although such a person may be able to read the fine print on a doctor's wall chart, he sees only such a small area that he cannot keep oriented.

Care for the newly blind

Failing, diminished, or lost sight requires the most careful medical consideration. After a thorough examination, a physician will inform the patient and his family of the exact nature of the blindness, and of the probable changes for the better or worse that may be expected in the future. Only with this complete information can the proper arrangements be made for the future life of the afflicted and his family.

When children are born blind, or become blind during infancy, proper early care prepares them for the years ahead. The approach of blindness in some aging persons is so gradual and expected that it does not create the problems that arise when blindness occurs suddenly. But when a person becomes blind within a relatively short period, the gravity of the event may understandably cause severe emotional strain. Both the afflicted and his family may feel socially and economically insecure. Often, it is almost impossible to console such a patient concerning his loss of sight. Courage and determination are greatly needed at such times, and there must be a realistic understanding that blindness is a common affliction and one that need not lead to despair and hopelessness. Indeed, the afflicted person must understand that with edu-

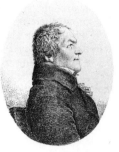

HAUY, Valentin (1745-1822) French teacher of the blind. Moved to begin his life work when he observed the brutal treatment of blind beggars in the Paris streets. In 1784 he founded the first educational institution for blind children at which they were taught to read raised letters embossed on paper, while learning music and trades, as well as formal subjects. His work set a pattern for similar schools founded throughout the world.

cation or reeducation he should be able to pursue an active and productive life. Such a possibility is now readily available to all blind persons. It is no longer necessary for the blind to be economically insecure. In most cases, local organizations for the blind are prepared to send similarly afflicted persons to talk with the newly blind. By discussing the effective manner in which he has solved his problems, the visitor can often convince the newly blind person that life will not be as gloomy as it seems.

With a little experience, the blind are able to carry on normal activities amazingly well. Usually, they do not want sympathy, and when in familiar surroundings, they neither require nor desire unnecessary guidance. The memory and senses of touch and sound become highly developed in the blind and take over many of the normal functions of the eyes. A feeling of independence develops, and there is no cause for undue solicitude on the part of others. As far as is possible, the blind should be treated much like other persons. Consideration must be given, however, to their few limitations.

A blind person will need some guidance when in an unfamiliar room for the first time. If led to a chair, he will seat himself. When led, he should be allowed to take the arm of his guide. He should not be grasped by the arm and pushed

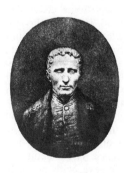

BRAILLE, Louis (1809-1852) French teacher of the blind. When he was but three years of age, Braille was blinded as the result of an accident, but this handicap did not prevent him from becoming one of the world's most famous pioneers in the teaching of the blind to read and perform many other useful occupations. He is most famous for the elevated print system that he perfected in 1837, some years after it had been suggested by Charles Barbier.

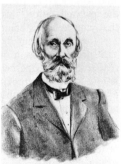

HIPPEL, Arthur von (1841-1917) German ophthalmologist. Provided the technical basis for modern keratoplasty, or corneal transplantation, an eye operation devised to restore the transparency of an opaque or clouded cornea. In 1885 von Hippel transplanted the corneas of lower animals with a successful graft. However, their surfaces shortly became opaque. Later he described a technique producing better results.

or moved about forcibly. When entering a room, a seeing person should speak to any blind individual present. He should also let the blind person know when he is leaving. Doors in the home of a blind person should be left open or shut, as found, since they are remembered by him as being in a certain position. Chairs and other objects should not be moved about. The blind keep their possessions in definite places, and achieve almost complete independence in their homes by so doing.

Education

Proper education can fit the blind to perform many of the activities of normal life. Training is of two kinds: all blind persons must develop certain basic abilities, such as reading, and traveling about in a strange place. The methods of achieving these have been available for some time. Of almost equal importance, however, is education to perform useful work and to participate in other more complex social activities. The most common means by which the blind are enabled to read is the *Braille system*. In the Braille system the letters are represented by various arrangements of dots punched in the paper so that they are elevated above its surface.

Modified slightly since its origin, Braille writing is an almost universal system. Special books, newspapers, and periodicals are now available in Braille. A second form of literature is referred to as *Moon's type*. It consists of raised lines and curves, and is chiefly valuable for the small percentage of persons who do not seem able to learn Braille. Books in Moon's type are both expensive and bulky, and so are rather scarce. Braille literature, by contrast, is available in most public libraries of moderate size. In addition to these methods, phonograph records and tape recordings have been used extensively in bringing education and material to the sightless.

Recent developments in electronics and radar give promise of major changes in reading for the blind. Scanning pencils which are able to pick up ordinary printed letters, just as radar picks up a ship at sea, have recently been developed. In addition, a probe-pin machine which transforms the printed letter, through vibrations, into one that can be felt is being tested. In another device for the "near blind," the letters are picked up and projected on a television-like screen. The reader can then perceive these highly magnified letters a few at a time. One experimental project is a tactile vision substitution system which enables the person to perceive images through his skin.

Traveling about is one of the first and greatest problems causing anxiety for a person who has recently become blind. Self-confidence and determination are among the major factors in the solution of this problem. Most blind persons eventually become adept in feeling their way with a cane. Many say that their sense of hearing is of even greater value than the cane, in this regard. The sounds of people, traffic, and nature may all help in confirming for the individual his location. The reflection of the sound of fast steps or of cane-tapping from some object aids greatly in avoiding collisions. Some sightless persons become so adept at traveling around that people observing them do not recognize them as being blind.

In 1929, a nonprofit organization, The Seeing Eye, was established in the United States for training guide dogs for the blind. The average working life of such a trained dog is about eight years. It is not considered advisable for most blind persons to attempt the use of a guide dog. Persons who profit by this means are those who, aside from being blind, are healthy and in the active years of their lives. The adaptation to a guide dog requires patience and intelligence on the part of the owner, and many blind persons apparently are not emotionally adapted to the use of such a guide.

By proper training, many blind persons are able to engage in sports. Blind persons are frequently able to play games of ball. Bowling is another sport the blind often enjoy. These seeming "impossibilities" are achieved by the extreme sharpening of the other senses after the sight has been lost. In addition to sports, a variety of other hobbies, such as molding, sculpturing, and weaving are open to the blind. Many such persons develop unusual musical abilities and become accomplished musicians on any instrument they may select. Even blind painters are not unknown. Determination and ingenuity have opened almost all of these fields of endeavor to the sightless.

Schools

All 50 states, plus the territories and protectorates, have facilities within their areas, or arrangements can be made with nearby states for education and training of the blind. Many of these schools are of the residential type where the board and tuition are free. Some cities also have day schools for the blind, in which the student attends along with children who are not blind. The success of blind students in both types of schools depends somewhat on the adequacy of their preschool training. Such training may be given at home in some cases, although special nursery schools are sometimes available.

Many public schools have "sight-saving" classes for pupils who are nearly, but not quite blind. The lighting in the classroom is particularly designed to provide easy paper work and reading. The books that are used have large print, and the students' working habits are closely

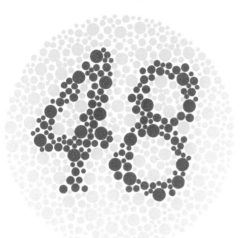

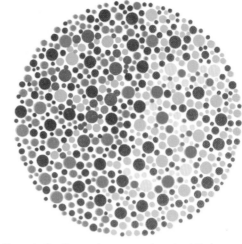

The numeral in this circle may be detected by persons who are either color blind or who have normal vision. To either group, the number is 48.

Some indication as to a person's color blindness may be obtained from this arrangement of colors red, brown, orange and green, to make 95.

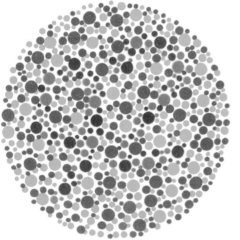

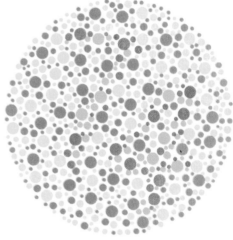

With a test chart made out in brown and red, a person who is not suffering from color blindness will be able to distinguish clearly the number 92.

When orange and yellow are grouped together in the pattern shown here, a person with normal vision should be able to recognize number 74.

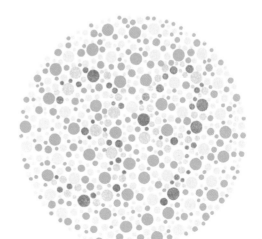

In still other types of color blindness, the number 56, shown here, cannot be distinguished for it is represented in dots composed of blue and violet.

Grouping of colors such as violet and blue makes it difficult for individuals suffering from some types of color blindness to distinguish the number 39.

DVORINE COLOR BLIND TEST. Devised and copyrighted 1944 by Israel Dvorine, O.D.

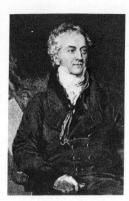

YOUNG, Thomas (1773-1829) English physicist, archeologist and physician. Wrote in 1793 the first description of astigmatism and the process of adjusting the eye for clear sight at differing distances, called the mechanism of accommodation. In 1803 he formulated a correct theory of color vision which was more fully developed later into the Young-Helmholtz theory; and he derived a mathematical formula for determining proper medicinal dosages for children.

supervised by special teachers. These students, too, do much of their recitation work in classes with individuals having normal vision, thus avoiding a feeling of social separation from other children.

Blind students attend most colleges and universities, where they are able to pursue successfully courses in many fields. Such students require someone to assist them in the preparation of their lessons, but this problem is not usually great. Many schools provide scholarships which supply the funds with which to hire assistants, or readers, as they are sometimes known, for blind students. In addition, many private organizations also provide such scholarships. Since 1943, the Federal government has encouraged such spending and furnished a part of the money, which is matched by various states, for this purpose.

Provisions for the training of the adult blind are of great importance in their rehabilitation. Although the blind can perform an amazing variety of types of work, they usually require special training. Most training agencies are closely associated with a program of vocational rehabilitation. At present, all states have training programs and many private agencies within each state which are concerned with these problems. The agencies not only provide training, but attempt to locate blind persons in some gainful employment, as well as to establish workshops where they may find employment. In many cases the training is given in the home of the student and is conducted by another blind person, who is on the staff of the agency.

Finding gainful employment has always been one of the major problems of the sightless. Through the concerted efforts of the various agencies that are concerned with the blind, many blind persons are now employed in this country. The number of positions available increases from year to year. The number of blind people engaged in operating retail businesses increases each year. Individuals who take the necessary

training may even be successful in one of the professions, such as law or teaching.

Many blind persons are not able to establish themselves in a business of their own, just as many people with sight are limited in this manner. In the past, the blind found it necessary to work at some simple craft in their own homes, or in some special workshop for the blind. One of the most important changes in vocational adjustment has been the success in finding employment for the blind in industries which also employ seeing people. There is a growing list of such types of work. Some skilled factory work can be done by the blind with as much efficiency, speed, and safety as by any other worker. In the United States during a single year the list of blind persons who were engaged in new positions included, among others, auto workers, typists, teachers, filling station attendants, carpenters, kitchen workers, and farmers. Other work carried on by the blind included that of the clergy, masseurs, textile weavers, gardeners, watchmen, vending stand operators, and janitors.

Many blind people feel more comfortable when working in public, if their blindness is not obvious. In some cases, when the blindness is due to loss or degeneration of the eye, it is desirable for the person to obtain prosthetic devices which decrease changes in the appearance of the face. Artificial eyes serve this purpose admirably, since they improve the appearance. In many cases agencies for the blind are able to give assistance in the procurement of artificial eyes.

Legal benefits

It has long been recognized that the handicap of blindness is so great that society must undertake certain added responsibilities regarding the afflicted. Special relief funds and pensions were begun by many states, and Federal legislation has provided specified amounts to be matched by the states for aid to the blind. Another Fed-

CHESELDEN, William (1688-1752) English surgeon. He originated the operation of iridotomy for the relief of a certain type of blindness, a contribution to ophthalmic surgery ranking second in importance only to the operation for cataract. He developed lateral lithotomy, another successful surgical method for which he was acclaimed. Serving his surgical skill was a tremendous knowledge of anatomy which he embodied in two books on the subject.

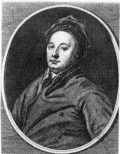

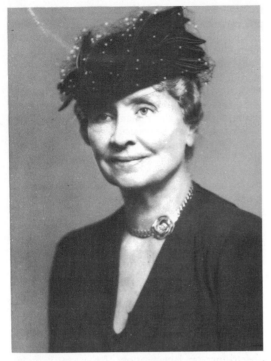

KELLER, Helen Adams (1880-1968) American author and lecturer. Although she became both deaf and blind as the result of illness at the age of 19 months, Miss Keller became famous throughout the world for her conquest of these handicaps and for her work in education of the deaf-blind.

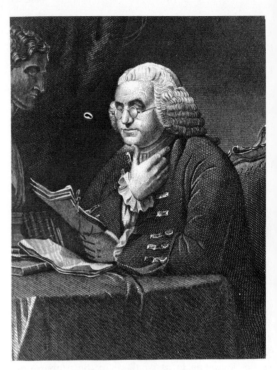

FRANKLIN, Benjamin (1706-1790) American scientist and statesman. Among his many achievements was the invention of bifocal spectacles which permit the wearer to read a book as well as to see objects at a distance. *Bettman Archive.*

eral bill permitted the establishment of vending stands in public buildings to be attended by the blind. The provisions of the Wagner-O'Day Act provide that the Federal government purchase many of its needs from organizations in which the blind are employed. Special exemptions for the blind are made in the federal income taxes.

More recently, the 1967 amendment to the Federal Vocational Rehabilitation Act attempted to aid the blind in reestablishing themselves in productive occupations. By its provisions, the Federal government pays for the cost of administration, vocational guidance, and placement in state programs for the blind. The government pays half of the costs for medical examinations and treatment, training, and living expenses during vocational rehabilitation. Under the provisions of this bill are also included the cost of artificial eyes, tools or equipment, a college education, training in Braille, and capital to set up a business. None of these provisions can be regarded as charity; rather they show a recognition of the special needs of a large group of able and conscientious citizens. With the assistance offered, many blind persons are able to become completely independent.

Public recognition of the handicaps of blindness is seen in many other activities of the state.

Workmen's compensation acts within each state provide a specified sum of money to be paid to persons who lose their sight in the course of employment. Likewise, government pensions are provided for persons who are blinded while in the employment of the Federal government. Many insurance policies provide payments for the loss of sight of one or both eyes.

The multiple handicapped

The problems of blindness are greatly increased when the affliction occurs in combination with some other physical deficiency. Most multiple handicapped persons are afflicted during early life so that treatment of the patient starts early in childhood. Blind persons who are also feebleminded are best cared for in special institutions for such mental infirmity, since their training is extremely difficult. They are seldom able to become self-sufficient. The blind-deaf are best trained in schools for the blind or deaf where many special techniques are now available for their instruction. When proper instruction is available, the blind-deaf often are able to become well integrated in society. Miss Helen Keller was both blind and deaf; yet she became one of the world's most famous and inspired educators.

EDUCATION OF THE BLIND

Each year there is a growing realization that the rehabilitation of the blind must include a great deal more than the learning of a useful trade. To be successful it must restore personal confidence and make the patient self-sufficient in the performance of the ordinary tasks of life. Great success has been achieved in meeting these needs. These photographs show activities in the Blind Rehabilitation Section of the Physical Medicine and Rehabilitation Service, V. A. Hospital, Hines, Illinois. Information from VA Pamphlet 10–32, "A New Approach."

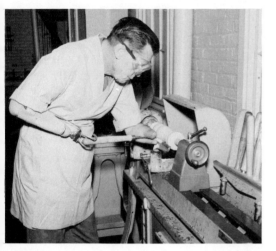

Wood turning is but one of the many useful activities that may be learned by the blind, but it requires a great deal of prior training in methods.

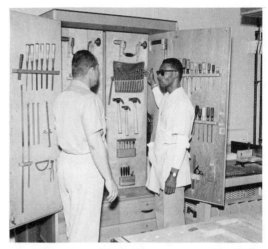

By keeping each item in its proper place, it soon becomes possible for a blind person to locate correctly any tool or device that he may require.

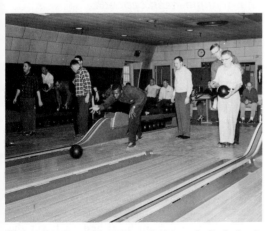

By learning to apply certain principles of physical orientation, the blind are soon able to participate in athletics with a minimum of sighted assistance.

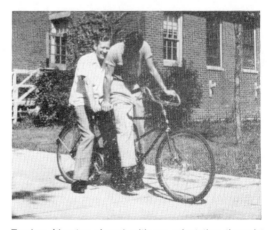

Tandem bicycles shared with an orientation therapist are used in out-of-doors reconditioning and also provide another of the available recreations.

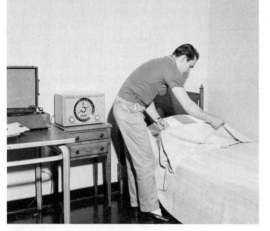

When the blind are provided with a room of their own, it rapidly becomes possible for them to locate necessary items and care for many personal needs.

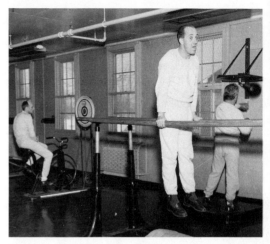

An important part of the rehabilitation of blind persons is the employment of exercise to insure the maintenance of a good physical condition.

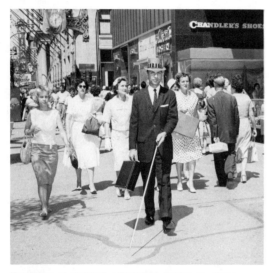

Teaching of physical orientation begins in simple surroundings where techniques are developed for use when travel situations become more complex.

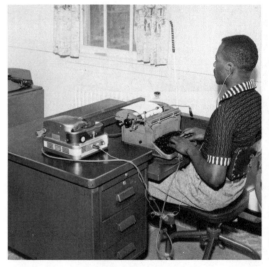

By learning the use of the typewriter, electronic recording equipment, and aids for handwriting, the capabilities of the blind person increase.

18 THE EAR

WHAT IT IS AND DOES

The ear is the organ concerned with the sense of hearing and equilibrium. It consists of three parts. The visible portion is called the *external ear;* the *middle ear* (*tympanic cavity*) is inside the head, just out of sight; the *internal ear* (*labyrinth*) is formed partly of one of the bones of the skull (*temporal bone*). Both the middle ear and the internal ear are essential for transmitting to the hearing center of the brain the vibrations which comprise sound. These vibrations are transmitted to the middle ear through the *external auditory canal.* An accessory part of the ear is the *auditory tube* (*Eustachian tube*), a canal which connects the back of the nose with the middle ear. Its function is to equalize the pressure between that of the middle ear and the external ear.

The external ear

The two parts of the external ear are: the portion most persons refer to as the "ear" (*auricle*), and the auditory canal (*external auditory meatus*), which is the opening leading to the eardrum (*tympanic membrane*).

The auricle, shaped somewhat like a shell, extends from the side of the head. This part of the ear receives sound waves and directs them into the auditory canal. It is composed of strong pliable tissue (*cartilage*), fatty tissue, and muscles, and is covered by skin.

The auditory canal is partly visible to a person looking directly into the ear. Its function is to guide the sound waves from the outside portion of the ear (*auricle*) to the middle ear. The canal is a tube-shaped opening approximately one inch in length. It is lined with fine hairs and small wax-producing glands on the outer half. The skin of the inner half is very thin. The hairs and wax help keep foreign substances out of the ear.

The middle ear

The middle ear (tympanic cavity) resembles a small odd-shaped box, and is located at the inner end of the auditory canal. It is separated from the auditory canal by a thin sheet of tissue, the eardrum (tympanic membrane). A thin wall of bone separates the middle ear from the internal ear. Inside the cavity of the middle ear is a series of small movable bones. They are named according to their shape: the hammer (*malleus*), the anvil (*incus*), and the stirrup (*stapes*). These small bones are connected to one another and stretch from their attachment to the eardrum, at the end of the auditory canal, to the beginning of the internal ear. Sound vibrations coming through the auditory canal are transmitted through the eardrum, across the small bones of the middle ear to the internal ear.

In the back part of the middle ear there is an opening into the porous part of the temporal bone of the skull. This opening leads from the middle ear (tympanic cavity) into the mastoid antrum. It is through this passage and cavity that middle ear infections may pass into the mastoid cells causing the disease known as *mastoiditis.* Through this same passage infectious organisms also may seep inward to the brain. Ear infections of any kind may not only present

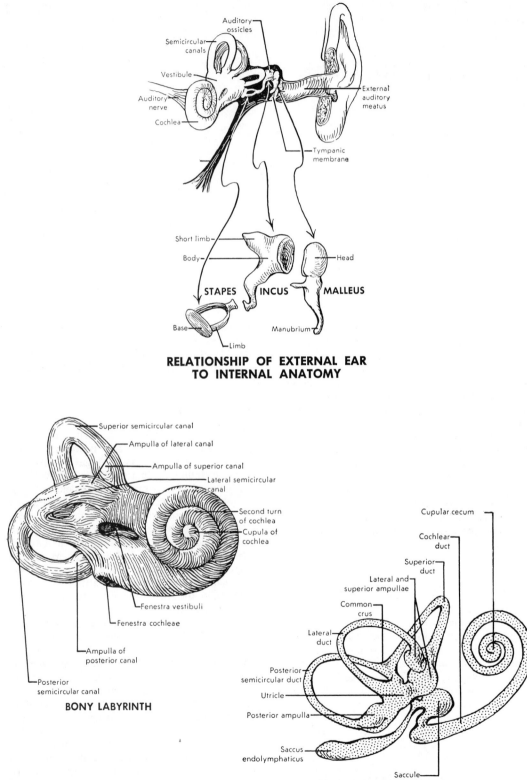

Auditory ossicles

Semicircular canals

Vestibule

Auditory nerve

Cochlea

External auditory meatus

Tympanic membrane

Short limb

Body

Head

STAPES   **INCUS**   **MALLEUS**

Base

Limb

Manubrium

**RELATIONSHIP OF EXTERNAL EAR
TO INTERNAL ANATOMY**

Superior semicircular canal

Ampulla of lateral canal

Ampulla of superior canal

Lateral semicircular canal

Second turn of cochlea

Cupula of cochlea

Fenestra vestibuli

Fenestra cochleae

Ampulla of posterior canal

Posterior semicircular canal

BONY LABYRINTH

Cupular cecum

Cochlear duct

Superior duct

Lateral and superior ampullae

Common crus

Lateral duct

Posterior semicircular duct

Utricle

Posterior ampulla

Saccus endolymphaticus

Saccule

MEMBRANOUS LABYRINTH

Anatomy of the Ear . . . Grace Hewitt

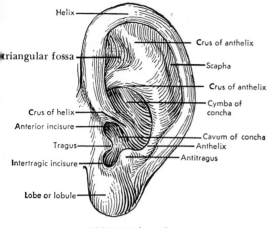

Helix

Crus of anthelix

Triangular fossa

Scapha

Crus of anthelix

Cymba of concha

Crus of helix

Anterior incisure

Cavum of concha

Tragus

Anthelix

Antitragus

Intertragic incisure

Lobe or lobule

EXTERNAL EAR

a hazard to auditory acuity, but they may spread to other critical areas with possibly grave consequences. Prompt attention to ear infections is of great importance.

The internal ear

The last and most essential part of the ear is the inner or internal ear. This portion of the ear is a series of connecting hollows and passages (*bony labyrinth*) in a portion of the temporal bone. This bony labyrinth encloses a much smaller *membranous labyrinth*, which follows its contour and is connected to the outer bony structure by fibrous strands. The space between this inner labyrinth and the surrounding bone is filled with a fluid, *perilymph*. The membranous labyrinth itself is filled with *endolymph*.

The three components of the bony labyrinth are named according to their shapes: the *vestibule*, the *cochlea* (from the Latin word for "snail shell"), and the *semicircular canals*. Of these, only the cochlea is involved with hearing;

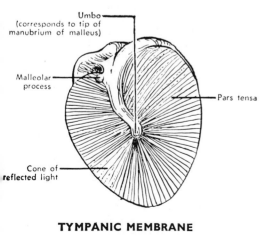

Umbo
(corresponds to tip of manubrium of malleus)

Malleolar process

Pars tensa

Cone of reflected light

TYMPANIC MEMBRANE

the others are essential to equilibrium and bodily orientation.

The *vestibule*, the central part of the bony labyrinth, is in contact with the middle ear along one side. Its membranous labyrinth is divided into two pouches or sacs containing endolymph, the *utricle* and the *saccule*. Along the inner wall of each pouch are small nerve cells. Also, the two sacs contain a gelatinous material in which are suspended tiny crystals containing calcium carbonate. These crystals are called *otoliths*.

The semicircular canals are above and behind the vestibule. They are called the upper (*superior*), the back (*posterior*), and the side (*lateral*) canals. These interconnected canals are arranged in three planes of space. They have five openings into the vestibule. Within the bony canals are the smaller membranous tubes, the *semicircular ducts*, which also have five openings into the vestibule.

The spiral-shaped cochlea, which is on the front side of the internal ear, is the essential organ of hearing. Two membranes divide the bony cochlea into three tubes. As with the other parts of the internal ear, the bony structure of the cochlea contains a smaller, similarly shaped membranous cochlea. Within this portion of the ear is a highly specialized structure, the organ of Corti, which contains hair cells. When stimulated by sound waves, these cells send impulses to the brain along the auditory nerve.

What it does

One major function of the ear is to convey the sound vibrations through the various channels of the ear to the portion of the brain (*cerebrum*) which controls the hearing. The external ear guides the vibrations toward the eardrum. When the sound waves reach the eardrum, it is set in motion. The waves are conducted across the series of small bones in the middle ear to the internal ear. From the internal ear, a cordlike band (*auditory nerve*) receives the vibrations from the small chambers in the cochlea. This nerve carries the waves to the center of hearing in the brain, the *temporal lobe*, where the sounds are classified and "registered." And thus we hear.

The ear has another important function. The semicircular canals are responsible for the individual's sense of balance, or equilibrium. The canals contain a fluid which remains at a certain level. When the body is off balance, this fluid is displaced over a series of sensory hairs. These hairs communicate with the brain, making it possible for the person to sense that he is off balance.

The otoliths of the vestibule's utricle and saccule respond to acceleration and deceleration. Since the advent of space travel, much more has been learned about their mode of action.

DISORDERS OF THE EAR: EARACHE

Earache may arise from many causes, and may occur in numerous forms. The most usual cause of pain in the ear, aside from mechanical injuries, is some type of bacterial infection. Each form of earache is characterized by a somewhat different type of pain and is accompanied by distinct symptoms. Although painful, most forms of earache are not dangerous, but because some types can become fatal, it is wise to consult a physician whenever symptoms arise.

Infection of the outer ear

In many cases, earache is caused by a foreign body that has become trapped in the ear. Children often deliberately insert objects into their own or another's ears. In all cases, such foreign bodies should be removed by a physician who knows the correct procedure to avoid injury to the delicate parts of the ear. Sometimes earache may be caused by hardened wax in the ear. This, too, should be treated by a physician. Foreign bodies occasionally cause inflammation of the ear (*otitis externa*). If the foreign body plugs the auditory canal, there may be a blunting of hearing or a temporary deafness which is relieved on removal of the object.

Boils or furuncles

Objects such as hairpins and metal clips used to relieve itching caused by wax in the ear may break the skin. Infection introduced through such a break may cause a boil or *furuncle* in the outer ear.

Boils in the external ear produce severe pain because the skin in this region normally adheres closely to the underlying cartilage and bone. The swollen ear is red and painful; the overlying skin is stretched and tender. Swelling may force the ear out of shape and cause it to lean forward. If the infection is severe, the swelling may extend to around the eyelid of the infected side. Since the joints involved in eating, talking, and yawning communicate with the ear canal, their movements may intensify the pain from the furuncle. The hearing is not affected unless the swelling blocks the ear canal. Perforations of the eardrum may occur. Through them, infection may spread to the middle ear, the inner ear, or the mastoid area. An x-ray picture may be helpful in determining the nature of any secondary complication.

Pain relief is the primary aim in treating patients with boils in the external ear. Antiseptic agents may be applied locally by the physician.

Antibiotic therapy is required in some cases. If a boil is about to rupture spontaneously, the physician will open and drain it. Proper cleansing of the ear is necessary to prevent a recurrence. If this infection recurs, an underlying physical disorder may be a causative factor.

Fungus infection

A *fungus* infection of the outer ear (*otomycosis*) and canal primarily affects the skin of the area. The inside of the ear appears dirty and crusty, and fluid seeps out continually. When the crusts and scales are removed, the skin beneath is raw and bleeds easily. Itching causes additional discomfort. In the majority of cases, pain is present because of the swelling of the canal. Hearing may be impaired. Various solutions and ointments have been found effective in the treatment of patients with this condition, which can be extremely persistent if inadequately treated by home remedies.

Inflammation of the eardrum

Sometimes following a cold or other respiratory infection, shooting pains are felt in the ear. The eardrum, which divides the outer ear from the middle ear, may become inflamed; this condition is called *acute myringitis*. The physician probably will use a medicated solution to clear the inflammation. Normal hearing may continue throughout the course of the disease.

Aero-otitis media

In this disorder, the structures of the middle ear are affected by changes of pressure which occur during airplane flights. In milder cases, there is a sensation of stuffiness in the ears, with a slight inflammation of the eardrum, and perhaps some minor hearing impairment. Excruciating pain and hemorrhages in the tympanic membrane may occur in more severe cases. During a flight, chewing gum or moving the lower jaw with the mouth open will usually prevent this disorder by opening the Eustachian tube, which will equalize the pressure. An individual who has any upper respiratory infection or severe nasal allergy should avoid flying.

Nondraining infection of the middle ear

Many disorders, both inflammatory and noninflammatory, may affect the middle ear. Often, bacteria from respiratory infections invade the middle ear through the Eustachian tube, which opens into the cavity (*nasopharynx*) behind the

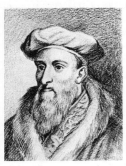

EUSTACCHIO, Bartolommeo, (ca. 1520-1574) Italian anatomist. Noted for his description of the auditory or *Eustachian tube*, the bony part of which was at one time known as the *Eustachian canal*. Also identified a number of nerves and muscles of the ear. Among his other contributions were his discovery of the thoracic duct and his description of the suprarenal or adrenal glands. One of the valves of the heart and a special catheter are also named in his honor.

nose. Bacteria may also enter the middle ear cavity through a perforation in the eardrum. Blowing the nose incorrectly is sometimes responsible for middle ear infections. Both nostrils should be blown at the same time, for blowing only one side at a time may force purulent material into the sinuses or the Eustachian tube.

Disturbances in the middle ear are often caused by infections in other nearby organs, such as the tonsils or nasopharynx. In these so-called "catarrhal" disorders of the middle ear, the primary problem is that the Eustachian tube is partially or completely closed.

In an acute middle ear infection (*otitis media*) of this type, sharp stabbing pains may shoot through the ear, and a heavy feeling is noticed on that side of the head. Momentary relief is achieved by yawning or blowing the nose. This kind of middle ear infection may last a few days or a few weeks, with healing slower in damp climates. Often, removal of the tonsils and adenoids is recommended after recovery as a preventive measure against further attacks.

Sulfonamide drugs, broad-spectrum antibiotics, or antihistamines are now used effectively to clear up this disorder and the underlying infection or allergy. After the inflammation subsides, it is sometimes necessary to remove or add air to the middle air chamber in order to attain the correct pressure there. Therapy should be carried out only by a physician.

A *subacute infection of the middle ear* is practically the same as the acute form except that it is not so severe, but may last longer. The cause may be enlarged or infected tonsils or adenoids. The Eustachian tube, through which the infection is carried, is usually swollen, although pain may be slight, and waves of deafness are intermittent. A ringing sound (*tinnitus*) may be heard, and a fullness felt in the affected ear. Further attacks often may be prevented by removal of infected tonsils.

A person's hearing may be impaired in later life if repeated attacks of otitis media persist.

Another danger is the possibility of the development of a chronic ear infection.

A *chronic middle ear infection* may develop as a result of persistent ear infections or from respiratory diseases. It may also be caused by diseases such as tuberculosis, measles, and syphilis. Other causes are obstructions in the nose, improper blowing of the nose, washing out the nose, or diseased tonsils or adenoids.

In these conditions, both acute and subacute infections begin with inflammation. After a varying period of time, the inflammation regresses, but a chronic change in the tissue takes place. The membrane becomes thicker and pale in color. The Eustachian tube becomes smaller but rarely closes completely.

One of the main symptoms of chronic middle ear infection is a ringing sensation in the affected ear. It comes at intervals at first, then gradually the ringing becomes constant. The sounds vary both in pitch and intensity. Nausea rarely accompanies the ringing. Hearing is usually affected, but total deafness seldom occurs. The only hope of complete recovery lies in early treatment. Draining of the middle ear can be accomplished successfully and safely by a surgical procedure by which a small incision is made in the eardrum. Eardrums that rupture spontaneously may become infected chronically, with a possibility of mastoid complication. If discovered early, the causative factor can be removed, and the progress of the infection can be stopped. Surgery of the drum membrane alone does not benefit most advanced cases. More radical surgery is required to clear up the disease.

Secretory otitis media (also called *serous otitis media*) is characterized by the collection of fluid in the middle ear. This fluid may be either clear (*serous*) or glue-like (*mucous*). The predominant symptom of the disorder is impaired hearing, which varies from slight to almost total loss of hearing.

Children who have secretory otitis media may be subject to frequent upper respiratory infections and often have enlarged lymphoid tissue in the nasopharynx.

If there is an underlying allergy or infection, appropriate antihistamines, antibiotics, or sulfonamides may be prescribed. Draining the fluid through an incision in the eardrum may relieve the condition. When there are repeated attacks, tiny plastic tubes can be inserted into the middle ear to provide adequate aeration there. These tubes are left in place for as long as three to four months.

Many cases of severely impaired hearing in adults can be attributed to middle ear infections in childhood. One reason such infections are so prevalent among children is that, in infants and young children, the Eustachian tube is shorter and more nearly horizontal. Thus, the tube is even more likely to become an avenue of infection in children than in adults. The prevention of chronic middle ear infection should be connected closely to the early hygiene of children. The child should be taught to establish good health habits which prevent low resistance to respiratory diseases.

Acute draining middle ear infection

Acute draining middle ear infection (*acute suppurative otitis media*) originates from the same causes as all middle ear infections previously mentioned. Respiratory infections, diseased tonsils and adenoids, and inadequate nasal hygiene may all be causative factors in this infection. Draining middle ear infection differs in the type of inflammation and the changes occurring in the tissues. A head cold may precede the infection. The attack of inflammation is, sudden and causes congestion in the linings of the ear spaces, Eustachian tube, and mastoid cells. The ear itself fills with fluid, which gradually becomes puslike.

Pain is the chief symptom. It is severe, radiating, and throbbing. In infants and young children, the early symptoms include refusal to eat, nausea and vomiting, rolling the head, or tugging at the ear. The patient's temperature rises to about 100° in adults, but may reach 105°

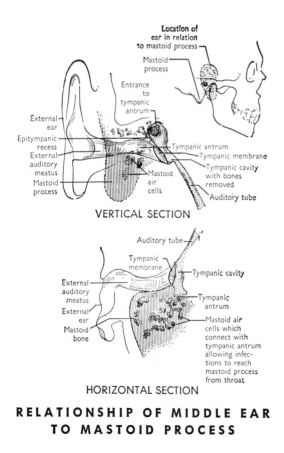

VERTICAL SECTION

HORIZONTAL SECTION

**RELATIONSHIP OF MIDDLE EAR
TO MASTOID PROCESS**

in children, with convulsions not uncommon. A ringing sensation and dizziness may be present. Hearing is impaired as long as pus remains in the middle ear.

After several days, the eardrum ruptures spontaneously. For as long as three weeks, the fluid seeps through the canal, then subsides, and stops. This perforation in the drum usually, but not always, heals over.

Early diagnosis of middle ear infection is extremely important. The parts of the ear are so intricate and delicate that infections spread easily. Possible complications of ear infection include mastoiditis, chronic otitis media with a permanently perforated eardrum, or even meningitis.

DISORDERS OF THE EAR: MIDDLE EAR AND MASTOID TROUBLE

The middle ear is generally involved when there is an infection of the mastoid process of the temporal bone. The acute form of this disease (*acute mastoiditis*) has practically been eliminated since antibiotic drugs have become available to combat middle ear infections.

The inflammation in mastoiditis involves the lining of the mastoid cells. The infection may enter the bone, which becomes soft and decayed. The causes of mastoiditis include respiratory infection, abnormal anatomy of the ear in infants and children, improper channels for ear drainage, and lowered resistance to infection. Mastoiditis may occur as a secondary infection to various diseases.

The predominating symptom of acute mastoiditis is pain, which may be either continuous or intermittent. If the patient is not treated, the intense pain could persist for six or more days, which may not be true for middle ear infection. Also unlike middle ear infection, mastoiditis is characterized by a definite, localized tenderness over the mastoid process.

Especially in *chronic mastoiditis,* which now occurs far more often than the acute type, drainage from the ear (*otorrhea*) is the principal symptom. Characteristics of this discharge vary somewhat with different types of mastoiditis.

Fever may or may not be present. In the early stages of mastoiditis, the temperature varies from 99° to 105° in children. Hearing may be impaired to some degree. Tenderness over the mastoid area is present, along with swelling behind the ear and an outward protrusion of the ear itself.

If acute mastoiditis does occur, the physician

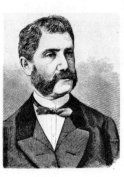

GRUBER, Josef (1827-1900) Austrian otologist. Famous for his many contributions to the study of the disorders of hearing. He devised a speculum known as *Gruber's speculum*. A hearing test known by his name involves placing a tuning fork near the ear until its sound becomes inaudible, inserting a finger in the ear and placing the fork against the finger at which the sound should again become audible. Gruber was a pioneer in the field of otology.

may perform a *mastoidectomy*. In this operation, the infected mastoid cells are removed through an incision in the area behind the ear, or in the external auditory meatus.

DISORDERS OF THE EAR: TINNITUS, A COMMON SYMPTOM

Most persons, at one time or another, experience *tinnitus*, a sensation of ear noise which is more noticeable in a quiet environment. These "noises" may seem to be in the head rather than the ear, and may affect one or both ears. This symptom is associated with many conditions, including middle ear infection, Ménière's syndrome, exposure to intense noise, circulatory disorders, otosclerosis, overbite, and neuritis of the auditory nerve. The symptom may also be caused by excessive amounts of coffee, tobacco, or alcohol. Quinine, certain antibiotics, or large doses of aspirin could also produce tinnitus. The incidence of tinnitus increases with age and the ear noises occur most often in persons between the ages of 50 and 70.

The reason for this sensation is not known. One theory is that some abnormal irritation causes a sequence of discharges along the course of the auditory nerve to the brain.

The patient's description of his particular tinnitus is of diagnostic importance. For example, noise resembling the ocean's roaring is characteristic of Ménière's syndrome, but a low-pitched buzzing sound might indicate otosclerosis or conductive hearing loss.

Since this symptom could be an early warning of hearing damage, it should be investigated by a physician. He will attempt to find the underlying physical disorder and initiate appropriate treatment. If no such cause can be found, there is no sure method for eliminating the symptom itself. If the tinnitus is extremely distracting, the patient often worries, has difficulty sleeping, and even becomes emotionally disturbed. Since the symptom seems intensified under conditions of stress and tension, sedatives are sometimes prescribed. Also, masking the tinnitus with everyday sounds (such as music or playing the radio) often provides temporary relief.

DISORDERS OF THE EAR: PUNCTURE OF THE EARDRUM

The eardrum (*tympanic membrane*) which divides the external ear from the middle ear is subject to puncture or rupture through several types of injury.

The most common cause of a punctured eardrum is the insertion of a sharp object into the ear. Violent explosions near the ear may cause the drum to tear or rupture. Decreased air pressure during or after descent from high altitudes, severe sneezing, diving, and increased pressure frequently are responsible for damaged membranes.

Diagnosis and treatment

Sometimes, the diagnosis of a punctured eardrum is difficult. The pain accompanying a puncture is sharp and intermittent. Blood may ooze from the injury, but this is not positive proof of a drum tear, because the same symptom may be present in a skull fracture. Dizziness, ringing sounds, and headaches also are significant symptoms, sometimes associated with a punctured eardrum.

A tear in the eardrum may heal without treatment within a period of a few weeks. But there may be aftereffects which may not be noticed for some time, even after a year.

When the bleeding stops, a small piece of sterile cotton may be inserted in the outer canal, but no syringing of the ear should be done. A grafting operation known as *tympanoplasty* can be employed in cases in which the tear does not close.

Growths on the eardrum

Following the rupture or perforation of the eardrum, small, chalky (lime) deposits may form at the site of healing as a result of repeated attacks of middle ear infection. The deposits form on the outer or middle layer of the drum. If they have formed from a healed perforation, they mark the path of least resistance for a future rupture. It is the general opinion of physicians that these deposits do not affect normal hearing. There is no successful method of removing chalk deposits without injuring seriously the eardrum or depressing the hearing. Hence, it is rarely attempted.

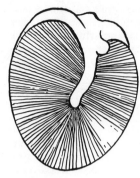

Drawing of the external appearance of the eardrum or tympanic membrane as it may be seen through the external auditory canal when healthy and normal.

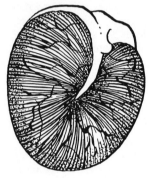

In the condition of *otitis externa* or inflammation of the outer ear, the tympanum gives the swollen and highly congested appearance shown in the drawing.

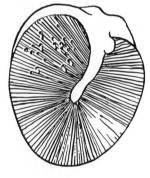

Illustration of the appearance of the tympanic membrane when, as a result of infection, it is disturbed by pin-hole perforations. Drops of pus exude from them.

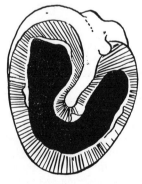

A loud gun blast or explosion may cause sufficient changes in pressure in the air to rupture the eardrums in what is called a *kidney perforation*, such as this one.

DISORDERS OF THE EARDRUM

DISORDERS OF THE EAR: MÉNIÈRE'S SYNDROME

Prosper Ménière described this malady in 1861 and correctly attributed its origin to the inner ear. Its characteristic symptoms are sudden, severe episodes of *vertigo* (dizziness), tinnitus (ear noises), and fluctuating hearing loss. As the cause and mechanism of this disorder have not been definitely established, the term "syndrome" is generally used rather than "disease."

Persons in the middle age group are more commonly affected by this syndrome. The vertigo associated with an attack may be so violent that the simplest activities become impossible. Usually, the patient has a sensation that he or objects around him are whirling. This same type of dizziness also occurs with certain cardiovascular disorders and middle ear infections. The attacks of vertigo last minutes or weeks. The tinnitus, usually a roaring noise, sometimes persists between attacks. Nausea and vomiting are also usual symptoms.

The course of this syndrome is unpredictable. Remissions of up to several years often occur. About two thirds of the patients improve or recover regardless of the treatment.

No single form of therapy has been completely successful. Certain drugs such as Dramamine often help control the vertigo. Sedatives or tranquilizers are occasionally helpful. Some doctors recommend a low-salt diet and prohibit smoking.

If the condition is disabling and unilateral, the diseased parts of the labyrinth may be surgically removed. This procedure does stop the vertigo, but balance is impaired and the hearing loss in the ear involved is total. Recently, ultrasound waves have been used to irradiate the labyrinth and destroy the diseased portions. This method apparently does not have as high a risk of damage to the cochlea as do other surgical methods. However, the symptoms do sometimes recur. For relief of severe vertigo, other surgeons now recommend the Tack operation to drain the saccule, which contains endolymph. A tack, a small pointed piece of metal, is placed through the footplate into the sac, thus allowing drainage. According to one theory, this syndrome is related to an imbalance of pressure between the perilymph and the endolymph. Another innovation has been the use of surgical instruments which are maintained at temperatures as low as −140° C. With these instruments, a surgical procedure seems less likely to damage the cochlea. Long-term results must be analyzed before any one of these new procedures gains wide acceptance.

OTHER EAR DISORDERS

An *abscess* is a central collection of pus in areas of inflammation. The pus is formed by dissolved tissue, bacteria, and the white blood cells involved in the destruction of the bacteria. Abcesses have various causes and, in the case of the ear, require skilled care.

In abscess of the external ear, there is pain and tenderness over the affected area. The auricle may enlarge to two or three times its normal size. If proper care is not given, the ear may be permanently distorted in shape.

Antibiotics and sulfonamide drugs may be used effectively. Surgical treatment may be required but only after careful evaluation by a specialist.

Cauliflower ear

Cauliflower ear *(hematoma of the auricle)* has long been recognized as the badge of the prize-fighter. It is caused by injury to the external ear. A hard blow may cause bleeding below the skin. If this accumulation of blood remains for some time it becomes *fibrous tissue* and eventually will be converted into a bonelike or cartilaginous substance. The ear will thus be deformed by this irregular mass of extra tissue. Treatment consists of removing the blood before it clots or begins to change into tissue. Usually, it can be drawn off with a large needle. If, however, the tissue has become hard, plastic surgery is required to restore the ear to normal.

Congenital malformations

Congenital malformations of the ear occur rather frequently. Generally, they are not gross enough to impair hearing but may be unsightly. Absence of the lobe or the outer rim of the ear *(helix),* large protruding ears, and irregular shapes are some of the malformations which occur. Plastic surgery can restore most of these to resemble the normal. Occasionally, a congenital defect, such as an obstruction in the canal, may have to be removed before hearing improves. In rare instances the ears may be displaced on the head, and in some extreme cases when the lower jaw is grossly misshapen, they may even be fused together *(synotia* or *otocephaly).*

MOTION SICKNESS AND OTHER DISTURBANCES OF EQUILIBRIUM

The semicircular canals of the inner ear are responsible for adjusting the body to changes in motion. The rate of these changes normally allows sufficient time for the canals to maintain bodily equilibrium. When rapid, irregular, and continuous waves of motion persist, the canals are not able to function properly, and *motion sickness* results.

Seasickness, airsickness, and *elevator sickness* are forms of motion sickness caused by irregular and abnormal motion which upsets equilibrium. The usual symptoms are dizziness, nausea, vomiting, and thirst. Despite the extreme unpleasantness experienced by the victims, motion sickness is often thought of as a trifling ailment. However, the number of deaths that occur from this disturbance is greater than would ordinarily be expected. Death does not occur as a result of motion sickness in itself, but rather from exciting a preexisting disorder.

During World War II, in an effort to prevent seasickness, many experimental tests were performed on troops going overseas in which a large number of drugs were investigated. *Dramamine* was found to be the most effective. More than half of the men who received this drug did not become seasick or were relieved of the symptoms of seasickness. In practically all the cases, the ordinary severity of the illness was lessened.

In discovering the relation of motion sickness to inner ear functions, the reason for dizziness *(vertigo)* in other diseases became clear. Some of the diseases in which dizziness may be a symptom are: Ménière's syndrome; diseases of the central nervous system; direct injury to the ear; malformation of the inner ear; syphilis; and alcoholism.

CAUSES AND TYPES OF DEAFNESS

The terms *deafness* and *hard of hearing* have different meanings. Deafness means nearly complete or total loss of hearing. There are two types of deafness: congenital and acquired. In the congenital type, the person is born deaf or later becomes deaf because of an inborn defect; whereas in the acquired type, the person is born with normal hearing but becomes deaf because of an accident or illness. Hard of hearing applies to those who lose some of the ability to hear later in life, but who may have learned how to speak before the loss occurred.

Deafness is caused by many conditions. The physician must determine the cause of the defect before he will know which type of treatment is best. The following are some conditions from which poor hearing may result: (1) temporary or chronic infections in one or both ears; (2)

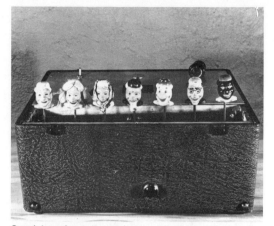

Special equipment must be used in testing the hearing of children. Puppets in box are made to pop out when child pushes button, indicating perception of sounds in tests of various frequencies.

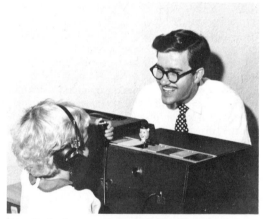

Friendly testing personnel convince the child that the test is a game, thus getting her co-operation.

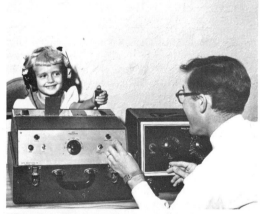

When the child hears the test sound, she pushes the button causing the puppet to appear and indicating her auditory acuity to tester. *Photographs by courtesy of C. Olaf Haug, Houston, Texas.*

secondary complications of disease elsewhere in the body; (3) direct damage or defect in some part of the hearing system; (4) aging; (5) occlusion of the auditory canal; (6) aero-otitis media; (7) Ménière's syndrome; (8) otosclerosis; (9) noise, and (10) certain ototoxic drugs, including Kanomycin and Streptomycin.

Also, there are many types and degrees of hearing loss. *Conductive deafness* results when sound waves are not transmitted properly through the outer and the middle ear. If the damage is to the inner ear or the nerve pathway to the brain, a *sensorineural* (also called *nerve* or *perceptive) deafness* occurs. The latter type is generally a greater handicap and usually cannot be reversed. In *mixed hearing loss,* there are elements of both the conductive and the sensorineural types of loss. Some deafness is caused by a disorder in the *central* nervous system.

Poor hearing caused by severe infection is common. Head colds, tonsillitis, measles, scarlet fever, mumps, and meningitis are some of the diseases which may damage part of the hearing system during childhood. These diseases may attack one or many parts of the ear. The degree of loss of hearing is dependent on the severity of the infection.

If a woman develops German measles *(rubella)* during the first three months of her pregnancy, the baby will, in at least 50 percent of the cases, be born with at least a partial hearing defect. This congenital deafness may be masked by even more severe birth defects resulting from the mother's infection. After a nationwide epidemic of rubella in 1964, many children were seen with this form of deafness. A similar outbreak occurred in 1969. The recent development of a rubella vaccine offers the hope that this disease will eventually be eradicated.

Old age may have some bearing as a cause of hearing loss. Serious infection with damaging consequences to hearing rarely occurs after a person has passed the age of 20. Later in life, however, usually after the age of 50, changes which lead to partial loss of hearing, especially for high tones, may occur in the auditory nerve.

Otosclerosis

Usually first detected during early adulthood, *otosclerosis* can cause a conductive type of hearing loss. Bony growths form just inside the inner ear where the middle ear's stirrup *(stapes)* enters it. Eventually, the footplate of the stapes becomes anchored and no longer conducts sound waves to the inner ear.

About ten percent of the population have otosclerosis to some extent, although they may have no noticeable hearing loss for many years. It seems that this disorder may become arrested at any stage.

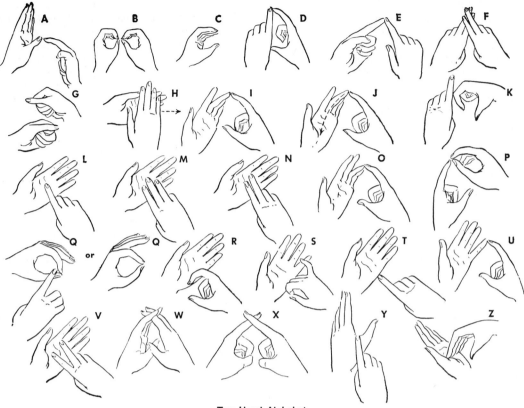

Two-Hand Alphabet

Heredity appears to be an important factor in most cases; middle ear infections are *not* a cause. The disorder occurs about twice as often in females as in males.

The chief symptom is the slowly progressive hearing loss. Tinnitus also occurs frequently, and usually increases with the deafness.

Remarkable advances have been made in surgery on the ear. Since 1952, an operation on the tiny stapes itself has been used for many patients with advanced otosclerosis. In this *stapedectomy,* all or part of the fixed stapes is removed and is replaced with an artificial device. Although at first successful in restoring the hearing, these early techniques sometimes led to damage of the cochlea. In other cases, the improved hearing was only temporary.

After 1962, a modification of the stapedectomy procedure was developed which seems quite effective, although long-term results are not yet available. By the new method, as much as one half of the thinnest section of the stapes footplate is removed. Through this opening, a piston is inserted into the labyrinth. Some surgeons use a Teflon piston, and others prefer one made of stainless steel or Teflon and wire. As the piston functions as a substitute for the footplate, sound waves can once more be trans-mitted to the cochlea. This operation does not stop the progress of the disease, but the piston resists the continuing bony growth for long periods of time. In a few such cases fenestration remains the procedure of choice. The fenestration operation bypasses the fixed stapes to substitute a new window to replace the immobile oval window.

Noise and hearing

Our modern industrial society is plagued with ever-increasing noise from traffic, machinery, rock-and-roll music, rocket and jet engines, and many other sources. The most obvious danger from excessive and constant exposure to noise is loss of hearing. Noise can also disturb sleep, impair efficiency, and produce drastic physical and psychological changes.

During wartime, military personnel often receive partial or total hearing loss after exposure to noises such as blasts or gunfire. More than 58,000 veterans of World War II now get compensation for ear damage considered to be a service-connected disability.

Occupational deafness (originally referred to as boiler maker's deafness) is a hearing loss resulting from prolonged exposure to industrial noise. The loss is permanent, and may be either partial or total.

Efforts have been made to determine which levels of noise are safe and which are harmful to the hearing mechanism. The intensity of the sound, the length of exposure to the noise, and an individual's age and his susceptibility to noise are factors other than loudness which must be considered.

The Walsh-Healey Public Contracts Act was modified in 1969 in an attempt to provide better protection for the hearing of industrial workers. All industries fulfilling government contracts must now meet rigid standards of noise control. Twenty-seven million industrial workers will benefit from such regulations.

Modern rock-and-roll music, with the type of amplification now popular, has been found potentially damaging to the hearing of the participants. These sounds usually exceed the levels considered safe for the hearing. Persons repeatedly exposed to the music could develop temporary or permanent hearing loss.

Many organizations are studying the problem of noise control. These include the National Council on Noise Abatement, the Acoustical Society of America, and a New York City group known as Citizens for a Quieter City, Incorporated.

OPPORTUNITIES FOR THE DEAF

An estimated 15 million adults and three million children in the United States have some degree of hearing impairment. Of these, 250,000 might be classified as deaf, that is, their hearing loss is either total or nearly so. Regardless of the extent of their hearing defect, their condition is not hopeless. Many opportunities are available for their training and special education.

If deafness is congenital or if it occurs before a child learns to talk, the handicap is even more severe. Early diagnosis is extremely important, so the child can be taught to communicate as soon as possible. Some children are considered mentally retarded until hearing tests show that their real problem is deafness and an associated inability to communicate. Special hearing tests have been designed for tiny infants, and a child may be fitted with a hearing aid before he is one year old.

Perhaps the greatest problem of the deaf person is the limitation of his ability to communicate. "Deaf-mute" is the term applied to individuals who have never heard and consequently have not used their organs of speech, which are probably normal. Helen Keller was a notable example of success in learning to communicate. Although blind as well as deaf,

she learned to speak through the patient but persistent work of her teacher.

Training for the deaf child begins in the home. He needs the stimulation of an environment with people who have normal hearing and speech. Parents can be of great assistance in special training programs for the child.

To learn what services are available to deaf persons, one should consult the May 1970 issue of the *American Annals of the Deaf*. This journal may be found in many of the larger libraries. Included are lists of private and government organizations which offer financial as well as other types of assistance to deaf persons, and also all schools and classes which offer special training. Help in locating schools may also be obtained from The American Hearing Society, 919 Eighteenth Street, N.W., Washington, D.C. 20006, and the Volta Bureau, 1537 Thirty-fifth Street, N.W., Washington, D.C. 20007. A free correspondence course for parents of deaf children below the age of six is available from the John Tracy Clinic, 806 West Adams Boulevard, Los Angeles, California 90007.

Several books for parents of deaf children are available, including "Your Deaf Child" by Helmer Myklebust, published by Charles C Thomas, Springfield, Illinois; "If You Have A Deaf Child" by the Illinois School for Mothers of Deaf Children, University of Illinois Press, Urbana; "What's Its Name?" by Jean Utley, University of Illinois Press, Urbana; and "Deaf Children at Home and at School" by D. M. C. Dale, published by Charles C Thomas, Springfield, Illinois.

Education of the deaf

Various methods have been used to teach the deaf person to communicate orally. As early as 1620, essentially the same one-handed manual alphabet used by some persons today was advocated by a teacher of deaf children in Spain. In the mid-eighteenth century, the Abbé de l'Epée of Paris considered a language of signs to be the natural language for deaf persons. He developed a more elaborate system than the one being used at that time. In Germany, an opposing view was developing at the same time. There Samuel Heinicke insisted that a spoken language must be used rather than manual signs.

A small institution established in 1817 in Hartford, Connecticut, was the first training school for the deaf in this country. The earliest schools of this type used manual communication to teach the deaf students. After 50 years, the German oral method began to gain favor. Currently, the oral method or some combination of it with finger spelling is preferred.

There are three types of schools or classes for deaf persons in the United States. At the 80 public and private residential schools, chil-

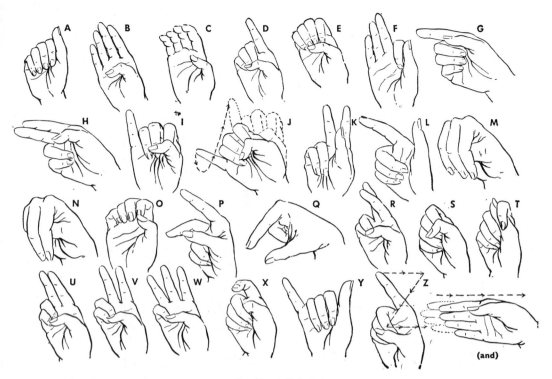

One-Hand Alphabet

dren live at the institution and are under the continual guidance of skilled instructors. In public or private day schools, the same type of training is given, but students live at home. Day classes are also available, usually as a part of the regular public school systems. The deaf children attend school with children of normal hearing, but have special classes to help them with their problem of communication.

Teaching speech, or the oral method, instead of the sign or finger-spelling method, has many advantages. It is a more natural means of expression to those with either normal or subnormal hearing, and it does not attract attention to the deaf child or pupil. The easier the communication between the pupil or deaf person and one with normal hearing, the more sincere the link between the two individuals. Confidence grows with accuracy and normality in speech. Therefore, the deaf person is usually more at ease in a business or social situation if he is able to speak.

Although not all deaf persons can acquire the ability to speak, the majority gain some knowledge of lip reading, which is a great asset when associating with the public. Both speech and lip reading are taught simultaneously in the schools. Even a small understanding of each is an advantage, because too few persons of normal hearing are able to "read" the manual signs. Also, persons knowing only the sign language find themselves segregated from normal activities.

Schools for the deaf admit all age groups. Some institutions begin the training of the child as early as two to three years of age, and it is desirable to start as early as possible. A child of two years who has not yet started to talk should therefore be examined for possible deafness. In special schools or classes, each child is treated individually. Specialists have found that many children who are supposedly "deaf-mute" actually can use a hearing aid and thus become able to speak. Also, many deaf children have some degree of residual hearing which may be amplified and used in teaching oral communication.

Physical education is provided in all schools for the deaf. Many such institutions have excellent football, baseball, and basketball teams. Athletic competition is important in the mental adjustment of deaf persons. Training of these students should compare closely to that of normal students in order that they may be free from feelings of insecurity.

Hearing aids

Many types of these intricate electronic instruments are now available. Since the transistor replaced the bulky vacuum tube of hearing aids in the 1950s, the devices have become tiny but

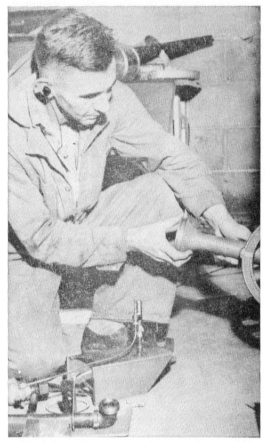

Many mechanical pursuits, such as that of a furnace installer, offer opportunities to the deaf. *Picture courtesy of Federal Security Agency, Iowa Division, Office of Vocational Rehabilitation.*

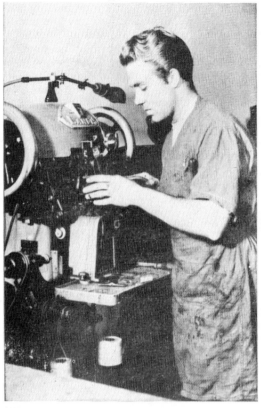

Shoe repairing is one of the many vocations that a deaf person may pursue successfully with profit. *Picture courtesy Federal Security Agency, Utah Division, Office of Vocational Rehabilitation.*

even more powerful. Further improvements have been made as space-age technology has advanced.

Almost five million Americans use hearing aids, and perhaps ten million others could benefit from their use. Of course, not all types of hearing loss are decreased by such instruments. Usually, persons with a conductive hearing loss can adapt more rapidly to hearing aids, since their primary need is for increased sound energy.

Persons with a sensorineural deafness have more difficulty. They require a more selective amplification of sound which hearing aids do not provide as well. Often what these persons are able to hear is distorted and they must adjust to the different type of hearing.

The individuals with a mixed type of hearing loss generally respond to the hearing aids less well than those with conductive deafness, but better than those with the other type of loss. In all cases, patience and persistence are necessary. The will to hear is vital.

The hard-of-hearing child should have a hearing aid fitted by his third birthday, or before, if practical. But it is not enough to give a child a hearing aid. He must be taught how to use it correctly so that later he may be able to attend

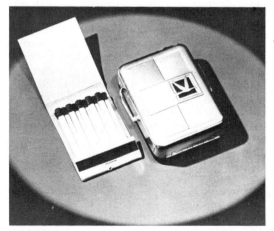

Developments in the hearing aids have made them less conspicuous and the power units of small size, such as this matchbox-size device. *Otarion, Inc.*

regular school with pupils who have normal hearing. At first there must be many brief acoustic training periods lasting from 10 to 15 minutes at a time. The sound must be carefully regulated; the hearing aid may be too weak or too strong. If insufficient attention is paid by parent or teacher to training in the use of the hearing aid, there may be further traumatic deafness caused by overstimulation of hearing.

There is often a tendency on the part of the child to hear only what he wants to hear. This cannot be permitted if he is to make the most of the hearing he has. He must strive to hear all the sounds that come to him and differentiate them as the child with normal hearing must do. Because the hearing aid catches background noises, he must exert a conscious effort to hear.

PROBLEMS OF THE DEAF

Most of the residential schools for the deaf offer only an eighth-grade education. For many, this ends their formal education. Whatever method is used in teaching the deaf child, he should learn to communicate in oral and written language well enough that he can continue his education in regular secondary schools and colleges. Gallaudet College, a federally supported institution in Washington, D.C., is the only college for the deaf in this country.

Deafness itself does not imply any mental deficiency, but there are cases in which the cause of deafness is also the cause of a mental deficiency. If learning among persons with this handicap seems slow, it is usually because of the difficult and slow process of mastering lip reading and speech. As with all learning, some individuals attain more proficiency than others.

An important phase of education or rehabilitation for the deaf is industrial training. A few colleges now offer vocational training programs for deaf persons. After taking aptitude tests, students are given training in the trade for which they seem best suited. Almost all deaf adults (five-sixths) work at manual jobs, as compared with 50 percent of hearing adults. Better educational programs and more sophisticated vocational training are needed to broaden the deaf person's ability to compete for a wide range of jobs and professions.

One of the major needs of handicapped persons is psychological rehabilitation. In patients who have lost their hearing after they reached maturity, there is a feeling of suspicion toward family and friends, and a period of discouragement and depression. The deaf person is unable to communicate easily with those of normal hearing; and as the disability becomes more apparent, some psychological changes occur in the personality of the handicapped individual. He may feel inadequate at social gatherings and gradually drop out of the group entirely.

In deaf children, the absence of communication with others is baffling and causes a feeling of insecurity. School children who are hard-of-hearing should not be segregated from normal school children. Special instructions may be given for lip reading, but they should continue their regular school routine. The feeling of "belonging" to the general group is essential for children.

19 THE MIND

THE HEALTHY MIND

The study of man would be incomplete if it failed to include the concept of man as a whole. All of the body systems are deserving of separate scrutiny, but the impression gained by considering these separate portions of the body is only a hazy one. In order to understand the composite picture of all these physical attributes working together in a unified whole, it is necessary to take a more comprehensive view regarding man through the unifying aspect of the mind.

The human brain contains an estimated 10 billion nerve cells (neurons). These neurons interact electrochemically one with another to produce the responses and reflexes, sometimes subconsciously and at other times by the desire of the individual. Such responses may save the person from a burn or injury or might even be lifesaving. Changes in the electrostatic fluid surrounding the cells or in the neurons themselves produce disease.

Foremost among the functions of the mind is *consciousness*. Consciousness includes the individual's awareness of himself and his environment, and the relationships existing between the two. It includes, moreover, a vast number of impressions, thoughts, words, and emotions. Only a small part of the material contained within the mind is in the focus of consciousness at any given moment. Surrounding that, there is an extensive field of experience which may be recalled at will. Yet, there is an even greater body of material which is totally inaccessible for conscious recall under ordinary circumstan-

ces of mental activity. Thus, there are three different *areas* of consciousness. These have been referred to by a variety of terms, but a convenient way to think of them might be: the conscious, the latent conscious, and the unconscious.

Besides the areas of consciousness, there are also varying *levels* of consciousness. When the mind is operating at its highest capacity, full consciousness prevails. It is only on this level that man's total mental potentialities can be exercised. Intelligence, insight, judgment, and constructive thinking must take place on this level. Structural damage to the brain, the action of depressant agents, and sometimes the inability to cope with emotional distress—all may bring about a recession to lower levels of consciousness. At the lower levels, vital processes of the body are maintained in the absence of higher states of mind.

A second function of the mind is *perception*. Sensory images received by way of the eyes, ears, nose, mouth, or skin arouse reactions in the mind. Not all of them, however, are consciously perceived. Reflex actions, in which a painful stimulus is received and the affected part immediately withdrawn, demonstrate the way in which impulses are assimilated into the mind and acted upon, even before the individual becomes aware of them. Those stimuli which do invade the consciousness are true perceptions, and are evaluated by the mind in terms of its past experience. The individual recognizes those perceptions which have been experienced before. Any new perception is judged by comparison with the old. Most perceptions are dismissed from conscious awareness quickly, as the need for attention to them recedes. The trivial, the irrelevant, the no-longer-significant sensations are not entirely lost, however, but instead are dropped out of the range of immediate consciousness, leaving the conscious portion of the mind free for more pressing activity.

Among the more pressing functions of the mind is *intellection,* which includes the powers of knowing, understanding, and reasoning—in fact, man's ability to think. Through the mass of his sensory experience, his memories, and the impressions gained from his relationships with others, the individual accumulates a sum of facts which constitutes his knowledge. He may accumulate a large body of knowledge, but unless he has the ability to comprehend the interrelation between these facts, he cannot be said to be intelligent. Intelligence, then, is the ability to understand and to apply the knowledge one has gained This has been suggested in another way by saying that man is distinguished not by the number of his thoughts, but by the quality of the thoughts he thinks.

The continuous flow of thoughts which occupy the mind has been referred to by William James as the *stream of consciousness.* He noted that within the stream there are changes in the type of thought, and significant groupings, or punctuations, in the stream itself. He insisted that it is these halting places which are most important, since all thought is fruitless until it reaches some conclusion.

A thought may arrive at a conclusion through any number of different routes. For example, one may be thinking in terms of visual images. The pictures formed within his mind then fuse one into another as the process of thought goes on. If the thought involved happens to be of a growing tree, the individual will picture in his mind the seed, the sprout, the tendril pressing upward, the sapling, and the tree. The same conclusion may be reached by thinking in words. Instead of thinking in images, a person may think in terms of the language he knows, or in any number of different languages. Still, so long as the thought is the same, it will arrive at the same conclusion. One's thoughts, then, may take a plurality of routes. The most effective route by which he can communicate his thoughts to other persons, however, is that of language. Through language—speech and the written word—communication with others reaches the greatest facility. Language communication may be interrupted by *aphasia,* a defect in the ability to express thoughts by words or to comprehend written or spoken language. Without language man benefits but little from the experiences of others, nor does he pass on to others his own thoughts, whether meaningful or seemingly *idle.* An example of idle thought is the flow of images comprising daydreams. Daydreams are most assuredly mental processes, yet they are not characteristically productive. For thoughts to become productive, the mind must classify them, compare them with other thoughts, in short, "make something" of them. In this effort, one experiences a feeling of having to make and of actually making a *choice* between various alternatives.

These thoughts and actions which one feels have been deliberately *willed* to occur are called *voluntary.* With constant repetition, what the individual *wills to do* gets established into set patterns which become his habits. Thereafter, they lose most of their voluntary character and are performed automatically, in a sort of economy of action. Through the economy of habit, many voluntary actions take place without simultaneous regulation by conscious thought. But the habits had to be created in the first place, through conscious effort in the *choices* of the individual. An ancient philosopher once said, "as a man thinks, so is he." He would have been equally accurate, and even more specific, had he said, "as a man chooses. . . ."

Inherent in the need to make a decision is the possibility of making the wrong one. Many factors in the experience of the individual converge to influence the direction his decisions will take. Thus, the desire to make a decision may be strong, and at the same time, the desire *not to* make the decision may be equally strong. This state of mental vacillation—one desire conflicting with the opposite—may evoke emotions which are painful to the individual.

Emotion, simply defined, is the way one feels about things. For centuries students of medicine and philosophy believed the emotions were centered in the heart. It is now understood, however, that emotions are a function of the mind. Sometimes emotions become so strong that they overbalance the power of decisive thinking. Violent emotion, and even petty emotional disturbances, if prolonged, take their toll on the whole person by interfering with logical thinking and also by interrupting the smooth functioning of the body processes. The interaction between physical and mental forces is complete and constant. Not only do disturbed states of mind become reflected in bodily reactions, but when physical needs are denied, strong emotional reactions occur. The awareness that something is needed, and that one is being deprived of it, becomes a basic driving force which impels the individual to action. The entire range of behavior is influenced by emotional factors, many of which are entirely unconscious.

Man has at his command a variety of unconscious devices by which he may defend himself from the pressure of the world without, and the inner pressures of his own making— pressures brought about through conflict between what he wants to do and what he feels he must do.

Mechanisms of the mind

Among the mental mechanisms which influence man's behavior, there are a few which are employed so universally that they will be recognized by all. A few of the unconscious mechanisms of the mind will be discussed in succeeding paragraphs; it is not within the scope of this book to treat this complex subject in its entirety.

One of the most common defense mechanisms known is *projection,* in which the individual attributes his own feelings to others, stating that they feel as he does. The secure individual should be able to face reality without having to project his own failings onto some outside object, but there are many instances in which this is impossible. For example, if a man has a deep feeling that he wants to do someone harm, this thought may be unacceptable to him. Hence, his mind projects this feeling into reverse: "I hate him" is changed to "he hates me." In like manner, morbid jealousy is a typical example of projection. If a husband has an intense desire to be unfaithful to his wife, he may, by projection, accuse his wife unjustly of infidelity, in an unconscious effort to banish his own feeling of guilt.

Another mechanism is known as *introjection,* by which the individual incorporates into himself the ideas and attitudes of others. One hardly realizes how many of his likes, dislikes, opinions, ideals, and prejudices are carried over from his parents, or some other influence in his environment, without any critical evaluation on his own part. Almost automatically, he absorbs the outlook of the group in which he lives. The process of introjection is useful from the standpoint of conformity, but if carried to an extreme, it may stultify imagination and prevent any originality of thought and action.

A third mechanism commonly employed by the mind is *identification.* This is familiar to all in the case of the little boy who insists that he is the current cowboy star. By means of identification, the adult comes to feel himself a part of the group in which he moves. This is a positive manifestation if it enables men to work together to a common goal, but when used negatively, it results in clannishness and unhealthy exclusion of new contacts and new ideas.

Still other mechanisms employed defensively by the mind are *compensation, rationalization, displacement,* and *reaction formation.* Everyone is familiar with the little bully, who tries to make up in overaggressive behavior what he lacks in size. This is easily recognized as *compensation.* A more beneficial use of the mechanism is seen in handicapped persons who accomplish outstanding feats with those facilities left unimpaired.

Probably no device is more universally employed than is *rationalization.* Through this mechanism, the individual attributes a conscious excuse for his unconscious motives, substituting some acceptable reason for his behavior for the real one, which he may only dimly sense. By fooling himself, the individual finds all manner of plausible reasons for doing what he does. The reasons he gives, however, are not his most compelling ones. An example is the salesman who says that his next client is "probably not in, anyway," when he dreads having to make another call that day.

Still another defense mechanism is called *displacement.* This consists of turning the emotion felt toward one object onto another object. Thus, the painful element in the emotion is reduced, since the immediate object of the emotion has been excluded from consciousness. If one is angry with his employer, but afraid to antagonize him, that person is quite likely to "take it out" on the first harmless individual to cross his path. This enables him to discharge the hostile emotion without incurring dangerous retaliation.

Reaction formation is a process of denying, through contrasting outward behavior, what one inwardly feels. It is the "whistling in the dark" of the emotional life. A typical illustration is the aloof, disdainful attitude sometimes adopted by those whose craving for affection goes unrealized.

These and many other mental mechanisms are employed unconsciously by everyone in daily living. They serve to keep the mind at ease. By making use of these mechanisms, yet without knowing he uses them, the individual escapes painful feelings of inadequacy, insignificance, and guilt.

Much that is understood of unconscious motivation is found in the work of Sigmund Freud, whose prolific investigations on the processes of the mind greatly influenced the course of psychiatric thought. While many aspects of Freud's

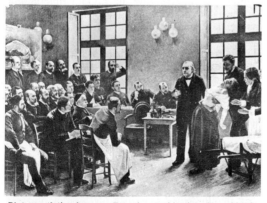

Picture of the famous French psychiatrist, Jean Martin Charcot (1825-1893), giving a demonstration of his methods for treating the insane. Charcot was a pioneer in this field. *Bettmann Archive.*

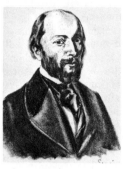

SEGUIN, Edouard (1813-1880) American psychiatrist. Regarded as the greatest figure in the nineteenth century in the training of mental defectives. Realizing the futility of trying to restore the feeble-minded to normal intelligence, he emphasized a "physiological method." which developed the motor and sensory functions for practical use. His work in the U.S. for the retarded blind accelerated greatly the growth of schools for the mentally defective.

teaching have been modified, he made many fundamental discoveries on the role of basic impulses in the development of emotional illness. He emphasized that as the child is molded into conformity with the demands of his environment, certain spontaneous feelings are necessarily suppressed. Most severely discouraged are those feelings of an aggressive and of a sexual nature. As a result of harsh parental restriction of such impulses, the child may react with fear whenever the impulses recur. A strong impulse complicated by intense fear concerning it produces conflict. These conflicts, which occur in childhood, are almost forgotten in adult life, but they can be recalled with psychiatric help. Sometimes, when the original conflicts can be uncovered and brought to light, the emotional disturbance may be dispelled. A great deal of controversy resulted from Freud's teachings, which were widely criticized and often misunderstood. Much of the criticism was unscientific indignation at the mere suggestion that mankind is motivated by sexual impulses, often expressed by individuals themselves well-suited to illustrate Freud's contention. Scientific objections to some of Freud's premises, however, were made on an entirely different basis.

Adolph Meyer, who died in 1950 at the age of 84, has exerted a far-reaching influence on psychiatric thought. The difference in outlook between Freud and Meyer is basically one of perspective. Meyer rejected the concept of Freud—that mental disorders result from unconscious repressions—on the ground that this explains only a small portion of man's emotional difficulties and fails to account for his total motivation. While acknowledging that sexual conflicts may be significant in causing some emotional disorders, he insisted that it is necessary to consider man *as a whole*, weighing the mutual interaction of his physical and mental functions and the influence of significant persons and things in his environment. By this approach, which Meyer called *psychobiology*, he contended that physicians could learn much of what is troubling a patient without having to probe into the deep unconscious processes. By regarding mind and body as an integrated unit, he has a broader basis for discovering the nature of the patient's difficulties. According to Meyer, a person may become physically or mentally ill as a result of faulty adaptation to the stresses of his environment. Since mental distress has a disruptive effect on the functions of the body, just as physical illness disturbs one emotionally, the goal of the well-adjusted individual must be a "sound mind in a sound body." The achievement of this is a lifelong goal, beginning in infancy.

Infancy

If the mind of the infant is to develop normally, it must have a warm emotional environment, a rich educational stimulation, and protection from such destructive feelings as excessive fear, doubt, guilt, and insecurity. As every stage of development has its own specific accomplishments, so each stage has its own particular pitfalls.

The act of being born has been called one of the greatest adjustments a human being is ever called upon to make. From the warmth and security of his mother's womb, the child is projected harshly into the world, where, cut off from his previous supply of oxygen, he first encounters physical tension. When the mounting tension impels him to breathe, the newborn baby achieves his initial victory over the environment. His first breath is thought to be emotionally satisfying to him because he has accomplished something essential to his existence. Adequate satisfaction of physical needs forms a preliminary basis for mental health.

As further physical tensions arise, the baby discovers a variety of needs and limitations. He becomes aware of the demands of his stomach, his bladder, and his colon. He soon finds that the momentary relief from emptying his bladder is supplanted by the discomfort of dampness and cold. By trial and error, he learns that crying brings attention. He becomes aware of his relationship to others who are necessary for the fulfillment of his needs. During his first year, the baby is completely dependent on those responsible for his care. The manner in which his needs are answered gives rise to his pattern of emotional response. Any baby who is repeatedly left hungry, wet, cold, and desolate will probably come to feel that the world is a hostile place. When he is forced to wait so long for his feeding that he suffers hunger pains, he will react with rage. When he is handled clumsily or without the proper support, he will feel afraid. When left in physical discomfort for long periods of time, he will experience anxiety, which can quickly become a habit of reaction. This is not to say that the baby should be permitted to tyrannize the household. The mother who is emotionally secure herself learns to recognize the tone of her baby's cry. The petulant lament which is a bid for further pampering usually sounds quite different from the frightened screams when something really hurts him. If there is any doubt in her mind, the mother can always pick him up and see whether the hubbub dies down. Then a few soothing words and reassuring pats will serve to let the baby know that mother is close by and will respond when he really needs her. This may spare him hours of fury and frustration. A little frustration will not result in any severe emotional disturbance; but prolonged denial, whether it stems from mere neglect or from deliberate unkindness, may give the child a feeling of insecurity which will stay with him throughout life.

Emotional stunting: In a private home, the baby gets a great deal of loving attention. He is played with, smiled at, talked to, and fondled many times a day. This stimulation encourages him to all kinds of responses which serve to identify him with his environment. Extensive studies of babies in institutions reveal that isolation during this crucial period can seriously inhibit a child's capacity for understanding the world he lives in. In understaffed foundling homes where one nurse has full responsibility for the care of a dozen or more infants, it is naturally impossible for each baby to receive the personal expressions of affection it needs. These children, deprived of warm, human contact, often fail to develop normally, either physically or mentally. Even though their bodily requirements are fully met, these babies do not gain weight as they should; and many reveal a shockingly lowered resistance to infections. They become listless and lack the alertness found in children raised in private homes. Indications that these children become both emotionally and intellectually retarded are shown by actual tests, comparing them with children from normal homes. These tests revealed that the institutionalized babies were much slower to learn stories

and songs, had greater difficulty in understanding and remembering things, and were slower to comprehend all types of situations.

Authorities feel that the earlier this emotional deprivation takes place, the more damaging will be the effects on the mind. If it occurs at a later stage than infancy—after the child has learned to speak—the harmful effects can be partially reversed by attentive foster care. Foster parents are therefore instructed that the young baby taken from a crowded orphanage needs more coddling and petting than does the average child, to give it the sense of security it so desperately needs.

It was assumed at one time that everyone was born with certain unchangeable natural endowments, and would reach the level of intelligence dictated by these endowments, regardless of his life experiences. This viewpoint, however, overlooked the close connection between emotional deprivation and intellectual retardation. Many tests are available for measuring the comparative intelligence of infants and children. Far from being static, intellectual capacity has shown a decided increase following the transfer of children from the barren emotional environment of institutions to new homes rich in positive emotional stimulation.

Similar increases are found in many cases where children from "culturally deprived" homes are exposed to esthetic and cultural environmental stimulation.

An all too familiar sight is the adult who has an open mind in all respects but one. His unreasonable emotional attitudes toward one particular subject make normal reasoning impossible in that particular field. Such a person is incapable of objective thinking on that subject. This is an example of stunting in but one area. Frequently it is traceable to some painful emotional experience in the background of the individual. It is easy to understand, therefore, that when the emotional background contains only painful deprivation, a corresponding stunting can take place in many areas of learning. The child deprived of affection cannot help feeling isolated and insecure, and a mind in which these emotions predominate is not a fertile field for developing one's full potentialities. Of course, even an ideal environment will not make a genius of the child with but average endowments, nor lead to normal development in one who is born mentally deficient. It is the responsibility of the controlling adults, however, to make every effort to insure that their attitudes do the child no harm, so that he may develop his own capacities up to the limits of his individual potentialities.

While he is in this early, receptive stage, the infant is capable of gaining his first faith in the world, provided he is handled with reassuring warmth and affection. He gains confidence from having his bodily needs attended to with reasonable promptness. The expressions of love and

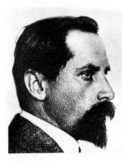

MEYER, Adolf (1866-1950) American psychiatrist. First to suggest the term "mental hygiene" to describe the worldwide movement toward the reform of asylums for the insane, which began in the early years of this century. During his time, Meyer was the leading psychiatrist in America. He taught psychiatry at Clark University, at Cornell, and at Johns Hopkins, and directed the Phipps Psychiatric Clinic at Johns Hopkins.

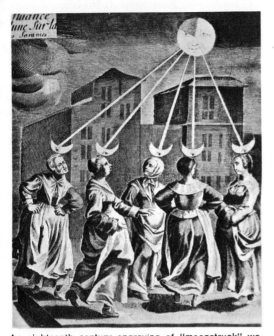

An eighteenth century engraving of "moonstruck" women, illustrating the old belief that the moon caused insanity. The word lunatic is derived from the Latin word meaning moon. *Bettmann Archive.*

tenderness he receives impart to him some warm sensation which is a forerunner to human affection. At the same time, they establish in his mind a groundwork of basic trust.

Orientation into the world of reality: While the baby is learning his first trust in the outside world, he begins to perceive his own place in that world. The capacity to distinguish internal sensations from external reality is taken for granted by the adult, but it must be learned gradually by the child. He may be but a few months old when he gains his first awareness that there is a difference between himself and the external environment. Just what that difference is remains confused to him throughout his early years.

Childhood

Gradually, the time comes when the nursing baby is replaced by the nursery child. The baby finds that he is no longer *completely dependent*. When he wants something, he can go after it, and many times he has to be restrained. With his growing need for self-assertion, the baby can find this constant prohibition most infuriating. At this early stage, he is still unable to compromise with the environment. The parents, however, can do many things to compromise with him. The rooms in which he plays can be "child-proofed," somewhat, by the removal from the child's presence of dangerous and breakable objects.

Development of self-assertiveness: The baby's awakening capacity to assert its desires are seen in many areas of behavior during the second year especially. The little individual feels a desperate need to make some *choices* for himself. With a little tact, this need can be exploited to the benefit of all concerned. The child can be asked, for instance, not whether he wants to eat, but which of two foods he wants to *choose* for supper.

Too frequently, during this period of seemingly willful resistance, toilet training becomes an issue surrounded with emotional strife. Parents do not always realize how important it is to a child to discover one area of performance over which he can exercise full control. For the first time in his life, the baby finds that *his* bowel movement is something *he* can hold on to or let go at will. If the mother demands unreasonable perfection, or shows undue impatience at his failures, the baby may refuse to co-operate just for spite, or he may become anxious, thus deepening his sense of inadequacy. It is important, therefore, that no disciplinary issue be allowed to grow up around bowel training—which it is best to postpone until the early part of the second year. Later, when the baby's seeming willfulness has subsided somewhat, the mother can obtain his co-operation by praising him and making him want to show how reliable he can be in this respect. Above all, the baby should not be punished and made to feel that there is anything shameful about eliminations, for shame and doubt are the potential pitfalls of this stage. The impatient mother who imposes unreasonable demands can create in the child a sense of self-doubt. This may create a pattern of overconscientious reaction. When such patterns are deeply instilled, the child may grow to adulthood with a rigid, unyielding attitude toward life.

During the period from the second to the fifth years, the wise mother will attempt to enlist on her side that new and powerful weapon—the baby's increasing self-assertiveness. It is best to avoid a clash of wills whenever possible, by using a little foresight and humor. The child needs to be guided, lovingly, firmly, and tolerantly, but allowed to feel that he stands on his own two feet. In this way, he is helped over the emotional crises peculiar to this stage of growth. And he is given a chance "to develop self-control without the loss of self-esteem." This is a highly important milestone in the baby's emotional life.

The awakening initiative and sexuality: The child of four or five has perfected locomotion and language to the point where he has a fair command of his surroundings. Walking and talking, instead of being ends in themselves, are now used as means to an end. This broadens the child's scope tremendously and opens new and limitless vistas for learning about the world. Prodded by insatiable curiosity, the little individual sets about with growing initiative to find out all the answers. He has to get under, behind, and into everything to see, to learn, to know. Also his verbal prodding never seems to cease.

Comparisons assume great importance in explaining the phenomena of reality. Such concepts as big or little, boy or man, girl or woman, and boy or girl, fascinate the child, and with good reason. A special interest in the difference between the sexes arises at this period, as well as a new awareness of the sensory function of his own genital zone. Both boys and girls usually discover that pleasurable sensations are associated with this area of their bodies. This is part of the normal sexual development and should not be regarded as cause for alarm by the child's parents. Above all, the child should not be made to feel guilty for indulging in natural experimentation characteristic of this period in life. Parents might find it reassuring to remember that genital manipulation is not physically harmful and can do no injury to the mind *unless emotional conflicts are artificially created*, surrounding the practice with fear and guilt.

The child at this stage is particularly vulnerable to feelings of guilt. He is extremely sensitive; he is beginning to distinguish right from wrong; and he is beginning to develop a conscience. And the conscience of a little child is more cruel and less flexible than that of the rationalizing adult. Therefore, it is all the more important that parents maintain a gentle and tolerant attitude to the child's natural tendency to sexual investigation.

The sexual role assumes significance in other ways, too, at this period. The little boy wants to be a grown man—the man of the house—and, as he may state, he wants to marry his mother. The little girl desires to be a woman and take full charge of her father. These budding emotions are sincere and strong. They merit respect, rather than thoughtless ridicule. A child can sincerely love both parents and at the same time feel painfully jealous of the parent of his own sex. This can heighten his feelings of inadequacy and guilt. Powerful and destructive emotions can thus be engendered.

The legend of King Oedipus, a classic of Greek literature, illustrates the guilt connected with conflict between father and son. When Oedipus was born, it was predicted that one day he would kill his father. To prevent this, the father decreed that the infant prince be killed. An attendant was instructed to take the baby to the forest and murder him. As the story goes, the man did not kill the child, but instead abandoned him in the forest. The child survived, grew to manhood, and became a powerful warrior. He overthrew and killed his father and married his mother without knowing their identity. When he discovered later what he had done, his guilt was so severe that he renounced his kingdom and blinded himself in atonement. No better illustration could be found for the conflict between love and jealousy which the little boy often feels toward his father. He cannot help it if, loving his father, he nevertheless wants him out of his way, so he can have his mother all to himself. He feels, however, that this desire is wrong. The normal child usually weathers this conflict with an adequate adjustment, but some children are unable to throw off the excessive feelings of guilt.

The child needs affectionate reassurance to help him overcome the distressing mental conflicts of this period. He can be helped through this highly impressionable stage if parental attitudes minimize, rather than accentuate, these potential dangers of sex. Emotional crises first encountered in the fourth and fifth years can remain fixed in the mind of the adult and jeopardize his chance for a serene and happy sexual adjustment.

The awakening of industry: Adults have often observed that children are remarkably "busy" when they play. Children themselves agree. Whatever the game, they pursue it with unremitting diligence. The three-year-old who lines up his cars must place every one "just so"; the six-year-old who saves paper dolls must complete her collection in minute detail. When interrupted, children frequently protest that they "have work to do." The significance of this "work" may be lost on the adult, whose own play is approached in a spirit of escape from life's daily chores. Play is important to the child, because as he plays, he achieves a sense of mastery over objects, time, and space. In play, he becomes "Superman." It is an accomplishment worth working for. The sense

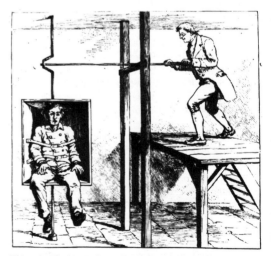

This circulating swing of 1818, which was supposed to bring the depressive back to sound reasoning, was considered at that time to be a great advance in treatment of the insane. *Bettmann Archive.*

of mastery, with its accompanying pride, motivates every meaningful contribution which man gives to the world.

With entrance into school, emphasis is placed on new attainments, which one day will serve the individual in fulfilling his life's vocation. It is important that the child's schooling proceed with about the same speed as his capacity for assimilating it. If his instruction is too fast, he will become frustrated and discouraged. If too slow, he will become bored and impatient. The importance of good teachers cannot be overemphasized, for the finest teachers impart not only knowledge, but also inspiration and zeal, which are powerful determinants in the individual's choice of a career. By giving genuine encouragement to work done well, parents and teachers alike can help establish positive attitudes toward learning in the child's mind.

The dangers of this period lie in the tendency of the child to develop inferiority feelings when it seems that his efforts go unappreciated and that his work is deemed not worthwhile. These inferiority feelings can be kept to a minimum if the child's favorite adults will emphasize his successes, rather than his failures. They should help him to learn that mistakes are normal and expected—even grown-ups make their share of mistakes.

By this time, the child's patterns of emotional reaction are fairly well established. The years of elementary schooling constitute a period of industry in which the child indeed has serious work to do to fit him for his role in life. Recognition of the value of his work implies recognition of his personal worth as well. This stimulates enjoyment of work and pride in accomplishment. And it may go a long way to create in the growing mind a desire to establish a sound position in the world of achievement.

Adolescence

At puberty, the youth relives some of the emotional upheavals of his earlier life. Again he encounters conflict in the realm of sex. In the years from three to five, he learned of the differences comprising the world of opposites. He was impressed with the fact that mother and father, men and women, boys and girls, were not alike. The little girl became aware of her own feminine traits which foreshadowed the passive role she would have in our society. The little boy exercised aggressive tendencies, laying the groundwork for his future status as an active male. With the physical changes of puberty, even their own bodies seem strange and unreliable. The girl is jarred from childhood irresponsibility by the onset and implications of menstruation. The boy is disconcerted by his awkward physique and the unfamiliar sound of his own voice.

At the same time that he must cope with the demands of an unstable body, the adolescent embarks upon a totally new social role. After the fantasies of childhood have been outgrown, his own position is still remote and undefined. Not content to be the make-believe head of his father's home, he seeks a satisfactory identity of his own. No longer a child, but not yet a man, he strives desperately to establish a sound feeling of personal identity. He seeks his own kind, who are also eager for reassurance. They band together in cliques and gangs and go to great lengths to maintain their identity as members of the group. They willingly adopt a rigidity of manner and a sameness of dress which never could be imposed on them from without. The most outlandish garb may be selected, but they will wear nothing different because in being able thereby to identify one another, they are aided in identifying themselves and their position in the world. This stylized sameness employed by the adolescent serves as a defense against his feelings of insecurity. He overcompensates by this desire "to belong," displaying a ruthless intolerance of all who differ from him.

The adolescent overcompensates in other ways as well. As a bid for his own acceptance, he accepts the current heroes of his group. Depending on his environment, these may range from movie stars or crooners to political leaders or militarists. His admiration for these idols is only excelled by the "crushes" he develops on members of the opposite sex. No longer happy with the exclusive company of his own sex, he agonizes in the throes of "puppy love," usually a form of intense but powerless yearning. His behavior may seem capricious as he alternates from hesitancy to brashness in the company of the opposite sex, but he should not be ridiculed, for he is in much the same position as a child groping with the burdens of a man.

The adolescent who cannot lose himself in the meaningful, though apparently shallow, fads of his age level may court disaster. For without this emotional support during the precarious years of adolescence, he may become the delinquent victim of his own impulses or the neurotic victim of his own inhibitions.

One of the most important things the adolescent has to learn is the desirability of foregoing immediate satisfactions for long-term goals. This may be particularly difficult for him in the field of sexual activity, since he is called upon to regulate the powerful pressures within his body with a mind which, in many respects, is unsure of itself. A broad and tolerant attitude on the part of his parents provides his greatest support in meeting the problems of this period and will help him to establish sound values in his approach to maturity.

Above all, the adolescent needs assurance of his place in the world. Mental health during this trying period rests upon the outcome of each previous crisis: trust of the environment learned in infancy; faith in himself gained in childhood; and confidence that the world will provide opportunities for the fulfillment of his natural aspirations. The normal youth eventually surmounts the trials peculiar to adolescence, emerging with a sense of self which assures the confidence necessary to a healthy adult mind.

Young adulthood

The life of an individual is filled with alternating periods of order and chaos. Youth is a time for gathering in and consolidating the experiences of previous stages. Dependence on the group for identification, so important in adolescence, is replaced in adult life by independent rivalry or voluntary co-operation. A task of young adulthood is learning to work and to love.

If he is self-assured, the young adult is capable of both competition and intimacy in his relationships with others. If his foundation of self-esteem is secure, he will adjust readily to the rivalry of the business world and to the necessary interdependence of the married state. Deep psychological value may accrue from the mutual experiences of marriage. The capacity to love and to be loved, mentally and physically, is of prime significance in evolution of the healthy mind. Mutually satisfactory marital relations, states Erikson, "somehow appease the potential rages caused by the daily evidence of the oppositeness of male and female, of fact and fancy, of love and hate, of work and play."

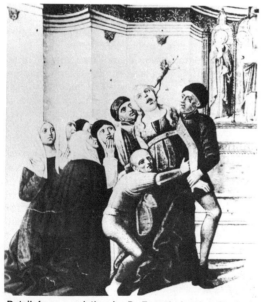

Detail from a painting by B. Fungai showing St. Catherine casting a devil out of a woman. This picture reflects the old belief that disease in humans was caused by devils. *Bettmann Archive.*

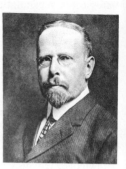

SACHS, Bernard Parney (1858-1944) American neurologist. Chiefly noted for his description of the prenatal degeneration of the macular region of the retina (1887) in amaurotic family idiocy, previously observed in 1881 by Tay. In this disease, which is believed to occur chiefly in Jewish children, Sachs further observed such other pathological effects as the progressive breakdown of brain and spinal cells, and atrophy of the eye.

Arising spontaneously with satisfactory sexual relations is the natural urge for procreation. This involves an interest which goes beyond merely "liking children," or the passive resignation to their accidental birth. Gradually, as his own life assumes greater meaning, the young adult comes to feel somehow that life is worth renewing. The desire for children is the conscious manifestation of this attitude.

As a parent, the individual becomes involved again in the struggles of a child for independence. But this time, he finds himself in a different role. If he has developed healthy emotions, he will be able to recognize the rights of his child as an individual. It does not occur to some parents that even a child has certain rights of his own, for example, property rights. When parents fail to respect the right of a child to control his own possessions, the child may never learn respect for the property of others. Recent studies of children apprehended for theft reveal a background in which parents failed to acknowledge the property rights of their children. It is the parent's responsibility to give the child all the care he needs, so long as he is dependent, but it is equally important for them to encourage the child to assert his independence in gradually expanding fields. This involves much guidance and some restraint. The restraints employed, however, should be kind and reasonable ones.

The emotionally immature parent sometimes lives vicariously through his child, to an exaggerated degree, making decisions for him, even when the child is well able to make them for himself. The parent who does this is working out the frustrations of his own life on the child. Although done in the guise of sacrifice and devotion, this actually is rejecting behavior on the part of the parent because it deprives the child of the opportunity to develop self-reliance. This is not to say that parents should permit their children to make all their own decisions, without any restraint. This would be as unfair to the child as overprotection, for then the child would never learn to conform to the standards of society. Between the extremes of neglect and domination, there is a middle ground of constructive guidance, which bolsters the child's incentive toward self-realization and independence.

Even if he does not produce children, the adult on the route to full maturity usually becomes imbued with the desire to contribute something of merit to the world. In wanting to originate something worthwhile, he is not giving way to petty vanity. The creation of ideas and things is a further means of satisfying the innate craving of the healthy mind for generative expression. Whatever means he selects, the young adult finds that his life holds greater significance if he is able to carry forward something to nurture and enrich his later years.

The mature personality

Maturity is not an absolute quality. There is probably no individual living who has a completely mature personality. Such a person undoubtedly would be all-wise, all-tolerant, and in emotional balance. He would hardly be human, for he would be beyond human frailties. Nevertheless, it is well for man to have the mature personality as his goal, to approximate as best he can.

Hardly anyone can be said to have a perfect body; yet everyone remains as strong and healthy as he can. So long as his body functions adequately, the individual learns to accept his physical imperfections. He must also accept himself as a whole, despite the minor imperfections of his mind. With the ability to accept oneself, there is increased ability to accept others; thus the individual enlarges his capacity for tolerance. He learns to tolerate his own weaknesses without shame and the weaknesses of others without contempt. He acknowledges that people can be different without being wrong. Also he can recognize a course of action as inappropriate for himself without deeming it worthless.

In his approach to maturity, the individual faces many decisions: when to adapt to, and when to effect changes in the environment; when to follow; and when to assume the responsibility for leadership. When he has a choice of going forward into self-expansion, or holding back in order to conform, he experiences normal anxiety at the threshold of each new venture. Working through that anxiety is a constructive process of growth to further maturity.

With growing maturity comes a sense of human dignity and admiration for one's fellow man, expressed first in comradship with one's contemporaries, and later in a common understanding with those who have left contributions to the world in the liberal arts, scientific discoveries, institutions, and traditions. The insecure and immature person will appraise the present through the distortions of the past. One who is more mature will try to appraise the traditions of the past in terms of present knowledge and requirements. No one lifetime is long enough for the individual to make his own discovery of all the great and basic truths available to man. The person who selects the best out of tradition to cherish for himself benefits from the thoughts and works of people in the past. He places value on great contributions which have gone before him without, however, accepting blindly all that former leaders have taught. He will reject those factors in tradition which hobble him too much and which if followed would lead to the stagnation of his mind. Whether in science, politics, religion, or whatever field, the mature man's quest for truth requires constant reevaluation and reissuing in more enlightened terms in the light of new experiences of the species.

Dreams

The dream has long been a subject of controversy among students of the human mind. Many took the view that a dream was merely an idle flight into fantasy, while others believed that it played the role of a "mental cathartic."

Studies have shown now that the average individual dreams several times during the night. The average length of the dream is about 20 minutes. At the University of Chicago, a team of investigators undertook to determine the importance, if any, of the dream. Volunteer subjects were used in the experiment which was designed to keep the person from dreaming throughout the night. Those individuals deprived of dreams for several nights became irritable, nervous, and upset. Some of them even began to hallucinate. The data accumulated from various studies such as this seem to indicate that if a person is deprived of his freedom to dream, he might suffer a nervous breakdown. It is believed that dreams are a natural release for simple frustrations and tensions stored within the mind during the process of daily living.

DISORDERS OF THE MIND: THE NEUROSES

One of the greatest obstacles to the achievement of maturity is chronic emotional disturbance. The person who is suffering from painful emotions constantly seeks some satisfactory way of dealing with this pain. Among the various solutions open to him are the so-called neurotic reactions.

Perhaps the most important aspect of Freud's work has been the explanations it provides for the origins of the common neuroses besetting man. Their cause, their purpose, and a clue to

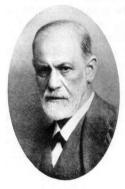

FREUD, Sigmund (1856-1939) Austrian psychiatrist. Founded the science of psychoanalysis, and is regarded as one of the great creative minds of the nineteenth century. His discovery of the unconscious mind has had a profound influence on modern life. His doctrines emphasize the importance which childhood impressions, stored in the unconscious, have on mental life; and the sexual root of many desires, dreams, and cultural and social activities.

their cure are believed by most authorities to be found in Freud's concept of repressed material disturbing the emotional equilibrium. According to his theory, neurotic conditions arise from old emotional conflicts, long buried below the level of consciousness. Emotional stress experienced early in childhood may be stifled and forgotten, yet the emotional responses of the child are distorted by these repressed impulses. The emotional conflicts often center around feelings of resentment, hostility, aggression, and guilt. The child comes to believe that these feelings are unacceptable and therefore represses them. These repressed impulses remain alive below the level of consciousness and interfere with his subsequent emotional adjustment throughout life. Whenever the buried emotional conflicts threaten to reach consciousness, the individual experiences anxiety and spontaneously attempts a solution which will put that anxiety to rest.

Regardless of the origin of neurotic reactions, it is clear that their purpose is an attempt on the part of the individual to deal with emotional pain. Emotional pain can be just as severe as physical pain and even more alarming because the individual cannot always localize it. He develops devious methods for dealing with this pain. As a simple reaction to emotional stress, the individual may give way to tears, or blushing, or he may break out in a sweat. These are universally recognized as physical accompaniments of emotion. They are involuntary and uncontrollable responses, yet they may be regarded as "normal" since they are common experiences of all. In some instances, however, when the emotional stress is greater, or the individual's power of resistance is weaker, he well develop imperfect, or neurotic, reactions for coping with this pain. The neurotic manifestations take various forms. One person may react to his emotional discomfort with generalized uneasiness, known to psychiatrists as the *anxiety reaction*. Another type of solution for dealing with emotional stress is the *phobic reaction*, in which the anxiety is attached to a specific object or situation which

the individual then scrupulously avoids, thereby avoiding the anxiety it symbolizes. A third neurotic solution is the *obsessive-compulsive reaction*, in which the persistent self-doubts are reassured by precise and ritualistic behavior. Still a fourth device is the *depressive reaction*, which is characterized by physical and mental inertia and a general sense of pessimism. A more serious neurotic manifestation is known as the *dissociative reaction*. This takes a variety of forms, but in each the patient loses awareness, for a time, of who he is. Still another neurosis is the *conversion reaction*, in which the anxiety is converted into apparent disorders of the sensory functions of the body. These and other neurotic reactions are merely attempts on the part of the individual to cope with the feeling of anxiety without having to face the underlying conflicts which actually cause it. By these measures, the neurotic is protected from total mental disruption. Although his emotional functioning is disturbed, these neuroses serve as unconscious safety devices and allow him to maintain contact with reality. He does not understand, however, how this machinery works.

Emotional stress

Emotional stress is as common to man as thirst or hunger. No generation in all of history has been free from stress. Past generations have had to fear plagues, wars, the king's tax collectors, and highwaymen, as well as the normal burdens of daily life. Today, especially in America, the normal problems of daily living should be lessened because of the high standard of living. Yet, approximately 19,000 people commit suicide each year in the United States because of intolerable stress. A breakdown of the causes of these self-imposed deaths reveals such factors as romantic quarrels, business failures, grief over the death of a loved one, excessive guilt feelings, etc.

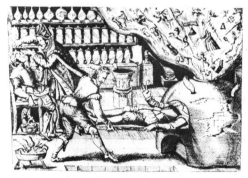

This old picture depicts a doctor of about the year 1600 treating a patient with heat, which was believed to be efficacious in driving out fantasies, hallucinations and melancholy. *Bettmann Archive.*

However, some individuals who are borderline neurotics attempt to assume the emotional burdens of the world, becoming excessively anxious over such matters as pollution, modern rocketry with nuclear warheads, and perpetual war. Depending upon the fragility of their emotional defenses, they may or may not be able to endure these burdens. There has never been a stress-free society and the immediate future shows no prospect of producing one. It is up to each member of society to yield just enough to the blows of life to keep from breaking and thus, in time, develop a mature personality.

Anxiety reaction

Anxiety has a beneficial function. Whether it warns of external threat or inner emotional stress, the function of anxiety is to alert the individual to danger. Some degree of anxiety is normally encountered by everyone in the process of growth, with each succeeding separation from familiar surroundings. The emotionally healthy individual is able to turn his anxiety into constructive use, recognizing it as a danger signal and following its warning by effecting changes in the disturbing life situations. The emotionally disturbed individual, however, may become the victim of a chronic state of anxiety which he cannot overcome because of his inner conflicts. This constitutes the neurosis known as the *anxiety reaction*.

In the anxiety reaction, the individual is conscious of his state of tension, but unable to locate the source of the impending threat. This has been described by psychiatrists as "free-floating" anxiety, because it cannot be pinned down to any particular source. The individual simply cannot find peace of mind because of a pervading sense of uneasiness. His symptoms of agitation are frequently apparent to others. He may appear frightened and excited. Among his physical responses may be a racing pulse, pounding heart, profuse sweating, and heavy breathing. He may feel weak and dizzy and complain of vague disturbance of the digestive tract. The patient sometimes will not know exactly what is the matter, but will fear that he is going to die. He may suffer nightmares which leave him with a feeling of nameless dread. These overt signs of apprehension indicate the presence of some emotional conflict of which the individual is not aware.

Most authorities hold that the roots of chronic anxiety are laid in childhood, often unintentionally, by overly rejecting or overly permissive handling on the part of the parents. Parents who are undemonstrative usually make a child feel unloved and insecure. An adult can often appraise threats to his emotional security and take measures to overcome them, but a child cannot do so as well. His feeling of insecurity is increased with each instance of unkind or unrealistically permissive treatment. The discrepancy between expectation and reality is a source of conflict and resentment in the child. He responds by a show of hostility directed against those he loves. The awareness of his hostility in turn creates feelings of guilt and fear. He may anticipate punishment and yet feel that punishment is deserved. Although he tends to repress his feelings of hostility, he may not be entirely successful in eliminating the accompanying guilt. The resulting anxiety becomes a pattern of reaction to many of his troublesome life situations. Emotional conflict is at the root of the anxiety reaction. According to May, anxiety always involves two contradictory desires within the individual. The anxiety reaction cannot be dispelled, therefore, without eliminating the source of inner conflict.

Phobic reaction

Unreasonable fear of a specific thing, such as the fear of closed places (*claustrophobia*), characterizes the *phobic reaction*. The object of fear is usually a thing or situation which the individual can avoid, and so long as he does avoid it, he is relatively free of anxiety.

This fear of certain objects is thought to arise as a substitute for some conflictive situation in the person's mind which he prefers not to face. This displacement of anxiety takes place in the unconscious level of the mind. The feeling of apprehension which stems from emotional conflict is detached from its painful association and placed instead upon some more or less harmless object in the environment. An outside situation thereby is made the symbol of the inner conflict. By avoiding the outside situation, the neurotic avoids some of the anxiety and at the same time saves himself from having to acknowledge what really troubles him.

The individual with a phobic reaction is not aware of the inner workings of his mind. He knows only that he is unaccountably overcome by dread in certain situations, and is thereafter compelled by an inner force to avoid them, even though he recognizes that his fear is unreasonable.

An example of the phobic reaction is seen in the child who grows up in fear of his father, whom he also loves. The resulting conflict creates uneasiness within him, unconsciously repressed. The presence of the father cannot be avoided, so to relieve his anxiety the child transfers his fear of his father onto something else, which serves as an unconscious symbol of his father. As a substitute for the towering stature of the father, he may come to fear high places. Or he may come to fear all men, developing a fear of crowds. By avoiding large crowds or high places, his feeling of anxiety is alleviated. He thus develops a complicated device to make himself more comfortable because he could not face the fact that he feared his own father.

Phobic reactions are tenacious emotional disturbances. They are exceedingly difficult to manage, but with competent medical help the individual may be brought to see the symbolism behind his unreasoning fears. If so, his phobic symptoms may lessen in severity or, in rare instances, actually disappear, if he faces and overcomes the painful memories attending the original conflictive situation.

Obsessive-compulsive reaction

Some persons are troubled by recurrent obsessive thoughts which they cannot stifle. Others are compelled by some inner force to perform certain apparently meaningless and repetitive acts. Although they may try, they cannot understand why they must do these things; they only know that they are extremely uncomfortable until they comply with this powerful impulse. The obsessive-compulsive neurotic is aware that his acts and ideas are irrational and sometimes bizarre, but his symptoms are usually more disturbing to him than they are to others. These symptoms cover a wide variety of manifestations, ranging from the seemingly innocent habit of having to check a locked door several times in the night, to the crippling extreme of constant motor activity. This reaction, like the other neurotic reactions, comes about as a result of repressed emotional conflict which leads to a state of tension. Like the phobic reaction, it also involves displacement of the original anxiety-causing thoughts. But instead of simply avoiding the substitute object, as in the phobias, the compulsives must *undo* the damage and *atone* for these emotional conflicts by an elaborate system of ritualistic behavior. Among the routes they hit upon to safeguard their peace of mind are such devices as perfectionist housekeeping; some people cannot sleep in a room in which one thing is out of place. Others must proceed to their homes always by a certain route; if they make one unaccustomed turn, they must go back and start all over again. The classic example is Lady Macbeth, whose compulsive handwashing was a fruitless effort to eradicate her feeling of guilt. This handwashing compulsion is shared by many neurotics who never took part in a murder, but who suffer from intense guilt feelings connected with their feelings of hostility. Indeed, the obsessive-compulsive is unlikely to commit any crime, for his extraordinary capacity for the displacement of dangerous desires will usually save him from any untoward acts.

The obsessive-compulsive reactions are often reminiscent of primitive, deep-seated responses shared by all. The rhythmic drum beats of the savage, the rocking of the baby, the rhyming of the child—all these repetitive sensations are agreeable and somehow reassuring. During childhood, most people become familiar with the ancient superstitions of the race, and indulge in such "safe" practices as knocking on wood, stepping on or avoiding cracks, walking around ladders, and playing "needles, pins, when a man marries, his trouble begins." These rituals serve a mystic purpose to the child—they placate the uncontrollable and mysterious powers and so protect the child from bad luck, or so he believes. The mature individual tends to outgrow these feelings, but the obsessive neurotic employs to excess similar mystic rituals to placate his own inner doubts and unconscious fears.

In extreme cases, the obsessive-compulsive neurosis can be among the most incapacitating of emotional disorders. Fortunately, however, most persons suffering from this neurosis do not progress beyond the eccentric stage. At times they are fussy and dictatorial, especially when a threat looms before their patterned behavior; but for the most part, they do not come into conflict with their fellow men. Desiring as they do to leave nothing to chance, they are usually superconformists. As a result, they retain high standings in their communities. With their orderliness and their proclivity for a rigid and repetitive activity, they excel in many types of precision and assembly work.

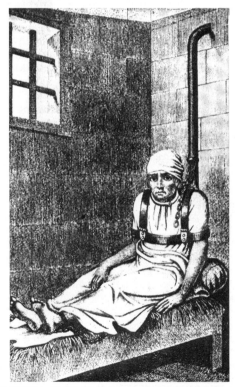

Illustration of one of the devices employed during the nineteenth century for forcibly restraining mental patients. *Copyright Ciba Symposia.*

Depressive reaction

A general slowing up of mental and physical drive is apparent in the *depressive reaction*. This method of handling anxiety is common among people of shy and pessimistic temperament, who allay their feelings of anxiety by excessive self-condemnation. In the depressed emotional state, they are dominated by feelings of worthlessness and guilt.

The feeling of sadness may be precipitated by life situations. The depressed person frequently places the initial blame for his anxiety on financial worries, marital difficulties, or the death of a loved one. Such external situations bring sadness to everyone, but in neurotic individuals the reaction is intensified and prolonged. This is interpreted by some authorities to mean that guilt is present because of repressed aggression. Guilt is especially apparent where the depressed individual held feelings of hostility toward the person he also loved.

Physical symptoms may cause the depressed person to seek medical aid. Though some physical disturbance actually may be present, the depressed individual may be unduly preoccupied with worries about his body. He may complain of insomnia, poor appetite, decreased sex drive, or constipation; often he also reveals indifference to his personal appearance.

Victims of the depressive reaction may respond favorably to reasonably sympathetic handling. They should not be coddled, however, as this may intensify their self-preoccupation. Frequently, they can benefit from guidance into new and interesting avenues of occupation and recreation.

Dissociative reaction

There are some conditions in which the personality becomes temporarily disorganized, the feeling of anxiety takes control, and the individual forgets who he is for a while. When he regains his self-awareness, he will not recall what has taken place. This unconscious flight from situations of intolerable emotional stress is known to psychiatrists as the *dissociative reaction*. It takes a variety of forms, including some kinds of amnesia, sleepwalking, automatic writing, and the extremely rare "dual personality" in which two mental selves exist within the same body at the same time. The most common example of dissociative reaction, of course, is amnesia.

In amnesia, anxiety has become so great that the individual is forced to forget it. In forgetting his anxiety, he forgets also a multitude of necessary associations, even including his identity. In spite of this inconvenience, the patient is well-oriented as to present time and place. He simply cannot recall anything about the past. His behavior appears so normal that he moves about

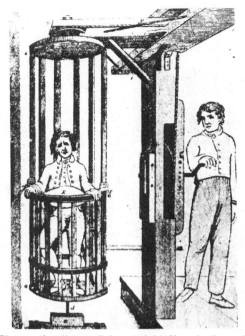

Picture of a "rotater," invented by Horn in the early nineteenth century, which was supposed to bring the insane to their senses. *Bettmann Archive.*

freely without attracting notice. In some instances he may wander restlessly from place to place, covering extensive areas in his travels. Recovery of the memory is sometimes spontaneous. If not, it may frequently be achieved with psychiatric help. Upon regaining his memory, the amnesic patient does not recall events which took place during his period of amnesia. Under hypnosis, however, he can bring forth these events in full detail. This indicates that the loss of consciousness in dissociation is different from that of the delirious states, for the patient who recovers from delirium cannot recall his experiences while unconscious even when hypnotized. Like the other neurotic reactions, dissociation protects the mind from having to face emotional pain, and supports the individual in his effort to surmount an intolerable situation.

Hypnosis

Hypnosis has a definite usefulness in the treatment for certain conditions of anxiety and emotional disturbances and as an aid in controlling chronic pain. It should be used under the supervision of a physician. Surgeons have found that it helps relax the patient before going into anesthesia. In one dramatic instance, a young boy who had been severely burned in an ex-

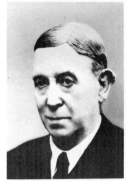

EGAS MONIZ, Antonio C. de Abreu Freire (1874-1955), Portuguese neurologist. Published in 1935 his important studies on the function of the frontal lobes of the brain; in it he described a new therapy, called frontal lobotomy, in which the lines of communication between the frontal lobes and the thalamus are cut to cure certain psychoses. He also introduced arteriography, which is widely used in diagnosing cerebral affections.

plosion kept having repeated dreams about the fire, to the extent that he was afraid to go to sleep and his recovery was threatened. Under hypnosis, the suggestion was made that he would never have this dream again. The suggestion proved effective and marked a turning point in his recovery.

An important role of hypnosis is in assisting to remove underlying neuroses which are reflected in psychosomatic illness, with such symptoms as bronchitis, asthma, neuritis, headaches, and some allergies. Often the phychiatrist or physician can convince the patient while under hypnosis that his disease has no organic basis. When the patient gains insight into his emotional stress, the symptoms begin to regress.

In some instances, it is possible for the psychiatrist to implant a "posthypnotic suggestion" in which he will establish certain words as a key for inducing the hypnotic state. If the patient needs help he can call the psychiatrist on the phone and upon hearing the key words, he will fall into the hypnotic state and accept needed suggestions to alleviate his symptoms.

Conversion reaction

One of the most dramatic forms of neurotic reaction to emotional pain involves the sensory organs under voluntary control. In this reaction, the individual converts his emotional conflicts into apparent disorders of the senses. For this reason, it is spoken of as the *conversion reaction.* Among the striking symptoms are blindness, deafness, and paralysis, all of which occur in the absence of any real organic damage. Frequently, however, the symptoms serve to prevent the individual from carrying out some unacceptable impulse or undesirable task. Since he is unaware of these motives, the conversion neurotic is not a deliberate malingerer. Nevertheless, his symptoms spare him from some distasteful situation. He reacts like a person who is hypnotized and told he has no feeling in a normal limb. Indeed, it may be said the conversion neurotic

unknowingly hypnotizes himself. An example is the soldier, who upon looking upon the dead body of his friend, is suddenly "struck blind." With nothing actually wrong with his eyes, he symbolically blinds himself by becoming unable to see something too painful for his mind to accept. The same mechanism is responsible for certain forms of paralysis in which no muscular or nerve damage exists. A neurotic dancer, for example, excessively fearful of unfavorable criticism, may become paralyzed and unable to take a step.

For many centuries this condition was known to physicians as hysteria. The extensive medical literature on "hysterical blindness" and "hysterical paralysis" referred to this phenomenon. The term *hysteria,* when used in this sense, was not the same thing as the so-called "hysterics" widely attributed to nervous women. This temporary loss of self-control with alternate laughing and crying is not unconscious behavior. Partly because of this confusion, the term *hysteria* is being abandoned in medicine in favor of *conversion reaction,* which more accurately describes the unconscious mechanism which takes place in the sensory field.

The symptoms of conversion, while impressive, give an imperfect imitation of the disorders they simulate. In his ignorance of anatomy, the patient mentally marks off a hand, or an eye, or some part which he conceives to be a physical unit, disregarding the actual relationship of nerves and muscles throughout the body. As a result, his reflexes usually respond normally, which is not common in the organically afflicted.

Once the conversion neurotic has been somewhat relieved of his anxiety by his physical symptoms, he may become reconciled to a condition which cuts him off from a normal life. The French psychiatrist, Janet, named this unusual attitude "the beautiful indifference." This indif-

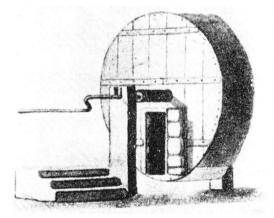

This eighteenth century rotating drum was used for calming mental patients. The patient was strapped in a seat inside. *Copyright Ciba Symposia.*

ferent attitude is closely associated with the factor of secondary gain. The patient evades responsibility and at the same time gains the center of attention. If the secondary gain is great enough, the patient may even resist treatment. He may not recover at all unless removed from the solicitous influence of members of his family. The physician familiar with the psychological mechanism involved, however, can often take the measures necessary to effect a cure.

DISORDERS OF THE MIND: PSYCHOSOMATIC DISORDERS

Certain forms of exaggerated physical reaction to emotional stress resemble the neuroses in the nature of their origin. These are the *psychosomatic* disorders, so called from the interaction of mind *(psyche)* and body *(soma)*. These disorders also resemble the everyday experiences of weeping, blushing, and sweating, to which people readily ascribe an emotional cause. If long sustained, transient disturbances of this kind may become permanent disorders of function, and eventually may result in real structural damage.

That there is an emotional component in illness has been recognized since antiquity. Hippocrates called attention to the fact that strong emotional experiences, such as fear and anger, were often accompanied by transient disturbances in some of the bodily functions. Not only are malfunctions caused when one is psychologically upset, but all illness can be made worse if the patient remains in a state of severe mental unrest. The interaction of mind and body is constant and profound, so that any major disturbance originating in the mind is quickly reflected in the workings of the body.

Unlike the conversion reaction which affects body systems under voluntary control, the psychosomatic disorders usually affect only the organs under the control of the involuntary *(autonomic)* nervous system.

Some psychosomatic disorders differ from the conversion neurosis in another important way. The conversion reaction is symbolic, substituting an apparent functional illness for repressed emotion. In contrast, psychosomatic reactions may occur solely as physical reaction to overstimulation. High blood pressure, for instance, though sometimes resulting from emotional stress, is not necessarily a substitute for the emotion. It may be only an exaggeration of the physical part of the emotion itself. This is commonly experienced in the increased heart rate accompanying sudden fear. Here the functional disturbance has no psychological meaning, though it is truly psychosomatic, having resulted from a mental state.

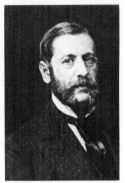

WESTPHAL, Carl F. O. (1833-1890) German neurologist. Westphal described pseudosclerosis, a form of hysteria which simulates multiple sclerosis. Multiple sclerosis is a disease characterized by hardening of patches of tissue in the brain and spinal cord. The disease is not curable, but pseudosclerosis, which is of purely mental origin, produces no brain damage, and is amenable to therapy.

The physical changes which accompany emotion were illustrated by the work of Cannon, who demonstrated that animals react to fear, rage, pain, and hunger by alterations in the gland secretions, blood circulation, and muscle tone. These processes are under control of the involuntary nervous system, which also controls the body systems most often disturbed by psychosomatic disorders in man.

Extensive investigations have revealed that emotional stress causes certain substances to be released during the process of metabolism, which, in effect, cause body and mind to interact. The process has the nature of a chain reaction producing shock and countershock, chiefly by activity of the pituitary and adrenal glands. Prolonged stimulation of these glands may cause high blood pressure, or other dysfunction, to which the name "diseases of adaptation" has been given.

It does not detract from the important research into physiological processes of emotion to emphasize that the *cause* is psychological. Only the embarrassed person knows why he blushed, and even he may not understand his unconscious reasons. The psychological component of emotion is a sensation experienced only by the individual himself. It gives him a distinct feeling of pleasure or pain. The psychological component may be easier to verify than the physiological, since the individual at times is able to describe his own reactions.

The fact that some disorders are emotional in origin does not minimize the value of medical treatment. Psychosomatic disorders may result from multiple causes where the emotional stimulus is combined with other factors, such as a physical predisposition. In disorders of multiple cause, for instance, asthma or colitis, the site of weakness may be physically predisposed, while the precipitating factor is emotional.

Psychosomatic disturbances may take place in any of the involuntary organs of the body systems. These include the digestive, the respiratory, the heart and circulatory, the genitourinary, and the endocrine system, and the skin.

Gastrointestinal reactions: Nervous diarrhea is an extremely common complaint, affecting various patients with different degrees of intensity. Symptoms may include abdominal pain, nausea and bloating, weakness, and diarrhea alternating with constipation; self-treatment may only serve to irritate the sensitive intestinal membrane further and interfere with the natural rhythm of elimination. It is possible that the patient is also seething with emotional conflict.

The emotional component of diarrhea has been recognized by medical men for centuries. Diarrhea occurring with tension states is more frequent than one might suppose. It is a familiar manifestation of fear, occurring frequently in combat and even in such minor situations as examinations in school. As a physical reaction to stress, it is of considerable annoyance to the patient. It may also lead to *mucous colitis,* a psychosomatic disorder which tends to become chronic.

Two factors contribute to the cause—an hereditary predisposition, plus the pressure of emotional stress. Everyone, at one time or another, undergoes periods of mental unrest. These crucial states are able to record themselves in the

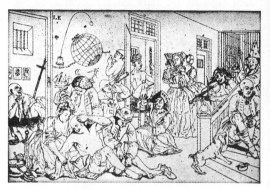

Picture by Hogarth depicting Bedlam, the London establishment for the care of the insane, during the eighteenth century. *Copyright Ciba Symposia.*

body in some way. Among that group of persons who inherit a sensitive gastrointestinal tract, the brunt of emotional crisis may be carried by the colon.

Analysis of many cases of chronic diarrhea has definitely established its close association with the discharge of emotional tension. Fear, rage, and resentment may bring on an acute attack. When mucous colitis is regarded as a bodily reaction to emotional disturbance, rather than a distinct disease, it becomes easy to understand that the symptoms cannot be eradicated in many cases without first improving the emotional status of the patient.

Skin reactions: The idea that an emotional element is present in certain skin disorders is not a new one. This has been recognized for centuries. Still, there are authorities today who minimize any relationship between the emotions and the skin. While acknowledging that mental distress and skin disturbances coexist, they will not agree that one results from the other.

Nevertheless, when no organic basis for an inflammation can be found, the patient's emotional adjustment should be studied for some internal conflict which may be finding expression through the involuntary nervous system. Frequently, in cases of this kind, it may be shown that the skin reaction comes on the patient "in spells," and that these occasions have coincided with specific instances of emotional upheaval.

Some people who have no serious emotional problem are nevertheless constantly torn with petty anxieties. These are the perfectionists. They are good candidates for psychogenic skin eruptions. Still other unstable people may find the obvious skin ailment a useful device for influencing others. This unconscious but effective method is sometimes seen in children.

In a survey of infantile dermatitis, evidence is presented of the interrelation between skin changes and emotional distress. Prominent among the complex causes of this disease, ma-

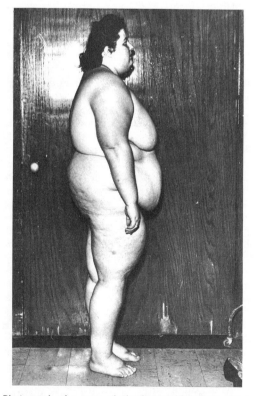

Photograph of a case of obesity resulting from excessive food intake. Certain individuals who feel deprived of love habitually overeat to allay the pangs of emotional hunger. *Courtsey of George J. Hamwi, M.D., Ohio State University, Columbus.*

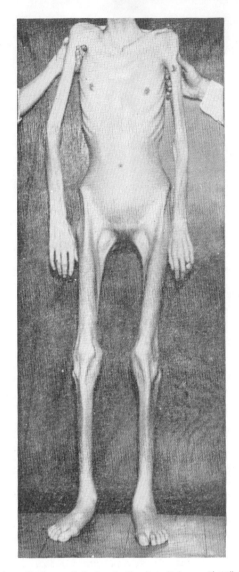

This patient on admission to the hospital was 5′ 11″ in height but weighed only 64 pounds. Although she presented many of the signs of an insufficiency of the pituitary gland, it was decided that the primary disturbance was *anorexia nervosa*, a mental condition in which there is a hysterical aversion for food. *Pictures by Courtesy of G. J. Hamwi, M.D., Department of Medicine, Division of Endocrine and Metabolic Diseases, Ohio State University Health Center, Columbus, Ohio.*

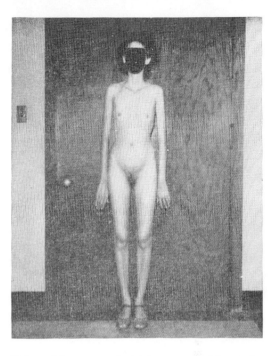

Picture of the same patient taken one year later, during which the only treatment was mental reassurance. As the result of treatment there was an increase in intake of calories and a gain in weight.

ternal rejection appeared to be a factor which all of the cases had in common. The reaction of the children to this rejection took two forms of expression: an emotional outburst of hostility to the mother, and a physical eruption of the skin. Treatment directed toward increased understanding between mother and child in many cases produced definite improvement in the skin.

In adults, dermatitis has been known to arise following threats to physical safety, blows to self-esteem, and bitter sexual conflicts. Fortunately, most patients who show the characteristics of a nervous dermatitis, like other psychosomatic patients, seem to carry their emotional problems close to the surface of their minds. This renders them more accessible to psychiatric treatment.

Respiratory reactions: Bronchial asthma illustrates the multiple factors at work in some psychosomatic disorders. Heredity, allergy, life situation, and, perhaps, deep internal conflict—all may be present and contribute to the illness.

The high incidence of asthma in certain families is striking, yet asthma is not one of the rare diseases which can be transmitted to the child by the parent. In asthma it may be the oversensitive bronchial system which is inherited. The victim is said, then, to have a constitutional predisposition for asthma.

When such an individual also has an intolerance for apparently harmless substances in amounts not harmful to most other people, he is allergic to that substance. When confronted with that substance, his body will display oversensitivity in its weakest point. Allergic reactions are commonplace. Hay fever, skin rashes, hives, or areas of unusual swelling are often seen.

If a child with allergic tendencies frequently witnesses attacks of asthma in his own household, he may come to associate the patient's discomfort with emotional strain. Thereafter, in his

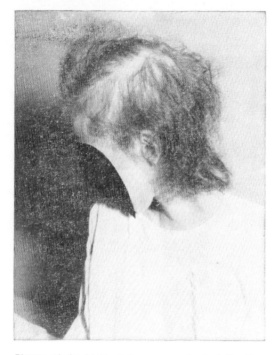

Picture of the head of the same patient at the time of admission to the hospital, showing the extent to which general debilitation affected the scalp.

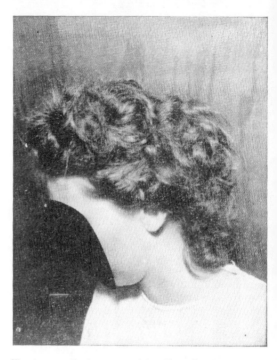

The same patient one year later. Note the dramatic improvement in her hair, that accompanied her increase in weight and general well-being.

case, emotional stress may unduly disturb respiration. Whether the initial attack of asthma comes on in response to allergy, emotion, or bronchitis, subsequent attacks may be precipitated by any one of them.

Some psychiatrists, especially those of the psychoanalytic school, interpret psychosomatic disorders in terms of deep emotional conflicts. They hold, for instance, that peptic ulcer—"stomach ulcer," one of the first structural changes to be positively identified with emotional stress—stems from a deep-seated desire to be babied or "nursed." The aggressive, driving conduct of the typical ulcer victim, they hold, is overcompensation for this unconscious desire. Thus, the businessman who develops ulcers, while striving desperately for success, may be trying unconsciously to prove that he does not need to depend on others. A somewhat similar reasoning is believed to prevail for the asthma victim. According to this theory, he is assumed to have deeply-buried hostility toward those on whom he is dependent. In the process of stifling his resentment toward these persons, he may partially stifle himself by means of an attack of asthma.

In psychosomatic disorders, a minimum of appropriate psychotherapy can often accomplish gratifying results. If specific physical techniques or drugs are administered, the patient should understand that these are but temporary measures which are used to obtain relief until the underlying emotional basis for the symptoms can be found and removed.

If the patient's history shows recurrent attacks of his disorder and these can be shown to coincide with periods of mental stress, these stressful situations may be suspected as the precipitating factor. If the patient can bring to light certain basic conflicts in his mind, his functional symptoms may be no longer needed to express bodily protest. It is important for such an individual to meet his problems squarely, since the worries one faces with frankness are less likely to take a physical toll. If he cannot fully resolve them, perhaps he can at least work out a suitable compromise with the troublesome situation, reasserting the control of his own mind, instead of permitting his body to control him.

DISORDERS OF THE MIND: PERSONALITY DISORDERS

Some people are emotionally maladjusted without suspecting it. Their entire personalities are dominated by some distorted perspective, and all their reactions in life are modified by this peculiar slanting of the mind. They do not bury their painful memories and endure the indirect consequences of anxiety, like neurotics or those suffering from psychosomatic disorders. Instead, they *act out* their protest in defensive patterns of behavior.

Although their neighbors may regard them as "difficult," they usually manage to pursue lives within a fairly normal range of activity. There are some who create rather troublesome social problems, while others go through life making only halfhearted and inadequate efforts. Still others prefer to confine themselves to narrow interests. There are some who become moody without due cause, and some who look with jaundiced eyes upon the motives of their fellow men.

RORSCHACH, Hermann (1884-1922) Swiss psychiatrist. Developed the Rorschach Test for examining the personality. This method, called "projective testing," measures the nonintellectual traits of a person by his interpretation of ten inkblots. It is based on the concept that a person projects his own inner feelings into perception of abstract designs. It has become a significant research device. *A.F.M.L.; Copyright 1944, Swiss Archives of Neurology and Psychiatry.*

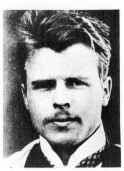

The social problem types

The *antisocial psychopath:* There is a type of person who seems incapable of developing any feeling of right and wrong. Consequently, he is not troubled by a sense of guilt. Intellectually, he comprehends *the theory* of such a difference. It merely fails to affect him or interfere with any of his acts. He frequently runs afoul of the institutions of organized society for which he has a sort of cold contempt. His most distinguishing characteristic is his inability to profit from past experience. These individuals are sometimes designated *psychopaths,* and they make up a considerable percentage of the convicts in our penal institutions.

The psychopath has been described by some authorities as a "moral inbecile," signifying that he fails to develop any moral sense in much the same way that the feeble-minded fail to develop in the intellectual sphere. Despite a normal, or even superior intelligence, the psychopath seems always to be getting into trouble, acting out a lifelong pattern of rebellion and defiant behavior. A past history which shows the recurrent pattern of failure to adjust to the demands of society is of value in diagnosing this personality disorder.

The psychopath is often charming superficially, since no pangs of conscience deter him from the use of hypocrisy and flattery. He is, however, undependable, unpredictable, and impulsive to an extreme. These persons are poorly equipped for enduring stress and are totally disinterested in postponing immediate pleasures for the sake of long-term gains. A typical psychopath is the heiress who rejects the obligations of her station and turns to a career of shoplifting, forgery, and sexual promiscuity. Many women of this personality type are prostitutes. The males often become swindlers, white slavers, gamblers, and confidence men, seeking devious routes to easy and effortless profit. Some show a history of petty scrapes with the law from which they were saved by the intervention of family or friends. Others make use of their disarming ex-

terior to talk themselves out of many incriminating situations, finding it easy to present a fictitious but convincing argument in their own behalf. Those who feel that society is aligned against them comprise a potentially criminal type. If their antisocial tendencies are overtly expressed, they may end in jail. This is one of the most difficult of all types to rehabilitate.

The *sexual deviate:* The most familiar example of such deviation is the homosexual, who chooses a sexual partner of his own sex. The average person, normally attracted by a member of the opposite sex, often finds it hard to understand the preferences and practices of the homosexual. But the average person may not have had to contend with the situations which obtained in the early life of the deviate. In some instances, early history has revealed that the homosexual's mother had wanted a girl, bitterly resenting the fact that her child was born a boy. Such mothers may attempt to compensate for their own disappointment by dressing their

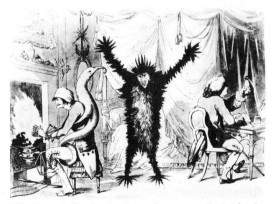

This cartoon by Rowlandson shows a patient who is suffering from hallucinations. Although hallucinations usually indicate mental disease, they can have a systemic origin. *Bettmann Archive.*

sons in feminine attire and encouraging them in girlish pursuits. The child grows up in the knowledge that his mother valued his feminine traits, and sometimes he learns to value them also. If so, it is possible that as an adult he will still think of himself in the feminine role. He may then find it extremely difficult to assume an aggressive, dominant sexual role toward women. A background of this type may not be common to all homosexuals, but it has been recorded in the history of an unexpectedly large number. Other environmental situations which surround sex with ideas of fear and shame may create emotional blocking which prevents the development of a mature *heterosexual* relationship. Similar deep-seated mechanisms are believed to underlie other sexual deviations. Psychiatric treatment aimed at reversing the tendency toward homosexual behavior has met with minimal success. However, the homosexual may be helped to overcome feelings of anxiety and guilt associated with his deviation. In recent years, organizations working in behalf of homosexuals have endeavored to lift the stigma attached to being "gay," as the homosexuals often refer to themselves, rendering them acceptable members of society.

The *drug abuser:* Drug abuse has been defined as loss of the power of self-control with reference to a drug, rendering the individual harmful to himself and to society. Many drug abusers suffer from some form of personality disorder. Of a group of 1000 patients admitted to a federal narcotic hospital, only 4 percent were found to be emotionally stable. The majority of these patients had personality disturbances of the antisocial type, while another large group were suffering from neurotic disorders. Drug addiction was but one manifestation of their lifelong history of maladjustment. Having failed to solve their emotional conflicts by any other route, they resorted to drugs to relieve their symptoms of anxiety. Occasionally, but by no means in all cases, drug addiction is seen in association with a major mental illness of which such addiction is but one manifestation.

Some of the oldest historical records of man contain evidence of the use of various extracts of berries, leaves, beans, roots, fungi, and tree bark for their mental and physiological effects in escaping the drudgery of life. Practically every society on earth today makes use of some drug to escape from reality or ease the tensions of daily living. Some are mild and beneficial in moderation, but dangerous when abused by overdosage. Others, such as the opiates, are treacherous from the beginning because their use produces an overwhelming physical dependency which can only be satisfied by larger and larger doses.

The opium derivatives, which include *morphine, codeine,* and *heroin,* are so habit-forming that once the craving for them becomes established, the victim's entire emotional life is subjugated to the drugs. Heroin is considered so dangerous a drug that importation into the United States for *any* purpose is banned. Morphine and codeine, however, are used by the medical profession in combating otherwise uncontrollable pain. The whole problem of addiction arises out of the nature of habit-forming drugs and the difficulty the human organism has in withstanding them. The addict's dependence upon his drug is twofold. He is prompted by a tremendous physical craving, and at the same time the feeling of elation derived from the drug provides temporary support for his emotional insecurity. Morphinism is unique among addictions in that sense perception remains clear. Drug tolerance is one of the features which complicates the problem. Increased resistance to the effect of drugs develops over a period of time, so the addict requires progressively larger doses to obtain satisfaction.

The cost of heroin is so prohibitive that the only known and recognized means of supporting this habit is to turn to crime. The narcotics user is more interested in rapid relief of his craving than he is in sanitary measures of administering the drug, so he frequently employs contaminated syringes for his intravenous injections. This often leads to hepatitis (or even malaria) contracted when an unclean needle is passed from one user to another. Since the sale of heroin is not controlled by law, the addict never can be sure how pure the drug he has purchased might be or whether it has been admixed with other substances, which may be even more lethal than the heroin itself. The rate of deaths from overdosage of heroin reaches its highest point in the overpopulated ghetto areas of America's largest cities.

Sometimes diagnosis is difficult for those skilled in the field and can only be positively made with the removal of the patient from all possible sources of supply. Then the characteristic withdrawal symptoms appear, during which the addict cannot conceal his acute physical pain. Among the withdrawal symptoms are severe cramps in the abdomen and legs, muscular twitching, vomiting, and diarrhea. The patient will be irritable, restless, and unable to relax. He breaks out in sweat and "goose pimples." Rest and sleep are difficult or impossible to attain.

The drastic treatment required for drug addiction should be attempted only by well-trained personnel with adequate facilities. Withdrawal of the drug may be abrupt, rapid, or gradual. Following withdrawal, a period of psychotherapy and rehabilitation is required. This is a most important phase of the treatment, for it has been found that without a minimum of four months of psychotherapy, most patients relapse.

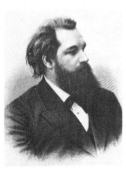

KORSAKOFF, Sergei Ser-geevich (1854-1900) Russian neurologist. Best known for his description of a form of polyneuritis with loss of memory called *Korsakoff's syndrome* or *Korsakoff's psychosis*. This condition was found by him to bring on gradual amnesia, with the patient at the same time displaying a tendency to chatter aimlessly. Korsakoff traced the causes to exces-sive drinking of alcohol and an inadequate consumption of food.

There has been much controversey over the practice of providing as a substitute for heroin another addictive narcotic drug, methadone, which can be obtained much more cheaply than heroin and thus can remove the incentive to commit crimes to support the habit. Not only methadone, but also scopolamine, can be given under the supervision of the medical profession to ease withdrawal agonies and act as a sub-stitute for the more devastating heroin. Objec-tions have revolved around the fact that this is merely substituting one addictive drug for an-other, but reports from some users who have made the change indicate that the relief of pres-sure to provide his own heroin more than justi-fies the method used. Many patients who obtain methadone at clinics regularly can maintain pro-ductive lives.

The United States Public Health Service main-tains two hospitals exclusively for the treatment of drug addicts. Most of the patients have been convicted under the Federal narcotics law, but private patients are also admitted at a nominal fee. Indigent patients receive free treatment. In-formation regarding these hospitals may be ob-tained from the Surgeon General of the United States Public Health Service, Washington, D.C.

In recent years, there has been an alarming increase in the number of youthful addicts. Eighteen percent of the patients admitted to the federal hospital at Lexington, Kentucky, in 1950 were under 21. The criminal element which traffics in narcotics could not resist the lucrative prospects of introducing many of these children to heroin, the most habit-forming drug of all. Some, however, were users of cocaine and mari-juana. Parents should be on the alert for possible signs of drug addiction should their teen-aged children suddenly withdraw from customary activities and become secretive and irritable. Many parents have overlooked such warning sig-nals as arms covered with needle punctures, long and unexplained absences, and the unac-countable disappearance of valuable objects from the home.

In recent years several private and state in-stitutions have come into being to help cope with narcotic addiction. Among the most successful is Synanon, a private organization using a unique self-help approach. The number of permanent cures far outnumber those of any other group, including the Federal program at Lexington, Kentucky.

Narcotics Anonymous, another private organ-ization, run very much on the order of Alco-holics Anonymous, also boasts of success in cases suited to their program.

Several states, notably New York and Cali-fornia, have instituted narcotics control pro-grams in which they control the addiction, offer psychotherapy and a planned program of re-habilitation.

Addiction to other types of drugs follows a somewhat similar pattern, modified only by the peculiarities of each drug. *Cocaine,* which is derived from the leaves of a South American shrub, is taken by sniffing through the nostrils. Unlike morphine, cocaine administration may be skipped for several days at a time without pro-ducing discomfort. It produces a feeling of ela-tion, and is commonly used by individuals whose pursuits require a false gaiety or sustained good humor for long periods of time. Its pleasurable effects are somewhat lessened, however, by the creation of hallucinations, especially the sensa-tion of insects crawling on the skin. The user refers to it as "snow" and he is known to the trade as a "snowbird." It is an extremely dan-gerous drug because it can produce psychosis, and an overdose can result in death.

Hallucinogens: Many of the primitive societies of the world have ascribed divine powers to various hallucinogenic agents available to them since prehistoric times. The use of these drugs is pursued with religious fervor and must, in

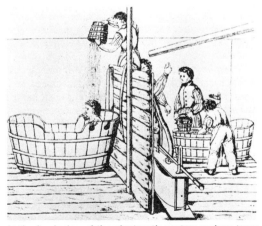

At the beginning of the nineteenth century various types of water therapy became popular in treating the men-tally deranged. *Copyright Ciba Symposia.*

fact, provide the only release open to them for the escape of the harsh realities of their daily lives. During the 1960's, however, usage of hallucinogens became suddenly widespread among young people throughout the world, producing a critical law-enforcement problem, and considerable controversy among users, police, legislators, and physicians.

They are particularly popular with rock musicians, hippies, high school and college students and youth elements which are in conflict with established society as a whole. A large variety of hallucinogens are available but the most popular by far are marijuana and LSD.

Marijuana is made from the dried leaves of Indian hemp, which grows wild all over the world. It is the same plant from which the drug, hashish, derives, but the effects of hashish are five to ten times as potent. Marijuana is rolled into cigarettes and smoked, often in a social setting where the cigarettes are passed from one person to another. Users refer to it by many names, including pot, grass, reefers, joints, and tea. It produces a sensation of floating, and a gross distortion of time and space perception, together with relaxation and euphoria, which lasts only a few hours. While clinical tests have indicated that marijuana is not habit-forming, it is still debated whether or not it is a stepping stone to the use of harder drugs. While under the influence of marijuana, reflexes and the ability for making decisions are decidedly impaired and driving a car entails a major risk. Mounting evidence suggests that long-term use may be associated with chromosomal changes which can possibly cause birth defects in future generations. Possession of marijuana is illegal in the United States and is accompanied by penalties in most of the states of the Union.

LSD (lysergic acid diethylamide) is an hallucinogenic agent derived from the fungus, ergot. It produces vivid and colorful imagery which combines visual, auditory, tactile, and olfactory sensations which are pleasurable to some and terrifying to others. There has been flamboyant publicity emphasizing the so-called mind-expanding properties of the drug, but aside from a temporary intensification of awareness, no one appears to have increased his usefulness to society as a result of its use. On the contrary, anxiety, disorientation, and impaired physical co-ordination are commonly experienced. There have been many reported instances of a bad "trip" in which the effects were more painful and anguished than pleasurable. Also there are instances in which the hallucinatory experience may recur without taking the drug again, for weeks or months after the last time LSD was taken. Some users of LSD have met their deaths by leaping in front of cars or out of windows in the mistaken assumption that they were invincible.

Another relatively new problem in the control of addiction is the widespread abuse of *bromides* and *barbiturates,* the sedatives and sleeping pills which were easily available to the public for some time. Legal control of these drugs, however, has recently been tightened.

Bromides are sedatives compounded from the element, bromine. Prescribed medicinally for a number of conditions, including convulsive disorders, they are also self-administered to relieve the effects of "hangovers." They do not cause physical dependence or call for increased dosages because of drug tolerance. The danger from continued use of bromides lies in the cumulative effects of the drug within the system. When bromide concentration in the blood rises to a dangerous level, bromide intoxication may result. The symptoms include unusual drowsiness, delirium, and hallucinations, and if not detected the condition may result in death. Bromide intoxication is readily determined, however, by tests of the blood serum. Upon diagnosis, hospitalization is advisable for elimination of the accumulated bromide from the system. This is done principally by continuous baths and the controlled administration of salt.

Barbiturates, widely used in sleeping pills, are derived from the organic compound, barbituric acid. They induce a feeling of relaxation usually followed by sleep. Barbiturates are advantageously used to provide temporary respite in times of unusual emotional stress. They should not be taken regularly as a substitute for a cure in chronic nervous tension. This will only prolong the stress and encourage the patient to continue his reliance on drugs instead of seeking a solution to his emotional problems.

The Expert Committee on Drug Addiction of the World Health Organization advised the United Nations that barbiturates "must be considered drugs liable to produce addiction." Some people do develop physical dependence on barbiturates. Others, however, remain able to abandon the drugs voluntarily. As in the use of other psychological props, the need for continued barbiturates lies in the underlying personality disorder.

Stimulants: One of the most popular stimulants is caffeine, found in coffee, tea, cocoa, and cola beans. It produces a mild euphoria and a rise in blood pressure. It is widely consumed in coffee in the United States and in tea in Great Britain. Another very popular stimulant is nicotine, found in all tobacco, especially cigarettes. It tends to become habit-forming, as millions of persons can testify who have tried to stop the habit of smoking. Also included among the stimulants are the amphetamines (benzedrine, dexedrine, and methedrine) which are taken to produce euphoria and drive, or release of fatigue. Amphetamines are prescribed by physicians in moderate doses for appetite depression for the control of obesity and for relief of mental depression. However, large numbers of drug abusers ingest extremely large amounts to achieve feelings of high exhilaration. Some dissolve the tablets in water and inject the drug directly into the veins, receiving a jolt far exceeding a recommended or safe dose. The user experiences an exaggerated feeling of euphoria and aggressiveness. It has been estimated that the life expectancy of one who "mainlines" (injects directly into the veins) methedrine (called "speed") is approximately five years.

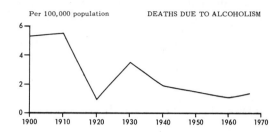

This chart shows the number of deaths in the United States resulting from alcoholism.

The alcoholic

Most persons can take a drink or leave it alone. They may get hilariously drunk now and then. But they are not alcoholics. The alcoholic drinks because he *has to*, and he is frankly incapable of leaving it alone. His drinking interferes with his family life and with his job, and therefore constitutes a social problem in the community. The alcoholic, however, is sick, rather than stubborn, and is thus a problem for the physician. Physicians realize that the compulsive drinker does not drink out of arbitrary willfulness. They know he cannot help himself; therefore, they employ a combination of physical and psychological therapies with which to overcome his addiction to alcohol.

Alcoholism is a manifestation of a disordered personality and a faulty method of adjusting to the environment. The emotionally disturbed individual was maladjusted before he began to drink; otherwise, liquor would not come to represent so much solace to him. He uses it as an escape and a crutch, and it is useless to deprive him of the crutch unless the underlying emotional disturbance is also attacked. If this is not done, he may eventually find another crutch on which to lean, which will not constitute an improvement. In one survey, 21 percent of a group of morphine addicts had previously been alcoholics.

Recent studies suggest that there is a physical as well as an emotional factor in alcoholism. Certain hormonal imbalances and a vitamin B deficiency have been found in large numbers of patients hospitalized for treatment of alcoholism. These, however, might be the result, rather than the cause, of excessive drinking. Many cases appear to be associated with a poorly functioning adrenal cortex. This provided a clue which has led to investigations into the use of hormones in treatment.

The medical profession is enlarging its body of evidence that alcoholism is an illness, rather than a form of social dereliction. Certainly, one has only to see the patient in the throes of *delirium tremens* to know that illness exists; the patient is seized with uncontrollable trembling, is unable to converse, and is the victim of terrifying hallucinations. The patient is also ill who cannot abstain from compulsive drinking.

Group therapy has provided a great measure of success in helping the alcoholic. There are many organizations devoted to the rehabilitation of the alcoholic. One of the best known is Alcoholics Anonymous. Composed of nondrinking alcoholics who endeavor to assist others to break the drinking habit, it has chapters in every large city. The sense of "belonging" engendered by this system is probably the most important factor in this organization's efforts to restore the alcoholic to a normal way of life. One big problem is to remove the element of remorse which rankles in the patient's mind and drives him to further drinking. Undoubtedly, there are many routes to the elimination of this illness. Many of them are based on sound psychiatric principles. Whether he receives it from the physician, the minister, or from the A. A., what the alcoholic needs most is understanding, tolerance, and guidance in getting at the root of his emotional disorder. Though viewed as a chronic disease, alcoholism should never be considered a hopeless one. When the will to recover is strong, there is no chronic illness from which the recovery rate is so high.

The inadequate personality

There are some people who give the impression that they were born tired. The dominant trait of the entire personality is inadequacy. Physically, mentally, and emotionally, they seem to fall short of their fellow men. Without actually being ill, they are yet listless, indecisive, and inept.

These are the partial failures who never seem to get anywhere. Their intellectual capacities lie within the normal range, but the output of their work is uncertain, since they lack the energy for sustained production. People of this personality type frequently become drifters, or financial parasites. They are harmless but impractical people who avoid responsibility and neglect the affairs of the world.

Socially, their inadequacy is also conspicuous. Their relationships with others are characterized by a hesitant approach and otherwise ineffectual behavior. They learned early in life that what was easy for others was difficult for them, and so they began avoiding those social contacts which call for competition. When even their vacillating and indecisive behavior fails to save them from situations of stress, they fall easy prey to the various neurotic disorders. Treatment directed to building up their self-confidence may help them to achieve some degree of success.

The lonely personality (schizoid)

Some people prefer to shut themselves away from others. They withdraw from associations with people whenever possible, and frequently go to great lengths to forestall intrusion. Whether clever or dull, gentle or mean, they are dominated by their desire for seclusiveness. These people are referred to by psychiatrists as *schizoid*, although different authorities have described them in various ways. Jung termed them "introverts," while Bleuler said they were "introspective." Meyer called them "shut-ins," and Kretschmer compared them to certain houses which "have closed their shutters before the rays of the burning sun; perhaps," he noted, "in the subdued interior light, there are festivities." The latter observation contains a clue to the schizoid personality, for the withdrawal of these individuals from the companionship of others is compensated to a large extent by the vividness of their imaginings and fantasies.

The schizoid finds many ways to justify his preference for solitude. He prefers books to people and is more concerned with abstract philosophies than he is with public opinion. He usually has few friends, and those he does have rarely know his intimate thoughts. Outsiders frequently resent the aloofness of the schizoid individual, and find it difficult to discover any common ground with him on which to base an exchange of mutual experience. Unencumbered as he is by the ordinary social demands, the schizoid usually has more time than the average person for contemplation and work. Left to select his own environment and choose amenable tasks, he is often capable of outstanding accomplishments in creative and intellectual fields. Many people of the schizoid type have made valuable contributions to research and to fields of thought in which solitary meditation becomes a significant factor. Others derive tremendous satisfaction from the fine arts, and if they possess creative abilities, their extraordinary qualities of patience permit them to pursue their chosen work with great diligence. Regardless of what type of occupation they select, they do their best work when a minimum of contact with people is required.

The schizoid individual may have been naturally shy and sensitive as a child, or feelings of inferiority may have been engendered in him during his early youth. As Karl Menninger says, "some parents frighten or bulldoze or shame their children into seclusiveness." This puts them at a great disadvantage socially, and may, in fact, warp the entire personality. Once a child's self-confidence is undermined, he is likely to establish a habit of avoiding contacts with people whenever possible. All schizoid persons seem to have a common need to shield themselves from contacts which threaten their feeling of security. To strangers, therefore, they may appear to be the most negative of people.

The child who wants always to play alone, who prefers the company of adults to that of other children, and who is so eager to please his parents that he is actually "too good," should be encouraged to enlarge his contacts with children of his own age group. The expenditure of his free time is of vital importance to the development of a healthy personality. He may need to be steered away from his books and into the playground, for a child of this type may be overstudious in order to hide his social insecurity. The child who invariably makes the best grades in school often incurs the resentment of his classmates as a result of his scholastic precocity. Their ridicule directed at "teacher's pet" will only doom him to further emotional distress. Such a child needs to be guided away from pursuits which tend to isolate him, and into activities which involve participation with others. Intelligent and affectionate relations between the parents and the child provide the best basis for the development of a personality free of excessive schizoid tendencies. The security of a happy home and continual encouragement to mingle with other children in agreeable pursuits will lessen the toll on the personality of the child who is naturally timid and retiring.

The moody personality (cycloid)

Some persons are always at the mercy of their own moods, and frequently their moods are not obviously related to the situations in which they find themselves. Some may appear to be always glad, while others seem unnecessarily depressed, and occasionally there are some who are unpredictably changeable, fluctuating from one extreme to the other. These people are known to psychiatrists as *cycloid* personality types. The cycloid who swings from one mood to its opposite without any apparent stimulus from his environment is a most confusing person to deal with. However, extreme fluctuations in one individual are rare. Much more common are the ones who seem always agitated or elated, known as *hypomanics*, and those who are always "feeling low," sometimes referred to as *melancholics*. Whether manic or melancholic, the persons who fall into the cycloid category respond to internal feelings

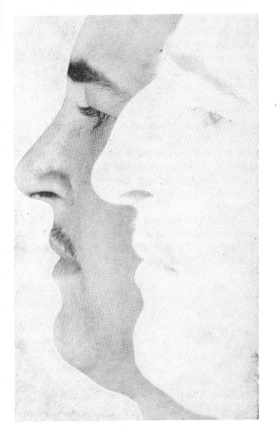

Rhinoplasty upon the nose shown in the foreground resulted in the changed appearance seen in the face in background. Facial appearance is often found to be the cause of a personality disorder. *Courtesy Peter Lund. Medical Illustration Lab., Veterans Administration, Hines, Illinois. Copyright 1952, Medical Radiography and Photography.*

without external cause, and are frequently impervious to attempts to cheer or to calm them.

The *hypomanic:* The hypomanic is always on the go. His overactivity is chronic. He is given to rash and impulsive decisions and goes to extremes beyond the imagination of the average person. Socially, the hypomanic finds time for innumerable contacts and extracurricular activities. His tireless energy makes it difficult for others to keep pace with many of his endeavors.

In the business world, the hypomanic may astound his associates because of his almost limitless energies. Frequently, however, the same qualities of restlessness and activity which underlie the energy will also create so much distraction that his working capacity is diminished. If the hypomanic does not control the frequent changes in the direction and content of his thoughts, he will be greatly handicapped in concentration and accomplishment. Despite phenomenal enterprise, these individuals often fail to remain with any one project long enough to make it successful.

Whether the hypomanic succeeds in life or fails is to a large extent dependent on his ability to discipline his thinking, direct his energies, and follow through his various enterprises.

Some authorities feel that there is a definite hereditary tendency at work in producing the hypomanic personality. However, early family environment and attitudes can do much to influence the factors which dominate a child's personality. It has been suggested that the hypomanic's habit of overreacting began as a defense against feelings of inferiority or guilt. If so, this form of denial becomes so ingrained that one would never suspect that it could be compensatory behavior. It has been said that, of all types, the hypomanic seems to have been most successful in vanquishing his conscience, and spends the remainder of his life in celebrating the victory.

The *melancholic:* In contrast to the hypomanic, an individual of melancholic personality is tyrannized by his conscience. Unreasonably shamed into a sense of guilt, he tries to placate his conscience, as well as the world, by assuming an ingratiating manner. He is constantly apologetic, pessimistic, and unhappy.

Both his mental and his physical activities are depressed. Often the physical symptoms predominate. He may consult a doctor about his vague complaints which shift from one part of the body to another, frequently centering on the digestive tract. He is chronically tired and unenthusiastic; consequently, he is inclined to spend much time alone.

When occasionally he goes out socially, he is quiet and retiring and accepts the lead of others with kindly resignation. When approached, he is diffident and lacking in spontaneity.

In the business world the melancholic person is inclined to be too serious. He is unsure of himself, vascillating when he should be decisive. He is often preoccupied with minor duties. Nevertheless, his conscientiousness makes him a

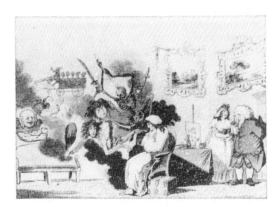

This illustration by the British artist Rowlandson shows his impressions of a patient who is afflicted with hallucinations. *Bettmann Archive.*

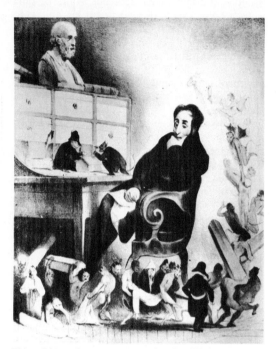

This eighteenth century engraving by Rowlandson depicts his impressions of a patient who is beset by hypochondriacal ideas. *Bettmann Archive.*

faithful, plodding sort of employee, meticulous in handling details.

Some authorities hold that the melancholic's low opinion of himself may be unconsciously deserved. They believe that guilt feelings arise from an unacknowledged tendency toward aggression. If this theory is accurate, then the self-depreciation of the melancholic person represents the turning inward of hostility which he is afraid to release against the world.

The moody behavior of the cycloid personality types, whether hypomanic or melancholic, is a faulty method of adaptation to life. Nevertheless, such patterns of behavior guard them from the consequences of their unacknowledged feelings of insecurity, without the distress of neurotic symptoms.

The suspicious personality (paranoid)

Some persons are dominated by the belief that others "have it in for them." Merely withdrawing from association with people does not satisfy them. They also feel the need of vindicating themselves. They are disdainful of others, yet they constantly worry about what people are thinking of them. They imagine that other individuals are talking about them behind their backs. They misinterpret casual words in terms of their own suspicious viewpoint. They are ab-

solutely convinced that they are the subject of uncomplimentary attentions. These people are referred to as *paranoid.*

At times, anyone may feel that he is unjustly persecuted. Usually, a period of bad "breaks" prompts such a reaction in the normal individual. In the paranoid personality type the same reaction becomes a habit of thinking, and persists even without experiences to precipitate it.

The paranoid person is an extremely self-centered individual. Excessive vanity is essential to maintain his unwarranted belief that he is the center of so much agitation and comment. The paranoid person is determined and ambitious and needs desperately to succeed. He hangs on to his ambitions with more than usual tenacity, refusing to realize that his stubbornness may bring him defeat. He rationalizes failure by placing the blame on others. These unfortunate qualities may greatly handicap an otherwise excellent mind.

The paranoid personality gets its orientation in childhood. Discipline is especially resented; a child of this type is easy to take offense at any criticism. An uncompromising attitude may cost him his popularity. As an adult, he becomes envious and unable to see why others should surpass him.

Some authorities hold that persons of this type have been unduly frustrated; all agree that such troubles arise from within.

Paranoid persons become cranks and reformers. They are somewhat difficult to get along with, as their unfounded suspicions and unjust accusations can make life miserable for their families and friends. Since they need an extraordinary amount of reassurance, those who live with them must learn to handle them gingerly and with great tact. Patience, understanding, and loyalty from those they love will help them more than anything else to gain a more normal personality adjustment.

KRAEPELIN, Emil (1856-1926) German psychiatrist. Kraepelin was a pioneer in experimental psychiatry, and introduced a simple classification of mental disease. He classified the psychoses as dementia praecox, and manic-depressive; and gave excellent clinical descriptions of these two mental diseases. His classification has been modified, and the psychoses of psychological origin are usually divided, at the present time, into schizophrenia, manic-depressive, paranoia and involutional melancholia.

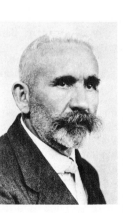

DISORDERS OF THE MIND: THE PSYCHOSES

When the personality disorders grow so severe that the individual can no longer cope with the demands of his environment, his impressions become distorted, and he loses contact with reality. The medical term for the severe mental illnesses in this category is *psychosis*. The legal term is *insanity*.

Throughout the centuries, men have stood in fear and awe of those unfortunate individuals who suffered from severe mental illness. As a result, these patients were inhumanly and unjustly persecuted by their fellow men whose lack of understanding prevented a rational approach to this unfortunate condition. As far back as the sixteenth century, Johann Weyer, a Dutchman, protested volubly against the practices of witchcraft directed toward exorcising demons from the mentally ill. Mental patients could expect no better fare than violent and brutal physical torture and harsh confinement. Weyer wrote extensively, advocating that reforms be instituted in the care of the mentally ill.

In the seventeenth century, a Catholic priest, St. Vincent de Paul, embraced the cause of the mentally ill. He instituted procedures for humanitarian treatment of mental patients in religious hospitals throughout France. Here, patients were treated with kindness and mercy and spared the brutal treatment and harsh confinement which was commonplace throughout Europe at that time.

Only small groups, however, could be accommodated in these humanitarian hospitals. By far the majority of mental patients were thrown into large asylums where they fared worse than criminals.

It remained for Philippe Pinel, an eighteenth century French physician, to bring about the far-reaching reforms which humanized the care of mental patients throughout Europe. Pinel contended that by treating mental patients as though they were criminals, a grave injustice was done them, and their chances of recovering were greatly reduced. He believed that with understanding and kindness many patients once considered hopeless might recover completely. Fortunately for mankind, Doctor Pinel was placed in the position of Director of the Bicêtre and later the Salpêtrière, two of the largest insane asylums in France. At each of these institutions, the conditions were appalling. The patients were confined in dark and humid dungeons, chained, and otherwise mistreated. No freedom, exercise, or sunlight was available to them. Pinel worked diligently to obtain permission of the authorities to remove the chains and permit the patients to go outdoors. His efforts were rewarded when he discovered that, true to his belief, many patients responded favorably to this kind and gentle treatment. The sweeping reforms instituted by Pinel revolutionized the entire hospital system of the European continent and England, and later their influence was felt in the United States. Pinel bequeathed to his fellow men the right to receive merciful and enlightened treatment when it is most needed.

With the rising young science of psychiatry becoming more influential in the nineteenth century, medical attention was directed toward discovering the cause and removing the source of acute mental disturbance. The nineteenth century also saw great popular interest in the phenomenon of hypnosis. It was a weapon in the hands of both earnest and unscrupulous practitioners, but it revealed the latent power of unconscious mental forces.

In this work the Salpêtrière maintained its pre-eminence among mental institutions, under the leadership of Charcot, first to advocate the importance of psychological forces in mental disorders. In addition to his brilliant neurological work at the Salpêtrière, Charcot is remembered for his scientific study of hypnosis and for the gifted pupils whom he inspired. Among these was Sigmund Freud. With other investigators, including Jung, Janet, and Bernheim, Freud demonstrated that the unconscious is not a static reservoir of dead material, but, like the conscious mind, is a dynamic, living source of emotional energy.

Work continued in the nineteenth and twentieth centuries on description, classification, and organization of knowledge of mental diseases. Kretschmer, Kraepelin, Bleuler, and Meyer were outstanding among those who helped to evolve present concepts of mental disorders of psychological origin.

Schizophrenia

Schizophrenia is the most widespread form of mental illness. Over half of all hospitalized patients in the United States are mental cases, and about half of those have schizophrenia. Consequently, approximately one fourth of all hospitalized patients are suffering from schizophrenia.

In schizophrenia, the mind turns away from reality into a world of its own creation. As a result, the patient's actions are often difficult to understand because they are dictated by the fantasies which rule his mind. The disease was formerly known as *dementia praecox*, which meant "a precocious demented state." While it is true that the disease frequently does appear in early adult life, this is by no means true in all cases, so Bleuler in 1911 advocated the substitution of a new term. He suggested "schizophrenia" for the reason that "schizo" (splitting) "phrenia" (mind) gave some indication of the "breaking away" of the patient's mind from its normal evaluation of reality.

There are many different froms in which the illness, schizophrenia, manifests itself. However, denial of reality and inappropriate emotional responses are common to all of them. The distorted content of his mind is revealed by the patient's behavior. He may be given to periods of wild behavior in which he breaks up furniture and throws his entire surroundings into disarray. He may rip off his clothes and go naked, or may decorate himself in all manner of fantastic dress. He laughs or cries without due cause and may use a language, consisting of jumbled fractions of words and phrases, which is incomprehensible to others. He may be confused as to his identity and make fantastic claims that he is someone else of wide repute. The actions and mannerisms of the schizophrenic patient appear bizarre and unintelligible when viewed in the light of reality. They are more easily understood when one realizes that they are products of a dream world, erected because the patient cannot perceive reality in a normal way.

When a person becomes unable to find any solution which will enable him to accept a painful situation, his attempted defenses break down entirely and he imagines reality as he would like it to be. He finds that his daydreams offset the poverty of his true relationships and thus become more satisfying than reality. The external world is thereafter distorted to conform to his dream world. When personality disorganization progresses this far, the patient no longer can distinguish facts from fancy. This is particularly likely to happen in persons of seclusive (schizoid) temperament. For, as Strecker and his associates state, "the roots of schizophrenia are firmly embedded in schizoid soil."

Schizophrenia cannot be fully comprehended in terms of one disease. Rather, it is a set of complex symptoms with manifestations so varied that it has been called "a group of diseases." Considered thus, it is reasonable to attribute to schizophrenia a plurality of causes. Some cases of schizophrenia, but not all, are found in conjunction with an emotional background which would foster the development of withdrawal tendencies. However, many individuals with just as detrimental a background fail to develop the symptoms of schizophrenia. This would suggest that a person's heritage may render him more susceptible to schizophrenia. There are, in fact, some cases of schizophrenia which are difficult to account for on any other basis than that of organic disorder. The factors at work in producing the psychosis are, of course, significant considerations in the treatment selected and in the outcome of the illness. Since both innate temperament and adjustment to life situations are involved in schizophrenia, Adolph Meyer has described it as habit disorganization on constitutional ground.

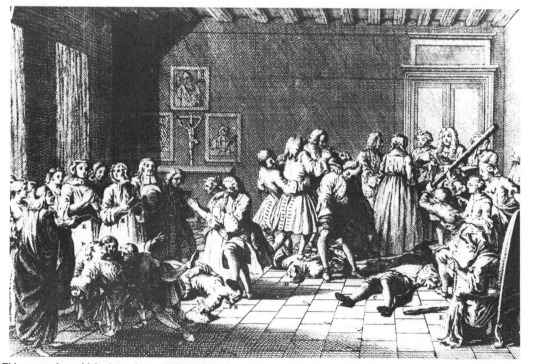

This engraving which dates from 1727 depicts the custom of the time of beating mentally deranged persons to their senses. At left doctors are stomping patients. *Courtesy of Bettmann Archive.*

Extensive research into the pathology in the families of schizophrenic patients shows that parental attitudes and interfamily tensions play a major role in the production of schizophrenia. Kanner is one investigator who has done much research on the early histories of schizophrenics. Looking into the childhood of these patients, he determined there was an extremely "close connection" between parental attitudes and the meaning attached to life experiences by the preschizophrenic child. Particularly the aggressively oversolicitous parent, who must direct all aspects of the child's life, leaving him no privacy of thought, may drive the child into a shell and so begin the practice of habitual recoil. Parents who make too many frustrating demands and show only impatience when their demands are not fulfilled engender lonely antagonism in the child. The child who feels he cannot depend on anyone erects a barrier of reserve to shield himself. He becomes a quiet, docile child, well-behaved until interruption diverts him from the consolation of his fantasies. For a time, he may try to compensate for his lack of adaptability by reading or studying, displaying to the officious adults his industry and knowledge. This is a dangerous symptom, for it is thought to result from a further withdrawal of the potential schizophrenic. The extra social demands which accompany the onset of puberty may prove too great for the youngster of this personality type and with this background. This is why schizophrenia frequently comes on early in life, when the budding adult begins to realize he is unfitted for normal competition in the external world.

Certain hallucinogenic drugs, such as mescaline and LSD, produce symptoms which closely simulate schizophrenia. Some of these hallucinogens are derivatives of substances found in brain metabolism. This discovery has led investigators to believe that schizophrenia may be, at least in part, a metabolic disease. As more has come to be understood about schizophrenia, the outlook for many of these patients has improved. Tranquilizing drugs offer hope of improvement to many patients, and have made treatment at home possible for many who formerly would have been hospitalized. Research into possible hereditary and environmental factors is continuing, as are studies of neurochemical substances that appear to play major roles in the physiology of brain functions.

Manic-depressive psychosis

Exaggerated emotional reaction dominates the thinking and behavior of the *manic-depressive*. He is apt to show extremes of mood and to display sweeping, unpredictable changes from one emotion to another. Some manic-depressives are unnaturally elated. Not even hospital confinement inhibits their vigor, aggression, and unjusti-

fiable optimism. Others are hopelessly depressed, so deep in melancholy that other people cannot cheer them. Still others have cycles, alternating from elation to depression. In mania, their excited mood carries thoughts and actions rapidly in a whirl of restlessness. In the depressed state, a mood of dejection retards both speech and activity. This is unlike the schizophrenic, whose mood and thoughts may not even coincide. Retarded thinking and gross protestations of guilt are classic symptoms of the depressed phase of this condition, which is sometimes difficult to distinguish from other depressed mental states.

Manic-depressive disorders are more common among people of the moody (cycloid) personality type. In gradual shadings of the behavior, some of them pass from normal moods into unwarranted moodiness. The temperament of the moody personality type remains much the same for a lifetime. In contrast, the emotions of the manic-depressive usually are periodically more intensified. Manic-depressive disturbances may begin early in life and are prone to recur.

Like other disorders of an emotional nature, the manic-depressive reaction is somewhat more common among women than among men. Also, it is found more often in cities than in rural areas. Some people appear to be predisposed by heredity to manic-depressive psychosis. The incidence in certain families is higher than in the general population, and the frequency among certain racial groups is a strong argument for this theory. In persons so disposed, guilt feelings, or other conflicts, may precipitate the illness.

Both the depressive and the manic phases are often accompanied by numerous physical complaints. In the depressive phase, the danger of suicide should not be overlooked. While the patient is in the manic phase, care should be taken by members of the family to prevent moral or legal complications. They may be warned that the patient is liable to be swept into irresponsible action by the force of his rash impulses.

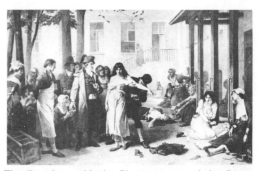

The French psychiatrist Pinel was one of the first to advocate treating the insane kindly and without force. He is shown here removing a patient's chains at Salpêtrière Hospital, Paris. *Bettmann Archive.*

Most patients tend to recover spontaneously from each attack within a period of 6 to 18 months. This period has been lessened through modern methods of treatment. Tranquilizing drugs have been used successfully in lessening the manic tendencies of some patients, while antidepressant drugs or stimulants have shown some improvement in cases of depression. Both types of drug treatment have replaced the use of electroshock therapy in some less severe cases.

Paranoia

Paranoia is a rare and insidious psychosis characterized by delusions of persecution. When the chronic suspiciousness of the paranoid personality type is exaggerated to the point of actual and disabling delusion, acute paranoia is present. Between the two extremes, there are many grades of paranoid reaction—some temporary, some partially justified, and some which appear as symptoms of other emotional disturbances. There is also a form of schizophrenia which is dominated by paranoid attitudes. As Strecker says, "the paranoid stream flows through the territory of every form of mental disease."

In true and acute paranoia, however, the patient is seriously and completely deluded on one particular subject, and the entire functioning of his mind is subordinated to his false belief. Usually he believes that a specific person, group of persons, or even an institution is bent on his destruction. The persecutory delusion may become so severe that the patient is dangerous to society. Political assassinations and mass homicide may seem to the paranoiac as completely justifiable and even necessary behavior.

In paranoia, contact with reality is not lost. Instead, reality is misinterpreted. Thus, the paranoiac will know who he is, yet consider himself a martyr; usually he will not "hear voices" but he will misconstrue everything he does hear. His emotional reactions, while inappropriate to his actual situation are completely in keeping with his own misguided impression of that situation.

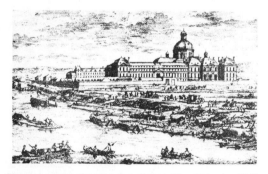

Picture of the famous Salpêtrière Hospital at which many improvements in the treatment of the insane were instituted. *Copyright Ciba Symposia.*

The suspicions of the paranoiac are often coupled with inordinate ambition. Failure to achieve success is met by placing the blame on others. Believing earnestly that someone, or something, is conspiring to keep him down, he decides that the world does not recognize his true worth. He may become haughty and disdainful with delusions of grandeur accompanying his delusion of persecution.

The paranoiac usually begins life as a sensitive child. He is emotionally insecure and lacking in self-confidence. As he grows older, he becomes resentful, frequently getting his "feelings hurt" at the hands of others. Over the years, he builds a logical structure of beliefs on his feeling that there are those whose prime desire is to do him harm. Trusting no one, he hides his sentiments so that many years may pass before his outward behavior betrays the extent of his delusion. In retrospect, however, it may be noted that his suspicious traits were present all the while. Between the chronic, but comparatively mild suspicions of the paranoid personality type and the disabling delusion of acute paranoia, there are many grades of paranoid reactions. Noyes states that the period at which the paranoid personality merges into the paranoid psychosis is only a matter of opinion. The paranoid reaction may become arrested at any of the intermediate stages. Acute paranoid breakdowns seldom occur before middle life. Once the delusions become fixed in acute paranoia, recovery is rare. Fortunately, however, cases of pure paranoia, uncomplicated by other mental disorder, are relatively infrequent, accounting for less than two percent of the total admissions to state hospitals in recent years.

Involutional melancholia

Some people are not emotionally equipped to absorb the combination of physical, mental, and situational changes occurring during middle age. A small percentage of them fall victim to a serious mental illness peculiar to this stage in life, known as *involutional melancholia.*

At this period, subtle adaptive demands are made upon the individual. Women, especially, when faced with the obvious physical changes of the menopause, may react with considerable emotional distress. The cessation of menstruation is sometimes accompanied by certain unpleasant physical symptoms. The "hot flashes" and heart palpitations resulting from minor alterations in the circulatory system may cause severe worry and distress, but these symptoms are not to be confused with involutional melancholia. Some women mistakenly confuse the physical symptoms of the menopause with early signs of mental illness. This has no medical basis whatever.

Adjustment to the normal slowing down of bodily functions at this time is often complicated by misinformation which causes the individual increasing mental concern and self-doubt. Many women mistakenly believe that the menopause marks the end of their active sex life and physical attraction, whereas all that is really ended is the childbearing period. Adequate medical care and information can do much to forestall a tendency to depression and apprehension by the woman who fears the loss of affection and love. The woman at middle life should normally find her sexual life even fuller and more satisfactory following the menopause, because of the freedom from the discomforts and responsibilities attached to menstruation and childbearing.

Emotional pressure which may be brought to bear on the woman at this period frequently involves her diminished usefulness within the home. Her husband is probably more settled and in less need of her encouragement and bolstering. Her children are too old to need help but still too young to provide her with grandchildren. With nothing to take up the slack in the receding demands of her household, many women feel lost and useless and in this frame of mind may sink into a state of serious depression.

In the absence of proper medical guidance at this important time of life, both men and women may "suddenly become aware of the fact that they no longer have the flexibility or the power that was once theirs to alter themselves and to adjust themselves to the environment." As a result, they experience extremes of apprehension, self-depreciation, and gloom which progress into the serious mental disorder, *involutional melancholia*. The onset usually occurs somewhat later in men than it does in women.

In the typical case of involutional melancholia, there is no history of previous attacks of depression. Involutional depression seems especially common to the strict, overconscientious type of person who has lived a rigid, self-effacing existence. Frequently, these individuals have made fairly successful adjustments in life up to this time. The extreme depression may come on gradually or suddenly, though careful questioning of relatives often reveals a warning period of vague symptoms such as insomnia, loss of enthusiasm, and mild anxiety. This gives way to an outburst of agitation in which the individual may wring his hands, moan, and weep. He may stride about restlessly, making outrageous charges against himself. The nature of the accusations may involve some actual but long-removed indiscretion of youth. The self-depreciation is so exaggerated that these patients are often convinced that they have committed "the unpardonable" and are therefore unfit to live. Suicide attempts are a grave danger of this state and should be anticipated; and, if possible, preventive measures should be taken. Delusions of a serious nature may be present. A common type of delusion concerns the body. The patient may seize upon the idea of the physical regression occurring at this time and distort the notion into exaggerated form. Thus, patients with involutional melancholia have been known to declare that certain internal organs are missing. Some patients may even decline food because they believe that they have no stomachs.

Formerly the outlook for patients with involutional depression was poor. Convulsive therapy in the hands of skilled therapists, however, and during the past few years, the newer anti-depressant drugs have been widely used with success.

Organic psychoses

According to many authorities, all of the preceding mental disorders have their bases in psychological forces which disturb the mind so severely that faulty reactions are employed for meeting situations of stress. Depending on the form the illness takes, symptoms consist of bizarre and inappropriate behavior, frequently unacceptable or even dangerous to the patient and society. The same disturbed and psychotic symptoms also occur in a variety of conditions which stem from structural damage to the brain. These physical, or organic, psychoses are much more resistant to therapy than those which are caused by emotional distress, for disturbed emotions often can be relieved, while destroyed brain tissue cannot be restored. However, physicians do have pharmaceutical and surgical measures for improving the condition of patients suffering from some of the organic psychoses.

Among the many physical conditions which damage the brain are injuries from external sources, and injuries sustained from within, such as a ruptured blood vessel and hemorrhage causing pressure on the brain. When the supply of oxygen to the brain is temporarily shut off, certain areas of brain tissue may deteriorate and soften, becoming incapable of function. Several of the infectious diseases are accompanied by high fever, resulting in delirious states and some-

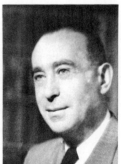

SAKEL, Manfred (1900-1957) American psychiatrist. Introduced insulin shock treatment for schizophrenia and other mental disorders. By this method, the patient is put into a state of coma for a specified length of time, following which the coma is terminated by the administration of sugar. Insulin shock is widely used in mental hospitals and has gained prominence, along with other forms of shock therapy, in the successful management of psychoses.

times in permanent damage to the brain. Cerebral arteriosclerosis, a condition which is extremely common in the later years of life, may be associated with areas of softening throughout the cerebral cortex; and the entire capacities and behavior of the individual thereafter become disturbed and enfeebled.

The commonest organic psychosis is that which results from senility and hardening of the arteries of the brain. The patient becomes confused and disoriented at times. Often, the first noticeable symptoms are in the field of memory. The patient's recent memory is poor, while his memory for things past is excellent. The onset of such symptoms is a warning to members of the patient's family. They should see that medical attention is made available to him immediately. With proper medical care, the patient may be benefited greatly and probably assured of many years of happy, profitable life.

Treatment for the psychoses

Treatment for the psychoses is of four principal kinds; psychotherapy, chemotherapy, shock therapy and psychosurgery.

Psychotherapy is concerned with discovering, through the medium of his own testimony, what is causing trouble in the patient's mind. Psychotherapy may be either deep or superficial. One form of deep psychotherapy is psychoanalysis, in which deeply buried unconscious repressions are drawn into consciousness through long and extensive interviewing. The theory behind psychoanalysis is that emotions which were once painful or inadmissible were repressed and forgotten, but nevertheless left their imprint on the mind, in the form of exaggerated emotional reactions and distorted thinking. Awareness of these heretofore unconscious motivations often helps to free the patient from many of the emotions and thoughts which are causing him trouble. Deeply repressed information may sometimes be obtained more quickly through the use of such devices as hypnosis or the administration of one of the hypnotic drugs, producing a semisomnolent state. This technique must be employed with caution, however, and preferably is reserved for those patients who cannot be successfully interviewed by other methods.

Much successful psychotherapy is conducted in discussion of problems of which the patient is fully conscious. The patient and the therapist seek together the means by which the patient's resources can be strengthened and the stressful conditions of his environment modified so that a more equitable balance between them will prevail. Employing enlightened persuasion and suggestion, the therapist leads the patient to discover, through a better understanding of the patterns of his own behavior, many of the forces operating within his mind.

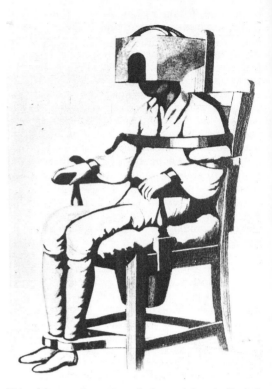

This picture portrays an early form of the straitjacket, long known as a "tranquilizer," used in the control of mental patients. *Bettmann Archive.*

Psychotropic drugs: Shortly after World War II, many new tranquilizers such as the phenothiazines and butophenones made their debut. The addition of these new compounds to the physicians' armamentarium made decided changes in the care and treatment of mental patients. Patients who, before the advent of tranquilizers for clinical use, would have required hospitalization in a locked ward with barred windows, could now be treated on an outpatient basis or at least allowed to roam the ward. *Chlorpromazine* and *reserpine* are two examples of the major tranquilizers available to the psychiatrist. Both reduce aggressive behavior to a minimum in test animals as well as hyperexcited patients. Siamese fighting fish (Betta), for instance, which normally fight to the death if two males are placed in the same tank, become as placid as goldfish when treated with chlorpromazine.

An array of less potent tranquilizers (such as alcohol and meprobamate) are used for keeping the hyperactive patient on an even emotional keel. Whether or not these drugs slow the reflexes to the extent that driving a car would be hazardous depends on the amount of the drug ingested.

In some cases, stimulating drugs are used rather than tranquilizers. Extracts of the coffee bean (caffeine) and coca (cocaine) as well as many synthetic products have to a large extent replaced electroshock. Results are obtained much more quickly and without the more undesirable discomforts. It is clear that extensive use of both old and new drugs has been a decided boon in the treatment of the mentally ill.

Shock therapy is a method by which patients are rendered temporarily unconscious, by controlled clinical measures. The unconsciousness is induced either by electric current or by drugs, such as metrazol or insulin. The muscular reaction to shock treatment is considerably modified by the administration of *anectine* or some similar preparation. The advantage gained by shock treatment is that it helps the patient suffering from delusion, morbid depression, or an abnormal sense of reality to forget for a while his unnatural fears and fantasies and return to a consideration of the real world about him. The actual mechanism through which this is accomplished is unknown, but shock therapy has proved remarkably effective in altering the outlook of mental patients. Through this means they can frequently be rendered accessible to interviewing, during which psychotherapy has in many instances been instituted with gratifying results.

In a small percentage of cases not benefited through other measures, *psychosurgery* is recommended. The usual operation is prefrontal lobotomy (also referred to as leukotomy) which involves severing nerves fibers leading to the frontal lobes of the brain. Following this procedure, patients who were formerly intractable, violent and uncontrollable often become sufficiently calm and docile to return home without posing a danger to other members of their families.

DISORDERS OF THE MIND: MENTAL DEFICIENCIES

Not only brain damage, but also congenital malformation of the brain may render the individual incapable of normal reactions. Even where no actual malformation is known to exist, there are some instances in which persons are born with inferior potentialities for normal mental development. This group comprises the mental defectives.

There are some children who are brought to clinics for examination because they learn slowly. These children may have posed behavior problems or health problems because of the difficulty with which they learn. Upon examination, they are found to be mentally retarded. The children with abnormally low intelligence ratings (*feeble-minded*) are not necessarily psychotic, although some may have mental disease in combination with mental deficiency. The feeble-minded are those whose intellectual capacity does not develop properly or has been retarded. The degree of adaptability attained by such individuals depends to some extent upon the wisdom with which they are handled by others. When neglected, their mental limitations can predispose them to emotional disturbance.

The movement for the care and training of the feeble-minded began in a French forest in 1792, when hunters encountered a wild youth, "The Savage of Aveyron." The story of this young savage, who for some time eluded capture, was taken up by newspapers of that day and aroused great public interest. Proper care of the child when captured was discussed by leading scholars, including Jean Itard, resident physician at the Paris school for deaf-mutes. Philippe Pinel, the French psychiatrist known for his humane treatment of the insane, held that the boy was unteachable. Nevertheless, Itard took the boy into his care. He had concluded from his work among the deaf that a child who appeared retarded might display normal intellect once his sensory handicap had been removed. Itard failed to stimulate the boy's intellect, but the *habit-training* which he accomplished provided a model for modern physiological training of mental defectives.

In training his little charge, Itard worked patiently toward a few simple goals. He attempted to cultivate the child's responsiveness, to awaken his sensory impulses, and stimulate his affections. Next he sought to enlarge the boy's capacities by increasing his wants and inducing him to indicate what he wanted. Finally, he endeavored to teach the child to apply what he had learned.

The work of Itard was carried forward by his pupil, Séguin, who fled France after the revolution in 1848 to finish his life's work in America. He inspired the founding of training schools for mental defectives. The first training school in the United States was opened as an addition

BINET, Alfred (1857-1911) French psychologist. Collaborated with Théodore Simon in developing a standard by which human intelligence can be measured. The famous I.Q., or intelligence quotient test, familiar to all military men and most civilians, is based on this standard. Called the Binet-Simon test, and revised by Terman in 1918, it is still in use for establishing one aspect of mental capacity, reasoning ability. A.F.M.L.; J. Consulting Psychology. Copyright, 1945, Amer. Psychological Assn.

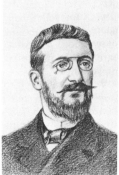

to the Perkins Institute for the Blind under Samuel Gridley Howe. Training schools for mental defectives have been in long and continuous operation at Waverley, Massachusetts; Elwyn, Pennsylvania; and Vineland, New Jersey.

Fernald, the "emancipator of the feeble-minded," was associated with the Waverley school for 37 years. He concerned himself with the social possibilities of mental defectives. Since intelligence is only one element of personality, Fernald insisted that evaluation should not rest upon the intelligence rating alone. He was responsible for shifting the emphasis to what the feeble-minded *could* do. To improve methods of diagnosis and treatment, he devised a classic test for examination of all phases of the patient's background.

Classifications within the feeble-minded group rest upon the work of Binet and Simon who were commissioned by the French government to study the conditions of mentally retarded children. Simon and Binet painstakingly examined hundreds of normal children in an effort to determine what an average child should be able to do at any given age. These tests were introduced in America at the Vineland Training School. With the Stanford-Binet "I.Q." test, the child's intelligence quotient is measured. The age level he achieves on the tests is divided by his chronological age and multiplied by 100. On this basis, an eight-year-old boy who passed examinations intended for the average ten-year-old would be given an I.Q. rating of 125, whereas the average child is rated at 100. Below the rating of 70, an individual was classed as a moron; below 50, an imbecile; and below 20, an idiot.

Although useful for measuring mental capacity, these tests do not give the complete picture, since only one quality—the reasoning intelligence—is measured. Consequently, retarded children are now examined by means of a series of psychological tests which often reveal special aptitudes which may be advantageously developed.

Custodial care is essential for idiotic children. They do not create a major social problem, since comparatively few of them live to adulthood. Those who do live are completely infantile and consequently do not perpetuate themselves. Imbeciles can be trained to perform a few tasks for themselves, but require protective supervision. Almost all morons can be taught to care for themselves and may even become self-supporting.

Training of the feeble-minded is based on sensory stimulation and muscular co-ordination. It is important to keep them in good physical condition to offset their other handicaps. They benefit especially from training which improves co-ordination.

Good results have been obtained by permitting retarded children to complete the maximum academic education they are able to absorb. When

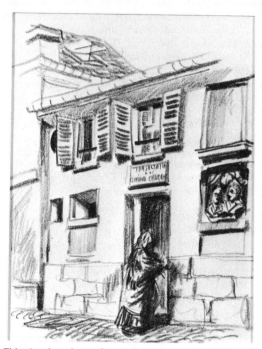

This drawing shows the consultation rooms of Charcot, the famous French psychiatrist and neurologist, in Paris. *Courtesy The Cancer Bulletin, Copyright 1950, The Medical Arts Publishing Foundation.*

this point is reached, however, they should be removed from competition with normal children. They do better work in ungraded sections of public school or in special training schools. Regardless of the chronological age, when they can no longer benefit from formal education, they should be transferred to a vocational training program.

Investigators have been surprised at the range of jobs which the feeble-minded can fill and at the minimum intelligence required to do certain types of repetitive work. Mental defectives have passed beyond their traditional jobs as domestics and are now widely employed in industry. Un-

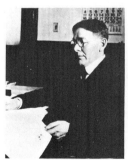

TERMAN, Lewis Madison (1877-1956) American psychologist. Prepared the most acceptable revision of Binet's test for intelligence, known as the *Stanford Revision*, and the most widely used of individual tests of intelligence. With Merrill he further revised it. Fascinated by unusual ability in some children, he wrote *Genetic Studies of Genius*, adopting to a limited degree Galton's view that superior intelligence is inherited.

der supervision they are able to perform many tasks.

In Minnesota, one survey disclosed a boy with an I.Q. of 51 working as a machinist's helper. He operated a drill press. A girl with an I.Q. of 70 turned out depth gauges in an ordinance plant. And another mentally retarded boy earned up to $45.00 weekly as a steelcutter.

Professional people who work with mentally retarded children frequently encounter feelings of self-blame in the parents, who state that in some way they must be responsible for the unfortunate condition of their children. They should be assured that this has no basis in fact. Research in recent years has demonstrated that some cases of mental retardation are caused by previously unsuspected factors which have come about through no fault of their own. German measles during a particular stage in pregnancy may retard the development of the unborn child. Injury during birth is another possible cause which may be taken into consideration. As research progresses, other reasons for mental retardation will probably be found. These situations are entirely beyond the control of the parents, and they should have no feeling of guilt. Parents who have a retarded child should seek competent medical advice. In this way, much needless doubt and worry can be avoided, particularly fear that future children in the family might be similarly afflicted.

Many biochemists and physiologists, among them Nobel prize winner Linus Pauling, contend that more exploration should be made relative to the association of metabolic deficiencies with mental retardation and mental illness. Dr. Pauling contends that such research, when coupled with data gathered by the geneticists, though it may take years, will have as its fruition a better and more scientific approach to a chemotherapy of mental illness.

Research on Brain Function

The study of the function of the human brain remains one of the most complex fields of investigation in the entire area of medical research. The development of sensitive electronic devices which can pick up the delicate electrical responses of the cerebral cortex has been one of the greatest advances in this field, because it is now possible to study the activities of very small areas of the cortex. The scientists who specialize in such investigations are known as *electrophysiologists* and *neurophysiologists*, and from their laboratories is coming a wealth of information that may be expected to aid greatly in the battle against neurological disease and many other disorders. While studies in neurophysiology may include the investigation of all parts of the nervous system, research on brain function is at present considered to be the most important

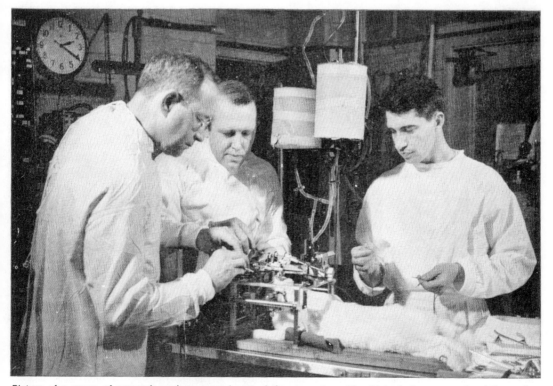

Picture of a group of research workers around part of the apparatus with which studies are made of the various parts of the brain. Rabbits and other small animals serve ideally for these studies.

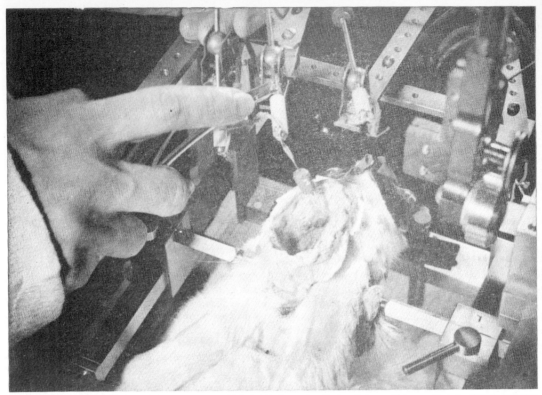

Close-up view of the portion of the apparatus which holds the animal's head securely in position so that electrodes may be placed accurately in position in various areas of the animal's cerebrum.

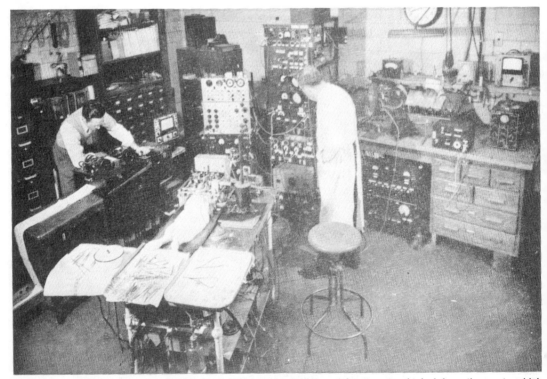

View of the electronic equipment that is used in the neurophysiology laboratory to obtain information as to which areas of the brain control such functions as vision, hearing, and touch.

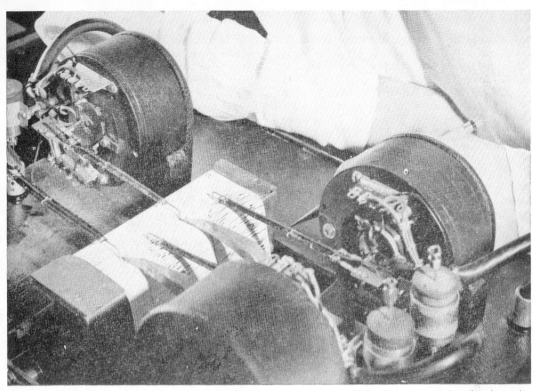

Close-up view of the low frequency ink-writing oscillograph, an instrument which, when connected to the electrodes in the animal's brain, makes a permanent recording of the electrical responses.

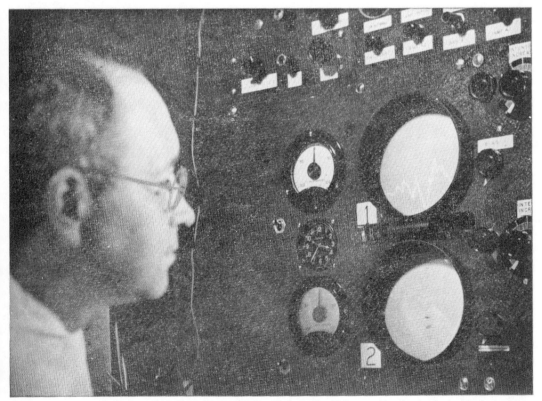

Photograph of the cathode ray oscilloscope upon the window of which may be observed electrical responses coming from electrodes which have been implanted in the cerebrum of the animal.

aspect of the field, for it is the brain that dominates the activities of most of the other areas of the body. An impairment of some small area of the brain may result in a complete loss of function of some organ or limb. Research on brain function may eventually provide a solution to many of these difficulties. There is no greater challenge to the neurophysiologists, however, than the problem of the causes of the many types of mental disease. There are those who feel that as more information becomes available, it may eventually become possible to combat successfully many of these strange maladies, that at present resist all efforts at treatment.

In the past, the machinations of the human mind were studied in the main only by psychiatrists and psychologists. Some time after World War II, however, biochemists and physiologists became interested in thought processes. This new laboratory approach to the "biochemistry of thought" has produced many unique discoveries. "Memory RNA and protein," for instance, can be transferred from a trained rat to an untrained rat, after which the untrained rat immediately acquires the training of the donor. Only the future can tell what these findings will mean in the human realm.

The photographs on pages 631-633 series depict some of the complex equipment which is required in the modern neurophysiology laboratory. Pictures courtesy of National Institute of Mental Health and National Institute of Neurological Disease and Blindness, United States Public Health Service, Washington, D.C.

20 THE LATER YEARS

PROBLEMS OF AN AGING POPULATION

Never before in history has there been so large a population of the aged as today. In ancient Rome, average life expectancy was about 23 years. In 1850 the life span in the United States was 40 years; by 1930 it had risen to 60 years. At the present time it has reached 74.39. This increase in longevity is paralleled in civilized countries all over the world. In the United States between 1960 and 1968, the number of persons over 65 was increased by three million.

From data compiled by scientists engaged in studies of the aged, a continuing increase of this group can be anticipated. Indications are that within the next few decades those in the older brackets will greatly outnumber the youth of the country. Already, the age distribution is showing the effect of this trend. In the United States, factors influencing this unprecedented age shift are a declining birth rate, the extension of life expectancy, and diminished immigration. In the last quarter of the nineteenth and the first quarter of the twentieth century, about 27 million immigrants were added to the population. At the time of admission to the country, these people were chiefly young adults. Only a negligible number of the younger adult level have been admitted to the United States since 1925, thus further affecting the age balance in population.

This preponderance of the aged has already caused many serious social and economic problems. In order to solve these problems, various community, state, and national groups are working on projects for the betterment of the aged. They realize that the difficulties and hardships which assail the older individual are of vital importance to the whole culture.

Dr. N. W. Shock in *Trends in Gerontology* says: "We are confronted with a situation which is wholly without precedent, namely, an ever increasing number of elderly persons who must either have the opportunity to work and support themselves or be supported by the proportionately dwindling group of younger people. Never before has such a grave social problem presented itself."

Social legislation has offered a partial answer to the problem. The Social Security Act, passed in 1936, provides retirement pensions for working people and sets the guidelines for old age assistance welfare. In 1965, Medicare and Medicaid were appended to the act to provide for medical care for the elderly and the medically indigent. Much of the impetus behind legislation for care for the elderly comes from the National Conference on Aging, a group of physicians and health-care professionals appointed by the President.

Among organizations working actively in behalf of the aged are two national professional groups, The Gerontological Society and the American Geriatrics Society. The United States Chamber of Commerce, the National Association of Manufacturers, and many other groups have set up committees to study and provide for the needs of the aged. Every state in the Union has a committee on aging.

The concept of aging as it affects the present culture is changing rapidly as more studies are being made in this fast developing field. The

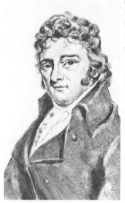

PARRY, Caleb Hillier (1755-1822) English physician. Noted for his confirmation and extension of the earlier work of Heberden on angina pectoris, which he considered to be the result of coronary artery disease. He later presented a careful description of a series of cases of toxic goiter which is sometimes spoken of as *Parry's disease*, but more often as *Grave's disease*. He described a number of other pathological conditions including facial hemiatrophy.

span of years lived after age 65 has increased so much that new stages in aging are being observed scientifically for the first time. These studies are based on different phases of aging such as physiological aging, psychological aging, and sociological aging. Even our terms for those over 65 recognize the spread. Terms used for subgroups among these people are senior citizens, the elderly, the aging, and the old.

The basic problems of an aging population are:

1. Emotional security and social recognition for the older individual.

2. A means of achieving financial independence.

3. Sufficient food, satisfactory living arrangements, and adequate health care.

Although older persons face many problems, they also have unprecedented opportunities. The chance for an enjoyable retirement is now available to many people for the first time. Insurance programs, company pension plans, and the development of resort and retirement facilities have opened new possibilities. The fact that many people begin a second career at 65 is adding to the work force of the nation in a significant way. A rewarding life, whether spent in work or retirement, can be a reality to those who· formerly looked forward to ill health and poverty.

PHYSIOLOGY OF AGING

Most normal people want to live a long time, but nobody wants to grow old. Yet aging is a continuous process beginning with birth and progressing throughout life.

The wise individual, before he reaches the later years, will rely on his physician to help prepare him for old age. Many changes occur in the aging process which, if neglected, can result in chronic physical illness or mental infirmity. With proper treatment, such deterioration often can be prevented or mitigated.

What is aging? It may be a gradual inability of the body's tissue to reduplicate. From laboratory attempts to grow human skin from a few cells, scientists conclude there is a mathematical limit to tissue reduplication that is about 100 to 120 years. Other researchers use the placenta within a pregnant woman to study aging and immunity. The placenta has the strength to ward off toxins and antibodies from the mother, but at the end of nine months shows extreme aging and loss of function. Is aging the loss of immunity? A clear answer has not been found. In general, we know that heredity contributes to longevity when combined with a healthful, well-ordered life.

With increasing age, there is a slowing down of all the functions and physiological reactions of the body. There is impairment of strength and motion and a general dulling of the senses. Also, there is usually some loss in weight, height, and sexual activity. There may be failing sight, deafness for high tones, graying hair, and loss of elasticity of the skin. These changes in themselves do not constitute disease processes.

Although all people do not age at the same rate, certain aging processes are inescapable. Changes occur in the body's tissues and in all its organs. The tissue cells of the kidney, liver, pancreas, and spleen lose weight and size because of aging blood vessels. These changes are primarily because of degeneration of the tissue in the walls of the blood vessels. The same is true of the thyroid and other endocrine glands. There are degenerative changes in the circulatory system, the respiratory tract, the eyes, the ears, the bones and joints, the blood, the skin, the hair, the nails, and the teeth. In old age, degeneration of the digestive tract is accompanied by diminished secretion of gastric juices, weakened muscle tone of the stomach and intestines, and a disturbed blood supply. Since the process of digestion is closely connected with the circulatory system, this diminished activity may seriously impair the entire gastrointestinal tract.

While these biological changes must occur if life continues over a sufficiently long time, they do not progress uniformly. In a man of 60 years, changes may have occurred in different organs in such varying degrees that he is, in some respects, 80, in others 40, 30, or even 20 years old.

General health rules

For contentment and continuing usefulness in the later years, the maintenance of good health is paramount. This is largely a matter of hygiene and common sense, barring the development of a crippling or debilitating disease. Of utmost importance is a yearly or twice-yearly physical examination. Almost all conditions of the elderly —hypertension, incipient diabetes, and cancer— can be prevented or halted through early detection.

Proper dental care is essential for older people. Regular checkups and immediate correction of ill-fitting dentures are important. Corrective glasses should be checked frequently and readjusted until comfortable. Good foot care is another common sense rule. Loss of weight and bone changes can result in aching feet and a strained back unless care is taken to find shoes that give adequate support and are comfortable.

In menu planning for the elderly, it is usually advisable to serve three meals daily, of almost similar size, rather than a large meal for the evening. Tea and coffee may be allowed in moderation if they are not harmful to the individual, and hard-to-digest foods should be avoided.

Obesity

Food requirements in adults are mainly energy requirements. As age increases, less energy is expended, and a smaller amount of food is required to maintain the body. Although less food is needed, the appetite usually determines the food intake. From habit, one is likely to continue eating the same amount of food consumed in earlier years. Thus, more food is used than the body needs, the surplus turns into fat, and obesity results. Fat increases the size of the capillary bed and greatly increases the amount of tissue to be nourished by the blood and through which the blood must be pumped. It is this increased and unnecessary load that makes obesity a decided health hazard and often the indirect cause of premature death. According to a life insurance statistician, "the longer the waistline, the shorter the life line." Overeating occasionally is caused by a neurosis or anxiety state. In some cases the overweight individual has lost interest in everything but food and literally "lives to eat." This condition requires counseling or special help.

At the first evidence of surplus weight, diet should be adjusted so that a normal weight can be maintained. Small dietary changes may achieve satisfactory results. Curtailment in the amount of bread, pastry, potatoes, and other carbohydrates, and a reduction in cream, butter, pork, and other fats may bring about gratifying results. Smaller portions should be taken at meals, thus preventing bloating or uncomfortable fullness after eating. A reducing diet should not be so restricted that loss of weight is rapid. A reducing diet should maintain a proper balance of foods to prevent nutritional deficiencies. A well-rounded diet should include meat, fish, dairy products, fresh vegetables, and fruits. If these foods are properly combined, the diet will contain adequate vitamins, iron, and calcium. Supplementary vitamins should be taken when prescribed by a physician for some specific deficiency.

Malnutrition

In contrast to the voracious eater, there are many aged individuals who eat too sparingly to maintain health. For these persons, menu planning is difficult because properly balanced meals may be refused. Because the sense of taste declines with age, food loses appeal for the appetite. The variety of foods formerly enjoyed becomes restricted. This restricted diet soon becomes monotonous, and a further distaste for foods results. In such cases, it is necessary to supplement the diet with vitamins. Important vitamins for the elderly are vitamin A and the vitamin B complex. The physician should determine the proper vitamins and dosage. In many cases, an adequate intake of vitamins over a prescribed period of time tends to delay the onset of some of the disabilities that come with age.

Another factor which restricts food consumption by the aged is impaired mastication because of diseased or lost teeth. Preservation of the teeth aids in averting many forms of indigestion and malnutrition. Teeth in bad condition should be repaired; if they must be extracted, properly fitting dentures should replace them. Teeth should never be extracted on the vague assumption that they might be foci of systemic infection. For further discussion of diets, consult Chapter 21, "Nutrition."

The use of tobacco and alcohol

Smoking and use of tobacco in other forms vary in their effects on different individuals. Many people have smoked for half a century without obvious ill effects. If tobacco is used excessively by the aged individual, the amount should be reduced gradually. It is perhaps not necessary to discontinue its use abruptly unless it has proved injurious. Smoking is harmful if it causes palpitation, dizziness, digestive upsets, and chest pains. If these symptoms are experienced immediately after smoking, tobacco should be banned. Patients with certain peripheral vascular disturbances, coronary or other heart disease, peptic ulcer, and bronchitis should refrain from smoking. The same reasons for other adults to avoid smoking are true for the aged.

Alcohol in moderation is regarded by some authorities as having distinct therapeutic value and may serve a beneficial purpose in the health requirements of the aged. In general ill health and malnutrition, alcohol may be helpful because of its food value. Often, it stimulates the appetite, dispels irritability, and promotes a sense

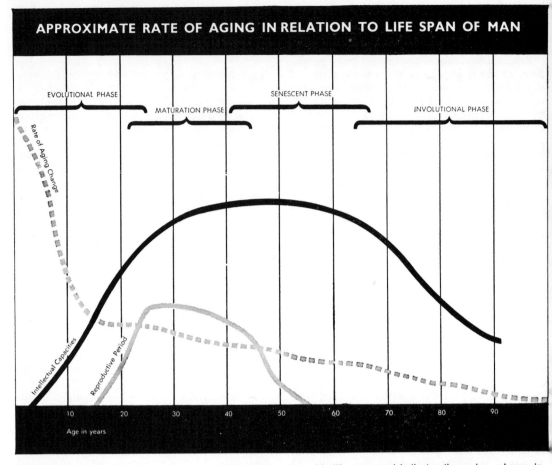

This chart compares the rate of aging in man in relationship to his life span, and indicates the various phases in his existence. *Adapted from Geriatric Medicine, edited by Edward J. Stieglitz, Copyright by Saunders Company, 1949.*

of well-being. Taken moderately before retiring, it may induce restful sleep. However, alcohol is dangerous in certain conditions such as peptic ulcer and liver disease.

Exercise

Differences in the physical condition of older persons make it difficult to specify a set schedule of exercise. However, some form of daily exercise should be taken unless it is prohibited by some impairment. Exercise should never be strenuous enough to cause exhaustion. Sudden spurts of effort, such as running, could be hazardous because they may put too great a strain on the heart. However, "jogging" for a few blocks each day is sometimes recommended by a physician if it is a supervised activity. Walking and light exercise are highly recommended. Stair-climbing is not dangerous if the climber has a healthy heart. Most important is the realization that the body and many of its organs lose their power to meet excessive strain. Therefore, the individual should recognize his

increasing limitations in order to avoid abusing weakened organs.

Of more value than physical exercise is a set of suggestions outlined by Doctor Martin Gumpert. Condensed, they are as follows:

1. Keep up social and mental activities. Try to acquire new skills, interests, and knowledge.
2. Plan to save energy in everything. Make a point of reaching the same end with a smaller expenditure of effort. Be aware of the danger signals of undue fatigue.
3. Do not long for retirement and *do not retire* unless it is required by urgent physical necessity. Then do so in order to pursue a better, more stimulating activity.
4. Plan to lengthen your intervals of rest and to shorten those of exercise.
5. Try to avoid boring situations.

Sleep

It is an old wives' tale that as one grows older, less sleep is required. Research data report that older people who sleep eight hours or more have fewer complaints. It may be more difficult for older people to get the necessary sleep. Those who do not sleep well suffer from tension and nervous exhaustion. In fact, some of the problems of the aged may simply be due to a lack of sleep.

Since the amount of sleep required varies with each individual, no arbitrary number of hours of sleep can be set. The prime requisite is that one should sleep enough to awaken rested and refreshed.

Many elderly people remain in bed eight or ten hours during the night even though they sleep but part of the time. This is advisable only if they are able to rest and feel invigorated upon arising.

In some individuals, sleeplessness may cause frustration, irritation, and nervousness. Often a glass of wine or warm milk may help to induce sleep. Chronic constipation may be a factor in insomnia, and changes in eating habits and fluid intake may be necessary. A study of the problem with the physician may lead to a solution.

Rest

Rest is a splendid restorative. Regular rest periods help to maintain health, and may even prolong life. However, physicians now advise that it is best *not* to lie down after eating. Moving around promotes circulation and digestion.

Prolonged bed rest for the ill can be harmful. Physicians now insist that their patients move about as soon as they can do so without danger.

Healing is promoted by the circulation of blood through damaged tissues. The more blood that is pumped through injured areas, the quicker wounds will heal. Inactivity slows the healing process. In many instances, *the longer the patient stays in bed, the longer it takes to get well*. This is especially true of the aged. For them, prolonged bed rest is hazardous, frequently causing heart, lung and circulatory complications. Wasting of the muscles may occur, and there may be a notable loss of calcium from the bones. Constipation, retention of urine, backache, pressure sores, and lowered morale often result. Too much bed rest is particularly bad for arthritic patients.

In certain diseases, this ban against bed rest does not apply. Patients suffering from tuberculosis, coronary thrombosis, pneumonia, and some other diseases must be governed by the regimen prescribed by their physician.

Elderly people who must maintain complete bed rest should change their positions frequently.

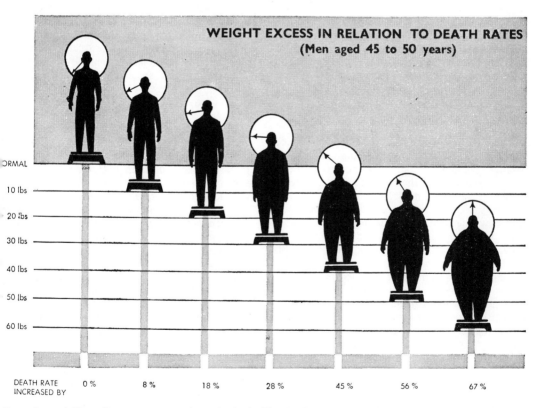

WEIGHT EXCESS IN RELATION TO DEATH RATES
(Men aged 45 to 50 years)

| NORMAL | 10 lbs | 20 lbs | 30 lbs | 40 lbs | 50 lbs | 60 lbs |

DEATH RATE INCREASED BY   0 %   8 %   18 %   28 %   45 %   56 %   67 %

Excessive weight predisposes a person to early death. The death rate for men between the ages of 45 and 50, who are 60 pounds overweight, is 67 percent higher than the death rate for men of normal weight who are of the same age.

Muscular exercises and massage of the lower extremities are helpful. The patient with a severe heart disability is an exception to this rule.

Sex

Although there is a gradual decline in sexual capacity after the age of 40, sexual activity is possible to a very advanced age. There is some evidence that moderate sexual activity tends to maintain normal endocrine balance, and that this in turn may inhibit or ameliorate the processes of aging.

Many older people, including those 90 years of age, continue to enjoy normal sexual relations. Their ability to do so depends on whether they have led an active, happy sex life and have no physical impairments. Those who are single or have lost a marriage partner tend to withdraw from sexual contact. People who have never adjusted to their sexual roles during the formative years will tend to have problems in old age resulting in a cessation of sexual interest and a rise in ailments of the sex organs.

A recent questionnaire found that 70 percent of married men over 65 engaged in sexual activities. Since only one third of all women in the United States over 65 are married, it is more difficult to assess the effects of age on their sexual activity.

Potency in old age is conditioned by frequency. Or, as one scientist put it, "nonuse, rather than abuse, causes impotency." Abnormal or prurient concern for sexual function usually signals mental distress. Such individuals may benefit from psychiatric or medical help.

Surgical operations

Old age brings constitutional changes which make surgical operations more difficult than in younger persons. An operation, however, should not be refused on the grounds of age alone. Medicine has made notable advances in the care of the aged, and improved surgical techniques and new anesthetic methods now make it feasible to operate on extremely old persons. Physiologic rather than chronologic age is the criterion for surgical treatment.

One of the main factors governing the decision for an operation is the mental attitude of the patient, which can be significant to the outcome. Those who are apathetic are not the best surgical risks; indeed, some surgeons maintain that if a patient lacks the will to live, his chances of surviving an operation are significantly diminished.

As a rule, both undernourished and obese persons are not good operative risks. In these cases, the operation should be deferred, if possible, until the patient has returned to a more normal weight.

Surgery is usually successful with any aged patient accepted for operation. The surgeon expects comparable results to those obtained in younger people, provided, of course, that the heart, kidneys, lungs, and other organs are functioning satisfactorily. Physical rehabilitation following an operation is feasible and desirable for older patients. It is important that the elderly patient be as well and ambulatory as possible. Artificial limbs, once given to younger patients only, are now available to older patients. Space is also reserved for them in the nation's growing number of rehabilitation centers.

PHYSICAL DISORDERS

During late maturity, a thorough physical checkup by a physician is a wise precaution against disease in old age. A certain amount of damage may already have occurred; but proper medical care may correct or ameliorate the condition. With increasing age, aches and pains may multiply. A sensible acceptance of this fact is important to happiness. The mental attitude toward the aging process has considerable influence on the rate of physical deterioration. Understanding and acceptance of this encroaching impairment postpones decline, while ineffectual hostile attempts to deny it may hasten the decline. However, physical infirmity is not an unfailing accompaniment to age; many people are physically quite sound in their advanced years.

There are no specific diseases caused primarily by old age. The maladies prevalent in older groups are not necessarily caused by the aging process. Frequently, these diseases result from chronic disorders which occurred years earlier. Many disorders can be traced to illnesses of childhood. Most old people die of degenerative diseases which had their beginnings between the ages of 30 and 40. These ailments, progressing into advanced years, result in illnesses generally regarded as "the diseases of old age." Although no such category actually exists, it is true that a general pattern of diseases is found which is common to this group. The diseases that take the greatest toll of life from the aged are heart diseases, cancer, and cerebral hemorrhage (also known as stroke). Also among the afflictions of the aged are arthritis, rheumatism, diabetes, prostatic enlargement, kidney, nervous, and mental diseases, as well as hardening of the small arteries (arteriosclerosis), deposits of fat in the large arteries (atherosclerosis), and high blood pressure (hypertension). The exact causes of senility are unknown, although it is known that excessive amounts of alcohol can produce premature senility. Further research into the aging process may reveal means of preventing many of the degenerative changes that occur in the later years.

These diseases and their treatment are described in detail in other chapters.

Fractures

Falls and bumps must be viewed seriously in the older person. Many kinds of fractures are peculiar to this age group. Because of the increasing brittleness of the skeleton, a minor trauma can result in a major health problem. A leading cause of fracture is *osteoporosis*, a disorder of bone metabolism that results in decreased bone mass.

The most common fractures seen in older patients are breakage of the hip (at the neck of the femur where it joins the pelvis), the wrist joint, and the upper end of the humerus (arm). These types of fractures are a result of falling. Those of the wrist or arm are caused by the patient extending his arm to break the fall.

If the femur is shattered, a piece of metal is inserted surgically to fix the bone to the joint. To get the patient walking again, rehabilitation begins as soon as he has recovered from the operation. First he walks through parallel bars. Then he graduates to partial weight bearing in a "walker," a framework of bars on wheels. Often, corrective shoes must be made to accommodate changes in bone length. After a few months, the patient is usually completely healed and can walk normally.

Fractures of the upper arm and shoulder, though not the most serious, are very painful and sometimes blood is lost. By immobilizing the arm with a sling, pain is relieved until a callus can be formed at the joint. Exercises begin as soon as the pain is gone entirely. The patient imitates the movements of a pendulum, "stirs the pot," pretends he climbs a wall, and uses pulleys. Local heat and ultrasound are comforting to remove soreness. Whirlpool therapy and paraffin baths are sometimes prescribed, especially for those with wrist fractures.

The damaged heart

As the individual grows older, physical fitness is most frequently dependent on the healthy heart. If hardening of the arteries develops, the arterial walls become narrowed and less elastic; hence, the heart must perform more vigorously to achieve the same work. As the heart adapts to the strain, and contracts and pumps more vigorously, it becomes enlarged. Eventually, when the organ reaches the limit of compensation, heart failure ensues. A person having a damaged or enlarged heart should remain under medical care. In the past decade, battery-operated pacemakers that regulate the damaged heart have extended the useful lives of thousands of older people. Such devices enable formerly incapacitated heart patients to live normal lives.

High blood pressure is not a disease, but is a symptom. The blood pressure normally fluctuates considerably and therefore is determined by repeated checks. If pressure continues to be elevated this is known as *hypertension*. After years of hypertension, structural changes develop in the heart and arteries. Even then, with proper medical care, the overtaxed heart can continue its work favorably. The hypertensive patient should have regular consultations with his physician and be governed entirely by his advice. Disorders of the heart and circulation are further discussed in Chapter 7.

Stroke

In the United States, approximately 100,000 people die annually of stroke (*cerebral hemorrhage*). About 98 percent of them are over the age of 50. Arteriosclerosis and hypertension are the chief causes of cerebral hemorrhage. Arteriosclerosis also frequently causes cerebral thrombosis of the smaller vessels in older persons. Approximately 40 percent of all cerebral vascular accidents are caused by extracranial vascular occlusion. Warning is frequently given by preceding symptoms. Sudden emotional changes from depressions to overexcitement, persistent, long-lasting headaches, dizziness, and impairment of vision or speech may indicate that brain arteries have been damaged. Measures should be taken at this time to prevent hemorrhage. The physician may recommend a few days "sleep and rest." Mild sedation is often valuable. After this, adjustment may be sought in the patient's mode of living.

In the event of a disabling stroke, rehabilitation must begin immediately in the weeks following the cerebral accident. Formerly, aging patients were not rehabilitated. Now it is recognized that restoring normal functions is a goal of geriatric medicine. The therapist's aim is to help the patient rejoin society as an independent and contributing member.

Cancer

Cancer is a disease characterized by abnormal growth of tissue. A tumor is considered malignant, and therefore a cancer, if it can spread to remote areas of the body. This spread (*metastasis*) occurs when a minute piece of the tumor breaks off from the growth and is carried by the blood or lymph stream to other body areas or nearby lymph nodes. The metastatic cells from the original tumor attach themselves and set up a "colony," which eventually may exceed the parent growth in size and destructiveness. The most frequent sites of metastasis are the lymph nodes in the region of the tumor, the lungs, long bones, the spine and ribs, liver, skin, and brain. The sexes are about equally divided as to cancer incidence, although the disease occurs in some sites more frequently in one sex than another. Men suffer most from cancer of the skin, lung, prostate, stomach and rectum. Women have cancer of the breast and womb more frequently than other types. Children have the highest incidence of brain tumors and leukemia. Thus, general incidence of cancer does not steadily rise throughout the life span. The principal sites of cancer in elderly people are the same for all adults except that older men are more apt to develop cancer of the prostate gland.

If a tumor does not spread but stays in its original area, it is known as a *benign tumor*. Another important difference between benign and malignant tumors is that the benign tumors grow locally by simple expasion of the mass, but cancers grow locally by extension of fingers of tissue into the normal surrounding tissues.

A cancer can arise in any of the body's tissues, whenever those tissues begin to grow wildly and uncontrollably. In general, cancer may be of two types according to the tissue of its origin; if the growth arises from epithelial tissues, it is a *carcinoma,* and if it arises from connective tissues, it is a *sarcoma*. Metastasis from a carcinoma usually takes place by way of the lymphatic system, while sarcoma spreads most often by way of the blood stream. The primary new growth may occur in a specific organ, such as the stomach or the rectum, or widely throughout the body, as in cancer of the blood (*leukemia*). In each case, it is an abnormal growth of the tissues already present, rather than of any new, previously absent tissues.

If the growth is not checked, a cancer will eventually spread to many parts of the body, invading and eroding the normal tissues and causing pressure against and within the vital organs of the body. Death will result unless a cure is effected.

Symptoms

The cure of cancer depends upon early recognition of the symptoms of the disease, followed by early, adequate therapy. The symptoms of cancer are innumerable, varying with the site of the original growth and any secondary growths. In general, however, there are seven "danger signals" which indicate that a malignant tumor may be present in the body. If one of these signs appears, it should cause no undue alarm, because in most cases it does not mean cancer. However, such a sign indicates that the patient is not well and should consult his physician in order that he may make the diagnosis and ascertain the true cause of the disturbance. Thus, an attitude of calm vigilance and serious inquiry when these symptoms arise is far better than a "cancer phobia."

The seven warning signals mentioned above

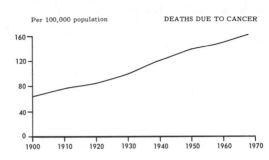

Per 100,000 population   DEATHS DUE TO CANCER

This chart portrays the increase during the first half of the twentieth century in the number of individuals who die each year as the result of cancer.

are: persistent hoarseness or cough, any sore that does not heal, any change in a mole or wart, unexplained bleeding or discharge from any of the body orifices, any change in normal bowel habits, a lump or thickening in the breast or elsewhere, and persistent indigestion or difficulty in swallowing. On appearance of any one of these, the physician should be consulted immediately.

The cancer danger signals are especially significant in persons over 40 years of age. However, the disease can and often does occur in persons of all age groups.

Diagnosis

During the past few years numerous new diagnostic techniques have been developed which enable the physician to determine whether a patient has cancer. These include: *mammography* (x-ray study of the breast), which may be helpful in the diagnosis of early carcinoma of the breast;

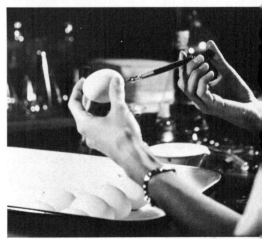

Cancer research involves the use of many types of animals. Here, fertilized eggs are being inoculated with cancerous tissue from a mouse. *Biochemical Institute, The University of Texas, and Clayton Foundation for Research.*

radioisotopes (swallowed radioactive dye that shows up on special x-ray film), used for the localization of tumors in various organs; *lymphangiography* (an x-ray technique for looking at the lymph nodes), used for the accurate diagnosis of metastases to lymph nodes; *exfoliative cytology* (microscopic study of sloughed-off cells), which is being expanded beyond its usual application in the diagnosis of cervical cancer to include analysis of the sputum, urine, and blood, for the detection of malignant cells; and *tomography*, which is the technique of making radiographs of plane sections of solid objects, in which the predetermined plane is shown in detail while images of structures in other planes are blurred.

Cause of cancer

The cause of cancer is unknown. It is generally accepted that some persons have a hereditary predisposition for cancer in certain sites. Also, chronic irritation of a body area over a number of years may produce cancer. Certain substances, called *carcinogens*, incite cancer after repeated exposure to these substances. Many persons are exposed to these substances or to irritation in their occupations. For example, sailors and ranchers have a high incidence of skin cancer, thought to be caused by chronic exposure to the sun's rays. Chimney cleaners in England often suffered from cancer of the scrotum, which is induced by the carcinogens in the soot (now rare).

Cancer also may arise from certain preexisting lesions, which are regarded as "premalignant." White patches on the tongue and vulva (*leukoplakia*), certain clear-colored warts on older persons (*keratosis*), large burn scars, and pendulous growths (*polyps*) in the rectum are some of the lesions which can undergo malignant change after several years. These lesions should be called to the doctor's attention.

Theories exist that cancer is related to diet and weight as well as to certain of the patient's habits, such as smoking. However, the evidence that any such factors cause cancer is still not entirely conclusive. One popular belief, that cancer is related to an injury, has never been proved. In recent years, evidence has accumulated that some types of cancer may be caused by viruses in persons already predisposed because of heredity.

Treatment

Despite sporadic reports and claims of "miracle cures," there are only a few established, effective forms of treatment for the cancer patient. Chief among these are surgical removal of the growth and radiotherapy. This can be accomplished best when the cancer is in certain areas and *when the disease is in an early stage*—that

is, while the growth is still localized and has not spread to lymph nodes or other body organs. The majority of cancers arise in accessible sites; if the individual obtains early diagnosis and therapy, he may be cured. However, his chances for cure decrease as each month passes.

Surgical treatment for cancer is no longer a fearful ordeal. With the use of modern instruments, individualized anesthesia, newer supportive procedures, and preventives of infection, nearly any patient can withstand the operation itself. Also, measures exist to avoid postoperative complications that plagued patients in former years. Most gratifying, deformities caused by wide surgical removal of malignant tumors can now be repaired with plastic surgery or corrected with specialized devices.

X-rays and radium can also eradicate many forms of cancer. The x-rays may be directed to a tumor on the surface of the body or beamed to destroy an internal tumor. Radium is used in the form of needles or pellets planted directly into the tumor tissue and left there until the killing rays destroy the cancer. The chief advantage of x-rays and radium is that their use will leave few or no deformities.

Among the recently developed materials for the treatment of cancer patients are the radioactive elements (*isotopes*), manufactured in the atomic pile or cyclotron. These compounds have proved to be quite effective in the treatment of patients with some types of cancer.

Certain generalized forms of cancer cannot be attacked surgically and are only temporarily affected by irradiation. Among these are some of the leukemias, some malignant diseases of the lymphatic system, and far-advanced forms of cancer in which the disease has spread throughout the body. Patients with these disorders often benefit from treatment with certain drugs. Although chemotherapy for cancer patients has been recognized since early times, its modern use was initiated with the sinking of the Liberty ship, the John E. Harvey, carrying 100 tons of mustard gas, during a bombing of Bari Harbor on December 3, 1943. A U.S. medical officer observed that the men on the ship who had survived the blast and fire were dying of mustard gas poisoning. All had profound decreases in their white blood cell count. This observation led to an investigation of mustard gas and related compounds in the treatment of patients with leukemia and other malignant diseases in which the white blood cell count is pathologically elevated. In succeeding years, numerous compounds have been studied. Although there are many new drugs being used, they fall into four general types. These are: (1) Alkylating agents, which affect tumor cells in much the same way as irradiation, and some of which produce full but temporary remission in chronic leukemia; these compounds include nitrogen mustard, triethylene

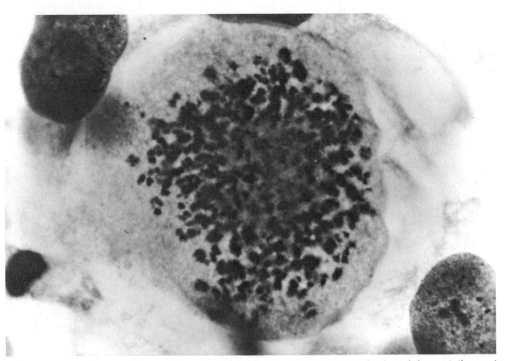

Photomicrograph of a tissue culture of liposarcoma incubated six days and stained to bring out the nuclear material. *Courtesy of Dr. T. C. Hsu, Tissue Culture Laboratory, The University of Texas M. D. Anderson Hospital and Tumor Institute.*

melamine (TEM), and triethylene thiophosphoramide (Thio-TEPA). (2) Antimetabolites. These compounds interfere with tumor metabolism by substituting a metabolic analogue for an essential amino acid, and cause remission in patients with leukemia; some of these compounds are Aminopterin® and Methotrexate®. (3) Cell poisons. These include urethane, which produces palliation in multiple myeloma; demecolcin, which has been described as beneficial in patients with some types of leukemia; and certain antibiotics, which are being used to treat patients with several types of cancer. (4) Hormones. Regulation of the gonadotrophic hormones has benefited patients with cancer of the breast and of the prostate gland; and administration of adrenocorticotrophic hormones (cortisone and ACTH) has helped some patients with cancer of the lymphatic system.

Research is continuing not only in an effort to find suitable therapeutic compounds, but also as to the best means of using them. At present, the chemotherapeutic agents are being used as the primary treatment in some disorders while in other conditions they are used as adjuvants to surgical treatment and radiotherapy. In recent years a technique known as *perfusion* has come into use. By this technique the body area in which the cancer is situated is partially isolated from the rest of the body by tourniquets or by ligating the blood vessels leading from the area; the area is then perfused with the chemotherapeutic agent.

In treating some areas such as the brain, perfusion is accomplished by injecting the drug for a few minutes and then injecting another drug to halt the effects of the first. This is done because some of the agents used to kill cancer cells are toxic to normal cells as well. The process is then repeated. Excellent results have been obtained in such cases using Methotrexate and its antidote, folinic acid (the compound used is known as citrovorum factor). Methotrexate causes a reaction with the body's supply of folic acid. Folinic acid dispels the reaction.

The above-mentioned methods are the only known means of treatment for cancer patients which can give the victims their best chances for benefit or cure. And these methods are administered only by ethical physicians. The unwary patient who falls into the hands of a quack is endangering his life. Not only are the pills, powders, or "treatments" dispensed by these unscrupulous persons ineffectual, but the time the patient spends trying them may allow his cancer to reach an incurable stage. One means of easily distinguishing the ethical physician from the quack is this: the quack advertises or promises a cure, the ethical physician does not.

Research is in progress which aims to perfect forms of therapy which can cure the patient more readily than those that now exist. However, until such time as a treatment method is announced by responsible members of the medical profession, the patient can obtain a great deal of benefit or even cure from present measures. Indeed, even if the patient is considered "hopeless," he can have his comfort greatly increased and perhaps years added to his life with proper treatment. The best way he can increase his chances for cure is to see his physician concerning any suspicious symptoms and to undergo the appropriate periodic examinations.

For information concerning the symptoms, diagnosis, treatment, and prevention of specific forms of cancer, reference should be made to the sections dealing with the disease in the organs concerned. For example, for cancer of the rectum, see Chapter 13, "The Digestive System: *Disorders of the Rectum.*"

Physical rehabilitation

The days are gone when older people were left to recover from surgical procedures as best they could on their own. Special attention is paid them in the recovery room, since the elderly can suffer shock easily. Special diets, exercises, and prosthetics are designed for them.

Elderly amputees are now being helped to walk again with artificial limbs, and are taught to use artificial hands and arms. This requires psychological preparation of the patient and general strengthening of body muscles. Such patients have the help of a hospital team consisting of a physician, prosthetist, and physical therapist. Some cases may require the aid of a psychologist, social worker, or vocational counselor. The doctor is in contact with all these professions, and directs them in helping his patient.

The dying patient

Death is the least studied phase of human life. Many doctors and nurses fear or try to ignore it since saving life is their business.

Helping a dying patient meet death with understanding can give dignity and peace to the patient. Too often, dying patients are left alone. Their baffled and hurt families are left with undeserved anger, fear, or guilt. Who can help them?

Dr. Elisabeth Kubler-Ross writes in her book, *"On Death and the Dying"* (Macmillan Co., 1969) that the living and the dying must help each other. She defines five psychological stages of dying, which if understood by the patient's family, might enable them to solve their own prob-lems and help their dying relative. They are: (1) Denial. The patient refuses to believe he will die. He seems to be collecting time. (2) Anger. He may turn against those dear to him because he cannot accept the fact that he, and not someone else, must die. This stage may be aggravated by weight loss and pain. (3) Bargaining. The patient believes he can "buy time," by being good, correcting his flaws, or perhaps by following his medical treatment compulsively. (4) Depression. To attempt to cheer the patient is absurd, warns Dr. Ross. This is a necessary stage to arrive at a more positive view. (5) Acceptance. This is sometimes mistaken for a sense of euphoria. It is instead a positive passivity. Although the dying patient may have found some peace, this is the time when the patient's family needs the most help. The dying person himself can often share his feelings best at this stage and does the most for his family.

It is a rare terminal patient, however, who abandons all hope. Many do not reach the stage of acceptance. All of these patients benefit greatly from talking about death. To continually divert them away from the subject may not aid them.

MENTAL HEALTH AND MENTAL DISORDERS

The concept that doddering, palsied senility must be the fate of the aged is disproved. The majority of those who have reached the later years are neither feeble nor decrepit. Poor mental health, as poor physical health, can be averted in most cases. Adequate medical supervision and pleasant surroundings will greatly retard mental deterioration in old age.

Two types of senility threaten the aged. These are *physical* senility and *psychological* senility. Although stemming from different sources, they create the same disorganized personality traits.

Mental impairment, in varying degrees, is found in senescent individuals in the following general pattern. Their interests frequently become narrowed to matters of self-concern. Their thinking may become sluggish. Fixed habits are stubbornly and tenaciously held, and new ideas are violently opposed. There is often a tendency to garrulous reminiscence, while attention to others is poorly maintained. Recent events may be forgotten, memory being usually the first function of the mind to wane. In many cases, however, apparent lack of memory is only lack of interest. With increasing senility, many undesirable personality changes occur. Seclusiveness, irritability, and depression develop. Outbreaks of temper are frequent. Hoarding is common. Tendencies to suspiciousness are exaggerated, causing the patient to fear bodily harm or even death at the hands of those dearest to him. As senility advances, the patient grows progressively more careless in dress, eating, and personal habits. He may suffer from disorientation, mental confusion, hallucinations, or phobias. Moral judgment may fail, and antisocial acts may be committed. Exhibitionism and abnormal sexual advances may be made. At this stage, institutional care is advisable.

The physician can help greatly in preventing premature senile changes. Attention to the control of nutritional deficiencies, the prevention of kidney and heart diseases, and care of infectious maladies in early life will postpone physical debilitation in the later years. Careful attention to mental hygiene may benefit the patient psychologically. It is of great importance that the patient continue to make successful social adjustments. Also, he should be aware that worry, fear, grief, and anger are disastrous. Effective control of the emotions helps guard against premature aging.

The elderly in the family

Younger people in a family sometimes have difficulties in getting along with the older relatives. Much family strife can be overcome by providing real functions for the elderly to perform, not just "busy work." Their independence should be encouraged.

Younger members may need counseling to show them the reasons behind old age antisocial behavior. Children should be given full understanding of the aging process. Efforts should be made to provide adequate living space for all members of the family so as to maintain privacy and allow teenagers to act as teenagers, married couples to enjoy themselves, and older members a sense of dignity. Social centers for "senior citizens" can help family mental health by providing recreation, friendship, and counseling for older members.

WORK OR RETIREMENT

Never before in history have people lived so long. The oft-quoted statistic that 90 percent of all scientists born are living today shows that the fruits of medicine and science flourish as never before to keep people alive and well.

Older people today are stronger and healthier. Thus the retirement at age 65 may be premature. There is even some evidence that intelligence influences longevity. Forced inactivity is a tragic waste. Scientists predict that by 1980, the man of 65 to 75 years of age will have the strength he had at 45 to 55.

People who reach the age of 65 have an important decision to make—how best to spend the remaining years of life, years that may be among the most productive and gratifying.

The older worker

According to the latest United States Census figures, there are more than 19 million people 65 and over. Less than 15 percent of them have jobs. Many of these people are physically and mentally able to work but have been forced out of employment by compulsory retirement. Failure to provide work for them constitutes a great loss of productive power for the nation. And loss of income for this age group constitutes the major welfare problem of the United States.

The problem of keeping older people employed is being approached from many angles. Through efforts of welfare workers, many industrial plants have lifted the ban against age limits for hiring.

Massachusetts has made notable progress in protecting the older worker. After many attempts to legislate against the discharge and nonemployment of the elderly, the state, in 1950, passed a law against age discrimination. This has now been made into a national statute. The elderly jobseeker, however, must meet the same qualifications required of the younger applicant.

In the industrial field, management and labor are now working in closer harmony for the betterment of the older worker. In a survey made

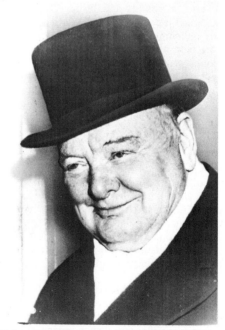

Winston Churchill, famous British prime minister and international statesman, was head of his nation at 79 years of age. *Photograph by Wide World Photo.*

by the United States Bureau of Labor Statistics, over 2000 agreements were analyzed. Pension provisions were studied, age limits investigated, and transfers to lighter work, when indicated, were provided for older employees. Though most labor unions oppose part-time work, some will permit an older worker to take such employment when it is necessary to conserve his strength and health. Many unions now allow the older employee to take a lower rated job at a lower wage scale. Seniority clauses in labor contracts protect older workers from discrimination in general layoffs. They also provide for better promotional assignments and other benefits applicable under seniority rights. In the building trades, the agreement between labor and management usually provides that at least one worker 55 or over must be employed to each five, seven, or ten journeymen hired. Some unions, notably the International Typographical Union, have contracts that forbid termination of employment because of age alone. These unions require medical examinations proving a worker's physical or mental inability to do his job before he may be discharged. At an executive level, it may be even more difficult to relinquish a job. Although places must be made for younger men and women, it is not necessarily true that an executive at 65 is old and slow. A study of 424 aging executives showed they possessed the over-all mental strength of 25-year-old medical students.

Recently compiled data indicate that industries in which one fifth or more of the work force consisted of men 55 years of age and over were finance, insurance, real estate, local and state government, and transportation, chiefly railroads. Also, a large percentage of this age group were found in agriculture, personnel, and professional services. The best chances for men 65 and over were in finance, insurance, real estate, agriculture, and professional services.

In industry, there are fewer available openings for older women than for older men. The greatest number of women 55 and older are employed in retail trades, public administration, and service industries.

New opportunities for employment are being opened for older people in most larger cities. State employment agencies are informed of union rules and laws on employment of those over 65. New careers are encouraged by state employment agencies. Many new openings for part-time workers are being created by state and federal commissions on aging. These are mainly in child care centers, agriculture, schools, and industry.

Retirement

Compulsory retirement affecting the mass of mentally sound, able-bodied older citizens, has long been recognized as one of the major problems of the later years. This forced retirement often predisposes the individual to disintegration of the personality and health. Many doctors, welfare workers, and organized groups are attempting to help the aging individual solve the problems of enforced leisure. They point out that those who face compulsory retirement at a specified age know well in advance this is in store and when it will occur. Therefore, the shock of dismissal should not be the turning point for physical and mental deterioration.

To enjoy a full and rewarding life in the later years, it is wise to begin preparing financially, physically, and mentally many years before actual retirement. There are, of course, many people with financial security to whom the future presents no economic problem; but for the majority a carefully planned budget is an absolute necessity. This budget should be planned to provide adequate living standards according to the ideas of the individual and the amount of life income available. Wise provisions for the future include privately purchased annuities, life insurance, and sound investment. Further, there will be available to most people pensions, social security benefits (including Medicare), and various industrial retirement plans. Also, for certain groups, there are civil service, state, municipal, and other benefits.

Paramount to a healthy body is a happy mental outlook. Those who achieve this have led an active productive life during earlier years. In making the transition from work to leisure, they

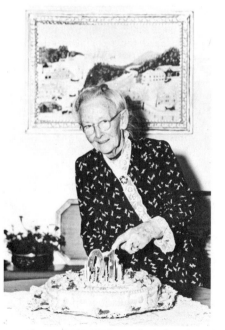

Grandma Moses (1860-1961), modern American landscape artist, is shown here as she celebrated her 91st birthday in 1951. *Wide World Photo.*

have new interests ready to take the place of old ones. They increase the scope of their hobbies and have many accomplishments of which they are proud. They have set goals for a long and healthy life. These people will go on *living* as well as *existing*.

After 60 years of age, many persons can learn as well as they did in earlier years, although they learn more slowly. What they learn they may retain better than things learned earlier. With age and experience judgment should improve. History demonstrates that the vitality of the human mind is not limited by age. Many able scientists are in their seventh decade, or even older. Many masterpieces of creative genius and other important achievements are the products of elderly persons.

Social facilities

In many communities there are activity centers which provide opportunities for the aged to associate with others in the same age group. Here the individual may enjoy social activities, make friends, and develop whatever creative talents he may have. The objective of such centers is not in doing things *for* the aged, but rather in giving them the chance to do things *for themselves*. Here, older persons find outlets for their needs for learning, companionship, and self-expression.

In these centers, educational opportunities are provided, and forum discussions are encouraged. Skills are developed in arts and crafts, and hobby shows are promoted. The task of finding employment for older persons is another vital service rendered by welfare workers who keep in close touch with employment needs and aid the applicant in securing work he is able to do.

One of the most noteworthy of these centers is the Hodson Community Center, New York City, which has a membership of over 3000. This center, opened in 1946, was one of the first established in the United States for recreational purposes. Diversions, games, and arts and crafts are provided. When other activities are desired, they are added. Programs now include poetry, painting, writing, dramatics, embroidery, woodworking, and choral singing. Lounges are provided for reading and group activities. Also classrooms, libraries, and workshops are available.

Almost every church, business or social organization, or special-interest club has a program for "senior citizens." Being over 65 is "in." Whole retirement communities are planned around the interest of the elderly. Newspapers written for this audience keep them informed of events and services. Civic centers offer legal and tax aid. No list of social facilities is necessary here, since anyone can call the Senior Citizen's Council, Chamber of Commerce, or local newspaper for a list of groups to contact.

Clubs

Old age clubs enjoy popularity in most parts of the world. There are differences in scope and facilities, governed by the requirements of the people. Flourishing clubs are maintained in the United States, Canada, England, Ireland, Australia, and New Zealand. They are also found in Belgium, Holland, and Austria. Finland has no clubs, but summer excursions are organized for the aged.

In the United States, Day Centers, McGuffy, Golden Age, Darby and Joan, Old Guard, and other old age clubs bearing various names dot the country from coast to coast. Abroad, the Darby and Joan Clubs are among the most popular. In England, clubs furnish activities of a useful nature as well as providing recreation.

One of the oldest organizations of this nature is The Recreation Opportunities for Older People of Greater Cleveland, Ohio, established early in this century by the Benjamin Rose Institute. The original club was started in a settlement house. Later branches were formed in churches, women's clubs, and other agencies. The formation of hobby clubs followed immediately. In 1948, The Rose Institute turned this work over to the Cleveland Welfare group.

Many foreign countries, however, have no organized activity facilities for the aged. Poland, Luxemburg, and Lithuania report that some recreational services are provided in the old age homes. In Denmark and Norway, old age pensioners form their own clubs. In Greece, as in Switzerland, there are no special activities provided for the aged. France claims that her highly individualistic population would not desire group activity. The French café, in many instances, answers the need for a social meeting place for people of all ages. In Oriental countries, the aged are held in high esteem. Their welfare is a family responsibility, and they do not form clubs or groups. There is a club in Tel Aviv for older persons, and Israel plans to build a "Village of the Aged" nearby, under the auspices of the Israel Ministry of Social Welfare.

SOCIAL WELFARE

The basic social needs of the aged have been defined as "somewhere to live, something to do, and someone to care." These needs meet with the wholehearted acceptance of groups working for those who have reached the later years. Welfare activities and facilities are planned to furnish all three of these requirements. If the aging individual is given pleasant surroundings, congenial companionship, and an occupation in which he feels useful, many of the problems of old age will be solved. The old person needs the security which comes from a sense of "belonging," of feeling he is needed. Abrupt realization that one is no longer useful may bring about disintegrating personality changes.

Welfare workers know this and are aiding older citizens in adjusting to their changed conditions. Practically every community has social agencies, citizens' committees, public health and welfare departments, church auxiliaries, and other organizations which are prepared to counsel this age group. They also establish rehabilitation and recreational centers.

Committees on aging

Although local community groups are closer to those they plan to serve, state and national services are also available for the aged. All states have special divisions in the health and welfare departments for old age assistance, aid to the blind, and aid for disabled persons. The New York State Joint Legislative Committee on Problems of Aging is probably the most active of all legislative committees interested in the enactment of laws to benefit and safeguard elderly persons. This group makes extensive studies of programs and activities available to the aged. These investigations cover work being done not only in New York but in other states as well.

On the national level, there are committies for financial aid, insurance, health, housing, nursing, institutional care, and other significant subjects. A National Conference on Aging is held in Washington each year. This conference meets to study the nature and extent of the problems confronting an aging population. Plans are made to set up voluntary and public organizations in each state, city, and community throughout the nation to help this age group. Measures are recommended to further research in health, recreation, rehabilitation, employment, education, and social and psychological fields; and programs are outlined to aid the older individual to adjust to environmental changes facing him.

Social security

The Social Security Act of 1936 set up a pension plan for retired people that forms the economic base for most older people today. Through regular payroll deductions, each person is eligible for a pension beginning at age 65. Widows may collect the pension granted to a deceased spouse. People who are employed on a casual basis are cheating themselves if they do not have deductions made for social security. They will not, under the present law, be eligible for a pension when they need it most.

The act also set up the nation's welfare program with an array of services adaptable to the needs of each state. There is a social security office and a welfare office in each county.

Medicare

Medicare is a medical insurance program for people over 65. Set up as Title 18 of the Social Security Act, it is financed by trust funds of federal tax money and by premiums paid by each person joining the program. Although the rules are changeable by Congress, those who are eligible must have worked a certain number of quarters of any year before reaching 65.

Medicare is divided into Part A for hospital benefits and Part B for outpatient care. Under Part A, Medicare (in 1970) pays for hospital bills except for the first $44. This includes inpatient hospital care for 90 days, posthospital extended care for 100 days, and posthospital home health care up to 100 days.

Part B pays 80 percent, or $4 out of each $5, of "reasonable" medical costs except for the first $50 in each calendar year. Part B covers physicians' fees, use of medical equipment and supplies, and home health care services.

Medicare exists in all parts of the United States. The program is administered in some states by privately owned insurance companies such as Blue Cross–Blue Shield, John Hancock, and Travelers', or by the Social Security division of the government. The operating agency, or carrier, sets what it considers "reasonable" medical costs for its particular area. Most ethical doctors' fees fall within the range set by Medicare.

A complete listing of what Medicare does and does not cover is given in the pamphlet "Your Medicare Handbook" available at the Social Security office or Health Department. Some of the things Part A includes are: bed in a semiprivate room and all meals, nursing services, intensive care nursing, hospital drugs, laboratory tests, radiology services, supplies, and equipment (such as splints and casts). These same services are covered if the patient leaves the hospital after a stay of at least three days to be placed in an extended-care facility or skilled nursing home. Part A hospital insurance also pays for home care beginning any time up to one year from the date the patient left the hospital or extended-care unit. Home-care coverage includes the following items if they are provided by a recognized health care agency, such as the home treatment unit of a hospital: part-time nursing; physical, occupational, or speech therapy; part-time medical aid services; drugs provided by the agency; and medical equipment.

Part B covers nonhospital fees owed to physicians. It will pay for dental surgery. Other services paid are tests, medical supplies, service of the doctor's nurse, and drugs administered in the doctor's office.

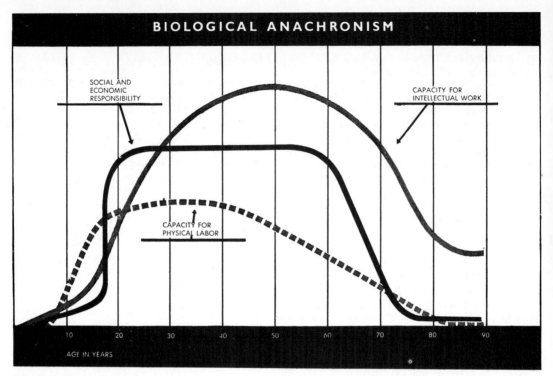

BIOLOGICAL ANACHRONISM

SOCIAL AND
ECONOMIC
RESPONSIBILITY

CAPACITY FOR
INTELLECTUAL WORK

CAPACITY FOR
PHYSICAL LABOR

AGE IN YEARS

This chart illustrates graphically one of the greatest problems of the aged, the fact that the capacity for intellectual work remains long past the time when other considerations make it easy for the individual to find a useful place in society. *Adapted from Geriatric Medicine, edited by Edward J. Stieglitz. Copyright, W. B. Saunders, 1949.*

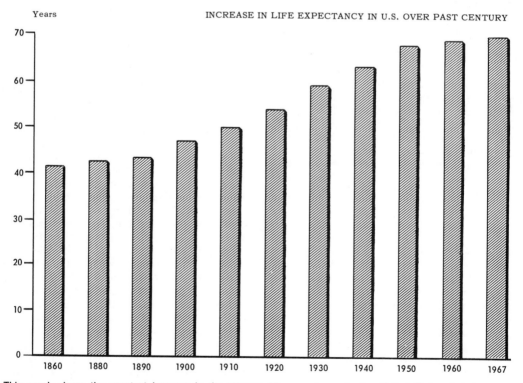

Years   INCREASE IN LIFE EXPECTANCY IN U.S. OVER PAST CENTURY

This graph shows the constant increase in the average life expectancy in the United States that has occurred during the period between the years 1860 and 1967. *Adapted from data furnished by the National Office of Vital Statistics.*

In general, Medicare does *not* pay for custodial, dental, or eye care. These items, of course, make up the largest medical expenditures of the aged.

Medicare provides another important service. A committee of the American Hospital Association grants accreditation to hospitals and extended care facilities that receive Medicare patients. Accreditation has undoubtedly improved care for the elderly in all institutions concerned. A list of accredited institutions in the area can be provided by the Social Security office or state welfare office. Most doctors can provide this information as well.

Medicaid

Medicaid is a federal-state program set up under Title 19 of the Social Security Act to give medical services to low-income or medically needy people. This is an important advance in caring for older people. All those receiving public assistance are eligible for Medicaid. Some states also include anyone falling below a certain level of income, whether they receive welfare or not. Although benefits and eligibility vary from state to state, the program is designed to eventually become uniform across the nation. Medicaid is in the form of a grant and is free to recipients.

Medicaid pays for inpatient hospital care, outpatient hospital services, laboratory and x-ray services, care in a skilled nursing home, and physicians' fees. In most states it also pays for dental care, prescribed drugs, eye glasses, home health care, and clinic services.

Medicaid was designed to help the elderly needy pay for what Medicare cannot provide. Thus many people receiving Medicare may be eligible for Medicaid benefits also. Medicaid will pay the premiums for a Medicare recipient in need as well as paying the $44 and $50 deductibles. In this way, a patient who receives Medicare who falls below a certain income level can be eligible for custodial, dental, and eye care. Most Medicaid state boards have ruled that recipients are eligible whether or not their relatives are financially secure. Medicaid and Medicare are administered by the Medical Services Administration, Social and Rehabilitation Service, United States Department of Health, Education and Welfare.

Homes for the elderly

The single most pressing need for the aged is some place to go when care at home is not enough. Many old people live in drab, rented rooms. Others are unwanted burdens in the homes of their children. Still others are in boarding or convalescent homes.

The advent of Medicare and Medicaid has spurred the development of a whole range of homes for the elderly, upgrading most public institutions and giving rise to hundreds of new private facilities. Twenty years ago, old age carried the threat of homelessness and poor medical services. Today, it should be possible to find a place for most older ill or incapacitated people regardless of whether they have a large source of income. In 1954, there were 180,000 beds in nursing homes. By 1967 there were more than 500,000. That year there were 2607 institutions with medical programs that qualified for Medicare, for a total of 188,998 beds. Of this number, 1968 homes were skilled nursing facilities, 351 were units located in hospitals, 139 were special sections of custodial institutions, and 9 were rehabilitation centers. The trend toward providing specialized medical care in nursing homes is increasing.

Types of homes

Classification of homes is difficult because most accept people from age 65 on and vary widely in their functions. Some take people of all ages who are ill. Many of the institutions for the elderly are special disease centers such as TB centers and mental hospitals. Public institutions for the blind and disabled have expanded into rehabilitation services in some areas. And the line between private and public homes has blurred since both depend on Medicare and Medicaid funds as the backbone of operating expenses.

In general, homes can be looked at as *public*, *nonprofit* (or *voluntary*), or as *proprietary* institutions. Public facilities are financed directly out of tax money. Nonprofit voluntary homes are managed by charitable organizations. Proprietary homes are managed by private individuals for profit. Although some doctors and professional groups are criticized for owning many of the homes for profit, it must be remembered that during the time when there was a dearth of legislation in the field, doctors built many of the few existing facilities for the aged. In defining homes, their function should also be considered. An *extended-care facility* is a nursing home that offers skilled nursing services to postoperative patients. Most *nursing homes* also provide custodial care for the aged and chronically ill. *Foster homes* are private homes that will board older and ill people. Institutions that do not include medical services state they give personal care rather than nursing care.

How to select a nursing home

Nursing homes are for people who because of illness or incapacity cannot be cared for in their own homes. Older people who are looking simply for a shelter had best seek aid through state public assistance. Most older people, of course, would prefer to stay in their own homes if at all possible. They fear loss of privacy and independence. It is wise to keep this uppermost in mind when it becomes necessary to place a relative in a nursing home, so that you may find one that gives the best service and treats its clients with dignity. Here is a checklist of important considerations:

1. Recommendations. Seek the advice of physicians (nonowners), clergy, nurses, or social workers who have access to homes during the course of their work.

2. License and ownership. Institutions certified by the Medicare committee of the American Hospital Association and the American Nursing Home Association are qualified to give adequate care. The Department of Health also grants a license to each institution. Any doctor can check the license of a home, and this information can also be obtained through a call to the Department of Health, a division of the city government.

3. Quality of care. Medical services should be looked at carefully. Are there skilled nurses available around-the-clock? Are there regular visits by a physician? Are there a sufficient number of practical nurses and aides? Also check the kind and quality of food and physical comforts. Are there regular calls by social workers?

4. Attitude of staff. This is difficult to judge, but a physician can be enlisted to aid you. The atmosphere of a home is generally provided by the aides who perform most of the daily chores. Are they warm, considerate people? Is their aim to keep each patient as active and well as possible or simply to keep them from being any trouble? What is the general philosophy of care? On a visit to a home, take care to speak to as many of the staff as possible to get to know them. Remember that rehabilitation, not just custodial care, should be their goal.

5. Costs. Question any contract carefully, checking for "extras." Public homes usually have *per diem* rates, but do not include all services in this fee. Find out which services are provided and which must be purchased individually, such as drugs, laundry, special foods, and entertainment.

Do not be afraid to ask very specific questions. Ask to see the rooms, patient beds, laundry facilities, kitchen, and grounds. Make more than one visit before deciding.

Many older people who do not require hospitalization or around-the-clock medical supervision can be cared for at home. Outpatient clinics and social service groups are experimenting with "meals-on-wheels," programs to bring hot food to shut-ins. Medicaid provisions can help with the costs of home care. Practical suggestions are made in Chapter 22, "Sickness at Home," on the care of home patients.

New housing projects

Old age homes, at the present time, are insufficient in number and lacking in facilities to meet the needs of all who seek shelter. However, the outlook for the future is brightening. Some areas have already constructed special housing for the aged, and other such projects are being studied in various parts of the country. In New York City, the Tompkins Square House, especially designed for the older citizen, is a model for the trend in this direction. Here, at low cost to the tenant, individual apartments are provided and self-service dining facilities are available. At Ft. Green, in New York City, a 53-unit project has been set up, and in Bridgeport, Connecticut, special housing for the aged has been constructed. In Millville, New Jersey, a cottage project, designed especially for older couples, has been built. The J. C. Penney Cottages in Florida follow the new trend in old age housing. In New York, the Desmond Committee on Problems of the Aging petitioned the legislature to consider a state loan for $50,000,000 for the construction of special homes, cottages, and apartments for the aged.

Investigators are continuing to learn what types of structures are best suited to older people, what architectural features are needed to eliminate accident hazards and to provide added comforts. Concerted efforts by groups interested in such housing projects will result in more adequate and desirable living arrangements for those who have reached the later years.

21 NUTRITION

FOOD AND FOOD DEFICIENCIES

Foods are the materials from which the body tissues are constructed and vital energy is obtained. The study of nutrition deals with the composition of the various foods, the amounts of their constituents that are required to maintain health, and the body processes by which they are utilized. The importance of correct nutrition to the individual is difficult to overemphasize. The person who eats properly not only feels better, but he is happier, is capable of more work and play, and is much less likely to suffer from disease.

Within the last 30 years there has been an increased public consciousness of many of the basic rules of nutrition. This has been brought about partly by educational programs and partly by the advertising of food manufacturers. Almost everyone has seen charts which show how much of each food component should be eaten. These charts may be complex and, in some instances, misleading. A simple understanding of the basic qualities of food, however, will permit one to improve the quality of his diet. Nevertheless, many people now suffer ill health, either from decidedly unbalanced diets, or from failure to recognize mild unbalances in a seemingly good diet.

The average person in the United States has available to him a large number of different types of foods from which he may choose. Even with a limited budget, a person should be able to maintain an excellent nutritional status if he will recognize certain basic rules for choosing his food. A high income and a large grocery bill do not insure good nutrition.

Chemists have discovered that all food contains only a limited number of classes of material which are essential to a good diet. These materials are *water, carbohydrates, fats, proteins, vitamins, minerals,* and *roughage* or residue. These materials are considered in detail below.

Besides choosing a diet that contains foods with all of the essential materials, one must bear in mind that individuals may vary greatly in their nutritional requirements. This variation is sometimes a general one. Thus, dietary requirements of any individual may vary with his age. Occasionally, individuals may have some unusual dietary requirement for no apparent reason, and a medical examination may be necessary to discover the exact nature of the requirement. When an individual becomes sick, his dietary requirements may be quite different from those during health. Special considerations in diet must also be made for pregnant women and nursing mothers. These special variations are discussed later in this chapter.

Another important consideration in choosing a diet is the manner in which the food is preserved, cooked, or otherwise treated before it is eaten.

Deficiency diseases

A *deficiency disease* occurs when one or more of the basic nutritional substances are not present in the food of an individual in amounts adequate to maintain him in a state of optimum health. Deficiencies of fats or carbohydrates may not be associated with disease if other elements of the diet are available to supply the necessary number of calories. During a period of starvation, most of the food elements are deficient, and there is a generalized breakdown of all of the tissues of the body. The majority of deficiency diseases, however, are caused by an inadequate supply of proteins, minerals, and vitamins.

Nutritional deficiencies are a major cause of disease and death in many parts of the world. This is particularly true in areas such as the Orient where food supplies are limited and dietary habits are poor. Even in the most bountiful countries, however, there is much suffering from deficiency diseases.

Many patients suffering from nutritional deficiency have indefinite symptoms which result from multiple deficiencies in their diet that have not developed to an acute stage. In other cases, well-recognized symptoms may appear which are attributable to a lack of some one substance. While a discussion of deficiency disease must center around these recognizable forms, it is important to realize that a diet which produces a lack of one substance may coincidentally bring about a deficiency of others. Persons suffering from vitamin deficiencies in particular may require a complete revision of their eating habits.

Deficiencies may be caused by factors other than the exclusion of proper amounts of a nutritional substance from the diet. The preparation of food may reduce the amounts of nutritional essentials which were originally present. Other substances in the diet may influence the amounts of a vitamin or mineral required by an individual; for instance, vitamin B_1 is needed by the body to utilize carbohydrates. Therefore, persons on high carbohydrate diets would become deficient if they attempted to exist on the same amounts of vitamin B_1 as do persons on low carbohydrate diets. Some individuals normally have much higher requirements for certain nutritional essentials than do others, and become deficient on what would be considered a *normal* nutritional intake. In some diseases, the nutritional requirements are increased either because of increased use, or great loss or destruction of some substance in the body. In these cases, deficiencies develop unless the appropriate substance is furnished in augmented amounts.

Essential food elements

Water: Almost all foods contain water. Meat, vegetables, fruits, and eggs all contain at least 50 percent water. Because over 70 percent of the weight of the human body is water, and because this water is constantly being lost though urination, respiration, defecation (particularly in diarrhea), and perspiration, the individual must consume water so that his tissues do not become dehydrated.

The average adult requires over two quarts of water a day to maintain a healthy degree of *hydration* in his tissues. About half of this is supplied from the water in the foods he eats. The remaining five to six glasses per day must be supplied in the form of drinking water or other fluids. This amount varies with different individuals. Those consuming large amounts of liquid foods, such as milk, cold drinks, or soup will not need to drink so much water. On the other hand, healthy individuals who habitually consume *diuretics* must drink more water. A diuretic is a chemical substance which has the ability to increase the amount of urination. Coffee, alcoholic beverages, and tea are common types of diuretics.

Carbohydrates: These are organic chemical substances containing carbon, hydrogen, and oxygen. They are important sources of energy for the body. Sugar is a common example of a pure carbohydrate. Most food contains at least a little carbohydrate in the form of sugar, starch, or "animal starch" (*glycogen*). Plant foods contain starch, whereas meats contain glycogen. Some foods have especially large amounts of carbohydrates, and often form the basis of the diet. Potatoes, rice, and wheat flour all are composed of approximately 90 percent starch, after their water is removed. As a rule sugars and starches are easily digested, and offer the body an immediate and inexpensive source of energy. They may also be stored within the body for future use, usually in the form of glycogen. When excessive amounts of carbohydrates are eaten, they may be changed within the body into fat and stored as such.

Too many starches and sugars crowd out other essential materials from the menu and are a common cause of nutritional deficiencies. Many carbohydrate foods are highly refined; sugar, for instance, comes in almost pure form. Flour is refined and rice is "polished" to remove certain portions of the grain. All of these procedures of refining may remove parts of the original grain which contain vitamins and minerals that are essential for health. Consequently, many manufacturers producing white flour add various vitamins and minerals to their product to restore, and in some cases surpass, their natural content. Since scientists are not sure that all the essential vitamins and minerals have been discovered, it might be a better policy to use unrefined carbohydrate products when carbohydrate foods form a large part of the diet. Thus, whole grain or enriched cereals and breads are recommended daily in addition to other foods such as fruits, vegetables, meats, etc.

Fats: These substances are found in almost all food material, but they occur in noticeable amounts only in meats, dairy products, and certain types of fruits and vegetables. They are a source of energy to the body, but cannot be the sole source. Fats are composed largely of carbon and hydrogen, and are capable of yielding considerable amounts of energy. However, they are not as readily absorbed as carbohydrate foods.

Fats contain both *saturated* and *unsaturated fatty acids*. Two of the unsaturated fatty acids are essential in the diet, whereas the saturated fatty acids (the animal fats) seem to play a role in the formation of cholesterol, and subsequently, hardening of the arteries. The human body also must contain at least small amounts of fat as insulation in the maintenance of normal body temperature. Fat is needed as a protective padding for many of the vital organs. Certain types of fats are also important components of vital organs. Another point in favor of including some fat in the diet is that some of the vitamins, particularly A, D, E, and K, are found in quantity in some natural fats.

Fats can be found in highly concentrated forms such as butter, lard, and vegetable oils and in emulsified forms such as in milk, salad dressing, cream, and egg yolks. The emulsified forms are more digestible. Consequently, *emulsified* fats and oils are sometimes regarded as a better source. Emulsified fat is fat which is broken down into small globules.

Proteins: Proteins are absolutely essential for general maintenance of the tissues of the body under normal conditions as well as following injury or illness. They are also required to combat infectious diseases. Proteins are composed of carbon, hydrogen, oxygen, nitrogen, sulfur, and often other elements. Proteins are extremely large *molecules* made up of smaller units which are called *amino acids.* Every amino acid contains carbon, oxygen, hydrogen, and nitrogen, and some also contain sulfur. Although called acid, they are actually almost neutral in nature. The amino acids found in the proteins from food are the same as those which must be present in the proteins of body tissue, although they may be arranged differently in the giant protein molecule. The body needs amino acids to replace parts of body protein which are constantly being destroyed or lost. Some amino acids can be manufactured by the body itself from other material. Other amino acids, however, cannot be manufactured in sufficient quantity to supply the demands of growth and repair. These *essential* amino acids must be contained in the proteins of the diet, if the individual is to survive.

The proteins in foods do not all contain each of the essential amino acids in adequate amounts. A *complete* protein is one which contains all the amino acids which are required by the human body, and in approximately the proper proportions. The proteins from animal sources, such as meat, milk, and eggs, are much more complete than the proteins obtained from plant sources, such as fruit, vegetables, and cereals. Therefore, when plant proteins offer the major dietary source of protein, the individual

FOODS AS SOURCES OF

PROTEIN

Animal foods are the best source of good quality protein

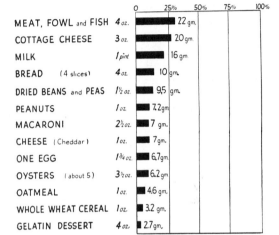

CONTRIBUTION OF SELECTED SERVINGS OF A FEW FOODS AS PERCENTAGES OF ADULT MALE ALLOWANCE (70 GRAMS)

Food	Serving	Amount
MEAT, FOWL and FISH	4 oz.	22 gm.
COTTAGE CHEESE	3 oz.	20 gm.
MILK	1 pint	16 gm.
BREAD (4 slices)	4 oz.	10 gm.
DRIED BEANS and PEAS	1½ oz.	9.5 gm.
PEANUTS	1 oz.	7.2 gm.
MACARONI	2½ oz.	7 gm.
CHEESE (Cheddar)	1 oz.	7 gm.
ONE EGG	1¾ oz.	6.7 gm.
OYSTERS (about 5)	3½ oz.	6.2 gm.
OATMEAL	1 oz.	4.6 gm.
WHOLE WHEAT CEREAL	1 oz.	3.2 gm.
GELATIN DESSERT	4 oz.	2.7 gm.

The serving which is indicated at the right of each food shows the amount required to give the stated percentage of the daily protein allowance which has been recommended for an adult male. *Courtesy Council on Foods and Nutrition of American Medical Association, and Food and Nutrition Board of National Research Council. Copyright American Medical Association.*

may not be getting enough of certain essential amino acids. In this case, the other essential amino acids which are supplied by the plants may be of no use to the body and may be discarded or burned as fuel. A simple way to eliminate the dangers of amino acid deficiency from incomplete proteins in the diet is to use two or more protein sources in substantial amounts daily. If there is little or no meat in the diet, the individual should eat a variety of vegetables and cereals to increase the probability that he will get enough essential amino acids to maintain his body tissues. An average adult should attempt to include from 65 to 100 grams (3 to 5 ounces) of proteins in his daily diet in order to achieve optimum health.

Persons who subsist on a high carbohydrate diet seldom have sufficient quantity and variety of proteins to supply the body with the amino acids necessary for good health. Protein deficiencies may also result from liver disease, difficulties in digestion and absorption, fevers, burns, surgery, etc.

Perhaps the most frequent and important

symptom of a marked protein deficiency is swelling of the body tissues (nutritional *edema*). In children, there may be an almost complete cessation of growth. The disease is widespread in famine areas, and is most dangerous during infancy, childhood, pregnancy, and lactation, when the protein requirements are highest. Possible future protein sources for persons living in such areas include leaf and fish protein concentrates. These concentrates may be used to enrich other foods, or may be processed and flavored, as in the case of leaf protein, to increase their palatability and acceptance. Studies have shown that fish concentrates produced normal growth in children when they supplied 70 percent of the total dietary protein.

In the normal healthy *adult,* the amount of nitrogen assimilated, largely in the form of protein, balances the amount excreted, largely in the form of urea in the urine, and the person is then said to be in "nitrogen equilibrium." Since body proteins are constantly being destroyed, the regular inclusion of protein in the diet is essential to prevent a negative nitrogen balance in which more nitrogen is lost from the body than is gained, and in which the tissues are unable to repair themselves and function normally.

Minerals: The essential minerals (calcium, phosphorus, iron, sodium, potassium, chlorine, sulfur, magnesium) and the trace elements (iodine, copper, cobalt, fluorine, manganese, and zinc) have several functions in the normal, healthy body. In the first place minerals are im-

FOODS AS SOURCES OF IRON

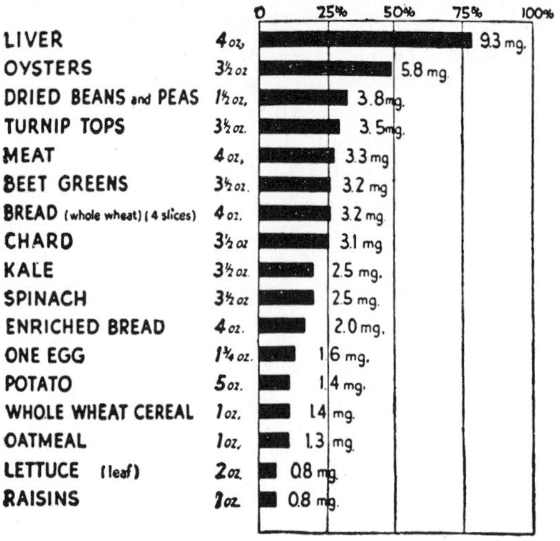

Food	Serving	Amount
LIVER	4 oz.	9.3 mg.
OYSTERS	3½ oz.	5.8 mg.
DRIED BEANS and PEAS	1½ oz.	3.8 mg.
TURNIP TOPS	3½ oz.	3.5 mg.
MEAT	4 oz.	3.3 mg.
BEET GREENS	3½ oz.	3.2 mg.
BREAD (whole wheat) (4 slices)	4 oz.	3.2 mg.
CHARD	3½ oz.	3.1 mg.
KALE	3½ oz.	2.5 mg.
SPINACH	3½ oz.	2.5 mg.
ENRICHED BREAD	4 oz.	2.0 mg.
ONE EGG	1¾ oz.	1.6 mg.
POTATO	5 oz.	1.4 mg.
WHOLE WHEAT CEREAL	1 oz.	1.4 mg.
OATMEAL	1 oz.	1.3 mg.
LETTUCE (leaf)	2 oz.	0.8 mg.
RAISINS	1 oz.	0.8 mg.

The serving indicated at the right of each food shows the amount required to provide the stated percentage of the daily iron allowance recommended for an adult male. Four slices of whole wheat bread give one fourth of the total daily recommended consumption. *Courtesy Council on Foods and Nutrition of American Medical Association, and Food and Nutrition Board of National Research Council. Copyright American Medical Assn.*

FOODS AS SOURCES OF CALCIUM

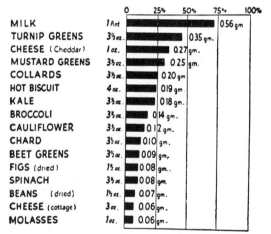

Food	Serving	Amount
MILK	1 Pint	0.56 gm
TURNIP GREENS	3½ oz.	0.35 gm.
CHEESE (Cheddar)	1 oz.	0.27 gm.
MUSTARD GREENS	3½ oz.	0.25 gm.
COLLARDS	3½ oz.	0.20 gm
HOT BISCUIT	4 oz.	0.19 gm.
KALE	3½ oz.	0.18 gm.
BROCCOLI	3½ oz.	0.14 gm.
CAULIFLOWER	3½ oz.	0.12 gm.
CHARD	3½ oz.	0.10 gm.
BEET GREENS	3½ oz.	0.09 gm.
FIGS (dried)	1½ oz.	0.08 gm.
SPINACH	3½ oz.	0.08 gm.
BEANS (dried)	1½ oz.	0.07 gm.
CHEESE (cottage)	3 oz.	0.06 gm.
MOLASSES	1 oz.	0.06 gm.

The serving indicated at the right of each food shows the amount which is required to provide the stated percentage of the daily calcium allowance that is recommended for an adult male. Biscuits are of the self-rising type. The calcium in spinach and green beans is poorly assimilated. *Courtesy Council on Foods and Nutrition of American Medical Association, and Food and Nutrition Board of National Research Council. Copyright American Medical Association.*

portant in the structure of the body. A large part of the bones and teeth is made up of various minerals containing calcium and phosphorus. Muscles and other tissues must also contain minerals so that they may function properly. Many of the vital chemical reactions in the body cannot take place unless certain minerals are present.

In many areas of the world, one or more vital minerals may occur in insufficient amounts or be entirely lacking in the soil. In such areas, the danger of developing a mineral shortage is particularly great, since the vegetation growing on this soil is itself low in mineral supplies.

When minerals are required for structural purposes, they are needed in relatively large amounts. For this reason, the diets of growing children must contain large amounts of minerals. Milk is among the best sources of calcium and phosphorus. Adults, however, need much less of the structural minerals, so that they seldom need to drink over one to one and one-half pints of milk per day.

Calcium deficiencies frequently occur in both children and adults because many foods lack appreciable amounts of calcium, and because calcium is the most abundant mineral found normally in the body. A diet containing large amounts of spinach, or some grains, which contain substances that are able to bind calcium so that it cannot be absorbed, may also cause deficiencies. A deficiency of vitamin D, the vitamin which is necessary for calcium utilization, may produce a calcium deficiency. Lowered activity of the *parathyroid* gland is also an occasional cause.

Calcium deficiency, like vitamin D deficiency, produces a condition known in children as *rickets* and in adults as *osteomalacia*. The bones and teeth of children with rickets are poorly formed and soft. A child with rickets frequently has malformed limbs, especially "bowlegs." Blood clotting may be impaired, and in extreme cases, there may be disturbances of the nervous system. An improvement in the level of calcium in the diet, along with vitamin D or parathyroid extract when required, brings about a hardening of the bones, but leaves them misshapen if deformity has already occurred. Various calcium salts may be prescribed by the physician as a rapid means of restoring the missing mineral to the body. Such supplements are also given pregnant women, not only because of the greater need at this time for calcium, but also for protein and other important nutrients. Nutritional changes are necessary to prevent a recurrence of the deficiency. The inclusion in the diet of moderate amounts of cheese, egg yolk, and milk or other dairy products is usually adequate to insure against a return of the deficiency.

While iron is not a structural mineral in the usual sense, considerable iron is present in the blood. The red pigment *(hemoglobin),* from which the blood gets its color, contains iron, and when iron is absent from the diet, the individual develops *anemia*. Children and pregnant women need more iron-containing foods than others, since their blood volume is constantly increasing. Liver, lean meat, and leafy greens are good sources of iron. Copper is needed for the normal utilization of iron. Iron deficiencies are discussed in detail in Chapter 6, "Blood and Blood-Forming Organs: *Anemia.*"

Salt *(sodium chloride)* is needed in the diet to the extent of about five grams daily for an adult. Most persons consume more than this, however. Under conditions of excessive perspiration, the adult needs an extra gram of salt each day. A salt deficiency occurs when the salt content of the diet is not increased to balance greater losses of salt from excessive perspiration, urination, diarrhea, or vomiting. The most common symptoms include nausea, fatigue, weakness, and cramps. Salt tablets may prevent the deficiency or restore the patient to a normal balance, but these should not be taken without the advice of a physician.

Iodine is used by the thyroid gland, and absence of it from the diet results in a disease called *goiter*. Iodine deficiencies are discussed in detail in Chapter 10, "The Endocrine System: *The Thyroid.*"

Fluoride deficiencies occur in certain areas where the fluoride content of the water is low. The only known symptom of this condition is an increased susceptibility of the teeth to cavities or *caries*. Treatment is almost entirely a community problem, involving the addition of minute amounts of fluoride to the community water supply.

Deficiencies of other minerals such as copper and phosphorus also may occur in rare instances, but they do not constitute frequent health hazards, as do those which have been discussed. Persons consuming a normally good diet need not worry about their requirements for these minerals.

Trace elements: Numerous studies have presented growing evidence of the importance of trace elements in human metabolism. Some, like copper, zinc, and manganese, are known to be essential to man; others are considered harmful, particularly in large amounts. Since the increasing use of metals has exposed man to an ever-growing number of these elements via food, water, and air, it is important to understand how they affect the human body.

Copper is widely available in foods like shellfish, liver, lean meat, green leafy vegetables, nuts, and cocoa, and in cooking utensils. For this reason, a copper deficiency is rarely found in man. Animal studies, however, show that such a deficiency results in loss of hair, abnormal bone formation, and aortic rupture. Above-normal levels of copper in human beings may indicate the presence of cirrhosis, tuberculosis, cancer, severe anemia, or other disease. Although copper toxicity is relatively rare in man, animal studies do show that excesses of copper may result in disease and sometimes death.

Zinc deficiency may manifest itself in growth retardation, delayed bone age, dwarfism, hypogonadism, and possibly failure of wounds to heal. Conversely, there is some evidence that cadmium-induced hypertension can be reversed by administration of agents which add zinc. Zinc is relatively nontoxic when compared with lead, mercury, and arsenic; however, poisoning may occur—with accompanying nausea, vomiting, stomach cramps, diarrhea, and fever—when foods have been stored in galvanized containers.

Chromium is of interest because this trace metal may prove of therapeutic value to patients with diabetes mellitus and other states with abnormal glucose tolerance tests. Adequate means of identifying those individuals who may profit from chromium supplementation need to be further developed, however, before any major medical benefit can be realized from the use of this element.

Manganese at present is inferred to be important to man mainly from studies with animals. These studies suggest that a manganese

VITAMINS KNOWN TO BE REQUIRED IN THE HUMAN DIET

Vitamin	Solubility	Daily adult male recommended allowance	Deficiency diseases	Good food sources
A	fats	5000 I.U.*	Night blindness Xerophthalmia Keratosis	Yellow vegetables, green, leafy vegetables, liver and liver oils
B₁ (thiamine)	water	1.8 mg.	Beriberi	Yeast, pork, whole grain cereals
B₂ (riboflavin)	water	1.8 mg.	Ariboflavinosis	Liver, yeast, milk, greens
Nicotinic acid (niacin)	water	16.0 mg.	Pellagra	Meat, whole grain cereals, peanuts, yeast
Folic acid and Vitamin B₁₂	water	unknown	Nutritional macrocytic anemia	Green vegetables and leaves, liver
C (ascorbic acid)	water	75 mg.	Scurvy	Citrus fruits, fresh uncooked fruit and vegetables
D	fats	variable	Rickets	Eggs, irradiated milk, fish liver oils, canned fish
K	fats	variable	Hypoprothrombinemia	Green vegetables such as lettuce and spinach

*5000 International Units (I.U.) of vitamin A is equivalent to 3 milligrams of beta-carotene.

deficiency may result in bone irregularities, ataxia, and sterility. Manganese intoxication often occurs in miners who breathe dust-containing manganese. Its onset is insidious, with eventual development of ataxia, tremors, and psychological disorders.

Vitamins: The vitamins are generally considered to be: vitamins A, C (ascorbic acid), D, E, K, P, and the members of the B vitamin group, B₁ or thiamine, B₂ which is also known as vitamin G, and riboflavin, nicotinic acid (nicotinamide or niacin), B₆ or pyridoxine, pantothenic acid, biotin, folic acid, B₁₂, choline, inositol, and para-aminobenzoic acid. These are special chemical sustances needed by the tissues of the body to carry out the many complicated chemical reactions associated with living. Fortunately, the same chemical substances are also used by plants and animals, so that many foods can offer sources of vitamins. For this reason, the unrefined plants and meats are the best sources of vitamins.

Although about 17 vitamins are known to exist, deficiencies of only eight of them are presently known to be common causes of human disease.

The symptoms of a deficiency of the various vitamins differ greatly, and require the careful evaluation of a physician. Treatment of a deficient patient with the appropriate vitamin prep-

arations is seldom adequate to produce a permanent cure. Measures must also be taken to ascertain and remove the original cause of the disease; this may be difficult.

Vitamin A is essential for most animals, including man. There are a number of different chemical substances which can be converted by the human body into vitamin A, and thus can substitute for the vitamin in the diet. These other materials are called *carotenes* and *carotenoids*. They derive their names from the fact that the carotenes are found in large quantities in carrots. Some of the vitamin A substances are colorless, but most of them are brightly colored, from yellow to red and purple. The yellow vegetables—carrots, sweet potatoes, squash, and the like—contain large amounts of carotenes from which they get their color, and consequently are excellent sources of the vitamin.

Vitamin A substances are found highly concentrated in the leaves of plants and in the livers of animals. Therefore, leafy vegetables, liver, and liver oil extracts are excellent sources.

Since vitamin A exists in different chemical forms and since some forms are less useful on a weight basis than others, the vitamin A value of foods and vitamin preparations must be given in *units* rather than by weight. Adults are thought to need about 5000 units of this vitamin a day. A generous helping of a yellow vegetable or a

FOODS AS SOURCES OF VITAMIN A

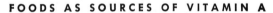

CARROTS	3½ oz.	12,000 I.U.
GREENS (beet, kale, chard, mustard, spinach, turnip)	3½ oz.	over 10,000 I.U.
LIVER	4 oz.	7,000 I.U.
SWEET POTATO	4 oz.	6,000 I.U.
SQUASH (Hubbard)	3½ oz.	4,000 I.U.
COD LIVER OIL	4 gm.	3400 I.U.
APRICOTS (dried)	1½ oz.	2,500 I.U.
PEACH (yellow)	3½ oz.	1,500 I.U.
TOMATO JUICE	4 oz.	1,400 I.U.
SUMMER BUTTER	1 oz.	1,200 I.U.
AVERAGE BUTTER	1 oz.	800 I.U.
PEAS (fresh)	3½ oz.	700 I.U.
PRUNES	1½ oz.	680 I.U.
MILK	1 pint	650 I.U.
GREEN BEANS	3½ oz.	600 I.U.
OLEOMARGARINE	1 oz.	560 I.U.
ONE EGG	1¾ oz.	500 I.U.
CHEESE (Am cheddar)	1 oz.	360 I.U.

The serving which is indicated at the right of each food shows the amount required to give the stated percentage of the daily allowance of vitamin A, that is recommended for an adult male. One International Unit of vitamin A has the same nutritional value as 0.6 microgram of pure beta-carotene. *Courtesy Council on Foods and Nutrition of American Medical Association, and Food and Nutrition Board of National Research Council. Copyright American Medical Association.*

FOODS AS SOURCES OF THIAMINE
(vitamin B₁)

Food	Serving		0	25%	50%	75%	100%	Amount
DRIED BREWER'S YEAST	1 oz.							3.4 mg.
PORK (lean)	4 oz.							1.5 mg.
WHOLE WHEAT BREAD	4 oz.							0.41 mg.
DRIED BEANS and PEAS	1½ oz.							0.34 mg.
CORN BREAD	5 oz.							0.30 mg.
ENRICHED BREAD	4 oz.							0.28 mg.
LAMB	4 oz.							0.27 mg.
PEANUTS	1 oz.							0.23 mg.
OATMEAL	1 oz.							0.23 mg.
POTATO	5 oz.							0.21 mg.
COLLARDS, KALE	3½ oz.							0.20 mg.
MILK	1 pint							0.18 mg.
BEEF, VEAL	4 oz.							0.17 mg.
ASPARAGUS, CAULIFLOWER, BRUSSELS SPROUTS	3½ oz.							0.17 mg.
MUSTARD GREENS, TURNIP GREENS	3½ oz.							0.14 mg.
WHOLE WHEAT CEREAL	1 oz.							0.13 mg.
ONE EGG	1¾ oz.							0.12 mg.
POULTRY and FISH	4 oz.							0.10 mg.

The serving indicated at the right of each food shows the amount required to give the stated percentage of daily thiamine allowance recommended for an adult male. *Courtesy Council on Foods and Nutrition of American Medical Association, and Food and Nutrition Board of National Research Council. Copyright American Medical Association.*

green leafy vegetable, other than cabbage, or a teaspoonful of fish-liver oil will insure an adequate daily supply of vitamin A. The use of butter or vitamin A-enriched margarine, cheeses, or egg yolk in the diet is recommended in addition to one or more leafy green and yellow vegetables.

Vitamin A deficiency may occur in persons who subsist largely upon a diet of white vegetables and grains. An equally important cause rests in disturbances of the intestinal tract which prevent the effective absorption of vitamin A. Diarrhea and an inadequate supply of *bile* may be two intrinsic causative factors. Excessive use of mineral oil may prevent adequate amounts of the fat-soluble vitamin A from being absorbed. Deficiencies may also occur during infancy, pregnancy, and lactation as the result of increased needs at these times.

Night blindness is probably the most common symptom of a mild vitamin A deficiency. Vitamin A plays an important role in the visual process, and when it is not present in adequate amounts, a person has difficulty in seeing in dim light. It requires considerable time for such a person to become accustomed to seeing in the dark, after being in bright light. When the deficiency becomes more severe, irritation, and inflammation of the eyes may occur.

Vitamin A is also involved in the maintenance of the normal health of the skin. A deficiency causes the skin to become rough, dry, and scaly. The oil glands of the skin become clogged, causing an inflamed "goose-pimple" appearance. The mucous membranes of the throat and respiratory tract are also affected, and are no longer able to provide an effective barrier against the invasion of disease-producing organisms. Consequently, the resistance against infection is lowered, and the vitality of the patient is decreased.

As early as 1850 B.C., the Egyptians recognized that liver was beneficial to persons who were night-blind. Today, the same form of therapy is used. Indeed, fish-liver oils are administered to children to insure improved general health. Similar treatment of adults is effective in curing vitamin A deficiencies, if the original cause of the deficiency is removed.

Toxic effects resulting from vitamin A overdosage *(hypervitaminosis)* have been recorded; these effects ranged from headache and double vision to stunted growth. The usual diets of most individuals meet or exceed recommended allowances of this vitamin, which is fat soluble and therefore is stored in the body. Vitamin A preparations should never be consumed over long periods of time except under a physician's orders.

There are eleven known *B vitamins,* and possibly others yet undiscovered. They are all different chemically and serve different functions in the body. They are all thought to be essential to all forms of life, because they perform basic processes in the body chemistry. Each has a different role in these processes, and a lack of one of them in the diet may result in a de-

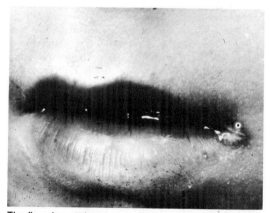

The fissuring at the corners of the mouth of this patient is known as angular cheilosis, and is one of the characteristic symptoms of a riboflavin deficiency. The symptom may also be caused by other conditions. Angular cheilosis is frequently difficult to cure, and does not readily respond to treatment in patients who lack a functional set of natural or artificial dentures, because of the distortions placed on the skin in these areas. *Copyright The Upjohn Company, 1943.*

ficiency disease. The vitamins are found together in nature to the extent that a food which is a good source of one of the B vitamins usually, but not always, contains large amounts of the others. The B vitamins are all relatively stable when cooked, except vitamin B₁ *(thiamine),* which is destroyed by alkali, and vitamin B₂ *(riboflavin),* which is reduced by acids. They can all dissolve in water, so that foods which are cooked in water and the liquid removed have a decreased B vitamin content.

B vitamins are found in all fruits, vegetables, meat, and whole grains. In corn, wheat, and rice, they are concentrated in the germ and bran so that refining of flours tends to decrease greatly the B vitamin content. But, most flours on the market in the United States have most of these compounds restored. When carbohydrates, such as bread, potatoes, and rice, comprise a large part of the diet, loss of B vitamins becomes a serious problem unless the starches are relatively unrefined or have had their vitamin content restored.

Thiamine or vitamin B₁ deficiencies most frequently result from diets composed largely of refined or polished grains. The resulting disease is known as *beriberi.* This deficiency is most common in the Orient where diets are limited almost entirely to polished rice. The bran of the rice grain contains adequate amounts of the vitamin, but it is usually discarded. Thiamine deficiencies may also occur in Western countries as the result of other inadequate diets. The deficiency frequently accompanies chronic alcoholism, when the drinker relies on alcoholic beverages as a major source of calories. It may also be caused by cooking foods with soda, which destroys much of the thiamine.

The symptoms of beriberi depend upon the extent of the deficiency. In severe cases, they include disturbances of the gastrointestinal tract and changes in the nervous system. There may be a generalized swelling of the body tissues in some cases, this edema being the result of an accompanying protein deficiency. The heart becomes enlarged and may assume a "gallop" rhythm. Unless promptly treated, the patient may die. Milder thiamine deficiencies occur throughout most civilized countries. In these cases, the most frequent symptoms are disturbances of sensation in the extremities, and various heart disorders. Loss of appetite is one of the earliest symptoms; indeed, vitamin B has been found helpful in restoring the appetites of many persons who have no other apparent symptom of deficiency. Fatigue, loss of weight, difficulty in breathing, and constipation are also frequent early symptoms.

Most of the symptoms of thiamine deficiency disappear upon administration of the vitamin in pure form or mixed with other vitamins. A recurrence of the deficiency may be difficult to

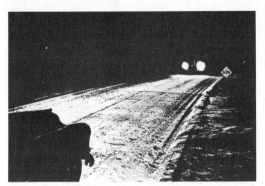

A vitamin A deficient subject, as well as a normal subject, both see the headlights of an approaching car in the manner illustrated in this picture.

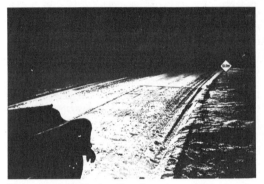

The normal subject, after the approaching car has passed him, will still be able to see before him, for some distance, a wide stretch of lighter road.

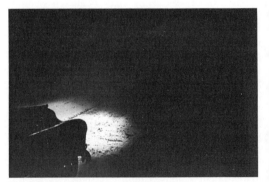

The vitamin A deficient subject, after passing an oncoming car, can see only a small area of illuminated road, as shown here. *Pictures in this series are copyrighted by The Upjohn Company.*

prevent. Yeast is a good thiamine source. Other good sources include most fresh meats and vegetables, eggs, milk, and whole grain cereals.

Vitamin B₂ (riboflavin) deficiencies are most frequent in persons who live on diets composed chiefly of such low riboflavin-containing foods as corn, rice, and potatoes. This deficiency is a relatively common affliction in the southeastern United States, the West Indies, the Orient, and parts of Africa and India.

A deficiency of riboflavin may produce a general body weakness and various forms of dermatitis. Other frequent symptoms involve the mouth, tongue, nose, and eyes. The tip and margin of the tongue become sore and inflamed (*glossitis*), and the tongue appears reddish purple in color. The tongue appears clean, but may have pronounced *fissures* in it. Painful cracks or fissures occur at the corners of the lips, but the mucous membranes of the mouth may be quite pale. A greasy, scaly condition of the face occurs.

The eye is one of the most sensitive organs to a riboflavin deficiency. The clear window of the eye (the *cornea*) may become cloudy, filled with small blood vessels, and ulcerated. Abnormal pigmentation sometimes appears in the *iris*, and *cataracts* form. Vision is considerably impaired, and the patient frequently avoids contact with any bright lights. There is a burning feeling in the eyes, and the mucous membranes about the lids are often badly inflamed. Many of these symptoms may become severe enough to produce damage that is irreparable.

Pure riboflavin is seldom effective in curing patients of this disease because of the absence of more than a single vitamin from most deficient diets. Preparations containing large amounts of most of the major vitamins generally bring about a rapid disappearance of those symptoms that have not been too long existent. The diet of patients must be permanently modified so as to contain adequate amounts of such high-riboflavin foods as liver, milk, eggs, and enriched cereals.

Nicotinic acid or *niacin* is one of the B complex vitamins. A deficiency of this vitamin results in *pellagra*. Most persons with pellagra also suffer from concurrent deficiencies of riboflavin and other vitamins. While pellagra occurs in most areas of the world, the disease has been particularly prevalent in the southeastern United States and in South Africa. It was the major form of acute vitamin deficiency occurring in the United States until recent years, and resulted largely from diets in which corn was the major item. Though better diets and the addition of vitamins to cereals have now made it much less common than formerly, pellagra has often occurred secondarily to alcoholism and drug addiction, and to various disorders of the gastrointestinal tract. Formerly it usually occurred in epidemic form in the spring of the year, probably as the result of deficiencies that accumulated during the winter months when food selections were less varied. In epidemic areas, the food often was so restricted that dogs suffered

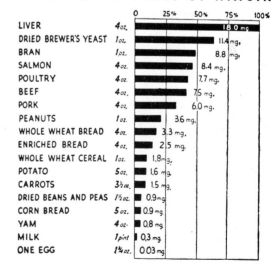

FOODS AS SOURCES OF RIBOFLAVIN

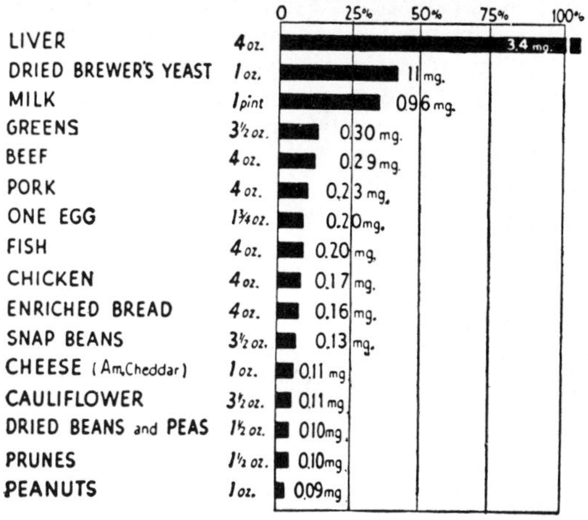

Food	Serving	Amount
LIVER	4 oz.	3.4 mg.
DRIED BREWER'S YEAST	1 oz.	1.1 mg.
MILK	1 pint	0.96 mg.
GREENS	3½ oz.	0.30 mg.
BEEF	4 oz.	0.29 mg.
PORK	4 oz.	0.23 mg.
ONE EGG	1¾ oz.	0.20 mg.
FISH	4 oz.	0.20 mg.
CHICKEN	4 oz.	0.17 mg.
ENRICHED BREAD	4 oz.	0.16 mg.
SNAP BEANS	3½ oz.	0.13 mg.
CHEESE (Am.Cheddar)	1 oz.	0.11 mg.
CAULIFLOWER	3½ oz.	0.11 mg.
DRIED BEANS and PEAS	1½ oz.	0.10 mg.
PRUNES	1½ oz.	0.10 mg.
PEANUTS	1 oz.	0.09 mg.

The serving that is indicated at the right of each food shows the amount required to give the stated percentage of the daily riboflavin allowance that has been recommended for an adult male. *Courtesy Council on Food and Nutrition of American Medical Association, and Food and Nutrition Board of National Research Council. Copyright by American Medical Association.*

from a canine form of the disease known as *black tongue*. Persons with pellagra usually improved spontaneously after a few months because of summer improvements in the diet; but the disease returned in ensuing years until the progressive weakening of the untreated patient resulted in death.

FOODS AS SOURCES OF NIACIN

Food	Serving	Amount
LIVER	4 oz.	18.0 mg.
DRIED BREWER'S YEAST	1 oz.	11.4 mg.
BRAN	1 oz.	8.8 mg.
SALMON	4 oz.	8.4 mg.
POULTRY	4 oz.	7.7 mg.
BEEF	4 oz.	7.5 mg.
PORK	4 oz.	6.0 mg.
PEANUTS	1 oz.	3.6 mg.
WHOLE WHEAT BREAD	4 oz.	3.3 mg.
ENRICHED BREAD	4 oz.	2.5 mg.
WHOLE WHEAT CEREAL	1 oz.	1.8 mg.
POTATO	5 oz.	1.6 mg.
CARROTS	3½ oz.	1.5 mg.
DRIED BEANS AND PEAS	1½ oz.	0.9 mg.
CORN BREAD	5 oz.	0.9 mg.
YAM	4 oz.	0.8 mg.
MILK	1 pint	0.3 mg.
ONE EGG	1¾ oz.	0.03 mg.

The serving indicated at the right of each food shows the amount required to give the stated percentage of the daily niacin allowance, recommended for an adult male. *Courtesy Council on Foods and Nutrition of American Medical Association, and Foods and Nutrition Board of National Research Council. Copyright American Medical Association.*

The symptoms of pellagra include diarrhea, mental unbalance, and skin manifestations. Loss of appetite, of weight, and of strength, accompanied by headache and gastric disturbances are among the earliest signs of the disease. The skin manifestations usually appear as deep red areas that gradually turn brown and become large, thickened, and scaly. The lesions are equally distributed on both sides of the body in most cases, and they are most pronounced about the neck and the backs of the hands and forearms. The lesions usually appear on those areas exposed to the sunlight and to chafing from the clothing. The tip and margin of the tongue and the lining of the mouth may also become scarlet, and there is an inflammation of the gums and lining of the stomach, and nausea.

The diarrhea associated with pellagra may be a fairly early symptom, and may become quite severe as the disease progresses. This further complicates the course of the disease and treatment, since it hampers effective absorption of essential nutrient substances from the intestine.

The mental symptoms in pellagra are quite variable, and in some cases may progress no further than sleeplessness *(insomnia)* and feelings of depression. In many instances, however, the patient may pass into a stupor, or become violent and completely irrational. Even the most severe mental symptoms disappear promptly following treatment with nicotinic acid. Any impaired sensation in the extremities is probably caused by a coincident deficiency of thiamine.

Until the discovery of nicotinic acid as a cure for pellagra, about 66 percent of all patients died from the disease. At present, the death rate has dropped to a low level. The vitamin must be given intravenously in acute cases, and must be accompanied by high levels of other vitamins. While nicotinic acid is essential, a well-rounded diet is equally so for recovery. Following treatment, the symptoms begin to disappear within a few hours, and relief is complete within a few days. As with all deficiency diseases, the original cause of the condition must be remedied to prevent a relapse. Meat (particularly liver), whole grain cereals, and peanuts are good sources of the vitamin.

Folic acid and *vitamin* B$_{12}$ deficiencies occur occasionally as the result of inadequate nutrition, but more often are the result of some impairment in the utilization of these vitamins after they enter the digestive system. The most typical deficiency symptom is anemia, which may occur in pregnancy. In addition, folic acid deficiencies undoubtedly complicate the symptoms of riboflavin and nicotinic acid deficiencies. *Tropical sprue* is a fairly common example of a disease which may result from impaired absorption of these vitamins, and causes impaired absorption of vitamins A, D, and K. This condition is characterized by anemia, diar-

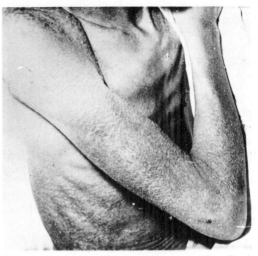

Photograph of generalized xerosis caused by vitamin A deficiency. *Courtesy Medichrome, Clay-Adams Co., Inc.; and Dr. Norman Jolliffe, Nutritional Division of City Health Clinic, New York.*

rhea, loss of weight, skin pigmentation, and inflammation of the mouth and tongue. An improved diet, treatment to relieve the diarrhea, and measures to permit proper intestinal absorption usually bring about an arrest or cure.

Other members of the B group, whose role as vitamins in human nutrition has not *as yet* been clearly defined, include vitamin B$_6$ *(pyridoxine), pantothenic acid, biotin, choline, inositol,* and *para-aminobenzoic acid.*

Vitamin C (ascorbic acid), like the B vitamins, is water-soluble, but it is also rapidly destroyed by heat or exposure to air. Its rapid destruction by heat or storage is an important consideration in choosing and preparing a diet containing sufficient amounts of vitamin C. Home-canned foods, in general, contain very little vitamin C because of the heat to which they have been subjected during the canning process. This is not necessarily true of fruits canned by the up-to-date canneries where methods of vacuum-packing and the exclusion of air prevent the loss of vitamin C. Under such canning conditions, citrus fruits contain practically the same amount of vitamin C as the fresh fruits, and sometimes more, because the fruits bought in the stores are not always as fresh as might be supposed. Frozen foods may gradually lose their vitamin C content unless they are vacuum packed.

Cabbage and related vegetables, and tomatoes contain large amounts of vitamin C. Cooking these foods, however, usually destroys much of the vitamin. Citrus fruits that are really fresh, as well as those that have been canned, contain the largest amount of vitamin C of any of the fruits. Tomatoes taken fresh from the vine usually contain one-third as much vitamin C as orange or grapefruit juice. Orange juice put in the refrigerator uncovered the night before may lose much of its vitamin C before breakfast the next morning. Likewise, a cabbage which has has been cut so that the interior is exposed to the oxygen of the air loses much of its vitamin C content within a few hours.

Vitamin C cannot be stored well within the body. For this reason, one should attempt to include some form of uncooked fruit (preferably citrus) or raw green vegetable in the diet each day. Frequent use of the especially good sources of the vitamin in most cases prevents a deficiency.

Vitamin C deficiency can cause *scurvy,* and occurs as the result of an absence of fresh fruit or vegetables from the diet. Scurvy has traditionally been most common in prisons and on ships, where fresh foods were not on the menu. When the explorer Jacques Cartier spent the winter in Canada in 1535, it is said that his men were saved from scurvy because the Indians showed them how to make a curative brew from the growing tips of branches of the spruce and other trees. About this same time the Dutch Boudewijn Ronsse described the disease and indicated that oranges were curative. An outbreak of scurvy occurred among the Pilgrims at Plymouth. The British naval surgeon, James Lind, caused the adoption of lime juice as a scurvy preventive by the British navy in 1795; from this custom arose the title "limey" for British sailors.

Among the most characteristic symptoms of scurvy are swollen and inflamed, spongy gums. Vitamin C is a necessary component of the tissues of the gums which hold the teeth in place; in a deficiency, the teeth become loose and may be lost. In children who lack vitamin C, the bones may be malformed. The disease is especially severe in infants, in whom there is likely to be a fever, diarrhea, loss of weight, and vomiting. Resistance to infection is reduced, and wounds take a long time to heal. The small blood vessels in the skin and other tissues become fragile, and slight blows may cause them to break and form bruised areas. In severe deficiencies, there may be considerable loss of blood from intestinal hemorrhages.

Most of the symptoms of vitamin C deficiency disappear rapidly when the vitamin is administered to the patient. All fresh fruits and vegetables contain vitamin C, and some of these must be included in the diet to prevent a recurrence of the disease. Citrus fruits are particularly high in this vitamin. Broccoli, Brussels sprouts, kale, mustard and turnip greens, and green peppers are high vitamin C foods, but lose much of their value when cooked.

Vitamin D is not a single chemical material, but comprises a group of chemically related and physiologically interchangeable substances. Vitamin D is essential to the proper absorption and utilization of calcium and phosphorus in the bones and teeth. When it is absent from the body, the bones become soft. Children, especially, need vitamin D because of bone growth. Adults, particularly pregnant or nursing women, also need this vitamin because calcium and phosphorus are continually dissolving from bones; and vitamin D is necessary for their utilization. Unlike most of the other vitamins, vitamin D actually may produce harmful effects when consumed in excessive quantities. Hence, large quan-

FOODS AS SOURCES OF VITAMIN C

Food	Serving	Vitamin C
GRAPEFRUIT (½ av.)	7 oz.	80 mg.
ORANGE (1 av.)	5½ oz.	75 mg.
CANTALOUPE (½ av.)	7 oz.	60 mg.
STRAWBERRIES	3½ oz.	50 mg.
TURNIPS	3½ oz.	32 mg.
SWEET POTATO	4 oz.	30 mg.
CABBAGE (raw)	2 oz.	28 mg.
POTATO (baked)	5 oz.	25 mg.
TOMATO JUICE	4 oz.	24 mg.
AVOCADO	2½ oz.	21 mg.
WATERMELON	11 oz.	16.5 mg.
PINEAPPLE JUICE	4 oz.	16 mg.
POTATO (American fried)	5 oz.	14 mg.
LETTUCE (leaf)	2 oz.	11 mg.
BANANA	3½ oz.	10.5 mg.
PEACH	3½ oz.	8 mg.
APPLE	4½ oz.	4 mg.
PEAR	3 oz.	3 mg.

The serving indicated at the right of each food shows the amount required to give the stated percentage of the daily vitamin C allowance recommended for an adult male. *Courtesy Council on Foods and Nutrition American Medical Association, and National Research Council. Copyright American Medical Association.*

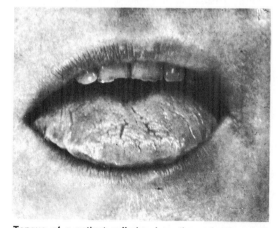

Tongue of a patient suffering from the early stages of nicotinic acid deficiency. The marks of the teeth may be seen plainly around the border of the tongue. *Copyright by The Upjohn Co., 1943.*

tities of this vitamin should never be consumed except on the advice of a physician.

Oddly enough, it is not necessary to have a dietary source of vitamin D in most cases if the individual is exposed to the sun's rays. The explanation of this lies in the fact that a chemical substance, probably *7-dehydrocholesterol*, is usually present in the skin. The light from the sun causes this substance to undergo a chemical change and the product is a new substance which functions as vitamin D. Negroes and persons who are heavily tanned, however, do not receive much benefit in this regard, because the pigment in the skin prevents entrance of the sun's rays.

Milk is normally a poor source of vitamin D. Since milk forms a major part of the diet of infants and children, however, evaporated milk and much of the milk sold by dairies contain vitamin D which has been added, usually in crystalline form.

Both vitamin D deficiencies and calcium deficiencies are called *rickets* when they occur in children and *osteomalacia* when in adults. Adequate amounts of both calcium and vitamin D are necessary to prevent these conditions. The diseases are most prevalent in parts of the world where the winter months are long, or where smoke and fog blot out the rays of the sun.

Cod-liver oil or other vitamin D concentrates usually bring about a rapid improvement in the child with mild rickets. Sunlight or other sources of ultraviolet irradiation are equally effective in causing a disappearance of the disease. Eggs, fortified milk, canned salmon and tuna are good dietary sources of this vitamin. In certain types of rickets, there may be a defective absorption of vitamin D from the intestine, and exposure to sunlight may be the only good means of bringing about a remission of the symptoms.

Vitamin E has been much heralded as helpful in the treatment of persons with a number of diseases but it is doubtful whether vitamin E deficiencies occur naturally in man. There is some indication that vitamin E may be beneficial in treating persons with certain forms of muscular degeneration and certain types of sterility. Vegetable oils, such as corn, soybean, peanut, coconut, or cottonseed, are the best dietary sources of vitamin E.

A deficiency of *vitamin K* is rare in normal individuals except in the newborn infant. It is common, however, in persons with certain diseases of the digestive tract. This deficiency is usually not encountered among persons whose diet contains adequate amounts of green leafy vegetables. Bacteria in the intestine generally supply the body with considerable amounts of this vitamin.

Vitamin K deficiencies occur most frequently in the newborn. Once the normal bacteria start to grow in the intestinal tract, they produce adequate supplies of the vitamin for most normal purposes; but in the first few days after birth, the infant is prone to become deficient in this substance. Vitamin K is essential for the clotting of blood, and in a deficiency the infant may develop hemorrhages which sometimes prove fatal. To prevent this, the physician usually prescribes vitamin K preparations for the mother during the last weeks of pregnancy and to the infant, after birth.

The result of vitamin K deficiencies, *hypoprothrombinemia*, in adults may be due to failure to absorb the vitamin, or to an inability to utilize it properly, as when the liver is damaged. In the former case, but not in the latter, vitamin K may be effective when it is administered by injection. The symptoms of a vitamin K deficiency in adults include a tendency toward hemorrhages, with the appearance of bruise-like areas under the skin. The vitamin is found in large amounts in green vegetables. Its beneficial effects are counteracted by the drug *dicumarol*, which is used in the treatment of patients with certain circulatory disorders.

Roughage

Roughage—also called residue or bulk—is defined as that part of the food which cannot be digested or absorbed. Nevertheless, this material must be considered in choosing a good diet. Roughage is helpful in giving the proper texture to the food, so that the stomach and intestines can function at their best.

The most common form of roughage in food is *cellulose*. Grain foods contain roughage, whereas meats and soft vegetables or fruits may contain little roughage. Most vegetables, fruits, and whole grain breads and cereals contain large amounts of cellulose.

A good diet, then, should contain adequate amounts of water, carbohydrates, fats, proteins, vitamins, minerals, and roughage. It should also

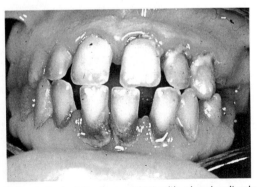

Picture of gingivitis in a patient with chronic vitamin C deficiency. *Courtesy Medichrome, Clay-Adams Co., Inc.; and Dr. Norman Jolliffe, Nutritional Division of City Health Clinic, New York City.*

be a varied diet. Such a diet is the individual's best single insurance against nutritional disease.

WEIGHT CONTROL

A person who exceeds by 15 to 20 percent the average weight of other persons of his height and frame may be said to be overweight. Persons who are as much as 25 percent overweight are classed as *obese*. Such a definition of overweight, however, is extremely unreliable. Many investigators have endeavored to list the most desirable weights for men and women of particular height, build, age, and racial stock; but the factor of individual and familial differences is impossible to include in any such listing. The individual himself is usually incapable of deciding just what is his most desirable weight. A physician, after conducting a thorough examination, is often the only person able to give an intelligent estimate of what the "normal" weight of any individual should be.

Persons who are overweight suffer many serious disadvantages. Muscular sluggishness, whether a cause or result of the obesity, may lead to a distinct impairment in working efficiency. The extra weight in obesity might be thought of as so much concrete carried around everywhere one goes. It may therefore be incon-

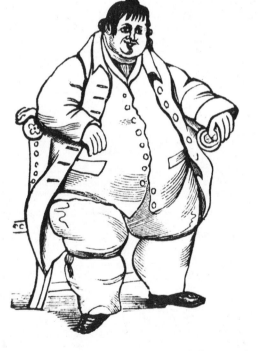

Daniel Lambert (1770-1809) was one of the most famous fat people of all time. His weight was 739 pounds at the time of his death. *Bettmann Archive*.

venient for these persons to get about and carry on normal activities. They frequently suffer considerable embarrassment and ridicule from others. Of even greater concern is the fact that obese people are especially predisposed to diseases of the heart, circulatory system, pancreas, skeleton, and kidneys. Hence, overweight persons usually live shorter lives than other individuals.

It is estimated that there are about 15 million persons in the United States who are at least 20 percent overweight. Indeed, this is the most common physical abnormality found within our population. There are two general categories of overweight persons. In the major group of obese persons are the heavy eaters. These are the persons who will most likely benefit from an understanding of the exact relationship between their diets and their excess weight. The second group of obese persons is rare and consists of those suffering from some organic disease which causes the accumulation of excessive weight. Thyroid insufficiency is thought by some physicians to be a common cause of this type of obesity. Proper management of underlying organic disturbance is an important step in reducing the weight of this type of patient.

Just as a machine must have fuel to burn for energy, so the human body needs fuel. This fuel comes in the form of carbohydrates, fats, and proteins obtained in the diet. The body employs complex chemical processes for "burning" these substances at body temperature to produce the energy needed for carrying out the innumerable life processes.

The amount of nutritional "fuel" the body requires can be calculated with surprising accuracy. The amount of exertion, the loss of body heat to the atmosphere, and the amount of internal work of the body must all be considered in computing the amount of fuel needed. The computations are made in terms of units called *calories*. One calorie is the amount of heat required to raise the temperature of one kilogram of water one degree centigrade. The complete utilization of one gram of protein or of carbohydrate by the body produces about four calories, while a gram of fat gives about nine.

A man of average size and activity should have about 3000 calories a day in his diet. If the diet includes more than the calories needed, the body stores the excess for future use. It does this by converting the dietary carbohydrates, fats, and proteins into body fat. This may be stored in the fat layer just beneath the skin, or in the more remote recesses of the body. If the individual continues to take in more calories than he needs, his fat supplies then grow until he has gained considerable weight. Consequently, the individual who maintains a fairly constant weight must consume approximately the right amount of energy-yielding foods in his diet.

An obese person has but one satisfactory way to prevent the gain of undesirable weight, and that is by cutting down his intake of food. However, this does not mean that he merely eats a much smaller amount. As has been stressed in the previous section, the body requires more from food than calories. It also needs proteins for replacement and repair of tissues, vitamins, minerals, water, and roughage. These needs continue, even though one wishes to cut down on caloric intake.

A rigid reducing diet is often extremely unsatisfactory, particularly if it lacks taste appeal. It can also be dangerous if it fails to supply the individual with essential dietary needs. Reducing diets which include only a few foods that must be eaten regularly are probably undesirable. Even though these diets appear to have the proper amounts of all the known vitamins, minerals, and amino acids, there may be undiscovered food factors which are lacking. Hence, the individual undertaking a reducing diet should eat as great a variety of foods as possible.

Foods to avoid

Those foods which contain large amounts of carbohydrates and fats should be eaten in small amounts by the obese person but must not be completely removed from the diet because of their source of energy. Carbohydrates are a more rapid source of energy than fats and, indeed, are necessary for the excess fat in the body to be properly utilized. If the individual desires to relieve himself of excess fat stores, he must plan to eat a few carbohydrate foods, but he must learn to eat them in much smaller amounts. A person eating six to eight slices of bread a day can cut down his caloric intake tremendously by decreasing his daily bread allowance to one or two pieces, providing he does not increase the amounts of the other carbohydrate foods in his diet.

A reducing diet should also contain small amounts of fatty foods such as butter or cheese, because many important food factors are found concentrated in these foods. However, since fatty foods have such high caloric value, their use should be restricted. "Hidden fats," disguised in the form of fried foods, salad dressings, gravies, sauces, etc., should be avoided. Bottled soft drinks and alcoholic beverages have a high caloric content, and should be replaced with unsweetened grapefruit or tomato juice.

Foods to include in the reducing diet

Although proteins constitute a major source of calories, no attempt should be made to reduce their amount in the diet below the level recommended for normal people (65 to 100 grams daily). A minimum is required each day to provide the essential amino acids for tissue repair. Any weight reduction gained from a pro-

RECOMMENDED FOOD QUANTITIES IN TERMS OF SERVINGS

Food groups and approximate number of servings per person, low-cost and moderate-cost plans

Food groups*	Number of servings per person	
	Low-cost plan	Moderate-cost plan
Leafy, green and yellow vegetables	7–9 servings a week.	10–12 servings a week.
Citrus fruit, tomatoes	Children, 7 servings a week. Pregnant and nursing women, 9–12 servings a week. Other adults, 6 or 7 servings a week.	Children, 8–9 servings a week. Pregnant and nursing women, 12–15 servings a week. Other adults, 7–9 servings a week.
Potatoes, sweet potatoes Other vegetables and fruit	10–12 servings a week. 7 servings a week.	7–9 servings a week. 10–12 servings a week.
Milk, cheese, ice cream (In terms of fluid milk)	Children, about 3½ cups of milk a day. Pregnant women, a little more than 1 quart daily. Nursing women, 1½ quarts a day. Other adults, 2½–3 cups a day.	Children, 3½–4 cups milk a day. Pregnant women, a little more than 1 quart daily. Nursing women, 1½ quarts a day. Other adults, 2½–3 cups a day.
Meat, poultry, fish Eggs Dry beans and peas, nuts	5 or 6 servings a week. 5 eggs a week. 2–4 servings a week.	7 or 8 servings a week. 7 eggs a week. 1–2 servings a week.
Flour, cereal, baked goods (Whole-grain, enriched, restored).	Bread at every meal and also a cereal dish once a day.	At every meal.
Fats, oils	Throughout the week as desired. Butter or margarine daily.	Throughout the week as desired. Butter or margarine daily.
Sugar, sirup, preserves	Throughout the week as desired.	Throughout the week as desired.

* In addition to the foods in the 11 groups, fish-liver oil or some other source of vitamin D should be allowed for small children, pregnant women, also for older children and adults who have little opportunity for being in sunshine. *U.S. Department of Agriculture, Miscellaneous Publication No. 662.*

DAILY RECOMMENDED ALLOWANCES OF SPECIFIC NUTRIENTS

	Infants	Children 1-5 years inclusive	Children 6-11 years inclusive	Children 12 years and over	Adults	Pregnancy or lactation
Vitamin A—*U.S.P. units*	1,500	3,000	4,000	5,000	5,000	—
Thiamine (B₁)—*milligram*	0.5	0.8	1.3	1.6	1.5	—
Riboflavin (B₂)—*milligram*	0.5	1.2	1.8	2.0	2.0	2.5
Niacin—*milligram*	4	8	13	16	15	15
Ascorbic Acid (C)—*milligram*	30	50	75	75	75	150
Vitamin D *—*U.S.P. units*	400	400	400	400	400	400
Protein—*gram*	35	50	70	85	65	100
Calcium—*gram*	0.8	1.0	1.0	1.4	0.8	1.50
Iron—*milligram*	6	7.5	10.0	15	12	15.0

* Cow's milk containing 135 units of vitamin D per quart, and evaporated milk containing 7.5 U.S.P. units per avoirdupois ounce, usually will prevent clinical rickets when fed to normal infants in customary quantities.

tein-deficient diet will lead to a loss of vital muscle tissues. If only the fats and carbohydrates are restricted, the fat deposits of the body will be consumed without damage to vital structures. By depriving the body of amino acids for tissue repair, the individual renders himself infinitely more susceptible to disease. The reducing person must continue to eat the same amounts of vitamins and minerals recommended for normal people. Persons attempting to use extreme reducing diets should plan daily supplementation of their food; prescribed vitamin and mineral preparations may be used.

Roughage is a great help to the reducing individual. In spite of the fact that it has little caloric value, it is capable of satisfying hunger. In some cases, the physician may prescribe various appetite depressants. The amphetamines often are used if the patient can tolerate them; also prescribed are amphetamines in combination with hormones, digitalis, diuretics, and other preparations. Such combination "reducing" preparations should be used with the greatest caution, since in a few instances their use has resulted in the patient's death. Use of any type of "reducing aid" may produce toxic side effects and should not be attempted without the examination and advice of a physician.

Weight loss

A gradual weight loss is most desirable from the medical standpoint. This gives the body an opportunity to become accustomed to its new state. When weight is lost too rapidly, appreciably more than two pounds per week, the individual should suspect that the diet he is using may be deficient in something besides calories. If the rapid weight loss is caused by a deficiency of vitamins, minerals, water, or amino acids, the individual may suffer serious consequences.

Other methods of reducing weight

The most widely used alternative to reducing diets is increased exercise; generally, this is far less effective than dieting. There are two important points to be made in this regard. First, the individual should not undertake violent exercise which might overtax a weak heart, or strain and permanently injure his spine, large joints, muscles, and tendons. Second, the individual should bear in mind that increased activities not only use up extra calories, but also increase the body demands for vitamins, minerals, and water. Thus, the diet should be increased to include these extra items used. Actually, most fat people are unable to take enough exercise to make them lose an appreciable amount of weight; a decrease in caloric intake is usually mandatory. Moreover, there is no accepted, reliable evidence to support the assertion that weight reduction may be effected by a diet rich in polyunsaturated fats; the obese person should always consult a reputable physician for competent advice on the safest and most effective manner by which to reduce his weight.

Hospitalization is a desirable practice for obese people who, for medical reasons, must undergo rapid weight loss. The diet can be more carefully controlled in the hospital, so that the patient may receive all essential food factors he needs, but only as many calories as the physician believes necessary. Such hospitalization may also provide a dietary education for the patient. Various drugs have also been used to bring about a rapid reduction in body weight by killing the appetite or increasing the rate at which food is burned. These substances are often dangerous, and must *never* be used except under the guidance of a physician. Total fasting is sometimes used in treating hospitalized patients for extreme obesity. Extended fasting (longer than 40 days) has produced electrolyte disorders, protein deficiency, and anemia; vitamin B_{12} malabsorption has been recorded in studies of such patients.

The importance of the mental attitude of obese persons is gradually being clarified by psychiatrists. They often find personality similarities among overweight people and believe that in some cases the individual's social or family life may be responsible for a desire to eat great quantities of food. Psychiatrists have found repeated indications that individuals who have experienced emotional deprivation sometimes try to satisfy the hunger for affection by eating as much food as possible. Many times this habit is continued throughout life. Overeating may become so habitual that an obese person may feel that he does not eat more food than the average person. By making careful notation throughout the day of everything he eats, including between-meal snacks, the obese person usually finds that he actually eats much more than he has realized. Such a realization is often an inducement to initiate a reducing diet.

Adherence to a reducing diet or a strict program of exercise is difficult for many persons. These individuals eventually may lose faith in any possibility of ridding themselves of their excess pounds. In recent years, it has been found that when these persons are organized into groups, they frequently can succeed in reducing. Such groups meet informally and discuss their problems in weight control, their successes, and their failures. By developing a feeling of common interest and competition, it is possible to overcome many of the psychological problems associated with overweight. Participation in such a group should be undertaken only after the approval of a physician.

Underweight

The problem of underweight individuals is occasionally as serious as that of obese persons. Underweight nearly always accompanies serious nutritional deficiencies or disease. Therefore, the treatment of the underweight person is often more complicated and may involve measures other than those that are strictly dietary.

When the lack of weight is caused by an insufficiency of calories, or by too active a life for the number of calories included in the diet, the problem may be strictly one of quantity. This condition most often results from poverty or inattention to the diet. Treatment involves a change to adequate, well-balanced meals. Supplementation with proteins, vitamins, and mineral preparations also may be helpful in speeding up the restoration of body tissues and the necessary fat stores.

Many underweight persons seem to lack an appetite. Loss of appetite (*anorexia*) may result from various factors, and its cause may be difficult to determine. Extreme nervousness, worry, or excitement may be instrumental in decreasing the interest in food. In such cases, the weight problem is not easily remedied until the nervous condition is brought under control. Mild vitamin deficiencies may also cause a loss of appetite. Supplementation of the diet with vitamins, and more specifically with *thiamine,* vitamin B_1, has been found helpful in many cases. Some persons who live a sedentary existence and get no outdoor exercise may also lack an adequate desire for food. Various common drugs such as nicotine and alcohol, when taken in excess, may eliminate the feeling of hunger.

When the cause of underweight has been discovered and corrected, a special diet is required to restore the patient to his proper weight level. For an adult, this diet should contain at least 500 additional calories a day and extra quantities of high-protein foods through the week. The increase should be gradual and the food simple in nature so as not to overtax the digestive system, which is not accustomed to the additional work and increase in metabolism. Ample rest must be followed with periods of exercise, so that the weight gained is not purely fat but also protein in the form of muscle. High caloric content foods should be used, and food provided between meals and at bedtime. If there is no contraindication to eating more food, the underweight individual should be urged to eat all he or she can and then just eat a few bites more at each meal. Incremin (Upjohn) taken before meals in doses of 30 to 60 drops is also very helpful in stimulating the appetite.

Underweight is a frequent reflection of many chronic diseases, such as tuberculosis, diabetes, and anemia. For this reason, a person who is underweight should seek medical attention if an improved diet does not cause a weight gain. Sudden loss of weight may be an indication of a serious disease, and should receive medical attention.

Other modified diets

Modified diets are often necessary in aiding in the recovery of patients. These diets usually contain all the normal amounts of the required nutrients and frequently increased amounts. Such a diet should never be undertaken except under the guidance of a physician. When a rigid diet is necessary, as for example following an operation on the intestinal tract, the diet may not be balanced and cannot be maintained more than a few days without risk of creating a nutritional deficiency.

A person may gain some idea of the adequacy of either his regular diet or of a special one by means of the charts provided in this chapter, the chart which lists the daily recommended allowances of the specific nutritional ingredients. According to this table, an adult should have at least three fourths of one gram of calcium daily. Smaller charts show the nutritional value of various foods, such as the one for calcium. From this chart it can be seen that the required calcium may be obtained, for instance, from less than a quart of milk, or from about three ounces of cheese. The amounts of calcium consumed in the various foods eaten during the day may thus readily be calculated, and an estimate made as to whether or not they meet the requirement. A glance at the smaller charts may be sufficient to determine what foods fulfill the needs for various vitamins and minerals.

Fevers are associated with an increase in the chemical activities of the body, and they frequently result in large amounts of perspiration. To replace water lost through sweating, the diet should contain liquids in excess of the normally required amounts. The caloric content of the diet must also be increased in order to provide replacement of the energy expended by the body in its increased activity. Fevers may also cause a depletion of body protein and the stores of vitamins and minerals, so that intake of these substances must be increased.

Gastrointestinal disturbances often call for a temporary change in the diet. When such disturbance is accompanied by vomiting or diarrhea, it results in unusual water and salt loss; consequently, water and liquid foods must be given to the patient. When it is desired to permit the patient's digestive processes to rest, a *smooth* or *bland* diet may be prescribed. These diets are composed of foods devoid of seasoning and of stems, seeds, peelings, cellulose, and other types of roughage. Eggs, milk, potatoes, soups, juices, and other fluids compose such a diet, as well as strained foods which have most of the roughage removed. For a bland diet, seasonings are kept to a minimum and alcohol is excluded.

When it is desired to stimulate the gastrointestinal tract, such as for the sufferer from constipation, roughage is one of the essential ingredients of the diet. The patient should also be instructed to consume greater amounts of fluids than he ordinarily requires. If organic disease has been ruled out, the control of constipation is largely dependent on the individual's attitude, the proper intake of fluid, and the adequate consumption of vegetables, fruits, and other bulk substances.

A SAMPLE REDUCING DIET

Meal	Food	Approximate Calories
Breakfast	1 cup coffee or tea 1 tablespoon milk 2 slices of toast 1 pat of butter 1 small orange	— 15 120 70 50
Midmorning snack	1/2 small head of lettuce	10
Lunch	1 lean pork chop 5 cooked Brussels sprouts 1 small peach 1 cup coffee or tea 1 tablespoon milk	300 60 40 — 15
Afternoon snack	1/2 small apple	30
Dinner	1 thin slice roast rib of beef 1/2 cup beets 1 slice bread 1 cup coffee or tea 1 tablespoon milk	70 30 50 — 15
Bedtime snack	1 fresh plum or 1/2 cup strawberries	25
		Total 900 Calories

The diet may be supplemented by adding to it any of the following indicated portions of food, each of which increases its energy value by about 100 Calories:

Fruit
1 large apple
6 apricots
1 small banana
2/3 cup canned blackberries
30 fresh cherries
1 cantaloupe
2 oranges
1 large fresh peach
1 cup canned pears
2 slices fresh pineapple
1 slice canned pineapple
2 canned plums
5 stewed prunes
2 cups fresh strawberries

Cereals
2 cups corn flakes
1/2 cup rolled oats
1 1/2 cup rice flakes
1 small roll

Vegetables
2 artichokes
12 stalks asparagus
1 cup broccoli
1 1/2 cups cabbage (cooked)
2 cups carrots (cooked)
2 large heads lettuce
3 medium size onions (cooked)
1 cup peas
1 cup spinach
1 1/2 cup canned tomatoes
4 small tomatoes (raw)

Liquids
1 cup grapefruit juice
1 cup orange juice
3 cups tomato juice
3/4 cup vegetable soup
3/4 cup milk
2/3 cup cocoa, half milk
1/2 bottle beer

1/2 cup dry wine
1 cocktail glass sweet wine

Meats
1/2 cup beef hash
6 thin slices dried beef
4 strips crisp bacon
1 small hamburger
1 pork sausage
1 broiled veal cutlet
1/4 cup chicken a la king
1/4 cup canned salmon
2 sardines in oil
7 clams
1/2 cup crab meat
3/4 cup oysters
20 small shrimp
1 1/2 egg

Special dietary attention may be required before and after surgery, depending upon the exact nature of the operation. In most cases, the patient should strive to achieve an excellent state of nutrition and a normal weight before an operation, in order to increase his body's ability to withstand the operation and to recover promptly. Immediately before surgery is undertaken, however, the patient may be put on a so-called "starvation" diet. The purpose of this is to relieve the gastrointestinal tract of its digestive duties, and thereby decrease its residue. After the operation, the patient may have to begin with a liquid diet, changing gradually to a soft diet, and ultimately returning to a normal one. High-protein diets are believed to be of special value in stimulating wound healing, and in counterbalancing the increased rate of protein destruction following burns, operations, and some of the infectious diseases.

Thyroid disease usually calls for special diets. When the patient is suffering from overactivity of the thyroid gland, he must be supplied with larger amounts of calories than usual. In addition, vitamins may be required by the body in increased amounts. Conversely the diet for the patient suffering from underactivity of the thyroid gland should not contain as many calories as for other persons of the same weight. Loss of appetite is a major symptom in patients with decreased thyroid activity, and additional efforts are often necessary to provide food that the patient will eat.

Diabetic patients may have particularly difficult dietary problems. A controlled diet is necessary throughout the life of the diabetic. Each patient will have a diet which is rather specific for his own case, and cannot be modified to resemble the diet of some other patient. This problem is discussed in Chapter 10, "The Endocrine System."

Circulatory disturbances of many kinds require special dietary measures for their alleviation. Diets in which the salt or protein content is severely restricted sometimes are of value in the treatment of patients with high blood pressure. Control of the consumption of fat and *cholesterol*, a complex chemical substance found in fats and in certain tissues of the body, is advocated in the management of patients with certain circulatory diseases. Many of these special diets are very restricted in their content of a number of vital elements, so that they can be maintained for only limited periods of time.

Gout is a disease in which crystals of *uric acid* are deposited in certain joints. Diets for persons with the gout are designed to exclude from the diet the substances which the body can transform into uric acid. These substances, called *purines*, are found in large amounts in association with protein in meat, fowl, fish, gravies, lima beans, peas, spinach, and whole grain bread and cereals. Hence, gouty patients are largely restricted to a vegetarian diet until the attack has subsided, although such short-term dietary measures are usually not long effective. Certain types of *arthritis*, affecting the joints, are sometimes more easily tolerated by patients on special diets.

Changes in nutritional requirements with increasing age

The mainstay of an infant's diet is milk. Milk is easily digested by the baby, while solid foods may pass through the intestinal tract completely undigested. The composition of milk varies with the source (human, cow, goat) and also with the state of nutrition of the animal giving the milk. Milk contains large amounts of calcium and phosphorus which the infant needs for manufacturing bones and teeth. It also contains easily digestible protein. Milk contains all the *amino acids* needed by the infant to manufacture new tissues, and these amino acids are present in approximately the proper amounts. Milk also contains liberal amounts of most of the vitamins needed by the child except vitamins C and D; hence, if milk is the sole source of nutrition, supplementation of these vitamins will be required. Milk also lacks adequate amounts of iron necessary for red blood cell formation, so that prolonged diets on milk alone are inadvisable.

As the child grows, he needs additional sources of energy. Milk is over 85 percent water. Solid foods, while having some water, contain more concentrated nutritional material, including carbohydrates, proteins, and fats. The child rapidly develops a need for roughage in the diet, as well as more concentrated sources of vitamins and minerals. Fresh fruits, vegetables, and meats provide most of these increases, while bread, potatoes, and other starchy foods supply him with increased sources of energy. Eggs supply protein, and dairy products provide vitamin A and essential fats.

At adolescence, the individual undergoes many important body changes, and these are greatly influenced by the diet. Development of acne, menstrual difficulties, and other disorders, may call for special diets or diet supplementation. Carbohydrate restriction, for instance, is helpful in treating acne patients. A sudden increase in height without accompanying increase in weight calls for a greater emphasis on the protein and caloric constitution of the diet, unless weight loss is desirable, as in overweight children.

With the advancement of adulthood, the individual finds many changes in his dietary requirements. His natural taste for foods may vary. His need for milk, dairy products, and eggs is greatly reduced, since large amounts of protein are no longer needed for growth. Many persons lead a sedentary life. This means that the requirements for energy foods are decreased. Unless these items in the diet are decreased, the individual may notice a gradual increase in weight.

As the adult grows older, his food requirements, including his needs for vitamins and proteins, are decreased. Older persons often develop food idiosyncrasies and exist upon a limited diet. As a result, some part of their nutritional requirement is frequently neglected. One of the most important aspects of the care of the aged is to maintain them on a balanced, varied diet which is sufficient for their energy needs.

The dietary requirements of the expectant mother and the nursing mother are somewhat different from those of other women. She must incorporate into her meals not only what she herself needs, but also what the developing child requires. Children need all of the classes of food, especially vitamins, minerals, and proteins. A special consideration for women during the final months of pregnancy and during lactation is their iron, calcium, and phosphorus intake. Building of fetal bones and manufacture of milk may rob the mother of calcium and phosphorus, with the result that her own bones and teeth may be depleted. Iron is needed for making red blood cells. It is desirable for these women to supplement their diets with iron and calcium as well as vitamins.

Dietary supplements

It has become increasingly common for persons to supplement their diets with concentrated vitamin or mineral preparations. The addition of various vitamins and minerals to refined foods, milk, and oleomargarine by food manufacturers may also be considered to be a form of dietary supplementation. Special protein supplements to the diet may also be purchased. There is probably little need for a healthy individual to supplement his diet in this manner if he is choosing the proper foods. Some individuals find that taking such preparations makes them feel better. In many cases, this is an indication that the dietary habits prior to their taking the supplement were not good.

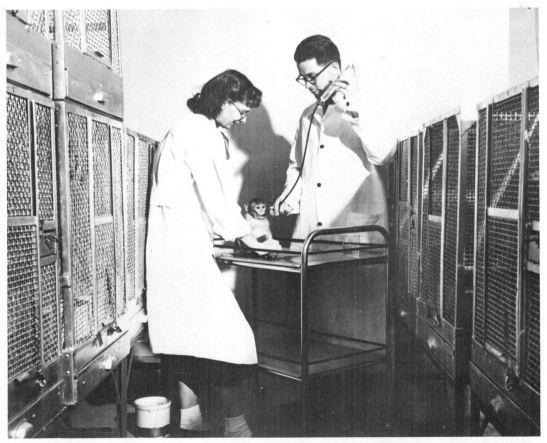

Studies on nutrition and the development of new drugs require the use of a variety of animals. The monkey shown here is being fed through a stomach tube to insure that the material is ingested. *Courtesy Stanford Research Institute.*

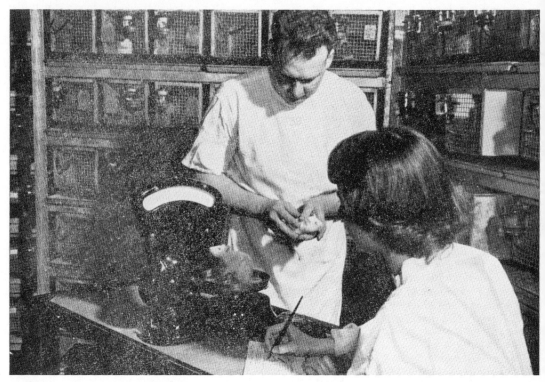

In following the course of nutritional experiments on white rats and other animals, regular recording of the gain or decrease in their weight is one of the common and most important means of assessing the animal's health.

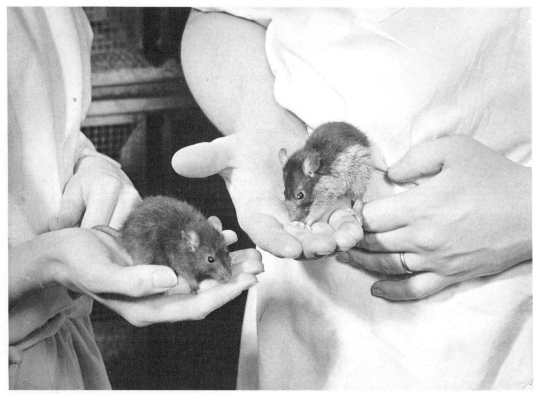

Dark rats are used in the study of pantothenic acid deficiency. Grey hair on animal at right indicates a deficiency.
Pictures in this series are by courtesy Federal Security Agency, Public Health Service, National Institutes of Health.

22 SICKNESS AT HOME

PREPARATION FOR BED REST

Most illnesses begin at home. The decision as to whether care should be given at home or in the hospital depends upon available facilities and the needs of the patient. Increasingly, physicians are recommending care at home rather than in a hospital if conditions permit, since in most cities, a shortage of hospital facilities and medical personnel exists. There also may be financial difficulties. Prolonged hospitalization, which may include special nurses during critical illness, often proves to be an overwhelming financial burden to the average family. The rising costs of hospital care account in part for the popularity of insurance plans that pay all or part of hospital expenses. If a family is unable to pay for a physician's services or hospitalization, medical care can be obtained through public or voluntary welfare agencies. Most large communities provide such medical care, and many private physicians serve the community without pay in certain situations. Information about local facilities for free care can be obtained from the Public Health Department. Information on hospital and medical insurance benefits available through Medicare is available from the local Social Security Administration office.

In many cases, the home is the natural and most desirable place for care of the sick. This is especially true for physically handicapped persons, convalescents, persons suffering from chronic illness, and the aged and infirm. The patient who must stay in a hospital for a long time often loses interest and becomes irritable and pessimistic. Most sick persons are happier at home because they can rest better, they like their own food better, and they benefit from the emotional support of family companionship. It is desirable to keep the family unit intact, and is easier to keep the patient interested and cheerful within the family group.

Obviously there are times when the home is not the best place for care of the sick. Such conditions as overcrowding, the status of the patient, and the excessive noise and confusion of too many household burdens make the home undesirable for certain types of illness. Fortunately, in most instances intelligent home nursing can be carried out successfully by a family member under the direction of the attending physician and the visiting nurse.

One trend in medical care is the community hospital, which uses the facilities of the home. The first experimental project in this phase of medical care was the program of home care developed at Montefiore Hospital of New York City. Most of its patients are those suffering from chronic or long-term diseases. There are a number of these programs now, scattered throughout the country. They range from intensive care programs with periodic visits from a physician or nurse to more simplified arrangements where only slight assistance to the family is required. These programs have proved to be unusually successful in many communities.

The medical and social services are coordinated to treat the patient and his family as an integral unit. The home is regarded as a department of the hospital and all special services or equipment that are mobile are brought directly to it. The medical service provides visits as frequently as needed by the physician, the public health nurse, and the physical and occupational therapist. If the patient must go to the hospital for treatment or examination, transportation is provided by ambulance or taxi. Housekeeping service is available to families who need it. Medications are dispensed by the hospital pharmacy, and equipment is borrowed from the hospital supply department. The social service worker maintains contact with the patient and helps to solve economic and other home problems. This community program not only recognizes the value of home care for the patient, but also utilizes home care to the fullest extent to help solve the problem of crowded hospitals. Furthermore, this hospital extension service is relatively inexpensive in comparison with the cost of hospital confinement. Additional information on this service can be obtained from the Public Health Service, either national or local.

The home nurse

A patient who is sick at home requires both mental and physical comfort. This necessitates consistency of treatment. For this reason, one person, preferably a family member, should assume the entire responsibility. In most communities, a Public Health Nurse, usually employed by the city or county, is available to instruct the family member who is to assume the role of home nurse. The Public Health Nurse should be consulted for a demonstration before attempting any unfamiliar procedure. The local Red Cross chapter also may be helpful; specific procedures are detailed in the "American Red Cross Home Nursing Textbook." The Public Health Nurse or Red Cross chapter personnel may know where special equipment, such as hospital beds, bed trays, etc., can be borrowed or rented.

The home nurse should exercise scrupulous

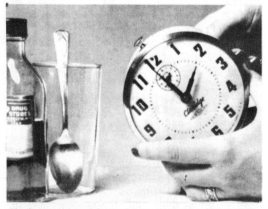

Clock too old to tick can be used as a reminder of the time medicine is to be given. After each dose, the hands may be set to hour for the next dose. *Copyright 1950, The American Home.*

attention to her personal cleanliness. She should be neat and well groomed. A serviceable apron is convenient when giving care to the patient.

The home nurse can win the respect and co-operation of the patient by the manner in which she treats him. The patient should not be forced to become the victim of the home nurse's personal moods, whims, prejudices, and moral judgments. A consistent, kind, and understanding attitude is important, and the nurse should not bewilder the patient by giving one kind of treatment one day and another the next. Respecting the patient as an individual and demonstrating her own emotional stability can help to develop the patient's sense of responsibility. Most ill persons will achieve satisfaction by doing as much as they can for themselves. This burden should not be greater than the limits of the patient's strength will permit. Thoughtfulness, consideration, and a cheerful attitude can evoke in the patient an interest and pride in maintaining his own schedule and participating in family activities even though he is bedridden.

Understanding the patient is much more important and constructive than pitying him. It is natural for an ill person to be apprehensive. Firm reassurance or simply allowing him to talk over his worries may lessen his disturbance. The patient will have confidence in the home nurse who promotes a sense of security and reduces his fears. It is of mutual advantage for both the patient and the home nurse to understand the orders of the physician. Except in special circumstances, forthright honesty usually is the best policy and will result in the most complete co-operation.

The atmosphere of the home

The atmosphere of the home should reflect kindness, optimism, tolerance, and sympathy toward the patient and his needs. Any illness creates problems, and confusion only intensifies them. When there is no definite plan for care of the patient, and several members of the family try to do the same thing at the same time, the patient is unduly disturbed and may feel that he has become an unbearable burden. Organization of the patient's daily care to co-ordinate with the household activities will prevent his feeling that he is seriously disrupting the family routine. A sick person who is confined to one room for a long time may become self-centered and over-sensitive to his surroundings and to the attitudes of those about him. An atmosphere of unnatural cheerfulness will only intensify such reactions. Similarly, oversolicitude may make the patient emotionally dependent, and indifference may cause him to make excessive demands during his illness. Sincere concern for the patient's welfare is desirable, and avoidance of overprotectiveness will best preserve normal family relationships and prove to be most conducive to the healthy home atmosphere. Such an atmosphere will help prevent the patient from lapsing into an enjoyment of invalidism.

The sickroom

The ideal sickroom is a moderately large room which the patient may occupy alone, and which preferably is located on the ground floor. The room should have a pleasant color scheme, adequate sunlight, and ventilation. It is better that the room be adjoining a bathroom. The sickroom should provide maximum privacy, and should not be a thoroughfare for family or visitors. The patient should be protected from drafts but provided with adequate fresh air. As far as possible, the temperature of the sickroom should be kept at a constant level, usually from 72° to 76° F during the day and from 68° to 72° F at night. The use of a room thermometer will help in maintaining a constant temperature. The floor of the sickroom should be kept free of dust and dirt with a vacuum cleaner. Advice can be obtained from the physician or Public Health Nurse concerning swabbing the floor with antiseptic solutions and the use of humidifiers such as cut flowers, potted plants, or jars of water. Suitable furniture should include a comfortable bed, two bedside tables, a straight chair, a dresser or chest of drawers, and an armchair.

The sickroom should be thoroughly cleaned in the morning and kept orderly at all times. Cleaning should be performed quietly and systematically, keeping the room as dustproof as possible. Cleansing materials with a strong or unpleasant odor should not be used.

Sick persons are very sensitive to odors; and antiseptics and disinfectants may be irritating.

Use of one of the chlorophyll or other deodorants, probably an odorless neutralizing agent, will help to keep the air of the sickroom fresh. By keeping the patient clean, making frequent changes of surgical dressings, and by keeping equipment clean, offensive odors will be better controlled. It will be of help to the patient if the home nurse finds out what odors are pleasant to the patient, and whether he objects to smoking in his room.

Sick persons are also sensitive to sounds. A quiet room does not mean absolute silence but it should provide freedom from loud, sudden, or mysterious noises. Family chatter, squeaky shoes, and slamming doors are unduly annoying. Strips of rubber or cardboard can stop windows from rattling. Doorstops can be made from covered bricks and door silencers can be made from old innertubes cut to fit around both doorknobs. Mumblings and whisperings in a far corner of the sickroom are especially disturbing.

An ill person has an acute perception of light. Glare may be disturbing or painful and should be regulated by shutters or shades. Sunlight is cheerful but should not be direct. Light fixtures should be shaded so that light will not shine directly into the patient's eyes. A bedridden patient should never be left with an unprotected light beaming into his face. For safety and the patient's mental security, a simply operated bedlight should be kept within easy reach at the bedside.

One of the most frequent problems of the sickroom is the disrupting effect of visitors. The home nurse should ask the physician immediately whether visitors are permitted, and then abide by his instructions. A sick person may feel that confinement is tedious and desire the stimulation of visitors. It will help the nurse to en-

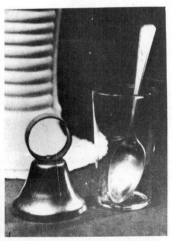
By placing a bell, or a spoon in a glass, at the bedside, the patient will find it easy to summon his attendant.

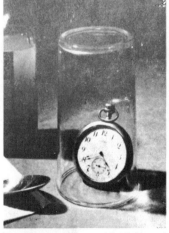
The annoyance caused by ticking of a watch by the bedside may be prevented by covering the watch with a drinking glass.

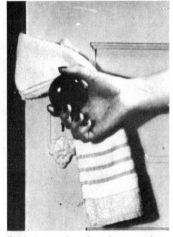
Folded towels placed over door knobs prevent accidental noisy slamming. *Copyright 1950, by The American Home.*

force the visiting regulations tactfully if the physician will tell her how long visitors should be allowed to stay. Visitors should not remain in the sickroom while the patient is eating, or when any treatment is being administered. Usually the best time for company is late in the morning, or after the afternoon nap, when the patient is likely to be rested and relaxed.

The patient's bed

The patient's bed, mattress, and pillows should be adequate to give proper support and insure maximum comfort during bedrest. In many communities a hospital bed can be obtained without charge. Such a bed is more comfortable because the patient's head and feet can be lowered or

How To Make a Backrest

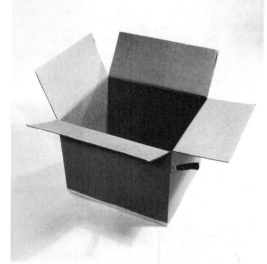

In preparing a back rest from a cardboard carton, the broad side must serve as the front. Two corners on one side are then cut, top to bottom.

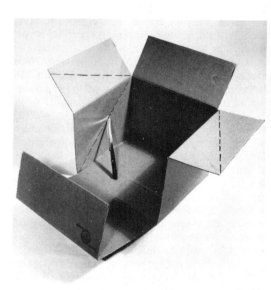

To prepare cardboard for bending, it should be scored along diagonal lines shown running from the top back to the bottom front inner surface.

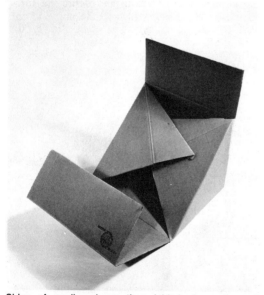

Sides of cardboard are then folded along diagonal lines as shown: top flap is brought down and front side and flap brought up over the folded sides.

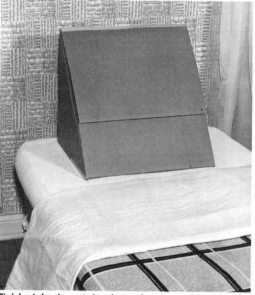

Finished back rest is shown in place. *Adapted from illustrations in Red Cross Home Nursing. Copyright, 1950, American National Red Cross.*

raised. Also, the height of a hospital bed prevents back and neck strain for the home nurse, and the bed can be easily moved because it is fitted with casters.

In case of a long illness, it is practical to use a plastic sheet to protect the mattress, and a draw sheet. If the sickbed is to be used for a short time, several thicknesses of newspapers, a table oilcloth, or a plastic sheet can be used under the draw sheet. This affords mattress protection when the patient is using a bedpan or urinal, or is being bathed. A draw sheet can be cut down from an old bed sheet, or a bed sheet can be folded and stretched over the plastic sheet. The draw sheet should extend from the patient's shoulders to his knees. A soiled draw sheet can be removed with little discomfort to the patient. It also helps the home nurse in turning an acutely ill person.

Making an unoccupied bed is simple, but when the sick person is not allowed to leave his bed, changing the bedding requires speed and skill to prevent discomfort. Making one half of the bed, moving the patient to it, and then making the other side is an operation that is easily mastered with practice. It is illustrated on the succeeding pages. The secret of good bedmaking is to tuck enough of the sheet around the head of the mattress to prevent wrinkling and crawling toward the foot of the bed. The patient should be kept warm during bedmaking. The necessary bedding and linens should be assembled at the bedside before beginning.

Bedrest equipment

The bedridden male patient should be provided with a bedpan and urinal and the female patient with a bedpan. These articles may be purchased or rented from a drug or medical supply house, or they may be borrowed from a local Loan and Gift Closet. The Sickroom Loan Closet is an accumulation of articles provided to facilitate the care and increase the comfort of the sick person in his home. Loan closets are made available by local social and welfare agencies, hospitals, and Visiting Nurse Associations. In some communities, the loan items include small articles such as thermometers, basins, and irrigating equipment; and large items such as beds, tables, and wheel chairs. The Closet often includes such articles as backrests, reading lamps, and small radios. The Loan and Gift closets maintained by the various agencies stock an almost endless variety of articles for the comfort and recreation of the patient.

A bedridden patient may need a backrest. The backrest on a hospital bed is the best type; however, a backrest may be purchased, rented or improvised. A folded card table or a washboard braced against the head of the bed and tied securely in place will serve as a backrest. Or, a back and headrest can be constructed from a pasteboard carton, as shown on page 676. A padded box or suitcase can be used as a footrest. Support for the patient's knees can be provided by a small rolled blanket. A bath towel, rolled and sewn, makes a satisfactory knee roll.

If possible, there should be two bedside tables, one on each side of the patient's bed. On one of these the home nurse can place the patient's personal toilet articles in a covered box, a call bell, and a shaded light.

Every home should keep at least a minimum stock of bedrest equipment. This should include a thermometer, bedpan, ice cap, hot water bottle, and a first aid kit. (See Chapter 23, "Physical Injuries and First Aid").

ROUTINE CARE OF THE PATIENT

The home nurse who has a definite plan of daily activity can complete her work with more efficiency, more ease, and less strain on herself and on the patient. If the patient is not acutely ill, he should assume as much responsibility for maintaining his own schedule as his condition will allow. The home nurse should change the position of the bedridden patient frequently enough to keep him relaxed and comfortable. Nourishment and medication should be given as ordered. The physician may request a record of the liquid intake and urine output be kept. An ordinary kitchen measuring cup can be used for accuracy. It may be necessary to collect a urine, fecal, or sputum specimen for laboratory examination. A small clean bottle can be used for the urine specimen. It should be covered and labeled. Unless the physician gives other instructions, a morning urine specimen should be collected. A covered plastic container can be used for sputum and fecal specimens.

The daily routine

Schedules for home treatment will depend upon the kind of illness and the type of treatment and medication. The following schedule can be used as a pattern for planning the daily routine.

7:30 A.M. Temperature, pulse, and respiration.
Morning care (bedpan, bath, care of teeth, change bed).
Rest.

8:30 A.M. Breakfast.
Rest.

10:30 A.M. Nourishment.

To noon   Rest.
               Diversional activity.
Noon: Lunch.
1:00 to 3:00 P.M. Rest.
3:00 P.M. Nourishment.
            Rest.
4:00 P.M. Temperature, pulse, and respiration.
4:30 to 5:00 P.M. Diversional activity.
            Rest.
6:00 P.M. Supper.
            Rest.
7:30 P.M. Temperature, pulse, and respiration.
            Evening care (partial bath, care of teeth, bedpan).
8:30 P.M. Lights out.

A more detailed schedule will be necessary for an acutely ill person, carrying it through the night to include medications and other instructions. Treatments should be dispersed at convenient times through the day to allow a period of rest following the treatment. The patient should be told in advance of any treatment or medication. It is disturbing to have any procedure thrust abruptly upon a person. The home nurse should not be mysterious or secretive about performing her duties.

Bathing and grooming the patient

The patient who is confined to his bed should have a bath at regular convenient times. The physician will indicate the number of full bed baths the patient may have. The bed bath is given to cleanse, to aid in elimination, and to refresh. A bath also provides passive exercise and stimulates circulation. Before beginning the bath, all the necessary articles should be collected at the bedside. The most important thing is to keep the room comfortably warm and avoid chilling the patient. The bath should be given in privacy; latching the door will prevent interruption and drafts. Two blankets can be used, one to protect the bedding, and the other to cover the patient. Warm water, at body temperature, should be used. The temperature of the water can be tested with the elbow. Only small areas of the body should be bathed at a time. As soon as any area is washed, rinsed, and dried, it should be recovered with the blanket. Special care should be taken to cleanse the navel and genital area. Also, the armpits should receive special attention. If the patient is an adult, an antiperspirant may be used.

The patient's mouth must be kept clean. Long cotton swabs dipped in a salt and soda solution can be used for cleaning the teeth if the patient cannot use a brush. A dry shampoo can be used to clean the hair. The male patient will appreciate a frequent haircut and having some type of hair conditioner applied.

Physical care and medication

Exercise, even of the most passive type, is essential in illness. For this reason, it is desirable that the patient's position be changed at least once every hour. Changing position not only helps prevent fatigue, but stimulates the blood circulation. This is especially important in obese or elderly patients. Depressed circulation in the skin causes the tissues to break down and bed sores will result. Before a bed sore is formed, the skin becomes reddened and will not blanch to touch. Such sensitive areas should be encircled by a "doughnut" of rubber foam, cut to size, which will elevate the affected area. The natural skin tone can be obtained with a lotion containing lanolin. Rubbing alcohol can be used if the skin is oily.

The physician may permit light massage or rubs of warmed alcohol or other lotion. Powdering the skin after a backrub or massage will of-

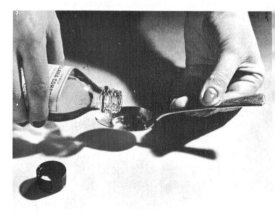

Bottled medicine should be poured with label on top to prevent its obliteration by fluids running down side. *Copyright 1950, The American Home.*

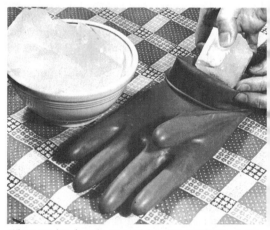

When an ice bag is needed but not available, a rubber glove filled with ice and tied at the wrist may serve. *Copyright 1950, The American Home.*

ten add to the patient's comfort. Massage should never be brisk enough to irritate the skin or cause fatigue. Gentle, long, steady strokes of the palms are most soothing. Massage lotion should always be warm and, in order to prevent chilling, the patient should not be unduly exposed during a massage.

Hot or cold applications are used only on the physician's advice to relieve pain, modify the blood supply to an affected area, give comfort, and promote healing. Dry heat is applied by hot water bottles, sun lamps, and electric pads. Any soft material can be used to apply moist heat. The physician will order a special solution if plain water is not adequate. A towel may be used to cover the compress and keep it in place, and a piece of rubber or plastic sheet may be placed around this to prevent rapid cooling. Hot compresses should be changed when they become cool, and care must be used to prevent burning the patient's skin. An ice cap is usually used for dry cold applications. A hot water bottle filled with finely crushed ice, a swimming cap, or a rubber glove filled and tied can be used. Wet compresses are prepared with ice water. Compresses should be changed about every three minutes and should be left uncovered unless the physician instructs otherwise.

Heat is sometimes given in the form of a steam inhalation to relieve hoarseness, coughing, or difficulty in breathing. A teakettle, commercial inhalator, or vaporizer may be used.

The urinal or bedpan should be offered to the patient on waking and at suitable routine intervals. The bedpan should be warmed if necessary. The patient should be cleansed and his hands washed after use of the pan. Newspapers or similar bed protectors should be used and the pan should be kept covered except when in use. Prepared enemas in adult and child sizes may be purchased at a drug store if needed.

Enemas and douches

An enema may be ordered to aid in elimination. Unless the enema solution is specified by the physician, pure warm tap water is the most practical liquid to use. The enema equipment includes an enema can or rubber bag, rubber tubing with a clamp, and a rectal tube or nozzle. A bed protector and a bedpan are also necessary. The container should be held or suspended about 18 inches above the bed. Some of the enema solution should be permitted to run through the tubing to expel the air. The patient lies on his left side, if possible, and the rectal tube is lubricated and inserted. The desired amount of fluid is allowed to run in slowly. The rectal tube is removed and after a few minutes the patient is allowed to attend to his own toilet. The procedure for the retention enema is essentially the same, except that the oil or other solution is not expelled as soon as the cleansing enema. A demonstration of these procedures can usually be obtained from the County Health Nurse.

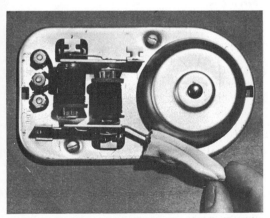

When ringing of a doorbell disturbs the patient, the finger of an old glove over hammer softens the sound. *Copyright 1950, The American Home.*

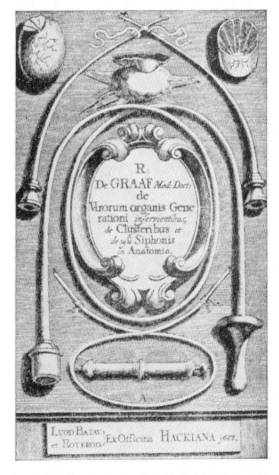

Title page of a book published in 1668 having as part of its design the newly developed flexible tube enema syringe. *Copyright 1944, Ciba Symposia.*

How To Improvise a Steam Tent

Many of the unpleasant symptoms of some respiratory disorders may be alleviated by the use of a steam tent. A satisfactory device to achieve such relief can easily be constructed at home with the use of a few common household items, as shown in the accompanying series of photographs. Care must be taken that the source of steam, such as a kettle, be placed on a protected surface and where it cannot offer a hazard to the patient. Care must also be taken to insure that the steam is directed toward the top of the steam tent directly away from the patient's face. Similar steam tents can be devised in various other ways, but the basic principle of insuring a warm moist breathing atmosphere while keeping the patient comfortable must always be observed. Patients who are severely ill and who cannot direct their own activities should not be left unattended in the steam tent, and the use of the tent should be restricted to those cases where it has been recommended by the physician. *Adapted from illustrations in RED CROSS HOME NURSING. Copyright 1950, American National Red Cross.*

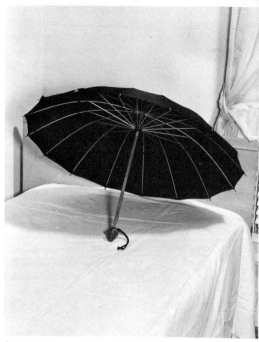

Support for the stream tent may be provided conveniently by an opened umbrella placed on the bed, over the patient's head and shoulders, in the position shown.

A vaginal douche is administered to a bedridden patient placed on the bedpan. Warm water or an antiseptic or douche powder prescribed by the physician is used. The appearance of the vaginal washings should be noted. The equipment should be washed with soap and water, and if necessary, sterilized, immediately after use.

Temperature, pulse, and respiration

The physician may request a periodic check of the temperature, pulse, and respiration. There are two types of fever thermometers. One is for taking the temperature by mouth only and the other for taking the temperature by rectum or mouth. Regardless of which type is used, the patient should not be left alone with the thermometer in place. The oral thermometer is cleaned by alcohol or antiseptic solution, and the mercury is shaken down to read 95° or lower. The bulb end is placed in the patient's mouth, under the tongue, and the mouth is kept closed. After a full three minutes, the thermometer is removed and read. The normal range of body temperature is from 98° to 99° F. The temperature is taken by rectum if the patient is too ill to hold the thermometer in his mouth, or if the patient is a small child or an infant. A rectal thermometer and a lubricant are used. The body temperature usually is one degree higher in the rectum than in the mouth. Therefore, the method used should always be noted on the patient's record.

The pulse rate should be taken while the patient is sitting or lying. The patient's arm is placed in a relaxed position with the thumb turned upward. With the index finger, the home nurse finds the pulse beat on the wrist near the thumb side of the hand. The beats are counted for one minute, using the second hand of a watch or clock. The normal pulse rate is 66 to 88 per minute, although there are individual variations.

Respirations are taken by observing the number of times the chest rises in breathing for one minute. The normal respiration count is approximately 16 per minute. The physician will probably wish to be notified of any sudden marked changes in either temperature, pulse, or respiration.

Medicines may be given in the form of liquids, powder, pills, tablets, or capsules. All medicines for use by the patient should be kept together on the medicine tray and out of children's reach. The label should always be read before medicine is given. Medicines should be given at the *exact* time, in the correct manner, and in the *right amount*. A prescription is always meant for a particular person with a particular condition. It should never be given to anyone else for any reason. There are other

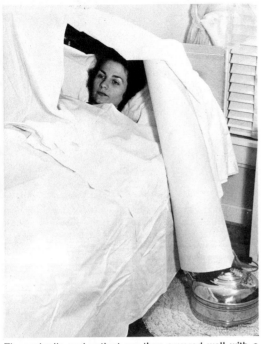

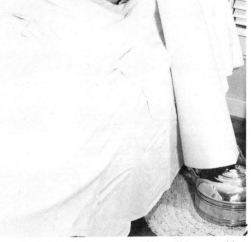

The umbrella and patient are then covered well with a blanket so as to leave an open air space in the front. Steam from kettle enters tent through the paper funnel.

Patient's hair may be protected from moistures with a towel. When tent is removed, damp bed clothing must be replaced and the patient protected from exposure.

ways of giving medicine, such as inhalation, irrigation, by rectum, and by absorption through the skin. Medicine given by hypodermic injection under the skin or into a vein is always administered by a physician or professional nurse. In diabetes, the physician or professional nurse may teach some family member or the patient himself to give medicine hypodermically.

When the home nurse has the duty of changing dressings, she will be given specific instructions by the doctor. Before and after changing a dressing, the home nurse should scrub her hands thoroughly with antibacterial soap and water. The skin surfaces around a dressing should be watched for signs of circulatory difficulties. When darkening of the skin or burning or tingling sensations occur in a limb, the bandage should be loosened.

Pain is an important sign in illness. No attempt to relieve a new and sudden pain should be made until the physician can observe the location, severity, and type of pain.

Rest is often the most important single healing measure during illness. There are many factors affecting the patient's ability to relax and rest. Everything possible should be done to prevent the patient from getting too tired during the day, because it may interfere with rest at night. If the patient is restless and unable to sleep, a warm sponge bath may prove helpful. A hot water bag at his feet or an extra blanket

may be needed. Sometimes a warm drink is soothing. A light back rub may help induce sleep.

The patient may come home from the hospital with an indwelling catheter for draining the bladder. Receptacles for receiving the urine should be sterilized daily and the amount of fluid checked periodically to insure proper drainage. The physician should be notified immediately if drainage stops.

Sanitary procedures

Cleanliness is a safety measure for both the patient and the rest of the family. The home nurse should be conscientious about washing her hands before and after giving any care to the patient. All equipment must be kept clean and disinfected if necessary. Boiling or sterilization, baking in an oven, or ironing, are forms of disinfection. Waste disposal is important. A medium-sized paper grocery bag makes an adequate waste bag, and is especially useful when pinned to the side of the mattress for the patient's use. Waste bags should never be used a second time and should be discarded promptly.

If the home nurse develops a cold or other respiratory infection, she should be relieved of her duties. If there is no one who can relieve her, she should wear a mask whenever giving care to the patient. Sterile masks can be purchased at local drug or medical supply stores,

How To Make an Occupied Bed

Good home nursing care requires knowledge of how to perform a great many menial tasks for the invalid in a manner that provides the least inconvenience. Changing bed linens often becomes a great problem, since it should be performed frequently and is a difficult task for the uninstructed. With training, however, it may be done swiftly and efficiently without disturbing the patient to any great degree. The following series of photographs show the precise method by which this may be achieved, and should be studied closely. *Courtesy Hermann Hospital, Houston. Photography by Bob Sallee.*

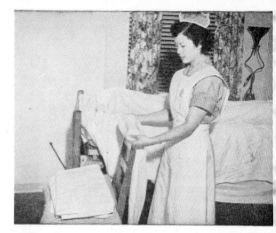

1. The first step consists in carefully removing the pillow from the bed, and hanging the dirty pillow case over a chair to serve as a laundry container.

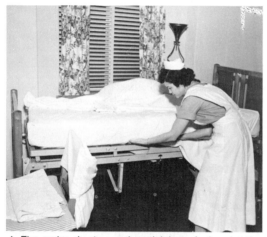

4. The under sheets are then tightly tucked under the mattress on this side of the bed so that they will be firmly retained and will not tend to form wrinkles.

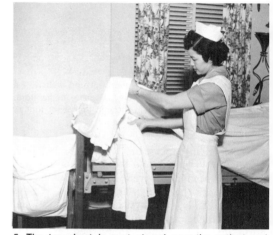

5. The top sheet is next placed over the patient and dirty top sheet removed from underneath it so that the patient at no time will be left without a covering.

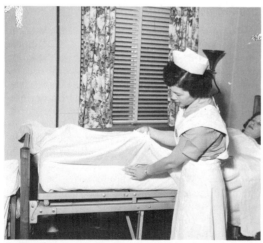

8. The flap in top sheet is then held out as shown in this photograph while the sheet is made level with the top surface of the mattress to make an even edge.

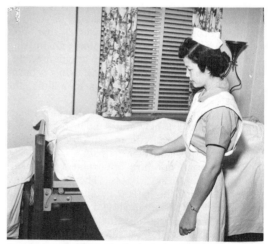

9. When both clean sheets have been properly placed on the bed and carefully tucked in as shown, the final result should have the neat appearance shown here.

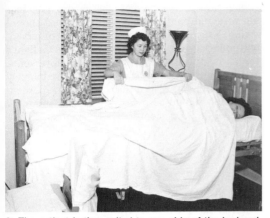

2. The patient is then rolled to one side of the bed and the dirty under sheets are rolled up to patient's back. Clean linens are lined up on the exposed mattress.

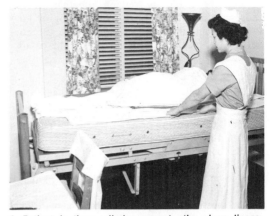

3. Patient is then rolled over onto the clean linens, thus permitting dirty under sheets to be completely removed and clean sheets to be spread on the mattress.

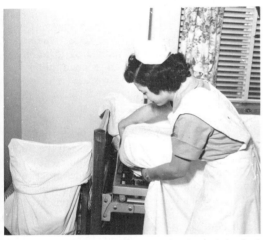

6. Tucking in of the top sheet at the foot of the bed must be done with care in order to insure that the patient will not pull it loose and suffer exposure.

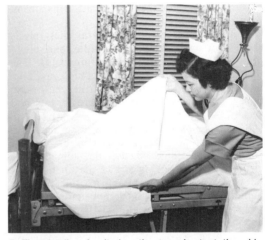

7. The details of mitering the top sheet at the side of the foot of the bed are shown here. A flap is lifted up first and the loose end is then folded under.

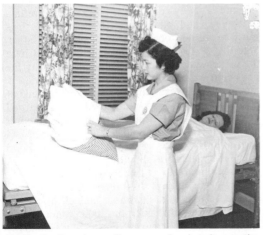

10. Finally the clean pillow case is placed over the pillow and smoothed out. Protective underpillow case should also be changed at this time if necessary.

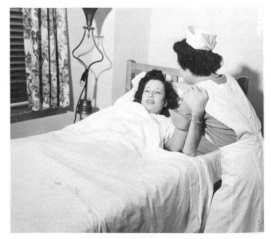

11. When removing and replacing the pillow, the patient must be carefully raised. This photo shows the proper method for supporting the patient's weight.

or may be made by sewing together at the ends several thicknesses of cloth. String or tape to tie around the head in attached to the corners. After each use, the mask should be disinfected or discarded.

Feeding the sick

The diet is an important part of the patient's treatment. If a special diet is required, this should be provided with as much care as that given for medication. If the home nurse needs help in planning meals that fill the patient's needs and fit the family's budget, the dietitian at the hospital can make helpful suggestions, especially if the patient is about to be discharged from the hospital. The home nurse also may request help from the visiting nurse at home, or the nutritionist at the local Red Cross headquarters, the local health department, or other community agency.

If the patient is on a general diet, meals should not only satisfy the appetite, but should also fulfill basic nutritional requirements. The diet should be rich in protein, vitamins, and minerals, and should include milk, fruit, eggs, vegetables, lean meat, breads and cereals, fats and sweets.

The patient's bed tray should be made as attractive as possible. Dishes can be brightly colored and should always be immaculately clean. Colored drinking straws may help to interest the sick child in taking his full quota of liquids. Dishes should be lightweight and easy to handle. For children, liquids in a thick tumbler or plastic cup are less likely to be spilled than in a tall glass. Food should be prepared so that it will be easy to handle in bed. Toast may be cut into finger-size strips and meat cut into bite-size pieces. Salads that can be picked up in the fingers are easier to manage than regular salads. The acutely ill person may have to be fed by spoon or tube. Straight or curved drinking tubes or straws can be used. Children often prefer to drink with straws or tubes.

The patient should be given sufficient time to feed himself, and should rest after each meal. If the patient's diet does not prohibit between-meal feedings, these may be given if they do not interfere with the appetite for regular meals.

The patient's record

The home nurse should keep a daily dated record of the patient's illness. The record should indicate how the patient feels, how he reacts to treatment, what has been done for him, and when it was done. The doctor will write his instructions for the patient on such a record if one is provided. When more than one person is giving care to the patient, the record is essential to avoid confusion. A simple record should include such entries as symptoms observed, treatments given, medicines given, the patient's reactions, nourishment, sleep, bowel movements, and liquid intake and urine output. The temperature, pulse, and respiration should be recorded. The hour should also be noted. The summary provided by the record can have great significance for the physician in prescribing treatments.

CARE IN COMMUNICABLE DISEASES

The method of caring for a person with a communicable disease is slightly different from that of caring for a patient with other illness. Communicable diseases are those diseases which can be transmitted from one individual to another. The means of transmission depend upon the type of germs causing the disease. The germs may be transmitted directly through contact with the patient's infected discharges, such as droplets coughed or breathed, or indirectly through contaminated water or food, or by insects. The attending physician will tell the home nurse what regulations are required by the health department and what home procedures should be followed. The home nurse must protect herself and see that other persons are not exposed to the patient's infection.

All equipment used in caring for the patient should be kept in the patient's room. The home nurse should wear a coverall apron when giving care to the patient. The apron should be left in the patient's room. The nurse's hands must be washed before and after caring for the patient. Infectious body discharges must be carefully destroyed, and all paper, tissues, or dressings must be burned or otherwise disposed of safely. Safe disposal of body discharges will necessitate the use of special disinfectants prescribed by the physician. Unless other precautions are ordered, inexpensive dishes and utensils composed of plastic or paper can be obtained and discarded after each use. If ordinary dishes and utensils are permitted, they should be thoroughly washed or rinsed in scalding or boiling water. Food from the sickroom should be disposed of immediately and never shared with others.

When the patient has recovered, he should have a tub bath, a shampoo, and clean clothes before leaving the sickroom. The room should then be aired and cleaned thoroughly. Hot soapy water will be sufficient to use, unless the physician states otherwise. Pillows, mattress, and rugs should be sunned outdoors for a period of six hours. All glassware and equipment must be washed in hot soapy water and boiled. Books, toys, or other nonwashable articles in most cases should be discarded.

In extremely infectious diseases, complete isolation may be required. To be effective, isolation technique must be taught. If isolation is required, the physician may request that a public health nurse visit the patient's home to give instructions in special procedures. This service is provided in most communities, without charge, by the Public Health Department.

Tuberculosis

Tuberculosis is one of the most prevalent of the serious communicable diseases. Because of the lack of adequate sanatorium facilities, many patients must be cared for at home. The majority of tuberculous infections occur in the lungs. The germs of tuberculosis are very resistant to cold, and can live for a year in water and for a long time in dried sputum. The dust in houses of persons with tuberculosis is particularly dangerous. The disease is transmitted by contaminated secretions, and germs may enter the body by way of the membranes of the nose, throat, or digestive tract. Infections may be caused from inhaling the breath, especially from the coughing of a tuberculous person.

The patient who is cared for at home should be isolated from the rest of the family as much as possible. Children are especially susceptible to infection and should be allowed to visit only a short period in the sickroom. The care of the patient will depend upon the stage of the disease; and rest, good food, and fresh air are the usual requirements. Since tuberculosis is characterized by copious secretion and expectoration, the safe disposal of sputum and the disinfection of hands are the most important protective measures. Any

article used by the patient or in his room must be disinfected. The family of the tuberculous patient should guard against all the things which lower natural immunity and vitality, such as inadequate diet, fatigue, and exposure to respiratory infections such as colds, measles, and influenza. Also the family members should have periodic physical examinations. A slight daily rise of temperature, usually in the afternoon, and a gradual loss of weight and strength are characteristic features of early infection. These symptoms often precede definite lung symptoms such as cough or expectoration. Tuberculosis is discussed in greater detail in Chapter 5: "The Respiratory System."

When a child is sick

When a child becomes ill, he should be put to bed immediately. It is especially important to watch for symptoms such as rashes, temperature, loss of appetite, and irritability. It will help the physician in diagnosing the disease if he knows how it began. The care of a sick child is different from that of the older patient. All medicines, antiseptic solutions, etc., must be kept out of the sickroom or at least out of the patient's reach. The greatest difference, however, is in the patient's mental approach to the illness itself. A child's initial attitude toward illness is fear and a feeling of loneliness. The young patient must be attended constantly at first to offset the feelings that the world is treating him unfairly. However, if the stay in bed is to be of long duration, the child can be gradually brought to occupying many hours with some simple game. Puzzles, crayons, cutouts, and magazines are interesting. A long stay in bed will be less lonely if the child has a doll or toy to share the sick bed, and if the child goes through the motions of treating the "sick" toy. Records and a radio are helpful and not tiring.

A child's temperature is taken rectally, and if the child is very young, the temperature is normally one degree higher than an adult's. The rates of the pulse and respiration are also higher in children. The physician will tell the home nurse what rates are normal for the age of the sick child.

When a child is bedridden with a chronic, long-term disease such as rheumatic fever, it may be necessary to teach him at home. The physician can request a home visiting teacher through the local school board. The physician can give specific instructions as to activities permitted. The local school board and the state department of education share the expense of home teaching in most communities. Home teaching not only provides instruction but also gives the patient a sense of security and accomplishment.

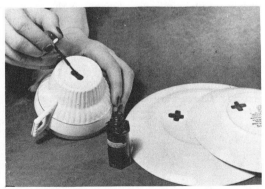

To prevent the spread of a contagious disease, the patient's dishes may be clearly marked with nail polish. *Copyright 1950, The American Home.*

CHRONIC ILLNESS

The term chronic illness is used to denote a prolonged disease process. Many chronic diseases are slowly progressive, and after arrest of the acute phase, there is never complete restoration to normal. The very length of time required for treatment of chronic illness creates many financial, social, and emotional problems. When the patient is the family wage-earner, the financial problems are greatly magnified. Either he must adjust to his illness and find a means of continuing to earn money, or other members of the family must provide for themselves and the patient. If neither alternative is possible, then assistance can be sought from community agencies. Emotional problems arise from the readjustment that must be made by the patient and his family. The chronically ill patient often develops attitudes of dependency and insecurity. With some understanding of the natural fears, irritability, discouragement, and loneliness which a chronically ill patient may feel, his family and friends can help him through his illness. Sometimes the patient and the family cannot make the adjustments by themselves. In such instances, both public and private social agencies, guidance clinics, psychiatrists, or vocational rehabilitation agencies can be consulted.

The aged patient

The aged patient is especially sensitive to cold and needs extra protection from chilling. The elderly patient's room may require extra heat and should always be protected from drafts. Adequate bedding and clothing should be provided. The aged patient must be protected from accidents, especially falls. With advancing age, there may be impairment of sight, hearing, and muscular co-ordination. Special safety devices such as handrails, adequate lighting, and protection on slippery surfaces may be needed. As in all illness, the home nurse should encourage independence as far as strength and safety permit. The aged patient should be helped to find some activity to occupy his time and prevent loneliness. Feelings of security are engendered by developing a hobby, and participating in family affairs.

The home nurse should give special attention to cleanliness. Elderly persons frequently develop excessive dryness of the skin. A daily rub with a light oil or lotion will relieve discomfort and help to prevent bed sores. A certain amount of exercise is necessary. Unless the physician prescribes otherwise, the patient should move around as much as possible. A wheelchair should be used to give the invalid a change of scene.

The home nurse should maintain a consistent daily schedule in caring for the aged patient. This will make it easier to accomplish housekeeping and nursing duties. Also, it prevents the aged person from feeling that he is neglected.

The diabetic patient

Diabetes is a long-term ailment which may occur in mild or severe form. The physician or visiting nurse will teach the home nurse or the patient how to give insulin injections and how to make a urine test. It is important that insulin injections be given in the proper dose and at the proper time to prevent shock. The home nurse should do everything possible to prevent bed sores or any abrasion of the skin. The diabetic patient is particularly susceptible to infection, and healing of the skin is often slow. The home nurse should never apply a heating pad or hot water bag except on specific instructions of the physician, as diabetics may be sensitive to heat. Adhesive tape should never be applied directly to the skin. The home nurse should give particular care to the patient's feet. Inflammation or discoloration of the feet should be reported to the physician immediately. Care of the diabetic patient is discussed further in Chapter 10, "The Endocrine System: *The Pancreas.*"

Heart disease

The bedridden heart patient must exert himself as little as possible. The home nurse must anticipate every need in order to spare the cardiac patient from unnecessary movement. The physician will give the home nurse special instructions regarding medication, bathing, and what to do in emergency. The patient's position should be adjusted so that he can breathe easily. Extra pillows, back and knee rests, and other aids can be used. The home nurse should see to it that the bed coverings are not too heavy. The patient should be helped to achieve a relaxed attitude and to avoid excesses in food and activity. Visitors should not be admitted without the doctor's permission, as conversation may be too tiring for the cardiac patient. The use of stimulants such as coffee, tea, and certain soft drinks is usually forbidden. The various heart disorders are discussed in Chapter 7, "The Heart and Circulation."

REHABILITATION

When the patient is pronounced convalescent by the physician, it means the acute phase of illness is over. During the period of recovery the duties of the home nurse will be lightened. When a patient reaches convalescence, he may become overambitious. An adult may want to rush immediately back to normal activities. The home nurse therefore must prevent the over-eager patient from straining himself. In contrast to the patient who is excited about recovery is the convalescent who has become depressed and discouraged about getting well. An adult who has been bedridden for a long time may be disturbed about the expense and time lost, and may lack the courage to face life and resume his ordinary responsibilities.

Nursing the convalescent patient will require scheduled treatments and meals, a daily bath which the patient can gradually take himself, and assistance in whatever activities he is allowed. The physician's visits will be less frequent, but instructions should be followed just as stringently during convalescence as during the acute phase. Medications and equipment which are no longer needed should be removed and the sickroom restored to normal as far as possible.

Rehabilitation does not begin after the patient gets well, but should be planned and begun while the patient is bedridden. The home nurse should seek expert advice about available resources for physical rehabilitation. The use of physical therapy is especially important in overcoming the complications of crippling illnesses. There are many types of physical treatment, including heat lamps, light therapy, diathermy, massage, hydrotherapy, and walking and posture exercises. Physical therapy is given on the prescription of the physician. The prescription is checked often and changed when necessary. Treatment must be given by a registered, graduate therapist. Most hospitals have physical therapy department which can treat outpatients, and many community agencies have therapists who visit the homes of patients to give treatments. The use of special appliances and devices prescribed by the physician can often help the patient overcome his disabilities.

Recreational facilities

After the acute phase of illness is past, it is important to prevent boredom. The recreational facilities of which the patient can take advantage, during convalescence, will depend almost entirely upon the nature of his illness.

Although activity may be greatly limited, even the slightest diversions such as light handwork, reading, and writing letters should be utilized.

In the case of chronically ill children, there are numerous special schools and clinics whose major purpose is to teach children how to play to the fullest extent and for the greatest enjoyment possible with their limitations. Adults usually face a greater problem if they are house-confined. Provision should be made for frequent visits by friends, and the diversions of a radio and a suitable hobby are time-consumers that provide some measure of recreation.

The individual with physical handicaps should be checked thoroughly for any defects of hearing or vision. If such are found to exist they should be corrected as nearly and as quickly possible. Poor vision or hearing, in addition to reduced physical activity, can force the patient into a void in which there is little possibility for any type of recreation.

Occupational therapy

Occupational therapy is a comparatively new field of medical science and has become increasingly important in rehabilitation during the last few years. Thousands of handicapped persons must be cared for at home. Patients crippled by accidents, persons born with defects, and the chronically ill must be helped to find suitable constructive activities. The home nurse, by use of common sense, may be able to help the disabled person find a new pursuit. Whenever possible, occupational therapy should be undertaken in terms of established interests. The first requirement of the new occupation is that it be within the ability of the patient. Most individuals may discover latent talents which they have never had the opportunity to develop. The matter of financial return is also important when the patient feels that he is a financial burden upon his family or society. Even the smallest additional income which can be provided by the patient will contribute to his self-respect.

A change in occupation for the patient may require reeducation along new lines. He may first have to attend a trade school, business school, or college. In many instances of long-term disability, it may be practical for the patient to take a university extension or correspondence course which can be followed at home. Various state and national organizations provide scholarships for this purpose. (For further information on this subject, see Chapter 9, "The Skeleton and Muscles," and Chapter 17, "The Eye,": *The Blind, Their Care and Opportunities.*)

Occupation for the chronically ill patient depends in many instances on the attitude of his family and friends. Honest encouragement may mean a great deal to the patient, but if encouragement is misguided, the patient will feel keen disappointment if he fails. The nurse, the family, and the patient himself must study occupational plans before they are undertaken. Many universities and social agencies maintain guidance bureaus that give vocational and interest tests that help in determining abilities and talents.

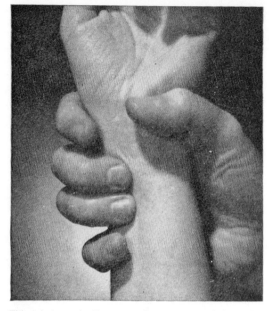

This photograph illustrates the proper technique for taking a patient's pulse, relying upon the finger rather than the thumb as a means of detecting it.

Many bedridden and seriously handicapped chronic invalids can be taught various handicrafts, such as sewing, knitting, weaving, modeling, and painting. Patients frequently prove to be enthusiastic workers but too often are unable to realize much income from their crafts. The problem lies almost entirely in finding a market for their wares. A number of social organizations maintain sales outlets for the products made by the chronically ill. Many communities provide workshops at rehabilitation centers for ambulatory patients. Handicapped persons often make better adjustments to their disabilities because of opportunities available to them in such centers.

NURSING FACILITIES

The amount of professional nursing required for the sick person at home will vary, depending upon the nature of the illness and the availability of registered nurses. If a full-time registered nurse is required, the physician will usually prefer that the patient be hospitalized. If this is not possible, for financial or other reasons, there remain a number of alternatives.

In most cities there are two types of professional nursing services available to the individual or family on a community basis. The Public Health Nurse is paid by the county or city while the Visiting Nurse is frequently supported by the United Fund. Both of these groups are staffed by professional registered nurses. Public Health Nursing in the home is primarily concerned with case reporting, teaching, and demonstrating nursing techniques. In the event of a reportable disease, the Public Health Nurse usually visits the home and in cooperation with the physician gives instruction in the home regarding skilled nursing care and special techniques. If further help is needed, one of the voluntary nursing services usually is called in to perform the actual bedside nursing.

There are over 8,000 Visiting Nurse Associations in the United States. These nurses are available for regular visits to the home. Any attending physician may request the services of these associations to give instructions and special nursing to a private patient. Thus, both Public Health Nursing and voluntary professional nursing are available to the physician in carrying out phases of treatment which the home nurse is not able to do. In addition to this, the visiting nurses instruct the family or home nurse. Although most of these associations are supported in part by the community, families of moderate or good income may be charged a small fee if they are in a position to pay. The name and address of the local Visiting Nurse Association can be obtained from the city health department.

Public Health Nursing is an integral part of the whole community health, medical, educational, and social welfare program. The Public

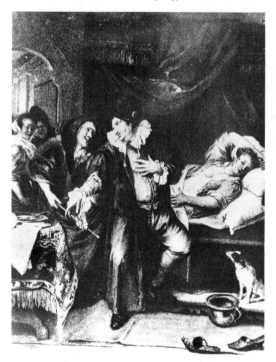

Reproduction of old painting by Jan Steen (1626-1679) entitled *The Sick Girl*, showing the appearance of an early sick room. *Bettmann Archive.*

Health Nurse is engaged in such services as health supervision, maternity service, industrial nursing, special immunization programs, and case-finding surveys. In many rural areas there are no health agencies, and the Public Health Nurse may be the only source of professional nursing service.

In many types and stages of illnesses a practical nurse is desirable. Hospitals for chronic and mentally ill patients have long depended on an attendant or practical nursing type of care. Persons ill at home often need and seek practical nursing care. They cannot afford the cost of professional nurses except for short intervals during acute illness or on a visit basis. Furthermore, in most sickness at home, professional nursing is unnecessary. The demand for qualified, practical nurses, trained for home or hospital service and licensed by the state to practice, has exceeded the supply in recent years. If professional help is needed by the practical nurse in the home, the attending physician can arrange for a professional Visiting Nurse Service to provide supervision and instruction.

In addition to practical nurses, another aid in sickness at home is the visiting housekeeper. A visiting housekeeper, supplied and supervised by a recognized welfare agency, often can supplement professional nursing and assume some of its simpler duties. Many communities have had such services for years. The housekeepers are trained by home economists, dieticians, and professional nurses to perform housekeeping and elementary nursing duties.

Medicare hospital insurance benefits help cover the cost of part-time nursing care. They also help pay for such items as physical, occupational, or speech therapy, part-time services of home health aides, medical social services, medical supplies furnished by the participating home health agency, and use of medical appliances. Full-time nursing care is not paid for by Medicare, nor are drugs and biologicals, personal comfort or convenience items, custodial care, or meals-on-wheels. The local Social Security Administration office should be contacted for complete information on eligibility and benefits.

23 PHYSICAL INJURIES AND FIRST AID

GENERAL CONSIDERATIONS

First aid may be defined as the immediate and temporary assistance given to a sick or an injured person before the services of a physician can be secured. In some instances, this immediate assistance may save a life. In any emergency, proper use of first aid techniques relieves suffering and assists the physician by preparing the patient to receive medical treatment.

Accidents and sudden illness occur without warning and it is important to know the proper thing to do if first aid is necessary. It is equally important to know what *not* to do.

The need for first aid

The need for first aid is very evident when one considers the opportunities for its daily use. The National Safety Council reported that 115,000 persons were killed in accidents during 1969 and that 11,000,000 more were disabled from injuries.

The statistics indicate that being "safe at home" is an inaccurate aphorism, since millions of accidents occur annually in American homes. Among the causes of home injuries, falls are by far the most common, then burns, followed by suffocation and poisoning. In industry, the handling of objects is the source of most injuries, followed by falls, machinery accidents, and falling objects.

These figures certainly indicate the need for widespread first aid training. Knowing how to find immediate medical aid may mean saving life or preventing permanent disability.

Purposes of first aid

Serious injuries and accidents usually happen where no professional medical assistance is readily available. Whether in the city, country, or on the highway, it may take considerable time to find medical help. Therefore, it is essential that every individual have a thorough knowledge of the basic rules of first aid *before* an emergency occurs.

There are three main purposes of first aid training. *First*, it enables the individual to determine the nature and extent of an injury. This does not mean that he will be able to make a full, accurate diagnosis that a physician can make; but it should enable him to make some intelligent decision as to the type of injury or illness occurring during an emergency. *Second*, first aid training enables the person to know the proper thing to do at the proper time, and also what not to do. *Third*, first aid training is one of the best means of preventing accidents. Obviously, the prevention of accidents is far more effective than first aid after damage has been inflicted. The American Red Cross, with its years of teaching and rendering of first aid has proved that accidents occur less frequently, and as a rule are less calamitous, among persons who have been trained in first aid. This is a logical result, since persons trained to understand the seriousness of injuries naturally keep in mind the possible causes of accidents and what should be done to prevent them. Emphasizing the importance of securing proper treatment will greatly enhance the success of any home safety program.

It is the responsibility of every individual to familiarize himself with the procedure to be followed in a critical situation and to teach such procedures to his children. Every family should have a first aid kit and a good first aid manual, such as the latest Red Cross Manual of First Aid, for ready reference. A chart of the poisons and their antidotes should be pasted to the medicine cabinet or in a handy place. Classes for first aid training are available from the Red Cross. Today, schools, the armed forces, the Boy and Girl Scouts of America, Camp Fire Girls, and many industries have classes in emergency aid. Civil defense organizations also educate citizens concerning first aid measures during natural disasters and warfare.

General directions in case of emergency

Common sense rules apply to any injury or illness. The "do not" rules are as important as the "do" instructions. The following considerations will be of help in emergencies arising from many different causes. Each treatment is given in further detail in this chapter.

Look for stoppage of breath: If the patient has stopped breathing from any cause, mouth-to-mouth respiration is the immediate treatment. Check pulse for presence, strength, and rapidity. If the patient has a blue color in his face, begin artificial respiration immediately, making sure nothing is blocking the airway. This can be done by a quick sweep of the finger around the mouth and down the throat.

Look for bleeding: Remove only enough clothing to ascertain the possible extent of the injury. It is preferable to cut clothing away, as removing clothes in the usual manner may cause pain and aggravate the injury. Stop bleeding by applying pressure directly to the wound. A tourniquet can be made above the injury if bleeding occurs in the arms and legs.

Look for medical tag: People with chronic illness often wear a tag around their necks, wrists, or ankles. Check wallet or purse for a card that might identify the illness.

Summon medical aid: Send someone to call the police and ambulance as soon as possible. Every city police force (and in some communities, the fire department) has a rescue and first aid unit with mechanical resuscitators, drugs, and trained first aid personnel. The first page of the telephone book has information on how to call the emergency rescue and ambulance units.

Keep the patient lying down: This prevents fainting and may help prevent development of *shock,* which will be discussed later. If the patient is vomiting, turn his head so that he will not become choked.

Keep the patient warm: This is also important in preventing shock. In cold weather, it is important that the patient be wrapped to cover under as well as over the body.

Never try to get an unconscious person to drink any liquid: Water or liquid stimulants should be withheld, since fluids may enter the windpipe and cause strangling.

Do not move the patient unless it is absolutely necessary: This is especially important in the event of injury; if it is necessary that the patient be moved, be certain that the method of moving him will not cause further injury. This is particularly important if a fracture of extremity or spine is present. Tests for such injuries are part of every first aid course and prevent complications that are hazardous to recovery or even to life.

Reassure the patient: Be reluctant to make a diagnosis to the patient or to bystanders. Before medical help arrives, the person rendering first aid should endeavor to maintain a composed and efficient attitude. Gaining the patient's confidence promotes his co-operation and aids his recovery by lessening the degree of shock. It is important to allay his fears, and also, in severe cases, it is important not to let him know the seriousness of his condition. Unless the patient is so reassured, he may become erratic in behavior and may even try to run away. This kind of violent action can, of course, be fatal to an injured person. In addition, by soothing and calming the patient, the person giving first aid may also overcome his own natural excitement or worry over the situation.

It is important to remember that first aid is only *first* aid, and in all but slight injuries or minor illnesses, the patient should be seen by a physician at the earliest possible moment. In addition to calling the police, or emergency ambulance, the patient's regular physician should be contacted. Prompt notification of the patient's family may avoid much confusion, since the family will know which physician to call. Furthermore, the family should be notified in any event, and should be advised as to where the patient is and whether he has been taken to a hospital.

The first aid helper should be prepared to give complete information concerning the emergency. The exact location of the patient; the extent of injury or nature of illness; what medical supplies are available at the site; and what first aid measures have been taken.

An injured person or a seriously ill person may be taken directly to a hospital. However, many hospitals do not maintain emergency service; the ambulance driver will know which hospitals do have such stations. Even those hospitals which maintain this service will admit only actual *emergencies* without the attendance of a physician. Therefore, in preparation for possible sudden illness which may not be of an emergency nature but which may require the services of a physician, it behooves the individual to be able to obtain assistance from some known physician. Much distress and confusion will be avoided if every individual and family has access to a personal, private physician upon whom they may call in time of emergency.

How to find a physician: A doctor can usually be found through the local medical exchange, a public service of the county medical society. The exchange lists all doctors in a community, their specialities, and which ones are available for emergencies. The exchange also is in contact with ambulance services. These bureaus can be located in the yellow pages of the telephone directory under the section devoted to "Physicians and Surgeons," usually displayed in a prominent place. These organizations are affiliated with the American Medical Association and offer their information free of charge.

Throughout this chapter, at the end of most sections are *"Do"* and *"Don't"* tables which contain short, easy-to-follow directions for quick reference.

First aid kits

A good first aid kit should be kept at home and in the automobile. The automobile kit need not be elaborate, but should be ample to allow treatment of several injuries. Around the house, first aid equipment is usually scattered and not readily available. A definite amount of first aid material should be kept in a metal box of convenient size, preferably in or near the medicine cabinet. Such an arrangement will keep bandages clean and safe to use.

A good first aid kit should contain most of the following articles:

1-inch compresses or adhesives.
Gauze squares—about 4″ x 4″ in individual sterile packages
Sterile triangular bandages
Burn ointment—nonoily, such as anesthetic jelly
Mild solution of iodine or mercurial antiseptic
Aromatic spirits of ammonia
A tourniquet
Scissors
Splinter forceps
2-inch roller bandages
Roll of adhesive tape
Roll of absorbent cotton
70% alcohol
List of poisons and antidotes
Snake antivenom for camping
Disposable sterile knife

How to transport the injured

In most situations requiring first aid, there is little problem involved in moving the patient to a place where he may receive medical treatment. Often the patient is able to walk, or he can be transported by ambulance. In serious accidents, it is always best *not to move the patient* until the ambulance arrives. Improper methods of moving an injured person may increase the severity of the injury and can even cause death. In many cases of automobile accidents, the patient is literally tossed into the first available automobile and driven at break-neck speed to the nearest hospital. This is a serious mistake and can result in death.

When moving an injured person, the rescuer must first think, *is this move necessary?* Then

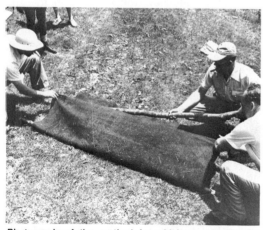

Photograph of the method by which a stretcher for carrying an injured person may be improvised. Use is made of a blanket which is properly folded over two wooden poles.

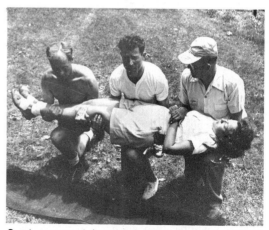

Great care must be exercised in placing an injured person on a stretcher. This photograph shows the approved method. *Courtesy of the American National Red Cross.*

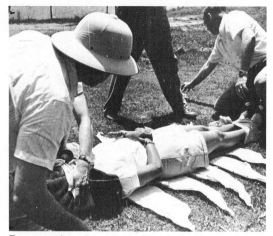

Transportation of a patient with a broken neck requires expert attention. The proper positioning of the body may be assured by securing the patient to a wooden plank.

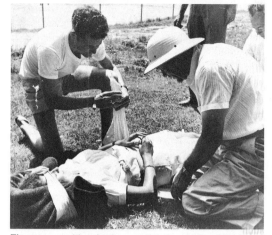

The person with a broken neck is immobilized by being bound to the board at several places. Hand towels make good bindings. *Courtesy American National Red Cross.*

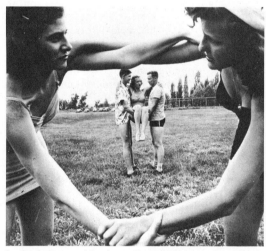

In the foreground is shown the proper method of interlocking arms for a two-man carry of an ill or injured person; the patient in a swing is shown in background.

the patient should be checked for all possible fractures. If a limb or bone may be broken, construct a splint so that there will be no movement of the injured part during transport. The rule is, *splint them where they lie.*

Occasionally accident or illness may occur far from the source of medical treatment, for example on hunting or fishing trips. In such instances *the kind of transportation should be determined by the injury.* In general, a stretcher is the desired method of carrying seriously ill or injured patients.

Short-distance transfer

When a rescue must be made from an accident such as a wrecked car, house, or place of

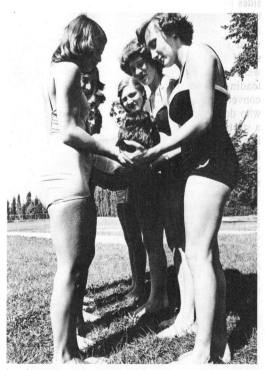

In circumstances under which strong people are not available to carry a heavier person, the eight-man carry is used. *Courtesy American National Red Cross.*

danger, the victim should be pulled to safety in the direction of the long axis of his body. He should never be lifted by head and heels (jack-knifed) or pulled upward by his belt. He should never be pulled sideways. The victim's entire body should be kept on a straight line and moved as a unit.

If the rescuer is alone and unable to use a stretcher, the injured person can be pulled carefully onto a blanket after splinting and first aid. The blanket is then wrapped around the patient and he is dragged to safety, with the rescuer pulling the blanket in an axis with the victim's head and spine. This method is the *blanket drag*. It can be dangerous unless carried out on very smooth ground and with great caution. It can also be used to transport an ill person from bed to a car or truck.

Long-distance transfer

The best method for moving an injured or ill person is a stretcher, cot, or large board (a door). A simple stretcher can be made by using two poles and a blanket. Articles of clothing such as shirts, skirts, or trousers may also be wound around poles if a blanket is not available. When no poles can be found, a stretcher may be made by placing the patient in the middle of a blanket and rolling the edges toward him. Then, several rescuers must stand on both sides to pull the blanket taut. This requires four to eight people all pulling on the blanket up and away from the victim. Whatever type of improvised stretcher is made, it should be tested to see if it is strong enough to bear the patient's weight. Extreme caution should be exercised in loading, carrying, and unloading a stretcher. A convenient method of carrying an ill person who does not have a wound or fracture without a stretcher is to seat the patient in a chair. This is particularly useful in carrying a patient to another floor level, where a stretcher cannot be used because of narrow, winding stairways or small elevators.

In some cases a patient may be able to support part of his own weight if one of his arms is placed around the neck of another person, who then offers further support by placing his hand under the patient's other arm. In the *pick-a-back* carry, the patient is transported on the carrier's back with his legs held through the carrier's arms, and his arms slung crosswise around the carrier's neck and held by the latter's hands.

In the *fireman's carry* the patient is carried with his torso across the carrier's shoulders. The patient's body is held in place by the carrier encircling one of the patient's legs and grasping the patient's arm which is thrown over his shoulder. By alternating one or several of these methods with frequent periods of rest, it is possible to cover a considerable distance even when the victim is a fairly heavy person.

Moving major fractures

The utmost care must be taken in moving patients with head, spine, pelvis, or major body injuries. If at all possible, do not move them. Only when medical help is not available for many hours or days should such patients be moved. In cases of spinal or head injuries, a soft stretcher or blanket should not be used. A board, such as a door, or several planks lashed together are the best stretchers.

The rescuer should try to enlist as many people as he can find to help him, instructing them to be as careful as possible. If six or more helpers are there, they should carefully insert their hands and arms under the patient until the hands are adjacent to the hands of the person opposite, so that all hands are in an alternating position forming a straight line from shoulders to heels. One person must hold the head and neck. If only three helpers are available, they should all stand on the same side.

To place the patient on the stretcher or board, all helpers must lift at the same time, holding the patient's legs as well. The head and neck must remain immobile. The patient should be lifted only enough to allow the slow insertion of a board, plank, or door under the patient. Any available cloth can be made into strips to lash the victim to the stretcher. In cases of head, neck, or spinal injuries the head should be gently but firmly tied to the board and sandbags or some kind of buffer placed around the head to keep it immobile.

People who have injuries of the pelvis, thigh, leg, arm, or torso should never be transported sitting up in a car. If a patient is being carried in a car or truck, the trip should be made as smooth and comfortable as possible.

COMMON AND UNCOMMON EMERGENCIES

Simple fainting is a common occurrence requiring first aid. The immediate cause of fainting is an insufficient supply of blood to the brain. Fainting may be the result of confinement in a close and poorly ventilated room, hunger, fatigue, severe pain, emotional shock, and many other causes.

If the person feels that he is about to faint, the best thing to do is have him lie down immediately. If this is not possible, have him bend forward at the waist with his head between his knees.

To give first aid to a person who has fainted, keep the patient lying down and loosen any tight clothing. The patient's head should be lowered or the legs should be elevated. Either procedure will help to increase the supply of blood to the brain. After the patient has regained consciousness, he may be given a stimulant such as coffee or spirits of ammonia. Even letting the patient smell spirits of ammonia may help to restore consciousness and normal circulation.

When the cause of unconsciousness is unknown, the first aider can give some care, depending on the type of unconsciousness. In "red" unconsciousness, the face is flushed and the pulse is strong. The patient should be placed in a lying position with the head and shoulders slightly elevated. Cold applications should be placed on the head. After the patient regains consciousness, *no* stimulants should be given.

In "white" unconsciousness, the face is pale, the skin is clammy, and the pulse is weak. The patient should be kept in a lying position with the head lowered. The patient should be adequately covered to insure warmth. The patient should not be given liquid stimulants, but inhalation stimulants may be used.

Common causes of unconsciousness are apoplexy (stroke), alcoholism, skull fracture, shock, sunstroke, heat exhaustion, poisoning, and diabetes or insulin shock.

In case of unconsciousness, treat according to type

In "RED" unconsciousness:
Chief symptoms: red or flushed face and strong pulse.
Treatment: lay the patient down; raise his head slightly; keep the patient quiet. Apply cold applications to his head. Loosen clothing. Give no stimulants—use just enough cover to keep the patient warm.

In "WHITE" unconsciousness:
Chief symptoms: pale face, weak pulse.
Treatment: keep patient quiet, in lying position with head slightly lowered. Apply heat. Give no liquid stimulants, but an inhalation stimulant such as ammonia may be used if there is no bleeding nor head injury.

In "BLUE" unconsciousness:
Treatment: if breathing has ceased, apply artificial respiration. Turn head to side, check with finger to see if the airway is clear; keep patient covered warmly.

Convulsions

Convulsions are never as terrifying as old wive's tales make them seem. The patient usually loses muscular control in a shaking movement, his eyelids flutter, and he may fall to the ground. Convulsions of themselves are not fatal. Since epilepsy is not a disease but a sign of any of several possible disorders, there is no single treatment. Convulsions rarely occur in people who are taking the proper daily medication. People whose disorders are under control drive automobiles, enjoy active sports, have no limita-

tion on their employment, and live long lives. Their main obstacle is the superstition of others.

If someone with an improperly controlled disorder has a convulsion, the patient should be helped by placing a firm but soft object between his teeth, such as a wallet or a folded washcloth. Never use a spoon or a stick since the contractions of the jaw muscles may cause the patient to injure himself on sharp objects. Loosen clothing around the neck. As soon as the convulsion has stopped, make sure with your finger that the tongue has not been swallowed and is blocking the airway. Keep the wallet between the patient's teeth at one side while you do this.

Care should be taken to avoid embarrassing the patient. If he is in a public place, the police will help move him to his home. If he is at home, let him lie where he is until he gains consciousness. Patients with convulsions often fall into sleep and are confused if awakened. Do not give any stimulants. Check to see if the patient has a medical tag or card with instructions to call a doctor.

Febrile convulsions sometimes occur in children with high fevers. A cool sponge bath may be given after the convulsions have ceased. Usually convulsions stop spontaneously. Poison can cause convulsions of a dangerous kind. If a child has a convulsion, check to see what he may have ingested.

Heart failure

Heart failure is a condition which frequently requires first aid. Usually there is no unconsciousness. The symptoms of heart failure vary, depending upon the cause. For practical purposes of first aid, the symptoms may be divided into three main types.

Heart failure resembling fainting: The patient may be conscious, the face pale, and the pulse weak. If no pain is present about the heart, the condition is distinguished from simple fainting by the failure to recover fairly quickly after lying down.

Heart failure characterized by pain: The patient may have an agonizing pain in the region of the heart, usually behind the breast bone (*sternum*) rather than on the left side. The pain may also go down the left arm. The patient is usually conscious and very apprehensive.

Heart failure characterized by shortness of breath: These patients cannot lie down and often there is congestion of the face. They are usually conscious and insist upon sitting up, leaning forward in order to breathe.

Treatment: The first two types of patients should be kept quiet and in a lying position. In the third type of heart failure, the patient should be propped up to allow him to breathe. If he insists on sitting up, he should be allowed to do so. With these exceptions, the first aid treatment is the same for all types. The patient's physician should be called or an emergency call to the police should be made. A stimulant, such as spirits of ammonia, tea, or coffee may be given. The patient should be covered to insure warmth. Keep the patient quiet and do not let him add to the strain on his heart by unnecessary motion. If the patient carries medicine for his attack, assist him in taking it. If the medicine is a vial, break it so he can breathe it.

Medical help must be sent for immediately. Police departments in many cities have access to special mobile coronary units that are set up to rush aid to a heart attack victim. If the patient becomes unconscious, mouth-to-mouth resuscitation should be tried if he is not breathing or is not able to inspire air.

If the heart collapses completely, the patient loses respiration, the pulse stops in all major blood vessels, and his pupils become dilated. In case of collapse, mouth-to-mouth artificial respiration should be given along with external cardiac massage.

To give cardiac massage, the patient must be placed on a firm surface such as the floor. If the rescuer is alone, the patient's lungs should be filled with three or four rapid mouth-to-mouth respirations before attempting to massage. Ideally, both artificial respiration and massage are performed at the same time by two rescuers. There is no need to co-ordinate the two activities between the rescuers. In massage, the rescuer puts one hand across the lower sternum (breastbone) of the patient. The other hand is placed on top to make a right angle. The full weight of the rescuer is applied rhythmically through the heel of the hands, at about one thrust per second. The sternum moves in about four or five centimeters, compressing the heart. When pressure is lifted, blood reenters the heart. If the rescuer is alone, several rapid mouth-to-mouth respirations should be given to the patient every 30 seconds.

If massage is successful, gasping and some movement may occur and the pupils will constrict. If no signs of reviving occur after three to four minutes, a sharp blow to the sternum should be tried. In any case, artificial respiration and external massage should be continued until medical help arrives.

Choking

Choking is caused when the act of swallowing becomes interrupted, by bone or food particles that will not dissolve. Although the obstruction is usually not total, a violent fit of coughing may be provoked. It is better for a person to cough up the obstruction than to pry the offending material loose with his fingers. Fingers may only force the blockage further down the larynx. Often a very sharp blow between the shoulders will dislodge the object. If the patient is a child or a small person, he may be picked up by the feet with the head held downward, and slapped sharply on the back.

If the airway is blocked, a *stridor* (a thin, shrill noise) may result which is loud enough to be heard across a room. The patient becomes *cyanosed* (turns blue) and becomes violent in his efforts to breathe, straining his neck and chest muscles. The victim's head and neck should be extended and the jaw pulled forward, as in mouth-to-mouth artificial respiration. This may free the obstruction. If breathing does not begin immediately, attempt mouth-to-mouth respiration. If the lungs do not inflate, the airway is totally blocked.

In cases of complete blockage, medical aid must arrive within four to seven minutes to be of help. *If all other methods have been tried to clear the airway and no help is near*, the skilled first aid practitioner can resort to opening the trachea. This can be done with little risk to the patient if the rescuer knows the proper procedure.

With the patient lying down, his head and neck extended (a helper's leg under the patient's neck will cause the patient's head to fall back, making the outline of the trachea clear), the airway can be established by locating with the fingers the *cricothyroid membrane*. It is in the middle of the neck between the two "bumps" of the larynx. It is the best place for puncture since there is little overlying tissue and chance of mismanagement is small. The space between the two "bumps" is larger in men than in women. The carotid artery and the jugular vein are not near the cricothyroid membrane. A sharp instrument should be used. There is no time to sterilize the instrument. It should be larger than a needle. A sharp kitchen knife or scissors will do. First, a one-inch incision should be made across the area between the two "bumps," to open the skin. If a scissors is used, the skin can be pinched up and cut. By placing his hand coming *down* the skin of the throat, the rescuer can then feel with his finger the U-shaped membrane through the incision in the skin. By pressing the index finger against the membrane and placing the other fingers on the sides of the windpipe, outside the incision, the instrument is guided to the point just at the end of the index finger. To puncture, the rescuer pushes the nail firmly into the membrane and slides the instrument over the nail into the membrane. The airway is opened by spreading the scissors blades in the wound, or turning the knife halfway around. Air may hiss out and coughing may start. The opening must be maintained until a doctor or ambulance arrives by putting a pen barrel (cut at both ends), tubing, a plastic straw, or even a couple of keys in the incision. Bleeding can be controlled by pressure or by packing the skin area with gauze. Keep the patient quiet and calm until medical help takes over. *This is strictly a life-saving procedure.*

Bleeding

This has been discussed in a previous section. See page 691.

Pain in the abdomen

Pain in the abdomen may be caused by a variety of disorders, many of which may be serious. Whenever there is persistent abdominal pain, tenderness, nausea or vomiting, appendicitis or obstruction should be suspected. *Never give a laxative to anyone having abdominal pain,* as the action of a laxative may cause the appendix to rupture, or an obstruction to become worse. Give nothing by mouth but water until the pain stops or until medical aid is obtained. If abdominal pains are severe and then suddenly cease, this may signify that the appendix has actually ruptured. Abdominal pain may not mean appendicitis; is is also a symptom of other disorders.

Hysteria

Danger, exhaustion, or tension may result in a state of *hysteria*. Two types of hysteria may be encountered. The first is a kind of tantrum, in which the patient cries, shouts, walks aimlessly about, cries for help, or may even attack his friends. The second type is a local or general paralysis, in which the patient may not talk or move or does not hear what is being said to him. There are many variations to the examples given.

First aid treatment of hysteria will, of course, depend upon the severity of the attack. If the patient is violent, he must be restrained to prevent endangering himself or others. In mild attacks of laughing or crying an abrupt action, such as throwing water in the face or a mild slap, may suffice. Ordinarily, however, the person rendering first aid will succeed better if he does not display hostility. The "crying child" attitude of a hysterical person seeks paternal help, not rebuff. Most persons can be quieted by simple means such as giving aspirin, coffee, or hot soup. These measures are really distractions. Occasionally, the hysterical person who seems to be paralyzed may respond to spirits of ammonia. After the patient recovers, he should rest or, preferably, sleep in a quiet room. If the symptoms are severe, relief is beyond the scope of first aid measures.

Nosebleed

Nosebleed may occur frequently in children. To give first aid, apply wet cloths over the nose. Pressing the nostrils together firmly often stops the bleeding and allows a clot to form. The pressure must be applied for four or five minutes to be effective. If the bleeding does not stop, take the patient to an emergency room of a hospital or clinic, or directly to a doctor. If the patient is in an area remote from a physician, pack the nostrils with strips of gauze bandage, taking care that at least an inch of the pack is left outside the nose. This packing should be done very gently. Never put the head in such a position that the blood will back up and go down the throat and thus not be seen. The bleeding is usually from one side and from the *septum* (middle partition). If the nosebleed victim has a history of heart disease or anemia, medical attention is urgent.

Hiccough

Hiccough or "hiccups" is a spasm of the diaphragm (the broad muscle that separates the chest cavity from the abdomen) caused by irritation of the *phrenic* nerve which controls it. Mild attacks of hiccough often may be stopped by holding the breath or slowly drinking a glass of cold water. Breathing into a paper bag will accumulate carbon dioxide which may prove effective in stopping the hiccough. Hiccoughs may become painful if they are prolonged over a period of time and are exhausting. In extreme cases, when hiccoughs persist for several hours, it may become necessary to hospitalize the patient.

Motion sickness

Motion sickness is a common occurrence in everyday life. Children are affected by "swing" sickness and motion sickness induced by various amusement devices. Adults and children are subject to this disagreeable condition by riding in automobiles, ships, trains, elevators, and aircraft. Probably the most notable and extensive investigation of motion sickness was carried out during World War II, when "Operation Seasickness" was made in 1948. From this and other experiments, the drug *Dramamine* was found to relieve symptoms of seasickness in a large number of instances. Another drug which is helpful in motion sickness is *Benadryl*.

Airsickness is an illness which is similar to seasickness, car sickness, swing sickness, and train sickness. While airsickness may occur during straight and level flight, it is noticed most frequently while flying through turbulent or "bumpy" air. Other factors which have an influence on the incidence of airsickness are emotional upsets such as fear or sorrow. Hot, humid, or ill-ventilated cabins or the presence of disagreeable odors may cause an attack of airsickness to develop (tobacco smoke is particularly bad). Airsickness is also brought on by digestive upsets, overindulgence in food or drink, or hunger. Infants practically never become airsick. The symptoms of airsickness are nausea, pallor, "cold" perspiration on the forehead, and, in severe cases, vomiting.

Recently, a number of excellent airsickness remedies have been developed and may be procured through the physician. The prescribed dose is best taken about one-half hour prior to a flight and may be repeated if necessary as directed by the physician. Other means of preventing airsickness consist of keeping the cabin cool and well ventilated and preventing disagreeable odors from entering the aircraft.

Airsickness, while disagreeable, practically never results in any serious consequences and clears up without treatment soon after the airplane has landed. Most individuals who become airsick during the first few flights are much less susceptible to airsickness on subsequent flights, and may have little further difficulty.

Aero-otitis media

Aero-otitis media is the medical term used to describe a painful condition of the ears which may develop during descent from high altitude. The cause of this pain is a difference in the pressure inside the middle ear and the pressure of the surrounding atmosphere as the airplane descends, causing the eardrums to bulge inward. There is a small tube extending from the middle ear to the throat (*Eustachian tube*) which is normally closed. If this tube is opened frequently during descent, no pressure difference develops between the middle ear and the surrounding atmosphere; and no discomfort or pain results. To open this tube, swallow or open the mouth widely as in yawning. If this is not effective, one may close the nostrils with the fingers and blow gently with the lips closed. If it is found difficult to swallow during a long descent, this can be aided by chewing gum or by taking sips of a liquid.

If one is suffering from an ordinary cold or sore throat, the opening of the tube which connects the throat with the middle ear is usually swollen shut and it then becomes impossible to open it by the means described above. In this instance, one should not fly until the condition has been corrected or unless the altitude to be flown is not in excess of 5000 feet. Many physicians recommend that flight not be attempted by persons with colds, sore throats, or ear infections.

If the pressure in the middle ear is not or cannot be equalized during a descent of 5000 feet or more, the individual will suffer discomfort and, in many cases, rather severe pain in his ears. This discomfort or pain may last several hours or even a day or two after landing.

Usually the pain may be relieved by taking one or two aspirin tablets. If this is not effective, a physician should be consulted. However, the condition in most instances will clear up without treatment if given time. It almost never results in any permanent injury to the ear but recovery should be complete before another flight is attempted.

There is another condition similar to aero-otitis media which occurs when the openings of the sinuses are blocked. In these cases, discomfort or pain may occur either during ascent or descent, and the location of the pain will depend on which sinuses are affected. If it is the frontal sinuses, the pain will be just above and on the inner side of the eyes; if the sinuses in the cheek bones are involved, the pain will be in that region. The sinuses are seldom so involved; but when this condition occurs, relief can usually be obtained by spraying the nose with a solution, or using an inhaler containing a drug which shrinks the mucous membranes of the nose; this can be obtained through a physician.

Oxygen lack develops as one ascends to high altitude because the air becomes less dense; and, accordingly, there is a decreasing amount of oxygen available to the individual. Ordinarily this does not cause any noticeable effect until about 8000 to 10,000 feet altitude. Even then the symptoms normally experienced do not occur until after several hours are spent at those altitudes. The symptoms consist of a feeling of fatigue and a headache. If one ascends to higher altitudes, unconsciousness occurs at about 18,000 feet; and, at about 25,000 feet and above, death will result after a short period of time. However, neither of these latter possibilities need concern the average individual, since commercial flying is never carried out at these higher levels unless oxygen or a pressure cabin is used to protect the individual from these effects.

SHOCK

The term "shock" means a condition in which essential activities of the body are greatly depressed, especially the volume of circulating blood. The vessels become dilated and do not respond to nervous stimuli. Shock may be caused by pronounced loss of blood. Shock may occur during times of stress, strong emotion, injury, pain, sudden illness, and accident. If a state of shock continues over a period of only a few hours, it may be fatal or cause permanent damage to essential organs such as the brain.

Measures which *alleviate* the shock state are equally useful in preventing it in situations where shock is to be anticipated.

Shock may begin with a sudden or gradual feeling of unusual weakness or faintness. There may be an accompanying pallor. Perspiration is increased and the skin may feel cold and clammy. The pupils of the eyes become noticeably enlarged.

Shock is also accompanied by changes in the mental state and in the pulse beat. The shock patient's mental attitude follows a pattern, ranging from a feeling of restlessness in the beginning to a gradual loss of ability to respond to stimulation, and finally stupor and unconsciousness. The pulse may seem weak or almost imperceptible; yet, it may retain a regular rhythm. However, when shock is accompanied by (or caused by) loss of body fluids, as in hemorrhage or in cases of severe burns, the pulse rate is usually rapid. Shock is accompanied by myocardial depression and a depletion of the compound ATP (adenosine triphosphate) that aids heart contraction. The physician counteracts this by administering ATP to restock the depleted store and to stimulate heart action.

Symptoms and treatment of shock

The symptoms of shock are caused to a significant degree by the decrease of the volume of blood in effective circulation and to a lowering of the blood pressure. Decreased blood supply to the brain causes mental apathy and may eventually lead to unconsciousness. Lack of blood in the capillaries near the surface of the body accounts in part for the coldness of the skin; evaporation of unusual amounts of perspiration also contributes to the lower body temperature. When the heart is only partly filled by the smaller amounts of blood, the beat will be noticeably weaker since less blood is ejected at each contraction. When the volume of blood becomes too small, as with the loss of one to two pints through rapid hemorrhage, the heart will compensate to some extent by beating more rapidly. Breathing may become rapid and shal-

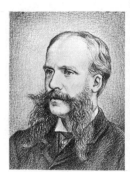

VOLKMANN, Richard von (1830-1889) German surgeon. Volkmann developed a splint, known as the Volkmann splint, which had a foot piece and two side supports, which could be used for fractures of the leg. He made several notable contributions to the study of cancer. He was the first person to describe cancer of the skin resulting from coal tar and paraffin irritation. In recent years occupational cancer has received much attention from industry.

low, because the brain is not being supplied with sufficient oxygen.

The physician is able to deal effectively with shock by administering blood or blood substitutes to increase the circulating fluid volume, and by treatment for the original cause. This original cause may be nervous in nature, stemming from the effects upon the circulatory system of a psychic reaction to pain and other factors; it may stem from the actual wounding, through accident or surgery, and may not appear for two to four hours after the injury; it may also, as mentioned before, be caused directly by loss of body fluids.

The shock victim should be made as comfortable as possible in a recumbent position. The head should be kept level. A pillow should not be used. It is better if the hips and feet can be raised higher than the head in order to facilitate the passage of blood to the brain. When an individual feels faint, he can utilize this principle by sitting down and lowering his head between his knees. Often, fainting will be prevented.

The patient should be covered with clothing or blankets to maintain body warmth. In cold climates equal care should be taken to see that he is protected from the cold ground. This can be done by placing newspapers or blankets beneath the patient or between the springs and mattress of his bed. However, it is undesirable for the patient to become too warm, since that would intensify the shock by dilating the blood vessels of the skin and thus would deprive other tissues of scarce, vital blood at a crucial time. In very cold weather, extreme caution should be used in providing hot water bottles for warmth, since the shock victim is exceptionally susceptible to burns because he may not be aware of the heat. Hot water bottles should be wrapped in cloth and should be examined frequently to prevent burning the patient.

Any constricting clothing, such as a collar or belt, should be loosened to avoid interference with respiration or circulation. Stimulants, such as hot coffee or tea without milk or cream, may prove helpful. However, if the patient is unconscious, no fluids should be given, since they may enter the lungs and cause "drowning." One or two aspirin tablets may be administered to a conscious patient to alleviate pain.

If shock occurs from serious burns, large amounts of fluid are lost from the tissues. These fluids are salty and must be replaced at once. Treatment for shock consists partially of infusing blood or plasma into the patient's vein. This must be done by a doctor, a nurse, or some other specially trained person. However, persons in shock can be given first aid. If the patient is conscious, have him drink a salt-soda solution slowly, and nothing else. If nausea or vomiting occurs, stop giving the solution.

When no physician is available for some

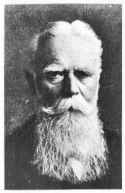

BARDELEBEN, Karl von (1849-1918) German anatomist. Bardeleben devised a dressing for burns which made use of starch, and was superior to other methods of treatment at that time. This method of treating burns has been supplanted in recent years, as a result of extensive research in prevention of burn infections, and the discovery of substances which both protect the burned tissue and promote healing. He also edited a handbook of anatomy.

Do not overheat the patient by excess covering.

Diabetic Shock: In diabetic shock the patient breathes deeply and rapidly, and his skin is cold and dry. The breath usually has an odor of acetone, which might be described as "sweet or fruity." In some cases this has been erroneously ascribed to alcohol and the patient treated for intoxication. Diabetics usually carry on their persons a card with instructions as to what to do in case of shock. There is no effective first aid treatment (except artificial respiration if breathing has ceased) other than following directions on such a card and calling a physician.

hours, as in isolated areas or during a disaster, the injured patient may drink as much as eight or ten pints of this solution. Do not force him to drink; his own thirst is the best guide. The salt-soda solution is prepared as follows:

In one quart of cool water, dissolve one level teaspoon of table salt and ½ teaspoon of baking soda (bicarbonate of soda).

In case of shock, do

Do put the patient on his back if he is unconscious. If there is head injury, keep the patient level. Keep the body warm, underneath as well as on top. If cold, apply external heat by use of hot water bottles, if possible, but be careful not to burn the patient.

Do, if the patient is conscious, place him on his back or stomach, with his head turned gently to one side.

Do keep air passages open. Clothing about the neck should be loosened to facilitate breathing. Mouth-to-mouth resuscitation must be given if the patient is not breathing.

Do raise the patient's hips and feet above the level of his head.

Do give the patient salt-soda solution to drink in shock following burns if the patient is conscious.

Do not

Do not move the patient unless it is absolutely necessary.

Do not have the patient sit up except in the event of chest injuries or nosebleed.

Do not use a pillow under the head.

Do not give a stimulant if there is severe bleeding, either externally or internally, or if the patient is suspected of having a fractured skull, or has a strong, rapid pulse and red face, as in sunstroke.

Do not attempt to make an unconscious person drink anything.

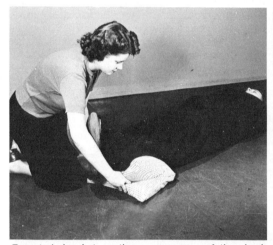

Except during hot weather, proper care of the shock patient requires that he be covered warmly, and that his feet be elevated. *Courtesy American National Red Cross.*

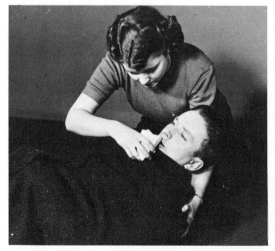

In giving fluids to a shock patient, the administrator must insure that the patient is conscious and that his head is raised sufficiently to prevent choking or strangling.

Insulin Shock: Diabetics are also subject to insulin shock, brought on by an overdose of insulin, by failure to eat enough food to neutralize the insulin, or by the accidental injection of insulin directly into a vein. If a person in shock can be questioned and it is found that he has failed to eat for several hours after a dose of insulin, he should be given an immediate source of sugar, such as a candy bar, any bottled or canned soft drink, or sugar itself. Caution must be used, however, since if the patient is actually in diabetic shock (failure to have sufficient insulin) instead of insulin shock (having an excess of insulin), his condition can be aggravated.

Electric Shock: A person suffering from electric shock must first of all be removed from contact with the current. The first-aider must use extreme caution in this procedure. He should not touch the victim directly, nor by means of a metal or wet object. Dry rope, a wooden stick (such as a broom), or a leather belt will serve best. If possible a switch should be thrown to stop the current, or the wire may be cut. In cutting the wire, one should use some cutting object with a dry wooden handle, such as an ax. He should protect his own face and person from the sparks which will fly when the wire is cut, and from contact with the live cut end of the wire. Clothing about the neck should be loosened to facilitate breathing. The patient must be given mouth-to-mouth resuscitation if he is not breathing. The victim is likely to be stiff because of the volume of electricity. Internal injuries and fractures may have occurred.

If the current passed through the central nervous system, the respiratory center of the brain may have been affected. If so, the patient will have ceased breathing. Artificial respiration should be begun at once and continued until the patient begins to breathe. This may take hours; hence, it is desirable to summon the Fire Department, or a First Aid Corps that has a *resuscitation unit.*

WOUNDS

A wound is a disruption of the outer or inner surface of the body. Wounds incur two dangers; infection and serious bleeding or hemorrhage. The danger of infection is present in every wound, but fortunately the danger of hemorrhage is present only in very severe wounds, or when a sizable blood vessel has been severed. Whenever the skin of the body is broken, germs may enter the break. These germs multiply not only in the wound, but also in the tissues surrounding it. Usually, these bacteria are of the *Staphylococcus* or *Streptococcus* groups of or-

ganisms, although many other types may be involved. Heat, pain, swelling, redness, and the formation of pus result. This is infection. The infection may enter the blood stream and cause *septicemia,* or *blood poisoning.* Many serious infections and cases of blood poisoning begin in very small wounds. Therefore, it is important to have each wound, no matter how insignificant it appears, properly treated *at once.* First aid treatment of wounds varies, depending upon whether the wound is bleeding seriously.

Wounds which bleed severely

Hemorrhage can usually be controlled by direct pressure applied to the wound by a thick sterile gauze. Application of pressure at the pressure points is an efficient method of controlling arterial bleeding in the arm or leg. Bleeding from a severed artery can be recognized by the spasmodic flow, which occurs in spurts of blood that correspond to each heart beat. If bleeding of an arm or leg cannot be stopped readily, a tourniquet or constriction may be used.

To apply a tourniquet, soft flat material at least two inches wide should be used. A tourniquet can be improvised from bandages, a necktie, stocking, or strip of cloth. The tourniquet is placed between the body and the bleeding point. Wrap the cloth around the limb twice, tie a half knot, and place a short strong stick or similar lever in the knot. Tie a square knot over it and twist the stick enough to tighten the tourniquet sufficiently to control the bleeding. The tourniquet should be loosened gently for a few seconds at 15 minute intervals. After 30 minutes, the tourniquet should be removed unless bleeding recurs. A tourniquet should never be left on for over an hour. The best places for applying a tourniquet are around the upper arm, about four inches below the armpit, and around the thigh about the same distance from the groin. The use of a tourniquet may be dangerous unless applied correctly. It cuts off the blood from the injured area, and if circulation is cut off for too long a time, the tissues are destroyed, and gangrene may develop. Gangrene is a serious complication, which may require amputation of the part or, if unchecked, may lead to death.

Bleeding from a vein is a slower and steadier hemorrhage than that from an artery and is much easier to control. Usually, venous bleeding can be controlled by placing a compress over the wound and bandaging it. A bleeding limb should be eleveated to help slow the blood flow.

In cases of bleeding, do

Do place thick, sterile gauze pads or a clean towel over the bleeding point and apply pressure.

Do apply pressure to the proper point. If the pressure points are not known, apply a tourniquet or tight band to the upper arm or upper leg, as the case may be, between the cut and the body. Elevate the limb.

Do not

Do not leave a tourniquet or band in place longer than 15 minutes at a time. After 15 minutes, the tourniquet should be loosened and then replaced if necessary.

Abrasions and cuts

Abrasions are wounds made by rubbing or scraping the skin or mucous membrane. The most common are "scuff-burns," "floor-burns," and "mat-burns." These are not really burns, but actual wounds that become infected easily. If the abrasion is extensive, simply cover the area with sterile gauze and let the physician do the rest. If the injured area is small, cleanse with warm water and soap or a mild antiseptic, and apply a light bandage.

Cuts are inflicted by sharp-edged objects such as knives or broken glass. These wounds usually bleed freely as the small blood vessels have been completely severed. Frequently, only a small amount of tissue around the cut is damaged, and cuts are not so likely to become infected as other wounds. Cuts should be treated in the same way as abrasions. If the cut has been made by a very dirty, rusty, or penetrating object, the physician may administer tetanus toxoid or antitoxin.

Lacerations

Injuries that are inflicted by blunt instruments, machinery, or falls against angular surfaces *tear* or *lacerate* the flesh. As a rule, bleeding is not so severe as in cuts. The danger of infection, however, is greater, because dirt and debris are often ground into the tissues, and damage to the surrounding tissue is more extensive. If the laceration is extensive or very dirty, the wound should be covered by sterile gauze and the cleansing left to the physician. If the wound is small, cleansing with soap and water, application of mild antiseptic solution, and bandaging should be done.

In case of cuts, do

Do wash well with soap and water and apply a sterile bandage, or a clean, freshly ironed piece of cloth if the wound is small.

Do cover with sterile gauze; press gauze firmly over wound to control bleeding, if wound is large, and hold in place until the doctor arrives.

Do not

Do not use strong antiseptics. Fresh tincture of iodine (half strength) or 70 percent alcohol may be used if desired. Soap and water is an excellent antiseptic.

Do not do anything if wound is large except cover with sterile gauze, control bleeding, and let the doctor do the rest.

Puncture wounds

Puncture wounds are caused by any penetrating object such as nails, pieces of wire, bullets, etc. Puncture wounds usually do not bleed freely. The edges of the wound tend to turn inward, making the wound difficult to clean. This tendency of puncture wounds to close makes the danger of infection much greater than in cuts and other wounds, since air cannot reach the injured tissue. Certain germs are *anaerobic* and grow only where no oxygen is present. This resultant lack of air in a puncture wound enhances the growth of those germs causing *tetanus* or *lockjaw*. First aid treatment of a puncture wound consists of inducing bleeding by the application of light pressure around the edges of the wound and then applying a mild antiseptic solution. In addition to treating the wound, the physician will often give tetanus toxoid or antitoxin to prevent lockjaw. However, before giving antitoxin, the physician should determine whether the patient has shown previous sensitivity to serum inoculations.

Powder burns and gunshot wounds are treated as other puncture wounds. Treatment to prevent shock and prompt proper transportation to a physician or hospital are the proper measures in such instances.

In case of puncture wounds, do

Do try to encourage bleeding by gently pressing again and again just above wound, and, in the case of a finger or toe, by gently squeezing or "milking" it.

Do ask the doctor in every case if he thinks tetanus toxoid or antitoxin advisable.

Do not

Do not ever try to close a puncture wound with bandage, adhesive, or anything else. A sterile gauze pad may be placed loosely over the wound until the doctor comes.

Do not forget to tell the doctor if the patient has had any kind of serum before and if the patient has any allergies.

Dog and cat bites

The wound made by a dog or cat bite is usually a puncture wound, but may be a lacera-

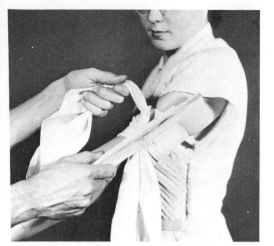

In applying a tourniquet, a triangular bandage may be tied around the limb with a single knot. The bandage is then tied around a stick which may be twisted to exert pressure.

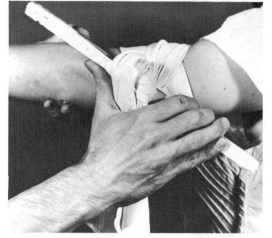

Pressure must not be exerted for excessive lengths of time; tourniquet pressure should be relieved from arm at regular intervals. *Courtesy American National Red Cross.*

tion. Many people have the mistaken idea that dog bites are serious only during certain seasons of the year, usually "dog days" in the summer months. Any animal bite may be serious in that it may cause tetanus or *rabies* (*hydrophobia*). The saliva of a rabid animal entering a scratch or abrasion can cause rabies. Once rabies develops, it is never cured, but it can be prevented by the Pasteur or vaccine treatment.

First aid treatment of animal bites consists of washing the saliva from the wound and applying a sterile gauze dressing over the area. The physician will give the wound any further treatment and give the Pasteur treatment if he believes it necessary.

The dog, cat, or other animal should not be destroyed immediately, but should be confined to a place where he cannot escape and should be observed for three weeks. If the animal does not develop rabies within this period, the patient is in no danger of the disease. If the dog must be shot, do not shoot through the head. Save

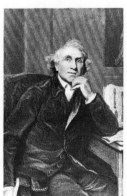

HUNTER, John (1728-1793) Scottish physician. Hunter had an active and inquiring mind, and made numerous investigations in anatomy, physiology, and experimental pathology. In 1784 he published a treatise on gunshot wounds in which he gave a classic description of inflammation. In attempting to differentiate between syphilis and gonorrhea, he inoculated himself with what he thought to be gonorrhea, and developed a primary syphilitic chancre.

the head so the physician can have the brain examined for evidence of rabies.

In case of dog bite, do

Do hold the wound under running water and wash it thoroughly. Dry it with clean gauze and cover it with gauze dressing. Since the doctor will probably want to cauterize the wound, do not use antiseptics before he arrives. The doctor will decide whether Pasteur treatment is to be given.

Do not

Do not let a well-meaning person shoot the dog. The dog should be caught and kept under observation for three weeks to determine whether it has rabies.

Insect bites

Many insect bites cause irritation, swelling, and inflammation. These stings may be painful and poisonous. Infection may occur from scratching. Remove the "sting" if it is still present and apply a paste made of baking soda. Insect bites about the face, especially the eyes, may require medical treatment. There are many people who are allergic to the stings of bees and wasps. Their breathing becomes difficult and shock sets in. If an allergy is suspected, call a doctor and treat for shock until he arrives, or until you can remove the patient to a hospital.

Spider bites

The most infamous spider in North America is the *black widow* or "shoe button" spider. A

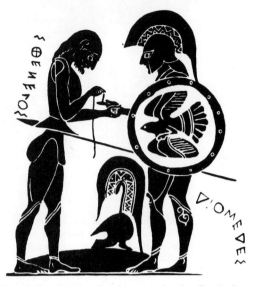

This painting from a Grecian vase in the Pembroke collection shows Sthenelos bandaging the hand of the Trojan war hero, Diomedes. *Bettmann Archive.*

characteristic crimson hourglass marking is found on the abdomen of the female, but black widows have also been seen with just a small red spot or no markings at all. Few first aid measures seem effective, besides those of keeping the patient quiet and warm until the physician arrives. Severe abdominal pain may develop. Death seldom occurs except in very young or very old and infirm persons.

A spider known as the *brown recluse* may be more deadly. A common spider also known as the "fiddler" because of a violin-shaped mark on its head, it is found in attics, closets, and barns. This ordinary-looking spider seeks dark corners and will not bite unless it feels threatened. However, babies have been bitten when they have inadvertently rolled over on a brown recluse. Intense pain occurs two to eight hours later with nausea, cramps, and a high fever. A blister may develop with hemorrhaging. In case of high fever and suspicious bite marks, consult a doctor immediately.

Woolly worm

There are several varieties of caterpillars that are poisonous to the touch. The most troublesome is the *woolly* worm, a caterpillar that grows into a kind of flannel moth. From brushing against the insect, a victim suffers severe pain and swelling, often accompanied by headache and swelling of the lymph glands. A few cases may go into shock. First aid can only rely on recognizing the cause and contacting the doctor promptly. The woolly worm is found primarily in the southern United States where it is vari-ously called the woolly slug, pus caterpillar, possum bug, Italian asp, or *el perrito* (little dog). In the north, the caterpillar of the common white moth may cause the same reaction.

Scorpions

Although common to the southwest regions of the United States and Mexico, scorpions are often inadvertently brought home by travelers. Some varieties found in desert areas are poisonous. They hide under rocks, debris, and in foliage. The immediate danger to the bitten person is from shock. Clean the puncture carefully, checking to see if the stinger has been removed. Swelling and redness may occur. If the bite is on a toe or finger, apply a tight band between it and the rest of the body for five minutes. The same is true for bites further up the arms and legs. Hold the limb downward to prevent rapid circulation. If the bite occurs on the torso, pack the area with ice. Consult a doctor.

Man-of-war

Bites from a poisonous jellyfish, the *Portuguese man-of-war*, are a serious hazard to swimmers in warm coastal waters. The *Physalia* group of jellyfish are under eight inches in width, purple-gray, irridescent, and have several tentacles as long as 50 feet. Unlike harmless jellyfish, the man-of-war carries a nerve poison inside its barbed tentacles. Shock is the greatest danger to a bite victim. The bite area should be washed with alcohol and shock treatment started. Pain lasts for several hours. Welts may linger for three months.

FOREIGN BODIES

A great variety of foreign bodies gain entrance into the body. Many of these are missiles or objects driven into the body by explosive force such as bullets, shrapnel, BB shots, arrows, and similar objects. Another group is made up of needles, splinters, pins, tacks, nails, and knife blades which are driven into the flesh. The third group is composed of those articles which enter the body cavities such as the mouth, nose, ears, rectum, and urogenital openings.

The location and depth of penetration of the object should determine the first aid measures. If the object penetrates only superficially, it may be removed safely with a pair of sterile forceps. A mild antiseptic or antibiotic solution should be applied to prevent infection and the wound should be loosely bandaged.

Foreign bodies in the eye

Most objects that enter the space between the eyeball and the eyelid may be removed by washing the eye or by everting the eyelid and locating the foreign matter, which may be removed with any clean soft substance. If the foreign object is embedded in the substance of the eyeball itself, no attempt should be made to remove it. The eye should be kept moist with warm weak *saline* solution until the patient is placed under the care of a physician. If there is a delay in getting to a physician, comfort may be given the patient by placing gauze or cotton on the closed eye and taping it on with adhesive.

If harmful liquids or chemicals have gotten into the eye, the eye should be washed out with dilute salt water, or with clean water, by as much as a quart. The water should be dropped into the outside corner of the eye while the head is tilted so that the whole eye will be bathed. If an eyedropper is not available, squeeze the water out of a clean cloth into the eye. The patient should be taken to a doctor as soon as possible.

Foreign bodies in the ear

Most foreign bodies may be removed from the ear by inclining the head so that the object can fall out. Insects are sometimes attracted by a strong light so that they will leave the ear. Warm mineral oil dropped into the ear will relieve the pain and also kill an insect. No hard object, especially such things as paper clips, hair pins, or matchsticks, should be placed in the ear. Such objects may penetrate the eardrum and cause permanent injury. Probing the ear may cause it to become swollen and thus make it more difficult to remove the object.

Foreign bodies in the nose

Solid objects are often introduced into the nose by children. A few drops of olive or mineral oil may help relieve the irritation and prevent swelling. Nose drops containing *ephedrine* or *neosynephrine* may prove useful, since they cause a shrinkage of the nasal *mucosa,* or lining. In case the object cannot be removed easily, force should never be used. The nose should not be blown violently, nor should it be blown with one nostril held closed. A physician can usually remove objects easily with specialized instruments.

Foreign bodies in the larynx, trachea, and bronchi

Many objects, such as coins, fish bones, and safety pins may become lodged in the voice box, *(larynx),* windpipe *(trachea),* and even deeper in the *bronchi.* Sometimes the introduction of the finger into the *throat* will enable the person to remove the *smooth* object or stimulate the vomiting reflex which will expel the substance. Care should be exercised to prevent pushing the object deeper into the larynx. Removal of *sharp* objects such as fish bones or pins may require use of specialized surgical instruments, and is, of course, beyond the scope of first aid. After the object is removed, the irritation may persist for several days and may lead the person to think the foreign object is still there.

Objects in the trachea are much more serious. If the trachea is not completely obstructed, the physician can locate the object by means of x-ray film or laryngoscopic study and remove it with special instruments. In a few rare cases an emergency opening into the trachea has been made with a penknife into which a tube (made from the barrel of a fountain pen) has enabled persons, in the last stage of suffocation, to start breathing and to survive. Such procedure is, of course, a last resort. (See page 696 for first aid in case of choking.)

Foreign bodies in the lung

If a person becomes choked on food or some other object, the violent choking may cause the

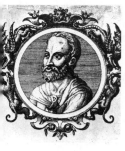

PAUL of Aegina (625-690) Famous Greek physician. Author of an *Epitome* of medicine. Paul gave many original descriptions of lithotomy, trephining, tonsillotomy, and amputation of the breast. He gave the best accounts of eye surgery and military surgery of any writer of antiquity. His tracts on pediatrics and obstetrics summarize all that was known on those subjects prior to the Renaissance.

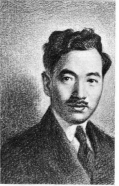

NOGUCHI, Hideyo (1876-1928) Japanese bacteriologist in America. Important early studies of the nature of the action of snake venom were performed by Noguchi in collaboration with Simon Flexner. In 1911 he succeeded in culturing the causative agent of syphilis, *Treponema pallidum,* and first obtained a pure culture of this organism in 1913, by culturing it from a syphilitic patient. He is also noted for his extensive studies on yellow fever and its etiology.

object to enter the trachea or windpipe. If the object does not become lodged in the trachea, it may be aspirated into the lung. After aspiration of a foreign body into the lung, the patient may or may not feel further discomfort. He may think he has swallowed the object. If the patient is not completely certain, then x-ray examination is necessary, because foreign objects lodged in the lung may become encysted and walled off or cause a cyst, abscess, *empyema* (pus), or pneumonia.

Foreign objects in the digestive tract

Fortunately, most objects swallowed pass through the intestine and one is seldom aware of them. Most round objects such as marbles, beads, buttons, and coins pass through the intestine without harm. However, some rounded objects will lodge in the base of the *esophagus* and cause erosion and eventual perforation of the tube. Removal of these objects requires the use of a long instrument, the *esophagoscope,* and special grasping devices. The removal of objects lodged in the stomach and lower part of the digestive tract may require surgery. Small objects may pass through the digestive tract without causing trouble, even in small children. Straight and open safety pins and other sharp objects are particularly dangerous because they may cause perforation and should be removed immediately. The x-ray picture and fluoroscopic study will reveal the exact location of many types of foreign objects.

Foreign bodies elsewhere in the body

Children occasionally insert objects in other openings of the body such as the anus, vagina, or urethra. In these cases, first aid measures should be restricted to gentle attempts to remove the object. The use of force or manipulation of the object should be avoided since it may serve to cause further injury and infection. Call a doctor to find out whether to place the child in his care.

INJURIES TO BONES, JOINTS, AND MUSCLES

A fracture is a broken bone. In a *closed fracture,* the bone is either cracked or completely broken in two, but there is no connecting wound from the break extending through the skin. In an *open fracture,* the bone is broken and bone fragments penetrate the surface of the skin, or an external object, such as a bullet, penetrates the skin and forms a connecting wound with the broken bone. Proper handling

of a fracture is essential. Rough handling may cause a simple fracture to become an open fracture; and it may cause the bone fragments to injure the blood vessels, nerves, and other tissues. General first aid measures are to prevent further damage, make the patient comfortable, and prevent shock. Do not attempt to set a broken bone, and never move a patient until splints have been applied to immobilize the broken part. If bleeding is present, control by applying pressure directly to the wound or by applying a tourniquet. Do not try to cleanse the fracture wound in any way; simply cover the protruding bone and torn flesh with a sterile bandage.

Splints can be improvised from many rigid materials and should be long enough to extend beyond the joint above the injury and below the fracture site. If boards are used, they should be as wide as the injured part. Pillows, newspapers, magazines, or blankets often can be used as splints for the arm or lower leg. All splints should be padded, at least on the side next to the body. The thickness of soft padding allows swelling of the injured part and reduces the danger of cutting off the blood circulation. Splints should be examined at short intervals to ascertain whether blood circulation is cut off. Splints should be loosened if the affected part becomes too painful or if the extremity becomes cold, pale, or blue.

Skull fracture and concussion

Injury to the head may result in these conditions: *a fracture,* in which the skull is broken or cracked; a *depressed fracture,* in which the skull is broken and fragments of bone are embedded in the brain tissue; or a *concussion,* in which the brain is bruised by swelling resulting from hemorrhage.

The person rendering first aid should not try to distinguish between fracture and concussion, since the first aid treatment is the same for both injuries. The patient may be conscious; there may be some external injury; and breathing may be unduly slow or rapid. Keep the patient lying down, with the head slightly raised if the face is normal or red, or keep level if the face is pale. Place the patient in a supine or lying position only. Keep the patient warm and do *not* give any stimulant. Pressure or strong antiseptics should never be applied to a head wound. Pieces of hair, bone, metal, etc., which penetrate the skull, should not be removed. If there is a watery discharge from the ear or nose, this is evidence of loss of the cerebrospinal fluid which fills the spaces in the brain. Bleeding from the ear may also be a sign of skull fracture. The ear or nose should not be washed out, but sterile cotton may be used to clean the organ externally. If the patient should cease to breathe, mouth-to-mouth artificial respiration should be given.

In case of skull fracture, do

Do keep the patient lying down with head and shoulders slightly raised if face appears normal or is flushed. If pale, keep head level or slightly lower.

Do move the patient only in a horizontal position and avoid unnecessary handling.

Do keep the patient warm.

Do control the scalp bleeding by applying a sterile gauze pad over the bleeding point.

Do lower and turn the head slightly to one side if blood or mucus collects in the throat or mouth.

Do examine the mouth and throat for swallowed objects, false teeth, tongue, etc. which might obstruct breathing.

Do institute artificial respiration immediately if breathing ceases.

Do not

Do not move the patient unless absolutely necessary.

Do not give stimulants or anything else by mouth.

Do not try to remove bone or foreign fragments embedded in the wound.

Do not apply antiseptics; simply cover wound with sterile gauze.

Do not exert pressure on head.

Fracture of neck and spinal column

A fracture or injury to the neck or spinal column is serious, and the first aid treatment can cause even more damage if not carried out properly. A fracture of one or more of the vertebrae results in intense pain to the patient in the area of the fracture. The pain in most cases radiates outward to other parts of the body, depending upon which of the vertebrae is affected. Fractures high on the spinal column may result in pain in the arms or chest, while fractures lower down cause pain in the abdomen or legs. When an injury has affected the spinal cord, the patient may suffer a loss of sensation and ability to move the part of the body which is supplied by nerves from the spinal column at the point of fracture and below it.

The patient suspected of a fractured spinal column, with or without injury to the spinal cord, should not be moved even to change the head to a more comfortable position unless it is absolutely necessary. If it is absolutely essential to transport the patient before the arrival of the physician, at least three or four strong people should be present to help in the transfer.

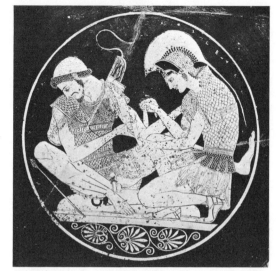

Painting from an ancient Grecian vase depicting Achilles bandaging the wounds that were inflicted upon the warrior Patroclus. *Bettman Archive.*

One person should hold the head steady on a line with the spine and not permit it to rotate. Two strong men may then lift the body, with perhaps a fourth supporting the legs. The patient must be placed on a firm support, such as a wooden door, with the head held steady by props or bags filled with sand. The patient must not be carried on an ordinary stretcher, bed, or other soft object, since this can result in extensive, permanent injury to the spinal cord which may even lead to death. (See page 692-694 for instructions on moving an injured person.)

In cases of fracture of the spine, do

Do keep the patient lying down.

Do maintain slight traction on the head in a lengthwise direction in the event that the patient must be moved.

Do place pillows or sandbags on either side of head after patient has been placed on a rigid flat surface such as a door.

Do place arms at sides and immobilize so no motion of the spine is possible.

Do not

Do not lift the patient's head.

Do not allow the patient to assume a sitting position.

Fractures of upper body

First aid treatment of fractures of the nose and jaw is very limited. If wounds are present, apply a compress and bandage loosely in place with a four-tail bandage. If a fractured lower

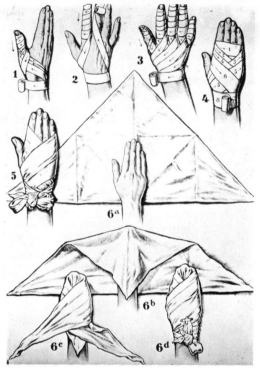

The series of pictures in this illustration portray the methods by which injuries of the fingers or of the whole hand may be properly bandaged.

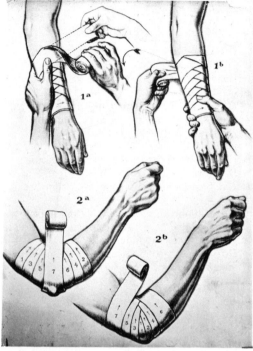

The problem associated with bandaging injuries of the wrist, forearm and elbow may be overcome by wrapping techniques shown in this illustration.

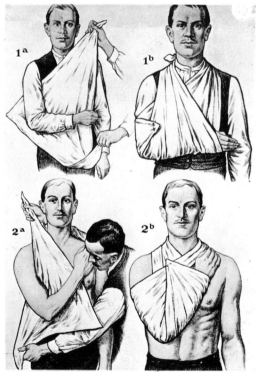

Illustration of the manner in which a triangular arm sling may be prepared either to support (above) or to raise (below) the patient's forearm.

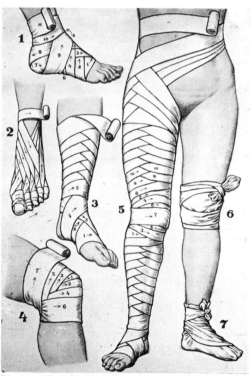

Diagram of various methods by which injuries of the lower extremities may be bandaged. *Medichrome, Clay-Adams Company, Inc., New York.*

jaw can be raised to bring the lower teeth against the upper teeth without discomfort, the jaw may then be immobilized with a bandage under the chin and over the top of the head. The jaw should *not be forced* in any way. If vomiting begins, remove bandage and support the injured bone with the palm of the hand. When vomiting ceases, reapply the bandage.

Fracture of the clavicle or *collarbone* usually prevents the patient from raising his arm above the shoulder. If the arm is hanging naturally, the injured shoulder is usually a little lower than the other. Put the arm in a sling made with a triangular bandage and secure the arm to the body by encircling the sling with a bandage tied around the chest. The bandage must not be tight enough to cut off the circulation in the arm. The fingers should be left free and the pulse should be taken at the wrist to determine whether circulation is impaired.

Fracture of ribs may sometimes be felt by moving the fingers gently along the rib. If a lung has been punctured by a jagged edge of broken rib, the patient may cough up frothy bloody fluid. Usually the patient experiences pain in the area of injury every time he breathes. Bandaging may relieve this pain by partially immobilizing the affected ribs. Two or three broad cravat bandages should be wrapped about the chest and tied loosely. Then the patient should expel air from his lungs and the knots should be tightened until suitable pressure is obtained. A pad should be placed under the knots so that the skin will not be bruised.

If the patient is coughing blood and puncture of the lung is suspected, *do not* apply any bandages. Keep the patient lying down with head and shoulders elevated sufficiently to permit comfortable breathing. Keep the patient warm and do not move him unless it is absolutely necessary, and then only in a lying position.

Fracture of the arm should be immobilized until it can be "set" or reduced. Fixed traction splints are effective in first aid work, but the person applying traction splints should have at least a superficial course in first aid and understand the principle of fixed traction. A good rule to follow in the first aid of fractures rendered by untrained persons is to "splint them where they lie." No attempt should be made to set the arm or to restore it to normal shape. If the arm is disfigured, a sling or support should be fashioned which will prevent any pressure being put upon the limb, especially at the point of fracture. A splint should be applied, but it should maintain the disalignment. The splint should be padded to absorb shock of movement. Obviously a fractured arm should be moved as little as possible until it can be x-rayed and properly set.

If the elbow is fractured and is in an extended position, simply splint the arm, applying padding over the fracture site. If the elbow is flexed, carefully apply an arm sling and bind the arm to the body. Further support may be given the injured elbow by using a sling around the neck and wrist.

Fractures of the forearm and wrist may be immobilized by making use of two light splints and padding the fracture site before the splints are applied.

If an injured person is found lying face down, he should be gently rolled into a face-up position. Such persons should be treated as though they suffered from head injuries, spinal injuries, and injuries to the lower body. The patient must be moved as a *unit* without sudden jerky movements and without bending the back or jarring the head. If the injured person is found in a crumpled position, he should be carefully straightened into a face-up position.

Fracture of the pelvis

Fracture of the pelvis is a serious injury; often blood vessels and organs within the pelvis, especially the bladder, are injured. There is usually severe pain throughout the pelvic region, and pressing the hip bones together usually produces pain if fracture of the pelvis exists.

The patient should not be moved unless it is absolutely necessary and then only on a rigid stretcher or board. Before moving the patient onto the splint, bandage the ankles and knees together and either flex or straighten the knees, depending on which position is more comfortable to the patient. Keep the patient warm and treat for shock, which may be severe.

Fracture of the hip and thigh

Fracture of the hip or thigh (*femur*) may occur from slight injury in elderly persons. With advancing age, the bones become brittle and often slight force will crack a bone. The hip and thigh are common sites of fractures among elderly persons. If the patient cannot lift his heel from the ground as he lies on his back, treat the injury as a hip fracture. If the foot on the injured side is turned outward or sideways, do not try to straighten it. Do not move the patient unless it is absolutely necessary and then only after the injured side has been immobilized. Steady the limb and gently bring it into normal position at the side of the other. A light bandage around the thighs and ankles will hold it there, using the uninjured limb as a splint. Begin treatment for shock immediately; it may be severe.

Fracture of lower leg

If the kneecap is fractured, the displacement can usually be felt as a groove of separation in the kneecap. The limb should be gently straight-

Splints

When accidents occur in the field, where the conventional methods of treatment for first aid are not available, it becomes necessary for the first aid administrator to improvise appropriate methods for emergency treatment and management of the patient. The following series of pictures illustrate how generally available items may substitute for the conventionally available first aid equipment. The support of a fractured limb requires that some firm material be secured, which will give the limb freedom from any pressures that might ultimately complicate the initial fracture. *Courtesy American National Red Cross.*

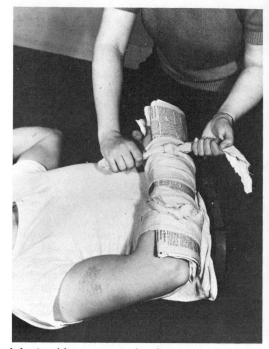

A fractured lower arm can be given temporary support by an arm splint made of newspapers and handkerchiefs.

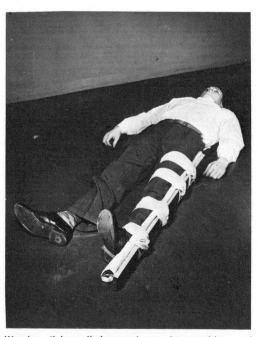

Wooden sticks or limbs may be used to provide an adequate splint for a break in the lower part of the leg.

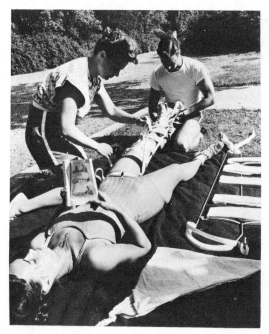

In this posed picture, two first aiders are applying a standard half-ring traction-type splint to a fractured leg.

ened. A board splint may be used and should extend from the buttock to the heel. A pillow wrapped and tied about the knee makes an excellent splint. Leave the kneecap exposed, as swelling may be rapid and the constriction painful.

One or both bones of the lower leg, the *tibia* and *fibula*, may be fractured anywhere from the knee to the ankle. If both bones are broken, usually there will be some visible deformity of the limb. A pillow or folded blanket may be used for splinting. If extra protection is desired, a stick or board can be used outside the pillow or blanket on each side. If a pillow is not available, padded splints may be used. These should extend well above the knee and below the ankle. The ankle should be padded to avoid bruising. Often, it will be desirable to tie the feet together to insure immobility of the limb.

If the foot or ankle is fractured, remove the shoe and stocking, cutting them if necessary. Place a large padded dressing around the ankle or foot and wrap a spiral bandage, beginning at the bottom going up. Do not bandage tightly. Keep the patient off the extremity. It is better that he try not to jump or hobble around even if he has assistance and holds aloft the injured member.

In case of limb fracture, do

Do keep the patient still and warm.

Do prevent movement of the part by applying a homemade splint. The simplest method is to use a pillow or blanket. To apply, slide the pillow under the limb, making certain that the pillow is long enough to include the joint at each end of the broken bone. Fold sides of pillow up over limb and secure by tying strips of cloth or bandage around the pillow at three to four-inch intervals.

Do cover any fragment of bone which is protruding through the skin with a sterile gauze bandage, and then apply pillow splint.

Do not

Do not let the patient walk on leg or use arm if fracture is suspected.

Do not apply splint or bandage tightly. To allow for swelling of the limb, provide adequate padding between limb and splint.

Do not try to "set" or straighten a fracture; simply "splint it where it lies."

Do not apply antiseptics to exposed bone and torn flesh. Cover with sterile gauze and let the physician do the rest.

Dislocations

An injury is termed a *dislocation* when a bone gets out of place at a joint. The joints are encased by flexible sacs held in place by ligaments. Ligaments are tough fibrous bands of tissue which extend from one bone to the other, entirely surrounding the joint. In a dislocation, the ligaments and sacs are partially or completely torn; the bony surfaces may be fractured; and the blood vessels and nerves may be injured or torn.

Dislocations of the shoulder and fingers are most common, followed by dislocations of the jaw, elbow, kneecap, and hip. A blow, fall, or violent muscular action may cause a dislocation. The symptoms are pain, deformity of the joint, and swelling which occurs rapidly.

Movement of the injured part is usually completely lost. Shock may be severe, and immediate measures should be taken to prevent it or to treat the patient for shock. The injured part should be padded and supported. No effort should be made to put the dislocated member back in place because there is danger of further injury to tendons, blood vessels, and nerves. If there is an open wound, cover it with sterile gauze. A physician should handle all but the most preliminary treatment.

Sprains

Sprains are injuries to joints in which ligaments are stretched or torn, usually caused by stretching, twisting, or pressure at a joint. The symptoms are swelling over the joint which occurs rapidly, inability to use the part without increasing pain, and often discoloration which may appear immediately. The affected part should be elevated and should not be used until properly examined, because the part may also be fractured. A sprain may be as serious as a simple fracture and in some instances may take longer to heal than a simple break. If walking is absolutely necessary in instances of sprained ankle, a bandage applied over the shoe and extended above the ankle will provide some temporary support. The patient should be supported on the injured side if this is possible so that he can hold his injured ankle above the ground.

Strains

A strain is an injury to a muscle or tendon which results from severe exertion. One of the main causes of strains is the lifting of heavy objects from an awkward position. The symptoms are pain and stiffness in the affected part. To give first aid, make the patient comfortable by placing him in such a position that the injured muscles are relaxed. Often heat applications and gentle massage will offer some relief by stimulating the circulation. Always rub the affected part in an upward direction. Application of liniments is of doubtful value, especially oil of wintergreen and such substances that tend to irritate the skin and make it especially sensitive to heat. Rubbing alcohol may be used to facilitate gentle massage which may aid in "loosening up" tightened muscles.

Bruises

A bruise is caused by a blow to some part of the body which breaks the small blood vessels under the skin (*subdermal hemorrhage*). As the blood collects in the tissues, it causes swelling and discoloration. Usually no treatment is required for minor bruises. Application of cold cloths may help to prevent discoloration, reduce swelling, and relieve pain. If the skin is broken, it should be treated as any other open wound. Minor bruises are usually tender, but are seldom serious.

Battered children

Doctors, teachers, and social workers sometimes find cases of cruelty and physical abuse to children. Apathetic or nervous children with unusual bruises and bumps are telltale signs. A concerned person who is not a physician should alert the Child Welfare Service of the state welfare department. There is an office in every county. In cases requiring emergency treatment, a call should be made to the police. Doctors have fought for and won the legal right to protect children from abuse.

INJURIES FROM HEAT AND COLD

Injuries caused by heat are *burns*; those caused by hot liquids or moist vapor such as steam are called *scalds*. Burns are caused by heat, flames, hot objects, intense flashes, electricity, and various chemicals. Burns are classified according to the depth or degree to which the tissues are injured. In a *first degree burn* the skin is reddened and tender; in a *second degree burn* the skin is blistered; in a *third degree burn* the tissues are more extensively damaged and may be charred and destroyed. In severe burns the tissue may slough away, a condition known as *eschar*.

In many cases first and second degree burns may be mixed. A third degree burn is the most serious, and involves damage to the entire thickness of the skin. Sometimes the underlying tissues such as fat, muscles, and bone are also burned. A third degree burn always requires medical attention. First and second degree burns may not, if they are small, but the size of the burned area is a more important consideration in determining its seriousness than is the degree. It is generally held that a first degree burn may

be fatal if it covers as much as two thirds of the body's surface, while second degree burns are equally grave if they cover only one third of the skin. Any third degree burn is serious, and any first or second degree burn that covers over one tenth of the skin requires medical attention. Burns on much smaller areas of the skin of children are dangerous.

First aid for small first or second degree burns involves easing the pain, protecting the burn from further injury, and preventing infection. A burned area of skin cannot offer its normal defense against infectious microorganisms, and so must be kept clean. A sterile bandage or a cotton cloth which has just been ironed to give it some degree of sterility may be used for a bandage. The bandage should not be too tight and it may be moistened with a cool solution of one teaspoon of baking soda in a quart of tap water, if cooling of the burned area seems desirable. Various medications which are available for the treatment of burns may be kept in the home, and aid greatly in relieving the burning sensation. Oily ointments should not be used. For burns covering less than 20 percent of the body, immersion in cold water is an acceptable first aid treatment. If immersion is difficult, ice packs or cold wet towels should be applied to the burned area. Very dilute silver nitrate in a .5 percent solution is used by some doctors. However, a stronger solution is harmful. *Large first and second degree burns should not be treated by first aid measures,* since the systemic effects accompanying them require treatment that is beyond the scope of first aid.

Victims of third degree burns, and first and second degree burns which are extensive in area, must be carefully watched for signs of shock. It is necessary to cover a burn victim with a blanket to maintain body temperature, except in hot weather. The first aid administrator is limited to giving one or two aspirin for the relief of pain, since stronger sedatives must be administered only after a physician can examine the patient. Methods which may be used to help prevent shock from fluid loss in burn patients are discussed under an earlier section, *Shock*.

Chemical and electrical burns

Chemical burns must be immediately treated by thorough flooding of the affected areas. A dilute baking soda solution (four tablespoons to a quart of tap water) may be helpful for acid burns, and weak vinegar for alkali burns, but thorough washing with water is generally possible more rapidly and therefore is more effective. A gentle stream of water directed into the eyes is necessary if these are affected, and eyes must be held open while this is being done. A weak solution of half a tablespoon of salt to a glass of water can be used to gently irrigate the

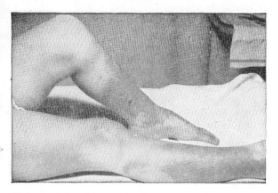

Picture of the skin on the legs of a patient suffering from *first degree* burns, showing the reddened areas and the absence of more extensive damage.

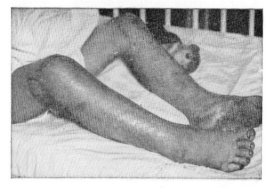

The burns shown in this photograph are both *first and second degree*. Extensive redness is present together with an appreciable degree of blistering.

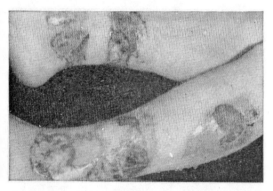

Second and third degree burns are combined on the legs of this patient, to produce blistering and a considerable amount of damage to deeper tissues.

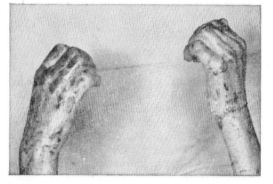

Photograph of *third degree* burns about the hands and forearms showing pronounced charring of certain areas of skin. *Photography by F. W. Schmidt.*

eye. Then close the eye until a doctor can be found.

Electrical burns may be misleading in their appearance, and may go much deeper than the surface area implies. Such burns generally are not as important as are the accompanying disturbances to the respiration and circulation. Artificial respiration may be necessary.

Sunburn

Overexposure to the sun's rays is harmful to most persons and dangerous to the few people who are sensitive to the sun's rays. These susceptible individuals are called *heliophobes* and usually are blonds or redheads with a clear pale skin. Because of their thin, nonpigmented skin, they absorb more ultraviolet light than does a darker person. They seldom tan. For persons who have pellagra, lung tuberculosis, high blood pressure, or hyperthyroidism, sunlight may be definitely harmful and sometimes dangerous. It is well to note that clouds do not remove all the ultraviolet light, so that severe sunburn may be acquired on a cloudy day. The ultraviolet rays may be reflected from the surface of snow (or water); such rays are the cause of snow blindness.

The symptoms of sunburn vary with the degree of exposure; in general, they consist of a redness and burning of the skin followed by blistering and peeling of the outer layers of the *epidermis*. If a considerable area of the skin is involved, there may be swelling, burning, and smarting, which may lead to generalized symptoms of fever, chills, insomnia, and varying degrees of weakness. Peeling and itching of the skin followed by variable degrees of tanning are some of the later symptoms of sunburn. Sometimes sunburn produces an inflammation of the eye and cracking or chapping of the lips. Severe sunburn may be complicated by infection of the hair follicles and sweat glands. Fortunately, these complications are relatively rare, and the person recovers quickly once the pain, burning, and itching subside. *Sulfonamides* often increase sensitivity to sunlight. Repeated exposure to sun, particularly by elderly blonds, may be a factor in the development of skin cancer. Signs of aging on skin may be due in large part to exposure to the sun.

The treatment of persons with sunburn depends upon the extent and the degree of the burn. For mild burns, various types of calamine lotion, some of which contain mild anesthetics or antihistamines, may be used. A powder preparation composed of boric acid, talc, and zinc oxide has been recommended. Persons with more extensive sunburn should be bathed in a tub of water containing about a pound of corn starch. Blisters should be opened only if necessary and then under sterile precautions, to prevent infection. Mild local anesthetic agents may be applied to stop pain and itching. A mild vinegar solution may be helpful.

Sunburn can be prevented by gradually exposing one's self to periods of sunlight. Sunbathing should be done in moderation with increasing daily exposure, starting at about ten minutes the first day and increasing the interval of exposure daily by seven to ten minutes.

There are various sunburn medications and ointments on the market which filter out much of the ultraviolet light from the sun. These preparations contain chemicals such as *quinine, titanium oxide, methyl salicylate,* or *para-aminobenzoic acid* in a liquid or cream base. Such substances, if applied before exposure, will often prevent or reduce sunburn. A thin film of olive oil will serve much the same purpose as the more expensive lotions. However, one should not rely on such applications for complete protection.

In case of burns, do

Do apply simple nonoily burn ointment, or paste made of baking soda and water, on clean gauze.

Do immerse in cold water if burns cover less than 20 percent of the body.

Do treat for shock if burns are extensive.

Do give a salt-soda solution if burns are extensive and only if help is not immediately available: 1 teaspoon of salt and ½ teaspoon of soda dissolved in a quart of cool water should be given if patient is conscious. Nothing else should be given.

Do wrap patient in cleanest covering available, such as a sheet, to prevent excessive contamination.

Do keep the injured person at rest.

Do not

Do not use oily substances on any burn.

Do not use absorbent cotton.

Do not underestimate a burn, especially sunburn. If skin is at all blistered, it is a second degree burn.

Burn Bandages

The theory of first aid is based on the principle that emergency treatment may be required at a time when it is least anticipated. First aid measures should, therefore, be learned before the emergency occurs. The following series of photographs shows some of the more important techniques that may be used in first aid. *Courtesy American National Red Cross.*

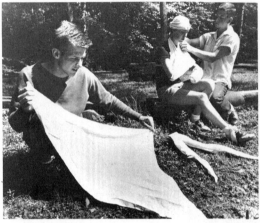

The triangular bandage is fundamental to many different types of bandaging technique. In the background it is shown applied to injuries of the arm, head, hand, and ankle.

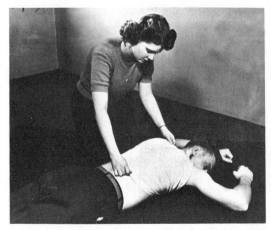

Injuries in the field or at home may be of a variety of unpredictable types. Here the triangular bandage is shown being applied to an injury or burn on the patient's back.

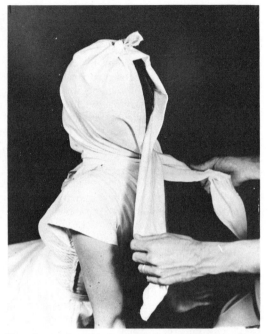

Many types of accidents, particularly burns, may affect the entire face of the victim, and thus require the use of an open face bandage with mouth and nose area cut out for breathing.

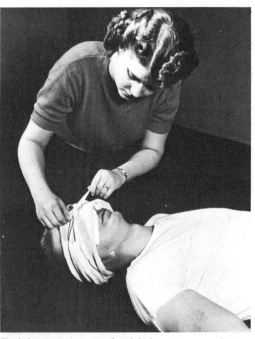

Flash burns and many other injuries may cause damage to the eyes and require some first aid protection such as the loose dressing and bandaging shown in this photo.

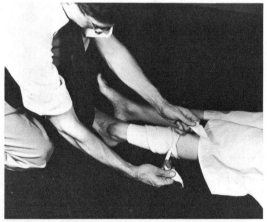

The bandaging of a dressing on a leg or arm requires spiral wrapping advancing up or down the injured part. The end is split and tied.

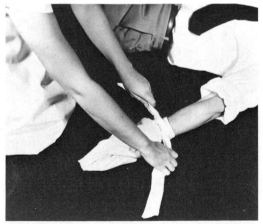

When injuries cover a large area of a limb and the dressing required is large, an open hand or foot bandage, which extends well above the injury, is often the most useful.

Bandage Techniques

Do not move a seriously burned person.

Do not remove burned clothing unless it lifts off very easily. Leave serious burns for medical treatment, but try to keep exposed burns from becoming infected by covering with sterile bandages.

Do not use antiseptics.

Do not give anything orally unless the doctor is far away and treatment for shock is necessary.

Sunstroke and heat exhaustion

The human body usually maintains a constant temperature of 98.6° F (37.5° C) regardless of the external temperature. This regulated temperature enables the various physiological processes within the body to proceed at a constant rate, and allows the body to remain active in all extremes of the earth's temperature. Body temperature from 111° to 113° F (45° C) quickly produces death in man. External temperature above 180° F may produce irreversible brain damage.

Excessive exposure to the sun may result in *sunstroke* and overexposure to any kind of excessive heat may result in *heat exhaustion*. Both are serious and both are preventable. In hot weather, especially during exercise, persons should drink water frequently. Adding a little salt to the drinking water is helpful. Light, loose clothing should be worn, and the eating of light, easily digested foods will help reduce the body heat. Iced drinks and alcoholic drinks should not be taken in hot weather if violent exertion or continued exposure to the sun is necessary.

Sunstroke is more common than heat exhaustion, and the first signs of each are similar—headache, dizziness, and nausea. However, the later symptoms and first aid care differ. In sunstroke, the face is flushed, the skin hot and dry, and the temperature is extremely high. The patient may become unconscious. To give first aid, move the victim to a cool shady place and lay him on his back with the head slightly raised. Cool the head and body with ice bags and cold cloths. Do not give any stimulants, and do not let the patient sit up until medical aid can be administered.

In heat exhaustion, the later symptoms are pallor, dizziness, palpitations, and weak pulse. The skin is moist and cool, the temperature usually normal or low. The patient may have abdominal cramps, but he is usually conscious. To give first aid, keep the patient quiet and lying down. Give table salt in several one-half teaspoon doses in water. After giving the water, give a stimulant such as coffee or tea.

Rashes can result from heat in children and adults. Prickly heat is the sensation of hot needles with or without a rash. Wear loose, cool clothing and bathe often without soap. Stay in a cool dry place. Too much powder on the body may become damp and clammy. Taking salt tablets during a heat wave is a good idea.

Prolonged exposure to cold

Overexposure to severe cold causes the individual to become numb and movement to become difficult; the victim becomes drowsy, and his drowsiness may be difficult to overcome. The person may stagger as he walks, his eyesight may fail, and he may become unconscious. First aid treatment consists of moving the patient to a cool room, and massaging the limbs briskly. If the patient has ceased to breathe, give artificial respiration. After the patient regains consciousness, the temperature of the room should be raised gradually. He may also be given hot milk, tea, or coffee. Then he should be put in a warm bed, if possible.

In instances in which the patient is chilled, no parts of the body are frozen, and he is conscious, put him in a warm bed and give hot stimulating drinks. Avoid placing hot water bags in contact with the patient's skin.

Frostbite

Frostbite is the term used to denote freezing of a part of the body. The nose, cheeks, ears, toes, and fingers are especially susceptible to frostbite. The frozen area usually becomes a peculiar pale gray, ashen color, because of actual ice formation within the tissues. First aid treatment consists of warming the affected area either by wrapping or bathing in cool water until the frozen part is thawed and circulation is restored. Do *not* rub the affected part, either manually or with snow. Frozen tissues bruise and tear very easily and there is danger of resultant gangrene. Do not expose to hot water, or heat from a fire or stove for some time, as this may cause severe pain and permanent damage to the tissues.

POISONING AND POISONS

A poison is any substance which produces a deleterious or lethal effect on living tissue. The effect of most poisons depends on the quantity consumed and the age and physical condition of the person. Substances which prevent the action of the poisons are *antidotes*.

Poisons may be classified in a number of different ways, but perhaps the most useful classification is on the basis of their physiological action. Under this simplified classification poisons fall into these classes: *corrosives, irritants, neurotoxins, hepatotoxins, hemotoxins,* and *nephrotoxins.* The corrosives include the strong acids and alkalis, the chief action of which is the local destruction of tissues. The irritants are those which produce congestion of the organ with which they come in contact. The largest group, the neurotoxins, affect the nerves or some of the basic processes within the cell. Neurotoxins include the narcotics, barbiturates, alcohols, and anesthetics. Among the hemotoxins, are carbon monoxide and hydrogen cyanide. These substances combine with the blood and prevent oxygen from forming hemoglobin. Thus death may occur from "internal suffocation," since the blood is deprived of oxygen that nourishes the tissues and brain.

General principles of treatment

The treatment of such cases involves the application of the following principles: First, the poison must be diluted. This is accomplished by having the patient drink as much water as possible. A large volume of water also promotes vomiting. Next, the stomach should be emptied. This is best done by stimulating the vomiting reflex.

Warm salt water, soapy water, or substances such as tartar emetic or prepared mustard will often bring on vomiting. Should this fail, the patient may gag himself into vomiting by holding his finger past the base of the tongue. After the patient has been induced to vomit, it is helpful to give milk, or general antidotes such as raw egg whites and olive oil. Finely divided charcoal, fuller's earth, or aluminum hydroxide antacids (e.g., Amphogel) might be given if available. By this time, the specific antidote should be administered.

Antidotes act in several different ways to counteract poison. They may combine *chemically* with the substance to render it harmless, as in the case of soda with an acid, or vinegar with lye; they act *physically* to coat the mucous membranes with a protective layer, as in the case of olive oil, or milk; or, the poisonous substance may be *absorbed* on the surface of finely divided particles, as in the case of charcoal or fuller's earth. Egg albumin (egg white) combines with many substances and is coagulated by them, making expulsion of the poison more effective. Some antidotes act *physiologically* to produce the opposite effect from the original poison, and therefore tend to counteract the action of the poison.

Another principle in the treatment of poisons is the elimination of the poison from the systemic circulation. This is a problem for the physician in charge of the case. However, in some cases of poisoning, as with ethyl alcohol, methyl alcohol, ether, benzene, and acetone, the elimination may be aided by breathing deeply in order to expel the substance with the exhaled air. Drinking as much fluid as possible will aid in excretion through the kidneys. The use of saline cathartics (e.g. Epsom salts, sodium sulfate, sodium phosphate) may aid in the elimination of some poisons from the blood by way of the liver, bile, and digestive system or prevent absorption by rapid evacuation by catharsis.

The emergency treatment of poisoned persons is aimed principally at keeping the patient alive until the poison is eliminated or neutralized. In the case of carbon monoxide, hydrogen cyanide, and any other poison that has been breathed, artificial respiration must be administered. Shock is often the cause of death in cases of poisoning; this may be prevented by warmth and stimulants such as strong coffee or tea. When possible, the patient should be kept conscious in order to aid in elimination by vomiting or other means.

If sleep-producing drugs have been taken, such as opium or morphine, it is best to keep the patient awake by giving strong coffee. In instances of strychnine poisoning, do not give any stimulant and keep the patient as quiet as possible.

A call should be made immediately to the doctor or to the police. Police rescue squads and physicians have access to poison information centers that are usually manned by the Public Health Service or state health department.

In emergency treatment of poisoning, do

Do dilute the poison by inducing the patient to drink a large amount of water.

Do bring about repeated vomiting by giving large amounts of soapsuds, warm salt, soda, or mustard water.

Do gag the patient by tickling the back of the throat with the finger. Then give more emetic fluid and do the same thing again.

Do keep up the vomiting until the fluid that is vomited is clear as when swallowed.

Do give artificial respiration if breathing ceases.

Do check chart in this chapter and administer specific treatment if the substance swallowed is known.

Do use the universal antidote given below if poison is not known.

Do call a physician or the police immediately.

Do not

Do not lose your head.

Do not waste precious time trying to look up an antidote when you don't know what has been swallowed. If you can bring about vomiting, it will greatly reduce the danger. The physician will give the proper antidote.

Universal antidote

Two parts of burned, powdered toast.
One part of milk of magnesia.
One part of strong tea.

The substances included above are found in most households. The burned powdered toast is the source of *carbon*, the milk of magnesia a source of *magnesium oxide*, and the strong tea a source of *tannic acid*. The carbon absorbs poisons, the magnesium oxide has a soothing effect on the mucous membranes of the stomach and a laxative action that tends to neutralize acid poisons, and the tannic acid tends to neutralize caustic alkaline substances.

Food poisoning

Food poisoning, erroneously known as "ptomaine" poisoning, occurs particularly during the summer months. It is caused by poison-producing bacteria in food. Certain poisonous plants may cause irritation. The symptoms are an uncomfortable sensation in the upper abdomen, pain, cramps, nausea and vomiting, and, occasionally, prostration. First aid treatment is the same as for chemical poisons.

Call local health department; save container (can, wrapper, etc.); save samples of vomitus and stool.

Metal poisoning

Poisoning can result from ingesting mercury, copper, lead, iron, cadmium, or their salts. Most metal poisoning is rare and occurs chiefly in cases of industrial carelessness. However, a common form of household metallic poisoning occurs in small children who nibble on peeling paint and plaster. The lead in the paint accumulates in their bones and eventually attacks the nervous system and brain. Exposure to sunshine increases the reaction. Since the poisoning occurs over a period of time, first aid consists of prevention and recognition. Unexplained anemia, cramps, nausea, lethargy, and convulsions are symptoms. Lead poisoning occurs from pottery finished with lead glaze, purchased outside the United States. Lead is a constituent in some foreign cosmetics, particularly eye makeup.

Iron poisoning can result when children accidentally take an overdose of iron tablets. If this happens, contact a doctor immediately. New drugs have been developed to attract metals and draw them out of bodies. Consult the chart of chemical poisons.

A kind of rat poison made of thallium sulfate also constitutes a danger to children. Rat poison is unfortunately put into cookie-like material and form and left around for vermin. The only treatment is prevention. Do not purchase anything poisonous that looks attractive to children. Do not leave any kind of rat or insect poison where children can reach it.

Chemical poisoning

There are several synthetic and natural chemicals that can cause poisoning. A chart of chemical poisons and their antidotes is included in this chapter. It should be noted that carbon tetrachloride can be taken into the system through the skin, mouth, or nose (inhaled). Many spray plastics and paints are poisonous. The user should keep his hands and body covered while spraying in a well-ventilated room. Chemical poisoning is often insidious and hard to detect.

Small amounts of carbon monoxide can be dangerous to people continually exposed to the fumes of cars and trucks, such as policemen and taxi cab drivers. Chemical poisoning can be heightened if the victim has recently had one or more drinks of alcoholic beverages.

Poisonous plants

Poisonous plants may be divided into two classes; those that produce irritation of the skin upon contact, and those that are poisonous if eaten. The most common of the skin irritant group is the poison ivy group of plants, which includes poison ivy, poison oak, and poison sumac. Poison ivy and poison oak may be recognized by their vinelike growth and the characteristic three leaves with white berries. Poison sumac has white berries, three to fourteen leaves, and forms a large shrub. All parts of these plants contain an irritating nonvolatile resin. Upon contact with the plant, the resin adheres to the skin and produces a swelling which forms small hard pimples that develop into tiny blisters. Scratching of the blisters may cause infection. To prevent "poison ivy" poisoning one should learn to recognize the plant and to avoid it. Protective clothing, such as gloves and leggings, gives much needed protection. Immediate washing of exposed parts of the body with strong soap and water serves to remove the resin. Lead acetate, tincture of ferric chloride, zinc acetate, thymol iodide, and tannic acid are substances that have been used successfully in treatment. Perhaps the safest procedure is to wash the inflamed part thoroughly with strong soap and water, cleanse with alcohol or other solvent, and apply a calamine lotion containing an antihistamine drug which will allay the itching and prevent scratching. Persons with bad cases of poison ivy dermatitis should be treated by a physician. An extensive discussion of poison ivy and other types of dermatitis caused by plants may be found in Chapter 8, "The Skin."

Some plants are poisonous only if eaten. Many common ornamental plants belong to this

TABLE OF CHEMICAL POISONS

Chemical Poison	Chief Signs and Symptoms	Emergency Treatment
Acetone Nail polish remover Paint and varnish remover	Nausea, vomiting, decreased pulse, difficulty in breathing, irritation to kidneys, stupor.	After patient has vomited, give stimulants such as strong coffee or tea.*
Acids Acetic Hydrochloric (muriatic) Nitric Phosphoric Sulfuric	Corrosion of membranes of the mouth and throat and esophagus. Vomiting, intense pain, collapse. Feeble heart beat, rapid pulse.	Give liberal doses of milk of magnesia, milk, soapy water, or egg whites.*
Alkalies Sodium hydroxide (lye, caustic soda) Potassium hydroxide (caustic potash) "Saniflush", etc.	Corrosion of mucous membranes of the digestive tract. Vomiting. Intense pain. Feeble heart beat. Rapid pulse. Blood often present in vomit and in stools.	Give strong solution of vinegar or citrus juice followed by olive oil, melted butter, or other nontoxic oil. Emetic contraindicated.*
Alcohol, Methyl Wood alcohol Paint or shellac thinner	Depression, muscle inco-ordination, headache, disturbed vision, nausea, blindness, delirium, collapse; often fatal.	After patient has vomited, give large dose of baking soda followed by a dose of epsom salts. Have the patient inhale spirits of ammonia if available.*
Amyl acetate Nail polish remover Banana oil Pear oil Lacquer thinner	Irritation of eyes, coughing, abdominal pain, vomiting, respiratory difficulty.	Give strong stimulants such as coffee or tea. Do not give patient anything to make him vomit.*
Arsenic Fly paper Fowler's solution Paris green Lead arsenate Ant or rat poison	Metallic taste, burning pain in esophagus or stomach, vomiting and diarrhea, thirst, choking sensation, garlic odor on breath, cold skin, rapid weak pulse, collapse, convulsions, coma.	Give strong stimulants, followed by castor oil or epsom salts.*
Barbiturates Barbital Phenobarbital Seconal Nembutal Amytal Pentothal	Small doses produce sleep. Large doses produce headache, mental confusion, coma, blue lips and fingernails, dilated pupils, slow or irregular breathing.	Administer strong stimulants. If breathing remains normal, patient will probably sleep off the effects of the drug.*
Benzene, Benzol Toluene Xylol Floorwax or polish Some shoe polish	Nausea, vomiting, headache, irregular pulse, dizziness, excitement, depression, coma. Heart failure. Damage to blood-forming organs.	Give large amounts of vegetable (cooking) oil, not mineral oil.*
Benzine Gasoline Kerosene Petroleum ether Cleaner's naphtha	Inhalation produces cyanosis, flushed face, coma, dilated pupils and respiratory failure. Swallowing produces burning of mouth, nausea, vomiting, drunkenness, thirst, slow pulse, difficult breathing, convulsions and coma.	Do not induce vomiting. Give large amounts of vegetable (cooking) oil, not mineral oil.
LSD *d*-lysergic acid diethylamide	Dilated pupils, exhilaration or extreme anxiety, delirium, muscle cramps, inability to move, convulsions.	Administer tranquilizers (chlorpromazine), and reassure the patient. Do not restrain physically.*
Carbon monoxide Coal gas Automobile exhaust	Dizziness, weakness, headache, stupor, throbbing pulse, increased blood pressure, skin dusky, lips pink, paralysis, coma.	Remove patient to fresh air and begin artificial respiration. Protect from shock.*
Carbon tetrachloride Noninflammable cleaning fluid Fire extinguisher fluid	Headache, drowsiness, confusion, coma. Abdominal pain, dilated pupils. Kidney and liver damage follows acute symptoms.	Give strong coffee or tea in addition to the treatment listed below for induction of vomiting and prevention of shock.*
Chlorine Sodium hypochlorite Bleaching solution of "Clorox" type	Inhalation produces irritation of the lungs and eyes, spasmlike cough, choking, vomiting, cyanosis, collapse. Swallowing produces irritation of the gastrointestinal tract and extreme pain.	If inhaled, remove patient to fresh air, give artificial respiration, and have the patient inhale spirits of ammonia. If swallowed, treat as listed below for production of vomiting and prevention of shock.*

TABLE OF CHEMICAL POISONS (Con't.)

Chemical Poison	Chief Signs and Symptoms	Emergency Treatment

Copper salts
  Copper sulfate
  Blue stone
  Blue vitriol
  Zinc salts
	Nausea, vomiting, purging, severe abdominal pains, cold clammy skin, delirium, coma, convulsions.	The patient should vomit repeatedly. Then, give egg white or magnesia followed by strong coffee or tea.*

Cyanides
  Hydrocyanic acid
  Cyanogen
  Some insect poison
  Gopher poison
	Large doses produce instant death. Small doses cause vomiting, diarrhea, difficult breathing, glassy eyes, pale face, blood-stained foam on mouth, stupor, coma.	After patient has vomited, give dose of hydrogen peroxide.*

Fluorides Cockroach or insect poison	Nausea, vomiting, abdominal cramps, weakness, fall in blood pressure, deep rapid respiration, convulsions, coma.	Give calcium tablets, lime water, chalk, or milk.*

Formaldehyde
  Home disinfectant
  Preserving fluid for natural history specimens
	Swallowing produces irritation of mouth and gut. Irritation of lungs. Severe abdominal pain, nausea, vomiting, rapid pulse, blood in urine. Intense irritation of eyes and lungs upon breathing fumes.	Before having patient vomit, give him dilute ammonia water, egg whites, or milk. After he has vomited, give large doses of baking soda in water.*

Iodine
  Tincture of iodine
  Iodex salve
  Lugol's solution
	Brown color on lips and mouth. Burning pain in stomach, vomiting. Bloody purging, heart depression, cold skin, convulsions, collapse.	Give large quantities of starch (bread, flour, corn starch, etc.) followed by strong coffee or tea.*

Lead
  Red lead
  White lead
  Paints
	Pain in stomach, thirst, blood in stools and vomit, weakness, paralysis, convulsions, collapse.	After patient has vomited, give him calcium tablets, powdered chalk, or milk, followed by epsom salts.*

Mercury
  Bichloride of mercury
  Corrosive sublimate
	Severe pain in mouth, throat, stomach, increase in saliva, blood and mucus in vomit. Watery bloody diarrhea, followed in 1 or 2 days by inflammation of colon, blood in urine, coma, collapse.	Give egg whites immediately.*

Opium
  Codeine
  Heroin
  Laudanum
  Morphine
	Mental exhilaration followed by drowsiness. Pupils of eyes pinpoint. Slow shallow breathing, slow onset of unconsciousness, muscles relaxed, skin pale, cold sweat, blue lips, irregular breathing.	After patient has vomited, give him a dose of charcoal and aluminum hydroxide. Follow this with strong coffee or tea, and keep the patient awake and warm until a physician arrives.*

Phenols
  Carbolic acid
  Creosote
  Lysol
	Burning pain from mouth to stomach, white patches in mouth, depression, weakness, nausea. Blood in urine, fall in body temperature. Pale, livid, clammy face.	Give patient large quantities of any nontoxic oil (olive oil, mineral oil, cooking oil, etc.). Also give lime water and egg whites. Do not give patient anything to make him vomit.*

Phosphorus
  Matches
  Rat poison (read label)
	Gastrointestinal pain, garlic odor, vomiting of blood, bloody diarrhea. If patient survives, remission of symptoms in 2 to 3 days. Later symptoms: skin eruption, enlarged liver, jaundice, pulse weak, heart weak, convulsions.	Give large amounts of mineral oil, followed by epsom salts.*

*In every type of poisoning, immediate medical aid is essential. Further, vomiting should be induced if the poison is swallowed (except in those cases noted where it is contraindicated) by causing the patient to gag or by administration of warm soapy water or a tartar emetic. Every patient must be kept warm until the physician arrives, and other standard means to combat shock should be instituted. Should the patient cease breathing before medical aid is available, artificial respiration should be given.

group. In case a person should eat some of these plants, the best first aid procedure is to induce vomiting. A specimen of the plant should be taken to the physician so that he may identify it with certainty. The following is a list of the most common poisonous plants, with the poisonous part indicated in parentheses:

Aconite, monks hood (all parts); *Atropa,* belladonna (all parts); *Cicuta maculata,* water hemlock (all parts); *Conium,* poison hemlock

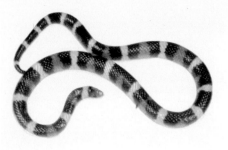

Scarlet King snake

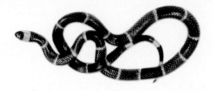

Coral snake

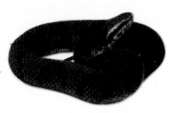

Water moccasin

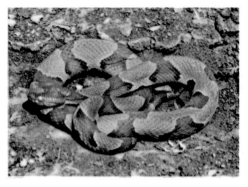

Copperhead

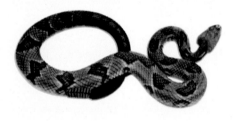

Timber rattle snake

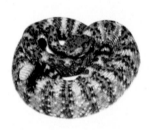

Southwest speckled rattle snake

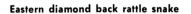

Eastern diamond back rattle snake

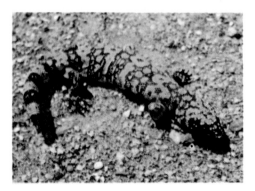

Gila monster

(all parts); *Datura*, Jimson weed (all parts); *Delphinium*, larkspur (foliage); *Dieffenbachia*, dumb cane, mother-in-law plant (stalks); *Digitalis*, fox glove (foliage); *Helleborus*, Christmas rose (roots); *Hyoscyamus*, henbane (juice); *Kalmia*, native laurel (foliage); *Laburnum*, golden chain (seeds); *Nerium*, oleander (all parts); *Phytolacca*, poke (root); *Prunus serotina*, wild black cherry (dried foliage); *Rhododendron*, all species (foliage); *Ricinus*, castor bean (seeds only); *Solanum nigrum*, deadly nightshade (foliage); and *Taxus* (all parts). Children often taste or chew the leaves of the elephant ear fern. Although this plant is not poisonous, chewing the leaves will cause a burning and painful tingling of the tongue.

Poisonous snakes

Four kinds of poisonous snakes are native to the United States and account for over 2000 cases of snake bite each year. These are the coral snakes, the rattlesnakes, copperheads, and cottonmouth moccasins. Cobras now live on the Louisiana coast.

The coral snakes belong to the cobra family. They produce a potent toxin that acts quickly on the nervous system. The bite of a coral snake may be quickly fatal. These snakes are small and are easily recognized because of colored bands arranged in the order of red, yellow, and black.

The other poisonous snakes belong to the pit viper group. These can be recognized by the presence of a pit between the eye and nostril. Like some nonpoisonous species, they are thick-bodied and have a flat arrow-shaped head. Also, they have two self-erecting hypodermic-like fangs in the upper jaw by which they inject poison into the wound. A large rattlesnake may inject about 200 milligrams of venom (approximately nine lethal doses); a water moccasin, 150; and a copperhead, 45. Incision and suction may remove as high as 100 milligrams, so a physician should be sought for an injection of antivenom for neutralization of the remaining toxin.

Emergency treatment of snake bites

Emergency treatment of snake bites is often necessary in the field because medical assistance frequently is not available. Speed is most essential to prevent the spread of the poison from the location of the bite.

1. A crosswise incision should be made immediately through the fang punctures. The incision should be as deep as the puncture (approximately one-fourth inch deep by one-half inch long), but care should be taken that a ligament or an artery is not cut. The knife used

Poisonous and Nonpoisonous reptiles.

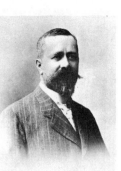

CALMETTE. Léon Charles Albert (1863-1933) French bacteriologist. In 1897, Calmette developed an antivenom for treatment of snake bite, now called *Calmette's serum*. He made several contributions to our present knowledge of immunization against infectious diseases. With Yersin, in 1895, he used antiplague serum, and in 1927 in cooperation with Camille Guérin he made a prophylactic antituberculosis vaccine, called *BCG* (Bacillus Calmette Guérin).

preferably should be sterilized first by a flame, or cleaned with iodine or alcohol.

2. Suction should then be applied to the wound by mouth or a suction cup. There is no great danger in sucking venom from the wound by mouth provided there are no sore places on the gums or mouth. This process may be repeated until blood in the immediate vicinity has been removed. If the wound is inaccessible for suction, then blood should be squeezed repeatedly from the wound.

3. An alternative plan, recommended by some doctors, is simply to cut out the flesh around the bite, taking care not to harm a vessel or ligament. Do not do this if the bite is on the head or neck. Pain is not a factor since snake venom usually numbs the area. Apply tourniquet and stop the bleeding. The size of the flesh removed is between that of a quarter and a half dollar.

4. A tourniquet should be placed just above the bite and should be tight enough to check the return flow of the blood, but loose enough to allow some blood to flow from the wound. The tourniquet should be loosened every 15 minutes for two minutes to restore circulation to the affected limb.

5. The limb should not be moved more than is absolutely necessary, as movement may spread the venom. The patient should be carried, if possible, on an improvised stretcher. The snake which bit the patient should be taken to the physician for identification in order that the right type of antivenom may be administered.

6. Antivenom should be given only by a physician; however, if it is necessary to administer it in the field, the directions on the package should be carefully followed. The antiserum should not be administered to a person known to be sensitive to horse serum. Alcohol or stimulants should not be given as they accelerate the circulation and thus increase the absorption of poison.

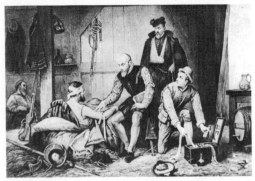

The French surgeon, Ambrose Paré (1517-1590), washing the wound of a soldier. *Bettman Archive.*

Prevention of snake bite

About 75 percent of snake bites occur on the lower leg. These could be prevented by the wearing of boots or leggings. In snake-infested country, one should watch where he steps and take particular care in picking flowers or berries. In climbing cliffs and ledges, it may be disastrous to reach the hand over rocks and prominences where a snake may be coiled. The arms and hands may be protected by the wearing of long sleeves and gloves.

In case of poisonous snake bite, do

Do begin first aid *at once*. Even a few moments delay may mean the difference between life and death.

Do have the patient lie down and keep quiet, for movement will only increase the spread of the poison.

Do apply a tourniquet at once, directly above the bite, using a handkerchief, necktie, or piece of cloth.

Do make crosscut incisions, using a clean blade, about one-fourth to one-half inch long and just through the skin, across the fang marks. The incisions should not be deep enough to sever tendons or veins. *Or* simply cut out the flesh around the bite.

Do use a suction cup to draw out the poison. If a suction cup is not available, the mouth may be used.

Do loosen the tourniquet and move it up a little if swelling causes too much constriction.

Do not

Do not delay giving first aid. Even a few moments delay is dangerous.

Do not let the patient move around, as this will only spread the poison.

Do not give the patient whiskey or any other stimulant.

ARTIFICIAL RESPIRATION

The Red Cross, the Y.M.C.A., the Y.W.C.A., and many other organizations give courses of training in life saving. Such training has saved countless lives. When an individual attempts rescue of a drowning person, his ability to think clearly may mean the difference between life and death, not only for the victim but also for himself. He should first of all never attempt to swim to the person's aid unless he himself is an excellent swimmer with *training in life saving.* The victim often is hysterical, and his behavior is erratic. Furthermore, the agitation of drowning persons causes even the frailest to exert tremendous muscular power, so that a very strong rescuer may be submerged. If a life buoy is not available, extend some floating object for the victim to grasp.

Often the victim will be unconscious and will be floating face down with his shoulders and the upper part of his back visible. Such a person should be brought to shore at once by any safe means available to the rescuer, keeping the victim's nose and mouth above water. Once ashore, the victim should be checked for swallowed objects or vomitus by swishing a finger through the mouth and throat. *When the mouth and throat are proved clear*, artificial respiration should be begun *at once*. This is true even though help may be very near. A few minutes spent in searching for someone with a pulmotor may mean death for the victim. Artificial respiration sometimes must be continued many hours before the victim shows any signs of life. Do not waste time "*jackknifing*" the victim's body in an effort to expel water from the lungs. The expulsion of air by artificial respiration tends to remove water from the lungs, but the fluid must be prevented from reentering the airways. This can be done by turning the victim's head to one side until the mouth touches the ground at intervals during artificial respiration. Or, if the person is small, he may be picked up by his heels.

There are two fundamental reasons for the cessation of breathing. The first reason to be sought by the person rendering first aid is mechanical obstruction. If the patient has swallowed some object, such as his tongue, false teeth, a large amount of water, etc., an attempt should be made to remove the obstructing material *if* it completely prevents breathing. If the patient is still able to breathe, even though with difficulty, it is often better not to attempt to remove the obstructing object, since such an attempt may only succeed in dislodging it into another position in which it obstructs breathing completely. In removing the foreign object from the throat or windpipe the first-aider may use forceps if they are available. Otherwise, he should attempt to remove it with his fingers, being very careful to hold the patient's jaw in such a way that he cannot be bitten. The fingers may be protected by placing some object such as a wallet at one side of the teeth or by wrapping the fingers in a handkerchief.

Breathing also may be stopped if there is functional injury to the brain. Any condition which cuts down the oxygen supply of the blood deprives the essential parts of the brain of their necessary oxygen and may thereby inhibit the breathing processes.

Many deaths occur each year as a result of suffocation or asphyxiation. Many of these lives could be saved by people present at the time of the emergency with just a little knowledge concerning artificial respiration. The procedure described here is the newest, safest, simplest, and most efficient procedure in use today. A pictorial illustration of this method will be found on the endpapers at the front of this book.

The *Journal of the American Medical Association* has published a detailed account of a new mode of artificial respiration. This technique, now known as "mouth-to-mouth resuscitation," has been proven far superior to all other procedures for the restoration of breathing. The untrained layman may at first revolt at the thought of placing his mouth over the mouth or nose of another person, but several hundred cases of successful oral resuscitation by individuals who just happened to be near when an accident occurred indicate that this concern is immediately forgotten when an emergency arises. In fact, the various devices currently being manufactured for placement between the mouth of the victim and that of the person administering resuscitation are not recommended unless one is *immediately* available and there has been previous training in its use.

The first step in oral resuscitation is to place the victim on his back and lift the neck with one hand while the other hand pushes the top of the head downward. When the head is tilted back as far as it will go, the mouth will usually open of its own accord. The hand beneath the neck is then brought around to pull the jaw upward, as far as it will go. This takes forceful pressure. Both hands may be needed. After the head and neck are extended, the rescuer's knees may be used to keep the head in position while raising the jaw. This opens the airway by making the tongue fall away. Keep holding the jaw up with one hand.

The rescuer then places his mouth over the open mouth of the victim so that a complete seal is obtained. The nose must be either pinched closed or blocked by the pressure of the cheek so there is no leakage of air. A seal can be made by making a circle with index finger and thumb, placing the circle around the mouth while pinching the nose with the same fingers.

Air from the rescuer's lungs is then exhaled into the victim's lungs without blowing until the chest expands visibly. The head is then raised slightly and tilted to one side and a new breath taken. In this brief instant, the rescuer should either feel or hear the air being expelled from the victim's lungs by the passive resistance of his rib cage. Or the rescuer may actually feel the air from the victim's lungs being expelled against his own cheek. If there is no such response, the resuscitation is not being administered properly. Either there is an obstruction in the air passage, the head is not tilted back far enough, or there is a leakage of air around the mouth or through the nose. The new breath of air is then exhaled into the victim's lungs and the procedure continued until the victim begins breathing of his own accord. It must be emphasized that the procedure should be continued at great length, even though the victim shows no signs of recovery.

In some cases where the heart has stopped beating, a procedure referred to as "closed chest cardiac massage" may restore the beat. The heel of the hand is placed on the center of the chest over the sternum and the other hand placed on top. A firm pressure is made downward followed by a sudden release 60 times a minute. If the pulse returns, the procedure may be stopped.

If the rescuer cannot or will not attempt mouth-to-mouth resuscitation, he should employ the manual method shown illustrated on page 726 or 727.

While resuscitation is being carried out, blankets or coverings should be used for protecting the victim. Wet clothing should be cut or torn away and the body warmly covered; however, this should be done during artificial respiration, which must not be stopped.

Other emergencies

Other circumstances besides drowning often necessitate artificial respiration. Whenever an individual stops breathing from any cause, *asphyxia* or *suffocation,* unconsciousness, and death occur unless atrificial breathing is carried on for him. The most frequent instances requiring artificial respiration are suffocation, heart attack, brain injury, electrical shock, and poisoning by gas. Pneumonia is the most dangerous afteraffect of victims of gassing, electric shock, and near-drowning. Such victims should not be exposed to infection from lack of proper warmth. Any patient receiving resuscitation should be kept warm.

Water Safety and Rescue

Few techniques in first aid are more important than the proper methods for rescuing a person from drowning. The individual victim and his emotional state dictate to a large extent the exact means that are employed, for the first aid administrator must insure that he will not himself be endangered in the rescue process. Many drowning persons become hysterical, and thus offer considerable danger to the rescuer. Extensive study has been devoted to the development of methods for effecting a rescue in the water with a minimum of danger, and a number of valuable approaches to this problem have been evolved. Each of these has its special application and advantages, and training is required before they can be applied with safety. It is axiomatic that a person who is not a reasonably good swimmer should not undertake the rescue of a drowning person, and thereby create two victims rather than one. The following series of pictures illustrates some of the more important methods by which a victim many be recovered from the water in an expeditious manner and with minimum danger to the person performing the rescue. *Courtesy American National Red Cross.*

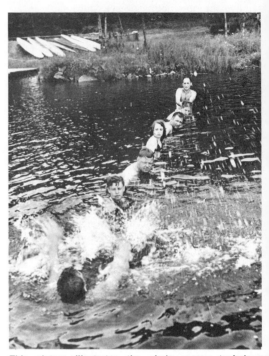

This picture illustrates the chain rescue technique which is used when the drowning person is near shore and a number of persons are present to help.

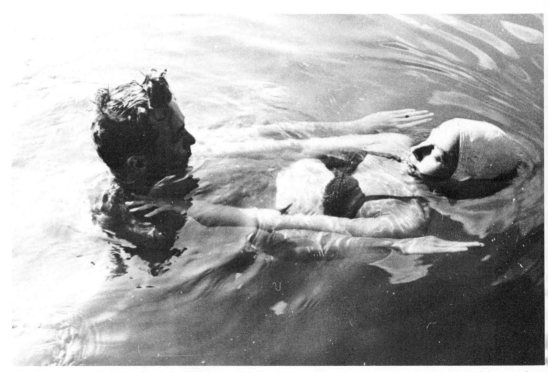

The tired swimmer's carry shown in this photograph is of value only when the person to be rescued is conscious and rational and can be counted on to give the rescuer maximum co-operation. The victim, who is floating on her back, is given support by the rescuer's shoulders as he swims with both arms to the nearest shore.

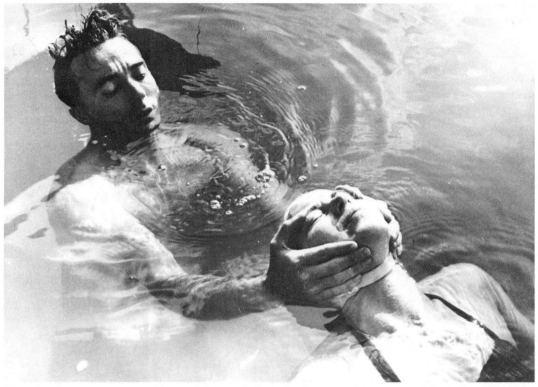

When the drowning person must be carried through the water for some distance, one of the better methods for pulling the victim is the head carry shown in the accompanying photograph, in which the swimmer grasps the victim's head and holds it above water as he travels through the water by his leg action.

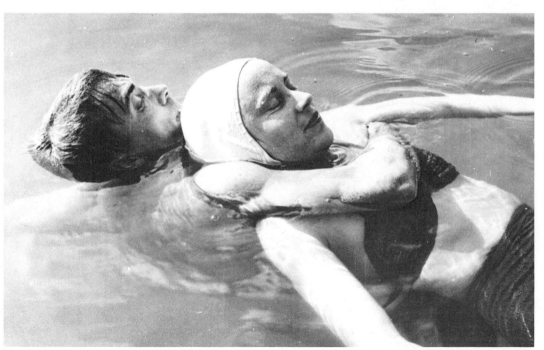

The drowning victim may be pulled to shore by means of the cross chest carry, shown above. This method keeps the victim's head safely above water and provides a firm grip for the swimmer, while at the same time it releases one arm of the rescuer to aid him in making his way through the water to the nearest place of safety.

Manual Methods of Artificial Respiration

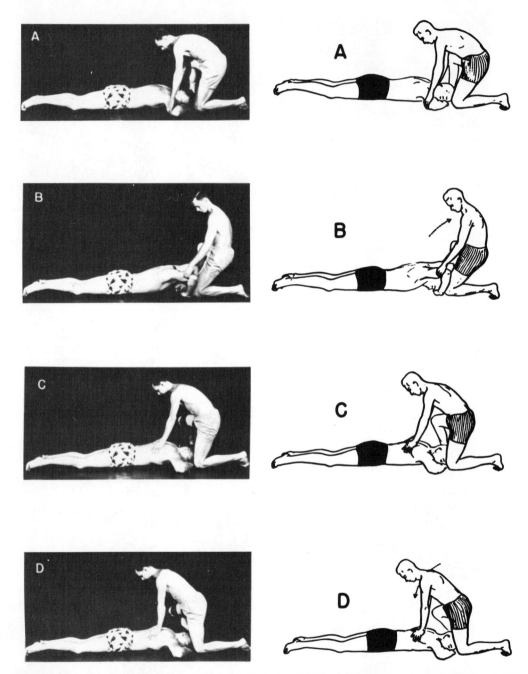

The back-pressure, arm-lift or Holger Nielsen method of artificial respiration is one of the types of push-pull methods that is considered superior to the older Schafer prone pressure method. In the above series of pictures, the hands are placed under victim's arms just above the elbows in A, then pulled upward and toward the operator in B. Next, hands are placed in position for back pressure in C, and pressure is exerted in D. This entire maneuver should be completed about twelve times each minute. Inspiration results from drawing back the arms, and expiration occurs when pressure is applied to the back. This method of manual artificial respiration is considered one of the best, and has been used in Scandinavian countries with success for over thirty years.

Photographs: A. S. Gordon, M. S. Sadove, F. Raymon and A. C. Ivy; University of Illinois College of Medicine, Chicago. By permission INDUSTRIAL MEDICINE AND SURGERY, 1952. Drawings: Copyright 1951, J. Amer. M. Assn.

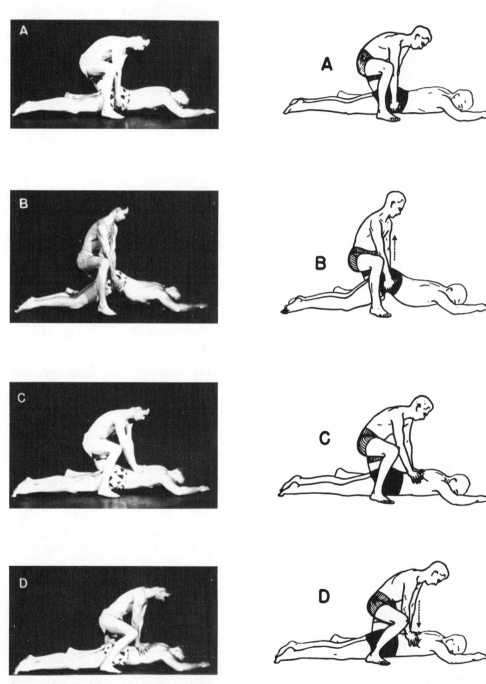

The above series of pictures shows the technique of administering the hip-lift, back-pressure method of artificial respiration. Identical steps are shown by posed models on the left and drawings on the right. This method combines alternately lifting the hips of the patient and then exerting pressure on the midback. In A the first aid administrator is placing his hands for the hip lift, in B hips are being lifted, in C hands are in place for back pressure, and in D the pressure is being exerted on the back. The operator rocks backward as he lifts the hips, and forward as he exerts pressure on the back. His arms are kept straight in both cases so that the work is imposed upon his shoulders and back rather than on his arms. As the hips are lifted there is an inspiration by the victim, and expiration results from pressure applied to the victim's back.

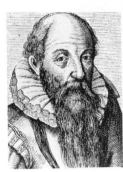

FABRICIUS, Hildanus (Wilhelm Fabry) (1560-1634) German surgeon. Fabricius recorded the first known classification of burns, and recognized that the severity of a burn is dependent on the body area involved as well as the depth of the burn. He is called the father of German surgery, and his writings reflect much practical experience in dealing with injuries. He published a book of case histories which was used for many years.

FIRST AID IN DISASTER

Catastrophes of varying kinds account for an enormous number of deaths in the United States each year. The Galveston tidal wave of 1900 alone claimed 6000 lives. Conflagrations, burns, and explosions account for the greatest number of catastrophic deaths, followed by tornadoes, floods, and hurricanes.

Such emergencies as the Texas City explosion and the Kansas City flood bring to the scene of disaster many emergency services such as the Red Cross and civil defense health services of the federal, state, and local governments. However, before these services can possibly reach the scene, there is much that should and can be done by the alert individual to reduce suffering and save lives.

Psychological reactions during emergencies

The effect of panic during catastrophe may result in disastrous consequences. The famous Orson Wells' broadcast of the "Invasion from Mars" indicated the reactions of a panic-stricken population. The resources of the population under stress will be the sum total of the individual resources. Therefore, if the individual will give some thought to a positive course of action beforehand, much tragedy will be averted. In general, a few over-all directions may prove helpful.

1. Do not lose your head; do not become panic stricken and run about blindly.

2. Take a moment to consider *what* you know concerning the situation. Recall *what to do* and *what not to do.*

3. After you have secured your personal safety and that of your family, then volunteer for rescue work. If no one is available to allocate responsibility, assume such responsibility and do what seems sensible.

4. Help, if possible, but do not crowd about any scene of rescue unless you can actually do something.

The greatest emergencies arising in disaster are burns, suffocation, hemorrhage, and shock.

Fires and floods

The first consideration during a fire is human life. However, if possible, rescue should be left to the well-trained firemen on the scene. Many persons have lost their lives in misguided attempts to save other people from a fire. A would-be rescuer should never rush headlong into a burning building to save another without first considering his own chances of survival; and then only when he is certain that someone is actually helpless within the fire. He runs the risk of being trapped in a collapsing building, as well as of being asphyxiated through lack of oxygen and an excess of noxious gases caused by the fire. A wet handkerchief over the mouth and nose may keep smoke out of the lungs, but it is *no* protection against asphyxiation. Doors should be felt cautiously before they are opened to prevent releasing a burst of flame. The purest air in a burning building is near the

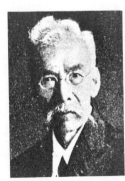

YAMAGIWA, Katsusaburo (1863-1930) Japanese physician. Yamagiwa conducted extensive research into the relationship of chemicals to incidence of cancer. In 1916, he successfully produced a so-called coal tar cancer, by painting the ears of rabbits with coal tar. This was the first cancer experimentally produced by coal tars. *From collections of Armed Forces Medical Library, and permission from The Wellcome Historical Medical Museum Library, London; British Medical Bulletin.*

ESMARCH, Johann Friedrich August von (1823-1908) German military surgeon. In 1869, Esmarch introduced a first aid packet for use on the battlefield, and a highly useful rubber tourniquet. He devoted most of his time and abilities to devising operations and equipment which would be of use on the battlefield, and to improving the effectiveness of the Medical Corps. He devised several operations, including a leg amputation.

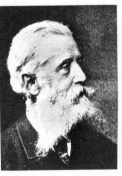

floor, so that keeping low may greatly facilitate breathing.

When an individual's clothing becomes ignited, a bystander is often in a position to save the person's life by acting quickly and intelligently. One of the greatest dangers of burning clothes is that the flames will be inhaled, causing irreparable damage to the lungs. Also, running fans the flames. Therefore, the first rule is to throw the person to the ground. The fire may then be extinguished by wrapping the burning person in a coat, blanket, or rug, or by rolling him on the ground. Flames may be beaten out by the hand.

In many cases, suffocation and the effects of noxious gases are greater causes of injury than are burns. For this reason fire victims should be given sufficient fresh air outside the burning building. Persons escaping a fire without burns still may suffer severely from shock or respiratory distress.

If the danger of flood is imminent, the preservation of life is more important than the preservation of property. There are on record countless tragic instances in which entire families have lost their lives in foolish attempts to save belongings by piling them in the middle of the house. The greatest immediate danger from flood is, of course, drowning. Once safety is reached, caution must be used in drinking water that may be polluted. As a general rule, do not drink water unless it has been boiled, or unless it is procured from some rescue source and is known to be pure. In most flood areas it is necessary to receive typhoid fever injections to prevent the disease. The danger of tetanus is also present in the event of wounds of any kind.

Warfare

Special weapons available for modern warfare fall into three groups: biological, chemical, and atomic. The United States government has made a positive move to prevent biological warfare by unilaterally dismantling production of material for germ warfare. But the possibility exists that another country might use biologicals. And while treaties to ban the use of atomic weapons might ease world tensions, nuclear accidents—the loss of bombs from armed planes or reactor explosions—have become a real threat.

Reasonably effective means of infecting human beings and their food sources, animals, and crops, with biological agents such as bacteria are well known. However, the danger of a widespread epidemic is thought to be minimal. Spread of diseases through whole populations requires a combination of many conditions, in addition to the successful spread of the germs, and this chain of factors has never been produced artificially. In other words, the individuals initially infected by a surprise attack with a biological weapon may require intensive medical care; but early detection of the source and nature of the infection by the Public Health Service and other organizations can reasonably by expected, together with specific action as to proper means of control.

Chemical weapons also have their limitations. During World War II, the Germans developed a group of so-called "nerve" gases, which are more toxic and rapid in action than substances previously used as weapons. Yet the Germans did not use these gases, even in desperation before defeat. It is conceivable that under special circumstances, chemical agents would be employed against limited key areas and personnel; but generalized use against large numbers of civilians seems both impractical and improbable at the present time.

The problems posed by the possible use of atomic weapons are somewhat different from those created by dangers from biological or chemical agents. Several countries now have the power to annihilate major populations with one or two explosions. Although an attacking power would hesitate to use uranium, plutonium, or hydrogen bombs because of retaliation, the danger of a power struggle is present. Nuclear accident, the accidental loss of atomic weapons because of a plane crash, has occurred. And, as peaceful uses of atomic energy increase, the danger of reactor explosions and radiation leakage must be considered. Nuclear accident—unlike biological warfare, which can be stopped—could be a limitless tragedy.

Effects of atomic explosions: Injuries produced directly by atomic explosions result from three types of physical forces released when bombs or reactors explode. *Blast waves* occur, which differ only in magnitude from those caused by more conventional explosive weapons. Intense *radiant* heat, a negligible factor in the older types of explosives, is sufficient to produce serious flash burns on surfaces exposed directly to an atomic explosion. Dangerous *radiations,* a new hazard in war, are emitted from the exploding bomb itself for a short time after the actual explosion. Under certain circumstances, similar radiations can persist in the area about the explosion for a limited period.

The effects of these three physical forces vary according to the manner in which a bomb is exploded. Bursts high in the air—as at Hiroshima and Nagasaki—produce the widest area of destruction but leave less significant radiations on the ground. Bursts close to the ground pulverize everything in a small area about the explosion and contaminate the ground with radiating material.

The injuries caused by an atomic explosion result in several ways from the three physical forces released. *Blast* was the direct cause of few of the injuries found among the survivors of the two explosions in Japan. It did great damage to buildings, however, and thus indirectly wounded thousands who were crushed by falling walls or were in the path of flying debris.

Radiant heat seared the skin and deeper tissues of many who were exposed to its action. In addition, it caused some materials to burst into flame and thereby contributed to the secondary fires which trapped many victims. Other fires were incidental to destruction of buildings by the blast.

Radiations from the bomb itself are dangerous for unprotected individuals within a mile of the explosion of the type of bomb used against Japan. Should a bomb be exploded near or under the ground, or under water, the area affected would continue to emit radiations for a time, but even these radiations rapidly cease to be dangerous *if* the material from which they come remains outside the body. However, should this material enter and remain in the body—such as dust drawn into the lungs, or a contaminant of ingested food or water—the diminished radiations can be dangerous by acting for a long period of time on the tissues. Escaping radiation is a hazard to workers near atomic reactors.

Prevention of injuries: Waves of blast, heat, and radiation generally travel in straight lines from the point of the explosion, although blast waves can sometimes be deflected freakishly by hills or other solid obstacles. Consequently, even a shallow ditch or curbstone can offer an amazing amount of protection for those who resort to them promptly after an explosion occurs. Any covering of the bare skin with cloth or other material, especially if it is light in color, will diminish the danger of flash burns from the heat wave. Breathing through a handkerchief, particularly a moist one, will reduce the inhalation of dust or mist which may be emitting radiations. Food and water in a bombed area should not be used until declared safe.

These elementary precautions can save many lives. More elaborate methods are being developed to fit the special needs of probable target areas. The individual's life and those of his family may depend on how well he keeps himself informed.

Treatment of the injured: Open wounds, hemorrhage, fractures, burns, and shock produced by atomic bombs do not differ from the same injuries caused in other ways. First aid skills discussed previously are of incalculable value wherever they are available to the victims. Control of serious bleeding, proper bandages for wounds and burns, and support of blood pressure with warmth and stimulants can keep many alive who would otherwise die before medical help could reach them.

The severity of injury from radiation is difficult to estimate immediately, but popular concepts of these "rays" have exaggerated their power. Many Japanese survived exposure to moderate amounts of radiation; and even though they suffered from temporary loss of hair, diarrhea, moderate decrease in weight, and other disorders, no permanent disability has been observed.

Effects of atomic bombs are discussed in greater detail in Chapter 29, "Medical Aspects of Atomic and Hydrogen Bomb Warfare."

ACCIDENT PREVENTION

Over 10 million persons in the United States suffer injuries from accidents each year. Over 100,000 are killed and there is an additional loss of billions of dollars in property damage. During the past half century much study has gone into the nature and causes of these accidents. Perhaps the most important fact that these investigations has established is that accidents can be prevented. Acceptance of this has resulted in the numerous "Safety First" programs which exist in schools, factories, and elsewhere. Laws have been passed to enforce accident prevention measures. Probably the major problem in accident prevention involves education of the public to the fact that accident prevention is everyone's business, and that it must be practiced continuously.

Safety organizations: In 1913 a group of employers organized the National Safety Council as an information center on industrial accident prevention. The activities of this organization, however, were expanded almost immediately to take in other phases of safety work, so that for many years the National Safety Council has been the center of accident prevention work in the United States. Similar organizations patterned after it now exist in most other countries. Accident prevention is taught in all grade

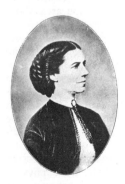

BARTON, Clara (1821-1912) American nurse and philanthropist. During the Civil War, Clara Barton recruited and trained nurses for use in the Army, and saw that the sick and wounded soldiers were provided with adequate shelter and food. Largely through her efforts, many soldiers were given a chance to survive. Her work is an example of the effectiveness of good nursing care. In 1881, she became the first president of the Red Cross.

schools through special classes, lectures, and devices; and many schools have special safety patrols. In most industrial organizations there is a safety director, who is responsible for accident prevention and safety education. That such efforts are valuable is indicated by the low number of accidents that occur in certain industrial plants as compared with others.

Prevention of traffic accidents: The major single cause of accidental death involves automobiles. In 1969, there were 55,200 fatal motor accidents. Deaths from motor vehicles are seldom caused by mechanical failure of the machine, but are usually caused by the drivers or by pedestrians. Pedestrians account for a large percentage of the traffic fatalities in this country, and in many cases it appears that the pedestrian is guilty of some violation of the law at the time he is killed. In the case of the drivers of motor vehicles, the two major factors in producing accidents are excessive speed and the consumption of alcohol. When the alcohol in the blood exceeds 0.15 percent per cubic centimeter, even the most inveterate drinker has impaired judgment and muscular control. Various types of medical equipment are now employed by the police to measure this blood alcohol level. It is emphasized in this regard that *drunken* drivers are seldom as great a hazard as *drinking* drivers, and that many accidents are caused by the split-second loss of acuity that may be brought on by drinking even small amounts of alcohol.

Aside from these factors, traffic accidents are caused by a lack of attention to details that are important when any machine the size of a modern automobile is propelled under human guidance. It is generally recognized that traffic accidents are among the most preventable of all accidents, and could be almost completely eliminated by adequate driver control. Certainly many fatalities and serious injuries could be avoided by the simple and habitual use of the two-point (lap) seat belt. It should be fastened at all times, no matter at what speed the car is moving. Even better protection is afforded by the three-point belt (a diagonal strap crossing the upper trunk and lap belt). The upper strap restrains the forward movement of the passenger in the event of a collision. Dashboards and sun visors now are usually padded to prevent head and chest injuries. Portions of the steering wheel are padded. Research underway indicates that the steering wheel will be completely padded. Installation of head rests has helped cut down on the severity of whiplash injuries.

Protective safety devices for future automobiles include an inflatable air bag, stowed in front of each passenger. In a collision, the bag rapidly inflates within less than a second. This air cushion will prevent serious frontal injuries caused by the passenger's impact with the steering wheel, dashboard, and windshield.

Research is also being conducted on a "collapsible front end" of the car, redesign of bumpers in order that they will absorb more of the impact upon collision, and improving the safety quality of the window glass.

Along with automobile accidents, accidents caused by motorized appliances constitute a hazard. Lawnmowers are too often used by young children or by careless adults. Snowmobiles have caused several accidents since some types have open motors and clothing can get caught easily in the moving parts.

Prevention of accidents in the home: About half of all accidental deaths in the home result from falls, and one-fifth from burns. Home accidents result from carelessness and also from hazards in construction and equipment of the home. To some extent building codes have helped to reduce home accidents, but carelessness will always be the major problem in reducing this tremendous number of accidents.

Many specific points may be mentioned regarding the causes of home accidents. Rickety furniture is a constant hazard, especially when it is used in place of a step ladder. Throw rugs and objects left on the floor often cause serious falls. Lack of adequate lighting causes many accidents, and placement of light switches so that they may be turned on without walking around in the dark is an easy method of preventing accidents.

Home workshops should be constructed with safety first in mind. All electrical equipment should be checked for frayed cords and be placed where children cannot reach them. Plastic goggles are a sensible piece of gear, whether one works with metal or wood.

Many substances, such as boric acid, are very useful and are seldom thought to be poisonous; yet boric acid taken internally can cause death. *Any household compound, however innocuous, should be checked to see if it contains a poisonous substance.* Liniments, floor waxes and cleansers, household liquids, such as household ammonia—all are poisonous if taken internally. Most parents keep rat and roach poisons out of reach of children, but they often overlook the ordinary seemingly harmless substances. Inflammable materials, such as cleansers and solvents, present two dangers: of poisoning and of fire. It is wise to purchase only noninflammable cleansers when there are children in the home.

Accidents in the home where there are children are much less frequent when the house is furnished with regard to the safety of the child. Efforts should be made to replace furniture that can be pulled over; light cords should be arranged so that they cannot be tampered with. Every stairway about which a child has access should have some kind of gate or barrier to prevent falls. Objects left on stairsteps are par-

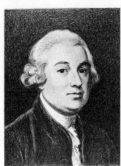

POTT, Percival (1714-1788) English surgeon. In describing chimney sweep cancer of the scrotum, Pott was able to trace the origin of this type of cancer to a specific environmental factor, thus giving the first description of occupational cancer. He advised early local excision of the affected portion of the scrotum. He is perhaps best known for his description of curvature of the spine which results from tuberculosis and is called *Pott's disease.*

ticularly hazardous. Hot dishes and liquids should be kept out of reach of small children even at the table. Small objects left lying on the floor or sharp objects that are kept in accessible places result in many serious accidents to small children who may swallow them. Kitchens should be reorganized if there is a toddler in the home. Canned goods, pots, and pans should be kept on the shelves near the floor. All liquids, soaps, and potentially dangerous items should be kept on the upper shelves.

Other major causes of home accidents include smoking in bed, firearms, carrying objects so that the carrier's view is obstructed, failure to dispose of rubbish adequately, and the lifting of heavy objects in such a manner that the back muscles rather than the leg muscles do the work.

Occupational accidents and disease: Industrial accidents have always been a major source of injury and death. Falls and accidents in handling objects account for about half of all industrial accidents. Training of workers in safe practices has been a major objective in industrial accident prevention. Protective clothing, which minimizes or prevents injury, is used widely. Attention to the construction of safer machinery has also been a great help, and most modern industrial machinery is equipped with safety devices. The introduction of workingmen's compensation laws makes the employer financially responsible for accidents. This responsibility has done much to make industry safety-conscious.

Accidents among people engaged in agricultural work occur at a fairly constant rate year after year, and in many instances tend to increase as a result of the mechanization of farm work. Intensive accident prevention training programs by local farm groups, however, offer an effective means for a material reduction in farm accidents. Some occupations obviously involve greater risks than others, and these risks are reflected in the greater costs of life insurance to miners, foundry workers, and lumber-

men as compared with professional persons. Life insurance companies have done notable work in accident prevention.

Industrial diseases: Industrial disease is defined as any abnormal condition of the body induced or aggravated by the occupation of the individual. With the increase in industrialization of the nation and the realization of the value of the individual worker, there has been a rising interest in industrial medicine (the science of keeping the worker physically and mentally fit to perform his work). The physician, chemist, and safety engineer have co-operated with management and labor to make the industrial plants of the nation safer. Basically, this requires a study of the causes of industrial diseases, their symptoms, treatment, and prevention. Occupational or industrial diseases may be classified, for preventive purposes, on the basis of the physical nature of the causative agent. These agents include:

1. Dusts, finely divided metallic and nonmetallic substances which are suspended in the atmosphere.

2. Vapors and gases, finely divided liquid particles or molecular substances that float in the atmosphere.

3. Skin irritants.

4. Abnormal surroundings, such as low or high pressure or temperature, high humidity, excessive noise or vibration.

5. Radiant energy, from the sun or from radioactive substances.

6. Infectious materials obtained from animal products that are handled.

Dust: These substances are breathed into the lungs with the air. Silicosis is a disease common among miners, glass workers, and persons employed in the manufacture of cement, abrasives, and ceramics. These workers breathe fine particles of *silicon dioxide,* the chief constituent of glass. The particles, which are less than one ten-thousandth of an inch in diameter, collect in areas of the lung and the injury forms fibrous tissue which appears as nodules. The

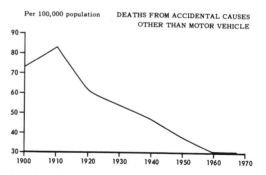

Per 100,000 population   DEATHS FROM ACCIDENTAL CAUSES OTHER THAN MOTOR VEHICLE

This chart shows decrease in the death rate in the United States from all accidents other than those in which a motor vehicle was in some way involved.

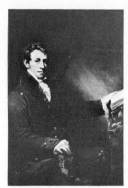

DAVY, Humphry (1778-1829) English chemist and physicist. Davy was the inventor of the miner's safety lamp, a simple device which prevents the explosion of accumulated coal dust and mine gases, ignited by the open flame of miner's lamps. This invention saved hundreds of lives throughout the world before the advent of electricity for lighting mines. He discovered the anaesthetic properties of nitrous oxide and proposed its use in surgery, in about 1800.

chief symptoms of silicosis are pains in the chest, difficult breathing, spitting of blood, and increased susceptibility to colds and other respiratory infections, but these are late symptoms.

Dust storms or short periods of employment in dusty locations do not produce silicosis. The disease seldom appears in individuals with less than ten years' exposure to a dust-laden atmosphere. Routine x-ray filming of the chest is the best method of detecting silicosis before it becomes serious. There are two means of prevention: by filtering the air, or by the wearing of masks. Asbestos dust produces a disease similar to silicosis. So does coal dust (anthrocosis) and fibers of dried sugar cane (bagatosis).

Finely suspended particles of metal may produce serious diseases. House painters and structural steel painters often contract lead poisoning by absorption through the skin. Manganese, cadmium, mercury, selenium, tellurium, and vanadium also are toxic. Practically all metallic dusts are mildly irritating to the upper respiratory tract, regardless of their systemic effect.

Poisonous gases and vapors: Many substances used in manufacturing produce poisonous vapors or irritating gases. Some of these substances are irritating to the membranes of the respiratory tract, while others may be absorbed by the blood and produce general systemic effects.

Acids and alkalis may be given off as gases. Some of these substances irritate the lining of the bronchi and the lungs, cause coughing and pain in the chest, and increase the susceptibility to respiratory diseases. Hydrochloric acid, perchloric acid, nitric acid, and ammonia are such irritating agents. Aniline and benzene compounds used in manufacturing processes produce many serious discomforts, and benzene can damage the blood-forming organs or may cause heart failure.

Amyl alcohol, benzene, naphtha, gasoline, pyridine, and turpentine are substances which when inhaled produce an inflammation of the respiratory tract, cough, and irritation of the

lungs. Many of these substances produce mental confusion accompanied by lack of coordination of the muscles. Methyl alcohol is dangerous in a gaseous state, and prolonged exposure may result in blindness and cardiac or respiratory failure. Carbon tetrachloride, an ingredient of some cleaning fluids, is a deadly poison when inhaled in excess or swallowed. The poison can seep in through the skin as well.

There are a few substances commonly used in manufacturing processes which are deadly poisons if inhaled or ingested. Hydrogen cyanide and its salts are lethal, and must be handled with extreme caution. Carbon monoxide, an odorless, colorless gas combines with the hemoglobin of the blood and is insidiously lethal. Chlorine, iodine, bromine, and fluorine are all dangerous gases.

Substances which produce skin irritation: Industrial dermatitis is any inflammatory disease of the skin for which industrial exposure can be a causative, or aggravating factor. Many of the agents mentioned in connection with dusts and vapors may affect the skin. The primary sore produced by the irritating agent may become infected with various fungi and bacteria which may spread to other parts of the body. It is often difficult to differentiate between true inflammations and the many other skin diseases that exist. People differ in their sensitivity to various substances. Some persons are sensitive to formaldehyde, a substance used in plastics and as a preservative or disinfectant. Chromates and chromic acids act directly to cause a pitting of the skin. Paraphenylenediamine, a common hair dye and photographic chemical, often produces a severe dermatitis. Barbers frequently become sensitive to quinine. Cement workers, tile setters, and bricklayers are subject to a dermatitis produced by cement.

Physical surroundings which produce industrial disease: High temperature and increased humidity frequently cause heat prostration. Con-

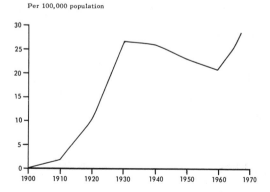

Per 100,000 population

This chart shows the changes which have occurred in the death rate, per hundred thousand population, in the United States, as a result of auto accidents.

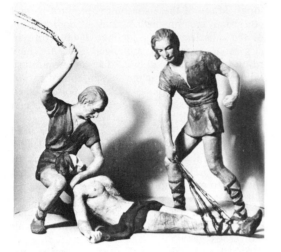

Centuries ago, the infliction of pain was regarded as a good method for reviving the unconscious. The patient was beaten with stinging nettles, hands, wet cloths, or anything else which might be expected to be sufficiently painful to revive him.

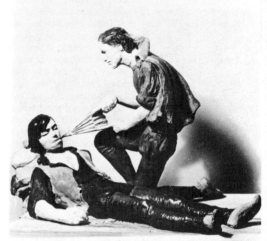

Paracelsus used bellows to introduce air into the lungs of apparently dead persons. *Courtesy A. S. Gordon, M. S. Sadove, F. Raymon, and A. C. Ivy, Dept. of Clinical Science. Univ. of Illinois College of Medicine. Copyright 1952 Postgraduate Medicine.*

stant loud noise and vibration in industrial plants produce a degeneration in the inner ear called "boilermaker's disease," which results in deafness to certain sounds. Noise has been shown to decrease the efficiency of the worker. Machines that require the worker to be in a strained or uncomfortable position also lower his efficiency. Persons working under changing pressures, as in the case of divers or subway builders, sometimes contract a disease called the "bends" *(caisson disease, compressed air illness)*. The condition results from the formation of bubbles of gas (nitrogen) in the blood and body tissues if the surrounding air pressure is too suddenly reduced. Aviators are subject to much physiological stress because of high altitude flying and resultant decreased air pressures.

Continuous exposure to the sun and the wind often produces cracking of the lips and drying of the skin. This leads to a thickened, brown or white horny deposit on the outer layers of the skin *(keratosis)*. Injury and formation of cataracts in the eyes often occur. These conditions are prevalent among sailors, ranchmen, and others who are constantly exposed to the elements.

Certain types of infection are common in industrial, medical, and agricultural work. In most cases these diseases are contracted from animals or animal products. *Anthrax,* a disease of domestic animals, is transmitted to human beings also, as are several *fungus infections* of animals, *undulant fever, ringworm, tularemia,* and *psittacosis.* These diseases are discussed elsewhere in this book; consult the index.

Control of industrial diseases: The control of industrial diseases is the responsibility of the worker, management, and the health services of the local community, the state, and the nation. Such control depends upon:

1. Education of the worker in realizing the hazards of his job, the prevention of disease or accidents, and the recognition of primary symptoms that might develop from prolonged exposure to working conditions.

2. Co-operation of management in providing adequate ventilation and air suction to remove dangerous particles of dust, gas, and vapor from shops, laboratories, and factories.

3. Proper facilities for application of first aid in plants where the danger may occur.

4. Adequate facilities for the diagnosis, treatment, and hospitalization of diseased persons in order that they may return to their positions in the shortest possible time.

5. Adequate insurance and compensation for workers who develop occupational diseases.

6. Provision of safety devices.

7. Counseling services for the discovery and aid of accident-prone individuals.

24 TROPICAL DISEASES

INTRODUCTION

Tropical diseases occur mainly in the broad equatorial belt extending from the Tropic of Cancer to the Tropic of Capricorn, but as will be seen later they are not necessarily confined to the torrid zone. The zone encompasses large segments of mainland as well as isolated islands. The illnesses found in this segment of the world can be divided simply into three basic categories: diseases caused by microorganisms, diseases caused by worms, and diseases caused by nutritional deficiencies.

Both diseases caused by microorganisms and those caused by worms are often spread by insects. The application of DDT as an insecticide since 1941 has led to a great reduction in insect-borne diseases, malaria in particular. (For further discussion of insecticides, see Chapter 25, "Environmental Health and Sanitation.")

DISEASES CAUSED BY MICROORGANISMS: LEPROSY

Leprosy is one of the oldest diseases described in the history of man. In fact, there are historical reports of the disease occurring in 1400 B.C. and perhaps earlier. It is caused by an infection with a bacterium, *Mycobacterium leprae,* sometimes referred to as Hansen's bacillus. Although the disease is found in many areas in the world, it is most prevalent in the tropics where it seems to be associated with low sanitary and economic levels. It is estimated that at least ten million people in the world have leprosy and that approximately four million of these suffer from some form of disablement as a result of the disease.

Leprosy is a chronic disease with an unusually long incubation period, often five years or more. It is thought to be acquired from prolonged and close contact with infected persons. It is probably one of the *least* contagious of all communicable diseases. Investigators have estimated that only three to five percent of the individuals exposed to leprosy actually develop the disease. Those who do contract leprosy have usually lived intimately in the same house with a leper for many years before symptoms have appeared.

Although proof is lacking, it is believed that the route of infection is the skin or the moist membranes of the nose and throat. Hansen's bacillus may invade any tissue or organ in the body, but it is found most often in skin and nerve tissue. The symptoms usually develop so gradually that they are seldom recognized. One of the common symptoms is the appearance of colored patches on the skin. These are red or brown at first but often develop pale white centers. Small hardened nodules may appear on the face or on the legs and feet. Often there is a loss of sensation of the hands or feet or of skin patches over the body, which may be first observed by receiving a burn or cut without experiencing any pain. Injury and infection following loss of sensation probably account for much of the disfigurement which characterizes the disease. Nasal obstruction, hoarseness, and loss of eyebrows, lashes, and body hair may also occur along with episodes of fever, neuritis, or eye complaints. As the disease slowly progresses, it tends to differentiate into one of two types.

Types of leprosy

The *lepromatous type* (or *cutaneous-nodular type*) involves the development of skin nodules and open sores in which large numbers of the bacteria are present. The nodules may occur anywhere but are most common on the face, ear lobes, and forehead. The general appearance of the skin is unhealthy and the open sores may penetrate deeply into the underlying tissues. In time, bodily mutilation may occur; fingers may drop off or destruction of the cornea may cause blindness. This type rarely shows spontaneous recovery. During the acute phases, transfer of the infection to other individuals probably occurs. In extreme, untreated cases, death may follow, but more often death results from a secondary infection, such as tuberculosis or pneumonia.

The *tuberculoid type* (or *maculo-anesthetic type*) is generally less destructive. Disfiguring skin sores are less common, but colored patches of skin develop which later lose all sensation. As a result of nerve involvement, there is a consequent atrophy of some muscle groups. The muscles of the hand are frequently affected and the wasting muscles gradually contract to produce the so-called "claw" hand. This type tends to become arrested spontaneously and is not believed to be important in the spread of the disease, since few if any bacilli are found in the skin lesions.

Diagnosis

The unusually long incubation period makes leprosy difficult to recognize in its early stages. As in other infectious diseases, the earlier leprosy is diagnosed, the greater are the chances of recovery. A positive diagnosis is established when the characteristic bacilli are found in skin lesions, but by this time the disease is well established. Although Hansen's bacilli are often found in large numbers in lesions and nasal secretions of patients with the nodular type of the disease, more than half of the actual cases of leprosy are of the *neural* type in which the bacilli cannot be found. In these cases, then, diagnosis must depend on the recognition of other important signs, such as loss of feeling in certain areas, enlargement of nerve trunks, skin thickenings and discolorations, as well as other evidences in the patient's past record which would suggest that he had once had symptoms of leprosy or had associated with lepers.

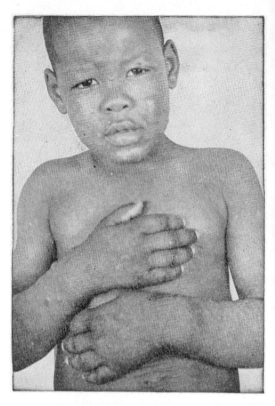

Photograph of a child displaying typical skin lesions associated with leprosy on the face, arms, hands and trunk. Such eruptions are present in only certain forms of leprosy, and closely resemble many other skin disorders which have no relationship to this disease and are of a less grave nature.

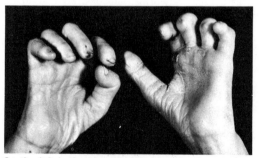

On the left is the characteristic claw hand appearance occurring in the neural form of leprosy, and on the right, degenerative processes that are seen in bone leprosy. The picture illustrates how various forms of the disease may progress in markedly different manners and with varying severity.

Treatment

Although many drugs have been tried in the hope of controlling leprosy, until about 1942 only one drug seemed to be truly beneficial. This was chaulmoogra oil, derived from the seeds of an East Indian tree—and its beneficial effects were slight. During the past fifteen years sulphone drugs (not the same as sulfa drugs) have largely replaced chaulmoogra oil. First tried at the National Leprosarium at Carville, Louisiana, the sulphones have been the most beneficial of any drugs tried so far. Clinical improvement is often quite rapid, but the failure of this drug to destroy Hansen's bacilli has been disappointing. Recent tests, however, indicate that combined sulphone-chaulmoogra therapy may be more effective than either one used alone. Further testing of other new drugs is also progressing rapidly and early evidence indicates that some of the antibiotics may be of value, particularly streptomycin and aureomycin, but Dapsone, DDS (Diamino-Diphenyl Sulphone) is the drug of choice at the present time.

The fear and suspicion associated with leprosy, dating back to Biblical times, are slowly being annulled by scientific study. Indeed, the leprosarium of today is far removed from the infamous leper colonies of a century ago. Modern leprosaria are designed to offer mental respite and to provide, in addition to medical treatment, adequate diet, rest, and suitable exercise. Physical therapy is being used to train the paralyzed muscles that result from nerve involvement. More important, many patients are being returned to their homes, freed of this, one of the most feared of all diseases.

DISEASES CAUSED BY MICROORGANISMS: JUNGLE ROT

Open sores of the skin are quite common in tropical climates. Some are caused by specific bacteria (e.g., *yaws*), others by parasitic molds (*madura foot*), a few by single-celled parasites (*leishmaniasis*), while still others are apparently results of the secondary invasion of the tissues by various bacteria which gain entrance through wounds or other small breaks in the skin. The expressive term, *jungle rot*, has been used as a general name for such sores, irrespective of their cause. It has probably been used most often for the disease known as tropical ulcer (or *phagedena tropica*) which occurs in warm, moist tropical areas.

Tropical ulcers develop almost exclusively on the feet and legs, usually following minor breaks of the skin such as insect bites, the tunnels of itch mites, the perforations of hookworm larvae, or some simple accidental abrasion. Tiny blisters first appear, and develop shortly into larger, foul-smelling sores. The ulcers become tender and painful, and spread rapidly in their early phases, with complete destruction of the skin and often of underlying tissue also. The diseased tissue gradually disintegrates and sloughs off, the eroded area becoming increasingly deeper. Unless the infection is stopped, muscles, tendons, and even bone may become infected. In severe infections an ulcer may penetrate completely through the foot. Usually, however, the infection heals spontaneously before it reaches such serious proportions.

In most of these cases, two kinds of bacteria predominate: a cigar-shaped bacillus and a spirochete (the two comprising the so-called *Vincent's organisms*).

Malnutrition is common among persons suffering from tropical ulcers. A severe deficiency of vitamins, especially of A, B, or C, is often a contributing factor. The ulcers usually occur on individuals who rarely wear shoes or stockings and whose feet are thus constantly exposed to injury.

Nearly all tropical ulcers will heal in time regardless of what treatment is used, but recovery is slow and disfiguring scars often develop. Skin grafts are frequently used to prevent the formation of scar tissue. Recently, promising results have come from the use of penicillin injections and aureomycin taken orally. These agents are usually able to destroy the Vincent's organisms within 24 hours. Complete recovery sometimes occurs in about three weeks.

DISEASES CAUSED BY MICROORGANISMS: MALARIA

Malaria is a disease confined largely to the tropics, although in the past many cases occurred as far north as the Great Lakes regions in the United States, and in other northerly areas throughout the world. Malaria is characterized by an alternation of chills and fever. It is caused by microscopic one-celled parasites living within the red blood cells of man. It was formerly believed to be associated with damp, "poisonous" swamp air. The name malaria is, in fact, derived from Italian words meaning "bad air."

In 1950, the World Health Organization reported that every year malaria killed three million persons and 300 million new malarial infections occurred. By far it was one of the most widespread of the tropical diseases. Until recently, malaria was responsible for more deaths per year than any other transmissible disease. Thus, in 1955 a global program of malaria eradication was launched, co-ordinated by the World Health Organization. During the early years of the eradication program spectacular progress occurred. The over-all new infections decreased from 250 million to about 50 million cases annually. For example, in India where it was estimated that there were ten million new cases per year in 1950, the number has now been reduced to approximately 150,000 cases per year.

Four species of parasites cause malaria in man. The most common and widely distributed is *Plasmodium vivax* which causes *benign tertian* or *vivax* malaria. Less common but in several respects more serious is *Plasmodium falciparum* which causes *malignant tertian* or *falciparum* malaria. The other two species are relatively uncommon and need not be discussed. Although infection with any of the malarial parasites brings about a sequence of periodic chills and fever, the course of the disease and the kinds of complications which may develop are dependent on the growth cycle of the parasites. It is necessary, therefore, to describe briefly the life history of a typical parasite.

Developmental cycle of the parasite

The form of the parasite infectious to man, called a *sporozoite,* is introduced into the body by the bite of a female mosquito of the genus *Anopheles*, the only type which transmits human malaria. The microscopic parasites migrate to various organs of the body, including the liver and spleen, where they infect certain cells lining the blood cavities. Within these cells they reproduce, forming in five to eight days a number of parasites, many of which break out of these cells and enter red blood cells. Each parasite lives and grows within a red cell, feeding on the material inside the cell. After several hours, it begins to multiply, producing (in *vivax*) 12 to 24 minute parasites in about 48 hours. The blood cell then bursts open, freeing these small parasites into the blood, where each has the ability to infect another red blood cell. Here it repeats its cycle of growth and division followed by rupture of the cell some 48 hours later. The number of parasites thus increases rapidly, while the infected red cells are constantly being destroyed.

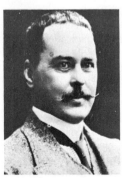

ROSS, Ronald (1857-1932) English pathologist and parasitologist. He is most famous for being the first man to demonstrate that mosquitoes are responsible for the transmission of malaria from person to person. He also made important studies on the life cycle of the malarial parasite, and was one of the first to demonstrate its complexity. For his many contributions to parasitology, he was awarded the Nobel prize in 1902. *Bettmann Archive.*

After several such cycles have passed, some parasites develop into different forms, called *gametocytes*, which grow more slowly and, when mature, are infective to *Anopheles* mosquitoes which bite the patient. Within the mosquito these parasites mature and develop into rounded cysts along the walls of the stomach. Within the cysts (and there may be several hundred of them on a single mosquito stomach) the parasites undergo rapid multiplication, producing as many as 10,000 sporozoites in about three weeks. When mature, the sporozoites break out of the cysts and wander about the body of the host mosquito, many of them coming to rest in the salivary glands. A number of these sporozoites will be injected into the blood stream of the human being the next time this mosquito bites, because of the insect's habit of injecting saliva under the skin when it bites. Not all of the sporozoites are injected at one time, however, so that a single mosquito may infect a number of persons during a period of a few weeks.

Chills and fever

Three types of parasites are present in the human host: those within the cells, lining the blood vessels in the liver and spleen; the developing gametocytes; and the red cell forms undergoing repeated multiplication. The first type is apparently responsible for new attacks after the disease is supposedly under control (relapses); and the second type is responsible for infecting more mosquitoes. Neither of them seems to be important in the production of malarial fevers. It is the third type which produces acute malarial symptoms. In *vivax* malaria there is a strong tendency for the various "broods" of parasites in the red cells to mature at about the same time, so that the bursting of the blood cells (and consequent release of young parasites, their waste products, and the remains of the parasitized cells) coincides with an "attack" of malaria. An attack generally begins with a shaking chill in which the patient's teeth chatter; his skin has "goose-pimples"; and his fever begins to rise. This is followed in one or two hours by a hot stage, the fever often rising to 104° or 105° F. This is accompanied by general body aches, severe headaches, and a rapid pulse. These symptoms last from four to six hours or longer. As the temperature declines, profuse sweating follows, the entire body perspiring freely. At the end of this stage the symptoms disappear, leaving the patient weak and tired. In *vivax* malaria, attacks occur every 48 hours if there is but a single brood of parasites; if several broods are present, attacks may occur at more frequent intervals.

In *falciparum* malaria there is less tendency for the rupture of the infected red cells to occur

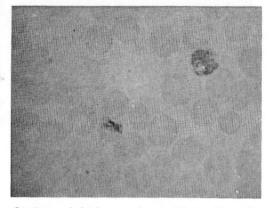

Quartan malaria in man is caused by *Plasmodium malariae*, shown in this photomicrograph, propagating in heavily parasitized human red blood cells.

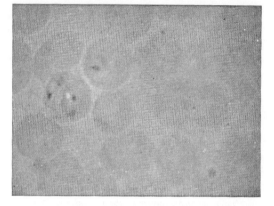

Photomicrograph of human red blood cells infected by *Plasmodium falciparum*, which causes malignant tertian malaria. *Photo by F. W. Schmidt.*

simultaneously, so that the chills and fever may occur every day or be quite irregular.

Complications of malaria

In *vivax* infections in which the patient receives no treatment, the acute stage may last for about two weeks, following which the patient may slowly recover and seem to be well. There may, however, be repeated relapses over many months or years. The attacks become less severe and there results the condition known as chronic malaria. Even after treatment, relapses may occur sometimes for as long as several years after the last acute attack. It is believed that the parasites living within the cells of the *reticulo-endothelial* system are responsible for relapses. Under conditions of body stress, such as a minor operation, seasickness, a battle wound, etc., these "hidden" parasites may break out of the liver cells and inaugurate a new cycle of red cell infections.

The acute phase of *falciparum* malaria is occasionally fatal. The parasitized red cells collect in the small capillaries within the body, sometimes in the intestinal tract but more often in the brain, producing cerebral malaria. The onset is sudden, with high fever, convulsions, and often unconsciousness followed by death. The number of parasites is frequently enormous and the number of red cells destroyed is therefore very great. Fortunately, early treatment can not only prevent cerebral symptoms but can usually bring about rapid and complete recovery. Relapses with *falciparum* malaria are quite rare.

Blackwater fever is a serious complication of *falciparum* infections, occurring most often in white men living in the tropics. Its cause is not certainly known. It seems to require a previous infection with *P. falciparum* which has been inadequately treated. Among the factors which may precipitate an attack are the administration of quinine, exhaustion, excessive intake of alcohol, and chilling. Frequently fatal, it is characterized by chills, high fever, jaundice, vomiting, severe anemia, and the production of dark red- or wine-colored urine which gives the disease its name. Internally, rapid destruction of red blood cells takes place and kidney and liver functions are impaired. Immediate transfusions of whole blood are often necessary to prevent death from acute anemia.

Antimalarial and suppressive drugs

In 1638, a Spanish official in Peru noticed that the local villagers treated persons who had fever with powders prepared from tree bark. Samples of the bark of these *Cinchona* trees were sent to Europe where it was shown that extracts of the bark had a powerful effect on malarial fevers. It was nearly 200 years later that the active principle of the bark, quinine, was isolated and prepared commercially; and until the outbreak of World War II in December, 1941, quinine remained the most widely used, and the most reliable, antimalarial drug. When the world's major source of quinine, in Java, was cut off by the Japanese, a tremendous effort was made to find new and better drugs, and this search is still continuing. Today, more than a dozen new synthetic drugs are in use in the malarial areas of the world.

The ideal drug would control the symptoms of acute malaria quickly, destroy the parasites in the red cells as well as the gametocytes and the parasites in the reticuloendothelial cells, and yet produce a minimum of undesirable side effects. It seems unlikely that a single drug will prove efficient for all these purposes. Of the newer drugs, atabrine hydrochloride (*mepacrine dihydrochloride*) has been widely used, since it, like quinine, is effective against the blood forms of malaria. However, also like quinine, it does

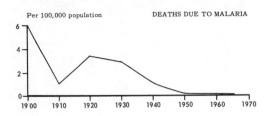

Per 100,000 population   DEATHS DUE TO MALARIA

This graph shows how the number of deaths in the United States caused by malaria has declined.

about a permanent cure. Since *falciparum* infections involve only one wave of blood parasites with no subsequent tissue forms, chloroquine alone will bring about a cure. One of the more effective therapies, at present, involves the use of both chloroquine and primaquine.

The therapy for malaria has been complicated recently by the appearance of a strain of *Plasmodium falciparum* that is resistant to chloroquine. These strains first appeared in South America and in Thailand and have been frequently encountered among American troops in South Vietnam. When cases of chloroquine-resistant malaria first appeared, it was found to be partially susceptible to treatment with quinine. This sudden new demand for quinine revealed the fact that the production of this drug had practically stopped and total stocks were virtually nonexistent. Repeated trials of different treatment regimens indicate that at this time these chloroquine-resistant strains are best treated with quinine combined with pyrimethamine. However, despite the growing concern over chloroquine-resistant infections, chloroquine remains the drug of choice for suppression of malaria in most areas of the world.

not prevent *vivax* relapses nor does it destroy *falciparum* gametocytes. Both quinine and atabrine are now being replaced by chloroquine, the action of which is similar, but which is rarely toxic.

Several drugs have been found useful in fighting the tissue forms of malaria which lead to relapses in *vivax* infections. Pyrimethamine is widely used, but has the disadvantage that, not only does it not control the parasite in the blood phase, but some strains may acquire resistance to the drug, rendering it worthless for future use. Primaquine is even more effective against the tissue forms of *vivax* and does not induce resistance in the parasite. Consequently, although chloroquine will control the acute symptoms caused by the blood forms of malaria, primaquine is often the most effective in bringing

In areas where malaria is endemic, it is advisable to use a system of suppressive medication, not to prevent infection but to control it as soon as it is acquired. Atabrine was used by the army during World War II and found to be effective on most forms of malaria. The main drawbacks to its use are the toxic side effects produced in some people and the yellow color it imparts to the skin. Chloroquine has now become the best choice for suppression, as it is not as toxic as atabrine. Also, it remains longer in the body; hence weekly rather than daily doses are effective.

When a person leaves a malarial area, it was formerly advisable for him to continue suppressive medication for as long as two years to prevent *vivax* relapse. With the development of drugs to attack tissue forms, this so-called interim therapy now usually involves about a two-week period during which daily doses of primaquine will usually destroy any residual tissue forms.

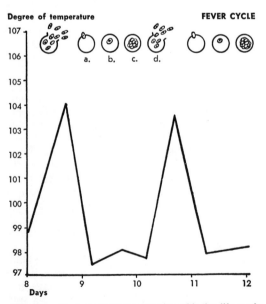

Degree of temperature   FEVER CYCLE

Diagram of how malarial fever varies with the life cycle of the causative agent, *Plasmodium vivax*. The *merozoite* stage of the parasite enters a red cell (a), develops into the "ring" stage (b), and produces more merozoites (c), which emerge (d) prior to the fever peak. The cycle is then repeated.

DISEASES CAUSED BY MICROORGANISMS: YELLOW FEVER

Yellow fever is an acute disease characterized by fever, jaundice, and vomiting. After an incubation period of three to six days, fever and headache appear suddenly. Usually on the following day the fever subsides but on about the

Research on Malaria

Research on tropical diseases, as on other diseases, requires the use of experimental animals in which the infection may be carried and studied. Studies on malaria, with particular reference to finding better antimalarial drugs, have been most successful when birds such as chicks and ducklings have been employed. General procedures involve the laboratory culturing of suitable insect vectors, in this case mosquitoes. Although the *Anopheles* mosquito is the carrier of human malaria, *Aedes aegypti* mosquitoes must be used to infect the birds with *avian* malaria; but the nature of the infection closely resembles the human form. Birds may then be treated with various drugs to determine the effect on the malarial parasite. Thousands of potential antimalarials were studied in this manner during World War II. The following photographs illustrate steps in this type of investigation. *Pictures courtesy United States Public Health Service, National Institutes of Health.*

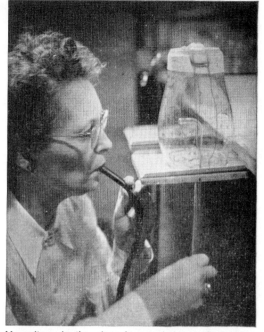

Mosquitoes in the glass jar are being sucked into a special container that can then be used in applying them to the skin of some infected animal.

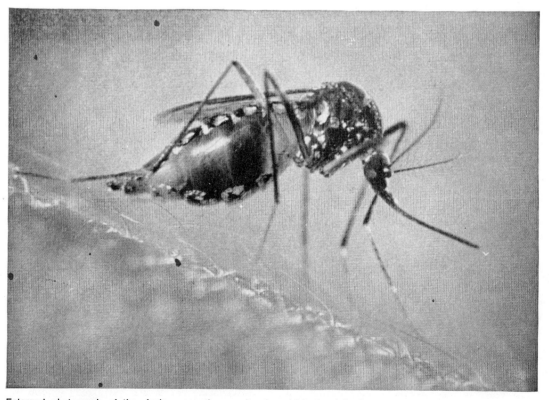

Enlarged photograph of the *Aedes aegypti* mosquito, by which the infection is carried from one experimental bird to another. After use, the mosquito is dissected under the microscope to assure presence of parasite.

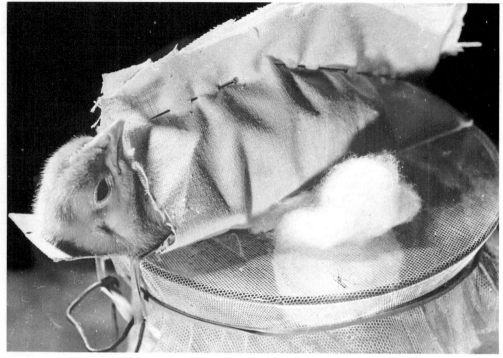

Photograph of a chick placed in contact with a container of infected mosquitoes. The malarial parasite can be demonstrated in the salivary gland of the insect, and it is injected into the experimental bird with the saliva.

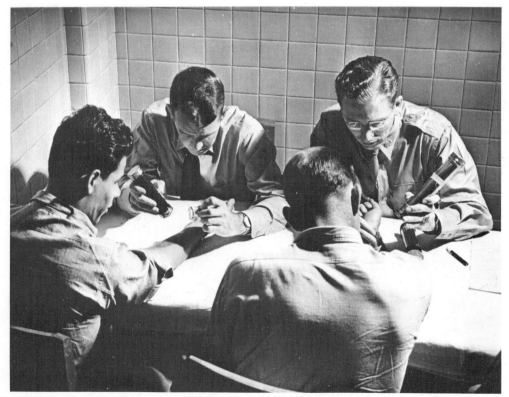

Ultimate testing of drugs must be done on human beings. Prisoners in a federal penitentiary who have volunteered for the test are shown being bitten on their forearms. Ten infected *Anopheles* mosquitoes bite each man.

third day it reappears, accompanied by jaundice, impaired kidney function, bleeding from the mucous membranes, and vomiting of dark blood. In isolated cases the attacks may be mild with recovery fairly certain, but in epidemics the course is frequently severe with fatalities of over 50 percent.

The infectious agent which causes yellow fever is a virus. This virus invades the liver principally, the extensive damage to the liver cells resulting in jaundice, especially noticeable in the skin. It is the characteristic yellow to brown color of the skin which gives the disease its name. When recovery occurs, however, it seems to be complete, with no evidence of former damage remaining.

The virus is transmitted from infected persons to uninfected persons by mosquitoes, principally *Aedes aegypti* (also by a few other species in Africa and South America). To transmit the virus, the female mosquito must suck the blood of a patient with yellow fever during the first three days after infection. After about twelve days, the virus in the mosquito becomes infective and a nonimmune individual bitten by this mosquito will develop yellow fever. The mosquito remains infective all its life.

Yellow fever was at one time a serious disease of the cities along the Atlantic and Gulf coasts of the United States, but at present it is largely confined to the tropics of Africa and the Americas. In Louisiana, in the last epidemic in 1905, there were nearly 8000 cases and 900 deaths. The French attempt to construct a Panama Canal failed in large part because of the disastrous effects of yellow fever among the construction crews. In 1900, Walter Reed and his colleagues in Cuba discovered that the disease is transmitted by a mosquito. This discovery enabled Gorgas and his fellow workers to complete the canal in 1914. So effective were the mosquito control measurers inaugurated by Gorgas that today, yellow fever is extremely rare in the Canal Zone.

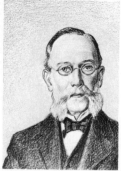

FINLAY Y BARRES, Carlos Juan (1833-1915) Cuban biologist and physician. In the year 1881 he first enunciated the theory that yellow fever, then common in most tropical countries, was transmitted to human beings by the bite of the mosquito. Since he could offer little real proof of this hypothesis, it was given no serious credence by medical authorities until the classical investigations of Walter Reed and his associates proved Finlay to be correct.

Jungle (sylvan) yellow fever

In 1933 yellow fever was found in some tropical areas of Brazil where *Aedes aegypti* does not occur. Now known in Africa as well as in the Americas, this disease, termed *jungle* or *sylvan* yellow fever, seems to be a disease of certain wild animals (howler monkeys, for example). It is transmitted by an entirely different type of mosquito which lives largely among the treetops. This form of the disease usually occurs in human beings who work deep in the forests. Individuals who climb into the treetops (nut pickers, for example) are most likely to be bitten by the mosquitoes. They may then return to their village, develop the disease, and, by infecting local *aegypti* mosquitoes, cause a full-scale epidemic to follow. Thus, yellow fever remains a potential menace in all of the jungle areas of the tropics, since control of "treetop" mosquitoes is quite impractical. Further, since wild animals may serve as reservoir hosts, there is the constant threat of future infections.

Prevention and control

Since no curative drugs have been found, prevention of yellow fever is most important. Preventive measures are of three kinds: immuniza-

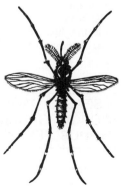

REED, Walter (1851-1902) American Army Surgeon. He is famous throughout the world for the discoveries concerning the cause and transmission of yellow fever made by the United States Army Yellow Fever Commission, of which he was the chairman. His publication in the year 1901, entitled *Experimental Yellow Fever,* first provided the medical world with absolute proof that the disease was caused by a virus transmitted to man by *Aedes aegypti.*

Drawing of the *Aedes aegypti* mosquito, much larger than its actual size. Many members of the genus *Aedes* are harmless except for their troublesome bites, from whence their name arose (a-, not; edos, pleasure). *A. aegypti*, however, is the principle agent responsible for the transmission of yellow fever, as well as another tropical infection, dengue fever. This species is quite widely distributed in nearly all tropical countries.

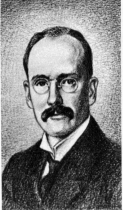

CARROLL, James (1854-1907) American Army Medical Officer. Noted for his distinguished services on the United States Army Yellow Fever Commission in collaboration with Lazear, Agramonte y Simoni and Reed. The historic investigations of this group on the causative agent of yellow fever resulted in the demonstration that it was transmitted to man by the bite of the mosquito, and thus provided an effective means for control of this severe tropical infection.

tion, precautions against the introduction of the virus into noninfected areas, and mosquito control. The general features of *immunization* (vaccination) are discussed in Chapter 4, "Disease-Producing Organisms." Acquired immunity to yellow fever may develop after having the disease, or by artificially vaccinating against it. Such immunity is of several years' duration. *Quarantine* measures are important in preventing the transfer of the virus into areas where it is not present. This could occur by the accidental introduction of infected mosquitoes (by ship or airplane) or of infected people into regions where *Aedes aegypti* exists. Quarantine stations in many countries are constantly on the alert for such unwanted importations. *Mosquito control* measures have proved to be important in the control of the disease. *Aedes aegypti* is a domestic mosquito, breeding mostly in water in artificial containers such as rain barrels, roof gutters, flower vases, old tin cans, etc. Such places are destroyed if possible, or oil is poured over the water to kill the mosquito larvae. A small amount of *DDT*, placed in all containers that can act as breeding places, has been found very effective in eradicating these mosquitoes over large areas. These measures, of course, will not control the jungle species. It is unlikely, however, that jungle yellow fever will invade urban areas in epidemic proportions if all workers in the jungle are vaccinated; if patients are isolated in a room protected by screening for at least the first four days of symptoms; and if local breeding of *Aedes aegypti* is eradicated.

DISEASES CAUSED BY MICROORGANISMS: TYPHUS FEVER

The typhus fevers are caused by microscopic organisms called *rickettsiae* which are transmitted to man by external parasites (lice, fleas, etc.). A person infected with rickettsiae develops severe fever, headache, and skin rashes, and may develop bronchitis or pneumonia-like symptoms. There are, in reality, three principal types of typhus fevers, differing markedly in their causative agent, transmitting agent, and distribution and severity of symptoms.

Classical typhus (also called epidemic, European, or louse typhus) occurs chiefly in Europe, Asia, and northern Africa. Not truly a tropical disease, it appears suddenly in epidemic form in populations weakened by famine or by disease, or in groups of people crowded closely together, as in armies, jails, concentration camps, etc. It is carried from person to person by body lice (*Pediculus humanus*), and frequently reaches epidemic proportions near the end of winter, since heavy clothing and crowding favor lice infestations.

The lice become infected by ingesting the blood of a diseased person. The rickettsiae multiply within the louse and pass out of the body in the excreta (*feces*) after the second day; infection is produced by rubbing the infective feces into wounds or other breaks in the skin.

The onset is abrupt, with fever, headache, and general body aches, followed by the appearance, on the eighth or ninth day, of a skin rash on the abdomen, chest, arms, and legs. Bronchitis and bronchopneumonia are frequent complications. The death rate in epidemics is often great; in Egypt, for example, there were 40,000 cases in 1943 with over 8000 deaths. In the Serbian epidemic, following World War I, the mortality rate varied between 30 and 70 percent.

Murine typhus (also known as New World, endemic, or flea typhus), caused by *Rickettsia mooseri*, is a disease of rats which is normally transmitted from rat to rat by several species of rat fleas (or rat lice in certain parts of the world). It is found in Europe, Asia, Africa, Mexico, and along the Atlantic and Gulf coasts of the United States. Human beings become infected when living in close proximity to infected rats, since rat fleas will bite man quite readily. Although the general symptoms of murine typhus are similar to those of the classical form, the clinical course is usually milder and the death rate lower.

Scrub typhus (also called tsutsugamushi, Japanese river fever, or mite typhus) is widespread throughout the Asiatic-Pacific region and has been carried to other areas by migrants. Probably a disease of field mice, it is caused by *R. orientalis* and is transmitted by several species of mites (*Trombicula*). The bite of the larval form of the mite, usually on the neck or in the groin, is often followed by the development of a small local ulcer, and the lymph nodes in the area become enlarged and tender. The fever in scrub typhus is similar to that of other typhus fevers but the death rate of scrub typhus is generally greater than that of murine typhus.

Control of typhus fever

Control of the transmitting agents is very important in controlling the incidence of these diseases. The body louse (the "cootie" of World War I) lives mainly attached to clothing worn next to the body. From this attachment it takes two blood meals a day, and lays eggs along the seams of the clothing. The "crab louse" lives attached to pubic hair; and the "head louse" lives among the hairs of the head. Destruction of the adult lice can be accomplished by the use of insecticide powders (DDT), and steam sterilization is effective on the eggs. Frequent bathing and changing of underclothes is also important.

The best control of rat fleas is by thorough eradication of the rats. Control of the mite vector of scrub typhus is extremely difficult and was a serious problem in the Pacific area during World War II. Infected mice and their parasitic mites are thickest in patches of tall grass; removing the clumps of grass from camp areas by bulldozers afforded considerable protection. Individual protection may be obtained through the use of a repellant such as *dimethylpthalate* for clothing, or an insecticide such as *benzyl benzoate* for buildings, tents, etc.

Within the past few years remarkable cures have been effected through the use of the antibiotics aureomycin, chloramphenicol, and terramycin. These agents apparently do not destroy the living rickettsiae but suppress their growth and thus permit the individual to develop immunity. Aureomycin also has the property of counteracting the toxic materials produced by the rickettsiae, bringing about marked clinical improvement within a few hours.

Prevention of typhus fevers by means of artificially acquired immunity is also possible; vaccines are now being prepared for use against the organism of epidemic typhus.

DISEASES CAUSED BY WORMS: ELEPHANTIASIS

Throughout the tropics and subtropics man is host to a variety of parasitic worms, some of which are transmitted by biting insects. The filarial worms are among the most important parasites which attack man; unlike intestinal parasites, these worms live deep within the tissues. *Filariasis* is a term referring to infections with filarial worms. Repeated infections with certain species of filarial worms may result in incredible enlargement of parts of the body. The legs, for example, may somewhat resemble the

legs of an elephant, and for this reason the condition has been given the name *elephantiasis*. Any part of the body may be affected, but the arms, legs, and scrotum show the enlargement most frequently. Less often, the breasts of women are so involved.

The worm responsible for elephantiasis in most localities where the disease occurs is *Wuchereria bancrofti*. Found in nearly all the tropics of the world, this parasite is especially prevalent in central Africa, coastal Asia, and the islands of the Pacific. To a lesser degree it is also present in the West Indies and in Central and South America.

If a mosquito, infected by these parasites, bites a man, the worms get under the skin and migrate into the lymphatic system, where they grow into adults. While living in the lymphatic system, the adult females produce large numbers of tiny larvae called *microfilariae* which are carried about in the blood. If the appropriate species of mosquito takes a blood meal at this time, some of these larvae will be sucked up and will develop in about two weeks into forms infective to man. These infective larvae crawl into the mouthparts of the mosquito and break out into the skin of a human host when next the mosquito bites. After penetrating the skin, they migrate into the lymph nodes and grow to maturity, thus completing the cycle.

Filariasis

When only a few worms are living in the human host, there may be no symptoms. A larger number may result in a series of local reactions. The adult worms, each about the size of a hair two inches long, lie in a tangled mass in the

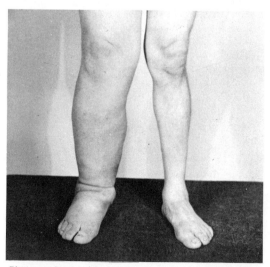

Photograph of legs of patient with elephantiasis, affecting right leg. *Photograph by F. W. Schmidt.*

lymph tissue, thereby causing some degree of mechanical obstruction. The area becomes inflamed, the infected nodes become swollen (*lymphadenitis*), and that part of the body may show temporary swellings. Red streaks along an arm or leg, associated with inflammation of the lymph vessels (*lymphangitis*), are common, while swelling, tenderness, and pain of the scrotum often accompany infection in the groin. Some investigators believe that this inflammatory reaction is not so much due to the filarial worm as to the presence of secondarily infectious bacteria, particularly *Streptococcus hemolyticus*. If the patient moves from the area, especially to a cooler climate, the worms eventually die and the symptoms of filariasis gradually disappear. The attacks may recur, however, for several years.

The production of gross deformities of the body seems to require frequently repeated infections, year after year. Although many features of elephantiasis are poorly understood, the onset is thought by some investigators to result from tissue changes brought about in response to the presence of adult worms in the lymph tissue. Probably the most widely held view is that the worms cause a primary obstruction of the lymph channels, causing some degree of inflammation; this, in turn, causes increased amounts of protein to enter the area, which stimulate excessive growth of connective tissue. Usually, too, streptococci invade the affected tissues, causing further inflammation. As more and more tissue develops, the affected part becomes larger and larger. In an individual who has lived his entire life in an area where filariasis occurs, a leg may have tripled in size by the time he reaches 40 years of age. Such deformities probably occur only in persons who have been constantly exposed to reinfection over long periods of time. Elephantiasis is rare among Europeans, even after they have lived for years in areas where the disease prevails; this is doubtless because they protect themselves from mosquitoes. Although elephantiasis interferes with the normal activities of the individual, it is not fatal; some patients are capable of living nearly normal lives.

Diagnosis and treatment

A positive diagnosis can be made when adult worms are found in the lymph nodes, or by finding the microfilariae in the blood. In some parts of the world the microfilariae appear periodically; that is, they are found in the circulating blood only during certain hours of the day or night. The local mosquito host usually feeds during this period, so the microfilariae are drawn up with the blood meal. The finding of adult worms or microfilariae in early cases is often difficult or impossible; indeed, in perhaps

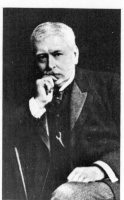

MANSON, Patrick (1844-1922) Scottish physician and parasitologist. In the year 1879 he demonstrated that the parasite that causes elephantiasis is transmitted to human beings by the bite of the mosquito, *Culex fatigans*. This is believed to be the first proof of the role of an invertebrate in the transmission of a disease to man. He studied intestinal schistosomiasis, Manson's disease, caused by the blood fluke, *Schistosoma mansoni*.

a majority of cases the microfilariae can never be demonstrated in the blood. Skin tests, therefore, have been devised which sometimes aid in establishing a diagnosis. Except in cases of obvious elephantiasis, diagnosis often depends upon transient swellings, lymphadenitis and lymphangitis, and a history of having been in a filarial region.

Simple filariasis seldom requires medical treatment. It is usually sufficient to prevent further contact between patient and infected mosquitoes by segregation or moving from the area. This, of course, does not rid the patient of adult worms already in his tissues. Tight bandaging and surgical treatment may reduce deformities of elephantiasis, but abnormal tissues cannot be removed medically. However, two drugs which aid in preventing the spread of the disease are worthy of mention: *hetrazan*, which destroys the microfilariae in the blood, thus making them unavailable to mosquitoes; and a compound called *MSb*, which kills the adult worms, thus preventing the further production of microfilariae. The use of these drugs will materially reduce the number of infected mosquitoes, and in that manner break the natural cycle. Eradication of the host mosquito is also important in long-range control.

There are many other diseases caused by both round and flat worms, in various areas of the world. Since these diseases are not necessarily tropical, they have not been included in this discussion. For further information relative to diseases of man caused by worms, see Chapter 4, "Disease-Producing Organisms."

DISEASES CAUSED BY NUITRITIONAL DEFICIENCIES

Many syndromes, often included in discussions of "island" or tropical diseases, are, in effect, nutritional deficiencies which are found in various degrees of severity in every nation in the world. These diseases are listed here followed by the deficient essential substance which causes the symptoms. These are *Kwarshiorkor* (protein deficiency), *beri beri* pellagra (vitamin B_2 deficiency), scurvy (vitamin C deficiency), and rickets (vitamin D deficiency). Although these diseases may seem to be more prevalent in the equatorial belt and certain remote islands, every person on earth is a potential candidate for any one of them. Prevention is usually rather simple: a diet containing adequate amounts of protein, vitamins, and minerals. However, treatment of established cases requires large amounts of these essential nutritional elements. In *severe* cases, the patient may have to be hospitalized. In *any* case, the patient should seek the advice of a physician. For further information regarding these metabolic problems, see Chapter 21, "Nutrition."

OTHER TROPICAL DISEASES

In the preceding pages some of the more important tropical diseases have been discussed. Many other tropical diseases are known, however, and some are worthy of mention. The following brief summaries will give an idea of the nature of the disease, the causative agent, and methods of control or treatment.

Diseases caused by bacteria

Weil's disease (spirochetal jaundice, leptospirosis) is an acute, infectious disease which may mimic yellow fever. The spirochete which causes it, *Leptospira icterohaemorrhagiae*, is present in rats throughout the world. The organism is usually transmitted to man through contamination of his food by the urine and excreta of the rats, or through immersion in water contaminated by rats. Workers in sewers, irrigation ditches, and rice fields are common victims. The onset is sudden, with chills followed by profuse sweating, fever, headache, and general body pains. Later, vomiting and severe jaundice appear, coincident with involvement of the liver and kidneys. The mortality may be as high as 30 percent in epidemics, but recovery confers long-lasting immunity, since specific antibodies are produced in the patient. The best treatment seems to be blood transfusions from patients convalescing from the disease. Their blood contains antibodies to the disease.

Relapsing fever, caused by *Borrelia* (or *Treponema*) *recurrentis* and several closely related species or strains, is commonly divided into two types: that transmitted by "soft" ticks (*Ornithodorus*), and that transmitted by head and body lice (*Pediculus*). Both types are characterized by recurring attacks of high fever (up to 105°

F.) accompanied by weakness and headache. After a few days there is a sudden return to normal, followed by a relapse in a week or so. Once universal in its distribution, louse-borne fever is now largely confined to Africa and Russia. Tick-borne fever is a local problem in many parts of the world, including the United States, its incidence being closely related to the distribution of the tick vector. Ticks become infected while still in the egg of the infected mother tick, or from feeding on various wild animals. They transfer the spirochetes to human beings by biting. Arsenic compounds have been used in treatment of patients with relapsing fever, although at present antibiotics, such as aureomycin, are being tried with considerable success.

Yaws (frambesia) is a disease of high incidence among children and young adults, especially of the dark-skinned peoples of equatorial Africa, South America, the Philippines, and the East and West Indies. It is caused by a spirochete, *Treponema pertenue*. It has been estimated that 80 percent of the rural population of Haiti are infected, and in other areas the figure is nearly as great. The disease takes the form of eruptions on the skin of the face, trunk, scalp, hands, and feet. The open, oozing sores may be painful, and if left untreated may penetrate the bones, producing body mutilation. The exact manner in which yaws is contracted is not certain, but bodily contact with infected persons is probably the most common method, since crowded living conditions and the custom of wearing little or no clothing are conducive to its spread. Flies may also aid in its transmission. In past years treatment has consisted largely of the use of arsenic and bismuth compounds. Penicillin seems to be highly effective, however, the lesions often drying up within 48 hours after the drug is administered. Aureomycin is also being experimented with, and at present it appears to be effective.

Oroya fever (bartonellosis) is a disease caused by a bacterium, *Bartonella bacilliformis*. It is confined largely to certain valleys in Peru, Ecuador, Columbia, and neighboring regions. The acute phase of the disease develops abruptly about 20 days after exposure, eventually producing high, irregular fever, severe anemia, and frequently death. The chronic stage (*verruca peruviana*) which may follow the acute phase, is accompanied by rheumatic pains, skin eruptions, hemorrhagic nodules, and often severe hemorrhages from the mucous membranes. The bacteria are probably transmitted by the bite of sandflies (*Phlebotomus*), which frequently bite at night. Native dogs, which have a similar disease, no doubt serve as reservoir animals. Treatment is still uncertain; a diet rich in protein and low in fat is recommended, along with preparations containing iron to combat the anemia. Recent experiments indicate that penicillin, aureomycin, and terramycin may be of value in treating patients with the disease.

Diseases caused by fungi

Madura foot (mycetoma, maduromycosis) is caused by a number of different fungi which produce a chronic, granulating infection of the lower extremities, less often of the hands or other parts of the body. The affected part usually becomes enlarged and develops many deep sores. Extensive bone destruction may occur, resulting in crippling deformities. The parasitic molds are believed to gain entrance through some minor injury to the skin, following which they grow subcutaneously. No adequate treatment is known; in most cases, amputation seems to be the only treatment possible.

Dhobie itch (Tinea cruris) is a type of ringworm infection usually located in the groin and inner surfaces of the thighs. Several different fungi may be responsible, but all produce a similar red rash which itches intensely. As in many fungus infections, treatment is difficult. Among the agents which are recommended are Whitfield's ointment and the newer chrysarobin ointment. It might be mentioned that the term "dhobie itch" has been widely used to identify practically any skin infection that is encountered in the tropics. Actually the term might have a more specific origin. In India, the Dhobie caste is the caste that does all the laundry. It is customary in marking the clothing to use a native nut. The juice of this nut makes an indelible laundry mark. The nut so used is derived from

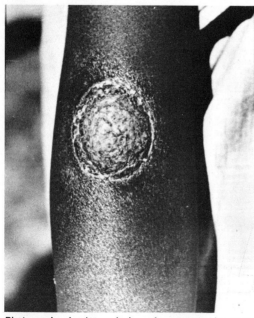

Photograph of primary lesion of yaws, on the upper arm. *(Armed Forces Institute of Pathology).*

a plant of the poison ivy group, and its juice produces severe itching and a rash. Some writers believe this to be the original "dhobie itch."

Diseases caused by protozoan parasites

African sleeping sickness (African trypanosomiasis—not the same as the sleeping sickness known as "encephalitis" and caused by a virus) is caused by two species of flagellated protozoa (one-celled animals called *trypanosomes*). *Trypanosoma gambiense* is prevalent in a broad belt across equatorial Africa while *T. rhodesiense* occurs in a limited area to the south. Transmitted to man by the bloodsucking tsetse flies (*Glossina*), the trypanosomes live at first in the blood stream, then in the lymph channels, and finally migrate into the cerebrospinal fluid of the brain and spinal cord. The first symptoms are remittent fever and swollen lymph nodes; during the second year a chronic state begins, with general physical and mental weakness. After an indefinite period of time the true "sleeping sickness" symptoms appear—a drowsy, dull, apathetic condition; the victim has a rapid pulse, low blood pressure, and becomes extremely emaciated. Unless treated early, death is nearly certain. The course of the Rhodesian form is more rapid and fatal, often terminating in death within a year. Arsenicals and antimonials have long been used, and newer preparations also contain these elements. One of the more promising drugs is the arsenical, *Melarsen B,* which is quite effective on the cerebrospinal parasites but is unusually toxic. More important, perhaps, is the prophylactic drug, *pentamidine,* which is believed to protect an individual from infection for about eight months following a course of injections.

Chagas' disease (American trypanosomiasis), caused by a related species, *T. cruzi,* is found in Central and South America, and is different from African trypanosomiasis. The disease is transmitted to man through the feces of a bloodsucking bug (and other members of the family *Reduviidae*) commonly referred to as the "kissing bug" because of its peculiar habit of biting people on the lips. The parasites undergo a transformation in man into minute, intracellular, nonflagellated organisms called *leishmania forms.* The symptoms of Chagas' disease often simulate those of heart disease, since the leishmania forms penetrate and multiply chiefly within the cells of the heart and brain. The tissue destruction produces general disability and frequently death. Mortality is highest in children. There is no satisfactory treatment; the trypanodical drugs used in African trypanosomiasis are largely ineffective, as are the antibiotics. Most promising results have come from use of a compound called *Bayer 7602* but a truly curative compound is yet to be discovered.

Kala-azar (visceral leishmaniasis), *oriental sore* (cutaneous leishmaniasis), and *espundia* (mucocutaneous leishmaniasis) are all produced by leishmanian parasites living intracellularly in man, gaining entrance through the bites of sand-flies *(Phlebotomus)*. *Kala-azar* caused by *Leishmania donovani,* is widespread in northern Africa, Asia Minor, India, and China. If the victim is untreated, the disease usually ends fatally within two years, since the parasites invade the liver, spleen, bone marrow, lymph nodes, and other vital organs. Oriental sore, caused by *L. tropica,* is found in middle and north Africa and Asia Minor. The parasites invade the skin and mucous membranes, producing ulcers which frequently become secondarily infected with bacteria. Uncomplicated sores usually heal within a year but leave disfiguring scars. Espundia, caused by *L. braziliensis,* is found largely in Central and South America. The mucous membranes of the nose, mouth, and pharynx are usually affected, the diseased areas often including the underlying cartilage. If the larynx becomes infected, the voice may be lost permanently.

Various antimony-containing drugs are used to treat patients with leishmaniasis. In *kala-azar, neostibosan* seems best, but relapses are not uncommon. *Stibophen* is the drug of choice at present in the cutaneous and mucocutaneous forms.

Tropical sprue is characterized by voluminous frothy diarrhea accompanied by soreness and erosion of the tongue and mouth. Other symptoms are severe anemia (resembling pernicious anemia), loss of weight, and the inability to absorb the products of fat digestion. The precise cause is unknown. Generally classed as a deficiency disease, it is believed to be caused by the lack of some substance in the food or the failure of the body to manufacture some essential material necessary for fat absorption. Sprue is prevalent in Asia, India, the Philippines, and the West Indies. Quite recently *folic acid* has been found to be beneficial in treatment, producing striking clinical improvement.

Dengue fever (breakbone fever) occurs in sporadic epidemics in all the tropical and subtropical areas of the world. *Aedes* mosquitoes are responsible for transmitting the virus which causes the fever. It is characterized by aches in the bones and joints, associated with headache and fever. Uncomplicated cases are probably never fatal, although the reduction in the number of white blood cells lowers the patient's resistance to other infections. No specific treatment has been found.

25 ENVIRONMENTAL HEALTH AND SANITATION

WATER PURIFICATION AND SEWAGE DISPOSAL

Water may be a carrier of disease-producing bacteria. Chief among the dieases that can be spread by contaminated water are typhoid and paratyphoid fever, cholera, and dysentery. Unpurified water may contain the cysts of amoebae that cause dysentery and the eggs of some parasitic worms.

Some persons do not have access to a dependable municipal water supply. Perhaps the simplest way to obtain safe drinking and household water in these instances is to boil it and then to protect it from contamination. As soon as water reaches the boiling point, practically all known water-borne, disease-producing organisms are killed; however, in order to be safe, the water should be boiled for ten minutes. The flat taste of boiled water may be remedied by pouring the water from one vessel to another until air again becomes dissolved in it. Unpleasant odors and tastes may be removed by passing water through a filter made of charcoal or by suspending a cheesecloth bag containing charcoal in the water for several minutes. Filter, cheesecloth, and charcoal should have been boiled previously.

Another method of purifying water is by the use of chlorine-containing tablets (*halazone*), which give off a small amount of chlorine when dissolved. The chlorine destroys most organisms that might be dangerous. If the odor and taste of chlorine are objectionable, they may be partially removed with charcoal. Sufficient chlorine is given off by halazone tablets so that in a pint of water treated with two tablets, there will be one

part of chlorine to 200,000 to 500,000 parts of water. Larger quantities of water may be sterilized by the use of chlorine gas, chlorinated lime, or a household chlorine disinfectant or bleach.

Water may also be purified with tincture of iodine: add two drops of tincture of iodine to each quart of water to be purified; mix and allow to stand 30 minutes before drinking. Certain porous filters are useful in removing suspended material prior to boiling or chlorination of the water. Properly constructed filters containing 24 to 30 inches of sand will remove many impurities and much of the bacterial flora. Such water, however, cannot be considered safe without further treatment. When traveling in many tropical countries, it is safer to consume bottled liquids, whether they be water, soft drinks, beer, or wine, rather than to depend on the local water supply. Ordinarily, most large cities throughout the world may be depended upon to have safe water supplies.

Sources of water

All surface water should be regarded as polluted, and no credence should be placed in beliefs that running water will purify itself. Such water is constantly being contaminated from many sources, and disease-producing organisms may survive in it for long periods of time. Spring water near populated areas is likely to be contaminated, since springs most often are derived from surface or near-surface water. A spring that becomes turbid after a rain is sure to be contaminated at times. Spring water should be consumed only after the spring has been cleaned,

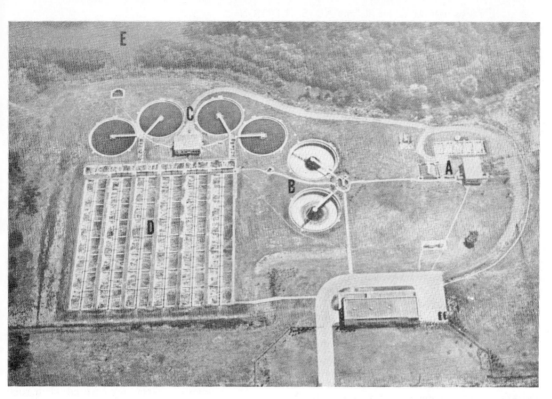

Sewage treatment plant. After screening (A) sewage is subjected to aerobic (B) and anaerobic (C) bacterial action in large tanks to reduce organic matter. Debris is then dried in beds (D) and used for fertilizer. Remaining clear fluid may be chlorinated and piped into stream (E). *Courtesy Department of Public Works, City of Houston.*

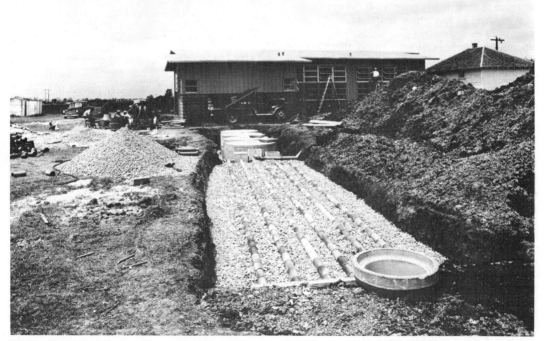

Photograph of a modern private sewage disposal system, in this case designed to serve the needs of two hundred school children. Sewage passes into the septic tanks in the background and eventually into the gravel filter; residue finally flows into sump tank in foreground, for chlorination. *Courtesy J. F. Smith and Sons, Houston.*

covered, and walled, protected against flooding by surface water, and has been tested for coliform bacteria following a rainy period.

All wells should be located as far as practicable from sources of contamination and at a higher level if possible. Shallow wells should be walled with a waterproof casing, and provisions should be made to prevent surface water from entering. A properly constructed pump should be installed. Construction of wells in conformity with recommendations made by the various state departments of health has proved desirable. Bacteriological testing is commonly advised, and a sanitarian should be consulted on the conditions surrounding the water source. Water from deep wells which are cased and grouted to the water-bearing strata is usually safe. These wells should be provided with a sanitary seal to prevent seepage of surface water but, in spite of all this, the water should be checked periodically for biological and chemical contamination.

Cistern water is sometimes the only source of water available. Cisterns are filled by rain water, usually from the residence roof. Since the roof is often contaminated by bird droppings and other material, a switch should be provided in the conducting pipe so that only the last part of the rain water is caught. The first part of the rain then washes the roof. Openings to the cistern should be screened to prevent mosquito breeding. While water from a properly constructed cistern is usually safe for household use, it still should be boiled or otherwise purified before drinking, for such water could hardly be regarded as sufficiently pure. Cisterns are in constant danger of pollution from disease-bearing organisms, insecticides and industrial effluents landing on the roof. They should therefore be checked constantly for biological and chemical contamination.

Municipal water supply

The problem of municipal water supply varies with the location of the community. Wells, streams, rivers, lakes, and melted snow are all sources that have been used. Almost any water can be rendered safe for consumption if properly treated. However, on a large-scale basis the cost may be prohibitive. The usual process begins with some type of filter to remove the larger particles. The smaller particles are removed by the addition of alum (usually about one grain per gallon) to the water, thereby producing a cloud-like precipitate which sinks and carries down with it the finer particles. The water is then allowed to settle for about four hours; then it is passed through sand layered over gravel for removal of remaining suspended material. Since some bacteria will have survived these processes, chlorine, approximately one

pound to a million pounds of water, is added for final purification. When desirable, the water may subsequently be sprayed through air or passed over activated charcoal to remove unpleasant odors or taste.

The disposal of wastes without water

To prevent water- and fly-borne diseases, the liquid and solid waste material of the body must be disposed of in a sanitary manner. In isolated communities, a flyproof pit toilet may be used. The simplest structure consists of a wooden building with a seat built over a deep pit (the old type privy). A satisfactory pit toilet may be constructed over a concrete, brick, or wood-lined pit with openings below the two-foot depth to allow the liquid material to escape. The pit should be at least five feet deep and covered with a concrete slab. The seat should be provided with a tightly fitting wooden cover. The pit should be ventilated with a flyproof pipe extending above the roof of the privy. Local health agencies and state health departments have available plans for building properly constructed toilets.

Other types of toilets may be used when running water is not available. One of these is the chemical toilet, whereby the waste material is disposed of by dissolution with a strong caustic soda solution. This solution will render all the substances liquid and will destroy objectionable odors. This method is suitable for use in trailers and summer cabins.

Septic tanks

Residences furnished with running water can have some type of water-borne sewage disposal system using flush toilets. Sometimes individuals or communities discharge untreated sewage directly into rivers, lakes, or the sea. This practice is now in violation of federal and state laws. The cesspool is another unsatisfactory method of sewage disposal. This is simply a deep hole into which the sewage is allowed to run. The liquid portions seep into the ground, thus contaminating the soil and making nearby well water unsafe. Since satisfactory systems can be constructed for approximately the same expense, cesspools are no longer tolerated by community health officers.

Septic tanks are in wide use and give satisfactory results when properly utilized. These consist of concrete or metal tanks with a baffle or partial partition extending down from the top. The sewage enters one side, is retained for a period of time, and then is discharged from the opposite side. The baffle board slows down the flow of the sewage and prevents passage of the

The municipal disposal of sewage

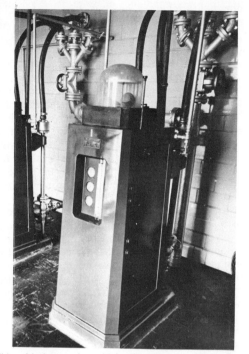

This chlorinator, by which chlorine is added to the water supply of a city to decontaminate it, may use over a thousand pounds of chlorine gas daily.

scum into the outlet pipes. Thus, both the scum which floats and the solids which settle are retained in the tank where the action of certain types of bacteria renders them less nocuous. The liquid sewage overflow from the septic tank, called *effluent,* contains bacteria, suspended particles, and dissolved gases, primarily methane, carbon dioxide, nitrogen, and the odorous hydrogen sulfide, and requires further treatment. This can be accomplished for a private residence by discharging effluent through loosely jointed tile pipe buried in the soil. The effluent escapes into the soil where oxidation destroys the organic material.

A septic tank for a single residence occupied by one family should have a capacity of at least 750 gallons. If automatic washing machines and garbage grinders are used, the capacity should be 900 or, preferably, 1000 gallons. Both concrete and metal septic tanks may be purchased preconstructed. Septic tanks must be cleaned at intervals by removing most of the scum and sludge which has accumulated; an adequate septic tank may not require cleaning for several years. Further information relative to the proper installation of satisfactory septic tank systems can be acquired from Public Health Service Publication No. 526; Superintendent of Documents; Washington, D.C.

Since many inland cities are located on rivers, the water supply for drinking and home use often is taken from the upper part of the stream and the sewage discharged downstream from the city. Because other cities downstream may get their water from the same stream, the sewage must be treated so that it is at least as pure as the original water.

The sewage as it comes from the homes, factories, and storm sewers often contains large objects which are removed as the sewage passes through screens which mechanically remove many particles and break up others.

The treatment of sewage after it leaves the screens varies with the different sewage disposal plants. In one of the most common kinds of plants, the sewage passes into one or more large circular or rectangular tanks, called "clarifiers," where the flow is slowed and much of the suspended solids settle to the bottom where a rake-like device moves the material to a collecting pitlike sump. From there, the solids are pumped to a closed, generally heated, tank called a "digester" where anaerobic bacteria break down the organic matter and produce methane gas and other by-products. The methane gas is usually used in the plant for heating and, in some plants, as fuel for engines. After the solids have been "digested," they may be safely discharged to drying beds. When dry, the digested solids may be used as a soil-conditioner, buried, or incinerated. The overflow, or effluent, from the clarifier passes to a trickling filter where the sewage is sprayed over a deep bed of crushed rock. On and between the rocks, there develops a mass of aerobic bacteria and other microorganisms which utilize the organic materials as food with more inert and innocuous matter as a by-product. The filter effluent is then passed through a final clarifier and then may be chlorinated prior to discharge.

Still another type of sewage disposal is called the activated sludge method. In this process, raw sewage is mixed with biologically active sludge, which is composed of large numbers of microorganisms. The sludge is prepared by passing bubbles of air through untreated sewage for several weeks. This causes the aerobic microorganisms in the sewage to multiply rapidly. When this "activated" sludge is then added to raw sewage and additional air is bubbled through the sewage, the materials in the raw sewage are utilized as food by the aerobic microorganisms. The rapid growth of the organisms results in more activated sludge, most of which is again mixed with raw sewage. A portion of the additional activated sludge is removed in a final clarifier and routed to a digester for the production of gas and inert materials. The digested sludge is dried and may then be used as a fertilizer or soil conditioner. The clear liquid from the final clarifier may be chlorinated and discharged.

POLLUTION

Pollution of land, air, and water became a major problem in the post-World War II era in the United States. The word "ecology," in the past generally familiar only to biologists, now is often seen on the front pages of newspapers and is used promiscuously by politicians and government officials. Basically, the term "ecology" means the interaction of all of the forces of the environment upon any organism (in this case, man) in its basic struggle for survival. The people in many communities began asking for pollution controls when monitoring systems revealed that certain industrial areas would soon be uninhabitable.

Water pollution does not mean that man will someday be without water for his own consumption, since it is possible, though at tremendous cost, to clarify contaminated water. Many cities today draw their entire water supply from grossly polluted streams and lakes. Many toxic substances find their eventual goal in bays and estuaries where commercial fishermen harvest seafood for the market. Water pollution has reached such an advanced state in some areas that large lakes and streams have been virtually destroyed as far as recreation and commercial value are concerned. It has been estimated, for instance, that restoration of Lake Erie would require 40 billion dollars and 500 years and only then if further pollution was stopped immediately. The Cuyahoga River which flows through Cleveland is so polluted with oil wastes that it occasionally bursts into flame, burning the bridges which span its foul-smelling waters. Biologists have reported that birds feeding on the fish in these waters have diminished and randomly selected specimens have shown concentrations of toxic substances in various organs of their bodies. Over 50 percent of the runoff from the largest watershed of the United States, extending from the east slope of the Rocky Mountains to the west slope of the Allegheny Mountains, drains into the Gulf of Mexico, carrying with it the effluents and waste products of industry as well as pesticides accumulated along the way. The pesticides most often accused of upsetting the balance of nature are the chlorinated hydrocarbons such as dichlorodiphenyl trichloroethane, commonly referred to as DDT. It might be stated, however, that there is no evidence that these compounds are responsible directly for human death.

Air pollution presents an even more dramatic picture than water pollution, since human health and life enter the picture more immediately. In some industrial areas, over two tons of air pollutants fall on each square mile annually. Air specimens may include such toxic substances as sulfur, carbon monoxide, and other engine exhaust fumes, as well as lead, zinc, copper, and many other chemicals known to be detrimental to health in varying degrees. If pollutants reach such a concentration in the air that birds leave the city and the growth of tender vegetation is thwarted, it is obvious that man will suffer too. Although the prodromal signs of decreasing wildlife were manifest, it was only after the death of several thousand people in England that Great Britain passed the Clean Air Act (1956). Now, London is one of the cleanest industrial cities of the world; lung and heart diseases have decreased immensely, and the birds have returned to Berkeley Square.

Pollution of the atmosphere is not confined to small industrial areas, however, but is progressing throughout the entire world. For instance, a superjet airliner dumps 100 tons of carbon monoxide into the air on each crossing of the Atlantic. Multiply this amount by over 200 flights per day and the enormity of the problem is readily seen.

Control of pollution is not just a matter for a few protest marchers or wrist-slapping health officials since industrial corporations soon find methods of postponement of litigation while continuing to discharge the effluents from their factories. One of the counterthrusts of the corporation lawyers is that the cost of installation of pollution control devices would be so enormous that manufacturers could better shut down their plants completely. Conversely, some industries are studying ways and means of reclaiming these waste materials as raw products in the industrial cycle. This seems to be a logical approach since it is obvious that polluted air is expensive air. It is apparent from all of the areas studied that air and water pollution are the problems of legislature on a world-wide basis, not merely for the conservation of wildlife, but for the conservation of man himself.

PREVENTION OF DISEASES TRANSMITTED BY FOOD

Food-borne diseases are divided into two main classes. The first is *food intoxication* (sometimes called *toxemia*) in which the poison or toxin is produced by the bacteria in the food and is present when the food is consumed; in other words, the bacteria do not grow in the body of the victim. The second type is *food infection* in which the living disease-producing organisms are present in the food, and upon entering the human body, multiply and cause infection. Food poisoning, of course, may occur from naturally poisonous plants such as some kinds of mushrooms, nightshade, or some of the holly berries. Arsenicals and other insecticides have been known to produce illness if used too abundantly on vegetables and fruits. *Ptomaines,* which result from putrefaction of food, were once believed to be the cause of "ptomaine poisoning." However, recent investigations have not confirmed the older view, but have shown that most cases of food poisoning are caused by some specific organism or toxin.

Food intoxications

Botulism is a specific disease, frequently fatal, caused by eating food that contains a potent poison produced by the growth of the organism, *Clostridium botulinum.* This organism lives in the soil and in decaying organic matter or animal excreta. The long rod-shaped bacteria form *spores* which are resistant to heat. Some spores withstand boiling temperature for several hours. Most outbreaks of botulism have been traced to home-canned vegetables or to improperly cured meats. Commercially canned vegetables do not usually cause botulism, because of the high temperatures and pressure and the rigid sanitation practices used in the canning industry. The toxin of these bacteria is one of the most potent poisons known to man, but is destroyed by maintaining the food at boiling temperature for 15 minutes.

Botulism may be controlled by avoiding home-canned food preserved by the cold-pack method. When home canning is done, steam pressure should be used, particularly to process vegetables, meats, and nonacid fruits.

Preserved fruits and jellies high in acid and sugar content do not cause botulism, even though spoiled by other kinds of bacteria. Nevertheless, foods that have the slightest spoiled odor or appearance should never be tasted, but should be destroyed at once, preferably by burning.

As a rule, foods containing *botulin* (the toxin causing botulism) neither taste nor smell spoiled, but the can may show bulging or leaking. For this reason, one should never taste home-canned vegetables or meats until they have been boiled for a full 15 minutes, which will destroy the toxin. A case on record describes the death of a woman by botulism who had eaten only one green bean taken from the jar as she opened it.

The second, and perhaps the most common type of food poisoning is a violent stomach and intestinal upset, of two or three days' duration, caused by small spherical bacteria called *staphylococci* (singular *staphylococcus*). They grow and multiply in improperly handled food and produce a toxin or poison. The foods most commonly associated with this disease are cream

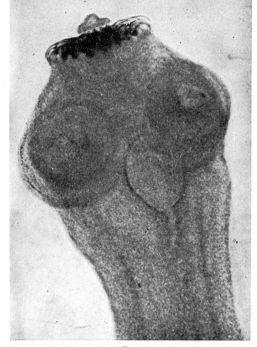

Photograph of head of *Taenia solium* or pork tapeworm, a human parasite, magnified 60 times. *Courtesy General Biological Supply, Chicago.*

puffs, pies, cakes with cream filling, and salads made from leftovers. Improperly handled meats such as hams have been involved in outbreaks of staphylococcic food poisoning. It has been observed that outbreaks most frequently occur after picnics and gatherings where the food has been prepared some time in advance of serving. Some outbreaks may be traced to boils or skin infections of the cook or other kitchen workers. Proper refrigeration, especially of starchy foods, and personal cleanliness appear to be the best methods of controlling this type of food poisoning.

Food-borne infections

The most common type of food-borne infection is caused by a bacterium called *Clostridium perfringens.* It is characterized by a sudden onset of abdominal colic and diarrhea, but thereafter is of short duration. The disease is transmitted primarily by improperly handled or prepared meat. The meat is contaminated by feces of infected humans or domestic animals or rodents. Control is accomplished by good hygiene of handlers and the proper cooking and refrigeration of meat.

The second most common type of food-borne infections is caused by a group of bacteria, *Salmonella.* In this group, there are more than ·60 different species of bacteria, and many of these produce some type of food infection. The symptoms, which consist largely of fever, diarrhea, and cramping, usually require several hours to develop and last longer than staphylococcic food poisoning.

This disease is transmitted by foods, milk, and sometimes water. Domestic animals, rats, mice, and cockroaches often carry the infection and contaminate foods. Eggs often contain *Salmonella,* which may be preserved in the preparation of egg powder. Salad dressing prepared from infected eggs has been known to cause food infections.

Most frequently, infections are transmitted by contaminated meat (especially turkey), vegetables, or egg products. Control of rats, mice, and flies, proper cooking and refrigeration of foods, and inspection of eggs and meat products aid in control of these infections. Personal cleanliness on the part of cooks and food handlers is another of the important preventive methods.

There are other bacterial diseases that are transmitted by foods. Typhoid fever is transmitted in the same way as *Salmonella* infection, with the carrier again playing an important role. Ice cream has been involved in some outbreaks of typhoid fever. Asiatic cholera also may be spread by food. Meat from cattle and hogs sometimes has been found to be infected with tuberculosis. Proper inspection eliminates most of the danger. For further discussion see Chapter 13.

Food-borne infections caused by animal parasites

Amoebic dysentery is an intestinal disease that is caused by the parasite, *Endamoeba histolytica,* which may contaminate food. Many individuals harbor these organisms and become carriers, without having symptoms of the disease. As high as 50 percent of the population in some tropical countries are infected. Since human waste is used as fertilizer in some areas, vegetables become contaminated. Careless domestic workers who do not wash their hands carefully after going to the toilet are often sources of infection. The control of this disease involves: boiling of questionable water, pasteurization of milk, the avoidance of native-grown raw vegetables where human excreta or fresh animal manure are used as fertilizer, and the proper cooking and handling of food.

A number of other animal parasites may be present in food. Chief among these is a small roundworm called *Trichinella,* which produces the disease *trichinosis.* This organism may be found in cysts in pork or the meat of other carnivorous animals, such as bear. Thorough cooking, or freezing for five days, will destroy the organism. Uncooked meat scraps should be

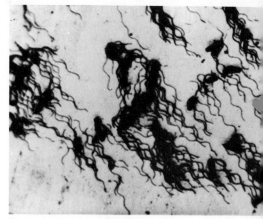

Photomicrograph of *Eberthella typhosa,* the bacterium which causes typhoid fever, magnified 1300 times. In this preparation the flagella were stained. *Courtesy General Biological Supply, Chicago.*

protected from rats and should not be fed to hogs.

Beef and pork tapeworms also may infect human beings, as well as dogs and cats. The infection is acquired by consuming improperly cooked beef and pork products. The inspection of meat and other food products aids in elimination of the diseases caused by parasitic or bacterial contaminants. The cost of meat inspection is less than one-tenth cent per pound; at this price meat inspection might be regarded as one of the best investments one can make in public health. The proper sanitary inspection of milk and milk products is equally important in control of milk-borne infections. (For further information concerning diseases transmitted by food, see Chapter 13, "The Digestive System," and Chapter 4, "Disease-Producing Organisms.")

FLY CONTROL

The most common fly found in the United States, Canada, and Europe is the housefly, *Musca domestica.* It is one of the most dangerous and troublesome insects that molest man.

The housefly is dusty gray in color. Its upper body is covered with tiny bristles and marked with four dark, longitudinal stripes. The lower part of its body is yellow and slightly transparent: its wings have a grayish cast and are yellow-tinged at the base. The legs of the housefly are covered with short hairs and are brownish-black in color; the feet are provided with hairy pads and exude a sticky substance, which enables the fly to walk on windowpanes and on ceilings. The spongy mouthparts of the housefly make it incapable of biting. Bites thought to have been inflicted by the housefly, therefore, may have been inflicted by the stable fly or biting housefly.

Stomoxys calcitrans, which closely resembles the common housefly. Adult houseflies feed chiefly on liquids from decayed vegetables and fecal matter, sputum, and foods such as syrup and milk. The fly dissolves dry substances before eating them; it does this with salivary secretions and with liquid regurgitated from its crop. Its feeding habits, sticky feet, hairy body, and ability to fly make the housefly an almost ideal animal for spreading disease-producing organisms from the filth on which it feeds and breeds into houses which it frequents in search of food and warmth.

The fact that houseflies commonly breed in human excrement and frequently in open privies makes them especially dangerous as carriers of diseases of the intestines. Eggs and embryos of wormlike parasites of the human intestines may be ingested by the housefly and later transferred intact directly to human hosts or indirectly through contaminated food and drink. Flies are known to be carriers of the causative organisms of typhoid fever, diarrhea, dysentery, and cholera.

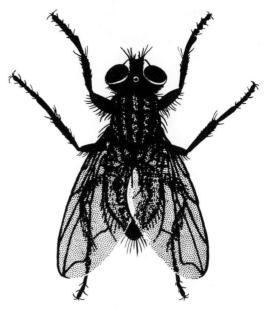

The common house fly, Musca domestica (8 x).

Life history of the housefly

Flies live relatively short lives. The entire cycle from egg to adult may be completed in 6 to 20 days; adult flies usually mate a few hours after reaching adulthood and start laying eggs within 2 to 20 days thereafter. Fly eggs are deposited in decaying or fermenting organic matter; in warm weather they hatch within 24 hours. The newly hatched young fly is a white, wormlike maggot; it is thought that it feeds on organic matter which causes fermentation and decay. The larva grows rapidly, increasing in length from one-twelfth inch to one-third or one-half inch within six or seven days. The skin of the larva gradually becomes brown, heavy, and contracted, and eventually forms an outer sac or case *(puparium)* for the young fly, or *pupa,* as it is called in this stage of development. The change into a winged adult fly takes place within the puparium. In cold climates, flies usually pass the winter as pupae; in warm weather, they become adults within three to six days. Adult flies soon leave their breeding place in search of food and new places to lay eggs; about 600 yards is the average life flight of a housefly, although some flies may fly much farther.

Elimination of breeding places

Since flies can fly from block to block and dwelling to dwelling, effective fly control must be carried out on a community-wide basis. Whenever flies are numerous in an area, the first thing to check is their breeding places. If the garbage and sewage of the community are not properly disposed of and dead animals are not promptly

buried or burned, ideal breeding places will become available to the fly. Outdoor toilets not only serve as sources of fly-borne infection, but may also be breeding places for flies. All toilets should be built as flyproof as possible, and the waste material in them should be covered with daily applications of crankcase oil or sprinkled with borax or lime.

Manure should be removed from barns and stables every two or three days to prevent flies from breeding in it. If manure is to be used as fertilizer, it can be spread thinly on the ground so that it will dry. In the northern part of the United States, compost piles of manure may be made during the winter months without much danger of serving as breeding places for flies. In warmer climates and in the summer, manure should be buried or treated chemically if it must be stored about the farm. Closely packed manure, covered with a foot of earth, generates so much heat that eggs and larvae of flies cannot live. One pound of borax to 25 gallons of water makes a solution which can effectively destroy

DARNALL, Carl Roger (1868-1941) American Army medical officer. Concerned with the many problems of sanitation confronting large bodies of troops in field operations. Darnell, like Lyster, developed a practical means of quickly purifying polluted water in the field. By Darnall's method, sodium hypochlorite is employed as the sterilizing agent.

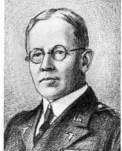

eggs and kill larvae of flies, yet not be dangerous to plants and animals. Concentrations of borax have an undesirable effect on plant growth; therefore, manure which is to be used as fertilizer should be treated with a solution consisting of one pound of *sodium fluosilicate* or *hellebore* to 20 gallons of water. Ten gallons of the solution is needed for every ten cubic feet (eight bushels) of manure.

Control of adult flies

The number of flies within a community may be significantly reduced with *malathion*. DDT (*dichlorodiphenyl-trichloroethane*) is no longer recommended because in many places the housefly and its close relatives have developed resistance to it; furthermore, the chemical is highly persistent and is accumulated in the fatty tissue of man and other animals. The clinical significance of such DDT accumulations is currently under study. *Pyrethrum* and malathion sprays (conveniently packaged in pressurized spray cans or aerosol bombs) and *vapona* (DDVP) impregnated strips may be used to kill flies about the home. With the possible exception of the pyrethrums, all of the insecticidal chemicals noted above are toxic to human beings in some degree, and the manufacturer's directions for use must be followed to the letter. In any case, chemical control of flies and other insects should supplement, not supplant, good sanitary practices. All windows and doors should be screened against flies. In areas where flies are prevalent, infants and invalids should be guarded by draping fine mesh netting over their beds. Food should be covered and stored in such a manner that it will not attract flies. Garbage and kitchen refuse should be kept in tightly covered cans; the can should be scrubbed frequently. Kitchen disposals that grind up refuse and discharge it into a sewage system aid in the elimination of materials that are attractive to flies.

MOSQUITO CONTROL

Mosquitoes transmit the organisms that cause malaria, yellow fever, dengue fever, and some forms of encephalitis and filariasis.

Mosquitoes belong to the same order of insects as houseflies (*Diptera*) but to a different family (*Culicidae*). This family includes a wide variety of mosquitoes and mosquito-like insects. *Culex, Aedes,* and *Anopheles* are the most important genera of mosquitoes from the standpoint of health and sanitation. These mosquitoes have slender bodies which may be as long as one-half inch; they have three pairs of long, delicate legs. There are scales along the margins of their long, narrow wings. The feeding organ

(*proboscis*) is slender and as long as the head and *thorax* of the insect combined. It is used by the female mosquito of many species to pierce the skin of man and animals and to suck blood; the male does not attack man or other animals but lives largely on nectar obtained from plants. The immature forms of mosquitoes are aquatic. *Anopheles* and *Aedes* mosquitoes lay their eggs singly, but *Culex* mosquitoes lay eggs in raftlike clusters of several hundred. Eggs are laid in water or in places where water is likely to accumulate; they will not hatch out of water. The wormlike, free-swimming *larvae* or "wigglers" which hatch from the eggs breathe by means of a syphon which carries air from the water surface to the gill of the insect. The syphon of the *Anopheles* larva is short; these wigglers stay close to the surface and feed on floating organic matter. The larvae of *Culex* and *Aedes* mosquitoes leave the surface of shallow water to feed on organic matter. However these, as well as the *Anopheles,* can be killed by the use of appropriate chemicals applied to the water. Larvae pass through four molts before the pupae or "*tumblers*" develop. The pupal stage is a short, quiescent stage during which the structures of the adult are organized.

Culex mosquitoes or "domestic" mosquitoes

Most house or "domestic mosquitoes" belong to the genus *Culex*. The majority of them are simply pests, but some species of *Culex* are carriers of minute worms which cause *filariasis,* a disease which is common in tropical regions. Filariasis is seldom fatal, but often produces enlargements of the legs and scrotum, resulting in a condition known as elephantiasis. *Culex pipiens* is one of the more common house mosquitoes in the United States; in Egypt, China, and Japan it is the usual carrier of filariasis. *Culex* mosquitoes are brown, and the abdomen is marked with whitish bands. Since they frequently breed near dwellings and have a short flight range, individual householders may do much to control them.

Aedes mosquitoes and yellow fever

Both yellow fever and dengue are tropical diseases which are spread by certain species of *Aedes* mosquitoes. Both of these diseases are caused by viruses which may be transmitted by the bite of a mosquito which has previously bitten an infected man or monkey. Once infected, mosquitoes retain the ability to transmit the disease-producing organisms as long as they live. *Aedes aegypti,* also called the "yellow jack" or yellow fever mosquito, is found in tropical and subtropical regions throughout the world. It is known to transmit dengue as well as yellow

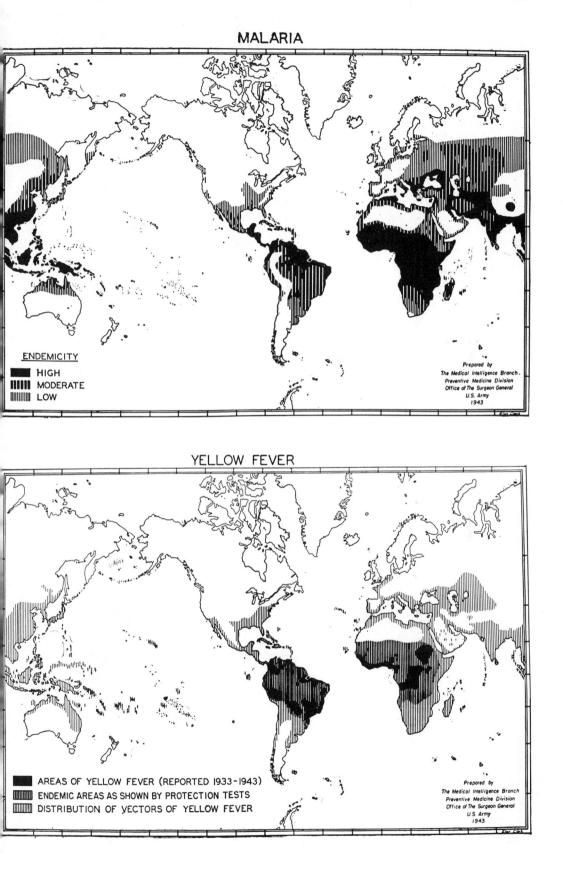

MALARIA

ENDEMICITY

HIGH
MODERATE
LOW

Prepared by
The Medical Intelligence Branch,
Preventive Medicine Division
Office of The Surgeon General
U.S. Army
1943

YELLOW FEVER

AREAS OF YELLOW FEVER (REPORTED 1933-1943)
ENDEMIC AREAS AS SHOWN BY PROTECTION TESTS
DISTRIBUTION OF VECTORS OF YELLOW FEVER

Prepared by
The Medical Intelligence Branch
Preventive Medicine Division
Office of The Surgeon General
U.S. Army
1943

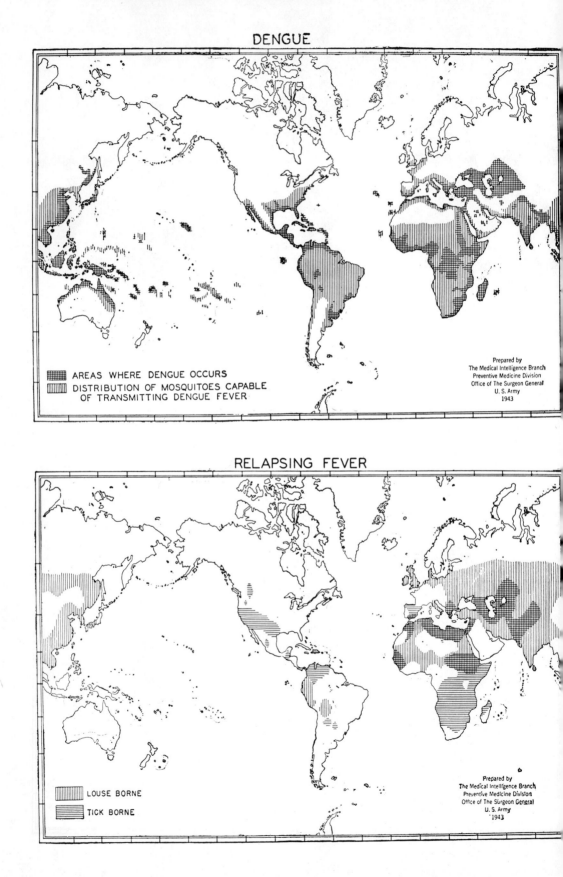

DENGUE

AREAS WHERE DENGUE OCCURS
DISTRIBUTION OF MOSQUITOES CAPABLE
OF TRANSMITTING DENGUE FEVER

Prepared by
The Medical Intelligence Branch
Preventive Medicine Division
Office of The Surgeon General
U. S. Army
1943

RELAPSING FEVER

LOUSE BORNE
TICK BORNE

Prepared by
The Medical Intelligence Branch
Preventive Medicine Division
Office of The Surgeon General
U. S. Army
1943

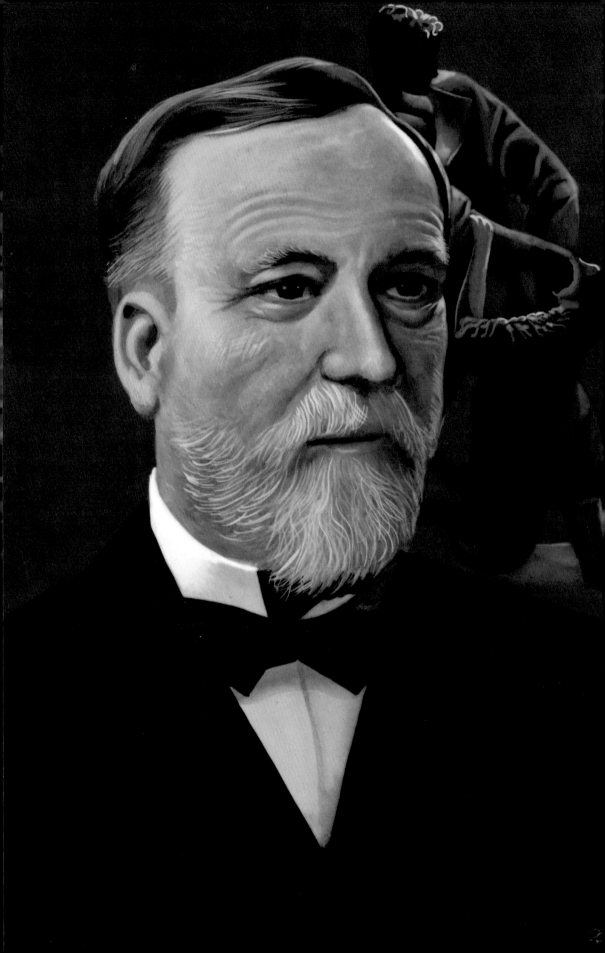

fever. Adult *Aedes aegypti* mosquitoes may be identified by the silvery, lyre-shaped markings on the thorax; they bite chiefly in the late afternoon and may attack without the buzzing hum usually associated with mosquitoes.

Aedes mosquitoes often breed along the banks of creeks and streams, in holes in trees, or in other natural depressions which collect water. Frequently, eggs are laid in dried-out pools and marshes. In warm weather, the eggs usually hatch soon after they are covered with water. Since the eggs may become submerged on the bottom of streams and lakes and not hatch until the warm days of spring, the *Aedes* mosquitoes are able to survive the wintertime in northern climates.

Anopheles *mosquitoes and malaria*

Mosquitoes of the genus *Anopheles* have been extensively investigated, because certain species are carriers of the organisms which cause malaria. Mosquitoes become infected with malarial parasites when they bite infected persons. The disease is not passed from man to man; a neces-

sary part of the life cycle of the parasite must be passed in the body of the mosquito. The parasite may remain dormant for many years in the blood of a person even though he has never had a malarial attack. The principle of malaria control is to break the line of transmission from the infected to the noninfected individual by eliminating the mosquito.

Most species of *Anopheles* have the wing scales arranged in a definite pattern; they are often referred to as spotted or "dappled wing" mosquitoes. The female may be distinguished by two long mouthparts, *palps*, which are as long as the proboscis. *Anopheles* mosquitoes usually bite in the evening and early morning. When biting, they hold their bodies at an angle to the surface on which they are resting; other mosquitoes hold the long axis of the body parallel to the surface on which they alight.

Anopheles mosquitoes usually lay their eggs in fresh water which has surface vegetation; however, some species will lay eggs in swiftly flowing streams with little or no surface vegetation, and others breed in polluted water or in salt water marshes. Their eggs may be distinguished from the eggs of other mosquitoes by the curious hollow chambers at the middle of each egg, which serve as floats and keep the eggs close to the surface of the water.

Control of breeding places

Nearly all of the *Aedes* mosquitoes which carry disease have been found breeding about dwellings, which is also true of many species of *Culex*. These mosquitoes may be partially controlled by efforts of individual householders in eliminating artificial breeding places. Wells and cisterns should be screened or otherwise protected to prevent the breeding of mosquitoes. Water which is to be used only for washing dishes and clothes may be treated with borax powder to keep it permanently free of larvae;

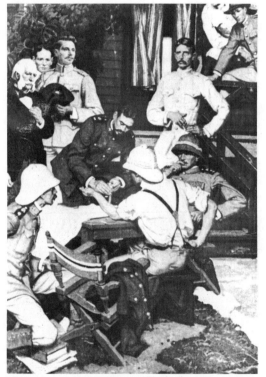

This painting shows the conquerors of yellow fever. Walter Reed stands at the stairway while Lazear performs an inoculation. Finlay (with white whiskers) stands at the left. *Bettman Archive.*

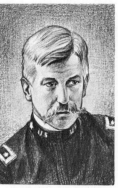

GORGAS, William C. (1854-1920) American Army surgeon. Directed the Panama campaign against yellow fever and malaria, controlling them in two years and making possible the completion of the canal. The basis of his control program was the eradication of yellow fever- and malaria-bearing mosquitoes. As director of the international health board of the Rockefeller Foundation, he extended yellow fever investigation through Central America.

ILLUSTRATION: Louis Pasteur . . . Joseph F. Doeve.
Louis Pasteur (1822-1895) French chemist and bacteriologist. Pasteur is generally regarded as the founder of modern bacteriology because of his many studies showing the relationship of bacteria to disease.

about two and a half ounces to a gallon of water suffices. Pools should be drained periodically; if mosquitoes are found to be breeding, the pool should be treated with a larvicide. Water-filled barrels, tubs, pots, and other containers should not be allowed to remain in the vicinity of houses; they should be drained and screened, or, if possible, discarded. Tin cans and other receptacles, including old automobile tires, often catch rain water and serve as breeding places; they should be emptied and eliminated. Poorly constructed cesspools and septic tanks may be breeding places for mosquitoes and should be repaired or replaced. Even water which collects in gutters and on flat roofs may serve as breeding places, if it is not drained.

Effective control of mosquitoes in large areas requires the supervision of public health engineers. It involves the elimination of breeding places wherever possible, as well as the destruction of larvae and adult mosquitoes. Marginal areas around lakes and rivers should be drained. If it is possible to control the water level of lakes and rivers, thus preventing the flooding of marginal lands, the edges of the waters that are thus established can be deepened and cleared. Streams should be cleared of heavy vegetation either by chemical or by mechanical means. Roadside ditches should frequently be cleared and drained.

Chemical treatment of waters to kill larvae may be necessary in many areas, especially where irrigation is required for agricultural purposes. Chemicals used in treating waters should kill mosquito larvae but not harm fish and other wildlife in the area. Dusts such as DDT or Paris green are effective in killing the larvae of mosquitoes. Oil emulsions of DDT, *toxaphene,* and *benzene hexachloride* are effective against the larvae of all mosquitoes, but are more toxic to wildlife than the dusts mentioned above. Airplanes are sometimes used to spray or dust areas.

Adult mosquitoes may be killed by spreading DDT from planes and on the ground. Sprays containing mixtures of *pyrethrum* and DDT or *chlordane* are effective in destroying mosquitoes which get into houses. Since mosquitoes often hide in closets, basements, and attics, these places should be especially well sprayed. If doors to rooms and closets are shut for a few minutes after spraying, the sprays are more effective.

Protection from bites of mosquitoes

People who live in regions where mosquitoes are prevalent should wear clothing which covers as much of the body as possible when outside. Effective protection against bites may be obtained by the use of repellents of which *dimethyl phthalate* is one of the most widely used. It is

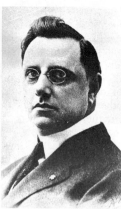

AGRAMONTE Y SIMONI, Aristide (1869-1931) Cuban parasitologist. Participated with other renowned medical officers Reed, Carroll, and Lazear in the brilliant work conducted by the U.S. Army Yellow Fever Commission in Cuba, from 1900 to 1902. The commission found that yellow fever is transmitted to man only by the mosquito, *Aedes aegypti.* This finding led to a rapid decline in the incidence of yellow fever in North and Central America.

available in creams which may be applied directly to the skin, and in solutions for impregnating clothing.

Well-fitting screens at windows and doorways are needed in most parts of the world to keep mosquitoes out of houses. The screens should be of 18-inch mesh; 16-inch mesh is fine enough to keep out most mosquitoes except the small mosquito which carries yellow fever. If a dwelling is already screened with 16-inch screening, the openings may be made smaller by painting the screens lightly with screen enamel. Screen doors should open outward so that mosquitoes resting on the screen will not be brought into the house as the door is opened.

In unscreened or poorly screened houses, mosquito nets may be needed at night for protection. They should be draped about the bed and tucked under the mattress at the edges. If the nets are impregnated with repellant, they provide added protection.

For further discussion of mosquito-borne diseases, see Chapter 24: "Tropical Diseases."

CONTROL OF LICE AND OTHER INSECTS

Aside from flies and mosquitoes, the most important insects directly affecting the health of man are lice, bedbugs, cockroaches, fleas, mites, and ticks.

Human lice are gray, wingless insects, varying in length from one-sixteenth to one-sixth inch. Two species of lice infest man. The head and body lice of man are different varieties of the same species *(Pediculus humanus);* the crab, or pubic louse is a distinct species *(Phthirus pubis).*

The head louse lives among the hairs of the scalp. It feeds on blood and cements its eggs, commonly called "nits," to strands of hair. The body louse is similar to the head louse, but it is lighter in color and larger. It lives and lays its eggs in seams of clothing; it is rarely found on the skin except when feeding or when infestation is extensive.

Crab lice usually cling to hairs in the crotch and armpits. They are sometimes found in the eyebrows and beard. They seldom move about, but remain attached by clinging to hairs with their crablike claws. Louse infestation is known as *pediculosis*.

Epidemic typhus fever and some forms of relapsing fever may be transmitted through the excreta of lice or when lice are crushed as a result of scratching, thereby releasing the disease-producing organisms.

Under ordinary sanitary conditions louse infestation is rare, but when people are forced to live in unsanitary places with few facilities for bathing or for cleaning clothes, louse infestation is common. The insecticide DDT is effective when used against lice. When it is not possible to change clothing often, a 10 percent dust of DDT applied to clothing worn next to the skin will give protection. Clothing, bedding, and luggage of infested persons should be fumigated or well dusted with DDT. Steam will also kill lice and destroy their eggs.

In mass delousing of populations, 10 percent DDT may be dusted on the hair or a 25 percent benzyl benzoate emulsion may be liberally applied, taking care to avoid contact with the eyes. A 24-hour contact time will insure a kill of adult and larval lice and will loosen the eggs as well. Vinegar or acetic acid will not destroy the glue which binds the eggs to hairs as was once commonly supposed. When DDT or benzyl benzoate are not available, 2 percent lysol or a mixture of 50 percent kerosene and 50 percent of any bland vegetable oil, such as olive oil, may be used. These substances are applied thoroughly to wet the hair, and the head is then bound up in a towel for at least an hour.

Bedbugs

The true bedbug, *Cimex lectularius*, often feeds on the blood of man. It also feeds on rats, mice, and poultry. Bedbugs are flat, dark brown insects about one-fifth inch long. They do not infest the body of man but live in cracks of furniture, along mattress seams, and behind loose baseboards and wallpaper. They lay their eggs along any convenient crack or crevice. A single female may lay from 200 to 500 eggs in a two- to three-month period. The eggs hatch in about ten days. Four generations may develop in a single year.

Both male and female bedbugs live on blood alone and feed chiefly at night. The bite of the bedbug produces irritation and swelling. No conclusive evidence has been found to establish them as important carriers of disease-producing organisms. If a house becomes infested with bed-

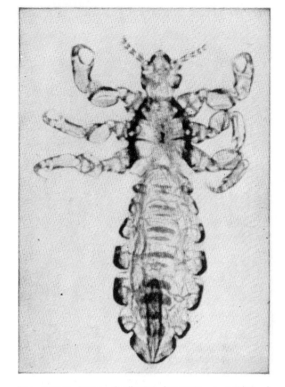

The human louse, *Pediculus humanus*, a carrier of typhus fever, magnified about 50 times. *Courtesy General Biological Supply House, Inc., Chicago Illinois.*

bugs, they may be exterminated by spraying with a household spray containing 5 percent DDT, or by dusting with a 10 percent DDT powder. Special attention should be given mattresses and springs and any cracks and crevices in the various parts of the bedstead.

"Mexican" and "China bedbugs"

The so-called "Mexican bedbugs" *(Triatoma sanguisuga)* and "China bedbugs" *(Triatoma protracta)* are not true bedbugs but belong to the *Reduviidae* family of insects. They are winged insects measuring in length from two-thirds inch to one inch. They have an elongated head and a beak of three segments. They are black, but some have pink or red markings on the body and wings.

Many species of the *Reduviidae* family feed on other insects and on plants; a few depend chiefly on the blood of wild animals for nourishment. In the southern and southwestern United States and in Mexico, the "Mexican bedbug," "big bedbug," or "kissing bug" frequently comes into houses at night to feed on human beings. The bite of these insects is painful and causes local swelling, faintness, and vomiting.

Triatoma megista, and several other reduviids found in Central and South America are carriers

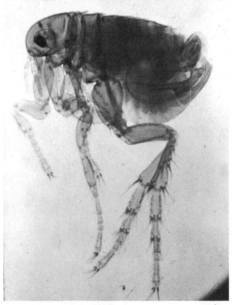

The human flea, *Pulex irritans*, a common parasite of the human race, magnified about 50 times. *Courtesy of General Biological Supply, Chicago.*

The wood tick, *Dermacentor andersoni*, the parasite through which Rocky Mountain spotted fever is transmitted to man. Magnified about 15 times.

of a human disease known as *Chagas' disease;* this disease is often fatal, especially to infants and young children. The causative organism, *Trypanosoma cruzi,* is a parasitic one-celled animal with a complex life cycle. It is carried from infested people or animals by the bite of the reduviids and transferred through the insect's feces excreted while feeding. Reduviids carrying *Trypanosoma cruzi* have been found in the southern United States as have nine-banded armadillos which are the *reservoir* for this parasite, but thus far fewer than a dozen cases have been reported.

No effective control measures for reduviids are known, for they seldom breed in dwellings, but come from out-of-doors to attack human beings. A tightly built, well-screened house is the best protection against them; mosquito nets also afford some protection.

Cockroaches

Cockroaches do not feed on human beings, as do lice and bedbugs. However, certain species feed on human feces as well as on foods. Cockroaches often become infected with disease-producing organisms, and may contaminate human food through contact or through feces which they excrete on food. Thereby they may spread the causative organisms of cholera and dysentery, as well as certain parasitic worms.

Cockroaches are world-wide in distribution; five to six domesticated species are common in the United States. They have flattened, elongated, oval, shiny bodies. They vary in length from one-half inch to over two inches, and in color from light tan to blackish brown. Adults of some species are almost wingless, while some are fully winged. Cockroaches hide in cracks and dark places during the day and are active chiefly at night. They lay their eggs in hard capsules, which are deposited in a corner or crevice before the eggs hatch. The life span ranges from two months to two and one-half years, depending upon the species.

Cockroaches may be brought into the home in grocery bags or boxes, laundry wrapping, and in furniture. They may come in through cracks, openings about pipe lines, or under doors. In poorly constructed buildings, reinfestation is inevitable.

Two percent chlordane (1068) and five percent DDT household sprays are effective in controlling cockroaches. Caution should be exercised in the use of chlordane, as it is very toxic, especially in enclosed areas. Both compounds should give control for as long as six months. All foodstuffs and utensils should be moved from kitchen cabinets and pantries. Shelves should be washed, then sprayed with DDT or chlordane household spray. Areas under the stove and refrigerator should be given a thorough cleaning and spraying. The rest of the house should be sprayed at the same time; crowded closets and basements are favorite breeding places. Sodium fluoride is highly effective in killing cockroaches, but should be used with great care since it is poisonous to animals and man. However, the old sailor's remedy of one part boric acid to one part sugar with a little water in bottle caps placed in areas inaccessible to children and pets still remains one of the most efficient means for controlling cockroaches.

Fleas

Fleas are commonly parasitic to mice, rats, cats, dogs, and many other warm-blooded animals; occasionally they also attack human beings. They are small, brown, wingless, laterally flattened, and possess mouthparts adapted to piercing the skin and sucking blood.

The female flea lays eggs in dust and dirt; eggs are often found in bedding in infested dwellings and in nests of rats and mice. The adult flea can live for long periods without food, but the female cannot lays eggs until it has had a blood feeding. The flea which most commonly feeds on human beings has a life cycle of from four to six weeks.

Various species of fleas show a preference for certain hosts but do not limit themselves to a particular host; thus, their potentiality as carriers of disease is great. Fleas are known to transfer the causative organisms of typhus fever and bubonic plague from animal to animal, animal to man, and man to man. The species of flea primarily responsible for the transmission of typhus and plague is the Indian rat flea (*Xenopsylla cheopis*). The dog and cat fleas (*Ctenocephalides canis* and *Ctenocephalides felis*) are not important carriers of known disease-producing organisms.

In tropical countries the *Chigoe,* or sand flea, is of medical importance. The impregnated female burrows in the skin between the toes, in the soles of the feet, or under the fingernails; here the female enlarges, causing much pain and itching.

Fleas are brought into dwellings chiefly by cats, dogs, rats, and mice. To prevent infestation, pets should be kept free of fleas by periodic washing with warm water containing an insecticide such as chlordane. Many good preparations can be purchased. Rats and mice should be exterminated.

Flea-infested dwellings should be thoroughly cleaned. Clothing and bedding should be sprayed with naphthalene or five percent DDT household spray and then washed in boiling water or steamed. Beds and other furniture should be sprayed with DDT. Rugs and floors may be sprinkled with naphthalene and the rooms sealed for several days, or they may be dusted with ten percent DDT powder or with sodium fluoride. Since basements are ideal breeding places for fleas and are frequented by rats and mice, they should be given special attention. Spraying with crude kerosene is an effective control measure; treatment with gaseous fumigants such as hydrogen cyanide and sulfur dioxide by an experienced person is also effective. Hydrogen cyanide and sodium fluoride are extremely dangerous poisons. Further information may be obtained by requesting U.S. Department of Agriculture Bulletin No. 121 "Controlling Fleas" from the Superintendent of Documents, Washington, D.C. (Price 5 cents).

Mites

Mites and ticks are not members of the large class *Insecta* to which the pests thus far discussed belong; they belong to the class *Arachnida,* which also includes the spiders and scorpions. There are marked differences between the various families of mites, but all typically undergo four stages in development: *egg, larva, nymph,* and *adult.*

Chiggers, or red bugs, are the larval stage of mites (*Trombicula irritans*) which usually lay their eggs in soil. Chiggers are barely visible to the unaided eye; they are egg-shaped, have six legs, and vary in color from bright red to light tan. They are parasites of many animals, including human beings. Chiggers do not burrow into the skin and die, as commonly supposed. Rather, they soften the skin with a secretion from their *pharynges;* the *serum,* oozing from the broken skin, hardens and makes a closed tube through which the chigger feeds. Once fed, they drop off their host and settle in the soil, where they may pass the winter. Two species of chiggers transmit scrub typhus (*tsutsugamushi* fever), a disease common in certain Pacific islands and Asiatic countries.

Chigger-infested lawns may be cleaned by dusting with ten percent DDT powder. The lawn should be closely clipped, and the DDT powder distributed as evenly as possible, using five to ten pounds per acre. Bathing with strong soap or medicated soap and sponging with alcohol immediately after exposure will often prevent the formation of the usual large red welts. In general, however, control of chiggers must be limited to preventing their bites. If chigger-infested areas cannot be avoided, a *miticide* (a compound which will kill mites) such as sulfur or benzyl benzoate should be applied to the skin and clothing, as a protective measure against chigger bites.

Scabies, a skin disease of man, is caused by the itch mite, *Acarus scabiei.* Several varieties of this mite are known, and will attack numerous animals. Man usually contracts the mite from other people, or from infested cows, sheep, goats, dogs, or cats. Miticides are effective in destroying the female mites which burrow into the skin and cause the disease. However, control of the mite is almost limited to avoiding infested animals, by isolating infested persons, and by sterilizing all clothing and bedding of infested individuals.

Ticks

Ticks belong to the same class (*Arachnida*) as mites. Like mites, they go through four stages of development and feed on the blood of man and animals. Ticks do not have a true head; the filelike tongue (*hypostome*) which is used to pierce the skin of the host is located in an anterior, median position on the saclike body. Ticks are divided into two families: the hard ticks (*Ixodidae*) and the soft ticks (*Argasidae*). The body of the hard tick is protected by a smooth, hard cover (*scutum*). This shield covers almost the entire back of the male, but only the forward third of the back of the female. Soft ticks of both sexes lack this shield.

The ticks *Dermacentor andersoni, Dermacentor variabilis,* and *Amblyomma americanum* are the known carriers of Rocky Mountain spotted fever, Colorado tick fever, and tularemia. The larvae and nymphs of these ticks feed on the blood of rodents. It is from the rodents that the disease-producing organisms are picked up. An infected female tick may transmit the disease-producing organisms to her offspring through the eggs. Later, adult ticks feeding on larger animals and man transmit the organisms.

The bite of the spotted fever tick, and of several other species of hard ticks, may cause paralysis. Ticks should not be carelessly pulled off the body. A drop or two of chloroform, gasoline, or turpentine applied to the tick will often cause it to retract its mouth parts so that it can be removed without danger of breaking off some of the mouth parts. Ticks may be dislodged with tweezers if the body of the tick is pulled gently but steadily.

Regions known to be heavily infested with ticks should be avoided as much as possible during the spring and summer. If it is necessary to walk through tick-infested brush or grass, rotenone dust or spray applied to clothing will be partially effective in preventing infestation. High grass should be cleared from campsites and dwellings, as it is often covered with "seed ticks" and adult ticks, and affords shelter for tick-infested animals. Thorough examination of the body after outings and removal of ticks before they have had a chance to feed may prevent some tick-borne diseases.

Soft ticks do not cling to a host and engorge as do hard ticks. They feed intermittently, night being the preferred feeding time. They live in nests of mice or other animal hosts. In some regions of Africa, they infest native huts, old campsites, and shelters along routes of travel. Some species of soft ticks are known carriers of *relapsing fever;* the disease-producing organisms may be transmitted by both adults and nymphs. In regions where these ticks are common, sleeping quarters should be kept as clean and as ratproof as possible. Beds should be away from walls and bedding kept off the floor. (For further information regarding diseases transmitted by lice and other insects, see Chapter 4, "Disease-Producing Organisms"; Chapter 8, "The Skin"; and Chapter 24, "Tropical Diseases.")

RAT CONTROL

There are several types of rats that have followed man throughout the world, that live where he lives and eat his food. Particularly important are the small Norway, or burrowing rat and the large brown roof or Alexandria rat. These rats cause a vast amount of economic damage. Furthermore, they are important health hazards, for they are known to harbor disease-producing organisms.

Rats as carriers of disease

Bubonic plague is primarily a disease of rats; man is an accidental victim. This disease is transmitted by the rat flea from rat to rat and sometimes to man. Bubonic plague is caused by small rod-shaped bacteria, *Pasteurella pestis,* which are present in the blood stream of animals having the disease. A flea biting a diseased rat obtains some of the bacteria which multiply to form a plug in the flea's gullet. This plug causes the flea to regurgitate some bacteria into the next rat it bites. When the rat dies of the plague, the fleas leave the dead animal to go in search of another host. If the fleas cannot find another rat, they will sometimes bite man, who in turn may become infected with bubonic plague. This is a serious disease, having a mortality rate of 25 to 50 percent.

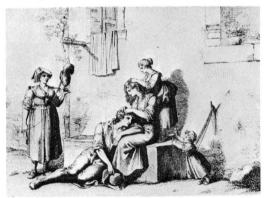

Flea hunting in Italy, by Pinelli. *Bettmann Archive.*

Another disease that rats and rat fleas transmit is *murine typhus,* a disease similar to typhus but usually not so severe. The infected rat shows few symptoms of the disease; but if an infected rat flea bites a human being, the disease may be produced.

The rat is also the carrier of Weil's disease, or *spirochetal jaundice,* an infection produced by corkscrew-shaped bacterial organisms *(Leptospira icterohaemorrhagiae).* This disease is acquired from food which has been contaminated by the excreta of rats that have this infection. Approximately ten percent of victims die. The rat also carries bacteria of the *Salmonella* type, which cause an intestinal infection when uncooked food that has been contaminated by the excreta from a diseased rat is consumed by human beings.

The rat is a carrier of the dwarf tapeworm *(Hymenolepis nana),* which is transmitted to human beings through food that is contaminated by the excreta of rats. Rat feces are also a factor in the spread of *Trichinella,* the organisms responsible for *trichinosis,* a disease of hogs and man. Other parasitic human infections have been traced to the rat.

Ratproofing

Since domestic rats depend on human habitations for food and shelter, premises of all types should be kept free of debris. Foods should be stored in tightly covered containers that rats cannot gnaw. Garbage cans should not be allowed to overflow and should be tightly covered. Kitchens and food-serving rooms should be kept clean at all times. No foods should be left accessible to rats between meal-service times.

Ratproof construction helps to keep rats out of buildings; but careful inspection often reveals holes large enough for rats to enter presumably ratproof structures. Many old, dilapidated buildings and barns provide easy access for rats. These structures can be ratproofed by thorough repair, using such materials as concrete, hollow tile, sheet iron, tin, and hardware cloth. Special attention should be given to breaks at the foundation and roof. Pipes should have tight-fitting metal shoulders at floor and ceiling levels. The use of hardware cloth on grain bins prevents rats from destroying grain.

Rat-killing

The rat has many natural enemies such as weasels, ferrets, skunks, hawks, owls, and snakes. Ferrets and dogs have been trained as rat-killers. Cats are often effective in controlling rats in a building.

Traps may be used effectively if only a few rats are present, but a rat soon learns to avoid traps.

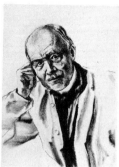

NICOLLE, Charles Jules Henri (1866-1936) French bacteriologist. He is famous for his many studies on the causative agents and carriers of human disease. Of his more important investigations, those on kala-azar and typhus are particularly significant in furthering our knowledge of sanitation procedures. With Comte and Conseil he demonstrated that typhus is transmitted by the body louse (1909). He received the Nobel prize for his work in the year 1928.

The best method of eliminating rats once they have become established is by the use of poison. The ideal poison is one that will kill the rats but be harmless to man and domestic animals. One of the most widely used poisons is *red squill,* an onionlike plant bulb, which causes heart failure and respiratory paralysis in the rat. A rat cannot vomit; hence it retains the poison, whereas a domestic animal or person will vomit immediately on eating the material. Red squill should be mixed with bait in the proportion of one part of squill to nine parts of bait material. The bait may be bacon grease mixed with oatmeal, lean meat, apples, or corn meal. Small parcels of the bait are placed in those areas most frequented by the rats, yet where children and domestic animals are not likely to find the bait. Phosphorus poison put up in small collapsible tubes is used to poison rats. It is effective, but poisonous to man and other animals. *Barium carbonate* is an effective poison and has the advantage of making rats thirsty. If their drinking place is outside the building, they usually will go outside and die.

Among the more recently developed rat poisons for professional exterminators is compound *"1080"* or *sodium fluoroacetate,* which may be used in water or bait. In water, it usually kills the rats so rapidly that they may be found within a few feet of the drinking place. They should be picked up and destroyed, since their bodies are

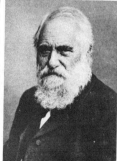

PETTENKOFER, Max Josef von (1818-1901) Bavarian biochemist and hygienist. First in Germany to develop practical instruction in hygiene. He carried on research on cholera, demonstrated the propagation of cholera by germs, and the effect of local conditions on contagion. His system of sewage disposal rid Munich of typhoid fever, a landmark in the history of sanitation.

also poisonous. Another compound, ANTU (*α-naphthylthiourea*), may be mixed with bait. Both these compounds are employed in large-scale rat control programs carried out by properly trained technicians. These compounds are violent poisons for all animal life. *Zinc phosphide* and *thallium sulfate* are useful in control of rats, but the surviving rats quickly become wary and avoid poisoned baits.

Two other poisons have real promise as rodenticides. They are *Warfarin,* developed in the United States, and *Toumarin,* a related compound from Switzerland. These compounds prevent the rat's blood from coagulating, and the rat dies from internal bleeding. One dose will not kill the animal, but, since the rat cannot detect the odor or taste, it will eat repeatedly on the poisoned bait. The rats usually die in about five to six days. If a person or animal eats the bait once, it is not likely to be harmful; and by proper medical attention the effect of the poison may be neutralized. These poisons are used in mixtures of one part of the poison to 19 parts of corn meal, brown sugar, and bacon grease or other fat.

INSECTICIDES AND GERMICIDES

Insecticides are often grouped into three general classes: stomach poisons, contact poisons, and gaseous poisons or fumigants. These classes are not rigid, as a substance may be effective as both a stomach and contact poison; also, the line between a fumigant and contact poison is finely drawn.

Stomach poisons and poison baits

Substances which kill insects by being ingested and absorbed through the walls of the digestive tract are called stomach poisons and are used primarily against insects with chewing mouthparts. They may be applied as dusts or sprays; often they are mixed with food or oils which attract insects.

Stomach poisons include a great array of highly toxic arsenic compounds, one of which is *Paris green.* This compound was originally used as a dye and was the first stomach poison applied to food plants to control insects. It is one of the quickest-killing insecticides, because it is absorbed by the digestive tract of the insect and has a high arsenic content. Paris green is used to destroy mosquito larvae; it is dusted on the surface of pools of water.

A large number of *fluorine* compounds, particularly sodium fluoride, are used as insecticides. In general, they kill insects quicker than arsenic compounds; they are toxic to plants and

higher animals as well as to insects, and should be used with caution. They are effective as both stomach and contact poisons.

Phosphorus is also used as a stomach poison. Yellow phosphorus mixed with syrup is an effective bait for cockroaches and rodents. The bait is highly poisonous and should be kept out of reach of children and pets.

Because of their high toxicity to human beings, the stomach poisons mentioned above are not highly recommended for household use. They are being replaced by synthetic compounds such as chlorinated hydrocarbons, organic phosphorus, and organic sulfur which are less toxic to human beings. These compounds act to some extent as stomach poisons but are mainly effective as contact poisons.

Contact poisons

Contact poisons do not have to be ingested to kill; they exert their toxic action by entering the insect's body through its outer covering or through its respiratory system. Some contact poisons leave residual films on surfaces with which they come in contact; these films may kill by acting on sensory organs present in the feet (*tarsi*) of the insect. Contact poisons are used mainly to control insects with piercing mouthparts, but they are effective against nearly all insects. They may be applied as dusts or sprays directly to the insects or as a residue in places where insects hide or breed.

Nicotine, in the form of finely ground tobacco or tobacco extracts, was one of the first materials used as an insecticide. Nicotine acts mainly as a contact poison and a fumigant, but it is also a stomach poison. It is used chiefly to control plant lice; however, solutions of *nicotine sulfate* are effective in killing sheep lice, ticks, and scabies mites.

Pyrethrum has long been used as an insecticide. It paralyzes insects rapidly and its low toxicity to higher animals makes it a valuable ingredient in household sprays. Most insects are killed by sprays containing as little as 0.002 percent pyrethrum; even sublethal doses paralyze insects for a time. Household sprays containing pyrethrum mixed with DDT or chlordane, or both, are more effective than sprays containing any of these insecticides alone. They will kill most insect pests, including houseflies, mosquitoes, cockroaches, and ants.

Sulfur may be dusted on clothing, particularly cuffs of trousers and socks, to repel chiggers. Liberal dusting of lawns with sulfur will keep them free of chiggers.

Rotenone is an insecticide which is isolated from the roots of certain leguminous tropical plants. It acts chiefly as a contact poison, but it is also a stomach poison. Since it is relatively harmless to higher animals, it can be used to

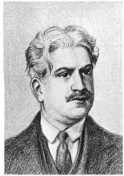

CRUZ, Osvaldo G. (1872-1917) Brazilian bacteriologist and hygienist. Cruz reformed the Brazilian public health service which had not been able to cope with the startling spread of disease, especially yellow fever, in his country. It was he who was largely responsible for freeing the capital city, Rio de Janeiro, from the grip of yellow fever. *American trypanosomiasis,* an infection in man caused by a parasite, is called *Cruz's disease.*

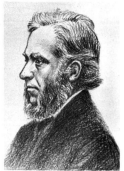

BUDD, William (1811-1880) English physician. Most famous for an important book on typhoid fever in which he insisted that the disease is carried within the contaminated waste discharged by infected individuals. In this same book Budd concluded that typhoid fever is spread by the consumption of water which is polluted by sewer seepage through soil and leaks in defective plumbing.

control parasites of domestic animals. Dust containing one percent rotenone is effective in killing lice and fleas; ticks can be killed with dust containing two to three percent rotenone. Since rotenone kills slowly, it is often mixed with quicker-acting pyrethrum.

Unlike the insecticides mentioned above, DDT and chlordane do not occur in nature, but are compounds which must be synthesized. DDT affects the nervous system of the insect, causing convulsions, paralysis, and death. It acts more slowly than most other insecticides; in some instances it does not cause death for three or four days. When applied inside the house, DDT may retain its ability to kill for as long as a year if not covered with grease and dust. This marked residual effect is one of the important factors contributing to its efficiency as an insecticide. It is slightly toxic to higher animals, but the possibility of acute poisoning of human beings is rather remote when used with caution and as directed. However, prolonged exposure to sprays containing DDT should be avoided, particularly oil-base sprays of DDT.

Two to ten percent dust of DDT may be used in the home to control cockroaches, ants, and lice. Aerosol "bombs" (a spray under pressure), which have come into common use, usually contain about three percent DDT in combination with chlordane and pyrethrum. These aerosols are effective against mosquitoes, stable and houseflies, bedbugs, and many other household pests. DDT dust and sprays are used to kill mosquito larvae.

Many organic phosphorous compounds were synthesized during World War II in research directed toward nerve gases and other chemical warfare agents. Continued research has led to the development of less toxic organophosphorus compounds such as malathion, diazinon, and ronnel which are widely used insecticides. All of them work as cholinesterase inhibitors and must be used with care; however, malathion is less toxic than DDT—and is one of the safest broad-spectrum insecticides in use. Malathion is effective against a wide range of mite and insect pests and is rapidly replacing DDT and other chlorinated hydrocarbons in household sprays.

Fumigants

Most fumigants are sold as solids or liquids which become gaseous when burned or heated. In general, fumigants must be applied with special equipment and by specially trained people. Most fumigants are toxic to higher animals as well as to insects. Some are explosive, and others are inflammable. Aerosols which disperse insecticides as fine mists capable of penetrating cracks and crevices are similar to fumigants in their effectiveness and can give satisfactory results.

Fumigants are sometimes used to kill microorganisms as well as insects; however, most materials which are used as insecticides have little value as germicides. When sulfur is burned, it produces a gas, *sulfur dioxide,* which is effective as an insecticide and to a limited extent as a germicide. It has largely been replaced both as an insecticide and as a germicide by more efficient materials. Aerosols containing germicidal compounds, finely dispersed, have been used to control air-borne disease-producing organisms. Hydrogen cyanide gas is widely used as a fumigant, but is quite dangerous, especially if used by untrained personnel. Methylbromide is also in use.

Germicides, disinfectants, and antiseptics

A *germicide* is by definition an agent which kills microorganisms. A *disinfectant* is an agent which kills or destroys organisms capable of causing infection. Both terms are partially synonymous with *bactericide* (bacteria killer). An antiseptic agent acts predominantly as an inhibitor of bacterial growth. Preparations which are in contact with body tissues for only a short time, such as gargles and douches, if they destroy bacteria in the dilutions recommended in a short period of time, really have germicidal as well as antiseptic properties.

Organic compounds of mercury (including *metaphen, mercresin,* and *merthiolate*) have been found to be better germicides than *iodine*. However, they have now been replaced in large part by *hexachlorophene,* cationic detergents, and the various antibiotics. Chloramine and other organic compounds containing chlorine and ammonium are used extensively, especially by sanitation crews. Solutions of bichloride of mercury are useful as general disinfectants; they are irritating to the skin if left in contact with it for long periods of time. All mercury compounds are poisonous and should not be taken internally. The soapless detergents, such as the sulfonated vegetable oils, are probably even better as skin disinfectants than most germicides.

Although they have been largely replaced by antibiotic preparations, compounds containing silver are used as disinfectants on *mucous membranes,* especially for the prevention of gonorrheal infection in the eyes of newborn babies. *Argyrol, protargol,* and *argonin* are commonly used silver compounds.

Phenol and *creosols* are coal tar products which are occasionally used as germicides. Five percent solutions of phenol are used for disinfecting a variety of materials. Creosols are usually emulsified with green soap and sold under the trade names of *Lysol* and *Creolin.* Creolin is about ten times more efficient as a germicide than phenol; and Lysol is about four times more efficient. Both are good general household disinfectants when used according to directions.

Soaps and *alcohols* are used to some extent as germicides. Both are only mildly germicidal, however. Alcohols are more effective when mixed with water; wood, grain, and isopropyl alcohols are usually used at approximately 70 percent strength. Soaps and alcohols also act through the removal of oily secretions of the skin in which the microorganisms collect.

Physical agents such as heat and light may also be used as germicides. Boiling of materials to rid them of infectious agents has long been practiced. The ultraviolet light rays are largely responsible for the germicidal action of the sun. Ultraviolet lamps are sometimes installed in schools and factories to check the spread of respiratory infections, such as colds, but the over-all benefits are questionable.

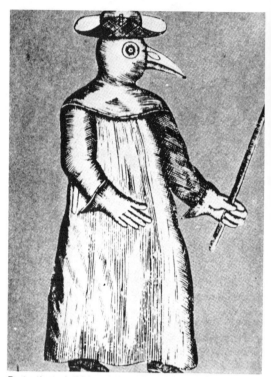

Protective clothing of leather used by 18th century doctors to avoid exposure to disease. *Courtesy of Armed Forces Medical Library, Washington, D.C.*

26 MEDICINE AND THE LAW

THE PHYSICIAN, THE PATIENT, AND THE LAW

When legal decisions affecting the life or property of an individual require expert medical evidence, such cases are termed *medicolegal*. Legal, or forensic, medicine (literally the medicine of the forum) deals with the application of expert medical knowledge and evidence in legal investigations. Medical jurisprudence deals with legislation governing the practice of medicine. Thus, these two sciences protect the health and safety of each individual in the community and assure persons accused of crimes of a fair trial.

The major part of forensic medicine is related to evidence given in courts of law. Since the practice of law is primarily concerned with the social health, and medicine with the preservation of physical and mental health, the two sciences are closely related and interdependent. Because law and medicine contribute to the discovery of truth and the administration of justice in civil and criminal cases, society bestows certain rights and privileges upon both professions, and it also exacts certain duties and responsibilities.

Licensing of the physician

At one time, any person who professed the ability to heal human beings was able to practice his art, and there were few restrictions upon the activities of such persons. Because of the increasing complexity of the medical sciences, society has sought to protect itself from incompetent practitioners. This is accomplished by the licensing of members of the medical and allied professions. This form of legal control is delegated to each state, and the regulations regarding medical practice therefore vary somewhat from one state to another. However, two general statutory requirements are followed by all the states: the general preliminary educational requirements, and the professional preparation. All states have examining and licensing boards. Passing a State Board of Medicine examination results in the issuing of a license to the physician to practice medicine in that particular state. Many states have *reciprocity rules* by which they recognize and license physicians from other states who meet their standards. Similar regulations apply to the licensing of dentists, nurses, technicians, and other members of the medical professions. In addition, examinations are also given by the National Board of Examiners which is made up of selected clinicians and scientists of high professional standing. The National Board was organized in 1915 with the aim primarily of establishing a comprehensive qualifying examination which would be generally acceptable to the legal agencies of the states. The Board itself has no direct legal status, except that its exam findings have been acceptable to the states. Virtually all states and territories of the United States accept the Board's examination results in lieu of their own.

A new medical licensure examination, called FLEX, was developed by the Federation of State Medical Boards and offered in June 1968, for the first time. Its purpose is to provide a uniform and valid examination to evaluate clinical competence and qualification for licensure. Under FLEX, one standard has been determined for reporting examination scores so that all candidates' grades will be comparable from state to state. The individual state, however, may still decide its own passing level on these standard scores. It is expected that within a few years all medical boards will adopt FLEX as their own qualifying examination. The states also license hospitals, medical laboratories, and other professional organizations associated with the practice of medicine.

Although medical practice is regulated by laws administered through the states, the medical profession itself exacts still further requirements of its members. Physicians recognize the complexity of their profession and the limitations of the ability of any one individual. For this reason the American Medical Association and its many constituent local medical societies, and the American Dental Association and its local groups set further standards of ethics and proficiency. A serious breach of the standards of professional conduct can result in the revocation of the license granted by the state and suspension of the physician from the association. The profession sets certain specific requirements for recognition of its members as specialists. Physicians who pass the exacting requirements and examinations of the *specialty boards* are qualified to establish themselves as specialists in certain branches of medicine. It is thus apparent that the qualifications of modern medical practice are regulated by members of the profession itself much more rigorously than by the state. The many criteria required by the medical profession thus provide the patient with a basis for confidence in his selection of a physician.

The physician as a witness

Under the Hippocratic Oath, physicians regard communications from patients as secret, or privileged. It is for this reason that physicians do not discuss a medical case with any person who is not directly concerned with it. This right of secret or privileged communication applies only to the information voluntarily given by the patient to the physician, and not to facts that the physician may observe for himself. English courts do not recognize privileged communication of patients, but in the United States, communications are made privileged by statutes in sixteen states. Under these laws the patient's consent is necessary for a disclosure of personal confidence. Seventeen other states have laws by which the patient waives privilege if he or his physician is presented as a witness.

When a physician is called as a witness in court to relate facts and events which he knows and has observed, he is governed by the rules applying to any other witness. As an ordinary witness, he is subject to subpoena as an ordinary citizen.

Under most circumstances, testimony in court is limited to *facts* of which the witness has personal knowledge; and other testimony gained indirectly, known as *hearsay* evidence, is inadmissible. Because of his specialized knowledge, however, the physician may testify as an *expert witness*, even in cases where he did not take part in the treatment of the patient. Persons other than members of the medical profession may also qualify as expert witnesses when their knowledge or skill is great enough to merit confidence in their specialized field. When the physician gives testimony to explain or interpret facts by reason of his knowledge, he becomes an expert witness. It is optional with the physician whether he acts as an expert witness. The adversary principle is the foundation of our jury system, and the physician, like any other expert witness, may be retained by either the defense or the prosecution. He also may be utilized by either in a civil action. Thus, at the present time, the laws provide employment of the physician by a particular litigant, and this involves the possibility of bias. Although there is definite basis for intelligent differences of medical opinion, the laws of the various states lag behind the progress of contemporary medicine since they require the expert medical witness to testify for one litigant or the other. Since physiological and biological phenomena are variable, varying in living material as much as several thousand percent, scientific testimony should be nonpartisan. Ordinarily, most expert witnesses, especially physicists, chemists, and mathematicians, work with great precision and a much lower order of variability, and thereby avoid criticism and challenge of opinion.

The physician-patient relationship

The physician who accepts a patient for treatment will normally follow the case until medical attention is no longer needed. He may refer the patient to a specialist during the course of treatment, or he may refuse to accept the patient because he feels the problems of the case are beyond his abilities to handle.

For these reasons, the law does not compel him to give treatment to any patient, regardless of the emergency nature of the situation. Obviously, the physician will administer first aid when the patient's life is endangered. Once a doctor undertakes to treat a patient, however, it is assumed that he will be compensated for his work, and that he will continue to care for the patient. By the acceptance of a patient for treatment, the physician therefore creates a legal *contract*. Either patient or physician may terminate the contract.

The *law of contracts* is therefore of great importance, because it provides the legal basis for mutual obligation. It assures the patient of the physician's attendance or referral to another physician. It further assures the patient that he will receive a standard of treatment equivalent to that available from any other physician of similar professional skill. The contract also implies responsibility of the patient to follow the physician's orders. Otherwise, the patient invalidates the contract. Failure to follow the physician's orders not only endangers the patient's health, but may forfeit the responsibility of the physician.

Legal permissions

By engaging the services of a physician, the patient authorizes the physician to carry out any reasonable treatment. A physician discovering an unconscious person who is obviously in need of medical attention may assume implied permission for treatment. Surgical treatment of patients, however, except in certain circumstances, requires specific personal permission, usually in writing. When a patient is unable to make a decision, his nearest of kin may give the necessary permission. Ordinarily, a minor cannot legally give such authorization, so that his parent or guardian must act for him. For surgery that involves both a husband and wife, the surgeon may desire the permission of both, particularly in operations affecting reproductive capacities. The acquisition of such permission is another important protection that medicine offers the patient, for it insures that some responsible person will be aware of the measures that the surgeon feels are necessary for the patient's safety. Failure to obtain proper care, whether through ignorance or neglect, can make the responsible relative subject to legal prosecution. When a patient requests medical attention that seems advisable to the physician, he may accept such permission even over the objection of relatives, since each individual has the right to act in his own behalf. In the case of hazardous diagnostic or therapeutic procedures, it may be debatable how much the patient should be told to constitute "informed consent." Similarly, it may be difficult for the physician to determine how much the patient should be told of his diagnosis when he is suffering from a lethal condition. In such cases the desires of the next of kin, who should be fully informed of the situation, should be followed.

Permission for autopsy

An autopsy or postmortem examination cannot be performed without written permission from the nearest of kin. In many states, if the surviving relatives are of equal kinship, permission must be secured from all of them. The only exceptions are mediocolegal cases in which autopsy is ordered by the coroner or medical ex-

aminer. In such instances, the family has no choice in preventing the examination. In cases of death from unknown causes, murder, or suicide, the medical examiner is authorized to order a postmortem examination. This legal authority operates to the advantage of the whole community, not only in the administration of justice but in protection of health. By medicolegal autopsies, plagues are prevented, infectious and contagious diseases or other dangerous conditions (as in workman's compensation cases) are accurately diagnosed, and proper control measures are instituted to protect the remaining populace.

Since autopsy permission must of necessity be secured at a time of extreme emotional upset, an understanding of what an autopsy is, its significance, and its value should be a part of everyone's knowledge. The importance of autopsies to the advance of medical science cannot be overestimated, since the beginning of modern medicine is marked by the allowance of the postmortem examination. In the period preceding the Renaissance, various superstitions and taboos had prevented the examination of bodies after death. This restriction resulted in many erroneous ideas concerning both anatomy and disease which were held by the medical profession for centuries. As late as the fifth century dissection was still forbidden, and medieval teaching was entirely from the works of Hippocrates and Galen. The first public dissection of a human body was not allowed until 1315, and this denotes the starting point of the science of anatomy. Still, dissection continued in disrepute until the sixteenth century, during which Vesalius published his great work on anatomy. Even then, Vesalius worked under a serious handicap, being forced to pillage the scaffolds to obtain cadavers. When the ban on examination of bodies was lifted, medical knowledge increased rapidly. Because of freedom to perform autopsies, the Viennese school of medicine was able to found the science of pathology. During the nineteenth century the famous Viennese pathologist, Karl von Rokitansky, performed more than 30,000 autopsies and prepared the way for clinical

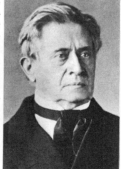

NÉLATON, Auguste (1807-1873) French surgeon. Nélaton devised a probe for locating bullets in the body of a wounded person. Noted for his many contributions to the treatment of patients with muscular and skeletal injuries and defects. Surgical operations that he devised for repair of calcified wrist, elbow or hip joints, and for excision of a shoulder are called *Nélaton's operations,* in his honor.

knowledge to become established on the basis of pathological anatomy. Rokitansky developed a method of performing autopsies that is still used in modified form today.

Often death occurs when the physician is at a loss to know the exact cause. Autopsy often will clear this problem and may save a life in some future situation of the same kind. When an autopsy is performed, the findings are correlated with the history of the illness as closely as possible. The treatment the patient received is carefully examined and the various tests given the patient can be evaluated. As a result, the course of the patient's disease becomes clear and the effectiveness of the various procedures can be determined. This results in an improved course of treatment for patients.

An autopsy is similar to a surgical operation and is performed in the same professional way. Only medical personnel are admitted to the autopsy room. Usually the autopsy surgeon or pathologist, his assistants, interns, resident physicians, and the patient's attending physician are allowed. An autopsy is performed with a minimum of disturbance of the body. Incisions are made in such a way that there will be no visible evidence of the operation when memorial services are held. Furthermore, a properly performed autopsy in no way prevents the satisfactory preparation of the body for burial.

Most hospitals maintain a staff pathologist, and the cost of autopsy is absorbed by the hospital. When a patient expires outside a hospital, a small fee may be charged by the pathologist for the postmortem examination. When the patient dies outside of a hospital, but under the care of a physician, and the circumstances of death are such that there is no jurisdiction for the coroner or medical examiner, the pathologist is entitled to a reasonable fee for the postmortem examination. A complete autopsy requires about three hours of the pathologist's time in the autopsy room. After this, a technician must spend hours preparing tissues for examination. Then the pathologist spends more time examining the tissue slides under the microscope. Finally, a report is prepared and becomes a permanent record for the physician and the hospital.

The autopsy procedure is valuable for both the physician and the surviving relatives. One of the greatest benefits derived from an autopsy is the knowledge gained concerning the nature of the disease and its relation to the survivors. Relatives will benefit by a knowledge of the disease as to its familial or congenital characteristics. In many instances, such knowledge may prevent early deaths in some of the surviving relatives, if proper treatment based on facts learned from autopsy can be given. An example of this is the case of death of a newborn infant. There may be some question of the advisability of future pregnancy if there is something

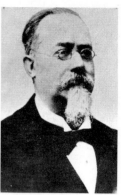

LOMBROSO, Cesare (1836-1909) Italian physician and criminologist. Noted for his extensive writings in which he advanced the theory that criminals constitute a definite physical and mental type of human being. Although this concept is no longer held valid, it was important because it stimulated thought regarding physical and mental influences in crime, a field still only poorly understood. Copyright CIBA SYMPOSIA.

"wrong" with the mother or the father which prevents normal birth. In many cases autopsy can determine the actual cause of death. If it is related to some condition of the parents, or if it is a matter of incompatibility of blood types, it is quite possible that autopsy not only will reveal the cause of stillbirth or early death but will also suggest the proper means for permitting a normal pregnancy or delivery at a later time.

Progress in diagnosis and treatment is largely dependent upon knowledge gained in the autopsy room. In spite of the most skillful antemortem examination of tissues, often the diagnosis in some cases remains unknown. The autopsy is the best approach for gaining a further knowledge of this unknown. Few religions have restrictions to autopsy, and the withholding of permission for autopsy from ignorance or superstition often denies the physician, the relatives, and future patients the benefit of further progress in medical care, early diagnosis, and treatment of disease.

MEDICOLEGAL ASPECTS OF IDENTIFICATION

Frequently a medicolegal autopsy is required to identify a corpse that is not recognizable. Autopsy is a valuable method of identification in noncriminal as well as homicidal deaths. Over 100 persons were burned beyond recognition during the Cocoanut Grove fire in Boston in 1942. Some of the bodies were identified by means of jewelry, shreds of clothing, and dental repairs. However, many could not be identified by external characteristics. All but one of the bodies were eventually identified by information obtained at autopsy. The discovery of various internal signs of disease, of pregnancy, or of past surgical treatment or dentistry or of old injuries or abnormalities made it possible for relatives to claim the bodies.

Identification is important when the body of an unrecognizable murdered person is found. Often the identity of the victim must be established before the criminal can be sought. Autopsy can disclose many facts that help in identification of decomposed, burned, and mutilated bodies. In some questions of identity, the pathologist may be able to determine the age, sex, and race from skeletal remains. Examination for signs of malnutrition, unusual habits, or physical peculiarities may be of value in determining identity.

Another problem of medicolegal autopsy is that of determining the approximate time of death. The time of death may be particularly important in deaths from unknown causes and deaths from violence. There are many means by which the pathologist can estimate the time of death; for example, by presence or absence of undigested or digested food and food residues and their location in the gastrointestinal tract, by chemical composition of the blood, and by determination of the presence or absence of *rigor mortis* (rigidity of the muscles after death). Rigor mortis usually begins within about five to six hours in healthy adult persons and usually disappears within 36 hours. In very young and aged individuals, rigor mortis appears fairly rapidly and lasts a short time. Another means of estimating the time of death is by temperature. It has been found that the body loses about 2.5° F. in temperature each hour for the first six hours after death. Thereafter from 1.5° to 2° may be lost each hour until the body temperature becomes the same as that of the surrounding air, or in case of drowning, the water in which it is immersed. This means may be useless when the body has been exposed to extremes of temperature, although even in these cases, at least some approximation may be ascertained.

Another widely recognized means of estimating the time of death, particularly after a period of weeks, is the chemical analysis of the body for *adipocere*. Adipocere is the word given to the form which the fat of the body assumes during decomposition. Chemically it involves a process whereby the soft and sometimes liquid fats of the body become hardened. In a temperate climate, it may require four to five months for this change to take place. In colder climates, the process may require longer periods.

There are many other ways of estimating the time of death, some based on knowledge of the changes taking place within the body after death, and some based on the particular circumstances surrounding any given death. If the examining physician discovers parasites on the body, he may call upon the *entomologist* (specialist in insects). Many body parasites die soon after the death of their host. Thus, their presence may help in determining the time of death.

Personal identification through blood tests

One of the most frequent problems in medical criminology is the determination of whether a substance or stain is blood. If the stain is found to be human blood, an attempt is made to determine its group.

When a stain is suspected of being blood, the *benzidine test,* or a similar test, is generally employed. A portion of the material containing the stain is placed in a mild salt solution to permit the bloodstain to dissolve. If the suspected blood is found on a hard surface, the stain may be scraped off and placed in a salt solution or the scrapings may be used directly for the test. When a proper solution is obtained, a drop or so of a solution of the benzidine reagent is added. If the stain is caused by blood, the solution will turn a deep green or blue color. In this test, as with all chemical tests of legal importance, the investigator maintains careful controls in order to avoid experimental errors. For instance, an unstained portion of the cloth or other material must be treated in the same manner to make certain that the material itself will not in some way form the blue or green color with the benzidine reagent. This test is so sensitive that it is usually necessary to dissolve the materials in glass laboratory vessels which have never before contained blood in any form or which have been thoroughly cleaned, as the slightest trace of blood may produce a positive benzidine reaction. These same precautions are also observed in any subsequent testing of the blood.

The benzidine test, although it is quite specific for blood when performed with the proper controls, will nevertheless give no indication of the source of that blood. Thus, not only human blood, but that of most other animals, such as dogs, chickens, cows, rabbits, mice, and the like, will also form the blue coloration characteristic of a positive reaction. Therefore, even if a stain is ascertained to be blood by the benzidine test, other tests are required to determine the source of the blood.

The *precipitin test* is used to determine the animal source of blood. This test is based on the same serological principles as those used in explaining such phenomena as the natural immunity to a disease. The principle, simply stated, is that if substances, particularly protein materials, are introduced into the blood stream of an animal which normally does not have that substance in his blood, he may develop *specific* antibodies apparently designed by his body to combine with and neutralize the foreign substance. The *specificity* of these combating substances or antibodies which are produced by the animal's body is important in the precipitin test.

Laboratory animals, usually rabbits, are used to supply the specific substances for the precipitin test for blood. Pharmaceutical houses prepare large quantities of the specific substances.

Even though a bloodstain may have been found to be human blood, as shown by precipitin tests, it is often necessary to determine more exactly the source of the blood. The individual accused of murder may, for instance, claim that his clothes are stained by his own blood, shed after a minor accident, and he may have a recent wound to support his claim. It is often possible, through proper tests, to disprove an alleged source of human blood, saliva, semen, sweat, or other excretions. It is not possible, however, to prove that a bloodstain or excretion came from one particular individual. The method for *disproving* the source of human blood is similar in principle to that for *disproving* parentage.

To disprove the source of human blood, and to settle disputes of parentage, it is necessary to determine the blood group. Details of this procedure are explained in Chapter 6, "Blood and Blood-Forming Organs." Not only may the blood groups which are important in blood transfusions be used in solving problems of this sort, but also other types, such as the MN, which are known to be hereditary.

Determination of the blood group of a stain is made directly from the stained material. If, for example, the suspect in a murder case has human blood of a known group on his hands, the defendant's claim of innocence may be upheld if the victim had blood of another group. Blood groups can be determined even days after the victim's death. If, however, the suspect's hands were found to bear stains of blood of the same group as that of the victim, very little has been proved, since not only the victim, but many other people, possibly including the suspect himself, may have that same blood group. If initial blood grouping (ABO) of a bloodstain fails to vindicate a suspect, the investigator may use the Rh and MN groups, in his efforts to prove the suspect innocent. The expert is limited here by being able to determine only the M factor of the MN group unless the bloodstain is very fresh. In fact, neither the Rh nor MN tests can be done reliably on dried bloodstains, especially if the stains are small and on contaminated materials. There are likewise several other known blood factors which can be determined, and there are probably others yet undiscovered. It is important to remember, however, that agreement of group between two specimens of blood does not prove that the two bloods came from the same individual. If it can be shown that the MN and Rh types agree, as well as the ABO type, the *probability* of the same source may be as much as doubled. Nevertheless it is never proved, since there can always be found a number of people with the same blood groups regardless of the variety of blood groups that are considered.

In the majority of cases, the blood group can be used only in offering negative identification. This means of identification is nevertheless valuable in many instances where other means of identification, discussed in the following pages, cannot be used. For instance, an individual may plot to defraud or escape punishment by "pretending" death. If he attempts to do so by arranging for a dead person to be found in his place, the deceit can often be discovered by determining the victim's blood group. Law enforcement agencies can call upon the armed forces, physicians, and hospitals who may have a record of the blood group. Since one's blood group never changes, blood group information retains its value, even though the determinations may have been made years previously.

Disputed parentage

In cases of disputed parentage, it is necessary to know the blood groups and types of the parents or parents-in-question and the child. Blood grouping offers a means of disproof of parentage but can never prove parentage. Suits often involve claims of a mother seeking support of a child by an alleged father. They also arise from husbands' claiming not to have fathered their wives' children. In other cases, the same procedures of blood grouping are carried out when it is suspected that infants, usually in a hospital nursery, have been accidentally exchanged. Any parents who suspect such an exchange may, through their physician, have the blood grouping performed. It should be pointed out that courts will not recognize positive proof in the form of probability of parentage in any of these cases. Many courts will, however, accept negative evidence from blood groupings as proof of a lack of parentage.

In order to understand the evidence given in cases of disputed parentage, it is necessary to consider certain basic concepts of heredity. It has been established that for the ABO blood group, there are three principal genes which may be effective. The gene producing the A blood group causes, among other things, a certain substance to be present on the exterior of the red cells of the blood; this substance is called agglutinogen A. The presence of agglutinogen A on the blood cells is detected with anti-A serum which causes such cells to clump together. The gene producing the B blood group acts in a similar way, but the substance agglutinogen B created on the red cell is slightly different chemically because of the somewhat different action of the gene. The gene producing the O group produces still another substance which is called O, because neither anti-A nor anti-B reacts with it.

The two genes producing A and B blood groups are approximately equal in their ability to act. This means that neither can overshadow the other, so that a person inheriting both genes A and B, one from each parent, is of the AB blood group. Conversely, the O gene is overshadowed by both genes A and B, so that to be group O, the individual cannot have inherited either A or B genes from his parents. It follows further from this, that a person found to be of group A or B may possess a hidden gene for O; or he may have two A or two B genes. By knowing the individual's blood group, it is therefore possible to know, or to estimate, which genes he possesses and, as a consequence, which he is able to pass on to his children. As an example, a man with blood group A can always pass a gene for substance A to his children, and also he may be able to pass on an O gene. However, he can never bestow a type B gene on his children, so that a child with group B or AB blood could not possibly be his *unless* the child's mother has group B or AB blood to pass gene B on to the child.

Although it might seem that many other inherited characteristics could provide a basis for disproving parentage, in actual practice, the blood tests are the most reliable; this includes, in addition to the ABO groups, the MN types and the Rh-Hr types, and at times also other types. The explanation for this lies in the fact that human genetics cannot be subjected to the careful scrutiny of science as can the genetics of lower animals with controlled breeding. As a result, human inheritance, which in many cases appears much more complicated than that of lower animals, is not nearly so well understood. Many other characteristics besides blood groups involve a number of sets of genes, or are easily influenced by their environment so that conclusions regarding their inheritance are usually subject to that "shadow of a doubt" which the law upholds as being all-important. *"Nemo dat, quod nemo habet"*—"One cannot give what he does not have."

Fingerprints

Fingerprints have for centuries been widely used as the basis for personal identification. Our earliest records of fingerprinting come from the Orient of ancient times. At a somewhat later date in Europe, the practice of sealing envelopes with wax upon which the sender left an imprint of his thumb was used to prevent forgeries. In modern times the fingerprint is often used in legal documents when the signee is illiterate.

Through careful research and tabulations it has been proved that in all probability each individual's fingerprints are different from those of any one else who has ever lived or ever will. Even in the case of identical twins, the fingerprints are not identical, though they may be as similar as the fingerprints from the right and

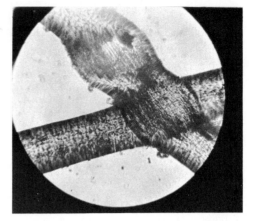

This photomicrograph of two human hairs shows the appearance of one crushed by a blow. *Courtesy of City of Houston Police Department, Houston.*

left hands of the same individual. This similarity of fingerprints and palm prints is indeed used to distinguish identical from fraternal twins in multiple births. Even in these cases, the differences may be such that an absolute determination of whether twins are identical is not always possible by this means alone.

Fingerprints and toeprints (the fine lines seen on the inner surfaces of the fingers and palms, toes and soles) are the outward manifestations of the interweaving of two layers of the epidermis. The projections exist elsewhere in the skin but only on the hands and feet are they so distinct. (For further details regarding the anatomy of fingerprints, see Chapter 8, "The Skin.")

Since the advent of the use of fingerprints for identification, notably of criminals, there have been developed several systems of classification. Four general patterns of fingerprints, however, are widely recognized. The *arched* fingerprint is composed of ridges running the width of the print, usually with more or less of an arch rising toward the tip. The *loop* type of print is characterized by the fact that some of the ridges turn without spiraling, to return to the same side of the finger from which they came. The *whorl* is seen as a print in which some of the ridges make a spiral or complete circle. The fourth and less definite type is termed the *composite* print and is defined as a print involving two or more of the other types or being too complicated to classify.

Pioneering work in the use of fingerprints in identification began during the mid-nineteenth century in India, through the efforts of Sir Edward Richard Henry, who developed the Henry system of fingerprint classification, and of Sir William James Herschel, son and grandson of the famous astronomers. These men, working independently in the Indian civil service, explored the method as a means of settling disputes in criminal cases. Sir Francis Galton, the famous English scientist and father of eugenics, made similar studies at about the same time. Through modern classification schemes, it is now possible for trained personnel to identify a given set of fingerprints in a matter of a few minutes—provided, of course, that the individual under examination had been previously fingerprinted.

Fingerprints are admissible as evidence in court subject to the usual rules of evidence. They are also of great value in identifying individuals who have a criminal record, but who are traveling under aliases or disguises. The armed forces recognize this form of identification as invaluable and attach no criminal connotations to it. Furthermore, many institutions and business organizations insist upon fingerprinting of personnel for various reasons implying no discredit to the individual. There are indeed many individuals and organizations who seek to promote universal fingerprinting to give positive means of identification to everyone. Such widespread fingerprinting would facilitate the work of identifying victims of accidents, amnesia, and other illnesses, and in times of regional crises, such as floods, wars, and earthquakes. The central collecting bureau for fingerprints in the United States is the Federal Bureau of Investigation in Washington.

The Bertillon system

The Bertillon system of personal identification is limited largely to use in criminology. It is based on physical measurements and was invented in 1886 by the French criminologist, Dr. Alphonse Bertillon. It is widely used today in combination with fingerprinting to identify criminals.

The system is designed to measure those characteristics which ordinarily do not change over the years, though many persons have been known to undergo various surgical procedures in order to escape their classifications in the Bertillon files. From the medical standpoint, the system is limited to men by virtue of the fact that these physical characteristics may change through the years in women. The measurements taken are those which are known to be relatively permanent after the age of 20. The principal measurement is that of head length. Each individual is classified according to small, medium, or long. Three similar divisions are made on the basis of length of middle finger, forearm, little finger, and height. The final subdivisions are made according to eye color and length of ear. Each individual's card, besides bearing these data, also presents photographs, full face and profile. Sitting height, extent of arms, length of forearm, and other measurements are also included. In addition, color of hair and location and descriptions of moles and birthmarks are also noted. By the use of such evidence, trained medical personnel are frequently able to identify bodies after the fingerprints have been destroyed.

Identification of hair

The medicolegal examination of hair has only limited value in personal identifications. This stems from the fact that not only does the appearance of individual hairs change throughout life, but also different hairs from the same individual may be very different, depending upon their location on the body. In spite of these limitations, evidence concerning hair is admissible in court records and is useful because it can serve as an important clue in various types of criminal investigation and in identification of unidentified persons.

When hair specimens are found at the scene of any crime, the police will often collect these for laboratory examination. Valuable clues can most often be found in crimes in which death was brought about through hand-to-hand combat, strangulation, or stabbing, in which cases the victim may have had opportunity to grasp his assailant's hair. In rape cases, it is also widely practiced to examine the victim's underclothing for pubic hairs of the assailant. The victim's hairs may also prove to be valuable evidence, for example, when found on the suspect's person or on the bumper of an automobile involved in a hit-and-run accident. Thus hairs may be used either in discovering the criminal's identity or in offering proof of his presence at the scene of the crime.

The study of hairs of a victim of violent crime can also yield important details of the crime. Under the microscope, hair which has been forcefully pulled out can be distinguished from hair which has fallen out as a natural course, by determination of the amount of follicular material adhering to the root of the hair. Hair which has been damaged, as by a blow, will have a "bruised" appearance microscopically, which the medical expert can identify. Torn hair can also be differentiated from cut hair. By examining the appearance of a single hair near a gunshot wound, it is sometimes possible to make a good estimate of the distance from which the shot was fired, since the appearance of a hair will change progressively with the amount of heat applied to it. Because hair is capable of yielding so much information, it can be seen that a study of the victim's hair may be of help in solving a crime.

Examination of hairs suspected of belonging to a criminal can yield clues concerning his identity. First of all, of course, hairs found near the scene of a crime must be definitely established as being human hair rather than hair from an animal or some other fiber which resembles hair to the naked eye. An expert can easily eliminate such a question by microscopic examination. Once a fiber is established by microscopic examination as being human hair, it is desirable to determine from what part of the body the hair came. Scalp hair, of course, is the longest, and the ends may show evidence of having been cut. Scalp hairs are more likely to be dyed or bleached than other kinds of hair. Eyebrows and eyelashes can be recognized by their thickness in comparison with their length. The ends of these hairs usually show no evidence of having been cut, but have smooth rounded tips.

When it is necessary to identify an individual with only a specimen of his hair as evidence, it is often possible to gain at least a general idea of his age. Children have very fine hair. In the course of time, however, hairs will fall out naturally, and the replacement hair is usually somewhat thicker. At best, of course, this means of age estimation is only approximate. When the person in question is of Negroid, Chinese, or Asiatic extraction, this can sometimes be detected through specimens of his hair, by its thickness and dark color. The hair of the Negro, further, is usually very curly, and the shaft of the hair may be quite flattened. The study of the pigmentation of a hair can often determine whether the individual has blond, dark, or red hair.

In addition, studies are now being conducted which deal with neutron activation of trace metals in the hair for purposes of identification. These studies attempt to characterize an individual's identity through the trace-metal profile of his hair—that is, the chemical, molecular, and anatomical configuration of the hair. It is believed that within a few years, this neutron activation procedure will be akin to present fingerprinting as a means of identification.

Other means of identification

There are many means for identifying individuals other than their fingerprints, blood groups, and hair. Chief among these other means is the study of the teeth. In cases of death from

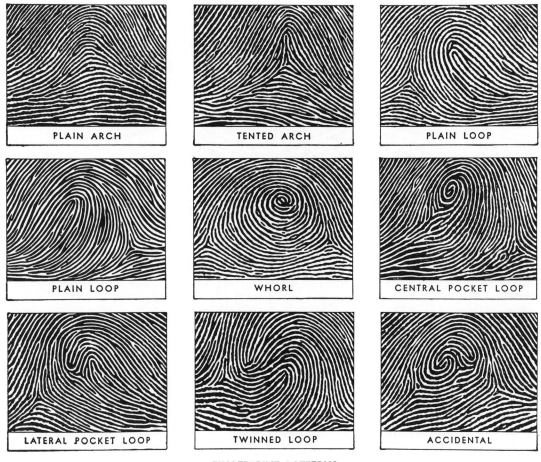

FINGERPRINT PATTERNS

Courtesy Faurot, Inc., N.Y. and City of Houston Police Department, Houston.

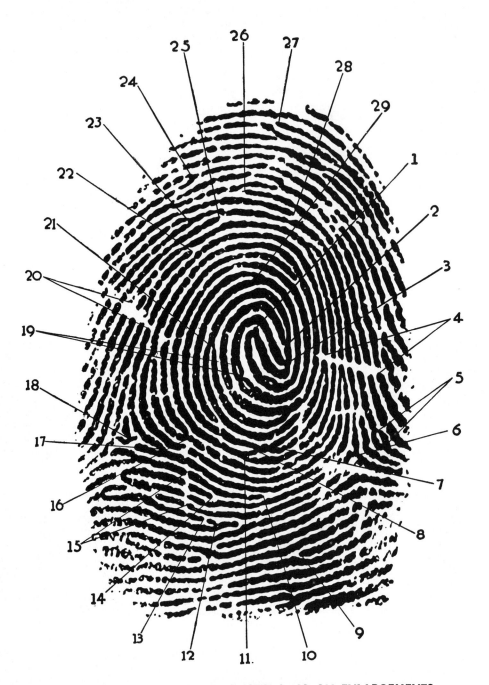

EXPLANATION OF CHARACTERISTICS ON ENLARGEMENTS

1 THE CORE	11 BIFURCATION	21 BIFURCATION
2 BIFURCATION	12 BIFURCATION	22 ABRUPT ENDING
3 BIFURCATION	13 ABRUPT ENDING	23 BIFURCATION
4 CICATRIX	14 ABRUPT ENDING	24 BIFURCATION
5 ENCLOSURE	15 CICATRIX	25 ABRUPT ENDING
6 RIGHT DELTA	16 BIFURCATION	26 ABRUPT ENDING
7 BIFURCATION	17 BIFURCATION	27 ABRUPT ENDING
8 BIFURCATION	18 LEFT DELTA	28 ABRUPT ENDING
9 ABRUPT ENDING	19 ENCLOSURE	29 BIFURCATION
10 ABRUPT ENDING	20 CICATRIX	

fire, the teeth may be the only remaining clue. The dentist, from a record of dental work performed on the individual, may be able to make the identification. If the dentist has ever made x-ray photographs of the individual's mouth, the task of identifying the teeth is greatly expedited. Sometimes the physician is also able to aid in identification of his patient; he can do so by means of the records of all operations and deformities of his patient, along with many of the bodily characteristics.

MEDICOLEGAL ASPECTS OF INJURIES

The practice of legal medicine is concerned mainly with the consideration of the various forms of physical, thermal, and chemical injuries with regard to evidence bearing on the agent of injury, the manner of injury, and the effects of injury. There is also the consideration of the various problems of the medicolegal autopsy, the identification of dead persons, the establishment of the time of death, and the recognition and preservation of biological traces of medicolegal importance. From the standpoint of justice, it is likely to be more important to know whether the decedent was shot from the front or from the side than to learn whether the bullet passed through a vital organ. When death coincides with violence, investigation may reveal a natural cause and thereby place the seemingly accidental death in its true causal relation. In insurance cases decisive proof may be vital.

Wounds and wounding

In cases of violent death, a physician, who may also be the medical examiner, is required to state the exact and primary cause of death. The medical examination of a gunshot wound can reveal clues regarding the crime, including the approximate size of the bullet, the distance from which the gun was fired, the probable time between shooting and death, and the approximate direction from which the gun was fired.

The exact appearance of a bullet wound will vary with the circumstances of the shooting. The wound caused by entrance of a bullet is usually round and clean-cut. In size it is often somewhat smaller than the diameter of the bullet. This is explained by the fact that the initial pressure of the bullet causes an indentation of the skin. The wound caused by exit of the bullet from the body generally is jagged and is somewhat larger than the diameter of the bullet.

The wound from a bullet's entrance will, as a rule, bleed less than the wound of exit which tends to bleed more profusely. Occasionally, a bullet wound will appear to be only a sharp cut

in the skin, so that an examination by a surgeon may be necessary to discover the bullet. In any case, final proof of the shooting, along with the determination of the caliber of the bullet, will usually depend upon recovery of the bullet either surgically from the victim's body, or from the vicinity of the crime.

A rough estimation of the distance from which the gun was fired can often be obtained from the appearance and nature of the wound. When a gun is fired with the muzzle in contact with the skin, the wound is generally larger than the diameter of the bullet and the edges of the wound are jagged and powder burned. When the gun is fired close to the skin, but not touching it, there is usually evidence of smudging and tattooing. The tattoo is caused by particles of metal and powder which are forced into the deeper layers of the skin by the impact of the discharge. Smudging may be wiped off, but the tattoo will remain indefinitely unless corrected by skin surgery. Tattooing occurs when the shot is fired from a distance of 18 inches or less.

When the victim of a fatal shooting is discovered at some distance from the scene of the shooting, obviously he did not die instantly, or he was transported from the scene. Such circumstances may create some confusion for the law enforcement agency in charge. A surgical examination, however, can usually determine whether the patient was actually able to transport himself. As an example, a bullet appearing to have gone through the heart and causing instant death may be found to have entered or been lodged in such a way that the victim might not die immediately. In these cases, an understanding of the circumstances surrounding the death becomes clarified.

It is often claimed that the angle from which a gun was fired can be shown by the angle through which the bullet penetrated the body. This is not always true, since the bullet will be deflected to some extent by the tissues. Bone will cause the greatest deflection.

The physician may be called upon to give his opinion concerning other types of bodily wounds, including knife wounds and wounds from blows with various types of instruments. He is also able to help clarify questions of legal importance by recognizing such things as wounds caused by hypodermic needles and other unusual instruments.

Homicide, suicide, and accidental death

Twenty percent of all deaths in the United States result from violence or occur suddenly from obscure causes. Each year, about 14,500 murders are reported in the United States. This is approximately 7.2 murders for every 100,000 persons living in this country. At the same time, about 10,000 additional murders go unreported every year in the United States. The medicolegal investigation of sudden death has five purposes: protection of the innocent, recognition of murder, recording of accurate medical evidence for civil and criminal courts, protection against public health hazards, and protection against industrial hazards.

In all cases where a violent death has occurred, the question of accident, suicide, or murder must be answered. This is determined by consideration of the cause of death, the nature and extent of injury, and by the circumstances of death. The position of the body, the kind of weapon, blood and its distribution, signs of struggle, motives, farewell letters, and actions of the deceased before death are all factors to be considered. It is often held that the more extensive the wounding, the more likely it is that death is caused by homicide. This is not true concerning wounds about the throat. The actual nature of the wounds may indicate suicide clearly. In the case of death from firearms, the situation of the wound and the direction of the bullet are most important. Often the position of the body may be indicative of the possible cause of death. The following case illustrates typical homicidal circumstances:

The body of a man was found lying in the road. His legs and pelvis were fractured, and one side of his chest was caved in. First investigators thought he had been struck by an automobile. Further examination, however, revealed a scuff mark on the man's shoe which contained gray paint, undoubtedly house paint. Across from the spot where the body was found was a window three stories from the ground, and on a gray ledge beneath the window was a scrape mark and a fiber of cloth identical with that of the man's sock. This, then, was murder. Witnesses were found who testified to having seen the man flung from the window. Experienced investigators knew that the body of a man could be thrown from a window to the far side of a road. A slanting ledge can deflect a body, causing it to roll far from the site of the fall. Also, the same fractures may be present in a victim of a fall that are present in a pedestrian struck by an automobile.

Often medicolegal investigations may save the expense of a lengthy search for a nonexistent murderer. This is illustrated in the case of a man found floating in a river. A rock was tied around his waist, his money was missing, and there was a bullet wound in the chest. The authorities thought it was murder. Doubt arose when the money was found hidden away and friends related the man's depressed mental condition. Examination of the man's clothing by infrared photography revealed a double smoke ring of powder residue about the bullet hole. X-ray examination of the cloth showed metallic fragments at the margins of the bullet hole characteristic of a close or contact shot. Such evidence suggested suicide and prevented a fruitless chase or a bungled trial.

An accidental death can be misleading as to the real cause, as illustrated in the case of the death of a child at a fair. The child suddenly toppled from a ferris wheel and fell to the ground. The examiners looked at her blood-stained hair and diagnosed a skull fracture. Autopsy revealed a bullet wound in the skull. The shooting gallery had a defective backstop and a stray bullet killed the child.

In cases of drowning, the appearances are the same whether the victim fell, jumped, or was thrown into the water. Only the circumstances of the case can decide the question. Suicide by drowning is common, but it is possible to drown a person without leaving any suspicious marks. Death by drowning is diagnosed by froth in the air passages, condition of the lungs, the character of the water in the stomach, and by signs of asphyxia. There is the famous case of Scotland Yard in which a man drowned three women in succession before he was caught. He would marry, take out insurance on his wife's life, and then drown her in the bathtub. The inquest verdict was always accidental drowning in the bathtub.

The high incidence of suicide makes it a strong possibility in sudden death. Often the very points which seem to rule out suicide to the lay mind are those which medicolegal experts recognize as strongly suggestive of self-destruction. More than 21,000 persons commit suicide in the United States each year. It is estimated from past data that 21 males and 7 females out of every 1000 born will eventually take their own lives. Male suicides outnumber females about three to one. However, women attempt suicide more often than men, but are less successful. The most common methods of suicide are by shooting, hanging, poisoning, and asphyxiation by gas. Women generally choose the less disfiguring means of suicide. There are more suicides in urban areas than in rural areas and suicides occur most often in spring and summer. There are many motives for suicide, and they are often obscure. The reasons most often indicated are ill health, economic distress, loss of a loved one, and domestic discord. The final circumstances leading to suicide may not be closely related to the underlying cause, but may point to a long chain of contributory events.

Poisoning

The study of poisons and their action is a major branch of medical science, and is referred to as *toxicology*. Toxicology not only includes studies of the physiological activity of poisons, but also their detection, particularly in biological material, and their antidotes. The toxicologist may be a pharmacologist, a physician, a chemist, or a biologist. His decisions with regard to illnesses and deaths in relationship to poisons are acceptable in court; hence, an injudicious decision could mean false accusations against the innocent as well as liberty for the guilty.

There are a number of situations in which it may be necessary to examine an individual or a body for the presence of poisons. In cases of death by poisoning, it is necessary to determine the exact poison in the body, and the approximate amounts. Such information may aid in deciding whether a crime has been committed. However, when death appears to be from unknown cause, examination for poisons in the body may uncover intentional or accidental poisoning. In cases of chronic poisoning, caused by occupational exposure to various chemicals, a toxicological examination of the body is usually necessary before claims may be made for damages or Workmen's Compensation.

In examining an individual for poisons, the physician or toxicologist will first make careful note of the appearance of the victim. If the mouth shows signs of burning, lysol, lye, or other corrosive poison may be suspected. If the skin has an unusual color, the presence of certain poisons may be suspected; for example, bright cherry red skin and mucous membranes of the victim indicate carbon monoxide poisoning. Furthermore, the position of the body and any unusual signs may indicate poisoning by specific chemicals.

Before chemical tests for poisons are begun, it is usually desirable for the physician or toxicologist to learn the symptoms of the victim. Many poisons produce specific symptoms, some of which may be sufficient for determining the poison used. When possible, this is learned from the victim himself; otherwise, witnesses may be able to describe the symptoms. In the absence of witnesses, an examination of the scene of the poisoning or the death may yield information as to vomiting, convulsions, and other effects.

After death, it is usually necessary to carry out an autopsy for chemical testing of the body for poisons. If the patient survives, tests are performed on various body materials which can be obtained. When the poison was taken by mouth, or thought to have been, the stomach contents are examined thoroughly. Moreover, blood, urine, vomitus, and various other body fluids may be tested. At autopsy, portions of the liver, kidneys, lungs, brain, or other organs may also be tested. This is necessary because poisons, having entered the body, may be found in several types of tissue.

There are many thousands of substances which can poison the human body, many having fatal effects. Besides those chemicals which are usually thought to be poisonous, and indeed may owe their primary importance to their use as animal poisons, almost any chemical taken in sufficient quantity can produce ill effects. Unusually large quantities of beverages or some normally harmless foods can produce symptoms of poisoning. A common cause of fatal poisoning is overuse or overdosage of drugs which may be ordinarily nontoxic, when taken in small amounts.

The poisoning of our land, food, and water as a result of increased industrialization and urbanization has caused lawmakers to give serious attention to ways this contamination can be stopped by legislative action. Conservationists cite areas, like the city of London, where enactment and strict enforcement of antipollution laws have succeeded in nearly eliminating the problem. In the United States, however, laws historically have developed with a strong tendency to protect rights to own and use (or abuse) private property. Thus, much reevaluating and educating must be done if our environment is to have any effective legal protection.

At present, control standards are established by the Environmental Protection Agency and enforced with varying degrees of efficiency by state and regional control boards. Legislation is pending which would provide stricter antipollution laws and require all states to at least meet, and ideally surpass, the federal standards.

Much effort is also being spent to educate the public about the dangers of continued contamination and to eliminate this health hazard.

The formulation of a procedure for the chemical isolation and identification of poison in tissues was proposed about 100 years ago. This procedure, now modified and widely used, permits the detection of most poisons. It consists of a stepwise elimination by groups of known poisons.

Toxicological tests cover five general groups of poison. Volatile poisons, or those which will evaporate upon heating, include such substances

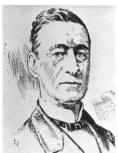

WORMLEY, T. G. (1827–1897) American physician. Author of the first American book on poisons, *The Microchemistry of Poisons,* which was published in 1867. He devised many new and important techniques for the identification of poisons, including the examination of their crystalline structure under the microscope. He served for many years as a professor of toxicology, during which he contributed many advances to this field. *Copyright CIBA SYMPOSIA.*

as alcohols, cyanides, phosphorus, ether, chloral hydrate, chloroform, phenols, acetone, and carbon tetrachloride (cleaning fluid). A second group of poisons includes barbiturates, hallucinogens, tranquilizers, salicylates, caffeins, antipyrine, and some sulfur compounds. The third group includes the various alkaloids, such as cocaine, codeine, morphine, heroin, quinine, and nicotine. The fourth group includes the heavy metals such as bismuth, mercury, arsenic, and lead. If these tests prove negative, other tests are made to detect the presence of the fifth group, the poisonous gases. If these fail, special techniques will be employed until the poison is identified.

Once the poison has been identified by these chemical tests, the actual amount consumed or breathed by the victim is measured, to make certain that a lethal or deadly dose was given and to rule out other possible causes of death.

Medical detection of rape

Examination by the physician permits proof of rape, particularly when the victim is a child or virgin. In these cases, the physician will note hemorrhage and damage to the hymen and vagina.

That rape has occurred can also be shown by laboratory examination for seminal fluid, and in court this is often essential. Swabs of the vagina and stains of the victim's clothing may show evidence of seminal fluid, final proof lying in microscopic recognition of individual spermatozoa.

Seminal fluid on the victim or at the scene of the rape can sometimes be detected by the use of ultraviolet light. Seminal fluid, when dry, shows a greenish fluorescence to ultraviolet or "black" light, although many other materials will also show this same reaction. The suspected seminal fluid is examined microscopically, either by placing a drop of vaginal washings upon a slide, or by mixing the stained material with a mild salt solution and examining the solution. The spermatozoa normally have a large "head" to which is attached a long thin thread-like "tail." When the specimen is old, or has been dried previously, the tail often becomes separated from the head, and the sperm are then more difficult to distinguish as such. When the specimen is very fresh, the spermatozoa may still possess their characteristic motility.

In detection of rape by the finding of spermatozoa, it is essential to have fresh specimens. Spermatozoa have been known to remain within the vagina as long as two days. When the victim is killed, spermatozoa within the vagina lose their motility very rapidly. Semen can be typed according to the ABO blood groups which can disprove but not prove that a suspect committed the crime.

Medicolegal aspects of abortion

The recent liberalization in many states of the laws governing abortions has created confusion and even disagreement among the general population and members of the medical profession as well. Until recently, the only abortions considered legal in the United States were therapeutic abortions. These included cases in which the continuance of a pregnancy was thought to be injurious to the life or health (physical or mental) of a woman; cases of rape or incest; or cases of malformation of the fetus.

The trend now, however, is toward more permissive abortion practices. Fifteen states now have reformed abortion laws—the most liberal being New York's which took effect July 1, 1970. This law permits abortions for any reason, up to the 24th week of pregnancy; it applies to all married or unmarried women 17 years old or older. There are no residency requirements; however, the individual performing the abortion must be a duly licensed physician and the procedure must be done in a hospital. Some insurance companies are revising their policies to pay costs of therapeutic abortions under maternity coverage. This still leaves the unsolved issue of whether to extend coverage to unmarried women, since most maternity benefits are presently covered only under family policies. Although supporters of the more liberal laws point out that they prevent births of millions of unwanted children who will be abandoned or placed in institutions, and that they save countless women from unskilled abortionists who may maim or kill them, there is still much opposition to the laws. Their staunchest opponent is the Roman Catholic Church which bases its opposition on the premise that an abortion destroys a life. There is also strong opposition in the larger cities from the major crime syndicates who often control the illegal abortion operations in the city. Also, many doctors and nurses who have been dedicated to the preservation of life believe the practice of abortion is exactly the opposite; for them, this change in medical practice is not easy to accept.

As more and more states take up the issue of legalized abortion, however, it appears that, in spite of strong opposition, such procedures will eventually become the most common gynecological operation, and that hospitals and medical personnel must be prepared to cope with these changes.

MEDICOLEGAL ASPECTS OF CRIMINOLOGY

It is difficult to make a precise definition of *crime,* since its meaning is constantly changing.

As a general definition, a crime might be said to be any act which fails to conform with the generally accepted social, moral, religious, or ethical customs of the time in any given community. With the advent of civilization, men have recorded definitions of crimes along with prescribed punishments. Obviously, an act which one civilization or group of people considers a crime is not necessarily a crime to all peoples at all times.

Medical studies of criminals

Medical criminology had its beginning around the turn of the twentieth century through the efforts of Cesare Lombroso, a learned Italian who undertook scientific study of criminals. The work for which he is most famous centered about the physical measurements and characteristics of criminals. He assembled evidence that criminals share many "primitive" physical and mental characteristics which relate more to evolutionary ancestors than to modern man. Furthermore, he showed that these backward traits were not nearly so predominant among the more law-abiding citizenry. Thus through analytical thought, scientific measurements, and statistical evaluation, Lombroso formulated the first principles of modern criminology.

Today many of Lombroso's original theories have been disproved by the evidence of modern biology. It is now generally believed that the physical and mental handicaps of the criminal are not necessarily the cause of his lawlessness, but rather a result of inferior training and environment. The physical disfigurement or drawbacks thus are linked with the crimes in that they both stem from the same cause. It can hardly be denied that low income, lack of education, poor nutrition, and lack of comprehension of law and society will tend to create an individual unable to conform to the demands of the community. Indeed, the rules of society are formulated by individuals who have decided advantages in each regard, and who might be regarded as incompetent to pass judgment on the conduct of the underprivileged.

Thorough physical examinations of criminals for detection and correction of defects and deformities is at present limited largely to experimental groups of criminals. Whenever this method has been employed, however, excellent results have been reported concerning subsequent rehabilitation of the individuals studied. It has long been known that correction of alcohol or drug addiction and the education of the criminal concerning his addiction do much to increase the chances of restoring the individual to society. Plastic surgery has also been used to improve the appearance of the criminal. Such procedures, though expensive in many cases, are frequently of inestimable aid in speeding the rehabilitation of the criminal who has suffered from extreme facial deformities. Provision of artificial limbs often helps the amputee who displays criminal tendencies.

When the criminal is examined thoroughly by a physician, he may be found to be suffering from some chronic disease which renders him incapable of earning his livelihood in a more acceptable fashion. In this case, treatment of the patient may permit him to engage in a more remunerative occupation and thus the necessity for him to steal or otherwise to disobey the laws is removed. In other cases, a chronic illness which keeps the individual in physical discomfort may lead to senseless crimes. Narcotics addicts are often driven to crime to pay the high cost of their habit. An individual suffering extreme pain may react violently, even criminally. Here again the medical examination of the criminal may lead to amelioration of the condition and rehabilitation of the patient.

When the examining physician discovers the criminal to be suffering from a chronic condition which does not respond to treatment, he may then advise occupational therapy. In this way the patient may be taught an occupation of which he is capable, and his need for criminal activity is reduced.

It is sometimes difficult to differentiate between physical and mental illness in a criminal. In this case, the psychiatrist can be of great help. Psychological examination of the criminal, which is now much more common than the complete medical examination, is often helpful in restoring the criminal to society, providing that the mental difficulties are not complicated by physical illness.

It has been estimated that 80 percent of all criminals are intellectually inferior. This mental inferiority is due in many cases not to an inborn or inherited feeble-mindedness, but rather to improper or insufficient training. It is possible that in the future all basically retarded children can be taught in special schools which can help with their specific problems. They may be trained in such a way as to decrease the likelihood of subsequent criminal proclivities.

Many criminals have average or even superior mentality. Among these people, the psychiatrist will find, in the majority of cases, an emotional immaturity which has led directly or indirectly to a feeling of contempt for the laws. Subtle psychiatric treatment and the intelligent cooperation of family and friends can usually aid this type of criminal in gaining social and personal acceptance. When the mental aberrations of the criminal come to the point where he is considered to be insane, he will require treatment of a much different nature. About 100 years ago there were introduced into England the *McNaughton rules* which provide for the recognition of insane criminals so that they may be confined, not in the penitentiary, but in hospitals for the mentally ill. These rules have now been generally accepted by law in most civilized countries of the world. Such laws recognize the fact that an insane person is not morally responsible for many of his actions, regardless of their consequences. The psychopathic patient as pictured by the psychiatrist definitely suffers from mental disease which results in his being completely unable to adjust to society and therefore requires hospitalization. However, persons with a psychopathic condition probably account for less than five percent of all crimes. Therefore, the legal considerations of the mental condition of the criminal probably should be expanded to provide at least limited psychiatric treatment for the criminal suffering from mild mental illness or maladjustment.

From the preceding discussion, it can be seen that the medical sciences have a great responsibility in the rehabilitation of criminals. Recognizing the basic mental and physical problems of the criminal, the medical profession also carries on extensive work in the prevention of crime. Provision of free or inexpensive medical attention, particularly for children in the formative years, will do much to prevent crime. Nationwide educational campaigns to disseminate information on narcotics, nutrition, and mental and physical hygiene similarly tend to prevent crime and receive the support of the medical profession as a whole.

In addition to crime prevention and the rehabilitation of criminals, medical science is also of aid in the problems of crime detection. The law enforcement agencies have utilized medical knowledge to devise scientific tests to aid in the investigation of individual crimes.

Lie detector tests

One of the most interesting of the recent developments in medical criminology has been the lie detector. The *polygraph* or lie detector has been developed on the basis of modern knowledge of the effect of emotions on the functions of the human body. The woman who claims to be able to tell when her husband is lying may well be depending on the same principle as does the lie detector. This principle, simply stated, is

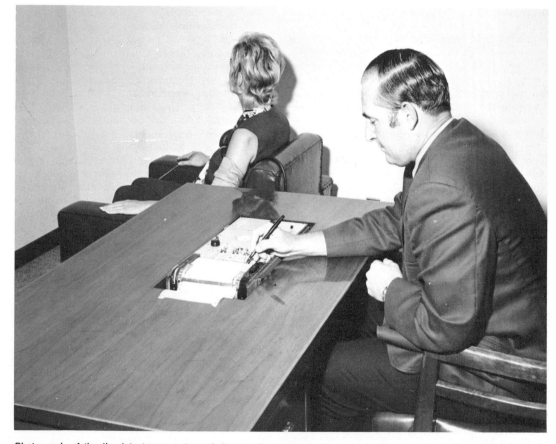

Photograph of the lie detector or polygraph in use. Pneumatic cuffs around the subject's chest and arm transmit pulse, blood pressure and respiration changes to the instrument where they are automatically recorded as a graph on a moving strip of graph paper. *Courtesy of the City of Houston Police Department.*

that an individual practicing deceit often shows changes in the physiological processes of his body. These changes may be evidenced by nervousness, blushing, dryness of the throat, and similar reactions. Moreover, there may be a rise in blood pressure and pulse, accelerated respiration, and increased activity of the sweat glands. These last variations, which can be measured with accuracy by machines, form the basis of the lie detector test. The limitation of the test is that the same reactions may result for reasons other than lying—and some hardened criminals can lie without any detectable emotional reactions. A man falsely accused of a crime has plenty of reason to be "nervous," and if he is uneducated and without a lawyer to help, is in a bad situation.

To carry out a polygraph test, the operator attaches to the subject the three recording parts of the machine, the *pneumograph* for respiration, the *sphygmograph* for blood pressure and pulse, and the *galvanograph* for measuring activities of sweat glands. Each part of the machine is so constructed as to trace a record of its values on a moving strip of paper. The length of the tracing is calibrated for time, and all three parts of the machine record simultaneously. The operator will ask the subject a series of questions, many of them having nothing to do with the topic under consideration. When the test is completed, the operator is then able to see from the tracings the changes occurring in the physiological responses of the subject and is able to correlate these changes with the questions or answers given at that time.

The operator of the polygraph should be thoroughly trained in the use of the machine, and have a thorough understanding of human psychology. The inexperienced or untrained operator would not only fail to comprehend the subject's reactions, but might report information which would be misleading or incorrect. He must be able to take into account the subject's natural nervousness during such an interview. For these reasons, persons giving polygraph tests generally have had extensive training in the use of this complex device.

It is always possible that the results of a lie detector test may not be a true reflection of the subject's reactions because of some unusual mental state of the subject. Persons working with the polygraph, however, have often reported that they themselves are only rarely able to "fool" the machine into telling a lie, and even then only after a great deal of practice.

The results of the lie detector tests are not generally admissible as evidence in court. Moreover, the test can be administered only after a written statement of consent has been signed by the subject. The chief value of this test lies in providing clues to evidence. The police, after being presented with the results of the test, are often helped in continuing their investigations. They can get some idea of an individual's innocence or guilt, though this cannot be used as even circumstantial evidence. They know from this, however, upon which lines of investigation to concentrate. In addition, new lines of inquiry are often opened as a result of information gained by the polygraph. For these reasons the

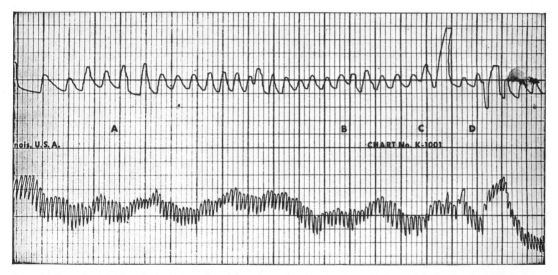

Reproduction of part of a typical recording taken in a lie detector test. Each modulation in the upper curve represents a respiration, while the more closely spaced peaks of the lower curve represent pulse beats. The more gradual undulations in the lower curve indicate blood pressure changes. These latter changes are relatively small when taken from a resting subject. A series of unrelated questions are given the subject to note his normal responses, and then a series of questions pertinent to the examination. Questions asked at points A and B produced only moderate changes in the chart when answered, but answers at points C and D caused elevation in blood pressure and changes in respiration, indicating a probable lie. *Courtesy Houston Police Department.*

lie detector is gaining increasing use in the investigation of criminal cases, such as murder, arson, rape, theft, and burglary.

Alcohol intoxication tests

Frequently the physician is asked to make an estimate of the degree of alcoholic intoxication in some individual. There are many instances in which it is necessary to determine whether an individual is intoxicated, and to determine the degree. Many communities, for example, forbid the driving of an automobile after drinking too heavily. Some cities prohibit the serving of alcoholic beverages to persons who are already intoxicated. Furthermore, it occasionally happens that an individual may be intoxicated at the time of the commission of a crime. Under these circumstances the law may rule that he was mentally inept and therefore willful intent was not probable.

Various law enforcement agencies, working in co-operation with the medical sciences, have developed a number of means for measuring alcoholic intoxication. The need for such scientific tests is based on a number of principles. Witnesses are not always good judges of the degree of intoxication, and, moreover, some persons are able to consume greater amounts of alcohol than others and yet retain their judgment.

Earlier tests for intoxication involved the measurement of ability to co-ordinate the muscles and of the action of the reflexes. The most familiar of these is the white line test, wherein the suspect is told to walk along a wide white line printed on the floor. This test along with others of a similar nature, including ability to answer simple questions or to repeat complex phrases, has, however, been subject to criticism. In the first place, judgment finally rests with the perception of individuals giving the test. Not only are they capable of error, but, all too often in court, they may be accused of personal bias in their rulings. A second and possibly greater criticism lies in the fact that failure to pass these

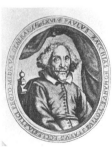

ZACCHIAS, Paul (1584-1659) Italian physician. Often called the father of legal medicine, he is noted for his important book *Questiones medico-legales* which was published in 1621. A personal physician to the Pope and an outstanding worker in public health, he was gifted in law as well as in medicine, and had many years of experience in legal medicine with the highest courts. He wrote a treatise on mental disorders. *Copyright CIBA SYMPOSIA.*

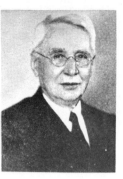

HEKTOEN, Ludvig (1863-1951) American physician and pathologist. Famous for his work in standardizing the immunological *precipitin* test for the identification of blood. His many other contributions to medicine and pathology included significant studies of infectious diseases. He was instrumental in the establishment of several research organizations and medical journals. *Copyright CIBA SYMPOSIA.*

mechanical tests may be caused by poisons, various diseases of the nervous system, fatigue, and other factors, such as tranquilizers or antihistamines, rather than alcohol. In automobile or other accidents, individuals with skull fractures have at times had their symptoms attributed to alcohol.

To determine accurately how much of an individual's condition is caused by alcohol intoxication, chemical tests for measuring the amount of alcohol in the blood have achieved wide use among law enforcement agencies. The analysis of blood for alcohol content can be carried out accurately and gives an excellent index of the amount of alcohol which is, at a given time, affecting the brain. The results of alcohol consumption depend on many factors, such as the size of the individual, and the dilution of the alcohol by the blood.

For direct measurement of alcohol in the blood, a blood sample must be obtained from the suspect. This is usually taken from the vein of the inner side of the elbow. Sterilization of the skin is achieved by materials other than alcohol lest the test value be altered by the antiseptic.

A simpler, indirect means of measuring blood alcohol can be achieved by analysis of the breath. The accuracy of this method is based upon the fact that alcohol evaporates readily and that its concentration in the breath is directly proportional to its concentration in the blood. As the blood passes through the lungs, a portion of the alcohol evaporates from the blood and is exhaled in the breath. The exact concentration of this alcohol vapor bears a precise relationship to the amount of alcohol in the blood.

A number of inventions have been perfected to carry out this chemical test of the breath. In one of the common types, the suspect is instructed to inflate a balloon. The gas within the balloon is then passed through a special chemical solution which is normally a deep purple color. Alcohol, however, decolorizes this solution, while other substances do not. The apparatus has a gauge for measuring exactly how much of the breath is needed to decolorize completely the purple solution. Obviously, the more intoxicated a person is, the smaller the volume of breath necessary to decolorize it.

Most states recognize a blood level of 0.10 percent, by weight, of alcohol in the blood as being definitely intoxicating. At this level, the driving ability of everyone is measurably impaired, no matter how experienced a drinker he may be. To reach such a level, the average person will imbibe three to four bottles of beer or three to four highballs in a relatively brief time and may expect to have an alcohol blood level of about 0.10 percent.

Instruments measuring breath alcohol are now used in many major cities in the United States. In some states the tests are admissible in court as evidence of intoxication. In others, where they are not yet accepted, police merely use the machines as a guide in determining the degree of intoxication. The test generally cannot be given without the consent of the suspect since such action would violate one of the oldest principles of English law—that of forcing an individual to testify against himself. In a few states, however, refusal to take the test may result in an individual's being booked on a DWI charge; or as in Texas, the prosecutor can comment on this during a trial, creating a presumption of intoxication in the minds of the jurors. It is physically possible to administer the test against the individual's wishes. Indeed the test should be performed upon unconscious persons in order to distinguish diabetic shock or other illness from alcohol intoxication. In these cases, the breath is collected in the balloon by the use of a hand pump or the test is done directly on the blood.

The odor of alcohol on the breath is an unscientific means of judgment, since some other factor may be primarily responsible for failure of the test, and the suspect may have consumed only a negligible amount of alcohol. A very serious aspect of the "alcohol breath" concerns the diabetic. Such a person may be far from friends or family when he suffers diabetic shock. In this instance, there may be the smell of acetone on his breath, brought about by incomplete oxidation (burning) of sugar in his blood. The average person cannot distinguish the difference between the odor of alcohol and acetone, so the victim is considered intoxicated and fails to receive vitally needed medical attention.

Drug abuse

The alarming increase in the number of drug addicts in this country has prompted lawmakers once again to look for a legislative solution to this problem. Historically, however, laws concerned with drug abuse have been far from effective.

The Harrison Narcotic Act, passed in the early part of the century, was intended to control the use of heroin. Even though the law was diligently enforced, the ratio of heroin users to the general population remains about the same now as then—1:400. This particular law failed because it was not enforced at the proper level, that of the organized crime syndicate.

The widely disregarded Marihuana Tax Act, passed in the 1930s, imposed extremely harsh penalties and permitted extraordinary inequities in the administration of justice. The act was overturned by the Supreme Court in 1969.

The Drug Abuse Control Amendments of 1965 were intended to prevent the abuse of sedatives, stimulants, and hallucinogenic agents. Concern about the growing number of ill effects and "bad trips," however, is credited with being far more influential in diminishing the use of such drugs than is any discernible effect of the law.

Those in favor of easing penalties for drug use believe that when the only "victim" is the user himself, no crime has been committed and no penalty should be served. They maintain that the use of drugs, like that of alcohol, should be punished only in order to protect other members of society from offenses to their sensibilities, morals, or safety. They add that there are usually laws, other than drug laws, that deal with such cases. They also cite the lower instance of drug addiction in the United Kingdom where addicts were registered and legally provided with drug dosages. They believe that such a program lessens the number of crimes committed to support a drug habit.

Opponents of more relaxed drug abuse laws contend that there should be further investigation into the possible harmful side effects of drug usage—birth defects, accident-proneness, impaired cognitive function, development of a psychotic syndrome—before the laws are changed.

It is generally agreed, however, that emphasis should be on curbing the manufacture, distribution, and sale of drugs, rather than on severely punishing the drug user. The sources, not the users, of drugs must be more stringently controlled.

MEDICOLEGAL ASPECTS OF CIVIL RIGHTS

Forensic medicine is not confined to criminal detection and cases of unexplained death. There is an equally broad field in civil law. So extensive is the scope of civil forensic medicine that it is possible to mention only a few of the phases. Of the many medicolegal problems concerning adoption, blood grouping tests in affilia-

Crime Laboratory

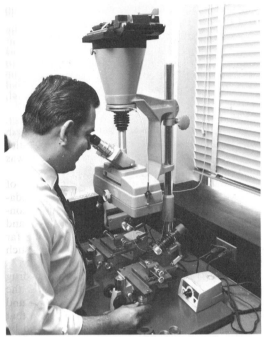

This comparison microscope is used to compare any two objects under high magnification. Actually two microscopes with one eyepiece, it allows the investigator to view two fields at one time. *Courtesy City of Houston Police Department.*

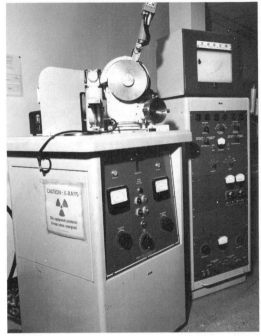

The X-ray defractometer is used for identifying crystalline materials by determining their intercrystalline spaces. Very small pieces of evidence such as smears, dirt, or dust can be compared. *Courtesy City of Houston Police Department.*

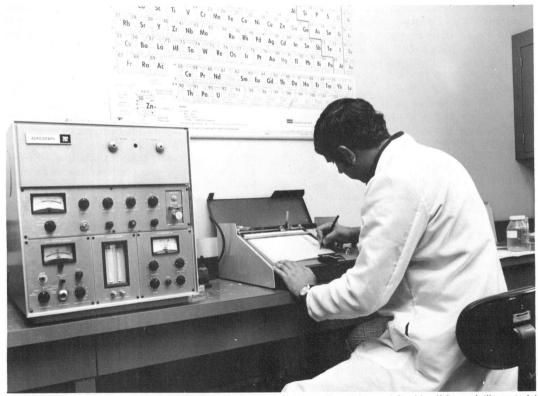

The gas chromatograph is used to identify liquid samples. Most often it is used for identifying volatile material recovered as evidence from fires in suspected arson cases. *Courtesy City of Houston Police Department.*

tion proceedings, artificial insemination, competence to draw up a will, or dying declarations, the average layman will need little knowledge. However, everyone should be familiar with the legislation pertaining to Workmen's Compensation and the role of the physician in its application.

Medicolegal problems of workmen's compensation

Workmen's Compensation is a type of insurance which provides medical care and wage compensation for workers or their dependents for economic losses caused by industrial diseases or injuries. The growing mechanization of industry has brought injury to millions of workers which has cost over two billion dollars per year. Workmen's Compensation laws are based on the theory that the expense of industrial injury should be borne by industry as one of the costs of production. The question of blame for accident or injury does not arise, and the employee is entitled to compensation if injury, accident or occupational disease occurs during the course of employment. All of the states and Washington, D.C., provide benefits covering Workmen's Compensation cases. In 1968, a total of $1,525 billion was paid in such benefits. Of this total, $1,360 billion was to cover disability and the remaining $165 billion, was for survivor benefits.

Every state now has compensation laws, but there are wide variations in the coverage of the laws. No compensation law covers all employment in a particular state. Some cover only employers who have a certain number of workers; others cover only the hazardous employments.

The amount of compensation is determined usually by a wage percentage, but the method of payment varies according to the type of injury. All the compensation laws require that medical aid be furnished to injured workers, and in 14 states medical benefits are virtually unlimited. To insure that benefit payments will be made, all states require employers to obtain insurance protection or to give proof of their qualifications to carry their own risks. In most states, employers are allowed to insure with private insurance companies.

The methods of settling Workmen's Compensation claims are by direct payment, by the agreement system, and by the hearing system. In many states a special agency, the Workmen's Compensation Commission, has been set up to administer claims. However, in six states, Workmen's Compensation is administered through court procedure. In states where the law is administered by a commission, the state agency has complete jurisdiction over the determination of facts, with appeals to the courts limited to questions of law. However, in some states the courts are allowed to reconsider the issues completely.

Although there are hundreds of thousands of industrial injuries each year, only a very small percentage ever reach the commission. The medical reports are sent directly to the employer or insurance carrier and are promptly settled. If proceedings are brought to the commission, all reports are filed with the agency. By special legislative provision these medical reports serve in lieu of oral testimony. This results in saving time, as it does not necessitate the physician's presence at the hearing. Thus the written medical report serves an important purpose and necessitates the strictest accuracy. Frequently an employee will be in apparent good health and sustain some impairment occurring during the course of employment. Only the physician can determine whether the man's condition resulted from employment or from some unknown disorder which existed beforehand. Also, an injury can be directly caused by an accident arising during the course of employment and it can also be the result of an aggravation of a preexisting condition, regardless of whether the condition itself was industrial in origin. Cases involving heart and cardiovascular disease and permanent disability are some of the many problems of forensic medicine in the application of Workmen's Compensation laws.

Medicolegal problems of life insurance

In most instances of death in which life insurance is involved, the establishment of the fact of death is all that is required. In instances in which accident indemnity is involved, the insurance company may require an autopsy. In one instance, a man was found dead at the wheel of his car which had rammed into a telegraph pole. The man carried a large amount of insurance with double indemnity for accidental death. Autopsy revealed that the man had a common heart disease capable of causing sudden loss of consciousness and death.

Among the younger age groups, a large number of persons are insured without medical examination. The insurance company merely takes a declaration from the insured that he is in good health. Some companies may then refuse claims in the event of death within a year after the policy is issued. It is obvious that many persons suffering from unknown serious organic disease may in good faith declare themselves healthy when insuring. Since most states recognize privileged communication, the family physician can refuse to issue any statement to an insurance company under such circumstances, except upon request of representatives of the deceased. When a physician examines a person for purposes of insurance, the position is different and he is ex-

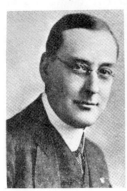

WEBSTER, Ralph W., (1873-1930) American physician. Long a clinical professor of medicine at Rush Medical College in Chicago, he was one of the outstanding authorities on medical jurisprudence. He made important revisions of Haines and Peterson's book on legal medicine and toxicology in 1923 and 1930, and these revisions along with the original edition were the standard text in this field for many years. *Copyright CIBA SYMPOSIA.*

pected to report to the company everything the examination reveals insofar as it affects the question of insurance.

Often in insurance cases, the ownership of x-ray films has been directly decided by a court of appellate jurisdiction. It is, of course, usually allowed to have films available for the future needs of the patient. When another physician follows up on a case, copies of the x-ray report and an opportunity to study the films are routinely allowed. It is held that, in the absence of any agreement to the contrary, x-ray films are the property of the physician who made them. Strictly speaking, the patient pays for a professional opinion, not an article of record or property. The physician is fully justified in refusing to surrender x-ray films, since it is a matter of common knowledge that x-ray films are practically meaningless to the ordinary layman. Further, the retention of films constitutes an important part of the physician's clinical record, differing little from microscopic slides or blood counts made in the diagnosis or treatment of a patient.

The questions of age, identity, feigned disability, and disease are also medicolegal questions that arise in insurance cases.

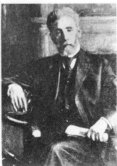

HAINES, Walter Stanley (1850-1923) Chicago chemist. While a professor of toxicology and pharmacy at Rush Medical College, he contributed many advances to the study of poisons and their detection. With F. Peterson he published the important *Textbook of Legal Medicine and Toxicology* in 1904. He is also known for the test that he devised for the detection of sugar in the urine. *Copyright CIBA SYMPOSIA.*

Medicolegal aspects of mental illness

Mental illness is as much a sickness as cancer or tuberculosis, and persons suffering from severe emotional or mental disturbance need medical help just as much as the patient suffering from appendicitis. Nevertheless, a large percentage of laymen continue to regard mental illness with superstition, prejudice, and fear. The care and treatment of mental illness are often medicolegal functions. In view of the legal formalisms necessary for hospitalization of the mentally ill and the custodial facilities that are utilized by some law enforcement authorities while awaiting action by the court, there is obviously a great need for correction of attitudes toward mental illness.

The process of securing hospital admission (often designated as commitment) varies in the different states. The states are vested with the power and duty to care for and control the insane. Legal inquiries into the sanity of a person are entirely governed by statute and the statutes vary in the different states. In most states when a person is judged to be of unsound mind, he becomes a ward of the state and administration of his estate is usually made through a guardian acting for the state.

In criminal law, insanity means such a derangement of mental and moral faculties as to render a person incapable of distinguishing bebetween right and wrong. Therefore an insane person cannot be legally charged with a criminal action.

Some states have laws which authorize county hospitals to admit persons for care and treatment of mental disorders as voluntary patients without the necessity of a court order. In such instances, the patient can be detained for a maximum period of 90 days in the county hospital. The patient, however, has the right to demand his release upon seven days' notice.

Another facility available in many states is the private psychiatric institution licensed by the state. Patients can be admitted voluntarily or upon the statement of a physician, for a limited time.

There is also the state hospital, which is frequently thought of as a place of last resort. Actually, the state hospitals are scientific institutions in which expert care and treatment are available. Usually there are methods other than court commitment permitted by the laws of the various states for admission of patients. Some states allow admission to state hospitals by the health officer application procedure which requires certificates from two physicians who have examined the patient and certify that he is mentally ill. The certificates are given by a relative or friend to the county health officer. The health officer completes the application and arranges for the patient to be admitted to the state hospital. In the health officer applications method, the patient is given treatment and provision is made for a review of the patient's progress within a definite time period. If the patient is not released, he may demand a court hearing. The legal rights of the patient are best safeguarded by such laws which enable the patient to petition the court for release at any time that he so desires.

In many states, no medical proof is required to establish that a person's mental condition needs supervision or treatment to the extent that the person should be deprived of his liberty and placed in restraint. Obviously such laws safeguard the patient only after he has been held in the county psychiatric hospital for a specified time. However, most states have safeguards concerned with court hearings for commitment which assure the person of having his day in court.

The use of general hospitals for patients suffering from mental disturbances would do much to overcome the superstitions, prejudices, and fears about mental illness.

Forensic psychiatry is concerned with the relationship of the law and the branch of medicine concerned with the treatment of mental disorders. Forensic psychiatry inquires into the status of feeble-minded persons, criminals, and social defectives. The laws concerning mentally deficient persons differ widely. Twenty states have laws authorizing sterilization of mentally retarded and criminally insane sexual psychopaths. These laws apply only to inmates of certain state institutions and have no application to the general public.

A few medicolegal problems

During the course of his practice the physician may be presented with several problems possessing medicolegal aspects. The legal boundaries in some of these cases are not clearly defined and so become intertwined with mores and religious opinion. *Therapeutic abortion,* for instance, may be lifesaving for a pregnant woman with a certain type of disease. Some of the conditions where an abortion performed by the physician may be indicated are malformation of the fetus, rape, heart disease, kidney disease, tuberculosis, and even some forms of insanity. The physician, to protect himself in such cases, must call in another physician as consultant.

Artificial insemination is a medicolegal problem quite often beset with religious and emotional involvements. In some cases, it is found that neither parent is sterile but that the husband is unable to deposit the seminal fluid near the ovum. In such cases, the husband himself can serve as donor. However, when the donor is an unknown third party the situation differs considerably from the foregoing case on legal, emo-

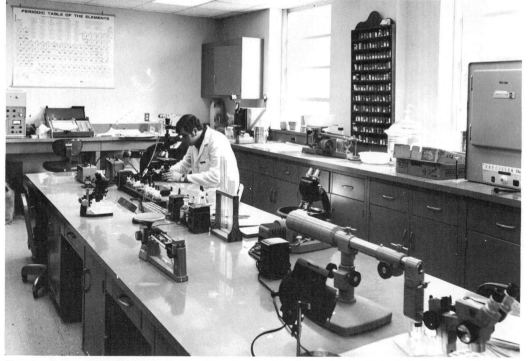

Photograph of a scientific crime detection laboratory in which tests of many kinds, including those of a biological nature, are performed daily. *Courtesy of the City of Houston Police Department, Houston, Texas.*

tional, social, and religious grounds. Some physicians feel that with the emotional impact involved, it might be far better for the couple to adopt a child.

Vasectomy and tubal ligation: There are no legal restrictions on these procedures, but there are strong emotional overtones which both the physician and the couple requesting them should consider. Vasectomies (sterilization of the male by removal of the spermatic duct) are usually done at the request of the individual, with his wife's consent. Whether a tubal ligation (sterilization of the female by tying the Fallopian tubes) is done often depends on hospital policy, and policies vary greatly. Hospitals are adopting a more permissive attitude, however, and more and more institutions now consider both vasectomy and tubal ligation a matter to be determined solely by the couple involved.

Battered child syndrome: During the past few years, there has been growing concern over the battered child. Legislators throughout the country are attempting to protect these juvenile victims by making compulsory the reporting of cases of child abuse. At present, it seems that the number of unreported cases of tortured and battered children far exceeds the reported ones, since physicians are often reluctant to consider this diagnosis and report such cases.

MEDICOLEGAL LEGISLATION

Medical legislation has only comparatively recently taken a prominent place among the statutes of most civilized countries. In 1798, the first federal medical act originated medical relief for merchant seamen. This service was originally known as the U.S. Marine Hospital Service. Legislation authorizing the appointment of a surgeon general was passed in 1870. The service was further enlarged from time to time until 1912 when it was reorganized and the name changed to the U.S. Public Health Service. The first Health Department for a particular area was established in the District of Columbia in 1822, and by 1913 every state had established a health department. All the states have legislation providing for licensing of physicians, maintaining academic and professional qualifications, and specifying causes and means for the revocation of licenses.

Federal legislation

In 1906 the Federal Pure Food and Drug Act was passed. This act makes it unlawful to ship in interstate commerce, to import, or to export "any article of food or drugs which is adulterated or misbranded." A federal act also provides for the purity of vaccines, serums, and similar products.

Federal legislation controlling narcotics dates from 1909, when an act was passed which prohibited the importation and use of opium for non-medical purposes. The Harrison Narcotic Act of 1914 legalized a system of registering legitimate dispensers of narcotic drugs. In 1929, two federal narcotic farms were established for the confinement and treatment of narcotic addicts. Every state has regulatory narcotic laws and laws forbidding purchase of many medicinal preparations except by the prescription of a physician.

Organ transplantation

The increasing performance of organ transplants has made it necessary to reevaluate present beliefs about these procedures. At present, there is little uniformity of rules among the 50 states in the United States with regard to donating bodies or parts of bodies for medical purposes. Thirty states allow any person of legal age and sound mind to donate all or part of his body; four states allow such donations for the eyes alone. Sixteen states permit the next of kin to donate all or parts of the deceased's body, while the laws of 18 states provide that the wishes of the testator shall outweigh those of the next of kin.

The Uniform Anatomical Gift Act is intended to standardize and clear up some of these points. The act, which has already been adopted by a few states, generally allows gifts to any hospital, surgeon, or specific individual and permits the gift to be made by will and acted upon without probate proceedings. It also permits gifts made by means other than a will and provides for simplicity of revocation of the gift.

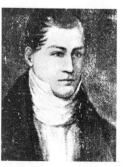

STRINGHAM, James S. (1775-1816). American physician. He is noted as the first professor of medical jurisprudence in the United States. With his medical background and an earlier experience as a professor of chemistry, he was able to combine the two fields to make a major contribution to this important field. Since his time forensic medicine has become an important area of study in all medical schools as well as in many schools of law. *Copyright CIBA SYMPOSIA.*

Determination of time of death has always been the legal responsibility of the physician. Since the advent of living organ transplants, however, questions have been raised as to how best to determine the exact time of death. Various criteria have been established for determining time of death; these include a 2-hour period in which there is no responsiveness to environment, no spontaneous breathing, no muscular movement, no reflex actions, falling arterial pressure, and an isoelectric, or flat, EEG. Determination of time of death must be made by two or more physicians, and these physicians, must be in no way immediately concerned with the care of the potential organ recipient or the performance of the transplant.

Notifiable diseases

Modern legislation in the various states provides a comprehensive system for notification of diseases. Most states require the reporting of all contagious diseases, and the regulations vary as to whom the reports are made. Venereal diseases are reportable in every state. The advertising and sale of cures for venereal diseases is forbidden in many states except on a physician's prescription. Almost all the states require a blood test for venereal disease before issuance of a marriage license.

Tuberculosis must be reported in every state. Many states have established tuberculosis hospitals and county sanatoria. Other types of legislation have been adopted which require sputum examinations, sanitation of premises, educational measures, and safeguarding of milk supplies.

Vaccination against smallpox

U.S. quarantine regulations provide for vaccination of persons entering the country from foreign countries where smallpox is prevalent. Compulsory vaccination is required in 13 states, and 18 states require vaccination of school children. When there is an epidemic of smallpox, unvaccinated children may be excluded from attending school in many states. Although there have been few cases of smallpox in the United States in recent years, vaccination of children is still recommended. The federal government also requires of persons leaving or entering the United States various vaccinations against typhoid, yellow fever, and other diseases.

Vital statistics

All the states now have laws requiring the recording of births and deaths. The usual requirement concerning births is that the attending physician, the hospital, or the parents shall report to a designated registry information regarding the child and its parents. The usual requirement concerning deaths is that a certificate giving the cause of death and other information shall be filed with a designated official. This requirement is usually necessary for the issuance of a burial permit. There is no right of property in a dead human body, but it is the duty of public officers and the next of kin to protect the body from violation and insure that it is properly disposed of and protected. If a person dies in one locality and transportation of the body is necessary, the officials in the locality of the death have jurisdiction over the body.

27 MEDICAL HISTORY

MEDICINE DURING EARLY TIMES

Medicine and other subjects associated with health have a fascinating story, reaching far into the past, and progressing with increasing speed after innumerable false starts and tragic disappointments.

Medicine deals with health and disease in men and animals. Four phases are discernible in its history: (1) primitive ignorance and superstition with resulting fear of disease; (2) accumulation of experience in managing disease, culminating in a professional group specially trained in ministering to the sick; (3) gradual growth of verifiable knowledge of the causes of illness, with recent application to the prevention of disease; and now (4), with knowledge applied to the control of disease, the effort to promote optimum health places emphasis on preventive rather than curative medicine.

Primitive medicine and fear of disease

Records from antiquity and from primitive peoples furnish proof that injuries from obvious causes, like fractures or bruises, were usually handled sensibly by splints and poultices. When the cause of sickness was not apparent, as in *metabolic* diseases, the illness was often ascribed to an evil demon which had to be driven away. Primitive surgery and obstetrics were usually sensible, but the primitive approach to infection or metabolic disease was generally superstitious.

Primitive peoples used many plant, animal, and mineral materials in relieving symptoms of disease. The American Indians used wintergreen for rheumatism. The Modoc Indians used cascara as a purgative. The early Chinese used ashes of sponges (containing iodine) for goiter. South American and African aborigines learned the poisonous properties of plant materials which were used to poison their arrows. However, native peoples never used poisons as medicines.

The medicine man of primitive peoples usually acted in some abnormal manner, as an epileptic, or one subject to trances. Often by frightening masks and dances, he would attempt to scare the evil spirits of disease away. This procedure was expected by the sick person, and probably comforted him. He would feel that there was someone with him to ward off the demon of disease.

Astonishingly, these magical rites seemed to help. The truth is that sick people often get well, regardless of what treatment is given them. Failure to understand this, however, results in thinking that whatever has been done for the sick person is responsible for curing him. These two facts—the healing power of nature, and the confusion between sequence of events and cause and effect—are responsible for the persistence of quackery and superstition in medical history.

Prominent healers from the past are preserved in legend. From the ancient Hindus come two names, Charaka and Susrata, who were revered as physicians. The Chinese revered Hua-Tó, who used pain-relieving drugs in operations.

The accumulation of experience in managing disease

China and Babylonia: The great static cultures of the past gradually permitted the rise of a

796

group of people skilled in treating the sick. This group preserved records of their experiences, and thus profited from the mistakes of the past. But without continuing experiment, even accumulated experience becomes rigid and uncorrected, and results in a ritualistic professional practice. This occurred in ancient China.

Lacking knowledge from direct study of the body, the Chinese developed a rigid system of medicine, based on impractical theories. There was an enormous drug lore, which was followed slavishly without correction for centuries. A similar situation arose in ancient Babylonia. There the medical group became so secure that large numbers were attracted to it. Inadequate training and poor results led to legal control. The Code of Hammurabi of about 2250 B.C. contains a section regulating medical practice. The code stipulated that if a physician killed the patient, then the physician himself must die. Later this principle was modified so that the offender could ransom himself by paying a fine. Although the old Babylonian physicians mixed superstition with medical practice, they had considerable hygienic skill.

Old Egyptian medicine: The most satisfactory medical records of ancient physicians are from Egypt. The pyramid tombs give a picture of the beliefs and customs of the people. Mummification, which was entrusted to priests, gave an opportunity to see how the body is composed, and afforded a background of medical knowledge.

Decomposition, putrefaction, pus, and decay were regarded as evil. These conditions were believed to prevail in sickness. The theory of medical treatment was to drive out foul material.

There must have been many injuries in the huge building activities, and in warfare. A systematic method was developed for treating injured patients. The accumulated surgical experience is recorded in the Edwin Smith Papyrus, an ancient surgical textbook now in the New York Academy of Medicine. The Edwin Smith Papyrus was written about 1750 B.C., when the arts flourished in Egypt. The scribe who wrote the existing document must have copied it from a much older papyrus, for he used archaic terms which date from about 3500 B.C.

A legendary medical figure in Egypt was Imhotep, physician to the Pharaoh Zoser, about 3500 B.C. His memory was revered long after his death; he became Egypt's first god of medicine. Priests and doctors gathered around temples erected in his honor and ministered to the sick. The temples were maintained by votive offerings. This worship was carried by Greek visitors to Hellas, where similar temples were built. Later, temples were erected in the Roman Empire.

Some authorities believe that Imhotep wrote the original surgical text preserved in the Edwin Smith Papyrus, although there is no evidence to show that this is so. The existing document is unfinished, stopping in the middle of a word in a case history. The Smith Papyrus was arranged by typical injuries from the head to the feet, and was used as a textbook. In each instance there is the title of the case followed by findings in the examination. There is a statement of the diagnosis, and indication of the probable course of the injury. The treatment recommended is practical, and involves splints, casts, and soothing applications.

Another medical text preserved from Egypt is the Ebers Papyrus. This is a medical teaching text, containing some 800 prescriptions for different diseases, with case reports.

In addition to these texts several papyri which were physicians' prescription books have been collected. The Hearst Medical Papyrus and the Berlin Medical Papyrus date from about the same time as the Ebers Medical Papyrus, 1700 B.C. Both contain some 200 recipes or prescriptions for various disease conditions.

Egyptian formulas were transmitted through Greco-Roman times to medieval Europe, and after translation into the different languages, remained in use until the nineteenth century. This slavish copying, originating in Egypt, led to a deterioration in the quality of medicine. The reasons for the original use of the various ingredients were forgotten. Medical knowledge began to include magical incantations, particularly regarding fertility, pregnancy, and cosmetics.

FROM HIPPOCRATES THROUGH THE DARK AGES

As recorded in the Homeric poems, Greece was the scene of many invasions. As the population became stabilized in Asia Minor and Greece, a free culture arose which developed a high degree of intellectual attainment. The fifth century B.C. was outstanding for geniuses.

Temples to the god of health, Aesculapius, were erected in many parts of the Greek world. The one on the Island of Cos was renowned. The medical leader there was Hippocrates (460–370 B.C.) The teachings of his school are characterized by high ethical standards, keen clinical ability, and critical evaluation of experience.

A clean break with superstition and religious involvement in disease was made by the Hippocratic writers in a remarkable treatise, "On The Sacred Disease" *(epilepsy),* which was stated to be no more sacred than any other disease, but instead, to have a physical cause. The statement is impressive for its declaration of principle. The Hippocratic writers particularly emphasized the importance of studying the natural causes of disease. They understood that sick people may get

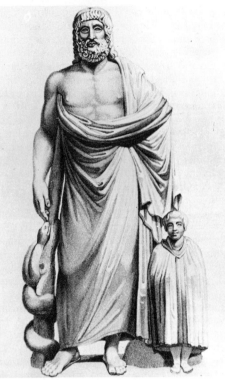

Drawing of a statue of Aesculapius, in Greek mythology, the son of Apollo, who was noted for his healing powers and became the god of medicine.

CELSUS, Aulus Cornelius. Roman physician and writer of the first century A.D. His *De Medicina*, discovered in 1443, provided most of the modern knowledge of medicine in ancient Greece, and a means of translating Greek medical terms into Latin. An operation he described for amputations of limbs resembles closely one still in use. He was the first medical historian of note.

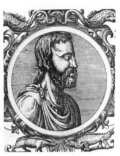

basic knowledge. Much activity was stimulated by Aristotle (384–322 B.C.) whose scientific studies laid the foundation for experimental biology. His investigation of animals was impressive for direct observations on the functions of the heart and the growth of the embryo.

Roman medicine

When Greece fell to Rome, the Greek culture and scientific spirit declined. There was no effective regulation of medical practice among the Romans, and quackery prevailed. The head of every Roman family was responsible for the health of the family. For proper guidance, a handbook of medicine was written by the Roman encyclopedist, Celsus, who lived during the beginning of the Christian era. Celsus' book is clearly organized and gives much helpful information on the management of ordinary injuries and illnesses.

The drug lore of ancient peoples, which came largely from Egypt, was organized by a Greek surgeon, Dioscorides. He studied each drug carefully and offered information on its medical uses and possible effects. He also discussed poisons and treatment of poisoned persons. His was a scientific approach, and formed the basis for the standardization of drugs many centuries later. Among the Romans, the practice of surgery flourished. Archigenes wrote about amputations and *ligatures*. Heliodoros described operations for *hernia* and *stricture,* and Antyllus operated on *aneurysm* and *cataracts*. Soranus wrote on *obstetrics,* and on diseases of women and children. Like most of the other skillful Roman physicians, Aretaeus came from Asia Minor. He gave excellent descriptions of diphtheria, diabetes, tuberculosis, tetanus, asthma, and mental disorders.

The outstanding Roman physician was Galen (131–201 A.D.), who was trained in Hippocratic medicine. He came to Rome as a surgeon for the gladiators, and later attended the Emperor Marcus Aurelius. In his writings, he systematized the earlier medical experience recorded by the Egyptian and Greek writers. He wrote on

well spontaneously; therefore, they curbed unwarranted claims for miraculous cures by medical men. They established high ethical standards for the practice of medicine through the "Hippocratic Oath." This was the first known ethical document for any professional group. Its principles are the basis of ethical medical practice today.

The Hippocratic writings are rich in detail regarding fractures and surgical conditions. They are noteworthy for their common sense procedures, based on practical experience. Case histories are included, as well as special treatises for instruction in anatomy and other fields of

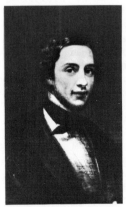

SMITH, Edwin. American Egyptologist of the nineteenth century. In 1862 he acquired a document now known as the *Edwin Smith Papyrus* which is the oldest known medical writing of ancient Egypt. Concerned largely with surgery, the document was written between 2500 and 1700 B.C., and is the source of much of our knowledge concerning the early practice of medicine. Many of the practices described are similar to ones that are still employed.

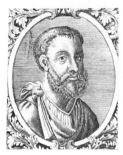

GALEN, Claudius (about 130-200) Mysian physician in Rome. Galen is one of the greatest figures in medical history, his authority being so great that few physicians dared to go against his writings until the time of Vesalius in the sixteenth century. Often referred to as the father of experimental physiology, he was probably the first to adequately describe cholera, hydrophobia, and malaria. He identified many anatomical parts.

nutrition, fevers, surgical conditions, and *therapeutics*. His writings were so well organized that they became the basis for medical teaching for 1500 years. Galen's works were developed into a system of medicine which persisted into the sixteenth century.

Galen's system of treatment for fractures and wounds was logical. However, his theory of disease was developed from the early Greek ideas of "humoral pathology." This was related to the Greek notion of the four elements: earth, air, fire, and water, with their accompanying qualities of dryness, coldness, heat, and wetness. There were thought to be four humours in the body: (1) blood, which is hot and wet; (2) phlegm, which is cold and wet; (3) bile, which is hot and dry; and (4) black bile, which was supposed to be cold and dry. Health was thought to consist in a balance of the four humours. If the physician thought there was an excess of any one of the humours, he attempted to get rid of it. If there was too much blood, the patient was bled; too much phlegm, the patient was made to sweat or vomit; too much bile, the patient was purged; and if there was too much black bile, all three procedures would be used. It was rough treatment.

With the decline of the Roman Empire, science and medicine also declined. The Romans had shown great practical ability in sanitation. They developed excellent methods of food and water supply, sewage, disposal of the dead (cremation), and even planned city recreation facilities and public baths. These facilities deteriorated with the fall of the empire.

Meanwhile, the Christian Church was developing. At the Council of Nicea in A.D. 376, the Trinitarian Creed was adopted, and the unitarian followers of Bishop Arius fled eastward. These refugees from the Roman Empire took into Persia and Arabia the medical books of Hippocrates, Dioscorides, and Galen. Translated into Persian, Arabic, and Hebrew, these works contributed greatly to the intellectual rise of the Mohammedan Empire.

Mohammedan medicine

Arabian and Jewish physicians made important contributions to medicine during the height of the Mohammedan Empire. They introduced distillation and prepared new types of drugs. Maintaining high ethical standards, they brought dignity to the practice of medicine, and promoted professional spirit. From Bagdad to Spain, they preserved the best medical traditions of the Greco-Roman world.

Important Arabic physicians were Rhazes (A.D. 850–923) and Avicenna (980–1037). Rhazes described smallpox and measles, used anatomy as a basis for medical practice, and introduced hospital organization. Avicenna, physician of the hospital at Bagdad, wrote the "Canon," a basic text for medical training for many centuries. In this he classified diseases thoroughly.

With the rise of Islamic culture in Spain, medical skill was promoted by Albucasis, Avenzoar, and Averroës. Albucasis invented probes and dental instruments, and first described the bleeding disease, *hemophilia*. With considerable foresight, Avenzoar described cancer of the stomach and esophagus. He recommended the use of *nutrient enemas*. Yet he claimed curative virtues for amulets and concretions from animals (*bezoar stones*). Averroës noted that smallpox never afflicts the same person twice.

In Cairo, Moses Maimonides (1135–1204) wrote treatises on personal hygiene, on antidotes for poisons, and on ethical medical practice. Other Arab and Hebrew physicians devised apothecaries' manuals, helping to standardize the use of various drugs. More than 700 drugs were used by the Mohammedan physicians, who exercised skill in their choice and preparation.

Medieval medicine

In western Europe, knowledge was carried forward through monastery instruction. The monks were the only teachers and the chief physicians. Important centers of learning developed in Italy as a result of trading at Salerno. A

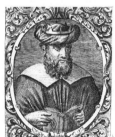

AVICENNA (IBN SINA) (980-1037) Arabian physician, philosopher and writer. One of the greatest of the Arabian physicians. Noted for his large volume on the medical knowledge of his period, which not only codified the information but correlated it with the systems developed by Aristotle and Galen. His work was considered authoritative for many centuries. This misplaced reverence retarded the development of surgery.

medical school there attracted students from all parts of Europe. Arabic and Jewish manuscripts were translated into Latin, and systematic instruction was developed in anatomy based on Galen's theories.

An important medieval medical translator was Constantine the African (1015–1087), who studied at Salerno. The formulary of Nicolaus of Salerno proposed anesthesia for the surgical work of Roger of Palermo and Roland of Parma. Both of these surgeons used improved techniques in removing cancerous growth, taught the use of *styptics* and ligatures in preventing hemorrhage, and are believed to have employed mercury in the treatment of syphilitics. Their work was followed by Saliceto (1201–1277) who wrote an important text on surgery. His pupil, Lanfranc of Milan, founded French surgery and wrote another important text.

Of far-reaching significance was the decree of Emperor Frederic II in 1224, that anyone practicing medicine for a fee must show a certificate of proficiency from the School of Salerno. This was the forerunner of licensing for the practice of medicine. Meanwhile, the rise of universities at Paris (1200), Bologna (1088), Oxford (1206), Cambridge (1229), and Padua (1228), contributed to the return to scientific methods. Hospitals were founded in the leading cities, which were the sites of recurring epidemics of the black death (bubonic plague), smallpox, and other serious infections.

Thirteenth century knowledge was epitomized by St. Thomas Aquinas (1225–1274), who endeavored to show that authoritarian faith could be reconciled with verifiable scientific knowledge. The cultural unity of the thirteenth century was revealed in learning, in medicine, and in religion, as well as in art and building. Medicine was based on galenic tradition, nothing having been found meanwhile to add to the knowledge Galen possessed. The Crusades had made contact with the eastern culture, and the Europeans learned that the Mohammedans possessed wide medical knowledge, having preserved some original Greek manuscripts on medicine preceding Galen. As these were brought into Europe, and were examined by scholars, doubts arose regarding the infallibility of galenic tradition.

THE RENAISSANCE OF MEDICINE

The revival of learning in Europe began when the examination of older documents in original Greek led to discovery of errors in the medical texts of Arabian and Jewish translators. Thus, Leonicenus (1428–1524) found mistakes in the standard works of Pliny, Galen, and Aristotle. In particular, he noted significant errors concerned with medicinal plants. Thomas Linacre (1460–1524), physician to Henry VIII, studied in Italy, and became the "restorer of learning" in England. His translations and comments were highly regarded. Francois Rabelais (1483–1553) made direct Latin translations from the works of Hippocrates. This physician was a pioneer psychologist, who recognized the therapeutic value of laughter for his patients. For this reason he wrote his novels "Gargantua" and "Pantagruel."

With the revival of learning, medical terms became more numerous and confusing. The first medical dictionary was prepared by Symphorien Champier (1472–1539) of Lyons.

The rise of science in the sixteenth century resulted in further improvement in medical knowledge. Direct investigation of the human body was undertaken first by Renaissance artists, stimulated by Leonardo da Vinci (1452–1519). Leonardo wanted to portray the human body as accurately as possible, but found that doctors could not help him since their anatomical knowledge was stereotyped from galenic sources. He undertook dissection himself and left a magnificant series of anatomical notes and illustrations which have only recently been published. His works undoubtedly stimulated other artists, and eventually physicians.

The founder of modern anatomy is Andreas Vesalius (1514–1564) of Brussels, who studied at Paris, and later became professor of anatomy and surgery at the University of Padua. With the artist, Jan van Calcar, he prepared a treatise on the structure of the human body. Vesalius also assisted in the standardization of drugs, and became court physician to the Emperor Charles V. He retired from teaching and research when his ideas were ridiculed.

Vesalian anatomy was incorporated in the surgical texts of the French surgeon, Ambroise Paré (1510–1590), chief military surgeon for the kings of France. Paré, a brilliant surgeon, revived the use of *ligatures*. His work helped to reestablish surgery as a respected field of medical practice.

The dissemination of new medical learning was accelerated by printing. It was already becoming difficult to find what was known in medicine. Indexes and bibliographies became necessary. The bibliophile, Conrad Gesner (1516–1565), filled the need with his *Bibliotheca Universalis* in 1545.

Emphasis on new discovery was dramatically shown by Paracelsus (1493–1541) who burned the books of Galen when he became professor of medicine at Basel. Paracelsus wrote on therapeutics, surgery, industrial diseases, psychiatry, chemistry, and philosophy. He was a skilled practitioner, who introduced simple chemicals and drugs in treatment. He opposed astrology and magical ideas in medicine. His contemporary, Valerius Cordus (1515–1544), discovered ether, and noted its sleep-producing properties.

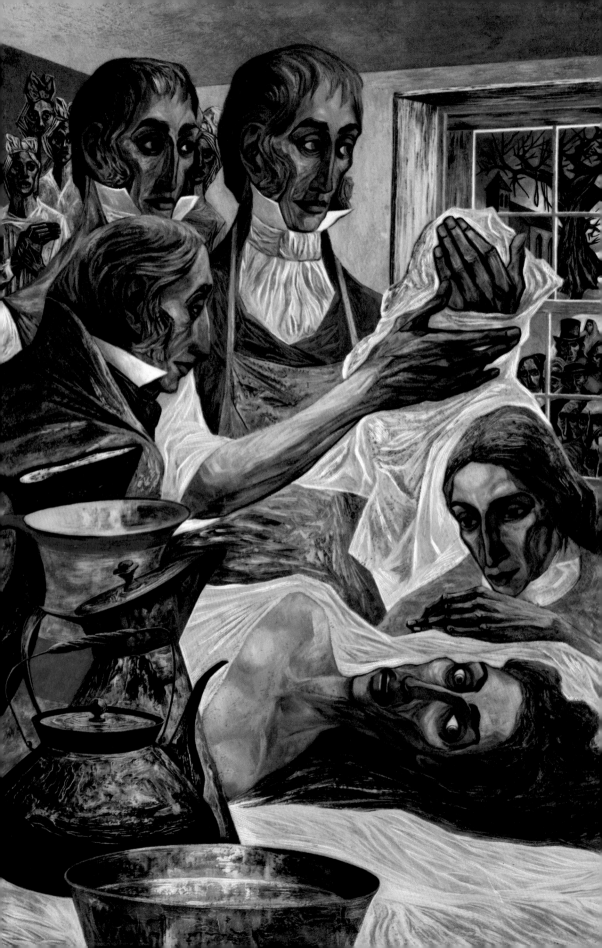

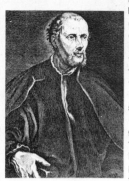

PARACELSUS, (AUREOLUS PHILIPPUS THEOPHRASTUS) (1493-1541). Swiss physician, chemist, and reformer. The pioneer of modern chemotherapy, he made many contributions to the treatment of the sick, including use of mercury in treatment of syphilis. He noted that the disease may be of a congenital nature. He observed that there is a relationship between cretinism and exophthalmic goiter, although the nature of these disorders was unknown.

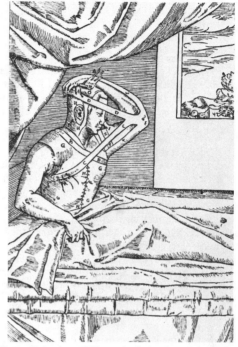

Illustration of a 1597 method developed by Gasparo Tagliacozzi for constructing a new nose from a flap of tissue grafted from the arm. *Bettmann Archive.*

He also classified medicinal plants, and prepared the first pharmaceutic formulary to receive legal sanction.

The most important disease of the sixteenth century was syphilis. It was thought that it was brought to Europe by the sailors of Columbus, but this has never been proved. The term was given by the Italian physician, Giralamo Francastoro (1483–1533), who classified and described the chief contagious diseases. His medical poem, "Syphilis Sive Morbus Gallicus" (Venice, 1530), describes the disease thoroughly, with regard to origin, symptoms, natural course, and treatment. "Syphilis" is the name of the hero of the poem.

New anatomical discoveries were made during the sixteenth century. Bartolommeo Eustacchio (1520–1574) first described the adrenal glands as well as the thoracic duct and the air tubes to the ears, which bear his name.

A successor to Vesalius at Padua, Gabriel Fallopius (1523–1562), described the ovaries, the Fallopian tubes which were named for him, the semicircular canals, and several nerves. His pupil, Fabricius of Aquapendente (1537–1619), observed the valves in the veins. He revived Aristotelian study of the growth of embryos and wrote extensively about muscles and surgery. Another pupil of Fallopius, Volcher Coiter

(1534–1600), studied the formation and comparative anatomy of bones and muscles. The school at Padua was the leading medical center during this period.

These anatomical advances were immediately important. Gasparo Tagliacozzi (1546–1599) of Bologna revived plastic surgery, but was reviled for meddling with divine handiwork. Texts on surgery were compiled by Felix Würtz (1518–1574), and by William Clowes (1540–1604), the outstanding English surgeon during the reign of Elizabeth I.

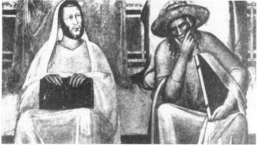

GALEN AND HIPPOCRATES. Fragment of a fresco by Gaddi in the cloister of Santa Maria Novella of Florence, Italy.

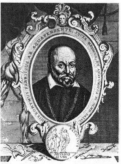

FABRICIUS AB AQUAPENDENTE, Hieronymus (1537-1619) Italian anatomist and surgeon. Famous for his investigations in embryology. He also studied the valves of the veins, and made numerous contributions to our knowledge of human anatomy. Pupils were drawn to his school from all parts of Europe, and many of them became masters of anatomy. The discovery of the circulation of the blood was made by his pupil, William Harvey.

Illustration: A Pioneer Surgeon . . . Reese Brandt. Ephraim McDowell, a physician of the Kentucky backwoods, first successfully removed an ovarian tumor in 1809. McDowell was assisted by his wife and a nephew. A mob threatened to hang him if the patient died.

SEVENTEENTH CENTURY MEDICINE

The greatest student at Padua was William Harvey (1578–1657), head of the English students at the School of Medicine. Stimulated by discussions of his teacher, Fabricius, on the valves in the veins, Harvey investigated the action of the heart and the motion of the blood.

Harvey's treatise, "De Motu Cordis," appeared in 1628. Reluctantly accepted after many years, this volume was a clear-cut refutation of galenic theory. It established the concept of the circulation of the blood and set a landmark in the history of science. It introduced the practical approach to clinical medicine on the basis of observation, hypothesis, deduction, and experimentation. Harvey criticized the inconsistencies in the galenic theory, gave a careful analysis of phenomena relating to the motion of the heart and blood, described experimental procedures to test his hypothesis that blood moves in a circle to and from the heart, and introduced quantitative reasoning to prove his theory. Harvey's scientific procedure is far superior to the laborious manipulation of data by cumbersome tables proposed by his contemporary, Francis Bacon (1561–1626), who is usually credited with introducing modern scientific methods.

Harvey's work was preceded by an account of the pulmonary circulation by the Spanish physician and theologian, Michael Servetus (1509–1553), who was burned at the stake for heresy by Calvinists. His book, practically all copies of which were burned with him, contained a description of the pulmonary circulation.

While Harvey's reputation suffered as a result of his criticism of galenic theory, he lived to see the acceptance of his work by the leading scientists of his day. His important study on the generation of animals was published in 1653.

Harvey could not furnish direct proof of the circulation of the blood, since he had no means

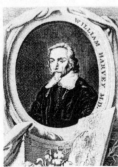

HARVEY, William (1578-1657) English physician. Famous in medical history for his original discovery of the circulation of the blood through the blood vessels. Various theories had previously been held with regard to the nature of the movement of the blood, but it had never been shown that the circulatory system was a closed one within which the blood continuously circulates. His discovery is said to have been the most important one in medicine.

of seeing the tiny junctions between arteries and veins. The physical studies of Galileo (1564–1642) led to the development of telescopes and microscopes. Microscopes were promptly applied to the study of living things. Robert Hooke (1635–1703) demonstrated the cellular structure of plants and began studies on the relation of respiration to blood changes. Jan Swammerdam (1637–1680) discovered red blood cells, and further investigated the movements of the lungs and muscles. These investigations prompted the work of Antonie van Leeuwenhoek (1632–1723), a janitor, who made his own microscopes and described his observations before the Royal Society of London. He discovered spermatozoa, protozoa, and bacteria, and completed Harvey's work by demonstrating the capillary union between arteries and veins.

Outstanding among the early microscopists was Marcello Malpighi (1628–1694), professor of anatomy at Bologna. He was famed for his studies of the silkworm and plants, and for investigations of the development of the chick. His study of the lung showed air tubes in close association with blood vessels, and proved the capillary junction between arteries and veins. Because of his studies on the liver, spleen, and kidney, he is considered a pioneer in microscopic anatomy.

The quickening pace of knowledge made it imperative for physicians to share their discoveries. During the seventeenth century, medical journals were published, and scientific academies were organized. Most important of these was the Royal Society of London. This began as an informal group that met once a week to talk over their investigations. The secretary of the group, Henry Oldenburg (1615–1677), collected the discussions, which were published as *The Transactions of the Royal Society*. Medical scientists from all over Europe contributed to the publication.

The influence of Galileo's discoveries was reflected in the application of physical principles to medical needs. The French mathematician and philosopher, René Descartes (1596–1650), wrote the first text on physiology ("De Homine," published by Elsevier of Leyden in 1662) in which Harvey's concept was stressed. Descartes gave a correct explanation of reflex action, and began the investigation of vision. The Italian mathematician, Giovanni Borelli (1608–1679), applied mechanics to muscular motion, analyzing movements of limbs in terms of levers. The Paduan physician, Santorio Santorio (Sanctorius) (1561–1636), described a clinical thermometer, and founded the study of metabolism by measuring water loss from the lung and skin.

Other seventeenth century physicians were interested in the chemical aspects of disease. Jean Baptiste van Helmont (1577–1644) studied digestive processes, the bile, and gastric juice. He

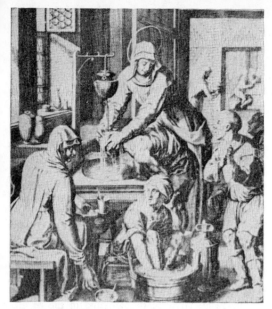

St. Ehrentrudid washing and caring for lepers. During the Middle Ages, such nursing as existed was usually performed by nuns. *Bettmann Archive.*

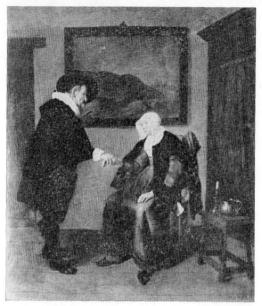

This old painting by Brekelenkam entitled *The Consultation* portrays a Dutch physician of the seventeenth century in attendance upon a patient.

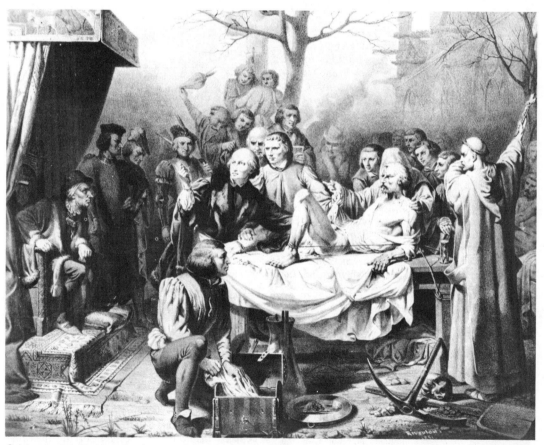

Colot removing bladderstone from a criminal in the presence of Louis XI of France. The operation was a success, the criminal freed, and Louis who also had stones, let Colot perform the operation on him. *Bettmann Archive.*

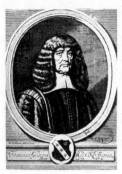

GLISSON, Francis (1597-1677) English physician. He is famous for the classic description of rickets (*Glisson's disease*) that he published in 1650, although the symptoms of this disorder had been recognized for centuries before his time. Among his many other contributions to physiology and medicine may be mentioned his studies on the anatomy of the liver, and the sling used in correcting spinal deformities, which has since been known by his name.

introduced the term "gas" and discovered what we call *carbon dioxide*. Franciscus Sylvius (1614–1672) began the study of ductless glands, and recognized the significance of saliva and pancreatic juice in digestion. Thomas Willis (1621–1675), one of the most prominent physicians in London, gave an excellent description of the anatomy of the brain with a classification of the cerebral nerves. He noted the sweet taste of diabetic urine, and studied puerperal fever and general paralysis. Regnier de Graaf (1641–1673), of Holland, made a systematic study of the pancreatic secretion. The Danish priest, Neils Stensen (1638–1686), described glands of the body and made important contributions to the understanding of muscular action. Francis Glisson (1597–1677), at the University of Cambridge, was first to describe rickets, and also gave a description of the liver and its blood supply.

The outstanding physician of the seventeenth century was Thomas Sydenham (1624–1689), who revived Hippocratic methods of observation and experimentation. He made extensive use of mercury in treating persons with syphilis, and of cinchona bark in treating patients with fever. Sydenham gave admirable first hand accounts of various diseases and described scarlet fever. His practical treatment methods supplanted the galenic tradition.

Obstetrics as a special field of medicine was begun in the seventeenth century through the in-

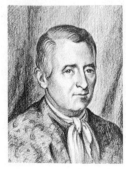

HELMONT, Jean Baptiste van (1577-1644) Belgian physician. He is noted for his introduction into medical practice of many new methods of urine analysis. They were important because they gave a great stimulus to the use of such data in diagnostic practice. He was the first man to recognize the physiological importance of the carbon dioxide that is exhaled.

fluence of François Mauriceau (1637–1709) and Hendrik van Deventer (1651–1724). Their well-written treatises on pregnancy and the management of labor resulted in midwifery becoming a recognized medical specialty.

Surgery in the seventeenth century was advanced by Wilhelm Fabry (1560–1634), who recognized the seriousness of gangrene and recommended amputation above the diseased part. He devised special tourniquets and reported an impressive series of case histories.

Medical education was widely extended in the seventeenth century, with leading schools at Leyden and Montpelier. Schools of medicine had already been established in the New World at universities in Lima and Mexico (1551). The first medical publication from what is now the United States was issued by Thomas Thacher (1620–1678) in 1667, to guard the English colonists against disease.

The rapid advance of medicine in the seventeenth century, together with pretension and fraud on the part of some of the European physicians, led to satirical attacks on the profession, particularly from the French satirist, Molière (1622–1673).

EIGHTEENTH CENTURY MEDICINE

In the eighteenth century, the tendency toward systematization was continued. The success of Isaac Newton (1642–1727) in bringing mathematical order out of chaos with regard to the movements of heavenly bodies stimulated similar organizing efforts in other fields of knowledge. The Swedish physician, Carl von Linné (1707–1778), presented a description of plants and animals, originating the binomial classification and grouping all living things into families and species. Medical men tried to classify disease along similar lines. George E. Stahl (1660–1734) began a classification of disease on the basis of symptoms.

The chief physician of the age was Hermann Boerhaave (1668–1738), who made Leyden the medical center of the world. His advances in chemistry are important in summarizing the knowledge of the period. He edited and translated the classics in medicine. Like Sydenham, Boerhaave insisted on practical experience in medical affairs. His chief pupil was Albrecht von Haller of Berne (1708–1777), who started systematic medical bibliography. Experimentally, he distinguished between nerve impulse (sensibility) and muscular contraction (irritability). He discovered that bile is necessary for the digestion of fat.

During the eighteenth century the tradition of

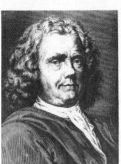

BOERHAAVE, Hermann (1668-1738) Dutch physician. Famous as a great clinician and one of the originators of modern clinical teaching. He was an advocate of discussion and consultation as measures to promote the patient's welfare. He made numerous contributions to physiology and was one of the first to describe the sweat glands. His book, *Elementa Chemiae,* was published in 1732, and was among his greatest contributions to medical science.

HALES, Stephen (1677-1761) English clergyman and physiologist. Famous as the first man to measure the blood pressure, having conducted his experiment on a horse. He was a pioneer in the use of artificial ventilation in mines, ships, etc. Hales is also noted for his early studies on the physiology of green plants. Although his versatility made him famous in many different fields, his studies on blood pressure were his most valued gift to science.

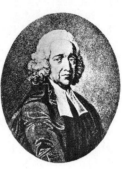

medical service was established. There developed a threefold division of responsibility between physicians, surgeons, and apothecaries. The apothecaries were directly sought by sick people for advice about their ailments, as well as for drugs. The practice of pharmacy was regulated by charter and license, and by membership in the guild. If a patient had a condition beyond the druggist's capacity to manage, it was the druggist's responsibility to refer the patient to a physician. The physician was an educated man whose independent means made it possible for him to obtain the M.D. degree. The physician might write a prescription, which was a legal order to a druggist. Since the physician would not undertake any work himself, he would refer the patient to a surgeon if an operation were indicated. The surgeon was usually a self-educated man of limited means, and did not hold the M.D. degree. He prided himself in *not* being a "doctor," and in England surgeons still insist on being called "Mister."

As a result of the industrial revolution, there was a mass movement of the population into the cities. It became necessary to establish hospitals for the poor. The rights and obligations of physicians, surgeons, and apothecaries had to be defined. Thomas Percival (1740–1804), a Manchester practitioner, proposed a "Code of Ethics" for governing the conduct of medical men. This "Code" established a basis for ethical standards of medical practice.

The rising industrialization during the eighteenth century was reflected in medicine by the work of Bernardino Ramazzini (1633–1714), who studied epidemics and wrote on trade diseases and industrial hygiene. Johan Peter Sussmilch (1707–1782) compiled medical statistics on public health. Johann Peter Frank (1745–1821) wrote a treatise on public health, covering sewerage, water supply, sex hygiene, and food and drug inspection. This was the beginning of public health.

The advance of scientific medicine was rapid in the eighteenth century, particularly in physi-

ology, biochemistry, and pathology. Stephen Hales (1677–1761), an English clergyman, began a systematic study of fluid pressures in animals and plants. He was the first to estimate the blood pressure, velocity of blood movement, and heart capacity. Another outstanding Englishman was William Hewson (1739–1774), who studied the lymph vessels and the coagulation of the blood. Lazzaro Spallanzani (1729–1799) discovered the digestive properties of saliva, experimented on respiration, and refuted the idea of spontaneous generation of animals and plants.

Gaseous interchange in the lungs was elucidated by Antoine Laurent Lavoisier (1743–1794), who thus initiated quantitative chemistry and biochemistry. Lavoisier demonstrated the biological significance of oxygen, which had been discovered by Joseph Priestley (1733–1804). Oxygen was promptly used in medicine in the treatment of respiratory disorders by Thomas Beddoes (1760–1808) at his Pneumatic Institution at Clifton.

Pathology was established as a basic medical discipline by Giovanni Battista Morgagni (1682–1771) of Padua, who wrote systematic accounts of a large number of autopsies on patients whose case histories had been prepared. He thus checked diagnoses made during life with the anatomical disorders observed after death. He gave authentic descriptions of diseases of the

SPALLANZANI, Lazzaro (1729-1799) Italian physiologist. He performed experiments that helped to disprove the theory of spontaneous generation. He is also noted for his investigations on the physiology of fertilization, circulation, and digestion. Spallanzani's studies on the nature of gastric juice produced many discoveries pertaining to its digestive function and the mechanism of its secretion.

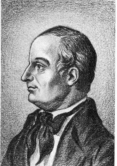

valves of the heart, atrophy of the liver, tuberculosis of the kidney, and lung involvements in respiratory disease. Leopold Auenbrugger (1722–1809) was the first to palpate the chest for diagnosis of disease.

Experimental pathology was developed by John Hunter (1728–1793), who collected pathological specimens, undertook experiments in comparative physiology, analyzed the process of inflammation, and described shock, phlebitis, and pyemia. John Hunter's study of the teeth established a foundation for dentistry.

John Hunter's older brother, William (1718–1783), developed an anatomical theater, museum, and medical school, where he trained the best British anatomists and surgeons of the time. Outstanding was his atlas of the pregnant uterus. William Hunter's efforts did much to establish the excellence of British obstetrics. His teacher, William Smellie (1697–1763), wrote the first treatise which explained the safe use of forceps and the measurement of the pelvis.

Modern embryology had its beginning in the work of Caspar Friedrich Wolff (1733–1794), who extended Harvey's doctrine of the gradual formation of tissues and organs, opposing the theory that the embryo is completely preformed.

A pupil of the Hunters was Matthew Baillie (1761–1823) whose "Morbid Anatomy" is the first modern pathology text. The diseases of each organ of the body were considered with case histories correlated with the results of postmortem examination. Baillie defined cirrhosis of the liver, endocarditis, gastric ulcer, and rheumatic heart disease.

Toward the latter part of the eighteenth century, the major advances in medicine and surgery were made by the English. Students from all parts of the world came to the schools at Edinburgh and London. Teaching was practical and based on experience. William Withering (1741–1799) observed that an herb preparation concocted by an old woman in Shropshire was effective in treatment of dropsical patients. By examining the leaf fragments in the mixture, he identified each plant. He discovered that the effective herb was foxglove, and thus introduced powdered digitalis for treatment of cardiac dropsy. His friend, Edward Jenner (1749–1823), observed that milkmaids who frequently had a mild skin rash (cowpox) were free of smallpox. He undertook the vaccination of patients, using material from the arms of the milkmaids. He demonstrated that vaccination with material from the sore of cowpox protects against smallpox. This idea was accepted in Europe and in America, and the incidence of smallpox declined. While there was opposition to the idea, it established the principle of immunity, and made preventive medicine a possibility.

The outstanding English clinical teacher of the eighteenth century was William Cullen

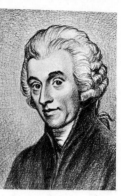

HEBERDEN, William (Senior) (1710-1801) English physician. Chicken pox and smallpox were once thought to be a single disease. It was not until the year 1767 that Heberden showed clearly that the two disorders are distinctly different, and thus paved the way for advances in the treatment of patients suffering from them. He is also noted for his description of angina pectoris, and for the accurate manner in which he described the influenza epidemics of his day.

(1710–1790) who helped to found the Medical School of the University of Glasgow. He introduced hydrotherapy.

William Heberden (1710–1801) wrote on arthritis, night blindness, and angina pectoris. The Quaker friend of America, John Fothergill (1712–1780), helped to found hospitals and wrote on the influence of weather on disease. Caleb H. Parry (1755–1822) gave a definitive account of exophthalmic goiter. Sir John Pringle (1707–1782) established basic principles of military sanitation and assisted in the improvement of hospitals, jails, and barracks. John Howard (1726–1790) made extensive reforms in the management of hospitals and prisons, and in the control of typhus fever.

Meanwhile, pioneering attempts were being made to control mental disorder. The idea that mental illness is a disease rather than demoniac possession was presented by Johann Weyer (1515–1588). The greatest philosopher of the century, Immanuel Kant (1724–1804) undertook a systematic classification of mental disease.

Outstanding in the development of humane psychiatry was Philippe Pinel (1745–1826) of Paris, who worked in hospitals caring for the mentally ill. He rejected the brutal treatment of the mentally ill and demonstrated the value of a kind approach. His contemporary, Anton Mesmer (1734–1815), used "animal magnetism," or hypnotism, with dramatic effects.

During the eighteenth century there were introduced new technical procedures in surgery. Surgery without anesthesia had to be extremely rapid. Percival Pott (1714–1788) made important innovations in surgical procedures, and described cancer resulting from exposure to soot. Jacques Daviel (1696–1762) originated modern treatment of cataract by extraction of the lens. Modern ophthalmology developed through the superb studies of Thomas Young (1773–1829). He described astigmatism, proposed a basic theory of color vision, and made fundamental contributions to optics.

There was also noteworthy progress in medicine in the United States during the eighteenth century. John Morgan (1735–1789) founded the Medical Department of the University of Pennsylvania, and acted as Surgeon General of the American Army. The greatest American physician of the period was Benjamin Rush (1745–1813), a signer of the Declaration of Independence. He gave careful accounts of disease, described dengue fever, and prepared a monograph on insanity. He was particularly interested in yellow fever. He showed that focal infection might cause severe sickness, finding that the extraction of decayed teeth sometimes would relieve distressing symptoms. Benjamin Franklin (1706–1790) also pursued medical interests, inventing bifocal lenses and a flexible catheter, and proposed the treatment of paralysis by electricity. In addition he founded the Pennsylvania Hospital and made observations on gout, sleep, deafness, and the death rate among infants.

NINETEENTH CENTURY MEDICINE

During the Napoleonic wars there was further scientific and medical development in Europe. Dominique Jean Larrey (1766–1842), the surgeon of Napoleon, helped to fill the need for military surgery. He originated first aid for the wounded, introduced army ambulances, and made a pioneer account of "trench foot."

The French clinical school in the nineteenth century was the center of a far-reaching controversy concerning the violent methods of treatment introduced by Francois Joseph Broussais (1772–1838). Broussais recommended such severe methods as vigorous bleeding with leeches, vomiting, purging, and sweating. This reaction was carried to extremes. In Germany, a homeopathic system was developed by Samuel Christian Hahnemann (1755–1843), who advocated the use of minute quantities of drugs.

In Paris, the reaction to the measures advocated by Broussais led Pierre Charles Alexandre Louis (1787–1872) to undertake statistical studies of treatment procedures. This was an important innovation, since it introduced clinical control. Louis proved that bloodletting is of little value in pneumonia, and revived the Hippocratic principle that sick people often get well without treatment.

A contemporary of Louis, René Théophile Hyacinthe Laennec (1781–1826), made extensive studies of the lung and invented the stethoscope in 1819. This instrument enabled Laennec to identify the diagnostic sounds of diseased heart and lungs, to describe pleurisy, lung gangrene, and emphysema, and to give accounts of bronchitis, peritonitis, pneumonia, and tuberculosis.

Laennec's teacher, Marie- François-Xavier Bichat (1771–1802), laid the basis for the study of tissue pathology. He dissected thousands of bodies and classified disease according to the various tissues affected.

The progress of French medicine was advanced by François Magendie (1783–1855), a vigorous investigator of physiology, nerve conduction, and the action of drugs. Magendie discovered the different activities of spinal nerves, showing that some transmit stimuli for sensation, and others, stimuli for muscular movement. In this work his name is associated with that of Sir Charles Bell (1774–1842). There was bitter dispute regarding the credit for this important discovery.

Under the direction of his teacher, Magendie, Claude Bernard (1813–1878) became the leading experimentalist in medical science in the nineteenth century. His outstanding discoveries were concerned with the liver, the pancreas, the sympathetic nervous system, and the internal stability of living bodies. He analyzed the toxic action of carbon monoxide, and investigated the functions of glands of internal secretion. An outstanding student of Bernard, Charles Edouard Brown-Séquard (1818–1894), investigated nerve

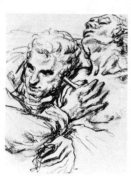

LAENNEC, René Théophile Hyacinthe (1781-1826) French physician. Famous for the invention of the stethoscope, reputedly by using a paper tube to observe the heart sounds of a woman. She would not allow him to place his ear on her chest. While he made other contributions to the knowledge of chest and abdominal disorders, his development of this instrument and its application to diagnosis of disease was his most important.

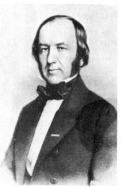

BERNARD, Claude (1813-1878) French physiologist. Famous as one of the greatest physiologists of all time for his introduction of the use of experimental methods. He made many of the first laboratory studies of the action of drugs on the body, and demonstrated the presence of nerves which dilate and contract the blood vessels. He showed that pancreatic juice functions in digestion and that the liver aids in blood sugar control in the animal body.

disorders and studied the effects of removing the adrenal glands. With his investigations on the internal secretion of testes and ovaries, he founded the specialty of endocrinology.

The greatest name in French medicine was Louis Pasteur (1822–1895), a chemist. Pasteur found that the spoilage of wine was caused by microorganisms that grow in the wine. Similarly, he found that beer spoils as a result of contamination with microorganisms. In both cases he observed that heating destroys the organisms. His work resulted in the "germ theory" of disease and the famous process of "pasteurization," which is now used everywhere to assist in preventing disease.

Pasteur made an extensive study of diseases of silkworms in southern France. He found that these diseases could be controlled by keeping the silkworms in a sanitary environment, which inhibited the growth of microorganisms.

Pasteur's first clinical demonstration was concerned with anthrax of sheep. He discovered a motile organism in the blood of diseased sheep and prepared from it a material for vaccination. He predicted that his vaccine could prevent the disease in sheep. The test was completely successful. Pasteur undertook to apply the same principle to rabies, and his success in preventing this disease was dramatic. His most famous case was that of an Alsatian boy, Joseph Meister, who had been bitten by a mad dog. Pasteur undertook the preparation of a vaccine from the brain of the rabid dog. Although filled with fear at the possibility of failure, he injected the vaccine. The child did not develop rabies. After this spectacular success, institutes for the preparation of antirabies vaccine were established all over the world. The bacterial origin of infectious disease was universally accepted, and a new science, bacteriology, was born.

An important result of the science of bacteriology was its application in surgery. Pasteur's discovery made possible the work of Joseph Lister (1827–1912), the Quaker surgeon who had been trained in Scotland. One of the memorable events of medical history was the acknowledgment by Lord Lister of his indebtedness to Pasteur. Lister recognized that pus and suppuration were the chief factors in death following surgery. He recognized that suppuration might result from the contamination of wounds. Accordingly he instituted "antiseptic surgery" in which all instruments were sterilized with carbolic acid. He also applied this disinfectant to wounds and sprayed it in the operating theater. As a result, infections were reduced, and death rates from surgery declined.

The practical success of Lister in reducing surgical infection attracted wide attention to new procedures. In the middle of the nineteenth century childbirth in hospitals was unduly hazardous. Thousands of women throughout Europe

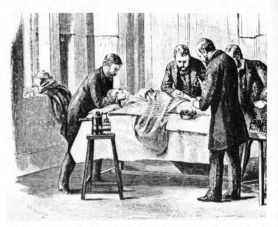

The antiseptic surgery first performed by Lister involved the use of a carbolic acid spray upon the area which was being operated. *Bettmann Archive.*

died mysteriously after childbirth. Women preferred to have their children at home or even in the streets. In Vienna, Ignaz Philipp Semmelweis (1818–1865) became convinced that the women were being infected by the physicians and students who attended them. He tried to institute a system of cleanliness in the obstetrics ward, insisting that all persons who were present at a delivery wash their hands with antiseptic solutions. There was bitter protest. Semmelweis persisted, and the results were startling. Whereas the mortality rate in the other wards continued high, in Semmelweis' group the mortality rate dropped to a low figure. Semmelweis had difficulty persuading physicians that he was correct. He had insulted the medical profession, and its members ridiculed him. Eventually, persecution led to his suicide.

The field of bacteriology was investigated widely by the Germans. Robert Koch (1843–1910) found methods for the isolation of specific microorganisms, so they could be grown in pure culture. Koch introduced the technical methods of bacteriology, and discovered the tuberculosis organism. His vaccine for tuberculosis, however, was not successful. Meanwhile Armauer Hansen

HANSEN, Gerhard Henrik Armauer (1841-1912) Norwegian physician. Hansen is known for his discovery of the microorganism known as *Mycobacterium leprae*, often called *Hansen's bacillus*. Discovered in 1871, it has long been thought to be the causative agent of leprosy. Absolute proof of this relationship is lacking because of the many difficulties attendant upon creating experimental human infections.

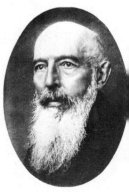

(1841–1912) discovered the organism causing leprosy, and Edwin Klebs (1834–1913) found the club-shaped bacillus which causes diphtheria. Joseph Leidy (1823–1891), of Philadelphia, described intestinal parasites, and began the study of their life cycles. His discovery of *Trichina spiralis* in the muscles of pigs, made possible prevention of trichinosis by cooking all pork products.

German precisionists

Two German workers, Matthias Jakob Schleiden (1804–1881) and Theodor Schwann (1810–1882), worked in the related fields of botany and zoology. They collaborated and published their theory of the cellular organization of living material, giving further impetus to research.

One of the leading nineteenth century microscopists was Johannes Purkinje (1787–1869), who developed the first physiology laboratory. He discovered sweat glands and ducts, and the flask-shaped nerve cells with their branches in the cerebellum. He introduced the classical techniques of microscopy, including the knife for making thin sections, photomicrography, and special fixing agents.

The outstanding physiological teacher of the early nineteenth century was Johannes Muller (1801–1858), professor of anatomy and physiology at the University of Berlin. His pupils were: Ludwig von Helmholtz (1821–1894), who formulated the principles of thermodynamics, invented the ophthalmoscope, and developed the theory of color vision; Emil Du Bois-Reymond (1818–1896), who experimented in electrophysiology and began the study of nerve-muscle physiology; Robert Remak (1815–1865), who found nerve cells in heart and other muscle tissue; Carl Ludwig (1816–1895), who developed graphic methods for recording physiological activity; Albert von Kolliker (1817–1905), who invented new methods for studying cells and organs; and Rudolf Virchow (1821–1902), who applied the cell doctrine to disease, thus making it possible to identify cancer histologically. Virchow showed how to recognize disease in various levels of living material: in cells, tissues, organs, bodies, or even societies. He founded the new science of cellular pathology and his journal, *Virchow's Archiv,* is still a leader in the field.

English medicine

Whereas in the eighteenth century, the major intellectual contribution was Newton's concept of mathematical order in the universe, the chief principle to develop during the nineteenth century was the idea of evolution and change. This theory was advanced in 1859 by Charles Darwin (1809–1882), who prepared his volume, the "Origin of Species," after 20 years of study.

Meanwhile, English physicians added greatly to understanding of special diseases. The London clinicians gave classic descriptions of disease. Outstanding was the discussion of nephritis, the disease of the kidneys usually associated with dropsy, given by Richard Bright (1789–1858); James Parkinson (1755–1824) described shaking palsy; and Charles Bell (1774–1842) defined peripheral paralysis of the facial nerves. Thomas Addison (1793–1860) gave the first clear account of pernicious anemia and tuberculosis of the adrenal glands. Thomas Hodgkin (1798–1866) gave a thorough account of malignant disease involving lymph nodes and the spleen.

It is frequently thought that superior hospital facilities are necessary for major medical advance. This is not always true, as was demonstrated in a Dublin school in the first third of the nineteenth century. With the limited facilities of only six beds in the infirmary, Irish clinicians observed and studied several important diseases. Here, Robert Adams (1791–1875) defined gout, arthritis, and rheumatism. Collaborating with William Stokes (1804–1878) he described the Stokes-Adams syndrome of fainting and heart block. With Robert James Graves (1796–1853) the symptoms of thyroid involvement were analyzed. Dominic Corrigan (1802–1880) described

SCHLEIDEN, Matthias Jakob (1804-1881) German scientist and botanist. He is famous for his important demonstration that the tissues of all plants are structurally composed of cells, and that an increase in the number of the cells brings about the growth process. Theodor Schwann, by analogous investigations performed on animal tissues, was able to show that this same phenomenon was true of animal life, and thus established the cell as the basic living unit.

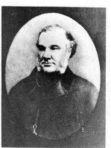

ADDISON, Thomas (1793-1860) English physician, diagnostician, and teacher. His classic description of pernicious anemia, which was published in the year 1849, was so accurate that the condition has since been known as *Addison's anemia.* He performed many important investigations on the nature and function of the ductless glands and contributed greatly to their elucidation. Hypofunction of the adrenal cortex is also known as *Addison's disease.*

insufficiency of cardiac valves and the peculiar pulse associated with it.

Modern surgery and obstetrics were improved by the discovery of anesthesia in the United States, the introduction of antiseptic methods by Joseph Lister in Scotland, and the development of nursing techniques by Florence Nightingale (1820–1910) in England. During the Crimean War, hospital conditions for English soldiers were shockingly inadequate. Dirt, neglect, and stupidity resulted in a heavy toll of life. Almost singlehandedly Florence Nightingale changed this situation, instituting practices of cleanliness, nutrition, and observational care, which have become standard.

Medicine in the United States

Medical progress in the United States developed rapidly during the nineteenth century. Many important surgical innovations were introduced from the new country. In the backwoods of Kentucky, Ephraim McDowell (1771–1830) successfully removed a giant ovarian cyst. One of the most difficult gynecological problems, an opening from the bladder into the vagina, which may occur as a complication of labor was first successfully treated by James Marion Sims (1813–1883), who developed gynecology into an important surgical field.

Extraordinary studies were made by William Beaumont (1785–1853), a U.S. Army Surgeon stationed at Mackinac. Here Beaumont had the opportunity to treat a Canadian voyageur, Alexis St. Martin, who had received a gunshot wound which penetrated the stomach. To Beaumont's surprise, the wound healed, but left an opening into the stomach. Beaumont used the opportunity to study the chemistry of human digestion.

Anesthesia was almost completely an American contribution. Sought by surgeons for centuries, it had been only inadequately provided by wine, whiskey, and opium. Ether had been discovered about 1540 by Valerius Cordus, who recorded its sleep-producing properties. Nitrous oxide was first described around 1800 by

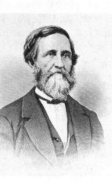

LONG, Crawford Williamson (1815-1878) American physician. Long employed ether in a surgical operation in the year 1842, four years before Morton reported its use in 1846, but failed to publish any reports of its use for many years. He continued to use ether for operative procedures, but did not reveal what he had been doing until 1852. Long's original operation with ether involved removal of a tumor in a man's neck.

Humphry Davy, who noted its pain-relieving properties on inhalation. Chloroform was discovered in 1831 by Samuel Guthrie (1782–1848) of New York. However, physicians failed to appreciate how helpful these anesthetics could be in surgery.

In the United States, chemical shows were popular. Nitrous oxide was used for "laughing gas" parties. Ether was also used for "ether frolics," especially in prohibition areas. In Georgia, the young Philadelphia-trained physician, Crawford W. Long (1815–1878), attended one of these "ether frolics" and noted that those who had inhaled the drug lost consciousness and were oblivious to hurting themselves. Long used ether on March 30th, 1842, during surgery in which he removed tumors from the neck of a friend, James M. Venable. Venable reported that he felt no pain during the operation.

In Hartford, the dentist, Horace Wells (1815–1848) witnessed a "laughing gas" demonstration and decided to administer nitrous oxide for extraction of teeth. Finding this successful, he arranged for a public demonstration of "painless extraction" at the Massachusetts General Hospital. Wells unfortunately had not adequately studied the method of administering nitrous

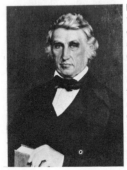

BEAUMONT, William (1785-1853) American Army surgeon. He was the first to be able to study the process of digestion in a living person by virtue of his observations on Alexis St. Martin. The latter had an opening into his stomach as the result of a gunshot wound. Beaumont's studies of gastric juice and the transformation of food in the stomach were of great value to physiology.

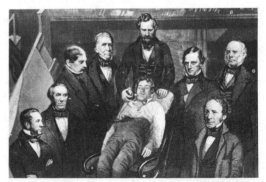

Dr. W. T. Morton, surrounded by the medical staff of Massachusetts General Hospital, demonstrates ether anesthesia in 1846. *Bettmann Archive.*

oxide and withdrew the anesthesia too soon. The patient struggled and screamed, and to the students' derisive shouts of "humbug," Wells withdrew in disgrace.

Wells' fiasco had been witnessed by his partner, William T. G. Morton (1819–1868), who was studying medicine at Harvard Medical School. Morton undertook experiments with ether. When Morton learned how to administer ether satisfactorily, he too arranged a demonstration at the Massachusetts General Hospital. The students had assembled to jeer, but the operation was carried out in complete silence, with the patient suffering no pain or distress. Morton and C. T. Jackson, a chemist (1805–1880), attempted to patent the use of ether, under the name of "Letheon." A bitter dispute followed during which Morton lost his professional prestige, and Wells committed suicide. The term "anesthesia" was coined by Oliver Wendell Holmes (1809–1894), professor of anatomy at Harvard Medical School.

The introduction of anesthesia created a sensation in Europe. The influence of the American surgeon, John Collins Warren (1778–1856), helped to assure Europeans that the procedure was sound. James Young Simpson (1811–1870) of Edinburgh tried ether for relief of pain in childbirth. He found that ether acts too slowly. Following experiments in his own home, using friends and relatives as subjects, he decided to use chloroform. This procedure was successful. Local anesthesia with cocaine was introduced by Karl Koller (1857–1944) in Vienna in 1884.

Outstanding among American contributions to medicine was the establishment of the Library of the Surgeon General's Office, now called the Armed Forces Medical Library. This was the creation of John Shaw Billings (1838–1913). The library contains over a million volumes, and a superb Index Catalogue, enabling physicians all over the world to find reports on medical matters.

The century after the studies of A. L. Lavoisier (1743–1794) was a period of significant advances in the field of chemistry. Humphry Davy (1778–1829) prepared potassium and sodium by electrolysis; Michael Faraday (1791–1867) developed electrochemistry; and Friedrich Wohler (1800–1882) isolated organic urea by synthesis from inorganic materials. The science of organic chemistry was made possible by this intensive experimentation which demonstrated that there is no significant difference between the chemical reactions which occur in living organisms and those which occur in lifeless matter.

The quantitative techniques developed by Lavoisier were applied to medicine by Friedrich Wilhelm Serturner (1783–1841). He extracted a pure crystalline substance from opium. Since this new compound produced sleep, Serturner named it "morphone" after the god of sleep, Morpheus. This was the first alkaloid to be isolated. After this work, François Magendie (1783–1855) analyzed other crude drugs, isolating emetine from ipecac. His associates, Joseph B. Caventou (1795–1877) and Joseph Pelletier (1788–1842) isolated quinine from cinchona bark, strychnine from nux vomica, and other alkaloids from crude plant sources.

James Blake (1815–1893) studied the effects of direct administration of inorganic salts into animals. He also showed that the elements could be classified into families on the basis of their biological action. Blake also studied the rates of absorption of drugs, and made preliminary investigations on the action of various dosages. These principles formed the basis of the science of pharmacology, which is concerned with the action of chemicals on living tissues.

Meanwhile, facilities for medical education in the United States had been expanded. Many medical schools were founded. Often these were staffed with insufficient medical faculties, and the physicians supplemented their incomes through student's fees. This practice resulted in exploitation of medical education and inadequate training. Samuel Brown (1769–1830), of Transylvania University Medical School at Lexington, Kentucky, organized a secret medical fraternity, the Kappa Lambda Society of Aesculapius, for improving medical practice. Chapters were formed in leading American cities. Unfortunately, the power thus assembled was misused, and by 1835 the society had collapsed. However, the need for adequate medical training resulted in the organization of the American Medical Association in 1846. This was accomplished chiefly by Nathan Smith Davis (1817–1904). The purposes of the American Medical Association were to improve the standards of medical education and medical practice. The new organization adopted a code of ethics and gradually exerted its influence to promote satisfactory medical schools.

Medical education had been improved by the

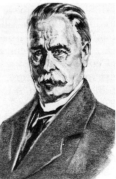

TRENDELENBURG, Friedrich (1844-1924) German surgeon. Noted for his operation for varicose veins of the leg in which the saphenous vein is ligated. He proposed an operation to correct obstruction of urine in the kidney pelvis, and in 1908 attempted to remove a pulmonary embolus, an operation which was not successfully performed until 1924. He devised a test for insufficiency of the valves in varicose veins. *AFML; Copyright 1950, Zeitschrift für artzliche Fortbildung 44:37.*

efforts of President Charles Eliot (1834–1926) of Harvard, who extended the period of medical training from two to three years. In 1893 Johns Hopkins University School of Medicine was established in Baltimore. This school afforded a four-year course of instruction, with a bachelor's degree as a requirement for admission. It set the standard for medical schools, and graduates from Johns Hopkins University became medical leaders in the United States.

The conquest of yellow fever was the most significant event during the latter period of nineteenth century American medicine. Yellow fever had been brought to the Americas by shiploads of infected African slaves. For many years it devastated coastal cities of the United States, and made pestholes of the seaports of Central and South America. During the Spanish-American War, yellow fever was a serious problem among American troops in Cuba. A special commission of the army medical corps was appointed, with Walter Reed (1851–1902) as chairman. Reed studied the theories of the Cuban physician, Carlos Finlay de Barres (1833–1915), who insisted that yellow fever was transmitted by mosquito bites. This theory was tested and proved to be correct. Immediate methods were instituted to control the spread of mosquitoes. The results were impressively effective.

Large-scale methods of mosquito control, by draining swamps and removing places where mosquitoes breed, resulted in the eradication of yellow fever from the New World. Under the direction of William Gorgas (1854–1920), a Surgeon General of the U.S. Army, mosquito control and the prevention of yellow fever made possible the building of the Panama Canal. Methods of sanitation introduced by Gorgas were based on accumulated knowledge of the prevention of infectious diseases, acquired during the nineteenth century.

The close of the century also was marked by the beginning of the conquest of malaria, which had taken a heavy toll of life all over the world for centuries. There is evidence that it may have contributed to the decline of some of the powerful Mediterranean civilizations. Medical writers have discussed this possibility frequently, and various theories have been developed. The introduction of cinchona bark in the seventeenth century, and the isolation of quinine from the bark in the nineteenth, had provided a semblance of control. However, such measures were effective only as a cure, but not as a preventive. Little was known of the cause of the disease until Ronald Ross (1857–1932) found malaria organisms in the red blood cells. He traced the course of the parasite, and confirmed its transmission by mosquitoes. Thus, mosquito eradication became one of the most important measures in the field of preventive medicine during the twentieth century.

TWENTIETH CENTURY MEDICINE

It has been said that there have been more advances in medicine in the past 100 years than in the 500 years before that, and that there were more advances in that 500 years than in the preceding 5000 years. The twentieth century may prove to be the golden age of medicine. The result of all this progress has been added years to the life of the individual. In 1900, for example, the average life expectancy in the United States was 47 years; in 1950, it was 68 years.

Today the danger of infectious diseases has been greatly reduced. As medical scientists have made discoveries to combat these diseases, the medical profession and public health agencies have applied the knowledge on a nationwide scale. For instance, when it was found that goiter was caused by a lack of iodine, authorities decreed that iodine should be added to table salt. Likewise, vitamins were added to bread, margarine, and other common foods.

Diagnosis and disease

Until 1900, bacteria were considered the prime causes of disease. Since then, research in biochemistry has uncovered elusive viruses and has separated disease-causing agents from harmless bacteria. Just as important, advances in the study of physiology have attained greater knowledge of the life processes in the cell, tissue, organ, and organism. Many inflammatory diseases have been clarified, genetic disorders found, and the metabolic factors in disease development recognized. The field of immunology, so important to transplantation as well as treatment of infectious disease and cancer, belongs to this century.

The development of the electron microscope has been a key factor in twentieth century discoveries. This instrument magnifies up to 60,000 times, allowing scientists to study viruses, details in cellular structure, and giant molecules.

Research in biochemistry and physiology has gained knowledge of the range of normal limits of metabolic reactions to many stimuli, thus making possible tests for hundreds of diseases and disorders. Analysis of body fluids, blood, urine, and amniotic fluid, yields information on present and past diseases as well as allergies and basic disorders. Knowing cellular structure enables doctors to gain genetic information that may aid in family planning.

Advances in diagnostic techniques

One of the major developments in diagnosis during the twentieth century was the test for syphilis devised by the German scientist, August von Wassermann (1866–1925), in 1906. This test has perhaps been more effective in the control of syphilis than any other single factor.

Of even more importance in diagnosis was the discovery and development of x-ray, which make it possible for the physician to observe disease processes located deep within the body; x-ray use in treatment is discussed in another part of this chapter.

Preoperative diagnosis of brain diseases was virtually impossible before the twentieth century. Then, W. E. Dandy (1886–1946), a Baltimore surgeon, developed a technique for localizing brain tumors in 1918; his method consisted of injecting air into the skull cavity, followed by x-ray studies of the brain *(pneumoventriculography)*. Injection of the brain arteries with an opaque fluid which can be discerned on x-ray film *(cerebral arteriography)* was done by the Portuguese surgeon, A. C. Egas Moniz (b. 1874), in 1927. Two years later, the German neuropsychiatrist, Hans Berger (1873–1941) introduced a method of recording electric brain waves graphically *(electroencephalography)*, thereby locating abnormalities in the brain.

Sophistication of these techniques has led to the use of radioactive isotopes, which, when injected with a dye into an organ or the circulation of the brain, gives an accurate picture on x-ray film of the smallest vessels. Isotopes can also be injected via the spinal column to watch the movement of fluid through the brain ventricles to differentiate circulating hydrocephalus, or blocked flow, from atrophy associated with senility.

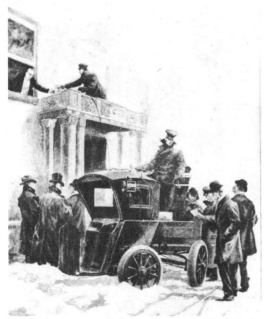

New York surgeons of 1903 using automobile batteries to run an x-ray machine in a patient's house that was without electricity. *Bettmann Archive.*

Of equal significance was the development of tubes *(endoscopes)* with which the physician is able to study various internal organs of the body. The use of endoscopes was popularized by a French scientist, Raoul Bensaude (1866–1938), and the American physician, Chevalier Jackson (1865–1957). Endoscopes were devised much earlier but were limited in their usefulness until proper lighting became available. Dr. Jackson devised an endoscope for study of the esophagus *(esophagoscope)* in 1902, and later one for the diagnosis of diseases in the lungs *(bronchoscope)*. A *sigmoidoscope,* through which the diagnostician can observe the large bowel, was perfected by Hermann Strauss (Germany, 1868–1944), in 1910. Intubation of the intestine was accomplished by a tube designed by Thomas G. Miller (b. 1886), and William O. Abbott (1902–1943), both of Philadelphia.

The early diagnosis of cancer has been a goal of medicine in the twentieth century, and the discovery of x-ray, of course, has been of invaluable aid. More recently, a method of smearing suspicious areas and studying the cells rubbed off has been introduced by George Papanicolaou (1883–1962) of New York. Of equal importance was the contribution of another American, Louis B. Wilson in 1905; he introduced a method by which pieces of suspicious areas could be frozen at operation and then studied under the microscope immediately. If the tissue proves to be cancerous, the surgeon may then carry out a radical operation.

Radioactive isotopes can also be traced by x-rays when injected into the blood system, through the heart and related vessels to provide an *arteriogram.*

Another diagnostic tool for cancer is the *thermogram,* a form of *mammography*. This means getting a picture of the soft tissue of the breast through heat intensity registered on heat-sensitive film. Tumors are warmer than normal tissue. A process called *xerography* will also take a picture of soft tissue through a special process based on the principle of the Xerox office machine.

Every doctor now has available a laboratory equipped to run hundreds of tests, primarily from samples of a patient's blood and urine. For some early stages of disease, such as diabetes, a urine analysis is the only way to get a diagnosis. For other diseases, the new tests give a more complete view of the patient's condition, or confirm diagnosis. It is now also possible to measure antibody levels (titers) in blood to determine whether the patient ever contracted or is immune to a variety of infectious diseases.

Blood tests can yield diagnosis of hepatitis and some forms of early cancer, as well as anemia and poisoning.

Tests run on newborn children also use urine to find inborn metabolic disorders such as phenyl ketonuria (PKU) which, if not corrected by diet, result in mental retardation.

Early diagnosis of pregnancy was made possible through the development of several "pregnancy tests." Chief among these is that developed by Bernhard Zondek (1891–1966) and Selmar Aschheim (b. 1878) in 1928, and modified by Maurice H. Friedman (b. 1903) in 1929. (See Chapter 1, "Life Begins," for modern pregnancy tests.)

More accurate diagnosis of disorders of the heart and circulatory system became possible in this century. The taking of a patient's blood pressure has become a routine procedure in the past 50 years, and this technique affords the physician valuable information about the patient's circulatory system. The *electrocardiograph*, a device which graphically records the patient's heartbeat and registers any abnormalities present, was invented by Willem Einthoven (The Netherlands, 1860–1927), in 1903. Walter Forssmann, in 1929, passed a catheter through a vein in the right arm into the heart in order to analyze the blood in the heart and to reveal any congenital defects. A technique which permitted calculation of the output and work of the heart *(ballistocardiography)* was developed by Isaac Starr (b. 1895) in 1937.

Advances in medical treatment

The twentieth century has been a period of revolutionary change in medical therapy. Before 1900, there were few drugs which were specific treatment for specific diseases. Moreover, the physician had to mix his own drugs in most cases. However, the drug industry has become one of the largest industries in the United States. Today, the strength and purity of drugs are rigidly standardized. Much of the research that goes into discovery of new drugs is carried on by the drug industry. After a new substance has proved useful in treatment, the drug companies

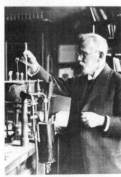

EHRLICH, Paul (1854-1915) German bacteriologist and pathologist. Ehrlich was a pioneer in the fields of bacteriology, immunology and chemotherapy. Ehrlich's discovery of the drug 606 or arsphenamine for the treatment of syphilis, marked the beginning of the long battle to eliminate venereal disease. Ehrlich made many other contributions to medicine, among which were his methods of tissue staining, and the differential blood-count. *Bettmann Archive.*

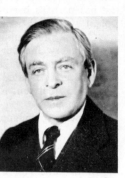

FUNK, Casimir (1884-1967) American biochemist. One of the first investigators of the vitamins and originator of the term because of his belief that the substance that he was studying was a *vital amine.* He investigated the nutritional basis of beriberi by carefully studying the deficiency produced by feeding pigeons upon a polished rice diet, and was able to isolate from rice polishings a curative substance which is now known as vitamin B1, or thiamine.

use their industrial skills to make the drug available at a practical price.

The method of research whereby most drugs are developed was introduced in 1910 by a German scientist, Paul Ehrlich (1854–1915). Dr. Ehrlich tested several hundred substances, all of which had similar chemical composition, in order to find a drug specific for syphilis. On his 606th attempt, he produced an arsenic compound which was effective against the disease; he called the new drug *salvarsan.* He continued his studies, and developed another antisyphilitic drug, *neosalvarsan,* which is less toxic than the original substance.

Hookworm disease is another illness for which a cure has been found in this century. Maurice C. Hall (1881–1938), an American physician, in 1921 found that carbon tetrachloride eliminates the hookworm parasites. At about the same period, scientists began to note that many diseases had a metabolic origin and could be cured by alteration of the diet or by administration of metabolic substances. The first vitamin was named by Casimir Funk (1884–1967) in 1911. Vitamins A and B were discovered as the result of investigations in the United States by E. V. McCollum (b. 1879), T. B. Osborn (1859–1929), and L. B. Mendel (1872–1935). F. Gowland Hopkins (1861–1947) of England and Christian Eijkman (1858–1930) of Utrecht shared the Nobel Prize in 1929, the former for his discovery of growth-promoting vitamins and the latter for isolation of the antineuritic vitamin. Today, more than 30 vitamins have been discovered. Pernicious anemia, a disease which was usually fatal, was successfully combated by three Americans, George R. Minot (1855–1950), George H. Whipple (b. 1878), and W. P. Murphy (b. 1892), who administered liver extracts to their patients.

Many therapeutic substances used today are either actual or synthesized hormones of the endocrine system. The science of endocrinology has had almost all of its development within this century. Researchers learned the secretions of the various endocrine glands, classified the actions of the hormones, and isolated and synthesized the hormones for use in therapy and for further research. Perhaps the most far-reaching discovery in endocrinology was made by two Canadians, Frederick G. Banting (1891–1941) and Charles H. Best (b. 1899), who in 1922 isolated insulin from the pancreas and used the substance in treatment of diabetic patients; for details on Banting's and Best's work, see Chapter 10, "The Endocrine System."

Another important discovery in endocrinology was the isolation by another Canadian, J. B. Collip (1892–1965), of a hormone of the pituitary gland which acts to cause secretion of an important hormone of the adrenal gland; this pituitary substance is called *ACTH (adrenocorticotrophic hormone)*. In 1936, the adrenal hormone itself was isolated by an American group: H. L. Mason, C. S. Myers, and E. C. Kendall; this hormone is called *cortisone*. The true significance of *ACTH* and cortisone has not yet been determined. At present they are being used as research tools and in the therapy of patients with such diseases as rheumatoid arthritis and rheumatic fever. Endocrine hormones are also used in treating cancer patients. An American physician, Charles Huggins (b. 1901), found that prostatic cancer growth was stimulated by male hormones, and he recommended the use of female hormones in treating persons with this disease. Likewise, male hormones may be employed to treat women with cancer of the breast.

Since ACTH was found, six other hormones in the pituitary have been isolated, including the growth hormone, and substances that stimulate the processes of the sex glands. Once the hormones are isolated and the molecular structure understood, the next step is artificial production of the hormones for treatment.

Several new drugs have been developed for palliative therapy of persons with another cancerous disease, *leukemia*. Alexander Haddow of England introduced *urethane* in 1946 for use in these patients, and the American, Sidney Farber (b. 1903), recommended *folic acid antagonists* for persons with specific forms of leukemia. Recently, *nitrogen mustard*, a chemical "cousin" of wartime mustard gas, has been administered to patients with leukemia and similar diseases.

Heart disease has become the leading killer among diseases in the twentieth century, so that a great deal of research has been undertaken to discover drugs to combat heart disorders. In 1912, James B. Herrick (1861–1954), an American, described the symptoms of heart attack (*myocardial infarction*). *Anticoagulant* drugs—that is, drugs which prevent clotting of the blood within the heart arteries—are important substances in therapy of patients with myocardial infarction. The first major anticoagulant, *heparin*, was isolated in 1917 by a Baltimore scientist, Jay McLean (b. 1890). An anticoagulant that can be taken orally was developed by an American, Paul Link (b. 1901), in 1941; this was *dicumarol*. Dicumarol was discovered as the result of an epidemic of bleeding in cattle. Dr. Link noted that the cattle which were bleeders all fed on a specific form of clover; he isolated the anticoagulant substance from the clover. Two other drugs important in heart disease are *quinidine*, developed by a Dutch physician, Karel F. Wenckebach (1864–1940), in 1903, and the drug *novasurol* for persons with dropsy (*cardiac edema*), perfected in 1920 by two German physicians, Paul S. Saxl (1880–1932) and Robert Heilig. An outstanding adjunct to the treatment of heart disease was the development of the electronic *pacemaker,* a device which keeps the patient's heart beating in rhythm.

Tuberculosis has eluded several drug treatments applicable only to certain groups of patients. Today, the drug *Isoniazid* is recognized as generally effective in treatment and prevention among high-risk people who are positive reactors to the tuberculin skin test but show no signs of the disease.

The phenomenon of *allergy* to specific substances was first recognized in this century. Jokichi Takamine (1854–1922), a Japanese-American, isolated *adrenalin* in 1901, and today this substance is widely used for patients with bronchial asthma. Another American pioneer in the study of allergy was Warren Taylor Vaughan (1893–1944), who studied especially the allergic causation of migrane headaches and food allergies. Perhaps the most publicized drugs for allergic patients have been the *antihistamines;* these drugs help relieve certain of the symptoms of allergy.

The symptoms of epilepsy, a syndrome without a defined disease entity, which accompanies a variety of illnesses, have come under effective control with a variety of drugs used in differing mixtures and strengths according to severity and type of symptoms.

In pediatrics, W. Gaisford and D. G. Evans in 1949 reported on the use of *hyaluronidase,* an enzyme which renders connective tissue more permeable. The substance is used as an aid to parenteral administration of fluids to infants and young children.

Many infectious diseases have been rendered harmless in this century, chiefly as the result of the discovery of the *sulfonamide* drugs and the *antibiotic* drugs. The first sulfonamide drug was synthesized by P. Gelmo of Vienna in 1908, but attracted little attention until used therapeutically by Gerhard Domagk (1895–1964) of Germany in 1932. Unfortunately, this group of drugs is highly toxic and must be given with the greatest of caution. The antibiotic drugs, however, have little toxicity. The first of these, *penicillin,* was

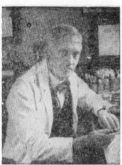

FLEMING, Sir Alexander (1881-1955) English physician. Famous for his discovery of penicillin and his isolation of it in the year 1929. The development of this substance, based upon studies of antagonisms between various microorganisms, initiated the vast research that has since been devoted to the search for new antibiotics. In the year 1945 he was awarded the Nobel prize with his associates, Drs. Florey and Chain.

discovered in 1929 by Sir Alexander Fleming (1881–1955) of London, who observed that the growth of a culture of bacteria was inhibited after the culture had been accidentally contaminated by a fungus growth. He isolated the antibacterial product of the fungus and named it penicillin. Little further work was done until 1938, when an Oxford pathologist, Sir Howard W. Florey (1898–1968) followed up Fleming's work and carried out research which has led to the discovery of other antibiotic drugs. Today, penicillin is used to combat a large number of infectious diseases. Before penicillin was discovered, the heart disease called *subacute bacterial endocarditis* was almost invariably fatal; today, 60 to 70 percent of patients with this disease survive. Penicillin is also used *prophylactically* to prevent infection during dental extractions, childbirth, or major or minor surgery. Another antibiotic drug, *streptomycin*, is used in treating patients with tuberculosis and various other infectious diseases. *Aureomycin, chloramphenicol,* and *terramycin* can all be taken orally and used in treating patients who do not respond to penicillin therapy.

One of the most widespread communicable diseases, *malaria,* was at one time thought successfully conquered in this century. *Quinine* was used to treat malaria patients for many years. Two other drugs were also developed, *atabrine* and *plasmochin*. However, drug-resistant strains of malarial agents have evolved in the Far East and South America for which drugs have not been found.

Nondrug, immunologic treatment of disease has been developed with new knowledge of the immunologic responses of the body. This has made possible reinforcing the body's reaction to antigens (disease-causing particles or their by-products) by strengthening the host response in cancer treatment, especially for cancer of the colon and skin (malignant melanoma). Some allergies can be overcome by desensitizing procedures aimed at stimulating the host-response mechanism.

Prevention of disease

Development of a strong public health system involving quarantine, early warnings of epidemics, and enforcement of immunization laws has greatly reduced the threat of worldwide pandemics. The World Health Organization, set up in 1948 by the United Nations members, has saved untold lives through its network of disease-reporting stations around the world. Headquartered in Geneva, Switzerland, WHO has five regional offices co-ordinating public health information and supplying medical staff and education for underdeveloped nations.

The prime weapon in prevention is vaccine for children. In addition to the classic vaccine for smallpox, developed in the last century, researchers have now perfected vaccines for typhoid fever, tetanus, whooping cough, cholera, some forms of influenza, rubella, mumps, poliomyelitis, and diphtheria. Immunization against diphtheria was developed by Emil A. von Behring (Germany, 1854–1917), Gaston Ramon (France, 1885–1963), and W. H. Park (United States, 1863–1939); and a skin test to determine diphtheria susceptibility was devised by a U.S. pediatrician, Bela Schick (1877–1967), in 1913.

Viral vaccine development has progressed most since the 1930s, after a yellow fever vaccine was produced by Max Theiler (b. 1899). In 1954, Jonas E. Salk (b. 1914) introduced a vaccine for poliomyelitis and an oral poliomyelitis vaccine was developed by Albert B. Sabin (b. 1906). Both mumps and rubella vaccines were developed by teams of virologists and tested by the U.S. Food and Drug Administration in the late 1960s. Measles vaccines were licensed in 1963.

Advances in surgery

With the development of measures to prevent and treat surgical shock, and measures to prevent infection made possible by the antibiotic drugs, many surgical operations that were not attempted in the previous century are being performed routinely today. Many patients who were formerly considered unfavorable surgical risks now undergo surgery with few undesirable consequences. Individualized anesthesia with newly developed substances has been a major reason for these surgical advances. Today, anesthetic substances are carefully mixed to fit the needs of each patient. Localized anesthesia, spinal and caudal anesthesia, and intravenous anesthesia are also products of the twentieth century.

Another reason for the improvement of surgical results has been the aseptic techniques developed in the nineteenth century. To these was added the use of sterile rubber gloves during operations; this practice was instituted by W. S. Halsted (1852–1922), a top-ranking American surgeon who also made many other contributions to surgical technique. Two other notable American surgeons of this century were W. J. (1861–1939) and C. H. Mayo (1865–1939), who founded an excellent clinic for all branches of medicine. They established the importance of a thorough general medical examination regardless of the patient's complaint.

Perhaps the chief reason for surgical deaths before 1900 was surgical shock. This phenomenon was carefully investigated by many researchers, including George Crile (1864–1943) of Cleveland, D. B. Phemister (1882–1951) and Alfred Blalock (1899–1964). These men noted that the addition of new blood by transfusion would often prevent shock. However, surgeons noted that death often resulted from the transfusion itself. In 1902, Karl Landsteiner (1868–1943), an Austrian-American scientist, described blood grouping and stressed the importance of having the donor and recipient of the blood be of the same blood type. Landsteiner was also codiscoverer of the Rh blood factor, with A. S. Wiener (United States, b. 1907) in 1940. The problem of clotting during blood transfusions was overcome by a method introduced by two Americans, A. R. Kimpton (b. 1881) and J. H. Brown (1884–1956), in 1913. Later Richard Lewisohn (1875–1961) of New York advised adding sodium citrate to the blood, which eliminated clotting. Another significant advance was achieved by an American biochemist, L. F. Shackell (b. 1887), in 1909 when he introduced a method of converting blood to powdered plasma. However, plasma was not used extensively until popularized by Max M. Strumia (b. 1896), an Italian-American, in 1938. The first blood bank was established in 1937 at the Cook County Hospital in Chicago.

Surgery of the lungs, heart, and other organs of the chest cavity was not feasible for many years, because the lungs would collapse immediately after the chest was opened. Ernst Ferdinand Sauerbruch devised the first low-pressure chamber to be used in thoracic surgery. In 1909, two Americans, S. J. Meltzer (1851–1920) and J. Auer (1875–1948), devised a technique which allowed respiration to be maintained by introducing air into the lungs under positive pressure through a tube in the trachea; anesthesia also may be administered intratracheally. Immediately thereafter, surgery of the chest and lung became routine. In 1931, Rudolph Nissen (German-American, b. 1896) was successful in removing a patient's entire diseased lung. Dr. Alexis Carrel (France) made heart surgery possible by perfecting a method of *anastomosis*, or joining of two ends of a blood vessel with very fine needles, and ·pointed the way to future transplantations by his experiments with dogs and cats in 1906.

Heart surgery techniques were developed in the next decades, based on more sophisticated methods of surgery. In 1938, Robert E. Gross, (United States, b. 1905) performed the first successful operation for an open ductus arteriosus; and two Americans, Helen Taussig (b. 1898) and Alfred Blalock (1899–1964) devised a procedure to correct a congenital heart defect known as the *tetralogy of Fallot,* in which the arteries supplying the heart are reversed.

Closed heart surgery, which did not touch the interior of the chambers of the organ, progressed into the 1950s with many new operations for artery and valve repairs.

However, the development of a heart-lung machine which pumped blood to the lungs and provided circulation to the entire body while bypassing the heart, eventually made *open heart surgery* possible. Although the concept of such a machine was recorded as early as 1813, actual clinical trials were first conducted in 1937 by J. H. Gibbon, Jr., of Jefferson Medical College of Philadelphia, and advanced, with modifications, by researchers at the University of Minnesota. Patches on the inside of chamber walls, placement of artificial valves, and ultimately, whole-heart human transplants became possible. Another technique for surgery, called *hypothermia,* where the patient's body temperature is lowered to utilize less oxygen, is also used for heart surgery as well as other major organ repair.

Several operations were developed at the same time for hypertension. Locating weak spots in vessel walls and repairing them was advanced by Michael E. DeBakey to prevent strokes. Several methods for reaming out vessels clogged with fatty deposits have been used, notably one by Dr. Adrian Kantrowicz, in which a balloon catheter is inserted into the vein or artery. Microvascular surgery was developed by Julius Jacobson, to repair the small vessels of the brain and eye. Dr. Charles Hufnagel developed plastic prostheses for correcting aortic insufficiency, as well as homologous, heterologous graft replacements for great vessels.

Organ transplants were first experimentally done on animals by a German, Emerich Ullmann, in 1902. However, not until extensive work was done by Willem Kolff of the Netherlands in 1944 on *dialysis,* or constructing an artificial kidney, did scientists explore human kidney transplants. Their knowledge of the patient's reaction to the graft was based on skin grafting, and new advances in blood and tissue typing.

The first series of kidney transplants was performed by David Hume, George Thorn, and John Merrill of Peter Bent Brigham Hospital in Boston. Since then, hundreds of patients have received human donor kidneys, as well as pancreases, livers, and hearts, with varying degrees of success. The first human heart transplant was performed by Christiaan Barnard (b. 1922)

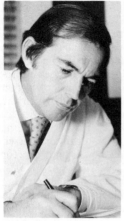

BARNARD, Christiaan Neethling (b. 1922) South African heart surgeon. He is most famous for his many transplantations of human hearts to patients in whom heart failure was imminent, and was the first in the world to perform the operation successfully. Advancement of surgical techniques in this operation are far ahead of intensive efforts to solve the perplexing problems of rejection of the transplanted organ by the patient's own immune defense mechanism.

COOLEY, Denton A. (b. 1920) American heart surgeon. He has written extensively on the development of a disposable heart-lung machine and was one of the first surgeons to institute the hemodilution technique for open heart surgery. Also, he was the first surgeon in the world to transplant an artificial heart into a human being (1969). Use of an artificial heart is so far only a temporary emergency measure used in patients who need a heart transplantation and for whom a donor heart is not immediately available.

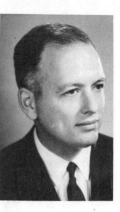

in 1967 in Capetown, South Africa. Drugs to combat the rejection of the transplanted organs have been developed, notably *Immuran* and anti-lymphocyte serum. But difficulties in finding and typing donors, cadavers for heart transplants and living relatives for kidney patients, has slowed the pace of transplantation. Lung transplants have never proved successful, because of that organ's extreme vascularity. Heart surgery has also developed the team method for operations in the past decades, a trend away from the single master surgeon concept of the nineteenth century.

Artificial assists for hearts during surgery and after have been pioneered by Michael E. DeBakey, Baylor College of Medicine, with the technical assistance of Dr. Domingo Liotta. In 1966, the first partial artificial heart, a left ventricular bypass machine, implanted half in and half out of the patient's body, was used. DeBakey also developed a total artificial heart. An artificial heart was first used briefly in a patient by Denton Cooley.

Another artificial organ, the *dialysis* machine, is now used widely to help kidney patients who have lost function in one or both kidneys. In

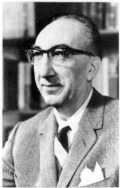

DE BAKEY, Michael Ellis (b. 1908) American cardiovascular surgeon. Most noted for his work in the development of an artificial heart, he also devised a roller type pump later used in heart-lung machines and he performed the first successful carotid endarterectomy in 1953. He pioneered in developing the use of Dacron tubing as replacements for blood vessels and surgical techniques for removing aneurysms from weakened aortas.

dialysis, patients are hooked up to the machine via a blood vessel in the arm or leg, and the blood is cycled through several membranes in the machine to remove waste products and then returned to the body through another vessel.

Because of the discovery of insulin, it has become possible to remove the pancreas, for cancer or other disease, and to keep the patient healthy on substitution insulin therapy. This operation was developed as the result of experiments and investigations carried out by the American surgeon, Allen O. Whipple (1881–1963) and his associates. The first total pancreatectomy was performed in 1943, by Alexander Brunschwig. Surgery of the thyroid was developed along the same lines, and the first excision of the thyroid gland was performed by Theodor Kocher (1841–1917), a Swiss surgeon.

Surgery of the brain is almost entirely a product of the twentieth century. The most eminent of all brain surgeons, Harvey Cushing (1869–1939), found that antemortem diagnosis of brain tumor was made in only 32 cases out of 36,000, before he entered the specialty; furthermore, most patients who did submit to a brain operation died. Cushing developed new techniques and instruments for brain tumor diagnosis and brain surgery, and achieved an operative mortality rate of only 8.7 percent. As the result of his work, brain surgery became practiced more widely, and patients who need brain operations are no longer regarded as hopeless. Another great aid to brain surgery was the development of an electric cutting instrument, which forestalled bleeding. Recent inventions, such as the use of Teflon for artificial shunts and surgical use of supercold probes (*cryosurgery*) have added to the sophistication of brain operations.

Delicate techniques for surgery of the eye have also been introduced in this century. At the turn of the century, Arthur von Hippel (1841–1917), Fritz A. Salzer (b. 1867), and S. Calderaro, each working independently, successfully carried out corneal transplantation. An operation for detachment of the retina was devised by Jules Gonin (1870–1935). Surgical operation for removal of a cataract was made possible by the development of specialized forceps with which the eye can be immobilized.

Many operations for the eradication of cancer have been developed; two of the most notable are the radical operation for cancer of the rectum, devised by the English surgeon, William E. Miles (1869–1947) in 1907, and the radical removal of the uterus for cancer of the cervix, worked out by Ernst Wertheim (1864–1920) of Vienna in 1900. Since 1940, massive visceral resections have been successfully carried out. The entire contents of the pelvis, that is, the bladder, rectum, vagina, uterus, and all soft tissues have been removed in cases of advanced cancer. Some of these patients have survived five years, without recurrence of disease.

Another recent surgical machine, the *hyperbaric chamber*, may improve the results of radiation treatment. A cylindrical chamber encloses the patient and saturates the tissues with oxygen to destroy organisms that only grow in the oxygen-free interior of the body (anaerobic organisms). Gas gangrene is an instance requiring the special chamber.

Advances in plastic and orthopedic surgery

The two World Wars afforded unusual opportunities for improvements in the field of plastic surgery. In 1917, the tubed pedicle flap, basis for most plastic operations, was devised independently by V. Filatov (b. 1875) of Russia and Sir Harold Gillies (1882–1960) of England. A practical *dermatome* to remove skin from one area for grafting on another was invented by E. C. Padgett (1893–1946) of Kansas City in 1939; and refrigerated skin grafts were first used by J. P. Webster (b. 1888) of New York in 1944. For arm amputees, an American, H. H. Kessler (b. 1896) developed an operation (the *cineplastic* operation) which permits the mechanical arm or hand to be manipulated by those muscles which performed the action of the normal hand.

Bone grafts were first brought into practical use by an American surgeon, F. H. Albee (1876–1945) in 1911, and today there are many bone banks. Other orthopedic developments include: an operation to lengthen the shorter of two uneven legs, devised by LeRoy Abbott (United States, b. 1890) in 1927; underwater exercises for poliomyelitis patients, advised by C. L. Lowman (United States, b. 1879) and made popular by Franklin D. Roosevelt; and the use of the *intramedullary nail* for long-bone fractures by Gerhard Kuntscher (b. 1902) in 1940 and a similar procedure for hip fractures by M. N. Smith-Petersen (1886–1953) of Boston.

Recently, several lightweight but strong materials have been developed to make prosthetics, or artificial limbs, with the greatest amount of natural articulation possible. An aluminum ball-joint has been constructed as an artificial hip.

Advances in radiology

Radiology is a science of the twentieth century. X-rays were discovered by Wilhelm C. von Roentgen (1845–1923) in Germany in 1895, and his great find was immediately pressed into use. The rays were first used in treatment by E. H. Grubbe (1875–1960) of Chicago in 1896 on a patient with breast cancer. Because Grubbe was a layman, credit for having treated cancer successfully for the first time is given to T. A. U. Sjögren (1859–1939) of Sweden, who applied the rays to a cancer patient in 1899. Guido Holzknecht (1872–1931) of Vienna, who later died of an x-ray-induced cancer, devised an instrument for measuring x-ray dosage and helped establish the measuring unit for x-rays.

Because so many bad results occurred after initial trials of x-rays, they fell into disuse for therapy. Then, in 1913, the American scientist, William D. Coolidge (b. 1873), invented a tube which better controlled the output, thereby reviving the therapeutic use of x-rays. The machine used by Roentgen to produce the first x-rays was probably a 50 kilovolt unit. The early units used in therapy involved an exposure period of nearly an hour and often as many as 80 sittings. A multisection type of Coolidge tube was developed, capable of operation at any

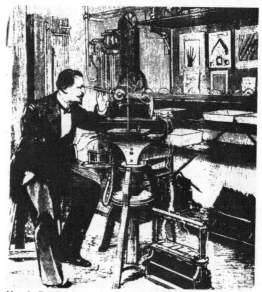

Henri Becquerel at work in his laboratory. He discovered the radioactivity of uranium and received the Nobel prize with the Curies. *Bettmann Archive.*

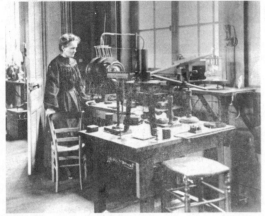

Photograph of the codiscoverer of radium, Madame Curie, at work in her laboratory in France about 1905. *Courtesy of Bettmann Archive.*

voltage, no matter how high, and this led to the development of higher energy units. In the 1920s, machines which produced hundreds of thousands of volts were developed, and by the end of the decade, there were several one million volt units in operation. Today, two million volt units are quite common, and a 70 million volt apparatus is available. X-rays are now being used to treat patients with diseases located in almost every organ of the body.

Shortly after Roentgen's discovery, a French physicist, Henri Becquerel (1852–1908), undertook several experiments to determine whether the fluorescent substances which glowed on exposure to x-rays might not themselves emit rays. In the course of these experiments, he found that radiation was emitted from uranium with or without previous exposure to x-rays or light. He mentioned this discovery to Marie Curie (1867–1934) and aroused her interest. She and her husband, Pierre (1859–1906), worked with uranium ore for some time, and finally succeeded in isolating a new element, *radium,* in 1898.

In 1901, Becquerel carried some of the radium salts in his vest pocket, and found that an ulcer was produced on the skin under the pocket. Pierre Curie was intrigued by this and purposely burned himself on the arm with radium. Believing the element could be used therapeutically, the Curies lent Henri Danlos (1844–1932) a supply of radium to be used for the first time in treatment. Then, in 1903, S. W. Goldberg and E. S. London announced that they had successfully treated a cancer patient with the new element. Two years later, Robert Abbe (1851–1928) of New York implanted radium needles into a tumor for the first time. Seeds containing the radioactive gas, *radon,* emitted by radium were first used in 1908. Later, large supplies of radium were placed in a radium "bomb," and the result was a beam of radiation similar to that of x-rays.

The most recent development in radiology has been the use of radioactive isotopes in research, diagnosis, and treatment. The use of these substances as a tool for the investigation of living organisms was begun nearly 40 years ago when a Hungarian-Swedish chemist, Georg von Hevesy (1885–1966), first used the naturally occurring radioisotope of lead (radium D) to find out how plants made use of this element. Irene Curie (b. 1897), daughter of Marie and Pierre, and her husband, Frederic Joliot (1900–1958), discovered in 1931 that ordinary elements could be converted into their radioactive isotopes. It was not long until radioactive isotopes could be formed from nearly all of the elements, including those that occur in biological material. Radioactive iodine was first used by the American researcher, Saul Hertz (b. 1905) and his associates, who showed that 80 times more iodine was concentrated in the thyroid than in any other normal tissue. Similar work was done by Mayo Hamilton Soley (b. 1907). J. H. Lawrence (b. 1904) and his co-workers used radioactive phosphorus in the treatment of a patient with leukemia in 1939.

Unfortunately, the production of these isotopes was highly expensive and had to be carried out with a cyclotron. In 1942, an Italian-American, Enrico Fermi (1901–1954) and co-workers devised the *atomic pile,* which made it possible to produce isotopes for a fraction of their former cost, and which led to the development of the atomic bomb. Radioactive cobalt has been used as a substitute for radium, and a cobalt irradiator was designed by Gilbert Fletcher (b. 1911) and Leonard G. Grimmett (1902–1951) of Houston, Texas, and Marshall Brucer (b. 1913) of the Oak Ridge Institute of Nuclear Studies. Their work in perfecting the design of the cobalt therapy machine opened a new era of cancer treatment; today there are more than 1200 refined cobalt-60 units in the world.

The linear accelerator, the latest and most powerful in cancer treatments, makes it possible to treat patients with large areas of malignancy. It can also be quickly adapted to treat either superficial cancers or tumors deep in the body. In addition, it makes possible treatment for malignant diseases with minimum damage to the surrounding normal tissues.

Advances in psychiatry

Psychiatry is another science which has had almost its entire development in the twentieth century. The most important single man in the history of psychiatry is Sigmund Freud (1856–1939) of Austria. Among innumerable other contributions, he developed the technique of *psychoanalysis* to treat emotionally disturbed patients. His work has been carried on and improved upon by his Swiss pupil C. G. Jung

(1875–1961) and by Alfred Adler (1870–1937) of Austria. Meanwhile, other investigators have contributed diagnostic tests, therapeutic methods, and theories of etiology to the development of psychiatry.

Shock therapy for mentally disturbed patients was introduced in this century. Electroshock was first used by two Italians, Ugo Cerletti (1877–1963) and Lucio Bini in 1938. Manfred Sakel (1900–1957), an Austrian-American, described the first successful treatment of a schizophrenic patient with insulin shock in 1937. Carbon dioxide inhalation was used by the Budapest psychiatrist, Ladislaus von Meduna (b. 1896) in 1935 as a means of shock therapy for schizophrenic patients. A. C. Egas Moniz employed surgical procedures on the brain of mentally ill patients.

The theory that some bodily disorders are *psychosomatic*—that is, they are physical manifestations of emotional upset—was first introduced by such investigators as W. B. Cannon, Helen Dunbar, Franz Alexander, and Eli Moshcowitz. Walter C. Alvarez (b. 1884), an American, described the nervous causes of indigestion, dyspepsia, and certain other ills; and the psychosomatic basis for peptic ulcer was explained by Sir Arthur F. Hurst (1879–1944) of England.

In the decade following World War II the use of *tranquilizing agents* became popular. There exists a considerable amount of disagreement among physicians concerning the use of these compounds. A number of patients experience side effects such as dryness of the mouth, blurred vision, nausea, and drowsiness. A few cases of liver damage have also been reported. However, for many patients who are prone to be nervous or "high strung," the tranquilizing drugs have brought about a serene way of life they could probably not obtain in any other way.

Population control

The greatest strides in science in this century and the greatest challenge of the next is the area of contraception and population control.

Several devices for preventing conception, such as the diaphragm and the many varieties of intrauterine contraceptive device (IUD), are now available. The first oral contraceptive drug, *Enovid,* was introduced in 1960. During the 1960s, scores of oral drugs were brought out, and large-scale testing for side effects began. Other methods for population control, such as vasectomy for men, gained acceptance.

28 THE MEDICAL PROFESSION

HERE IS YOUR DOCTOR

Not so many years ago, when a person became ill, he depended entirely upon his family doctor, the talents and knowledge of one man, to aid him in returning to health. Often, the same doctor brought an individual into the world, treated him for childhood and adult diseases, and perhaps presided at his deathbed. The pioneer physicians deserve great credit, but certainly their patients did not live the long, comfortable life in store for the average person today.

The modern patient is served by the skills of a large medical team, composed of literally hundreds of persons. The family physician, after a physical examination and study of the case history, may call in specialists in various fields as consultants to help determine the best treatment for the patient. Should surgery be advised, a surgeon and anesthetist are added to the team, or a radiologist for x-ray therapy. The patient may have to be moved to a hospital, in which case the large staff of that institution becomes part of the team: the resident physicians, hospital administrator, interns, nurses, laboratory technicians, dietitians, and physical and occupational therapists. The pharmacist and the entire drug industry supply the patient with the best drugs and medicines, and in addition, constantly conduct research for better materials. Surgical appliances, medical instruments, braces, etc. are the contributions of another large industry. Certain health organizations attempt to control the patient's disease on a local, state, or national scale. These organizations also engage in research

for better methods of prevention and treatment.

When the time comes to pay the bills to other team members, there are several voluntary health insurance plans—the Blue Cross and Blue Shield plans in particular—which assume part or all of the financial burdens if the patient is a member. Indeed, there are many more persons and groups on the medical team than is generally realized, and their combined efforts have added healthy years to the life of the average citizen. Some of these members are discussed in this chapter, beginning with the most important member, your doctor.

When a patient consults a doctor for diagnosis and treatment, he has a great deal of confidence in him. That confidence is well-placed, because to achieve the ability to give proper treatment, the physician has had to devote many years of his life to the intensive study of medicine. And the knowledge he received from that study was gained from hundreds of years of medical research and investigation on the part of his predecessors.

Among the professions, medicine today has the most stringent educational qualifications for practice. Perhaps no other group is so constantly striving toward professional improvement as are today's physicians. Throughout history, America has had reason to be proud of her doctors. But never before has the medical profession possessed the skill and knowledge held today by its members. There was a time when any young man could become a doctor by serving an apprenticeship to a practicing physician, meanwhile taking a few night courses in anatomy. Today, the future doctor must pass successfully through 8 to 13 or more years of the most demanding, intensive, and exhaustive study before setting up his practice.

The first stage of the future medical student's training takes place in an accredited college or university, where he spends from three to four years under the guidance of a special "premedical committee" composed of certain members of the faculty. This committee assists the student in the selection of his curriculum which is comprised chiefly of basic science and liberal arts courses. He must maintain during this period a record of high grades (a "B" average is required by most medical schools today) and retain enough information from his courses to pass the entrance examinations. The number of students applying for entrance to any medical college in any given year may determine the grade average required.

However, even though the medical curriculum is arduous, one of the foremost problems relative to this long-term training program is the cost. It is very difficult for a student to work part-time and maintain the academic pace of the medical college. Scholarships and long-term loans are available at many schools, but generally it is necessary to have the finances available in the family, and to show the medical school that adequate resources are available.

Training at medical schools

During the first two years of the four-year medical school curriculum, the student must master the laboratory sciences. To learn the structure of the human body, he studies *anatomy,* both gross and microscopic. Thorough training is given in the subject of *biological chemistry,* which is the basis for clinical laboratory diagnosis and medical therapeutics. The functions of the body are learned from books and by laboratory experiments in classes in *physiology.* Because he is to deal intimately with people, the student must have a working knowledge of *psychology,* the science of human behavior. In his *pathology* classes, he will learn about diseases and diseased tissues; and in *bacteriology* classes, the causes of the infectious diseases will be made clear to him. Studying *pharmacology,* he will learn about drugs and medicines. Usually, all this study is done before he ever treats a patient.

In his third and fourth years, the student receives instruction and practical experience in the actual care of patients. The organization of the course work may vary considerably from school to school in this phase of the training, but certain basic studies are common to all. Included among these are: the study of anesthetics (*anesthesiology*), the study of skin disorders (*dermatology*), the study of the glands of internal secretion (*endocrinology*), *forensic* or legal medicine, internal medicine, the study of the nervous system and its diseases (*neurology*), the sciences pertaining to childbirth and diseases of the female reproductive system (*obstetrics* and *gynecology*), *radiology, surgery, psychiatry, ophthalmology, otolaryngology, preventive medicine, orthopedics, pediatrics, proctology* and *urology.* During this time, the student frequently has the opportunity to spend considerable time in a hospital and acquaint himself with many of the more basic procedures and common disorders. While making the rounds of the wards with his instructors, the student will learn to develop the judgment and bearing necessary to mark him as a competent practitioner of medicine.

The medical school itself is organized into a considerable number of different departments, each of which teaches one of the previously mentioned subjects, or one of the branches of clinical medicine. The faculty of the school is composed of eminent members of the medical or allied professions, and in addition to teaching, this faculty usually engages in furthering medical progress through research. The clinical faculty also takes care of their own patients. A great many of our present advances in medicine come through the efforts of such teachers, who are also eminent research scientists. A list of approved medical schools can be obtained by writing the American Medical Association, 535 N. Dearborn Street, Chicago 10, Illinois.

After graduation from medical school, the student has the title of Doctor of Medicine in most states. However, he is still a student. Next comes one to two years of internship in a hospital. During this period, the intern usually lives at the hospital and receives some pay. While caring for the hospital's patients, he should develop more and more skill and knowledge, transposing the theories learned in medical school into practical use. Most states have a licensing board, which gives the prospective physician a thorough examination after internship is completed. If he passes the examination, he is allowed to practice medicine within the state.

At the end of this phase, the new physician may desire to specialize his practice. If so, he should obtain a *residency* or *fellowship,* lasting three to five years, through which he is guided in his study by capable and experienced men in the field of his chosen speciality. He may take an examination by a National Specialty Board on completion of this training.

A doctor cannot cease his studying even after he has "hung out his shingle." Medicine is ever changing and progressing, and he must keep abreast of this progress. His learning is augmented through careful reading of various medical journals and the taking of special postgraduate courses. There are over 2000 medical journals published in the United States, some dealing with general medicine and some with specialized fields. As new methods, drugs, and instruments are tested or proved, or as new knowledge is obtained, the results are reported by the researchers in these periodicals. Postgraduate medical courses are offered by medical schools, hospitals, and medical organizations in order to keep physicians abreast of new developments. In a sense, the doctor is always a student, and always is improving.

Specialization

With the acquisition of new knowledge of the body, new techniques of diagnosis and treatment, and new instruments and drugs, medicine has developed to the point where one man no longer can absorb all its teachings. Therefore, there has been a rise in specialization. In the United States, at least 45 percent of the physicians could be termed specialists.

The specialist must have an adequate background in all medical fields, but he concerns himself chiefly with diseases in one particular set of organs or with one disease or with the use of one set of techniques. The specialist in *internal medicine,* for example, is most interested in disturbances affecting the heart and lungs, the circulation, the organs within the abdomen, stomach disorders, diseases of old age, and other closely related problems. The *surgeon,* of course, is most concerned with the performance of operations on various parts of the body. Care of the child comprises the work of the *pediatrician.* The eyes, ears, nose, and throat are included in a specialty; and the eye alone is the concern of two other specialist groups.

The *obstetrician* handles prenatal care and childbirth. Nervous and mental diseases fall under the care of *psychiatrists.* Diseases of the skin are diagnosed and treated by *dermatologists,* pathological conditions of the teeth and mouth by *dentists* and *orthodontists. Anesthetists* are responsible for the proper administration of anesthesia during operations and special problems of resuscitation and gas therapy. The diagnostic and therapeutic methods requiring the use of x-rays or radium are items assigned to *radiologists.*

Each major field is further subdivided into more specialties. In internal medicine, the cardiologist is an expert on heart conditions, the hematologist on the blood, the gastroenterologist on the organs of the gastrointestinal system, and so on. Likewise, surgeons are divided into: general surgeons and abdominal surgeons; orthopedic surgeons, who are concerned with disorders of the bones and joints; neurosurgeons, who operate on the brain; gynecologists, who specialize in disorders of the female reproductive system; urologists, who specialize in conditions of the genitourinary system; and proctologists who are concerned with the lower bowel. The complete list of specialties is too lengthy to be presented in the limited space available here.

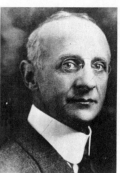

FLEXNER, Simon (1863-1946) American pathologist and bacteriologist. Made numerous contributions to knowledge of transmission of infectious diseases. With Noguchi, Flexner studied the effects of snake venom. Developed *Flexner's serum* for cerebrospinal meningitis. With Paul A. Lewis, he transmitted poliomyelitis to monkeys by means of cultures of a filtrable virus.

But despite the rapid rise of specialization, there is still one man who signifies "Doctor" to most Americans—the family physician, the general practitioner. This man still makes up a large part of the medical profession and holds a place of high esteem in the eyes of the public. A general practitioner treats the patient for most disorders from birth until death. When some condition arises for which he is not trained, such as a necessity for major surgery, he refers the patient to some specialist in the particular field indicated.

Because of the shortage of physician manpower and the extremely heavy workloads of many physicians, a new program of "doctors' helpers," called Medex, was established in 1968. Designed to utilize the training of former military medical corps personnel (medics), the program was conceived by Dr. Richard Smith of the University of Washington.

Before the establishment of Medex, a medical corpsman might have from 600 to 2000 hours of formal medical training and as much as 20 years' experience and still find it difficult to obtain a job in a health-related field upon leaving the military service. In the Medex program, former medical corpsmen undergo three months of training, with emphasis on skills not covered in their military training. After this three-month training period, each corpsman is assigned to serve a one-year preceptorship with a selected general practitioner. Upon completion, they are eligible to work as full-time physicians' assistants. As physicians' assistants they take patients' histories, help give physical examinations, suture minor lacerations, and apply and remove casts. Estimates of physician time saved by such assistants vary from 33 percent to 100 percent.

So far, 6000 former military medics have enlisted in Medex, and the program continues to grow.

Another means by which the family physician or the specialist makes use of other members of the medical team is by calling in *consultants.* For instance, the family physician may call in a radiologist and a gynecologist to give their opinions in the diagnosis of a woman with some disorder of the reproductive system. If the trouble is in another area of the body, the woman may be referred to a surgeon for operation. The surgeon, however, may wish to have the opinion of a specialist in internal medicine as to whether the woman's circulatory system is physically able to withstand the operation. At the time of surgery other assisting surgeons and anesthetists may be required in the operating room. Each of these consultants must be paid by the patient, and professional ethics do not permit the referring physician to accept a rebate from any one of them.

In recent years, a three-year residency program in family practice has been set up, in which the doctor spends three years of additional study after graduation from medical school. He is then eligible to take a specialty board examination in family practice and become certified as a specialist in his field.

Fees

The fees charged by a physician are usually reasonable, and represent what he believes to be a just price for the use of his time and extensive knowledge, which has taken so many years of his life to gain. Unfortunately for the physician, a smaller percentage of his "customers" pay him than in any other business or profession.

Sometimes persons do not wish to pay their physicians because they think the fees are exorbitant. If this should occur, the individual should contact the medical society in his county, giving this group full particulars in regard to the services rendered and the fee charged. The county medical society has a "Grievance Committee," which is set up to handle the complaints of patients against physicians. These committees are known for their fair decisions, and will not hesitate to defend the patient if he is in the right.

Medical organizations

It is the organizations within the profession of medicine itself which have kept the profession on the high plane that it is. There are two major types of medical organizations. First, there is the large group to which a majority of physicians belong, the American Medical Association. The AMA, along with the Association of American Medical Colleges, sets the standards for entrance to and graduation from medical schools. It also governs the conduct of its members and disqualifies those whom it considers unethical.

Other types of medical organizations are the specialty societies. Chief among these are the American College of Surgeons, the American College of Physicians, and the American Academy of General Practice. In order to become a member of these groups, the physician must be engaged in the practice of that particular branch of medicine, and must meet all of the previously established requirements, as well as agree to abide by the standards set up by the group. Further, each of the more "specialized specialties" has one or more organizations representing it. Gynecologists may belong to the American Gynecological Society, skin specialists to the American Academy of Dermatology and Syphilology, brain surgeons to the American Academy of Neurological Surgery, pediatricians to the American Academy of Pediatrics, chest surgeons to the American Association for Thoracic Surgery, plastic surgeons to the American Association of Plastic Surgeons, radiologists to the American Roentgen Ray Society, psychiatrists to the American Psychiatric Association, physiotherapists to the American Academy of Physical Medicine and Rehabilitation, etc. Some specialties have several societies, each one having certain membership requirements. Each holds sectional and national meetings to exchange new information gained in its particular field. Many of these societies and associations have periodicals which are sent not only to the individual members but to medical schools and libraries throughout the country and, in some instances, throughout the world. *The Journal of the American Medical Association,* for instance, probably has more subscriptions than any other medical journal in the world.

These organizations have as their goal the improvement of the practice of medicine, and each has a code of ethics which the members of the organization must follow. The most important of these is the code adopted for the American Medical Association.

The principles which the AMA has encouraged its members to follow include several sections devoted to various aspects of medical ethics. Three of the sections are quoted below as they appear in the *Principles of Medical Ethics* as revised by a two-thirds majority vote of the House of Delegates at a recent session of the American Medical Association.

Sec. 5—A physician may choose whom he will serve. In an emergency, however, he should render service to the best of his ability. Having undertaken the care of a patient, he may not neglect him; and unless he has been discharged he may discontinue his services only after giving adequate notice. He should not solicit patients.

Sec. 7—In the practice of medicine a physician should limit the source of his professional income to medical services actually rendered by him, or under his supervision, to his patients. His fee should be commensurate with the services rendered and the patient's ability to pay. He should neither pay nor receive a commission for referral of patients. Drugs, remedies or appliances may be dispensed or supplied by the physician provided it is in the best interests of the patient.

Sec. 9—A physician may not reveal the confidences entrusted to him in the course of medical attendance, or the deficiencies he may observe in the character of patients, unless he is required to do so by law or unless it becomes necessary in order to protect the welfare of the individual or of the community.

The physicians are further admonished to report to their local society any infractions of these rules of ethics by other members. Occasionally it has been the decision of a specially appointed committee composed of local members to expel a physician from the society for unethical practices.

Hippocrates, a Greek physician in the fourth century before Christ, is called the Father of Medicine. He formulated an oath for his students to take on going into the practice of medicine. Today, many young physicians on graduation repeat this oath and promise to follow its principles. With this oath as the foundation of their ethics, the members of the medical profession are pledged to a lifetime of service to mankind.

HERE IS YOUR NURSE

The nurse has closer contact with the patient than any other member of the medical team. She is responsible for carrying out the physician's orders. She administers the medicines and other treatment prescribed, and cares for the patient's comfort and physical needs. She teaches him how to care for himself. Furthermore, she observes the patient's course carefully and reports any unusual change to the physician. She must have a knowledge of psychology, medicine, practical hospital and home economics, and teaching techniques.

The majority of nurses are women. Throughout recorded history, there seem to have been women responsible for the care of the sick. In early Christian days, a group of charitable women, known as deaconesses, helped the poor and visited the sick—the forerunners of the modern visiting nurse. Phebe, mentioned by St. Paul in the Bible, was a deaconess. Christian Rome had the first free public hospitals and established the first systematic training of nurses. Roman nurses were recruited from those women of the upper classes who were interested in doing charitable work.

After Rome fell and throughout the Middle Ages, the Catholic Church was the only institution that was capable of any sort of organized effort in patient care. Consequently, the care of the sick was assumed by the monks in the monasteries. Such nursing as existed was performed by various orders of nuns which were associated with the monks.

With the coming of the Reformation, church property was confiscated in many countries, and the monastic brotherhoods were no longer allowed to care for the sick in many locales. As a substitute, city hospitals were built. These new hospitals were victimized by graft and public indifference, so that they were left in filth and disrepair. This is considered the dark period of nursing history. The nurses at the city hospitals were usually male servants, who were ignorant of medical knowledge and lacking in humanitarian ideals.

After about 100 years without nursing progress, a Frenchman, St. Vincent de Paul, founded an organization of religious women for the purpose of providing care for the ill and needy. This group was called the Sisters of Charity, and is considered to be the organization which revived nursing. Shortly after the Sisters began their work, there was a rebirth of the deaconess movement by Protestant women.

However, nursing still was nowhere near the professional status it holds today. Charles Dickens describes the nurses of his day in several of his books. According to him, they were dirty, harsh, and sadistic, enjoying a deathbed scene more than seeing a patient returned to health. The occupation remained in disrepute until the middle of the last century.

Florence Nightingale was the founder of modern trained nursing. Throughout her youth, she had always desired to be a nurse, but her upper-class family blocked her efforts to enter such a distasteful occupation. As she became older, she became more convinced that nursing was her calling. In 1854, she prevailed upon friends in the British government to allow her to reform the hospital system of the army, which was fighting the Crimean war at that time. Permission was granted, and she organized a group of 38 women to go to Crimea and tend the sick and wounded. On their arrival there, she was placed in charge of a hospital with four miles of beds

NIGHTINGALE, Florence (1820-1910) English nurse. Famous throughout the world as the founder of modern nursing. During the Crimean War she organized a woman's nursing service at Scutari and Balaklava (1860), the results of which were so sensational as to completely revolutionize earlier concepts of nursing and the role of women in medicine. Her devotion to her cause made her legendary and she became known as the Lady with the Lamp.

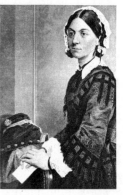

set 18 inches apart. The wards lacked ventilation and were dirty and unsanitary. Part of the filth was caused by a shortage of water.

The death rate at this hospital was 42 percent when Miss Nightingale and her nurses arrived. They cleaned the place, established diet kitchens, and undertook better care of the wounded soldiers—not without opposition from the army physicians. Within six months, the death rate had fallen to 2 percent. More nurses were then sent to Crimea, and Miss Nightingale was placed in charge of other hospitals.

Her work received wide publicity in England, and created an improved public attitude toward nursing. When Miss Nightingale returned home, she worked for the establishment of nursing schools. The first school was begun at St. Thomas Hospital in London in 1860, and nursing began to become professionalized.

Since the work of this woman, nursing has grown to become one of the most important elements in the medical team. Indeed, in 1969 there were 1308 nursing schools in the United States with a total of 144,024 students.

Nursing as a profession

There are distinct advantages for the woman who wishes to enter nursing. The cost of training is low; there is always a certainty of work for competent nurses; and the profession offers women unlimited opportunity to do service for mankind.

The woman who desires to be a nurse must first be in good health. Before entering an accredited nursing school, a high school education is required, but some schools limit their admissions to those women who have had some college work. If the prospective nurse goes to a collegiate school of nursing, the curriculum will include those courses required of all academic students.

The nursing school itself is usually associated with a large hospital, a medical center, or a university. A list of approved nursing schools may be obtained from the American Nurses' Association, 2 Park Avenue, New York, New York 10016. During the course, which lasts at least three years, the student nurse will wear the uniform of her particular school. She will attend classes in anatomy, physiology, chemistry, microbiology, nutrition and cooking, psychology, education, liberal arts subjects, and nursing arts and science. Forty hours a week are divided between classroom and clinical experience in the hospital.

Upon graduation, the nurse earns the right to wear the uniform of a graduate nurse and the pin and cap of her school. She takes State Board of Nurse Examinations, the passing of which grants her the title of Registered Nurse (R.N.) and licenses her to practice her profession. She also takes the Nightingale Pledge, which is similar to the Hippocratic Oath taken by physicians:

"I solemnly pledge myself before God and in the presence of this assembly:

To pass my life in purity and to practice my profession faithfully.

I will abstain from whatever is deleterious and mischievous, and will not take or knowingly administer any harmful drug.

I will do all in my power to elevate the standard of my profession, and will hold in confidence all personal matters committed to my keeping and all family affairs coming to my knowledge in the practice of my profession.

With loyalty will I endeavor to aid the physician in his work, and devote myself to the welfare of those committed to my care."

Specialization

Immediately after becoming an R.N., the new nurse usually registers with a local nursing registry. She may enter any one of several nursing fields, some of which require further training. The major fields are private duty nursing, institutional nursing, public health nursing, and industrial nursing. Each of these is further subdivided.

The private duty nurse may function as a private nurse for one patient, either in a hospital or at home. She also may become a nurse in a physician's office, in which case she may function also as the physician's secretary.

Institutional nurses are those who continue working in a hospital. Such a nurse may become a ward or a clinic nurse, or specialize in a particular branch. There are operating room nurses whose duties are limited to the operating room. Obstetrical nurses aid physicians in delivering babies. Pediatric nurses specialize in the care of sick children; and psychiatric nurses care for mental patients. Nurses also specialize in nursing administration, becoming head nurses, supervisors, and administrators. Some nurses enter the field of education, teaching student nurses and auxiliary personnel in hospitals.

The public health nurse may work for the city, state, or federal government in one of their health programs. She may be a visiting nurse, who goes to the home of the patient needing a limited amount of skilled nursing and health teaching in the home. Another field for the public health nurse is school nursing.

The graduate nurse may also enter one of the armed services and hold the commission of an officer.

Industrial nurses serve in factories, offices, and department stores. They also may be employed by airline, railroad, or steamship companies.

Male nurses

Although nursing is generally thought of as being a profession for women, it offers many opportunities for men. The male nurse must have the same educational qualifications and the same training as women nurses. Their duties differ in that male nurses usually work with male patients or as psychiatric nurses. More recently, opportunities in administration, operating rooms, industry, prisons, and public health programs have been developed for male nurses and they may now be commissioned officers in the armed services.

Practical nurses

Besides the registered professional nurses, practical nurses also serve with the medical team. These are nonprofessional workers who are trained to do less technical tasks in the patient's care. Most states now license schools of practical nursing. The length of time required for practical nursing preparation varies from 30 weeks to 18 months, the usual duration being one year. The demand for qualified practical nurses, licensed by the state to practice, has exceeded the supply. In 1969, there were 1120 approved schools of practical nursing in the United States. In 1968, there were 91,359 requests for services of licensed practical nurses.

In the past ten years, the activities of nurses have been studied to discover which may be safely and adequately carried out by nonprofessional personnel. Many housekeeping, clerical, administrative, purchasing, and maintenance duties have been placed in other departments. Within the scope of direct patient care, the professional nurse has become the head of a nursing team consisting of orderlies, aides, practical nurses, student nurses, clerks, and volunteers.

Volunteer hospital work

Because of a shortage of graduate nurses, a program was begun during World War II to secure volunteers with minimum training for hospital work. These volunteers are still being used and will continue to be needed. There are probably as many as half a million volunteer workers now employed in hospitals, and even more are needed.

In most cases, these workers are women who desire to do some form of altruistic work. They give one or two days a week of their time as either nurses' aides, dietitians' aides, occupational therapy assistants, or ward secretaries. They wear a uniform and are trained for their tasks by physicians and nurses on the hospital staff.

Women who wish to co-operate with a humanitarian profession may investigate the possibility of their doing volunteer hospital work by calling the administrator of a local hospital or contacting the county nursing registry.

HERE IS YOUR HOSPITAL

Before the time of Pasteur, when a person was sent to a hospital, he was almost always sent there to die. The hospital was the last resort, and only a few fortunate patients were discharged disease-free. The physicians of the time had good reason to postpone hospitalization as long as possible, because the hospitals were filthy, overcrowded, poorly ventilated buildings. Sometimes as many as four patients had to share the same bed for a few hours, and then alternate with four patients on the floor. There were no isolation wards for those with contagious diseases, and the patients received little or no medical or nursing care.

Since the discovery of the importance of antiseptic techniques, and since the work of Florence Nightingale in the field of nursing, hospitals have become a place of hope for the patient, instead of a last resort. The modern hospital is a complex organization which offers its patients the utmost in diagnosis, treatment, and care.

In the United States in 1872, there were less than 200 hospitals listed by the American Medical Association. In 1969, there were 7144 hospitals in America. Indeed, hospitals are the fifth largest industry in the United States.

In order to provide the best care for the patient, the American College of Surgeons, a professional medical organization, set up a standard for hospitals. In past years, this group has inspected the majority of hospitals in the United States and Canada, and if a hospital conformed adequately to the set standards, it received a certificate of approval. The burden of hospital standardization has become too great for this organization to carry alone, so that hospital inspection is now the joint responsibility of the American College of Surgeons, American College of Physicians, American Hospital Association, and the American Medical Association.

Among many other requirements, a hospital seeking approval of the Joint Commission of Accreditations of Hospitals of the above groups must have an adequate system of medical records. It is extremely important that accurate records be kept on each patient in the hospital's files. This record includes the patient's medical history before entering the hospital, the results of physical examination and laboratory tests, any x-ray findings, the diagnosis, type of treatment given, course in the hospital, condition of the patient at intervals after leaving the hospital, etc. These records are usually kept by a medical record librarian, and she classifies them according to many criteria. Thus, for example, if a physi-

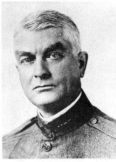

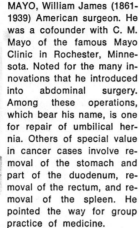

MAYO, William James (1861-1939) American surgeon. He was a cofounder with C. M. Mayo of the famous Mayo Clinic in Rochester, Minnesota. Noted for the many innovations that he introduced into abdominal surgery. Among these operations, which bear his name, is one for repair of umbilical hernia. Others of special value in cancer cases involve removal of the stomach and part of the duodenum, removal of the rectum, and removal of the spleen. He pointed the way for group practice of medicine.

type of patient; this is the most common form of hospital. A surgical hospital specializes in care of patients undergoing surgery, an obstetrical hospital in maternity patients. There are children's hospitals, and orthopedic hospitals for crippled children and adults. Some hospitals specialize in treatment of patients with particular diseases, such as mental diseases, tuberculosis, venereal diseases, gynecological disorders, cancer, epilepsy, heart diseases, contagious diseases, chronic disorders in aged persons, neurological diseases, and disorders of the eyes, ears, nose, or throat. One of the most important types of hospitals is the research hospital, wherein particular patients are accepted and studied closely while being cared for; laboratory research also is conducted in such a hospital.

cian wishes to know what type x-ray therapy for patients with a specific disease has proved most beneficial at that particular hospital, the records of those patients receiving x-ray therapy can be reviewed. Another manner in which medical records are essential is in checking the type of therapy given a patient on any previous stay at the hospital to determine if the new therapy planned will be detrimental or beneficial.

Another standard for approval is that the hospital must have monthly staff meetings to review medical records and summarize experiences. This allows the staff to avoid repeating mistakes and to take advantage of techniques which have proved useful.

Types of hospitals

Hospitals are usually owned and operated by the local, state, or federal governments, or by nonprofit organizations such as religious, fraternal, or philanthropic groups. Some hospitals are operated by industrial companies for their employees; and others are institutional hospitals, operated by schools, prisons, etc.

Hospitals are classified according to the type of patients that are accepted. A general hospital is a large hospital which cares for nearly every

Components of a hospital

Although there are differences according to type, most hospitals have the same basic organizational plan. The majority of the floor area is taken up by wards and rooms where the patients stay. These wards are divided according to the type of patient—that is, maternity patients occupy one floor or wing, mental patients another, etc. There is also an area for patients who do not stay at the hospital but come in for treatment (outpatients). Rooms with special equipment include those for diagnostic or therapeutic x-ray, surgical operating rooms, examination rooms, and rooms for other specialized procedures. One or more laboratories of various kinds are found in nearly every hospital. In addition, space must be set aside for administrative offices, diet kitchens, library and records library, laundry, and nurses' quarters.

The staff of the hospital is usually large. Besides the personal physicians of the patients, there are interns, resident physicians, nurses, and nurse's aides. There is the dietitian and her aides, and the housekeeping department with its maids. And there are social workers, laboratory technologists, and x-ray technicians. In addition, there is a hospital administrator and his staff of assistants, bookkeepers, and secretaries.

PHYSICIANS AND DENTISTS, AND MEDICAL AND DENTAL SCHOOLS IN THE UNITED STATES: 1920 TO 1966

Item	1920	1930	1940	1945	1950	1955	1960	1965	1966
Physicians, number	144,977	153,803	175,382	*	209,040	241,711	260,484	292,088	300,375
Medical schools:									
Number	85	76	77	77	79	81	81	83	83
Graduates	3,047	4,565	5,097	5,136	5,553	6,977	7,081	7,409	7,720
Dentists, number	56,152	71,055	70,601	*	86,876*	94,879	101,947	109,301	111,622
Dental schools:									
Number	46	38	39	39	42	42	46	48	48
Graduates	906	1,561	1,757	3,212	2,565	3,081	3,253	3,181	3,264

*Not available.
Source: United States Public Health Service.

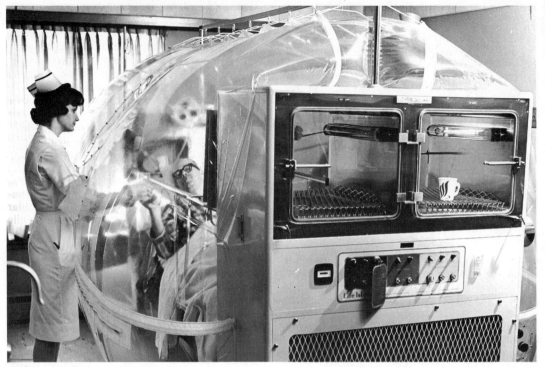

Life Island protects patients from the dangers of infection. Air, food, water, and medicine are sterilized before entering the isolated environment. Copyright 1970 Year Book Medical Publishers, Inc., courtesy E. J. Freireich et al., The University Texas M. D. Anderson Hospital, Houston.

Hospital professions

The *hospital administrator* is one of the more important members of the medical team. He is in charge of the business administration of the hospital, its personnel, and the carrying out of hospital policies. In addition to seeing that the patient has the best of care and that there is close co-operation between the professional and nonprofessional staffs, he must keep the hospital on a sound economic basis. To enter this profession, a person must be an organizer and have an educational background in business administration. At present, twelve universities in the United States offer a degree in hospital administration on completion of four years' college work.

The *dietitian* is another important member of the hospital staff. She must oversee the buying and preparing of food for patients. Not only must she have adequate knowledge of nutrition and cooking so that the food is both nutritious and appealing, but she must also possess a keen sense of economics so that she may stay within the budget allotted for food. A college degree in dietetics is usually desirable for persons entering this profession.

One of the important staff members of the hospital is the *social worker*, who interviews the indigent patient upon admission. This person assists the hospital staff in identifying relevant social, emotional, and economic factors of the patient. She also helps the patient and his family plan to meet the expenses incurred by a hospital stay; often she can secure financial aid for indigent patients from philanthropic groups. With Medicare and Medicaid now available, the social worker must now also assist private patients in finding nursing homes, etc. To become a social worker, a person must have extensive training, beginning with four years of college where she specializes in social sciences and liberal arts subjects. Then, she must apply at one of the 24 schools offering accredited medical social curricula. There she will obtain a familiarity with medicine and psychology—in particular, how the individual responds to illness. The first year of the two-year course is devoted to theory; she will receive field work practice two to three days per week during the second year.

Hospital costs

With so many competent, highly paid, professional staff members, it is obvious that the cost of hospitalization cannot be low. Further, a hospital is a sort of American Plan hotel, and cost must include food and lodging, as well as service. Today, hospital costs have risen, both because of the general rising cost of living, and because of new knowledge and methods, which demand more attention for the patient, and consequently, more personnel. Twenty-five years ago, the average cost per diem of a hospital stay was about $5.00; but the average hospital stay was 30 days. Today, the cost is $40 to $100 a day; but the average stay is only four to six days. Consequently, the total cost is often less, and the patient is more likely to return to his job at an early date and in good health.

Even so, the cost of hospital care can be a burden to the average family. Therefore, more families are securing medical and hospitalization insurance. In 1946, the American Medical Association sponsored the expansion of the Blue Cross and Blue Shield insurance plans. These are nonprofit plans, whereby the individual may have a small premium deducted from his monthly paycheck; should he or one of his dependents need medical care or hospitalization, it is paid for in great part by the Blue Cross or Blue Shield. These organizations, along with other ethical insurance plans, have a total membership of over 82 million persons and are adding about 28,000 new members each work day.

The insurance plans approved by the AMA must allow for free choice of physician and hospital. In the Blue Cross–Blue Shield plans, 82 percent of the money taken in is used to pay physicians and hospitals, 12 percent pays the expenses of administration, and the remainder is kept in reserve.

National health insurance

This country's first government-financed health program for the aged and the needy was signed into law on July 30, 1965, and became effective on July 1, 1966. Even though proposals for such a program had been made as far back as the Roosevelt administration in 1935, the plan is considered a legislative landmark in this country, since it is a departure from historical American views of financing health care. The program is divided into two parts, known as Medicare and Medicaid.

Medicare

This part of the health care program originally defined as elegible all individuals over age 65. In May, 1968, however, a new law was enacted which required individuals born after 1903 to have paid into the Social Security fund for at least six quarters—1½ years. Women who have never worked at a job outside the home or held a social security number may apply on their husband's number, provided he has paid into the Social Security fund for at least six quarters. Coverage under Medicare is divided into Parts A (hospitalization) and B (doctor's care).

Part A provides the following:

Inpatient hospital care for 90 days for each illness, with the patient paying a $60 cost for the first 60 days and $14 per day for any days over 60, up to a total of 90 days. When there is a 60-day period between hospitalizations, the entire 90-day period is renewed. In cases where the hospitalization period may be for longer than 90 days, the individual has 90 "grace" days from which he may borrow.

Post-hospital care for 100 days in an extended-care facility affiliated with a general hospital, with the patient paying $5 per day for the first 20 days.

Post-hospital or post-extended home health care up to 100 visits.

Part B is, in effect, a health insurance plan whereby an individual, on reaching 65 years of age, applies and then pays a "premium" of $5.80 per month which makes him eligible for coverage. The individual must apply for Part B coverage within three years of his 65th birthday. This part of the plan pays 80 percent of an individual's approved physician costs, after an initial $50 deductible per year. This means, for example, that even if the individual is hospitalized six times in a single year, he still pays only the initial $50 deductible. This part of the plan also pays on diagnostic x-rays, laboratory, and other tests; x-ray, radium, and other radioactive isotope therapy; ambulance service; surgical dressings, splints, casts, and other medical equipment.

Medicaid

Medicaid insures health care for the needy, the partially or totally disabled, and the blind of any age under 65, as well as for needy dependent children under 21 years of age. Needs of the aged are covered in conjunction with the Medicare plan. Medicaid pays as follows:

Hospitalization. The plan pays 30 days of in-hospital care per benefit period (a benefit period requires that there be 60 days elapsed between hospitalizations). It also covers the full cost of a semi-private room or the full cost of a private room, if deemed medically necessary by the attending physician. Also included are the full costs of usual and customary maternity care, all outpatient services (diagnostic, therapeutic, and rehabilitative), and all normal hospital services.

Physician. Medicaid covers all physician's charges (based on his usual and customary fees) regardless of whether services are performed in an office, a home, or a health care clinic.

Admission to a hospital

Usually a person will not go to a hospital unless referred by a physician. Indeed, most hospitals will not accept a patient who has not been so referred, except in cases of emergency. Consequently, if at all possible, the patient should seek a physician's advice as to referral before going to a hospital. However, if the patient needs immediate hospitalization and his physician is not available, a call should be placed to the prospective hospital to make certain that emergency patients are admitted there. If an ambulance is used, the driver will probably know which hospitals are open to the patient. But, when possible it is far more advantageous for the physician to decide when another member of the medical team, in this case the hospital, should be utilized.

YOUR TECHNOLOGISTS

Nearly every hospital and clinic employs medical technologists and x-ray technicians. A medical technologist, often called laboratory technician, aids the physician in making a diagnosis by performing several laboratory tests. The technologist may test a portion of the patient's blood to see if the patient has a venereal disease or is suffering from anemia. He also may examine swabbings and scrapings from diseased areas to determine the presence of pathogenic viruses or bacteria. The urine may be tested for foreign substances or for the amount of sugar or albumin contained. Microscopic examination of the feces by a medical technologist may reveal the presence of blood, intestinal parasites, or the eggs of parasites. A test of the blood serum may reveal an abnormal portion of some particular element which is significant—for example, a high level of acid phosphatase which often indicates that the patient has cancer of the prostate. Indeed, the services performed by these members of the medical team are innumerable; without them, diagnosis would often be impossible. They are under the guidance and supervision of physicians who have specialized in this field.

A person desiring to enter the field of medical technology should first enter an accredited college and there take courses in biology and chemistry, as well as general liberal arts subjects. A college degree is required by some schools of medical technology for admission, but two years of college is usually a minimum.

In 1969 there were 777 schools in the United States offering instruction in medical technology which had been approved by the American Medical Association. A list of approved schools can be obtained from the American Medical Association, 535 N. Dearborn Street, Chicago, Illinois 60610. These schools are most often affiliated with medical schools, large hospitals, or state and federal health laboratories. Once accepted at one of these schools, the student will spend a minimum of twelve months taking practical hospital training in the following subjects: the study of chemical reactions within the body *(biochemistry); the study of normal and abnormal conditions of the blood (hematology), and blood serum (serology); the study of cells, their origin, structure, and functions (cytology); the sciences dealing with identification and study of disease-producing bacteria (bacteriology), viruses (virology), and internal parasites (parasitology); the microscopic identification of normal and diseased human tissues and cells (histology);* and the techniques of making basal metabolism tests, electrocardiograms, etc.

Upon graduation from a technology school, the prospective medical technologist must pass an examination given by the Board of Registry of Medical Technologists of the American Society of Clinical Pathologists. Then, he is registered with this board and is allowed to enter practice at a hospital or laboratory. Should he decide to specialize in a particular field, he may have to take further training at a hospital or public health laboratory. Specialty fields open to medical technologists include: pathology, virology, bacteriology, parasitology, hematology, biochemistry, toxicology, and biophysics.

In the United States, there is an acute shortage of adequately trained medical technologists. In 1970 it was estimated that there will be 200,000 clinical people needed by 1975.

The x-ray technician aids the radiologist in making diagnostic x-ray films and in the application of x-ray and radium therapy. This field also has a shortage of trained personnel.

In most cases, a high school education is the usual entrance requirement of most schools of x-ray technology. In 1970 there were 1169 of these schools in the United States approved by the American Medical Association; a list of these can be obtained by writing the AMA at the address given in a previous paragraph. The average course lasts from twelve months to two years, and includes study in anatomy, physiology, physics, x-ray equipment, dark room chemistry

COHNHEIM, Julius (1839-1884) German pathologist. A pupil of Virchow, he wrote a textbook which completely revolutionized the teaching of pathology. He explained the processes of inflammation and suppuration and produced experimental tuberculosis in rabbits. Cohnheim produced an experimental salt frog, a living frog whose blood had been completely replaced with physiological salt solution; this experimental frog is known as *Cohnheim's frog.*

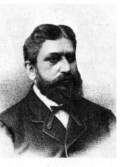

Illustration: Impressions of Disease . . . *Harold Laufman, M.D., Copyright 1947, Abbott Laboratories.*

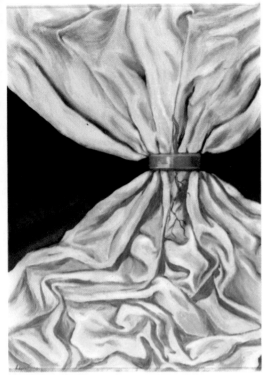

Coronary Heart Disease

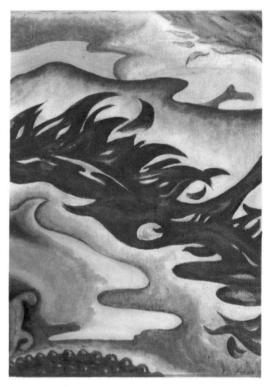

Scarlet Fever

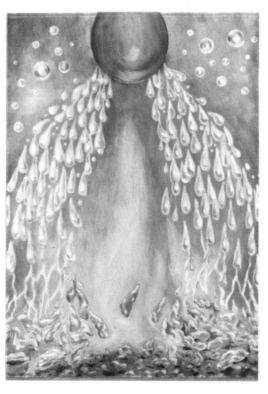

Common Cold

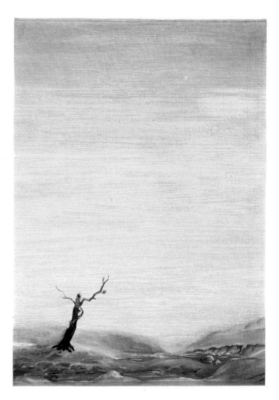

Shock

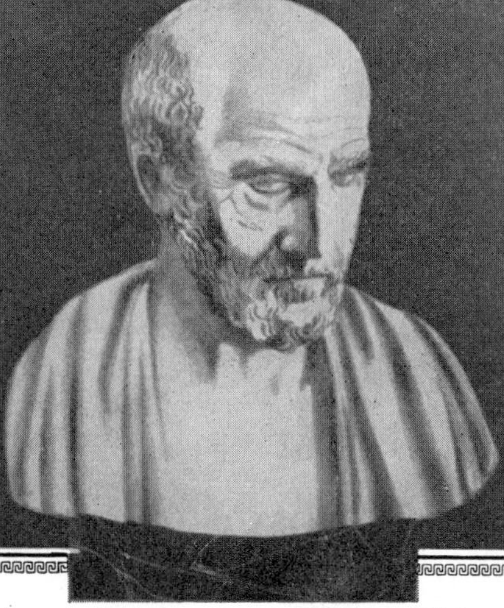

The Hippocratic Oath

"I swear by Apollo the physician, by Æsculapius, Hygeia, and Panacea, and I take to witness all the gods, all the goddesses, to keep according to my ability and my judgment the following Oath:

"To consider dear to me as my parents him who taught me this art; to live in common with him and if necessary to share my goods with him; to look upon his children as my own brothers, to teach them this art if they so desire without fee or written promise; to impart to my sons and the sons of the master who taught me and the disciples who have enrolled themselves and have agreed to the rules of the profession, but to these alone, the precepts and the instruction. I will prescribe regimen for the good of my patients according to my ability and my judgment and never do harm to anyone. To please no one will I prescribe a deadly drug, nor give advice which may cause his death. Nor will I give a woman a pessary to procure abortion. But I will preserve the purity of my life and my art. I will not cut for stone, even for patients in whom the disease is manifest; I will leave this operation to be performed by practitioners (specialists in this art). In every house where I come I will enter only for the good of my patients, keeping myself far from all intentional ill-doing and all seduction, and especially from the pleasures of love with women or with men, be they free or slaves. All that may come to my knowledge in the exercise of my profession or outside of my profession or in daily commerce with men, which ought not to be spread abroad, I will keep secret and will never reveal. If I keep this oath faithfully, may I enjoy my life and practice my art, respected by all men and in all times; but if I swerve from it or violate it, may the reverse be my lot."

and procedures, x-ray techniques, and general office work. A school of x-ray technology usually is connected with a medical school; however, some are affiliated with large hospitals and medical centers. The medical technologist and x-ray technician perform highly specialized tasks and the medical team would be sorely handicapped without their services.

YOUR PHYSICAL AND OCCUPATIONAL THERAPISTS

Two members of the medical team who are important in the rehabilitation of the patient are the physical therapist and the occupational therapist.

The *physical therapist* deals with patients who have had injuries or diseases which leave them wholly or partially handicapped. Besides massage and therapeutic exercises, the physical therapist employs specialized water baths and underwater exercises (*hydrotherapy*), ultraviolet and infrared irradiation, stimulation of muscles with electrical devices (*electrotherapy*), and application of heat.

In order to enter a school of physical therapy, the applicant either must have two years of college with courses in biology and the physical sciences or must be a graduate from an accredited nursing school. Some schools require a college degree.

In 1969 there were 49 schools of physical therapy in the United States, approved by the American Medical Association.

The average length of study is one year, some schools requiring up to four years. The student will take courses which give him a general scientific and medical background, plus theoretical and practical work in procedures of electrotherapy, radiation technique, hydrotherapy, massage, and therapeutic exercise. Physical therapy schools are usually affiliated with medical schools, hospitals, or universities connected with hospitals.

An *occupational therapist* has twofold duties. First, he attempts to find some sort of activity for the convalescent patient or the patient who is a permanent invalid. Also, he determines new occupations for the patient who is unable to return to his regular job because of some physical or emotional limitation.

In 1969 there were 35 schools offering courses in occupational therapy, approved by the American Medical Association. A high school education is usually sufficient for an applicant to enter one of these schools. The schools are most often affiliated with medical schools. In many of the schools, the course lasts five years and is divided into theoretical instruction, technical training, and practical hospital practice. The theoretical and technical instruction deals with general anatomy, anatomy of the brain and nervous system, study of muscular movements, physiology, psychology, the sciences, arts and crafts, education, and recreation.

YOUR PHARMACIST AND THE DRUG INDUSTRY

The pharmacist compounds drugs and medicines for the patient according to the prescription of the physician. He may be a pharmacist in a hospital or in the local drug store. In his tasks he must be exceedingly exact, because any mistake could have grave consequences. Consequently, his training must be thorough.

There are approximately 75 schools of pharmacy in the United States which are accredited by the American Council on Pharmaceutical Education; a list of these schools may be obtained by writing the Council at 77 West Washington Street, Chicago, Illinois 60602. Pharmacy schools are usually subdivisions of universities. The student enters the school of pharmacy after graduation from high school. There he studies for four years, receiving a degree of Bachelor of Science in Pharmacy on successful completion of his work. His studies include courses in physics, biology, chemistry, pharmacy, microscopic technique, toxicology, hygiene, the legal aspects of medicine, botany, mathematics, and disinfection and sterilization techniques.

After graduation, he must take an examination from a state board. Some states require that he serve an apprenticeship to a registered pharmacist for a period of time before he is granted a license to practice pharmacy on his own. He may also take graduate courses leading to the degrees of Master of Science or Doctor of Philosophy in Pharmacy. But whether he takes further training or not, the pharmacist must always keep up with new development in drugs and therapeutics.

The present-day pharmacist is the descendant of the medieval alchemists, and much of modern chemical and pharmaceutical knowledge has been the by-product of their efforts. The pharmacists branched from the alchemists when the former decided that their work should be done only under the authority of a physician. Indeed, the symbol Rx, which the physician writes at the top of every prescription, is taken from the Greek symbol for Jupiter; thus, the symbol proclaims that the prescription is written under the auspices of Jupiter, who was the ancient symbol for authority.

The authority under which drugs are dispensed goes beyond the authority of the individual physician. For instance, the American Medical As-

(Continued on p. 835)

Antibiotic Production

The production of vast quantities of antibiotics from molds is one of the great triumphs of the modern drug industry. A great deal of research and development is required to convert the synthesis of test tube quantities of these substances into the manufacturing process that will supply the health needs of the world. Moreover, the care and precision that must be employed in the production of drugs for use on human beings must be maintained at the highest standards. Modern factories in which these substances are prepared are therefore kept spotlessly clean, and the manufacturing process is carefully checked at each step by extensive laboratory tests. The purity of each batch of the material must meet the standards set by medical authorities, or that batch is discarded. The assiduous application of these safeguards guarantees the patient that the medicine supplied has its proper effect. *Photos from Merck Co., Inc.*

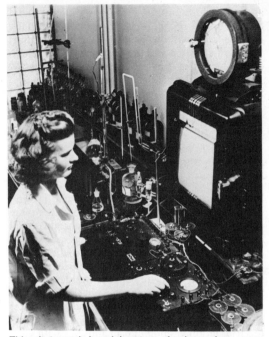

This photograph in a laboratory of a large drug manufacturing plant shows the use of a polarograph, an instrument used in the analysis of drugs.

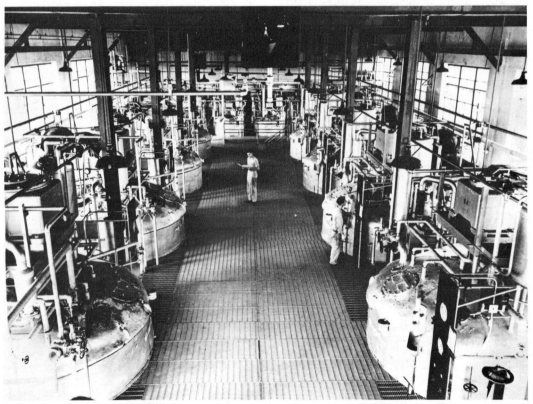

Partial view of the fermentation tanks in a large streptomycin manufacturing plant. Test tube amounts of the organism, *Streptomyces griseus,* are permitted to grow into larger quantities, which produce the antibiotic in these tanks. The drug streptomycin is then extracted by a lengthy process from the liquid fermentation medium.

sociation has a committee, the Council on Drugs, which extends control over new products and will not publish its acceptance of a new drug until it has been meticulously tested and has proved to be effective and nontoxic. The federal and state governments also exercise control over drug products, particularly requiring that container labels be consistent with the contents and that habit-forming or harmful drugs be dispensed only by authoritative prescription. Further, national and international meetings are held to standardize the manufacture and dosage of drugs.

Perhaps the closest control over the dispensing of medicines is exercised voluntarily by the drug industry itself. This large industry observes the strictest precautions in the manufacture of medical products. They also conduct research for new and better drugs, as well as research for better and cheaper means of production of drugs developed by other researchers. Besides producing the drugs which eventually are dispensed by the pharmacist to the patient, the drug industry manufactures laboratory materials, processes blood plasma for civilian needs and for the armed forces, and makes vaccines and antidisease serums for use in preventive medicine.

One of the most important functions of the drug industry is keeping the other members of the medical team informed as to new developments in the field of medicines. When a new or improved drug is developed, proved, and produced, the manufacturer conveys this information to the physician by means of a personal representative, a *detail man*. This representative calls on the physician and explains the new development, but he does not try to sell the physician supplies of the product. He also calls on other members of the medical team and then sees that the pharmacists in the area have a supply of the new drug available. Some persons who have taken premedical work in college but did not go to medical school become representatives for drug houses. However, the field is open

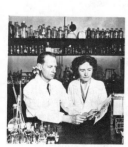

CORI, Carl Ferdinand (1896-) and wife, Gerty Theresa (1896-1957) American biochemists. Working as a team, the Coris have investigated a large number of the important steps in the metabolism of carbohydrates in the animal body. They have discovered evidence concerning the mechanisms of endocrine control of metabolism, by insulin and secretions of the adrenal and pituitary. In 1947 they were Nobel Laureates, with Dr. B. A. Houssay. *Chemical and Engineering News.*

to all qualified persons with good scientific backgrounds who wish to become members of the medical team.

HEALTH ORGANIZATIONS

To assist and co-ordinate the efforts of the members of the medical team, there exist several health organizations, some governmental and some private. These organizations attack health problems on a city, state, or national basis. Included are local, state, and federal health departments and voluntary health agencies. Most commonly, local organizations are on a city, city-county, or district basis.

The local health department is among the most active of health organizations. This agency may examine and establish the purity of water supplies and oversee the disposal of sewage, or it may secure such services from the state health department. In most cases food sold in the city is inspected by this group, as well as those places wherein food is processed, dispensed, or cooked. This department provides services to aid in the diagnosis, control, and treatment of communicable diseases and certain noncommunicable diseases which are of community interest, such as industrial diseases, the diseases of old age, and chronic diseases. These services include promoting, assisting, or directing programs which disseminate and also programs which provide for the early finding of disease conditions, particularly among infants and children of preschool and school age. The laboratories of the local health department are often responsible for the production or provision of diagnostic, prophylactic, or therapeutic products, such as sera, antitoxins, vaccines, and whole blood or blood plasma.

Further, the local health department attempts to control diseases occurring among animals which are transmissible to man. There are more than 80 such diseases, including rabies, Q-fever, brucellosis, tuberculosis, anthrax, and tularemia. Sometimes these diseases are transmitted by direct contact of persons with diseased animals, and at other times the diseases are contracted by human beings through consumption of meat, milk, and other food products of animal origin. Consequently, all animals and animal food products are inspected by a sanitarian or sanitary inspector with direction or consultation from a *veterinarian* in the local health department. To become a veterinarian, a person must attend college for one year or more, taking general liberal arts and scientific courses, and then must spend from three to four years at an accredited school of veterinary medicine. Upon graduation, he receives the degree of Doctor of Veterinary Medicine (D.V.M.). He may enter private practice and care for animal pets and livestock, or he may enter a health department or find employment with a school, college, or biological supply house.

Local health departments are often headed by a board composed of local citizens among whom are usually physicians and dentists. Local health departments usually have a physician as director or health officer either on a full-time or part-time basis. Usually there are public health nurses and sanitarians on local health department staffs and there also may be sanitary engineers, health educators, laboratory and x-ray technicians, and members of other specialties.

State health departments

Public health laws and organizations vary from state to state, but in each there has been extensive legislation specifying the health activities to be carried out by the state government. Most states have a state health board whose members are appointed by the governor of that state. Usually, the majority of the board is composed of members of the medical profession. This board, in turn, hires a state health officer to administer the health program and oversee the activities of the state health department.

The average state health department is divided into bureaus or divisions, each concerned with a particular element of public health. Usually, these divisions are concerned with: vital statistics, environmental sanitation, public health laboratory services, communicable disease control, maternal and child health, services for the physically disabled, public health nursing, health education, industrial hygiene, mental hygiene, and the administration of local health services.

The minimum functions of the state health agency are defined by the American Public Health Association. These are: the study of state health problems and planning for their solution; co-ordination and technical supervision of local health activities; financial aid to local health departments; the enactment of communicable disease and sanitary regulations applicable to local health programs; the establishment of minimal standards for local health work; the maintenance of central and branch laboratory services including diagnostic, sanitary, chemical, biological, and research activities; the collection, tabulation, and analysis of vital statistics; the collection and distribution of information concerning preventable disease; the maintenance of a safe quality of water and the control of waste disposal; establishment and maintenance of minimal standards of milk sanitation; provision of services to aid industry in the control of occupational hazards; the establishment of qualifications for health personnel; and formulation of plans in co-operation with other organizations for meeting all health needs.

State health departments are always available to answer questions regarding health and disease. Upon written request, they will supply pamphlets and other educational matter regarding specific health problems.

Federal health services

The federal health organizations of the United States are under the supervision of the Department of Health, Education and Welfare. There are four important subdivisions which are concerned with the public health services:

Environmental Health Service deals with the growing problem of contamination of our air, water, land, and food.

Food and Drug Administration is concerned with the problems surrounding the traffic in illegal narcotics; foods, pesticides, and product safety; and veterinary medicine.

Health Services and Mental Health Administration deals with community, regional, and federal health programs; research, development, and statistics; mental health; and family planning.

The National Institutes of Health carry on scientific research in specific fields and give financial grants-in-aid to private researchers. They also engage in educational activities for the medical profession and the public. The National Institutes of Health include:

Bureau of Health Professions, Education and Manpower Training, National Cancer Institute, National Heart and Lung Institute, National Institute of Allergy and Infectious Diseases, National Institute of Arthritis and Metabolic Diseases, National Institute of Child Health and Human Development, National Institute of Dental Research, National Institute of General Medical Sciences, National Eye Institute, National Institute of Environmental Health Sciences, National Library of Medicine, and the Fogarty International Center.

The Bureau of Medical Services administers a wide program of hospital and medical care, while the Bureau of State Services provides consultation, technical assistance, and financial aid to state and local health services.

Voluntary health organizations

Voluntary health organizations are private agencies, each interested in some particular aspect of health. Many are concerned with the control of a specific disease or group of diseases, while others are interested in the actual care and rehabilitation of patients. A partial list of health organizations in the United States follows.

1. Alcoholic Foundation—P. O. Box 459, Grand Central Station, N. Y. 10017.

2. American Association for Health, Physical Education and Recreation—1201 16th St. N. W., Washington, D. C. 20007.
3. American Association to Promote the Teaching of Speech to the Deaf—1537 35th St. N. W., Washington, D. C. 20007.
4. American Cancer Society—219 East 42nd St., N. Y. 10017.
5. American Eugenics Society—1790 Broadway, N. Y. 10019.
6. American Foundation for Mental Hygiene—1790 Broadway, N. Y. 10019.
7. American Foundation for the Blind—15 W. 16th St., N. Y. 10011.
8. American Hearing Society—817 14th St., N. W., Washington, D. C. 20005.
9. American Heart Association—1775 Broadway, N. Y. 10019.
10. American Mission to Lepers—156 5th Ave., N. Y. 10010.
11. American National Red Cross—17th and E Streets, N. W., Washington, D. C. 20006.
12. American Social Hygiene Association—1790 Broadway, N. Y. 10019.
13. Child Welfare League of America—130 E. 22nd St., N. Y. 10010.
14. Federation of the Handicapped—241 W. 23rd St., N. Y. 10011.
15. Industrial Hygiene Foundation—4400 5th Ave., Pittsburgh 15213.
16. Jewish Braile Institute of America—1846 Harrison Ave., N. Y. 10013.
17. John Milton Society for the Blind—156 5th Ave., N. Y. 10010.
18. National Foot Health Council—321 Union St., Rockland, Mass. 02370.
19. The National Foundation—800 2nd Ave., N. Y. 10019.
20. National Health Council—1790 Broadway, N. Y. 10019.
21. National Rehabilitation Association—411 7th Ave., Nashville 37203.
22. National Research Council—2101 Constitution Ave., Washington, D. C. 20037.
23. National Society for Crippled Children and Adults—11 South La Salle St., Chicago 60603.
24. National Tuberculosis Association—1790 Broadway, N. Y. 10019.

The American Heart Association is an example of a voluntary health organization. The activities of this agency are devoted to the control of diseases of the heart and circulation. The membership is composed of physicians and lay persons. Funds are solicited by public subscription in an annual national campaign. The American Heart Association has a threefold program, consisting of research into better means of prevention, diagnosis, and treatment of heart diseases; education of the public and the medical profession; and community service to victims of heart and circulatory diseases. They publish pamphlets and books for nonmedical persons and medical journals for physicians. The National Advisory Heart Council, which advises the governmental National Heart Institute on the making of grants, draws a large portion of its membership from officers of the American Heart Association.

This agency is much like other voluntary health organizations, all of which perform a vital service on the medical team.

HERE IS YOUR DENTIST

One of the most important members of the health team is the dentist. He is responsible for the diagnosis, treatment, and prevention of diseases of the teeth and mouth. He must have a thorough knowledge of the structure, origin, growth, function, and diseases of the organs of the mouth, as well as medical, surgical, and mechanical treatment in this area. He also must realize the relationship of the mouth to other body areas, and must know how general body diseases may be reflected by disorders in the mouth.

There have been dentists for as long as there have been physicians. Indeed, one of the world's most ancient civilizations, located between the Tigris and Euphrates rivers, left documents which cited some 52 rules for care of the teeth, including bleaching of discolored teeth and the prevention of bad breath. The Talmud contains specific rules of oral hygiene, and the Koran gives instructions in the use of a "toothbrush." However, the modern toothbrush was not invented until 1498, when a Chinese "dentist" developed such a brush for the royal family.

Little knowledge of the teeth was gained until recent years. In ancient Greece, infants were drugged during the teething period, and as late as the eighteenth century, dentists were advised to plunge a red hot knife into the gums for toothache. Much of the rudimentary information about the teeth was gathered in the sixteenth century by Bartholommeo Eustacheo, who studied the teeth, their blood and nerve supplies, and the phenomenon of first and second dentition.

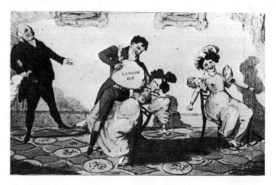

A 19th century caricature by Cruikshank suggesting the use of nitrous oxide or laughing gas as a cure for scolding wives. *Bettmann Archive.*

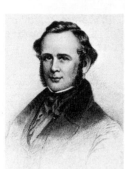

WELLS, Horace (1815-1848) American dentist. Nitrous oxide gas had long been a curiosity because of its strange effects when Wells put it to work to produce surgical anesthesia in the year 1844. It was two years later that Morton demonstrated the use of ether in producing general anesthesia in surgical patients. Wells' application of "laughing gas" was one of the milestones in medical history because it suggested the use of vaporous anesthetics.

One of the persons who contributed to the discovery of anesthesia was a dentist, Horace Wells, who in 1844 attended a demonstration on the effects of nitrous oxide or "laughing gas." Intrigued with the possibilities of this gas, he administered some to himself and had a colleague extract one of his teeth. The operation was entirely painless. Consequently, Doctor Wells employed nitrous oxide in his dental practice.

A little over 100 years ago, a person could become a dentist by serving an apprenticeship to a practicing dentist. In 1840, the first college for the systematic education of dentists was established, the Baltimore College of Dental Surgery. The history of dentistry as a profession may be said to have begun at this date.

Today, a person desiring to enter the dental profession must first spend from three to four years at an accredited college as a predental student. While there, he will take courses in mathematics, chemistry, physics, biology, English composition and literature, a foreign language, history, philosophy, and other social sciences. In his last year of predental work, the student takes a special aptitude test to determine whether he is a suitable candidate for dental school. Among other elements, this test measures the student's dexterity; this is an important quality for one who wishes to do dental work.

From the top level predental students, the dental schools select their student body. There are 59 approved dental schools in the United States, and these are usually branches of large universities; a list of these schools may be obtained from the American Dental Association, 222 East Superior Street, Chicago, Illinois 60611.

The dental school course takes four years to complete and leads to the degree of Doctor of Dental Surgery (D.D.S.). The curriculum includes many of the subjects studied by prospective physicians at medical schools. However, more hours are spent studying the anatomy of the head and neck areas and diseases and problems of the mouth and teeth.

After the student has received his degree from a dental school, he must pass an examination given by a state board of licensure before he is given a license to practice. If he does not go into practice, he may return to school to take advanced work leading to other degrees, or he may elect further study in a specialized field of dentistry.

The average practitioner of *dentistry* is not a specialist. His work consists of cleaning, filling, realigning, extracting, and replacing teeth. Until recent times, tooth extraction itself was one of the most crudely done operations of minor surgery; now it is scientifically performed and virtually painless. Indeed, as has been mentioned, the development of anesthesia had its origin in the offices of dentists who searched for a method to ease pain during tooth extraction.

The trend toward specialization among dentists has become increasingly apparent in recent years. Some of the specialty fields include *oral surgery,* which embraces procedures from tooth extraction to major surgery on the mouth and jaws, and *prosthodontics* or *prosthetic dentistry,* which implies the making of artificial replacements for facial areas removed by surgery. *Orthodontics* is another dental specialty which has to do with the prevention and correction of abnormal positions of the teeth and jaws by means of braces and other mechanical devices. The dentist who specializes in diseases of the supporting structures of the teeth, gums and gingiva, is a specialist in *periodontics. Pedodontics* is a dental specialty concerned with oral diseases in children, and a dental *roentgenologist* specializes in dental diagnosis by means of x-ray films.

The dental profession, like the medical profession, has its standard of conduct which its practitioners are required to follow. The official organization which formulates and maintains professional ethics is the American Dental Association, with its affiliated and local societies. Nearly every dentist belongs to this group, which has done much to equip the dentist to perform a vital function on the health team.

29 MEDICAL ASPECTS OF ATOMIC AND HYDROGEN BOMB WARFARE

ATOMIC WEAPONS

An atomic bomb having an energy release equivalent to 20,000 tons of TNT was exploded in the air over the city of Hiroshima in Japan on August 6, 1945, producing an estimated 120,000 casualties among the 300,000 inhabitants. A second bomb, exploded over Nagasaki three days later, produced another estimated 65,000 casualties, and contributed to the surrender of the Japanese government on August 14, 1945. About one sixth of the casualties were killed instantly in both cities, and later deaths brought the total to around 120,000. That these estimates of casualties were low is evidenced by the fact that in 1960, the U.S. Atomic Bomb Casualty Commission reported that 230,000 persons still suffered physical effects ranging from burns to cancer as the result of the two bombings. Certainly the casualties were great. Both in number and kind the casualties differed from anything in human experience, and they signaled the advent of a new and vast area in medical science. The experimental hydrogen bomb was exploded at Eniwetok on March 1, 1954, and had a power many times greater than that of the Hiroshima bomb, once again changing the magnitude of the medical problems of atomic warfare. While much of atomic medicine is devoted toward the prevention and treatment of atomic and hydrogen bomb casualties, a second aspect of the subject is concerned with the applications of radioactive materials in medicine and industry for the improvement of human welfare. An understanding of the fundamental nature of the bomb and its contents is essential for an appreciation of the facts of atomic medicine.

Principles of atomic energy

An atomic explosion is based upon principles *very different* from those in all other types of bombs, because it involves the conversion of matter into energy. Conventional explosives are effective because they are suddenly converted by chemical reaction from one physical form, generally liquid or solid, into gases which, because of their greater volume, create a high pressure wave. These changes from one physical form and substance to other substances in gaseous form are also accompanied by the release of large amounts of energy in the form of heat. Nevertheless, the weight of all of the products of the explosion is exactly equal to the weight of the exploding materials. This is *not* true in the case of an atomic explosion, because the products always weigh less, and the difference rests in the amount of material that has been converted into energy. One pound of uranium yields about 10,000,000 kilowatt hours of heat energy. This energy would be equivalent to that obtained from about 3,000,000 pounds of coal; the atomic blast at Hiroshima was close to the equivalent of 20,000 tons of TNT. Only a portion of the material in an atom bomb actually is caused to react in this fashion. In order to understand how so much energy can be stored up in one ounce of material, something must be known concerning the fundamental structure of matter.

Atomic structure

Matter consists of all of the physical things of which the universe is composed. It is made up of exceedingly minute particles known as *atoms*. There are 92 different kinds of atoms in nature, known as elements. Nine others are not known to occur in nature, but have been prepared artificially. These elements, totaling 101, have different chemical properties, and combine with each other in different ways to form the various compounds or *molecules* that give our physical surroundings their characteristics. Some common molecules composed of various combinations of atoms are: water (hydrogen plus oxygen), salt (sodium plus chlorine), sugar (carbon plus oxygen plus hydrogen), and TNT (carbon plus oxygen plus hydrogen plus nitrogen).

Most molecules are so small that they cannot be seen with even the most powerful microscopes, and the atoms of which they are composed are of course even smaller. If atoms could be enlarged to a size at which they were visible, it would be possible to show that they are composed of particles of energy. In the center of the atom is a core or *nucleus,* bearing a positive electrical charge, and around this in concentric shells would be found a variable number of negatively charged particles of energy known as orbital *electrons*. The ability of atoms to combine with other atoms to form molecules depends upon reactions involving the orbital electrons. The major particles of energy in the nucleus of an atom are called *nucleons*. Some of these, called *neutrons,* bear no electrical charge, while others, the *protons,* carry a positive charge. The nucleus of a hydrogen atom contains only one proton or positive charge; an oxygen nucleus contains eight; a nitrogen atom seven; a uranium atom ninety-two.

All of the atoms of any given element have the same chemical properties because they have the same number of protons in the nucleus (or electrons in their orbits) but they may differ from each other in relative weights because of a different number of the neutral particles or neutrons in the nucleus. The forms of an element having different weights because of different numbers of neutrons in the nucleus are known as the *isotopes* of an element. Thus the nucleus of the atom of ordinary hydrogen con-

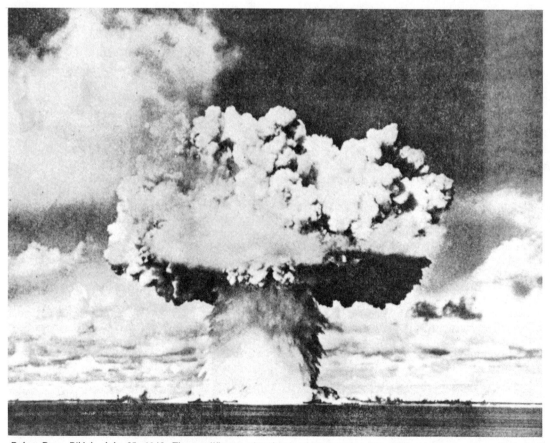

Baker Day—Bikini—July 25, 1946. The cauliflower aftercloud, after dumping two million tons of water, which had been sucked up by the underwater explosion. *Courtesy Joint Task Force One.*

tains only one proton and no neutrons. A rare isotope of hydrogen found in nature to the extent of 0.0156 percent has a nucleus with one neutron and one proton. The chemical properties of this isotope, known as deuterium, are still those of hydrogen, but it weighs twice as much as the common isotope because of the presence of the two particles in the nucleus. It is deuterium that combines with oxygen to form heavy water. Its *atomic weight* is therefore said to be two. A third and even rarer isotope of hydrogen, tritium, contains two neutrons in the nucleus, and therefore has an atomic weight of three. Some elements may have many different isotopes, all having the same chemical properties, but different relative weights. Common tin, for instance, has ten different naturally occurring isotopes.

Radioactivity

During the Dark Ages and for centuries thereafter it was the hope of the alchemists and chemists to be able to convert baser metals such as lead into gold. Such a type of change was finally realized following the discovery of the phenomenon of radioactivity.

The discovery of x-rays by Wilhelm C. von Roentgen (1845–1923) in Germany in 1895 led to the study by Henri Becquerel (1852–1908) of whether substances made phosphorescent by visible light emitted a penetrating radiation sim-

ilar to x-rays. Becquerel found that rays given off by uranium salts were capable of exposing a photographic plate, even though the uranium was separated from the plate by a piece of paper. Subsequent studies of this phenomenon by Becquerel, Marie Curie (1867–1934), Pierre Curie (1859–1906), and others showed that penetrating radiation was given off by a number of elements, and that in the process these elements were converted to completely different elements. Some isotopes found in nature are stable, giving off no radiation, while others are naturally radioactive, being continuously converted to other elements, which in turn may be either stable or radioactive. The isotope of hydrogen with an atomic weight of three is radioactive, while the other two hydrogen isotopes are stable. Radioactive decay of hydrogen three (tritium) converts it to helium, and is accompanied by the emission of beta rays or electrons. The property of radioactivity is much more common among the isotopes of the heavier elements. Radioactive decay may be associated with the ejection from the nucleus of *beta* rays composed of negatively charged particles identical with electrons, *alpha* rays composed of positively charged helium nuclei, or *gamma* rays which are high energy radiations similar to x-rays. Gamma rays have high penetrating power, beta rays much less, and alpha rays may even be stopped by a sheet of paper. Because these radiations act on matter to form pairs of positive and negative ions, they are known as ionizing radiations, al-

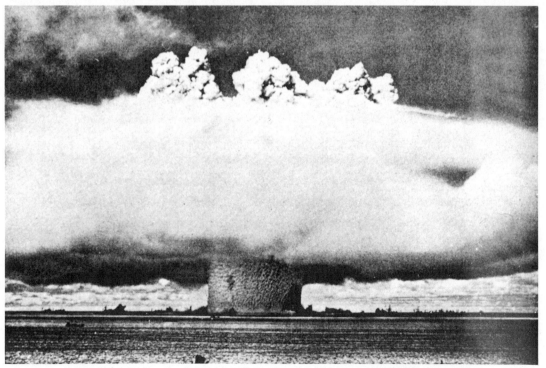

Formation of the plume (column) in the "Baker" test. *Courtesy Joint Task Force One.*

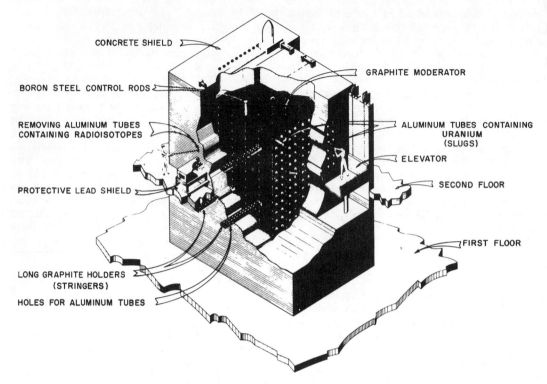

CONCRETE SHIELD

GRAPHITE MODERATOR

BORON STEEL CONTROL RODS

REMOVING ALUMINUM TUBES
CONTAINING RADIOISOTOPES

ALUMINUM TUBES CONTAINING
URANIUM
(SLUGS)

ELEVATOR

SECOND FLOOR

PROTECTIVE LEAD SHIELD

FIRST FLOOR

LONG GRAPHITE HOLDERS
(STRINGERS)

HOLES FOR ALUMINUM TUBES

Nuclear Reactor-Uranium "Pile." *Courtesy Isotopes Division, U.S. Atomic Energy Commission.*

though x-rays, gamma rays and neutrons produce ionization indirectly.

The rate and characteristics of radioactive decay vary from isotope to isotope, and have immense practical importance. The rate of decay or conversion to another isotope is measured in terms of the time required for a sample of the material to lose one half of its radioactivity. This rate is characteristic of each isotope and unalterable, and is known as the *half-life.* It may vary from less than one millionth of a second to billions of years. Of the ten natural isotopes of ordinary tin, one isotope is radioactive and constitutes about six percent of the tin. Its half-life is nearly one billion years.

In relatively recent times methods have been found for bombarding the nuclei of atoms with neutrons, protons, and alpha particles and thus producing nuclear instability and radioactivity. Examples of instruments used for the acceleration of particles to sufficient speed to insert them into the nucleus are the cyclotron and betatron. Capture of neutrons by a nucleus is generally associated with the instantaneous emission of gamma radiation.

Nuclear fission

In the case of some of the isotopes of the heavy elements, induced changes in the nucleus may cause the atom to break up into much smaller fragments of matter. This phenomenon is known as *nuclear fission,* and is accompanied by the release of large amounts of energy. The isotope of uranium having an atomic weight of 235, and the isotope of plutonium of atomic weight 239, have properties that make them undergo fission. They are therefore of value in the preparation of an atomic bomb.

Free neutrons, which exist in the atmosphere, may strike the nucleus of an atom of uranium 235 and cause it to undergo fission with the formation of lighter elements. Along with this, several free neutrons would be released, and would be able in turn to cause the fission of more atoms of uranium 235. By continuing this sort of a *chain reaction,* all of the atoms in a piece of uranium could eventually be induced to undergo fission. If the piece of uranium were too small, however, many of the neutrons might escape from the surface of the material before being captured by a nucleus, and the chain reaction would fail. An atomic explosion can therefore not ensue unless there is a large enough mass of uranium to capture enough neutrons to propagate the chain reaction. The *critical size* of fissionable material is that piece just large enough to retain more neutrons than can escape, and in an atom bomb is consequently one of its most important aspects. An atomic bomb works by

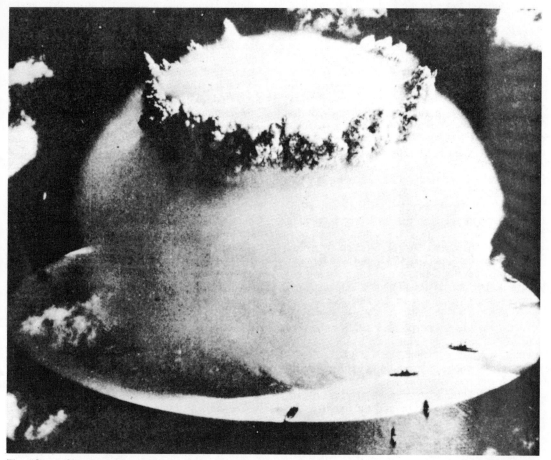

The "Cloud Chamber" effect observed after the underwater explosion at Bikini, July 25, 1946. *Courtesy Joint Task Force One.*

bringing into contact two subcritical sized pieces of the fissionable material to produce a piece exceeding the critical size. The magnitude of the critical size of fissionable material has been one of the great secrets of the atomic bomb. In order to achieve an effective explosion, the two pieces of material must be brought together rapidly. If the speed of this process is not sufficiently great, a *fizzle* will result with most of the material remaining intact. In an atomic explosion, the two portions of fissionable material are rapidly blown apart, and only a small portion of the total material actually reacts. Means for keeping the two portions in contact for a few millionths of a second longer greatly improve the magnitude of the explosion. Present atomic bombs are said to be over 25 times as powerful as the first models. The first atomic bomb was exploded at Alamogordo, New Mexico, on July 18, 1945. Between then and 1970, four other nations had mastered the technology of producing and detonating atomic weapons: They are Russia (1949), England (1952), France (1960), and Red China (1964).

The explosion resulting from the chain reaction-induced fission of heavy atomic nuclei involves the formation of isotopes of lighter elements and the loss of nuclear particles in the form of a tremendous amount of energy. The equation for the amount of energy formed from the disintegration of matter was first proposed by Albert Einstein (1880–1955), and is stated

$$E = mc^2$$

This expression states that the energy released (E) is equal to the weight lost in the process (m) multiplied by the square of the speed of light (c^2). This energy is released in the form of heat, light, and various other forms of radiation. The heat generated at the time of the explosion is enough to raise the temperature of the fission products to nearly two million degrees F.

The theory of the hydrogen bomb is quite different from that of the atomic bomb, in that it involves putting lighter atoms together to make a larger one, a process called *fusion*. Under suitable conditions, with the intense heat generated by an atomic bomb explosion, atoms of hydrogen isotopes may be condensed to form an atom of helium. When properly sparked, this *thermonuclear* reaction results in the release of a tremendous amount of energy, equivalent to over a million tons (megatons) of TNT. The test bomb exploded in April of 1954 was said by some writers to have had a power of 45 megatons. In October of 1961 Russia exploded what they stated to be a 50 megaton bomb; United States scientists estimated it to be 62–90 megatons.

The ability of atomic nuclei to undergo fission was first reported in Germany by Otto Hahn in 1939. In this case fission was demonstrated in the laboratory on a small scale. Controlled nuclear reactions have since been found to be of great value in the preparation of radioactive isotopes, and are carried out in a chain-reacting *pile* or nuclear reactor. The first of these, constructed at the University of Chicago, was first operated on December 2, 1942, and was a major step in the development of the atomic bomb because it first demonstrated that a self-sustained nuclear chain reaction was possible. Since then over a score of atomic piles have been constructed for various purposes, including the production of power and the manufacture of plutonium 239. In principle, they contain a neutron source such as uranium, a *moderator* to slow down the neutrons such as graphite or heavy water, and adjustable metal rods to capture some of the neutrons and thus control the rate of the reaction. The production of plutonium 239 in reactors for use in atomic bombs is much simpler than the long and expensive process of separating uranium 235 from its other isotopes for this purpose. Continued production of atom bombs is essential since they are an integral part of the hydrogen bombs.

Major United States government installations for the study and production of atomic weapons and radioactive isotopes are at Oak Ridge, Tennessee; Los Alamos, New Mexico; and Hanford, Washington, with many other distributed throughout the country. In addition, many studies are conducted under government contract by universities, hospitals, industrial laboratories, and other similar institutions. Control of all such activities is vested in the United States Atomic Energy Commission, which is concerned with the development of atomic energy for peace as well as for war.

Measurement of radioactivity

The problems of atomic medicine in both war and peace involve the accurate measurement of radioactivity. Standard units are in use for the expression of the strength of radioactivity and the biological effects of radiation. The unit of radioactivity is the *curie,* and is the amount of any radioactive material that undergoes the same rate of radioactive decay as one gram of radium. (One million curies is known as a *megacurie*. In medicine, much smaller amounts of radioactive material than a curie are often used. One thousandth of a curie is called a *millicurie,* and one millionth of a curie is known as a *microcurie*.) Expressed differently, in one curie of any radioactive substance, 37 billion atoms are converted to some other isotope each second. One minute after the explosion of an atomic bomb of nominal size, the gamma ray-emitting fission products have a strength of about one million million curies, but through radioactive decay this decreases after six months' time to about 260,000 curies. Since devices for measuring radioactivity are generally designed to measure the number of disintegrating atoms in any given time, the radioactivity is measured in curies, but this gives little specific information with regard to biological effects. The radioactive decay process itself is a harmless one. The dangerous effects associated with radioactivity are due to the rays that are emitted from atoms as they undergo decay, and depend entirely upon the type and strength of these rays. Two different isotopes having the same disintegration rate (strength as measured in curies) may give off different types of rays, and therefore have vastly different effects on living tissues. It is consequently necessary to be able to measure the effect of this radiation.

The unit of radiation is called the *roentgen,* and often abbreviated R. The roentgen is a measure of the amount of radiation energy available to produce electrical charges, or ions, in air that absorbs the rays. This type of change is known as *ionization*. For medical purposes, it is necessary to know the amount of damage produced by ionizing radiation in tissues. A dose of one roentgen will produce a certain amount of change in the body, just as a dose of one aspirin tablet will produce a specific effect. Unlike most drugs, however, doses of radiation may be restricted to only a portion of the body. A sudden dose of 600 roentgens, such as might be received from an atomic bomb, is considered fatal to human beings, if directed at the entire body. When directed at a finger, or a small cancer, however, this dose would affect only the irradiated area, without any other specific effect on the body. Just as with most drugs, a single fatal dose would not be harmful if received over a long period of time. The medical result of a given number of roentgens being absorbed thus depends upon the amount and type of tissues exposed and the length of time of the exposure. In general, it may be said that total body exposure to as much as 25 roentgens in a short period of time may not produce any apparent symptoms or detectable damage. A second dose of this size, repeated too soon thereafter, however, might produce injury.

The ability of a ray to produce damage depends to some extent on its capacity to penetrate tissue. This penetration in turn depends on the kind of ray and its energy. The energy of radiation is expressed in *millions of electron volts* (*Mev,* one of which is equivalent to 0.000000000000038 gamma-calorie). High-energy radiation has a much greater penetrating ability.

Instruments for measuring radiation are of two general types, measuring either the ionizing effect of the rays or their effect on a photographic plate. The latter type of device is particularly simple, and is convenient for personnel to carry with them on their clothing. It consists of one or more small pieces of covered photographic film, such as dental x-ray film, attached to the clothing in a convenient badge. The film is removed and developed in the laboratory at frequent intervals, and the amount of blackening of the film is an indication of the amount of body radiation. Such a film badge weighs an ounce or less, is inexpensive, and is capable of measuring both beta and gamma radiation over a range of from 0.010 to 10,000 R.

Of the instruments for measuring radiation based on ionization, the most familiar is the Geiger-Muller counter. In this and similar counter instruments, ionization of a gas by the radiation causes the formation of an electrostatic charge which can be detected by its effect on the counter tube. Intensity of radiation may be

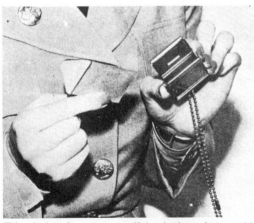

This device is a new, self-developing photographic dosimeter, used to measure the extent of exposure of individuals to atomic radiation. Readings can be obtained from the dosimeter in one minute after exposure to atomic rays. The device consists of a small metal case containing a flat paper package, which in turn contains photographically sensitized film and a pod of developing solution. Exposure to gamma radiation causes the center strip to turn light—the greater the exposure, the whiter the strip. Since gamma rays are the ones to be reckoned with in an atomic exposure, shielding in the case blocks out alpha and beta radiation. The dosimeter, simple and inexpensive to produce, is made to be worn about the neck. *Official Department of Defense Photo.*

indicated in various ways, depending on the exact type of instrument. Commonly it is reported in terms of the number of times that the tube discharges (counts) per second or minute. These counts may be indicated as sounds or flashes of light, or recorded on dials that read directly in number of counts. Some counters are so simple and light in construction that they may be portable and used in outside work, while others are quite complex, and adapted for the sensitive measurement of radioactive isotopes in the clinic and research laboratory.

Employment of atomic weapons

The problems of civilian defense and medical treatment in an atomic disaster are closely related to the type of weapon employed and its mode of delivery. The energy, radiation, and materials resulting from nuclear fission have been proposed as the basis for a number of different types of weapons. Most familiar is the atomic bomb based on uranium 235, or plutonium 239, and the hydrogen bomb. The size of the bomb blast at Nagasaki and Hiroshima, the equivalence of 20,000 tons of TNT, is described as *nominal,* and much more effective weapons have since been developed. The H-bomb is far more effective than any of the earlier types of atomic bomb. Artillery shells for use in warfare have also been developed and tested. Long-range rockets having an atomic head have been developed for use against civilian populations. Harbors might easily be mined with atomic weapons.

It has been suggested that a cloud composed of radioactive dust might be directed against personnel, but the practicality of this is uncertain. The soil of agricultural areas might be seeded with radioactive material that would contaminate the crops and make them unsuitable for human consumption, but this also seems remote at present. The problem of deliberate soil and air contamination is closely related to the question of whether such an event might not occur as the result of the explosion of too large a number of bombs. It has been estimated that the hazard of worldwide radioactive contamination of fatal intensity would require the explosion of a mi lion or more bombs of the size used in Japan. Similar considerations indicate the great improbability of any effect of a moderate number of atomic explosions on the weather.

The most probable means of delivery of atomic weapons on a civilian population is by long-range air attack. Southern areas of the United States, more remote from an attack via the Arctic route, might be more conveniently attacked by submarine-launched aircraft. Bombs may be delivered by rocket or by robot planes, and may be planted anywhere by espionage workers. There is therefore no safe area against attack. Detection of raiding bombers by a screen of radar stations surrounding the North American continent is possible but far from certain, and interception of raiders by planes of the United States Air Force Air Defense Command is likewise uncertain. These considerations are important to civilian defense against atomic attack because the disaster may come either with or without warning, and in either case preparations for the emergency must be made in advance.

The effects of an atomic or hydrogen bomb explosion depend upon whether the burst occurs in air, on the ground, or in water. The point directly beneath the detonation is known as *ground zero*. The explosions in Japan were of the air-burst type. Damage can conveniently be classified as resulting from air blast, heat, and radiation. Most of the effects considered here refer for purposes of simplicity to bombs of the size released in Japan. The range of injuries from more powerful bombs would not, however, be directly proportional to their increased power. Thus, to double the radius of blast and burn damage would require a bomb about eight times more powerful, but this would only increase the radius of radiation injuries by about one third.

Blast effects are caused by the shock waves that result from the sudden expansion of gaseous material at the center of the explosion. The front of the shock wave travels at a speed of about 1200 feet per second and acts like a moving wall of highly compressed air or water. As the shock wave moves, it loses its force. After ten seconds, when it is at a distance of about two miles from the ground zero of a nominal sized atom bomb, it is still strong enough to break windows. Blast damage from recent types of hydrogen bombs would extend to over 25 miles. The shock wave is the most effective damage-producing agent of the air-burst bomb. Most man-made structures are damaged by an air shock pressure of 2 to 15 added pounds of pressure per square inch. Maximum damage from a nominal atom bomb results when it is exploded at an altitude of about 2000 feet, and the pressures directly below this will be from 25 to 50 pounds per square inch. Buildings can be made to withstand this quite readily, but not the explosion of a hydrogen bomb. Following the aerial explosion of a nominal-sized atom bomb, blast damage will cause almost complete destruction for a radius of about one-half mile, severe damage to one mile, partial damage to two miles, and some light damage to eight miles. Complete destruction from a hydrogen bomb could extend for a radius of about seven miles or more. The shielding effect of buildings or hills may modify the shock wave. In a surface burst, of a nominal bomb, total destruction or severe damage would be limited to a much smaller area if there were sufficient high buildings. A subsurface explosion would cause strong earthquake-

LETHAL EFFECTS OF 20 MEGATON BOMB
(From Garb, *Missouri Medicine*, 1962)

Effect	Ground Burst No Shelter	
	Probable Lethal Radius in Miles	Probable Lethal Area in Square Miles
Crater	0.35	
Absolute destruction of underground shelter	1.0	3.14
Initial nuclear radiation	2.5	20.0
Blast effects	10.0	314.0
Flying missiles	10.0	314.0
Initial heat radiation	12.0	452.0
Firestorm*	Up to 20	1,250.0
Radioactive fallout	140 (oval)	10,000 to 20,000

*This effect is unpredictable.

type damage to walls, foundations, and buried utilities, but the over-all blast damage would be far less than in other types of burst. *Direct* blast effects from the nominal bomb are relatively harmless to personnel, the total injuries resulting from it in Japan being limited to less than 200 ruptured eardrums. *Indirect* blast effects, however, such as falling buildings and flying debris, accounted for a tremendous number of injuries. Over 30,000 persons are believed to have been killed in this way in Hiroshima, and an equal number injured.

Heat radiation from a subsurface explosion would be almost completely absorbed by the earth and water. The intense heat at the moment of the explosion of an atomic bomb is of short duration, and in surface or air bursts produces

HEAT EFFECTS PRODUCED IN VARIOUS MATERIALS AT DIFFERENT DISTANCES FROM AN ATOMIC EXPLOSION
(Values are for an average clear day)

Distance (feet)	Material	Effect
2400	Lucite	softens
	Bakelite	chars
4300	Black Maple Wood	burns
5100	Cotton twill	burns
5400	Worsted (tropical khaki)	burns
5900	Douglas fir	burns
6300	White paper	burns
	Cotton shirting (gray)	burns
	Gabardine (green)	burns
7000	Synthetic rubber	burns
	Rayon lining	burns
	White paper	chars
10000	Human skin	moderate burns
	Black paper	burns
	Nylon (olive drab)	melts
12000	Skin	slight burns

Distances are to the explosion, rather than ground zero.

RADIATION DOSAGE RATE ON GROUND ONE HOUR AFTER EXPLOSION OF A BOMB AT A HEIGHT OF 100 FEET

Distance from Ground Zero (feet)	Dosage Rate (R per hour)
0	8000
300	5000
600	600
900	150
1200	30
1500	10
2250	5
3000	.3
3750	.07

Residual radiation would be much lower for bombs burst at higher altitudes to achieve greater blast and thermal effects.

the effect of a flash burn. Most burns are produced within the first second following the explosion. Almost any material, however, will provide some shielding against this thermal radiation. In a surface atomic bomb explosion, inflammable materials will be ignited within a half-mile radius unless shielded by buildings or hills. In an air burst, fires may be started by the heat for a radius of about three miles. Some exceptions may occur in this instance, as with blast injury. In any case, many secondary fires are caused as a result of the air-blast damage. After the initial blast the winds then reverse and blow from the outlying edges toward ground zero and the central "chimney" through which the winds rise. The secondary fires that have been formed move together centrally with the wind in a devastating *fire storm*. Over half of the Japanese injured by the atom bomb suffered burns, but many of the flash burns were limited to areas of the skin not covered by clothing. The radius of thermal injury from a hydrogen bomb is of course much greater.

Radiation effects are due either to the initial radiation of the bomb burst or to *residual* radiation coming from the fallout of radioactive substances formed by the bomb. Because of shielding and absorption, initial radiation effects are of most importance in an air burst, in which case they may be fatal to unprotected persons within a radius of 4200 feet or four fifths of a mile from a nominal atom bomb. Initial radiation is harmless at a mile and a half from an atomic blast or several times this from a hydrogen bomb. Residual radiation is usually harmless in an atom bomb air burst. In a ground burst, residual radiation may be a hazard over a large area, and in the case of a subsurface blast, dangerously radioactive materials may be dispersed for great distances, particularly downwind. Residual radiation was not a significant factor in Japan, and only about 15 percent of the fatalities there resulted from initial radiation. Radiation injuries are the only type of injury unique to the atomic

bomb as contrasted with older weapons. The residual radiation from a hydrogen bomb may be greater than from an atom bomb. Even though the isotopic products of the thermonuclear reaction are not radioactive, the induced radioactivity may be very high. A hydrogen bomb could be specially constructed, however, to furnish large amounts of residual radiation in addition to the products of the atom bomb that sparks it. Radioactive fallout has produced accidental casualties, however, in the bomb tests in the Marshall Islands.

When a hydrogen bomb explodes, millions of tons of earth are sucked up and become radioactive. This material is carried through the stratosphere by winds, and falls back to earth at widely varying distances from the point of explosion. The fallout pattern will usually be cigar-shaped, and the area of most intensive fallout will be within less than 150 miles from ground zero. Persons within this area will probably receive lethal doses of radiation unless they have shelter.

Radioactive fallout is the major hazard of the hydrogen bomb. In the table relating to the lethal effects of a 20-megaton bomb, the radioactive fallout area is estimated to be 10 to 20 thousand square miles. If people are equally distributed throughout this area and have no shelter, 1 percent will be killed in the area of absolute destruction; fewer than 1 percent will be killed by initial nuclear radiation; perhaps 2 percent will be killed by blast and flying debris; another 1 percent might die from initial heat radiation, and if a firestorm occurs, another 5 percent would perish. The remaining 91 to 96 percent will die of radioactive fallout.

CASUALTIES OF ATOMIC WARFARE

Knowledge concerning atomic bomb casualties is largely derived from experience in Japan, where medical observation teams are still maintained. Other data have been obtained from observation of accidental radiological injuries (as in the Marshall Islands), and from studies on experimental animals. The destructive effects of the atomic bomb in Japan are believed to be indicative of what might be expected in the United States. The damage in Japan was more extensive because of the enormous number of shacks and flimsy living structures there. Some reinforced concrete buildings in Japan were designed to withstand earthquakes, however, and therefore offered as much protection as would most similar buildings in the United States. Since the types of casualties resulting from a hydrogen bomb would be the same as from an atom bomb, they require little specific consideration. The radius over which death and injury occur would simply be greatly increased.

Wounds, burns, and radiation injury, singly or combined, characterize the atomic bomb casualty. The relative frequency with which these injuries occur depends upon where the bomb is exploded, the distance of the patient from the explosion, the shielding provided the patient, and the degree of destruction of materials in the patient's vicinity. While wounds and burns generally develop immediately, much of the radiation injury is a delayed effect. The immediate casualties are therefore quite similar to those sustained from any large bombing attack. The total number of casualties is much greater, however. In addition, the total area of the destruction is such that the evacuation of wounded persons is particularly difficult, and many seriously injured patients die before aid can be reached.

Blast injuries

Blast injuries are caused by the shock waves that result from the atomic explosion. They occur for a radius of about two miles from the point directly beneath the air burst explosion of a nominal size atom bomb, and for a radius of over twenty miles from a hydrogen bomb. Shock waves may cause primary or direct blast injury by their effects upon persons, or they may act indirectly by destroying nearby structures, portions of which strike the individual. Direct blast injuries were rare in Japan, accounting for only a few ruptured eardrums. Indirect blast injuries were found in about 70 percent of the casualties in Japan. Collapsing buildings and flying debris are therefore the major casualty-producing agents of the atomic bomb. The injuries include crushing, fractures, lacerations, hemorrhages, scratches, and bruises. Of the injuries in one Japanese hospital, bruises accounted for 52 percent, lacerations for 37 percent, and fractures for 11 percent. Most of the lacerations were due to flying glass. Glass fragments penetrated up to an inch beneath the skin, and clothing offered protection only against the numerous minute fragments. Although most fatal injuries occurred among those persons in native Japanese buildings, due to collapse of the buildings, nonfatal injuries were greater among those in concrete buildings, partly because of the greater number of glass windows in these.

Successful treatment of blast injury patients depends upon the rapid administration of first aid by survivors, and subsequent evacuation of more seriously injured cases to emergency medical centers. The techniques of first aid for atomic bomb casualties differ in no way from those employed for the casualties from any other type of disaster. Artificial respiration may be necessary to keep the patient breathing. Hemorrhage must be stopped, wounds must be dressed, and the

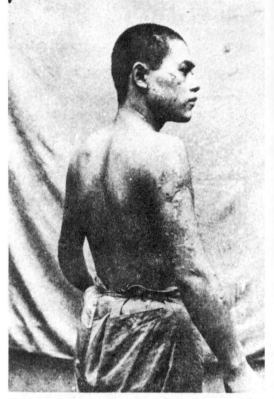

Multiple injuries by flying glass. Patient was standing approximately 5 feet from the window, indoors, in a military barracks. His upper torso was nude, but he was wearing trousers, which were not penetrated by the glass. *Courtesy Armed Forces Institute of Pathology.*

physiological shock that accompanies severe wounds must be minimized. Following a ground or subsurface explosion, early washing and dressing of open wounds may be necessary to prevent the entrance of radioactive materials into the body through the break in the skin.

One of the major medical problems following an atomic bomb explosion is the large number of trained persons and the vast amount of medical supplies that are immediately required to treat the thousands of blast injuries that occur. As an example of the enormity of this requirement, about 50,000 pints of blood or blood derivatives are required for the treatment of the casualties that result from a bombing such as that of Nagasaki. The total estimated collection of blood in the United States for civilian use is about 96,000 pints per week, of which about 74,000 pints are collected by the Red Cross, but only a small portion of this would be available for disaster use.

Burns

Flash burns result from the brief, highly intense thermal radiation given off with the initial flash of an atomic explosion. They occur within a radius of about three miles from the point of explosion of a nominal size atomic bomb. From 65 percent to 85 percent of the casualties in Japan suffered burns, but about 5 percent of the burns resulted from fires that destroyed large areas of the affected cities. These latter burns are similar in appearance to the flash burns, and therefore require no special consideration in this discussion.

Depending upon exposure, flash burns cause reddening of the skin (first degree burns), blistering (second degree burns), or damage to deeper layers of the skin (third degree burns). Close to an atomic bomb blast, burns and blisters appeared on the skin within five minutes. At about one mile, burns appeared in two hours and blisters in four to six hours. At a mile and one-quarter, burns appeared in three hours and blisters after ten hours. The initial redness of the burns in many cases changed after a few days to a walnut stain in appearance, known as the "mask of Hiroshima."

The thermal radiation that causes flash burns has poor penetrating power, and even light clothing offered excellent protection against it in Japan at a distance beyond three quarters of a mile. The image of protecting material was therefore often clearly outlined on the skin, producing a *profile* characteristic of the atomic bomb flash burns. An ear may have been burned, while the skin behind it was left intact. Since darker cloth absorbs more heat than lighter shades, black polka dots were burned out of clothing, leaving the lighter surrounding material intact, and a polka dot profile burn on the underlying skin. Floral designs on cloth were similarly affected, and the burned areas were often traced on the skin of the patient. Some of the most severe burns of all were caused in this manner. Tightly worn clothing was more dangerous than loose clothing from this standpoint, and double thicknesses of cloth, such as occur at seams, were especially protective and created a characteristic protected profile area on the skin. Hair was sometimes singed or burned off, and baldness resulted when the hair follicle was destroyed. In this case a cap would create a profile burn by restricting the area of hair loss.

A further characteristic of the burns that resulted from the atomic blasts in Japan appeared following healing, when many patients showed an unusual overgrowth of scar tissue, known as *keloid* formation. While malnutrition, irritation, infections, and other factors may have caused this, a Japanese racial characteristic may also be involved, since such keloids were observed following the healing of burns from fire-bomb raids over Tokyo.

Because of the large number of flash burn casualties from an atomic explosion, the demands for medical personnel and supplies are

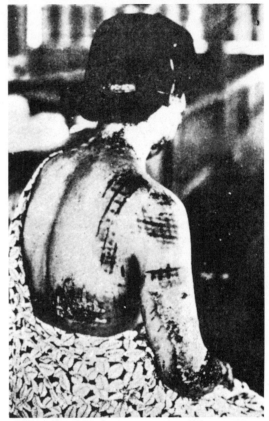

Flash burns. The darker portions of a striped pattern of cloth that the patient was wearing absorbed more heat and produced gridiron burns of the skin. The arm below the sleeve and the unprotected face were severely burned. *Courtesy Armed Forces Institute of Pathology.*

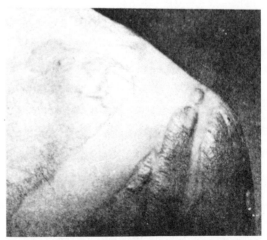

Keloids following flash burns. Protective effect of shoulder straps of slip and of sleeve seam. Pigmentation at margins of the burns. *Courtesy Armed Forces Institute of Pathology.*

great, as in the case of blast injuries. Many burns are delayed in appearance, however, so that there is less urgency in supplying treatment. Methods of first aid and medical treatment are the same as for ordinary flame burns. Few patients suffering third degree burns live long enough to receive medical attention. Uninfected first degree burns heal promptly if not irritated. In persons suffering concurrently from radiation injury, however, the danger of infection is greater than usual, so that added precautions must be directed toward protecting the burn from infection.

Radiation injury: cause

Radiation injury is caused by the damaging effects on the body tissues of penetrating radiation. Examples of such radiation are beta and gamma rays, neutrons, and x-rays. The rays may be given off during the explosion of an atomic bomb, in which case gamma rays are of major importance. Radiation may also originate from the radioactive materials that are formed as products of the atomic explosion.

Casualty-producing radiation is active by virtue of its ability to produce chemical changes (*ionization*) in the constituents of the cells of the body. These changes are dependent upon the total amount of radiation which the cells or tissues absorb. As the result of cosmic radiation from outer space, and radiation from natural radioisotopes on the earth, the average person at sea level normally receives about 0.002 R of radiation each week throughout his life. This is about one percent of the safety level of 0.3 R per week. Full body exposure to a sudden dose of radiation of 50 R or more produces injurious effects on the body, however, and doses of 600 R are thought to be generally fatal.

Effects in Japan

Over 30 percent of the atomic bomb casualties in Japan suffered some degree of radiation injury. Appreciable injury was limited to those within a distance of about one mile from the point directly below the explosion. Many of those who received the greatest radiation were killed almost immediately by blast and burn injuries which were severe in this area.

Symptoms

Radiation injury represents the only unique casualty-producing effect of the atomic bomb, but is not its major source of casualties. Clothing offers little protection against radiation, so that the casualties generally suffered full body irradiation, the symptoms of which are known as *radiation sickness*. Previous to the explosion

of the atomic bombs, accidental overexposure to x-rays and radioactive materials had been nearly the only source of knowledge of the effects of ionizing radiation on the body. In most of these instances only a small portion of the body was exposed and affected, and the resulting damage was known as localized radiation *injury*.

The specific effects of radiation injury depend not only upon the exact area of the body exposed, but also upon the fact that certain kinds of tissue are more susceptible to injury than others. An example of the variation in sensitivity to radiation may be seen in the observation that guinea pigs are twice as sensitive to x-rays as are mice, and over three times more sensitive than rabbits. In man, sensitivity of tissues to radiation decreases in the following order: lymphoid tissue and bone marrow; epithelial tissue such as the testes and ovaries; salivary glands, skin, and mucous membranes, endothelial cells of blood vessels and peritoneum; connective tissue; muscle, bone, and nerve tissue. It is in this general order, therefore, that the specific effects of exposure to ionizing radiation might be expected to appear and to do the most harm.

Blood changes are among the earliest to appear, and may occur as the result of doses of radiation that produce no other effect (25 to 50 R). If the white blood cells manufactured in the lymphatic tissue (lymphocytes) do not decrease in number within 72 hours following exposure, no serious dose of radiation has usually been received. Increase in the number of lymphocytes is almost the first symptom of recovery from radia-

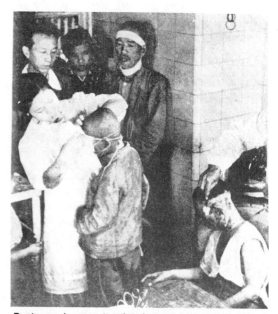

Doctor and nurse treating burned patients. Treatment Room, Post Office Hospital, Hiroshima. *Courtesy Armed Forces Institute of Pathology.*

tion sickness. Other white cells, manufactured in the bone marrow, and blood platelets, decrease in numbers in the blood somewhat later. Since the platelets are concerned with blood clotting, the low platelet count may be associated with severe hemorrhagic tendencies. Because the red ceils have a longer life span in the blood than these other cells, they are the last to show a reduction in number following radiation. All blood cells are thus reduced in number if the radiation dose is large enough. It has been stated by Japanese physicians that patients with white cell counts of less than 500 per cubic millimeter were in gravest danger. In general, the greater the radiation dose, the greater the damage to the blood, and the more slowly the recovery.

It has been recognized for some time that leukemia, a malignant disease in which there is a considerable increase in the numbers of white blood cells, may be induced by overexposure to x-rays. The incidence of leukemia in radiologists is said to be nine times as high as it is in other physicians. Careful studies of the incidence of leukemia among the population of Hiroshima and Nagasaki over a period of years have now shown that there has been a significant increase in this disease among the survivors of the bombs in these two cities. The peak incidence of leukemia was reached in 1961. In all age groups among the exposed people, acute leukemia still occurs at higher-than-usual rates. The rate of occurrence of chronic granulocytic leukemia, which also increased, has now dropped to rates found in the unexposed population.

Thyroid cancer also has been reported more frequently among the atomic bomb survivors than among those Japanese who were not exposed to the bomb. The frequency is higher in women and in those who were subjected to more intense radiation doses. This is a long-delayed effect of radiation injury.

Radiation-injured lymphatic tissue tends to swell due to the accumulation of serous fluid (*edema*), and this effect explains the early appearance of sore throats in many radiation casualties. Wasting away of the lymph glands and tonsils is a common later symptom. Because the cells of the *reticuloendothelial system* (lymph nodes, bone marrow, liver, spleen, and connective tissues) are also concerned with resistance to attack by microorganisms, severe infections may result from even weakly invasive microbes. Boils, infected ulcers, and systemic infections are common in severe radiation injury.

Skin changes due to ionizing radiation were not pronounced in Japan. Small hemorrhages beneath the skin were common, however. Loss of scalp hair due to radiation (*epilation*) was pronounced, and commenced at the end of the second week. This ceased after about 3 or 4 weeks, and in no case was permanent baldness caused by the ionizing radiation. In one group

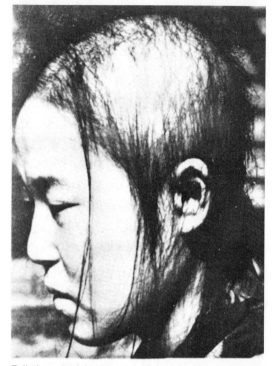

Epilation of scalp (removal of hair by the root). Scattered long hairs of the original growth remain. Patient was in a wooden building in Nagasaki, Japan, at time of bombing. *Courtesy Armed Forces Institute of Pathology.*

of patients who suffered epilation, 65 percent lost scalp hair, 12 percent lost hair from the armpits, 10 percent from the pubic areas, 6 percent lost eyebrows, and 3 percent lost hair from the beard. A few rare cases of edematous swelling of the skin may also have been due to ionizing radiation.

Gastrointestinal symptoms are among the earliest indications of radiation injury, and include nausea, vomiting, diarrhea, cramps, and later, bloody stools. In very severe cases ulcers appear on the tongue, gums, lips, and skin of the face. Inflammation, ulceration, and hemorrhage in the gastrointestinal tract are common. Subsurface hemorrhages tended to occur in certain portions of the urinary tract and other tissues. These brought about fatal consequences in many cases when they occurred in the heart, brain, lungs, or kidneys. Pneumonia occurred in some cases, but was not a common symptom.

The intense brightness of the flash of the atomic bomb caused blindness of only a few minutes to a day or so, even among those looking directly at it. The eyes of all but a few persons were protected from thermal radiation burns in Japan due to the natural resistance of the eye, its recessed position in the head, and the blink reflex. Eye injuries resulting from ionizing radiation were common, however, among those who received a high dose of radiation. Direct injury commonly involved degeneration of the lens, but many other symptoms resulted indirectly from infection and anemia. Radiation was also probably responsible for a relatively high incidence of cataract that appeared later among the exposed population.

Effects of ionizing radiation upon fertility in Japan were manifest in several ways. The testes were profoundly affected in men receiving high dosages of radiation, but the amount of radiation required to produce permanent sterility is in most cases also lethal. Temporary sterility was common among those receiving lower doses of radiation, but permanent sterility was rare. Women were similarly affected, although the ovaries are less sensitive. Various temporary menstrual disturbances were also observed. There was an increased neonatal and infant mortality rate. Microcephaly with mental retardation developed in some children exposed *in utero* to the atomic bomb, occurring most frequently among those who had been in the first trimester at the time of exposure. The frequency of evidence of such intrauterine injury appeared to be related directly to the distance from the hypocenter at the time of the bomb; it was greatest among those closest to the hypocenter. In children conceived subsequent to the bombings, any influence resulting from exposure of their parents to the radiation remains questionable at the present time.

Because of the well-known genetic effects of irradiation, the children conceived after the bombs and born to the survivors have been extensively studied. Six indicators of genetic damage were investigated: congenital malformation, stillbirths and neonatal deaths, birth weight, physical measurements, sex ratio, and childhood mortality. No effect attributable to radiation was demonstrated in relation to five of these six indicators; only in sex ratio (male/female) was a slight change noted. These shifts in sex ratio occurred in the first ten years following exposure to the bombs, but not thereafter. Thus, the exact significance of this one finding remains equivocal.

Persistent and complex chromosome abnormalities have been demonstrated in the white blood cells of bomb survivors. The frequency of such abnormalities was greater in those over 30 years of age at time of exposure, and in those who received greater amounts of radiation. Similar chromosomal changes were present with increased frequency among children exposed *in utero* to the bombs. No such abnormalities were found in children who were conceived and born after the atomic bomb to parents, one or both of whom had been exposed to the bomb.

Studies of growth of the exposed children have indicated a small but significant decrease in the body measurements compared to nonexposed children. Although these differences occurred at all ages and could be related to increasing radiation exposure, other factors such as nutrition and economic loss must be considered.

Radiation sickness

Any of the symptoms of radiation injury previously discussed may appear singly or in combination when only a portion of the body is exposed to ionizing radiation. These symptoms appear together in varying degrees of severity in radiation sickness following full body exposure. Their intensity will vary appreciably with the amount of radiation that has been received and with the individual.

A dose of several thousand roentgens will produce death in several days, but such exposures unaccompanied by grave blast or burn injuries are quite rare. Persons receiving a whole body lethal dose of about 600 R manifest nausea, vomiting, indefinite discomfort, and often shock after the first two hours following exposure. This may or may not be followed by a symptomless latent period of two or three days during which grave changes are occurring in the body. Fever, an inflamed mouth and throat, general pallor, and wasting away follow the latent period. Diarrhea, at first watery and then bloody, also appears as a symptom. There is a stepwise increase in temperature, severe degeneration of the internal organs, and in the later stages a tendency toward hemorrhage and infection. The more rapidly the initial symptoms develop, and the shorter the latent period, the sooner is the patient likely to die. Delirium, coma, and death generally follow exposure within a two-week period.

Doses of radiation of 400 R, which produce about a 50 percent mortality, are also marked by the appearance after two hours of nausea, vomiting, loss of appetite, and an indefinite feeling of discomfort. These symptoms remain for a day or so, and then disappear for a longer latent period of from several days to two weeks. At the end of this time the initial symptoms reappear, along with a stepwise increase in temperature, diarrhea, hemorrhaging, and inflammation of the internal organs. The hair may fall out, and the mouth and entire gastrointestinal tract becomes infected and then inflamed and often ulcerated. Severe general infection is frequent. Emaciation, delirium, coma, and death may follow in from two to six weeks or sometimes longer. Patients who survive for three or four months gradually recover when their condition is not aggravated by some complication such as tuberculosis, pneumonia, or malnutrition.

Moderate doses of radiation (100 to 300 R) generally produce no definite symptoms of radiation sickness at all for the first two weeks. Starting at about the third week, however, a sore throat may appear, along with diarrhea, pallor, a loss of appetite, and general weakness. The hair may fall out, and small hemorrhagic areas (petechiae) may appear in the skin. When these symptoms are uncomplicated by poor health or by other injuries, gradual recovery from these relatively mild effects may be anticipated. The speed of recovery will be greatest when the early symptoms are milder. Malnutrition due to impaired ability to assimilate food from the damaged intestinal tract may complicate the picture in many cases.

When nausea and vomiting are not present as an early symptom, the probability of survival from ensuing radiation sickness is good. When they are present, and the latent period does not appear or lasts only a day or so, the prognosis is very poor, since the patient will probably have received a lethal dose of radiation. When the latent period lasts for more than a few days, survival of the patient will depend to a considerable extent upon his individual constitution, concurrent disorders that he may suffer, and adequate medical treatment.

Experience with regard to radiation injury from radioactive fallout is largely limited to that gained from the accidental exposure of a number of Marshall Islanders during tests in the Pacific Ocean. Because of an unpredicted shift in the wind, radioactive material fell like snow on several inhabited atolls, approximately 100 miles east of the explosion, and was deposited on skin, clothes, hair, and the environment. It was estimated that people occupying these islands were exposed to about 175 R whole body radiation from penetrating gamma rays. In addition, they received superficial doses to the skin from fallout deposits. They also absorbed radioactive fission products internally from ingestion of contaminated food and water. The islands were evacuated within 72 hours.

During the first 24 to 48 hours, about two thirds of the people experienced anorexia, nausea, irritation of the eyes, and itching of the skin. The early symptoms disappeared within a few days. Radiation burns of the skin and epilation became apparent about two to four weeks later. Healing of the skin took place in a few weeks, with practically no residual changes; hair regrowth was complete by six months. Blood value alterations characteristic of radiation injury were also noted. These signs and symptoms were more frequent and more severe among children than among adults. No infections or bleeding tendencies were seen. There were no deaths attributable to the fallout radiation exposure. The contaminated islands were not considered habitable until three years after the fallout; return to the home island then took place.

Regularly conducted medical examinations of these people indicated a retardation in growth and development of some children—particularly boys exposed to fallout at less than five years of age. Beginning about ten years after the exposure, abnormalities of the thyroid glands became detectable. As of 1969, more than one third of the native people most heavily exposed to the fallout had developed thyroid abnormalities. Almost all of the children who were exposed to the fallout at ages younger than ten years have also been affected. While most of these abnormalities are benign nodules in the glands, several instances of cancer have been found.

Radioactive iodine was present in the 1954 fallout and was ingested in the drinking water and food prior to evacuation of the contaminated islands. The iodine was then concentrated in the thyroid glands. There seems to be little doubt that this led to damage of the gland, eventually causing the formation of nodules in many, and the development of cancer in some. The thyroid glands of young children were most intensely damaged and the tumor development as well as the growth retardation are now attributed to the thyroid injury. The evidence of this radiation effect became detectable after a latent period of ten to thirteen years.

Treatment

There is good reason to believe that, as medical research workers discover more facts concerning the exact nature of radiation injury within the cells of the body, it may be possible to treat successfully persons receiving presently lethal doses of radiation. Effective measures of treatment at present are limited to those persons receiving fewer than 600 R. Immediate hospitalization and avoidance of exposure or fatigue are essential, despite the appearance of the misleading and asymptomatic latent period. The principal direct causes of death from radiation sickness are the anemia, hemorrhagic tendency, gastrointestinal disturbances with attendant malnutrition, and infection. Whole blood transfusions must therefore be given until the bone marrow recovers sufficiently to restore the various types of blood cells to the circulation. The bleeding tendency also presents a therapeutic problem. In order to provide adequate nourishment, sugar, amino acids, vitamins, and minerals may have to be administered intravenously for some time. Extensive use of antibiotics to prevent and control infection is necessary until the integrity of the disease-combating reticuloendothelial system has been restored. Careful attention to other injuries is also of major importance. Extended bed rest, along with good medical and nursing care, would undoubtedly have greatly increased the number of survivors of radiation sickness in Japan. The facilities and training that would have made this possible, however, were generally lacking.

CIVIL DEFENSE MEASURES

The problems of civil defense against hydrogen bomb attack largely differ only in degree from the problems of atomic bomb attack. Since a much greater number of persons in the center of any populated area would be beyond all medical help, it is apparent that large population centers must be evacuated if possible when there is an attack warning, or otherwise protected in suitable shelters. The problems of civil defense and casualty handling in the large area outside the 14-mile-diameter core of complete destruction still remain similar to those encountered with the atomic bomb, but fallout radioactivity could be a great problem for many square miles downwind. Since the exact location of ground zero will remain unknown until after the explosion, there is a possibility for everyone that he will be in this surrounding zone of partial destruction. Therefore, when an attack is immediately imminent, people must take the same precautions that they would had the bomb been a small atomic weapon.

According to the best estimates, with presently known defense measures only three out of every ten missiles that might attack the United States in an air raid could be shot down before they reach their target. In the event of a war, therefore, and in view of the fact that the Soviet government is known to have exploded test hydrogen bombs as early as August 1953, extensive measures would be necessary to limit and handle the magnitude of bomb casualties that would result. The responsibility for defense measures is included in a Civil Defense program in which at least 15 million trained persons should be active participants. Hiroshima and Nagasaki had virtually no civil defense organization, and needless thousands consequently perished through fire, exposure, and neglect after the initial damage was done. Of equal importance to a nation at war, these cities could not have been restored to productive capacity for extended periods following the bombings.

Organization

The Civil Defense organization consists of existing civil authorities concerned with the public welfare supported by vast numbers of volunteer workers. Existing authorities consist of federal, state, and local officials, and members of the armed forces. In many areas, volunteer forces are as yet unorganized.

The role of the armed forces in civil defense is in detecting and repulsing the attack, and in warning the appropriate civil officials when an attack is expected. Adequate warning of an attack to permit evacuation from target areas is crucial to present defense plans. In addition, the armed forces may supply some technical information regarding defense measures, and a limited number of technicians to assist with special problems. They also decide on such matters as blackouts, dimouts, camouflage, and radio silence. They operate the radar ground observer system. The military services are not concerned with the details of local civilian defense. They may, however, assist local militia or police in insuring law and order if martial law is declared.

The Federal Civil Defense Administration is responsible for contributing technical information and some kinds of emergency supplies in civil defense, and pays part of the cost of equipment and shelters. It acts primarily as the basic planning unit in civil defense, but it does not run the civil defense program. The federal government merely supplies the defense plan upon which the states organize and operate.

The governor of each state appoints a state civil defense director, who is responsible for the program in that state. A continuously staffed civil defense control center in each state receives attack warning alerts from the Air Force, and acts as an operations headquarters for the direction and control of activities during an emergency. It is the communication center of the state, and is responsible for co-ordinating the activities of all communities and facilities in lending assistance to an emergency area.

Civil defense centers have been set up in most cities and communities, and particularly in major target areas, under the mayor or his local civil defense director and staff. This group is responsible for evacuation of the area and for the direct fight against fire, damage, injury, and death following an atomic or hydrogen bomb attack. While the community must depend as much as possible upon its own resources, some aid will undoubtedly be available through the state and federal agencies. Many communities have set up agreements with neighboring communities for mutual aid in the event of a disaster. Some areas have special mobile units that can move rapidly and lend aid on a state-wide or interstate basis.

It is manifestly apparent that the local civil defense director along with the usual public employees could not meet the emergency demands that would arise in an atomic disaster. Volunteer workers thus become the major key to the entire problem. It is said that public education, training, and organization are the biggest civil defense problems. In each area, volunteer workers are organized into ten major volunteer services to work for the public welfare.

The Warden Service is the backbone of civil defense because it is the source of neighborhood leadership before, during, and after an attack. A warden is usually responsible for a city block or factory area containing about 500 persons, and has records of all persons in his area. He helps to evacuate persons from the area or otherwise to prepare them for an attack when this is impossible; he conducts them to safety during the attack, and helps to restore order later. The warden is the link between the family and the city level of defense. Women make excellent wardens because they are usually at their home post night and day.

The Fire Service is concerned with preparations and training for fighting fires. Fire is a major cause of death following an atomic or hydrogen bomb blast. Aside from the numerous large fires that would be fought by local fire departments and volunteer auxiliary units, a great many smaller fires break out. These latter must be combated by persons in the locality who have been previously trained in the proper methods. In Japan, only limited equipment for fire fighting was available, and much of this was destroyed by the atomic bomb blasts, so that many of the casualties died in the fires that eventually consumed much of Hiroshima and Nagasaki.

The Police Service is concerned with two major problems in civil defense, the control of traffic and the maintenance of law and order. Following any major disaster, positive efforts are necessary to prevent pilfering, and in time of war, sabotage. Many police departments now have auxiliary police to aid in handling crowds, but these must be aided with further volunteer forces. Traffic control in an emergency area is fundamental to the success of all other efforts, both in evacuation of an area before an attack, and in establishing communications following one.

The Health Service has the responsibility for all matters dealing with health and medicine. Doctors and nurses are only a very few of the total number of persons required. Thousands of first aid workers, litter bearers, ambulance drivers, supply handlers, food inspectors, radiation monitors, clerical workers, dish washers and others are needed to handle the inevitably large numbers of casualties, and to provide for sanitation measures which are vitally needed in any disaster. First aid and home nursing training are essential aspects of this service.

The Welfare Service is concerned with providing food, clothing, money, and shelter to the helpless following a bomb blast. They would also care for infants, the aged, and the infirm, and help to locate missing persons. It may be quite necessary for those whose home and belongings survive an attack to give emergency food and shelter to many persons who have been less fortunate.

The Engineering Service must restore a bombed city to working order as soon as possible by clearing away debris and repairing damaged facilities. Existing engineering groups and utility personnel, assisted by other skilled workmen and by labor unions, would perform much of this service. Following an atomic or hydrogen bomb explosion, the rubble makes the movement of casualties to medical centers very difficult, so that the engineering service, aside from its reconstruction activities, is vital to the reduction of the mortality rate.

The Rescue Service must liberate persons trapped by debris following an attack. Rescue teams must include hundreds of first aid workers, aside from hospital staffs. The number required would be much greater for a hydrogen bomb explosion. The injured could not even be reached, however, until hundreds of trained members of the engineering service had cleared the way. The tremendous number of skilled persons required can only be attained by a large-scale training program prior to an emergency. For this reason, civil defense authorities schedule such training in most communities. Some courses are offered through the Red Cross, schools, and various other agencies, while many courses are sponsored directly through the Office of Civil Defense. Every person can and should volunteer for such training. Information with regard to its availability may readily be obtained from the top administrative office of the city or community, from the Civil Defense Director at the State Capitol, or from the Federal Civil Defense Administrator in Washington, D.C. Numerous instructive booklets are available from this latter organization or from the local office of civil defense.

Supplies

Following the explosion of an atomic or hydrogen bomb, there will arise as the result of the destruction a tremendous immediate need for medical supplies, food, water, engineering materials, and other items. Much of the available stock will have been destroyed, the demand will be greatly increased, and transportation facilities to deliver it will be impaired. The demand for blood and blood derivatives for the casualties from one atomic bomb would be about 50,000 pints a week for the first three weeks, and this amount would have to be pooled from the entire country. Many other requirements would be similarly enormous.

The major solution to this problem is in the stockpiling of many items as a civil defense measure. First aid supplies may be stocked in federal and local warehouses away from the target area. Additional hospital beds and equipment of that nature would probably be requisitioned from private homes. On the family level, food and first aid supplies should be available. Several days' supply of canned goods and well-sealed staples should be kept on hand in the home, and a complete emergency first aid kit should be sealed up in a moisture-proof covering and kept in the home shelter area. Persons living near a target area should establish contact with someone in a local community 30 to 50 miles distant with whom they could stay if evacuation became necessary.

Provision of a water supply for drinking, sanitation, and fire fighting following an atomic bomb explosion is a major problem. Water works may be destroyed, pipelines broken in houses and buildings, and what running water is available is frequently contaminated with sewage. All water for human use must therefore be sterilized. Restoration of water service will depend upon the problems encountered by engineers in the process, but will be a *top priority* undertaking. Individual fire fighting techniques may therefore have to depend on special techniques. For health purposes it is generally estimated that a gallon of potable water per day per person is the minimum requirement, but for one or two days this might be cut severely. Men die from lack of water, however, much more rapidly than from lack of food. Consequently, a supply of cans of juices should be kept available for such an emergency, and water should be similarly stored if at all practical. Many American homes have an adequate temporary reservoir in their hot water heaters.

Warning systems

Warning of an atomic or hydrogen bomb explosion is of the greatest importance in reducing the casualties that will be produced. Prompt action following the flash of light accompanying the bomb will even save lives, since the speed of light is much more rapid than the shock wave which follows it and which requires about five seconds to go one mile. Moreover at one second after the flash, only half of the gamma radiation will have been received so that instantly ducking into a slit trench or convenient building might well save the life of a person who otherwise would receive about 400 R and possibly die. Flash burns are not avoidable on this short notice, as shown by the fact that profile burns caused by the shielding effect of a moving object such as a leaf make it appear the leaf was standing still.

A warning of a minute or so could offer considerable protection to most persons beyond a seven-mile radius of the anticipated ground zero who had made previous arrangements for such an event. A longer period of warning would permit evacuation. The first line of defense against invading aircraft is the radar screen around the coastline, and this is supplemented with a ground observer system. This is broken up into air defense divisional units, each with a military control center. At this center aircraft are identified and military action is ordered. Also present is a civil defense air-raid-warning officer, who communicates by telephone or radio with key points in the area. The civil defense attack-warning controller at the key points relays the warning to his city, the surrounding counties, the hospitals, police, fire departments, and the public through local warning devices.

Outdoor sound devices for air raid warnings should be located at appropriate places throughout any populated area, and are centrally controlled. They are a community responsibility, although technical advice concerning them is supplied by the Federal Civil Defense Administration. The official sound signal for an impending attack (*red alert*) is a modulating sound of three minutes' duration. This may consist of a varying pitch or loudness, or of a series of blasts. The official signal for an *all clear* is a one-minute blast, a two-minute silence, a one-minute blast, a two-minute silence, and a final one-minute blast.

Radio has become a major medium of communication in many countries, and warning, as well as subsequent instructions, may be expected through the normal broadcast band. Special communications in an emergency would be broadcast at one or both of the extreme ends of the broadcast band, depending upon various factors. Evacuation instructions would be transmitted in this manner. Following the radio silence often observed during a raid, both ends of the radio dial should be periodically checked for important civil defense instructions. Public, commercial, and amateur short wave radio transmitters and receivers also play important special roles in civil defense activities.

Population evacuation and public shelters

Proper procedure following warning of an impending atomic or hydrogen bomb attack depends entirely upon the amount of time available. Proper public signaling systems to indicate this are arranged by the local civil defense authorities. When an hour or more is available, as may be the case when warnings originate from the far northern radar screen, target area populations will be evacuated to outlying districts. Extensive plans to expedite this massive type of move are the responsibility of the local authorities, and in many areas practice evacuations have already been held. All means of transportation are used in an integrated fashion to achieve efficient and rapid movement. Because of the tremendous traffic load placed on the limited number of roads leading from any given city, persons residing in any area are assigned a specific evacuation route. Some roads will be reserved for special civil defense purposes, and all traffic movement will be rigidly controlled.

Immediate shelter of some sort must be taken following warning of an imminent air raid. When away from home, availability will be taken of public air raid shelters. Public shelters may be either inside or outside of existing buildings, with the former predominating in the United

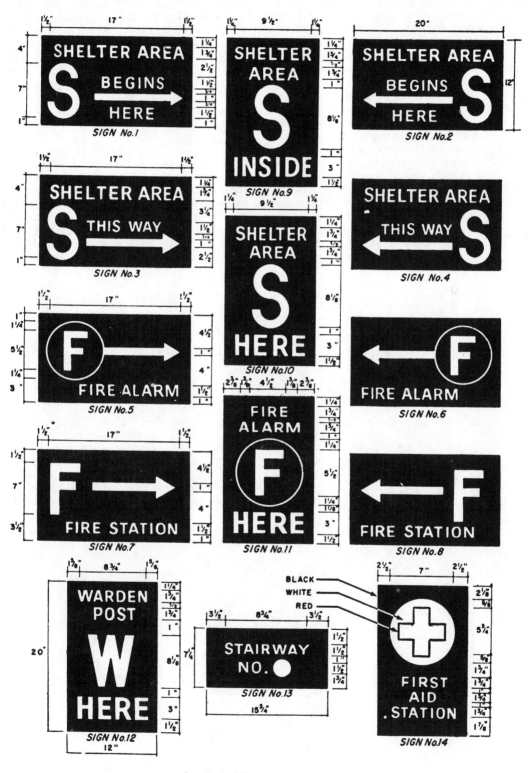

Standard civil defense signs.

States. Many existent American buildings would provide protection against blast, flame, and radiation at distances of over one-half mile from ground zero. Relatively few would be effective within this area, and construction of such buildings is largely impractical, although not impossible. It might be noted, however, that some Japanese in Nagasaki found protection in hillside tunnel shelters within a few hundred feet of ground zero.

Inside shelters should be adequately marked by Civil Defense signs. They should be located on the lower floors and halls or interior portions of fireproof, reinforced-concrete or steel-frame buildings that are resistant to collapse. They should be protected against falling plaster or flying glass. Outside shelters should preferably be buried or semiburied, so that an added cover of dirt will give protection against radiation. Some buildings require additional strengthening before they would provide sufficient resistance to blast. Ideally, shelters should be provided with a ventilating system, self-contained power system for lights, a telephone between the inside and outside, emergency rations, first aid equipment, water, benches, blankets, and chemical toilets. Frame buildings would provide little shelter within a radius of about one and one-quarter miles, but their cellars would provide better shelter than none at all despite the probability of being trapped there and injured by falling debris or fire. It is anticipated that new buildings will be constructed with higher blast resistance properties than those now in existence, but these will never provide a major source of shelter.

Home shelters

In constructing shelters for protection from the effects of explosions of nuclear weapons, radioactive fallout is a particularly important consideration. The reason for this is the great distance which the radioactive dust from the explosion travels through the atmosphere, a distance which may reach many hundreds of miles. Thus the area of exposure to the toxic effects of

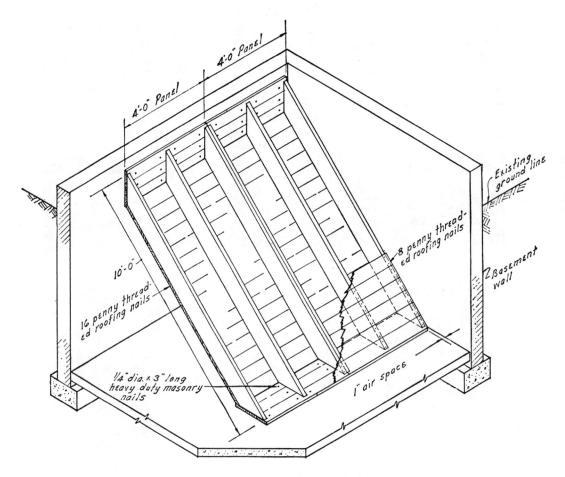

The basement lean-to shelter.

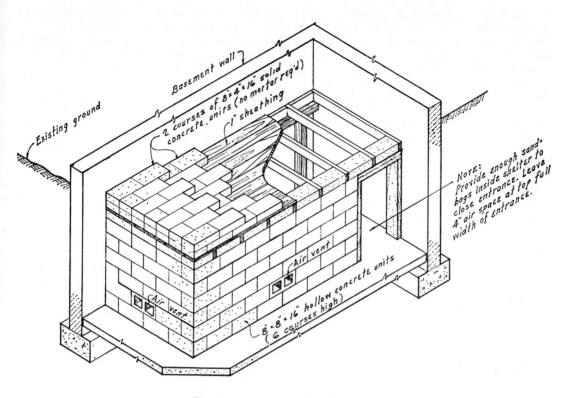

The basement concrete block shelter.

radioactivity is many times as large as that in which serious injury is likely from the effects of blast and shock wave. Therefore shelters should be constructed and equipped to make provision for fallout as well, as far as possible, as for blast.

These needs may be met, in large centers of population, by the construction of public shelters, or by the adaptation of cellars of large buildings and other available structures. For the many smaller communities, and for the smaller home areas of large communities, obviously other types of shelter are necessary. For that reason the U.S. Department of Defense and Office of Civil Defense issued the booklet, "Family Shelter Designs," which is available throughout the nation from local Civil Defense authorities,

and which gives directions for the construction of various types of shelters.

The *basement lean-to shelter* can readily be constructed by the homeowner, and provides a considerable degree of protection at minimum cost. It is designed to provide protection from the effects of radioactive fallout in the below-grade basement of an existing structure. Its advantages are low cost, simplicity of construction, general availability of materials, and the fact that it may be easily disassembled. An isometric view of it is shown. In the size shown, it provides 128 cubic feet of space—sufficient to shelter three persons, although it can be extended by the use of more materials. As shown, it requires the following materials:

2″ × 12″ × 10′ rough or surfaced lumber	6 pieces
1″ × 6″ × 4′ rough or surfaced lumber	50 pieces
1″ × 6″ × 8′ rough or surfaced lumber (for top covering)	20 pieces
¼″ diameter × 3″ long heavy-duty masonry nails	2 pounds
Sixteenpenny threaded roofing nails	6 pounds
Eightpenny threaded roofing nails	3 pounds
Dry sand	5½ tons
Sandbags	30
Building paper or polyethylene sheet	150 square feet
Water repellent* (5 percent pentachlorophenol or equal) toxic to wood-destroying fungi and insects.	1 quart

* Optional.

The shelter is designed to provide a fallout protection factor of at least 100 in most residences. It also provides some protection from flying debris associated with blast. Natural ventilation is obtained by omitting two sandbags from the top of the entranceway closure and by leaving a 1-inch gap between the end of the shelter and the basement wall. Construction time should not exceed 20 man-hours when all the materials are on hand at the shelter location. The use of precut panels would reduce the erection time. When this shelter is erected in a dry basement which is kept free of vermin, its life expectancy range should be from 10 to 15 years.

The construction sequence for building this shelter is as follows:

1. Brush-coat all surfaces of lumber with water repellant solution; double brush-coat all cut edges. (Optional.)
2. Cut 45° bevels on 2″ × 12″ stringers. Arrange in 4-foot panels. Using sixteenpenny threaded nails, attach bottom boards on the beveled ends first.
3. Fit in and nail remaining bottom boards.
4. Turn this panel rightside-up and place it in its permanent position. Fasten the panel to the wall and floor with heavy duty masonry nails, leaving a 1-inch gap between the end of the shelter and the basement wall.
5. Construct and fasten in sequence as many panels as are to be used.
6. Line the panels with building paper or polyethylene.
7. Using eightpenny nails, begin attaching top boards at the floor first. Keep the spaces thus formed filled with loose sand as the top-board application progresses. (Building paper or polyethylene sheet should also be applied between the sand and top boards.)
8. Thirty sandbags, each filled with 30 pounds of sand, should be placed in the shelter for emergency closure of entranceway.

The *basement concrete block shelter* also provides low-cost protection from the effects of radioactive fallout. It is intended to be installed belowgrade in a basement. Its principal advantages are simple design, speed of construction, ready availability of low-cost materials, and adequate protection against fallout radiation. By increasing the ceiling height to 6 feet or more, it could also serve as a dual-purpose room. An isometric view of it is shown.

In the size shown, it has 260 cubic feet of space—sufficient to shelter four persons. This model requires the following materials:

8″ × 8″ × 16″ hollow concrete masonry units*	65
8″ × 4″ × 16″ solid concrete masonry units*	135
Mortar (prepared dry mix)	5 cubic feet
Sand or concrete (for filling cores)	1 ton
Sandbags	30
4″ × 4″ × 3′8″ wood posts (structural grade)	4
2″ × 8″ × 3′8″ wood posts (structural grade)	2
2″ × 8″ × 2′4″ wood beam (structural grade)	2
4″ × 4″ × 10′3″ wood beam (structural grade)	1
1″ wood sheathing	52 board feet
2″ × 4″ × 4′8″ wood joists (structural grade)	8
4″ × 4″ × 10′3″ wood beam (structural grade)	8
2″ × 4″ wood bracing (structural grade)	10 linear feet
⅜″ × 7″ expansion bolts	12
Sixteenpenny nails	2 pounds
Sixpennny nails	2 pounds
Water repellent (5 percent pentachlorophenol or equal), toxic to wood-destroying fungi and insects.**	1 quart

* Units should be made with concrete having a density not less than 130 pounds/cubic feet.
** Optional.

In most residences, the shelter provides a fallout protection factor of at least 100. It would also provide some protection from flying debris associated with blast. Natural ventilation is provided by the airspace left at the entranceway after emergency closure, and the air vents in the shelter wall. Estimated construction time for the basic shelter is less than 20 man-hours. The life expectancy of the shelter would be about the same as most types of residences.

1. Lay out guidelines with chalk on basement floor for shelter walls. (See floor plan.)
2. Lay first course of block in a full bed of mortar. Vary thickness of mortar bed if basement floor is not level.
3. Continue to lay wall blocks. Corner of wall should be built up first, about three or four courses high, before laying blocks in remainder of wall. All blocks should be laid in a full bed of mortar. Where 8-inch blocks

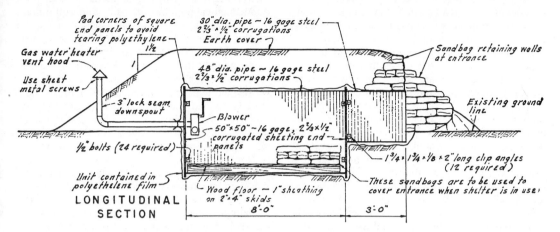

Belowground corrugated steel culvert shelter.

are required, cut 16-inch units in half with a hammer and chisel.

4. Fill cores of blocks with sand (or concrete) after three courses have been laid up.

5. Continue procedures indicated above in steps 3 and 4 until walls have been laid up to a height of 4 feet (six courses), and all cores have been filled with sand (or concrete).

6. Brush-coat all surfaces of lumber with water-repellent solution. Double brush-coat all edges. (Optional procedures. Desirable for wood preservation.)

7. Fasten wood posts and doorjambs to existing basement walls and shelter walls with expansion bolts. Use two bolts per post. (See side elevation.)

8. Place wall beam and door lintel beam in position and secure to posts with nails.

9. Place wood joists and bracing in position and secure together with nails. (See roof framing plan.)

10. Place portion of wood sheathing on top of joists. Nail wood sheathing to joists. (See isometric view.)

11. Place solid concrete masonry units on top of wood sheathing. No mortar is required between these units.

12. Continue procedures indicated above in steps 10 and 11 until roof covering has been completed.

13. Bags of sand or additional solid concrete blocks should be stored near entrance for emergency closure, but airspace of at least 4 inches should be left at top of closure for ventilation and air circulation.

The *belowground corrugated steel culvert shelter* is designed to provide low-cost protection from the effects of radioactive fallout. Its principal advantages are that most of the structure is lowered into an excavation and that it requires only simple connections and covering to complete the installation. A sectional view of it is shown below. In the size shown it has 120 cubic feet of space (including the entranceway). It provides space for three persons, although larger sizes are available.

As shown it requires the following materials:

Prefabricated steel culvert shelter (with bolts and clips supplied, if unit is not spot welded).*	1
Galvanized steel lock-seam downspout	6 feet
Elbow for steel lock-seam downspout	1 foot
Ventcap (gas water-heater type)	1
Intake air blower (optional for 3 persons or less)	1
Scrap lumber	9 board feet
6 mil. polyethylene film (20′ width)	30 feet
Sandbags (to hold 75 to 100 pounds each)	18
Sandbags (to hold 15 to 20 pounds each)	30
Flyscreen 7″ × 7″, for ventpipe	1
Entranceway insect screen 36″ × 36″	1
Soil or sand (for shelter cover)	5 tons

* Fabricators should treat spot-welded areas with bitumastic compound or other approved waterproofing material.

When the entranceway is properly shielded as shown in the drawing the fallout protection factor should be greater than 500. This shelter could be expected to withstand a limited blast overpressure of 5 pounds per square inch. A sheet metal ventilation intake vent 3 inches in diameter is provided together with a manual air-blower for more than three persons. Air is vented through the sandbag closure at the entrance. One man working with hand excavation tools should be able to complete the excavation in less than 2 man-days. Two men will be needed to roll the shelter structure into the excavation from the point at which the shelter has been delivered. If lifting rather than rolling is necessary to transport the structure, four men will be required. The estimated life of this galvanized steel shelter will be at least 10 years under most soil conditions. Under normal conditions highway culverts of similar material have been known to last indefinitely with little maintenance. The general construction sequence is as follows:

1. Select well-drained site. The total area required, including the mounding, will be approximately 15′ ×20′.
2. Use stakes to mark the corners of the area, and excavate. The hole required for the main shell is 5′ × 9′ × 2′ deep, and the entrance requires an additional 2½′ × 4′ × 6″.
3. Line hole with plastic film wrap.
4. Lower galvanized steel shelter into place on supporting wood strips.
5. Assemble and install the vent pipe.
6. Cover shelter with plastic wrap.
7. Backfill and mound. Be sure the shelter is covered by at least 2 feet of packed earth. Depth may be checked with a wire probe. The mound should be covered with grass as soon as possible by sodding or seeding to prevent the protective soil from being eroded.
8. Place small sandbags inside the shelter. These are used to fill the entrance completely after the shelter is occupied.
9. 1-inch boards may be used on 2″ × 4″ blocks to provide a floor.

Other types of shelters are described in the Department of Defense booklet cited earlier. Whatever type of shelter is used, however, provision should be made for certain supplies and equipment for the occupants. A radio receiver should be available to receive CONELRAD broadcasts, and a check of reception should be made in advance so that an outside antenna can be installed if necessary.

Lighting is an important consideration. Continuous low-level lighting may be provided in the shelter by means of a 4-cell hot-shot battery to which is wired a 150-milliampere flashlight-type bulb. With a spare battery, a source of light for 2 weeks or more would be assured.

The housekeeping problems of living in a shelter begin as soon as the shelter is occupied. Food, medical supplies, utensils, and equipment, if not already stored in the shelter, must be quickly gathered up and carried into it. Sanitation in the confines of the family shelter requires much thought and planning. Provision for emergency toilet facilities and disposal of human wastes will be an unfamiliar problem. A covered container such as a kitchen garbage pail might do as a toilet. A 10-gallon garbage can, with a tightly fitting cover, could be used to keep the wastes until it is safe to leave the shelter.

Water rationing should be planned carefully. An adequate supply of canned or tank water is the best source; if it is not available, then water in pails or other containers must be carried into the shelter quickly at the time of emergency.

A portable electric heater is advisable for shelters in cold climates. It takes the chill from the shelter in the beginning. Even if the electric power fails after an attack, any time that the heater has been used makes the shelter that much more comfortable. Body heat in the close quarters helps to keep up the temperature. Warm clothing and bedding, of course, are essential.

Protection of the home

A number of simple preparatory measures can reduce greatly the danger from an atomic explosion to both the home and its occupants. Since fire is one of the major hazards of an atomic explosion, fireproof housekeeping provides an important protective step. Trash should not be allowed to accumulate in closets, attics, and basements, and useless odds and ends should be eliminated. Yards, alleys, and vacant lots should similarly be cleaned up. Homes that have an air space between ceiling and roof should have a trap door into it and a ladder handy to enter it in case of fire. Nothing should ever be stored in such spaces. Wiring systems and heating plants should be checked periodically to insure that they are safe. An emergency first aid kit and three days' supply of food and water should be maintained at all times.

When an alert sounds and time is available, doors and windows should be closed, and blinds, shutters, or drapes drawn. Close all fuel and draft doors on furnaces, open the electric switch on oil burners, and extinguish other open flames. Unless instructions are received to the contrary, one should *not* shut off pilot light or utilities at the source. When there is not sufficient warning of a raid, these same precautions should be taken immediately afterwards when practical. A flashlight, rather than matches, should always be used because of the danger of leaking gas lines. When warning is available, the automobile should be moved off the street and if possible away from buildings that might fall on it. Car windows should be rolled down. The battery-powered car radio may prove to be the only one available after an attack, if electric power is not functioning.

Prevention of fires is greatly facilitated by the use of fireproof materials. This is particularly true of fabrics. All materials not injured by water can be easily and inexpensively given considerable resistance to burning by treatment with a special rinse each time they are washed. A simple and effective solution of this type consists of nine ounces of borax and four ounces of boric acid in a gallon of water.

Protection of food and water

The major danger from the food and water that is available following an atomic explosion is that they will be contaminated by radioactive dusts. Following an air burst, the danger from this is negligible; ground or subsurface bursts, however, may present a considerable hazard in this regard. A tightly closed house is considerable protection against such dust, and food within it will probably be safe. Packaged and canned foods offer complete protection, especially when the container is washed off prior to opening. Nearly any form of tight covering provides such protection, so that no special measures are necessary to protect food from residual dust. This is similarly true of fluids. Following an atomic attack, several quarts of water may be drawn from the household pipes for drinking purposes, but more extensive use of water from the municipal system may be hazardous until it has been officially reported to be safe. Since supplies of milk may not be available for some time following a disaster, canned milk should be stored for the use of children. Special attention must also be directed toward preventing small children from putting contaminated objects in their mouth, and teething rings and bottle nipples should be thoroughly cleansed before use.

What to do in an attack

Prompt personal action in an atomic or hydrogen bomb attack is essential for survival. Whether a person moves rapidly and properly determines in many cases whether or not he is among the survivors in each area. The Civil Defense Administration lists six important steps for surviving an atomic attack.

1. Try to get shielded. If time is available, get into a basement or subway. When out-of-doors, shelter alongside a building or in a ditch or gutter offers some protection.

2. Drop flat to the ground or floor in order to avoid being thrown about and to decrease the chances of being struck by debris. It is better to flatten out on the ground along the base of a wall to give added protection.

3. Bury your face in your arms to protect it from flash burns, prevent temporary blindness, and save your eyes from the danger of flying debris. At home, work, school, and in vehicles, when there is no warning, one should also drop to the floor and protect the face. Taking cover under a desk, bench, heavy table, or bed gives added protection. In any case, these first three steps must be taken instantly when the first warning of an attack is the flash of the bomb or immediately precedes it. With warning, a few more moments are available to seek a properly designated or more suitable air raid shelter.

4. Do not rush outside after a bombing. Following the air burst, one should remain inside for a few minutes, and then go outside to help fight fires or perform other civil defense work.

5. Do not take chances with food and water in open containers. Restrict consumption to canned and bottled materials if there is any chance of contamination.

6. Do not start rumors. A panic capable of costing many lives might be caused by a single rumor in the confusion following an atomic bomb disaster.

In addition to these major points for survival, a number of other observations, derived from the bombings in Japan, are pertinent. The confusion that follows an attack slows down all attempts at a rapid institution of civil defense measures. During this period, many injured persons will bleed to death and others trapped in buildings will be burned or smothered to death. Any measure that will restore order and organize every physically and mentally capable person into rescue and fire-fighting teams will greatly reduce the total number of fatalities. Immediately after an atomic bombing, there will be many small fires that can be put out with a minimum of effort. An hour later, these will have become large fires or fire storms that will burn out the entire area, as they did in Japan. It has been pointed out that immediately following an attack most persons suffer severe emotional disorganization, during which they require direction to insure their own safety, as well as that of others. Anxiety, fear, and anger are psychological enemies of civil defense that must be controlled by those few who remain in control of their faculties. One calm and informed individual at this time may therefore be able to take rational control and bring about a great saving of property and life. Following this initial period, uninjured persons should accept life-saving duties in the previously planned activities of the organized civil defense units.

RECOVERY FROM ATOMIC ATTACK

The major immediate steps necessary for the prevention of further damage following an atomic or hydrogen bomb attack involve the administration of first aid, the evacuation of injured to treatment centers, and the fighting of fires. Each of these may depend to a considerable extent upon individual action, as contrasted to the action of civil defense units. Failure to be able to perform any one of these tasks may greatly magnify the extent of the tragedy.

First aid for atomic casualties

Immediate first aid must be administered to bomb casualties by the first capable person who encounters them. First aid stations can perform only less immediate and more detailed steps. The most important measures in first aid include the stopping of hemorrhage, prevention of suffocation, extrication of a limb caught by fallen timbers or debris, supporting of broken bones, treatment of shocks, and assistance of persons with burns and other painful injuries. Individual first aid measures are *only* for emergency action to maintain life until further action can be undertaken at first aid stations.

Hemorrhage is among the most common dangers seen in atom bomb casualties. Bleeding may be stopped by the application of pressure on arteries and veins at the proper pressure points to stop the flow of blood out through the wound. Attempts to use such techniques by untrained personnel may be very dangerous, however. Pressing a pad or cloth directly upon the wound is much safer for the untrained, even if it is not as effective. A large wad or pad of cloth pressed firmly against wounds is usually successful, and when it does not work, more pads and firmer pressure are better measures than an unskilled attempt at the application of a tourniquet.

Electrocution, gas, smoke, dirt, and water may all cause suffocation in atomic bomb casualties. In each case the first step is to remove the impediment to normal respiration. Persons in contact with live wires should not be touched until the current is turned off, or unless dry gloves, wood, paper, or other insulating material is available for protection. When the source of respiratory difficulty is removed and it is ascertained that the patient's mouth and throat are clear of obstruction, artificial respiration may be instituted. Every person needs training in the proper administration of this technique.

Broken bones resulting from atomic bomb blast injury may be visible or may be indicated by pain, tenderness, or inability to use a limb. Fracture patients should not be moved if trained first aid workers can safely be brought to them. The greatest danger from leaving a broken bone unattended for a short period is that of shock, while unskilled attempts to support a fracture in a splint may injure important nerves and other tissues. When it is absolutely essential to move a fracture patient, a splint should be used. A splint is a support to prevent any movement of the fractured ends of bone. No attempt should be made to correct the fracture. While a splint must be firm, it should not be too tight. Movement of persons suspected of having a broken neck or back should not be attempted unless it is essential to avoid certain death from other causes such as fire.

Atomic casualties frequently suffer shock as the result of burns, fractures, and other injuries. Pallor, cold moist skin, a rapid pulse exceeding 100 heartbeats a minute, and fainting are common signs of shock. The patient should be made to lie down and remain quiet. He must be kept warm. Development of severe shock can often be delayed by giving the patient, when he is conscious and able to swallow, a drink made from one teaspoonful of salt and one-half teaspoonful of baking soda, dissolved in a quart of water. This solution is particularly good for victims with mild to moderate burns, who may consume six to seven quarts of it in a twelve-hour period.

The proper handling of bad burns is a complex medical problem that is severely hampered when it is first necessary to remove grease, oil, and other materials placed on the burn by inexperienced first aid workers. Burns should not be cleaned in emergency first aid, nor blisters broken. A clean dry compress or pad may be placed over the burn and held snugly in place with a bandage. Such dry dressings must not be too tight, but should fit well enough to keep air from easy access to the burn.

Evacuation of atomic casualties

The activities concerned with the safety of atomic casualties are of necessity dependent upon the plan of organization of medical services in the emergency areas. This organization will vary with the previous planning of individual local civil defense programs and medical societies, but in general will include three major parts. First, patients must be transported or walked to first aid and ambulance stations, depending upon their ability. From these points, they would be carried to existing or improvised hospitals in the general area. Finally, it would be necessary to evacuate patients from these hospitals to private homes, emergency centers, convalescent homes, or hospitals in other communities.

It is estimated that about 35 percent of the civilian casualties that survive an atomic bombing would have to be carried by litter to a first aid or collecting station. The average first aid station should care for about 600 casualties in a

24-hour period. Such care would be solely of an emergency nature, and would include the screening of casualties to determine further disposition, arranging for transportation, and treatment of patients suffering from shock, severe pain, and unarrested hemorrhage. The minimal requirements for staffing such a first aid station for 24 hours would include about 175 persons, 150 of whom would serve as litter bearers. On the basis of experience in Japan, it is evident that first aid stations can be established only at some distance from the point of the explosion.

Fixed first aid stations in permanent buildings are not practical for handling the casualties resulting from an atomic bomb, because of the concentration of damage. Mobile stations provide the ideal solution. These are set up along a circle centering on the point of explosion, and at a distance from this point such as to escape the area of major damage. Thus in a bombing such as that in Japan, mobile stations would be placed at intervals of about one sixth of a mile, and at a radius of one and one-half miles from ground zero. The radius would be considerably greater for the explosion of present-sized atomic bombs or hydrogen bombs. The total number of stations around such a larger circle would be greater to meet the larger number of casualties in the area.

Mobile first aid stations would rapidly be assembled around the damaged area. They would consist of a basic staff stationed in moving vans, panel trucks, or similar vehicles. An outer ring of first aid stations about one-half mile further out could support these. Smaller vehicles would be required to provide communication between the mobile first aid stations and the hospital systems.

Emergency ambulance service would require the use of a variety of vehicles, both because of the limited number of conventional ambulances and because of the problems of getting through severely damaged areas. Passenger vehicles, commercial trucks, and buses would all be useful. In addition to transporting casualties, ambulance service personnel would be responsible for keeping a record of available hospital beds, informing first aid stations of where to forward casualties, and otherwise providing a supply liaison between these stations and higher units.

Hospitals for treatment of atomic casualties would be of three major types: existing hospitals in the immediate community, hospitals improvised from other kinds of buildings, and hospitals in surrounding areas. In the event of an impending emergency, most hospitals would move as many patients as possible to noncritical areas, and provision could also be made for a considerable expansion in the number of patients that could be handled. Such hospitals and their staffs would be fundamental units for the treatment of critically injured atomic casualties. While some improvised hospitals might be set up in

tents, the use of schools and hotels would better provide a more uniform distribution throughout the community, have utilities, toilets, and often cooking facilities, and are characterized by a large amount of floor space and broad halls and stairways. Hotels and similar buildings have the advantage of being already equipped with beds, kitchens, and laundry facilities.

Fire fighting at home

An atomic bomb burst will start secondary fires in many homes that would otherwise withstand the attack. These fires are major casualty-producing agents, and are said to have caused 80 percent of the bomb damage in World War II conventional bombing attacks. *Every householder should have equipment and training for putting out fires.*

The three things required to make a fire are: some fuel to burn, heat to make it burn, and air to keep it burning. Most small home fires can be put out by cooling the fire with a stream of water, or by smothering it to keep out the air necessary for its continuation. Burning fluids must be smothered in most cases. Basic home fire-fighting equipment includes a garden hose, a hand pump, and some buckets for water and sand. Other equipment of value includes a wet mop or broom, or even a burlap bag or small carpet soaked in water. A hand water-pump extinguisher can be used beyond the range of a hose, and may use stored water in case there is no water in the pipes for use with a hose. A good ladder is also an essential part of the household fire-fighting equipment.

Immediately after an all clear signal has been sounded following the raid, the entire house should be carefully checked for fires, with particular emphasis on the attic, roof, and side of the house nearest the bomb. Help should be summoned immediately if there are more fires than the householder can handle. One should not wait for help to arrive, however, since it may not materialize. Immediate steps should be taken with the available tools and should continue until the fire is out, or too big to handle. When the burning material is removable, it should be taken from the house. If this is not possible, it should be doused with water or other available material. Dirt, sand, or even a rug are useful in smothering small fires. If the house is nearer than 50 feet to another frame building that is burning, there is a good chance that fire will spread, so the walls and roof nearest the fire should be carefully watched and when possible kept wet with a hose, or with buckets of water.

When the fire in a building gets completely out of control, one should immediately get away from it before he is trapped. If there is thick smoke, a handkerchief, preferably moist, placed over the mouth and nose, will make breathing easier. Crawl on the hands and knees, and follow walls to the door, since the center of the floor may cave in. Tread lightly on stairs in a burning building, feeling for each step to insure that it will bear the full weight. If it is necessary to drop from a window, a person should first lower himself out as far as possibile, since this will reduce the fall by about seven feet. From a second or third floor, one can slide down a makeshift rope assembled by tying together the corners of sheets or blankets with square knots and securing one end to a heavy piece of furniture. When it is impossible to escape from a burning room without help, close the door to hold back the heat, flames, and smoke, and call for help from a window.

If it is necessary to search a burning building it is best to work as a team with another person. The search should preferably be conducted from top downward, looking under beds and in closets and other possible places where frightened persons may have hidden. A door that is hot will have fire back of it. If it opens toward the searcher, it should be braced with the foot since an explosive back draft may occur. If it opens away, the searcher should duck to one side as he pushes the door open. Avoid the centers of rooms, but if they do appear safe, a smoke-filled room should be crossed from corner to corner to discover if someone is lying in the center. The air in a burning building may be dangerous because of gases given off by some burning materials, because of the heat, and because of the low oxygen content of the air. The air is best near the floor, so that creeping to safety may be advisable when breathing is difficult. Fire fighters must give this ample consideration in making an allowance for the time they will require to escape to safety.

Radiological decontamination

The closer to the ground that an atomic explosion occurs, the greater will be the degree of contamination with radioactive materials. Much of this residual radioactivity will be lost within an hour or two after the explosion, in which case decontamination procedures may not be necessary. The decision with regard to the measures that will be undertaken must rest with the local civil defense authorities. Radiological monitoring teams with special training and equipment will make accurate measurements of the amount of residual radioactive material in the area. Based upon these findings, the authorities may need to undertake necessary general decontamination procedures, and publish instructions for such individual action as is necessary.

Decontamination procedures include all methods for removing the source of materials of hazardous radiation. There are four general types of procedure. *Surface decontamination* includes measures to reduce the radioactive material on surfaces to a safe level, but is of little value to the householder. *Aging* involves letting the natural rate of radioactive decay decrease the amount of radiation to a safer level, and is probably the most useful method. *Sealing* consists of covering the radioactive material with a sealing material, and has only limited value. In some cases, *removal* of the contaminated material and storage or burial of it on land or at sea are the only practical measures.

Surface decontamination methods may include washing, steaming, burning, vacuum cleaning, or sandblasting. Washing and vacuum cleaning are the measures most available to the individual householder, and are capable of reducing contamination on most surfaces by a large degree. Soap and detergent solution are better than plain water, because they help to release the radioactive dust held by fine invisible layers of grease and grime. Prolonged hosing is capable of reducing surface contamination by only about 50 percent, but the water will also tend to carry contamination deeper. It seldom warrants the effort, therefore, or the use of the water. When painted surfaces are badly contaminated, it may be necessary to remove the paint with caustic. About one pound of lye is necessary to remove the paint from 100 square feet of surface. The radioactive material removed must be disposed of with care.

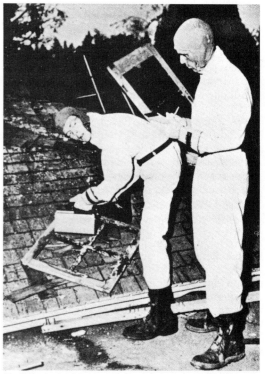

Radiological team examines debris for lingering radioactivity. *Courtesy Castle Films, New York.*

Sealing up of radiation hazards prevents further dispersion of the material and provides shielding against the alpha and low-energy beta radiations. Asphalt, paint, and grout—a thin mixture of sand, cement, and water—are the most common sealing materials. Sealing methods are seldom completely effective, and must be checked at intervals as to their adequacy.

Radiological decontamination procedures are dangerous when performed by untrained persons without the necessary equipment for measuring radioactivity and for protecting themselves against hazardous body exposure to the radiation. Decontamination crews wear special clothing, and work in conjunction with monitoring devices so that the radiation hazard in their work is accurately assessed at all times. Individual measures should therefore be restricted to items within the home that are badly needed and that probably have only low levels of contamination. The body and hands should be protected from contact with the wash water from the contaminated object. It is important to remember that radioactivity cannot be destroyed, and that all procedures simply remove or cover radioactive materials until they decay to stable isotopes at their own natural decay rate. A closed house should offer good protection against radioactive dust, but when the residual contamination is high on the outside, inside objects may also require decontamination. When possible, individuals who are exposed to such dust should bathe with soap and approved water supplies to reduce the contamination to their skin. Clean clothing should also be acquired at an early moment, and contaminated clothing sent to special laundry facilities that will become available for this purpose. Since considerable contamination may be introduced into a house on the shoes when a person has been in a contaminated area, the shoes should be removed before entering the house.

RADIOACTIVE ISOTOPES IN MEDICINE AND INDUSTRY

Death, destruction, and human misery are not the only consequences of the atomic age. Were this so, there would be few scientists who would be willing to direct their energies to the study of nuclear fission and its developments. Although the major advances in the field of atomic energy were the result of planning for the purposes of war, wonderful weapons against human disease have also appeared as an outgrowth of the development. The peacetime use of the products of the atomic energy program has rapidly expanded into a major effort in medicine, science, and industry. Radioactive materials are now widely used in the diagnosis and treatment of disease, in the search for new facts about the human body, and in industrial research. These areas of development are of inestimable value to mankind, and may eventually be expected to more than balance the destructive effects of atomic weapons. The humanitarian advances which have resulted from the employment of radioactive materials are a major area of interest to the Atomic Energy Commission. However, widespread use of radioactive isotopes creates additional problems in medicine, particularly from the standpoint of the radiation hazards involved. With the increasing industrial use of materials from nuclear reactors, intensive education is necessary concerning the hazards of ionizing radiation, the proper methods of handling isotopes, and the safety precautions that must be taken.

Procurement and use of radioisotopes

The major useful products from atomic piles are the purified radioactive isotopes. Most of the materials that have been employed for peacetime purposes have been obtained from a nuclear reactor of the Atomic Energy Commission at Oak Ridge, Tennessee. These isotopes are purified and standardized by the government, and shipped to responsible research and medical centers for use. All handling of such radioactive materials requires great caution, and shipment is in heavily shielded containers. Research workers and physicians who employ radioactive materials require special training for the work. Since the hazards to health are great, protective devices of many kinds are used. Extensive facilities are generally required for the disposal of waste from radioisotope studies.

Radioisotopes in biology

The development of new methods of treatment of disease depends to a considerable extent upon basic knowledge concerning the reactions that normally proceed in the healthy body. The difficulties involved in the study of these reactions are great. It is desirable to know, for instance, precisely what happens to all of the atoms in a molecule of sugar, from the time the sugar is consumed until it is excreted as carbon dioxide and water. With the increased availability of radioactive isotopes from nuclear piles, it has become possible to obtain substances, such as sugar, in which selected atoms are marked or *labeled* by being radioactive. These can be detected in very minute amounts by the use of Geiger counters or similarly sensitive electronic devices. By feeding labeled materials to experimental animals and determining which excretory products are radioactive, it is possible to trace the exact pathways by which the animal body utilizes various nutrients. Analysis of the organs

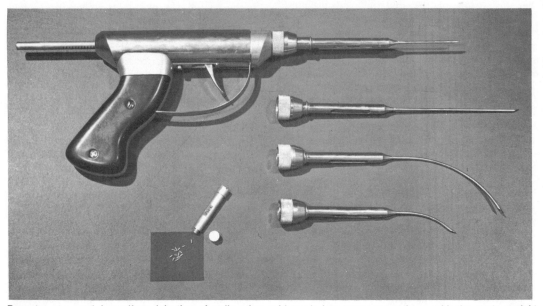

Repeater gun used for uniform injection of radioactive gold seeds into tumor mass shown with the gun's straight and curved needles and, lower left, platinum-coated gold seeds. *Courtesy The University of Texas M.D. Anderson Hospital, Houston, Texas.*

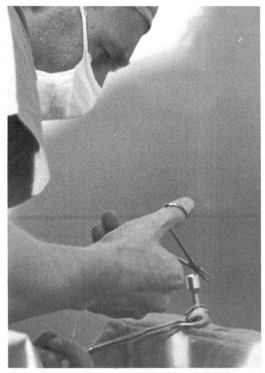

The physicist, who works in collaboration with the radiotherapist and who usually estimates dose and distribution is shown loading gun with radioactive gold seeds. *Courtesy The University of Texas M.D. Andersan Hospital, Houston, Texas.*

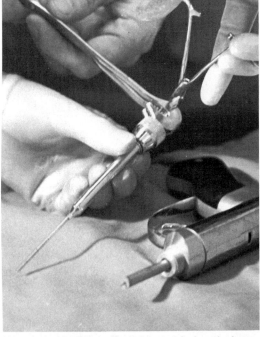

Magazine with gold seeds is inserted in barrel of gun. 15 seeds can be placed evenly and unerringly in tumor mass, one centimeter apart, without reloading gun. *Courtesy The University of Texas M.D. Anderson Hospital, Houston, Texas.*

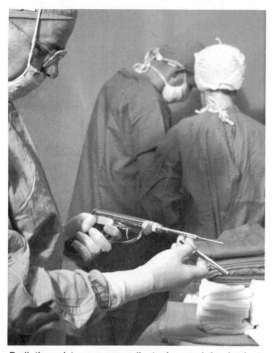

Radiotherapist uncaps needle to be used for implant. The gun does not present a radical departure in treatment, but is an improved method of implantation. *Courtesy The University of Texas M.D. Anderson Hospital, Houston, Texas.*

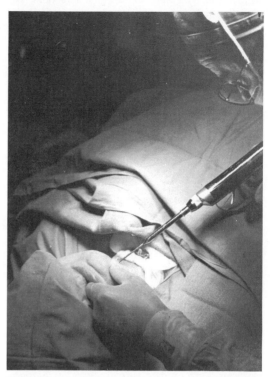

The tumor mass is held rigid by the radiotherapist's finger inside the mouth while the needle is inserted and the gold seeds injected from the gun. *Courtesy The University of Texas M.D. Anderson Hospital, Houston, Texas.*

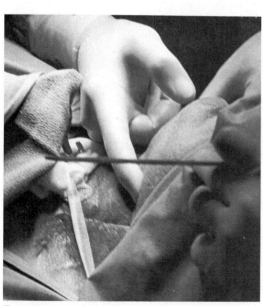

Tumor mass underneath chin is felt by radiotherapist before beginning the gold seed implant. Next, the insertion points will be marked. *Courtesy The University of Texas M.D. Anderson Hospital, Houston, Texas.*

of experimental animals fed radioactive isotopes may also show just which structures are involved in the metabolism of various foodstuffs or drugs. Hundreds of valuable studies on the chemistry of the human body have already been performed in this fashion. Because it is possible to detect exceedingly minute amounts of radioactive elements, the radiation given off by the isotopes in these studies is not sufficient to cause any injury to the tissue in which it is emitted.

Other fundamental studies give an indication of the rates of change in the body. Thus, in studies with radioactive iron, it was possible to measure the rate at which new red blood cells are formed, since these cells use iron as a part of the red blood pigment, hemoglobin. By measuring the rate of disappearance of radioactivity (or radioactive iron) from the blood, it was found that the average life of a human red blood cell was from three to four months.

Biological studies of agricultural importance have also been made possible through the products of atomic piles. Studies with milk cattle have resulted in valuable knowledge concerning the nutrition and metabolism of this species. Valuable agricultural information has been obtained regarding the function of fertilizers and minerals in the soil, by employing readily detectable radioactive materials.

Suitable isotopes have also been studied as potential agents in the fight against plant parasites, with the theory that the ionizing radiation from these isotopes might selectively destroy the disease-producing agents.

Radioisotopes in medicine

Because of their biologically active and easily detectable radiation, radioactive isotopes have found extensive use in the diagnosis and treatment of disease in human beings. Although the properties of radioactivity and its potential use in medicine have been known for almost 75 years, the naturally occurring radionuclides were of such limited value that they were not widely used until recently. Not until the development of cyclotrons in the 1930s and reactors in the 1940s, which made a great variety of artificially produced radionuclides available to physicians, did they come into widespread use in medicine. In the last 25 years, however, the internal uses of nonsealed sources of radioactivity have so increased in number and complexity that a new discipline of medicine has had to be established to assure that these agents, called "radiopharmaceuticals," are used to gain the greatest amount of information at the least risk to the patient. This new discipline is called nuclear medicine.

Basically, nuclear medicine is defined as the application of radiopharmaceuticals and nuclear instrumentation to the solution of biomedical problems that occur in patients. Although all diseases are of potential interest to physicians of nuclear medicine, cancer is the main disease presently under investigation.

In the beginning, users of radionuclides and labeled compounds in medicine hoped to find many *therapeutic* radiopharmaceuticals which would localize in tumors selectively and destroy them. This has not happened so far, but the increasing use of radionuclides in *diagnostic* procedures leaves little time to brood over this yet unrealized hope. Radiopharmaceuticals are almost ideal diagnostic tools because radioisotope tracers do not alter body physiology, and they do permit external monitoring with minimal instrumentation. Various diagnostic approaches have been developed—some have become routine procedures, others are useful only in special circumstances, and still others are too experimental to be recommended for use at this time. All, however, must be carefully integrated with other available diagnostic techniques.

Although therapeutic nuclear medicine procedures are much more restricted than those of diagnosis, they may still be useful, and a number of promising therapeutic techniques have been developed. As with diagnosis, however, therapeutic procedures using nuclear medicine

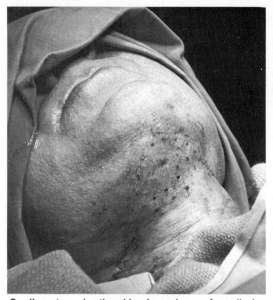

Small spots under the chin show places of needle insertion. Since the seeds have a short radioactive half-life, 2½ days, a secondary operation for their removal is eliminated. *Courtesy The University of Texas M.D. Anderson Hospital, Houston, Texas.*

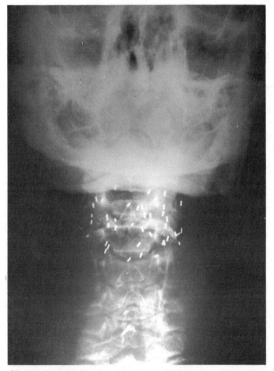

X-ray picture showing location of the gold seeds. The x-ray film is used by physicist and radiotherapist to compute the distribution of radiation dose. *Courtesy The University of Texas M.D. Anderson Hospital, Houston, Texas.*

must be combined with other methods of treatment to be most effective. There are presently three major areas of nuclear medicine procedures: (1) physiological function studies, (2) radionuclide imaging procedures, and (3) therapeutic techniques.

Physiological function studies

One example of physiologic function testing is the assay of thyroid hormone levels in the blood which, in turn, can aid in the assessment of thyroid function. The radioactive iodine uptake test, which involves the administration of a dose of iodine-131 to the patient, is also a most valuable procedure in assessing thyroid function. At present, however, it is best reserved for problem cases rather than used as a primary screening test. The main disadvantage of this test is the effect of the dietary intake of iodine, which reacts in various ways in different individuals.

Pulmonary testing with radionuclides has increased in the past several years, particularly since the introduction of xenon-133 for use in ventilation and perfusion studies. Such studies are useful in evaluating pulmonary function in patients with lung cancer and in selecting suitable candidates for surgical procedures.

Another complex piece of equipment currently in use in nuclear medicine is the gamma camera with computer-assisted data analysis which is used, together with ^{131}I-hippuran, to measure renal function. The renogram is of most clinical value in the assessment of ureteral impairment in pre- and postoperative patients with carcinoma of the cervix and other pelvic and gynecological tumors.

Radionuclides are also highly useful in assessment of hematological status to detect anemia and iron deficiency, and in studying radioactivity in feces in order to detect significant blood loss through the gastrointestinal tract. In addition, radioisotopes show promise of facilitating differentiation between well-vascularized and ischemic tumors and organs—although much more work remains to be done.

Radionuclide imaging procedures

Brain tumors can now be detected by external counting of radionuclides; this procedure came into general clinical use in the late 1950s when advances in instrumentation and radiopharmaceuticals gave dramatic demonstrations of brain tumors. Another significant advance in brain tumor imaging was the introduction of the gamma camera, which permitted more rapid studies with multiple views, as well as dynamic cerebral blood flow assessment. The brain scan is now fully established as a routine procedure in the evaluation of cerebral lesions, and it frequently provides information not available from other sources.

Another tumor localization technique that has been helpful clinically is ^{85}Sr scanning of metastatic bone disease. Since metastatic lesions of bone are frequently associated with new bone formation, there is usually a significant localization of several radioisotopes in the general vicinity of the metastasis. Early metastatic lesions will often go undetected on roentgenographic examination because a 30 to 50 percent change in bone density is required to produce visible changes on x-ray examination; bone scans, however, are generally positive quite early in the development of metastasis. Patients with prostatic carcinoma and carcinoma of the breast are most often candidates for study with this technique.

The liver scan, using radioactive colloids, utilizes a slightly different approach to tumor detection. In this scan, the radioisotope concentrates in the normal tissue, and the tumor appears as a nonradioactive, or "cold" area. This procedure is often an indicated procedure in the cancer patient because of the frequency of liver metastases, and because the liver is not easily visualized using routine radiographic techniques. There are limitations to this approach, however; lesions that are smaller than 2 centimeters in diameter generally go undetected because of limitations of resolution of scanning devices. Also, many other disease conditions may interfere with localization of radiocolloids, producing defects on the liver scan that are indistinguishable from neoplastic disease.

Lung scans can also be useful in checking for changes before and after radiation treatment of carcinoma of the lung. A technique for detecting bronchial obstruction has been developed using inhalation of radioactive aerosols, but is not widely used at the present. In addition, a liver-pancreas scan can also be performed, although interpretation of pancreatic scans is often difficult because of normal variation in size and shape and in trace concentration. When the scan appears to be within normal limit range, however, the presence of disease is unlikely.

Thyroid scans with ^{131}I are useful in determining the activity of thyroid nodules in the intact thyroid gland. A nonradioactive, "cold" nodule indicates a higher risk of thyroid carcinoma, but the scan alone is not recommended as a technique of selecting patients for surgery. After removal of a thyroid carcinoma, a scan of the neck may demonstrate areas of increased activity in the cervical lymph nodes and other organs, indicating metastatic disease.

Scintigram techniques of the kidney can be helpful in distinguishing between cysts and neoplasms, and salivary gland scanning can be useful in confirming abnormality in the salivary gland where tumor is suspected. Lymph node scans with the radiocolloid injected subcutaneously on the dorsum of the feet can be used as screening procedures for lymph flow.

Perhaps the greatest interest at the present time, however, is in the search for a general tumor scanning agent. Although several radionuclides have been found to localize in tumors of widely different types and regions of the body, most current interest is in the use of ^{67}Ga-citrate, which is presently undergoing a wide clinical trial and promises to be useful in the localization of lymphomas as well as some adenocarcinomas.

Therapeutic techniques

The most prominent therapeutic use of radiopharmaceuticals is radioactive iodine in the treatment of metastatic thyroid cancer. Iodine-131 has a half-life of about eight days and emits gamma and beta rays. When iodine salts are taken into the body, most of the dose is concentrated in the thyroid gland. A dose of radioactive iodine salt similarly concentrates in the thyroid gland. When there is a cancer in the thyroid gland, or the gland is overactive (hyperthyroidism), the excessive tissue may be destroyed by the radiation from the radioactive iodine that has been administered. Although removal of metastatic thyroid cancer is not always achieved with ^{131}I therapy, significant palliation

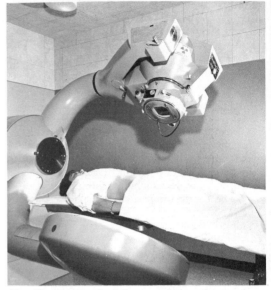

The Theratron unit delivers radiation therapy in a rotational fashion for the treatment of patients with cancer. *Courtesy of The University of Texas M. D. Anderson Hospital, Houston, Texas.*

can occur. In some instances of lung metastasis and lymph node metastasis in the neck, patients may show no evidence of recurrence, even many years after treatment.

Another therapeutic use is radiophosphorus in the treatment of patients with a number of diseases. This element has a half-life of about 14 days and emits beta rays; it is taken up in the body in the greatest quantity by those tissues

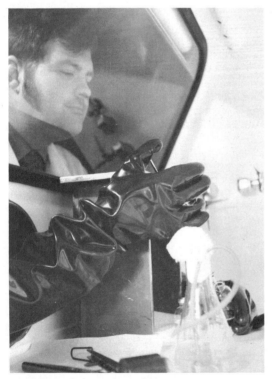

Radioactive isotopes used in the laboratory are handled behind heavily leaded glass shields. *Courtesy of The University of Texas M. D. Anderson Hospital, Houston, Texas.*

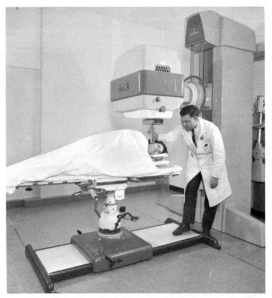

Another type of radiotherapy is delivered by the Siemen's betatron unit in order to give megavoltage doses of irradiation. *Courtesy of The University of Texas M. D. Anderson Hospital, Houston, Texas.*

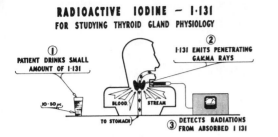

RADIOACTIVE IODINE — I·131
FOR STUDYING THYROID GLAND PHYSIOLOGY

① PATIENT DRINKS SMALL AMOUNT OF I·131

② I·131 EMITS PENETRATING GAMMA RAYS

10·50 μc

BLOOD   STREAM

TO STOMACH

③ DETECTS RADIATIONS FROM ABSORBED I 131

SHOWS:

1- THYROID GLAND TAKES UP MOST RADIOIODINE RETAINED BY BODY
2- IODINE ABSORPTION PROPORTIONAL TO PRODUCTION OF THYROXINE
3- RELATIVE ABSORPTION SHOWS PHYSIOLOGICAL ACTIVITY OF GLAND

Courtesy Isotopes Division, U.S. Atomic Energy Commission.

which manufacture blood cells. In polycythemia vera, a condition in which too many red blood cells are formed, the radiation from this isotope very often brings about a sufficient suppression of the blood cell-making tissues to alleviate some of the symptoms of the disease. Leukemia patients, in whom there is an excessive production of white cells, are offered added comfort— and in some instances prolongation of life—by the use of radiophosphorus. This element may also be used in treatment of metastatic cancer to the bone, and while this treatment is never used in an attempt to eradicate cancer, it can result in significant palliation of pain in some patients.

Gold-198, in the form of a suspension in water, has found increasing use in the treatment of certain types of cancer. Isotopes of gallium, sodium, arsenic, and other elements have been tested for possible uses in medicine, and show some promise. Other methods for using internal

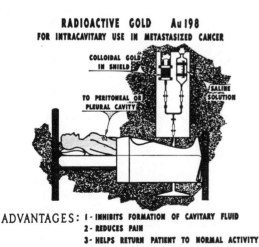

RADIOACTIVE GOLD   Au 198
FOR INTRACAVITARY USE IN METASTASIZED CANCER

COLLOIDAL GOLD IN SHIELD

SALINE SOLUTION

TO PERITONEAL OR PLEURAL CAVITY

ADVANTAGES: 1- INHIBITS FORMATION OF CAVITARY FLUID
2- REDUCES PAIN
3- HELPS RETURN PATIENT TO NORMAL ACTIVITY

Courtesy Isotopes Division, U.S. Atomic Energy Commission.

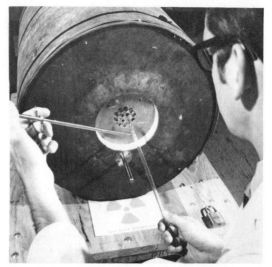

One of the newest isotopes, Californium-252, is stored in heavily leaded containers, until samples are taken out for research studies. Note caution sign denoting radioactive material. *Courtesy of The University of Texas M. D. Anderson Hospital, Houston, Texas.*

nonsealed sources include arterial therapy of liver cancer, endolymphatic therapy of lymph node cancer, and intracavitary therapy of pleural and peritoneal cancer. The basic principle behind the internal use of all radioactive isotopes depends upon the concentration of the isotope in some particular tissue. The search for elements that are concentrated in each of the organs by the selective abilities of the tissues, or elements that concentrate in tumor tissue as contrasted with normal tissues, is the key to all techniques in radiodiagnosis and radiotherapy.

Many radioisotopes emit beta and gamma rays and these rays are quite similar to the x-rays which have been used for years both in making x-ray pictures and in the treatment of patients with cancer. A number of radioactive substances therefore offer important possibilities as external radiation sources in medicine. Thus a small x-ray emitting source in the form of a suitable isotope has been suggested as a device for obtaining dental x-ray pictures in place of the conventional large x-ray apparatus. The advantages of such an application to both dentistry and medicine are apparent, but at present the details are incompletely developed. More important, and already in use, is the employment of powerful radioactive materials as external radiation sources in cancer therapy. Cobalt-60, a gamma and beta ray emitter with a half-life of about 5.3 years, is ideally suited for this purpose. Small pieces of radioactive metallic cobalt, made radioactive in an atomic pile, are placed into a proper shielding device and the radiation from them used in place of a high-powered x-ray machine (2 mil-

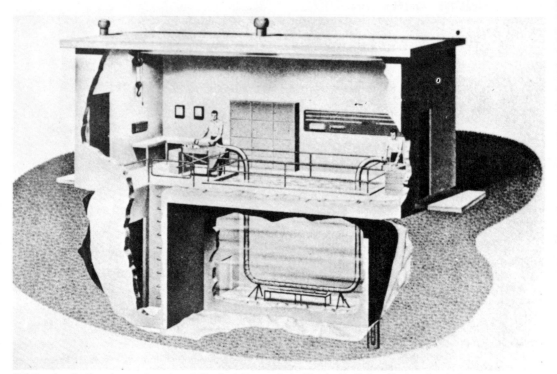

Artist's visualization, to exact scale, of Stanford Research Institute's Radiation Engineering Laboratory setup for cold sterilization of heat-sensitive materials by gamma rays from a radiocobalt source. *Courtesy Stanford Research Institute.*

lion volts) or radium implantations in treating patients with localized cancer. Thousands of cobalt-60 irradiators are now.in use. The most significant advance in radiotherapy since 1925 has been the development of supervoltage equipment, such as the millivolt x-ray generators (the betatron, etc.) and the cobalt-60 megavoltage units. The latter are the most suitable, since they are compact, have high activity source in a small volume, are flexible and adapt to many geometric patterns for therapeutic use, and are easy and economical to maintain.

With the cobalt-60 isotope, supervoltage is now made available throughout the world, and at a very low cost when compared with the cost of radium per se, or the x-ray generators. Cesium-137 units are also in use, but do not have the same therapeutic usefulness as the cobalt-60, and the activity cannot be concentrated as easily as with the cobalt.

Radioisotopes in industry

The present commercial application of the products of the atomic energy program is in an early stage of development, although many good suggestions have been made for the industrial use of isotopes. Whenever radioisotopes are used in industry, there arises the important problem of training personnel to appreciate the magnitude of radiation hazards involved. The use of radiation sources in industry thus involves the simultaneous adoption of additional measures for industrial safety.

Nuclear reactors, which have been used for some time as sources of energy, have become a reality within the past few years. There are approximately seven such power sources in the United States at present, with an estimated two to three more reactors being completed in this country each year.

A nuclear reactor produces energy in the following way: When a single, slow-moving neutron collides with an atom, the atom becomes suddenly so unstable that it may split violently, releasing, as it does, large amounts of energy which are quickly dissipated as heat. The energy release is so large by ordinary standards that the heat from the fissioning of all the atoms of just one pound of U^{235} is as great as that from burning 1500 tons of coal. It is possible for one fission to initiate another, and this still another, thus creating a chain reaction. The nuclear reactor is intended to effect such a continuous, controlled chain reaction, and the heat from the reaction is then used to heat water to steam and this, in turn, to drive an engine.

Although the cost of nuclear power was at

first prohibitory, it is now becoming financially competitive with other sources of power. In fact, in areas where there are no immediate supplies of coal, oil, or gas, nuclear energy is proving to be less expensive per kilowatt hour than other forms of energy.

This new source of power is also gaining in importance because sources of hydroelectric power have been nearly depleted; at the same time producers of energy from coal, oil, and gas are being strongly criticized for their pollution of the environment. While nuclear reactors eliminate the immediately obvious dangers and irritations of these other sources, they, too, are meeting considerable opposition from some critics who are concerned about the possible radiation pollution from such power plants.

Since there is a tremendous amount of energy stored up in even a small piece of fissionable material, a small piece of uranium or plutonuim can be used to drive an aircraft, ship, or submarine great distances without refueling. This attractive possibility is being explored, but presents many difficult problems. A very heavy weight of shielding material is required to protect personnel from the reactor, and this decreases the advantage to a considerable extent, particularly from the standpoint of aircraft power. An added problem resides in the radioactive contamination that may be spread by the system that transfers the power from the nuclear reactor to the engine. Special transfer materials are required that can withstand the high temperatures of the reaction and yet not become radioactive themselves through contact with the power source. Many of these problems can be approached more practically in larger seagoing vessels. The submarine *U.S.S. Nautilus* was the first vessel of any kind whatsoever to be powered by nuclear reactions. In 1960, the United States had 13 atomic-powered submarines. The aircraft carrier *U.S.S. Enterprise,* an 83,350-ton vessel, is propelled by eight nuclear reactors. Merchant ships, cruisers, and destroyers propelled by nuclear reactors are now being built. Atomic energy as a major power source is therefore possible, but it still requires extended technical development.

The radiations from radioactive isotopes have five main properties that may make them of value in industry. The rays can kill organisms, induce chemical reactions, ionize gases, activate phosphorescent compounds, and penetrate solids. Whereas in medicine the isotope used must be highly purified, this is not necessary in industry. Consequently, industrial radiation sources may be quite inexpensive, since many are now useless by-products of military atomic energy processes. Several excellent industrial applications of radioactive isotopes have already been developed.

The ability of ionizing radiation to kill organisms suggests the possibility of sterilizing foods and drugs without the deleterious effect of heat on these substances. In this regard, Trichina larvae, found frequently in pork and the causative agent of trichinosis, have been shown to be indioisotopes. Routine application of this principle capable of reproduction after exposure to rato meat is being developed.

Isotopes have proven a valuable tool in the study of the wear and corrosion of metals. Radioactive piston rings, made of the very best metals, show the presence of friction with the cylinder walls of an engine as indicated by the presence of measurable radioactivity which has rubbed off on the latter. Isotopes dissolved in the water exposed to metals in corrosion tests give an indication of the presence of even minute amounts of moisture on the metal, because of the extreme sensitivity of methods for detecting radioactivity. In the oil industry, radioisotopes have been used for studying the flow of fluids through petroleum-bearing formations. They are also used in assessing the nature of geological formations through which an oil well drills, by dropping a radiation source down a well hole, and recording the ability of various strata to absorb the ionizing radiation. When different lots of petroleum are pumped in sequence through the same pipeline, a radioactive material may be injected at the boundary of the two lots, and the radiation of this interface may be followed from outside the pipeline with radiation counting devices. The different batches of material may thus be sharply separated at their destination. The ionizing effect of the radiation from active isotopes may also be useful as to source of rays for industrial radiography, for stimulating certain types of chemical reactions, for improving fluorescent lights and luminescent paints and tiles, and in the manufacture of static eliminators. It provides the basis for different types of thickness gauges, since the radiation reaching a counting device from a radioactive isotope placed at a fixed distance from it will depend upon the thickness of intervening shielding material. Measurement of the depth of snow has been made possible by planting radioactive cobalt in the ground and setting a radioactive counting device high above it. Any intervening snow will diminish the actvity reaching the counter, and the results, readily converted to depth of snow, are transmitted automatically by radio to a central weather station.

The relative proportion of various isotopes of an element that exist on the earth is constantly changing due to radioactive decay of certain of these isotopes. Since isotopes of an element may have different physical properties, one isotope may become concentrated in certain places. The relative amounts of the various isotopes of carbon in living tissue are an example of this phenomenon. By careful measurement of the amounts of carbon-14 in once-living material, such as wood, shells, or petroleum, it is possible to form an estimate of its age. *Carbon-14 dating* has therefore become a valuable tool in assessing the age of geological and archaeological materials.

All of the commercial applications of radioac-tivity that have been mentioned have been proposed or developed within a short period of time. With increasing availability of isotopes and better understanding of their potential use, it is readily apparent that a vast requirement will develop for their use in peaceful pursuits.

30 SPACE MEDICINE

A key point in the space age is the penetration of space by man himself and his visit to another celestial body. This poses a tremendous challenge to the life sciences, particularly to *medicine*.

The role of medicine in this effort can be explained by the definition of its pertinent branch —*space medicine*—as the science and art of preserving man's health and well-being in space and on other celestial bodies. In brief, it is responsible for the lives of the astronauts and therefore more or less identical with what is now also called *bioastronautics*.

Because space medicine is actually a logical extension of aviation medicine or aeromedicine, and in certain problem areas they overlap, both are frequently combined in the term *aerospace medicine*. But space medicine in its own right has its place as a nucleus of scientific attraction and as a counterpart to space technology. In fact, while in the fifties attention centered almost exclusively around the technical aspect, the rocket, the sixties and seventies brought a shift to the medical and biological aspects of space. The reason: Man himself had already become an active participant in the exploration of space, as evidenced by the suborbital flights of Alan Shephard and Virgil Grissom, the orbital flights of Yuri Gagarin, Gherman Titov, and John Glenn, and finally the series of Apollo flights dedicated to landing a man on the moon.

After an on-the-ground tragedy on January 27, 1967, in which astronauts Virgil Grissom, Edward White II, and Roger Chaffee were killed in an oxygen fire in the space capsule, man finally fulfilled his dream of reaching the moon. On July 20, 1969, Neil Armstrong of the United States became the first man to set foot on the moon; with him on that historic Apollo 11 flight were Edwin Aldrin and Michael Collins. Five months later, the second moon landing was accomplished by Apollo 13 crew, Charles Conrad, Alan Bean, and Richard Gordon. After an aborted, but safely returned, Apollo 13 flight, man walked upon the moon still another time— on February 5, 1971, during the Apollo 14 flight of Alan Shephard, Edgar Mitchell, and Stuart Roosa.

Apollo 17 took place in December, 1972. Commander Gene Cernan joined by the first Astronaut-Geologist, Jack Schmitt, returned some 250 pounds of lunar rocks to the commandship, piloted by Ron Evans.

The moon has not been an end in itself however; even now, scientists and astronauts continue to plan, work, and train for future adventures in space.

In its efforts to cope with this unique task, space medicine, of course, depends to a great extent on its parent discipline, aviation medicine or aeromedicine; but it also has, like the latter, a close relationship to almost all other branches of medicine and biology. This relationship is by no means a one-way affair; rather, space medical research produces by-products which are of benefit to almost all branches of medicine.

We comprehend the immensity and novelty of the challenge to medicine in the space age by realizing the following facts:

1. The environment in space is characterized by the absence of a life-supporting, life-protecting, and flight-supporting atmosphere.

2. Travel through such a vacuum environment requires a sealed cabin with an artificial atmosphere, surrounded by a hull having life-protect-

ing capabilities against radiations and meteorites.

3. The astronauts occupying this isolated synthetic little earth in space represent, psychologically, a world of their own.

4. The physical environments on the target celestial bodies, such as the moon, are qualitatively and quantitatively different from that of the astronauts' home planet, thus requiring special biotechnical measures for their survival.

5. They may discover on the target celestial bodies, other living worlds with strange, exotic flora and fauna. This may pose important problems of useful and harmful biotic interrelations, such as contamination.

6. During the greater part of the space flight trajectory, the vehicle itself behaves like a celestial body, following the laws of celestial mechanics. This condition, and the transformation of an earthly machine into a celestial body, and its retransformation into an aerodynamic vehicle, together with the gravities found on the targets, such as the moon and Mars, subject the astronaut, who is basically a 1-g(ravity) creature, to a large spectrum of g forces from zero to various multiples of 1 g.

These, briefly, are the strikingly novel situations with which the life sciences are confronted in this space age.

The involvement in these problems puts medicine, to some extent, into the category of industrial medicine, and in other respects into that of environmental medicine. If we subdivide the mission of space medicine into more detail, these are the various tasks:

1. To implement medical requirements in the designing and engineering of space vehicles.

2. To provide medical ground support at launching sites and at tracking stations.

3. To evaluate ecologically the physical environment in space, its regional variations, and temporal fluctuations; furthermore, to determine the physical and possible biotic environments on other celestial bodies.

4. To provide life-support and protection in these environments.

5. To facilitate the tolerance of the g-spectrum encountered in the motion dynamics of the space flight trajectory and in the gravities on other celestial bodies.

6. To study the psychophysiological behavior, performance capabilities, and the potentialities of an active role of the astronaut in space operations, and to develop pertinent equipment.

7. To contribute to rescue and recovery operations.

8. To continue to select astronauts.

9. To continue to provide theoretical indoctrination in, and experimental familiarization with, space flight conditions in a simulated form.

10. To take care of preflght preparation of the astronauts and postflight observation and medical care.

11. To evaluate medically the actual space flight experiences made by astronauts for further programming of future space projects.

12. To have eventually a space doctor or physiologist participate in space operations.

It is impossible to review here the whole scope of the space medical problems; instead, remarks will be confined to the *environment of space* and *biodynamics* in space flight, which are focal points in space medical research and have relations to all other space medical problems and tasks.

A space medical task of the first order is to *evaluate ecologically the environment of space* in its basic structure, and especially in its regional variations and temporal fluctuations. This leads to a kind of ecological "geography" of space— more accurately called *spatiography*. Such a spatiographic study must include the earth's atmosphere in order to determine where above the earth's surface space actually begins.

From a medical point of view, the first 4000 meters (12,000 feet) above sea level represents the physiological zone of the atmosphere in which most of the world's population lives, except the Andes in Peru and the Himalayan Mountain area. Above this altitude, hypoxic effects are observed which require, as a countermeasure, the use of oxygen equipment. Without it the situation above 7 kilometers (21,000 feet) becomes dangerous or critical to life, whereas the

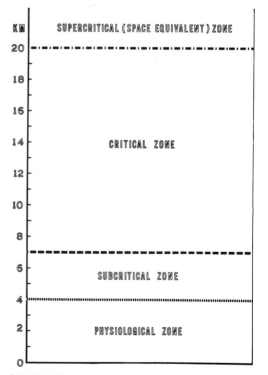

Atmospheric zones considered from an aerospace medical aspect. *Official Air Force Photo.*

region from 4 to 7 kilometers can be regarded as subcritical. A new pathophysiological effect at 20 kilometers (65,000 feet), namely, ebullism, or "boiling" of body fluids, makes the atmosphere a supercritical one because it produces the same pathological symptoms as a vacuum. For all practical purposes, the atmosphere at this altitude is *space-equivalent* so far as its physiological pressure functions are concerned.

Vehicles flying in these altitudes technically may be aircraft, but physiologically they are aerospace craft and their flights are of the space-equivalent type.

At still higher altitudes, with the cessation of scattering light due to the rarification of the air, leading to a black sky despite a bright, shining sun; with the gradual appearance of the whole solar electromagnetic radiation spectrum; with the occurrence of particle rays in their primary form, and meteorites; the environment, although still atmospheric, becomes more and more space-equivalent until, with the disappearance of air resistance at about 200 kilometers (120 miles), the environmental picture of space is practically complete.

The medical evaluation of this true space beyond the "mechanical border" of the atmosphere, where the Kepler regime begins, must be concentrated upon the regional variations and temporal fluctuations as they are found essentially in the radiation climate, because knowledge of these is decisive in choosing the safest routes and times for the various space operations. They even set definite regional and temporal limitations to manned space flight.

So far as *hazards from particle rays,* including cosmic rays, are concerned, the arena for manned satellite flight will have to be confined to the region from 200 to 800 kilometers (120 to 500 miles)—the lower border of the inner zone of Van Allen's Radiation Belt. This is a belt of particle rays (electrons, protons) trapped by the earth's magnetic field above the equatorial regions and consisting of two zones.

Only low orbits—as we might call orbits below this radiation belt—are relatively safe for manned flight. Higher orbits within the radiation belt, extending at the times of high solar activity, from 800 kilometers to 80,000 kilometers (500 to 50,000 miles) are hazardous. We do not have yet sufficient evidence to make definite statements as to what degree of shielding will be required for protection from the basic particle ray flux, and especially from those particles trapped and concentrated in the earth's effective magnetic field, now called magnetosphere. The same is true of the jet streams of solar plasma ejected from the sun, especially during solar flares. These flares have been studied by astronauts on the moon's surface, and these studies, no doubt, will continue. Certainly, however, the radiation doses inside the cabin have to be kept below the permissible maximum level, which is determined by a significant health or performance decrement.

The ecological evaluation of the topographical distribution of the particle rays and their temporal fluctuations continues to be an important and difficult task of space medicine. The task is somewhat simpler with regard to solar *electromagnetic radiation,* as its intensity distribution follows a fixed pattern; namely, the inverse square of the distance law. Because of this, we find a more or less stable intensity pattern within the solar system. High intensities of these wave radiations may be harmful for manned space flight; however, moderate intensities may be put to helpful use. The following table shows the total solar irradiance, expressed in cal cm^{-2} min^{-1}, in the third column, and solar illuminance, expressed in lumen per m^2, or lux, in the fourth column, for the mean distances of the various planets from Mercury to Pluto.

Using the values at the earth's distance as a baseline, we find that the intensity factor for total solar irradiance and illuminance nearly doubles at the orbital distance of Venus, and at the mean orbital distance of Mercury it is more than six times as high. At the distance of Mars, it decreases to less than one-half; at Jupiter's distance, to one twenty-seventh; and in the remote region of Pluto, the intensity drops to one sixteen-hundredth of the terrestrial value.

In the first place, we think of *heat radiation* in connection with the temperature control of the space cabin. Heat transfer in space, of course, is achieved only by radiation.

We immediately recognize that there is a zone in our solar system in which heat radiation is not too different from that at the earth's distance, that is, from the so-called terrestrial solar constant, and therefore, not too hostile to space operations. On both sides of this zone, however, it turns to extremes. We can, therefore, differentiate between a euthermal zone (from Venus to somewhere beyond Mars) adjoined by a hyperthermal and a hypothermal region.

SOLAR IRRADIANCE AT THE MEAN DISTANCE OF PLANETS

Planet	Mean Solar Distance 10^6 km	Intensity Factor	Total Irradiance cal cm^{-2} min^{-1}	Illuminance lux
Mercury	57.9	6.67	13.3	935,000
Venus	108.2	1.91	3.8	267,000
Earth	149.6	1.00	2.0	140,000
Mars	227.9	0.43	0.86	60,300
Jupiter	778.3	0.0369	0.074	5,170
Saturn	1428	0.0110	0.0022	1,530
Uranus	2872	0.0027	0.0054	380
Neptune	4493	0.00111	0.0022	155
Pluto	5910	0.00064	0.0013	90

The space medical conclusions from these extreme variations in solar thermal irradiance are obvious. It makes a great difference in cabin temperature control whether a space operation is planned into the furnace-like radiation conditions within the orbit of Venus or into the sparsely irradiated environment beyond Mars or Jupiter. The temperatures measured within the Explorer and Vanguard satellites were well within the physiologically tolerable range, around 77°F. Similar temperatures have been experienced in manned orbital flights in 1961 and 1962. But a space ship penetrating the intramercurian space would inevitably run into a kind of solar heat barrier, as symbolized by the legendary flight of Icarus, whose "wax" wings melted; and a trip into the region of the outer planets requires temperature control measures vastly different from those in the realm of the inner planets.

We find a similar zonal pattern in solar *light irradiation,* or solar illuminance. And, again, we might speak of a euphotic belt some 100 million kilometers (60 million miles) on both sides of the earth's orbit, adjoined by a hyperphotic and hypophotic zone.

This zonal pattern in the photic environment of space is significant in two respects: first, with regard to *vision,* and, second, concerning the utilization of light in *photosynthetic regeneration* of metabolic waste products in the closed ecological system of the space cabin.

With regard to the latter problem, solar illuminance drops with increasing distance from the sun below the effective minimum required for photosynthesis, and this limit may be reached somewhere in the region of the belt of the asteroids.

Concerning *vision,* there is one impressive feature in space; specifically, that there is always a black sky despite a bright shining sun, because there is no light-scattering medium similar to our atmosphere. This means there is only direct sunlight and no indirect sunlight or skylight. As a result, an extreme contrast between light and shadow dominates the visual scenery in space. Looking into the brilliant sun has a blinding effect; in fact, it can even produce in a relatively short time—less than 10 seconds—retinal burns of the kind observed after atomic flashes, or when a solar eclipse is observed with an insufficiently smoked glass. The retina-burning power of the sun might extend as far as Saturn. These conditions necessitate protective measures for the eye in the form of automatically functioning light-absorbing glasses.

Concerning ultraviolet and x-rays in space, not enough physical data are available at present for a complete or conclusive biophysical evaluation.

The best indicators for the regional difference in total solar radiation are the comets which hi-bernate, so to speak, in the remote regions of the solar system as icy mountains of dirt, frozen water, ammonia, and methane (F. Whipple), and come to life by displaying gigantic tails as soon as they come closer than three astronomical units to the sun [astronomical unit (AU) = the earth's distance from the sun = 149 million kilometers (93 million miles)].

All in all, we find only in the region from Venus to somewhere beyond Mars, a zone in which solar electromagnetic radiation is not too different from that found on earth, and which is more suitable for space operations and, therefore, does not have excessive protection requirements in this respect.

Finally, in all discussions concerning environmental hazards in space, *meteoritic material* attracts greatest interest. This matter in space occurs in a great variety with reference to chemical composition (iron, iron-stone, and stone) and size. Grain-sized meteoritic material, called micrometeorites, may produce erosion on the surface of space vehicles. This can, in the long run, affect their heat-absorbing characteristics and the transparency of optical surfaces. Collisions with meteorites with puncture capabilities seem to be not too great a problem as indicated by recordings from satellites and information from the Apollo moon flights; but there are also meteor streams moving in former orbits of disintegrated comets, and probably greater concentrations of meteoritic material in the belt of the asteroids. In an emergency caused by a meteoritic hit, the space suit, which must be always readily available, can provide immediate protection before the leak is sealed. For extended space operations, provision of bumpers is indicated, which might be combined with appropriate shielding devices against radiations.

All of this demonstrates clearly that, for the purpose of continued manned space flight, we need a more complete geographic approach in the medical evaluation of the environment of space or, in other words, an ecological space map or a spatiography. Spatiography, of course, refers only to the space between the celestial bodies. The description of the conditions found on these celestial bodies is called planetography. Both spatiography and planetography are parts of an all-embracing cosmography of our solar system.

On the *moon,* space, with practically all of its properties, immediately touches the moon surface. On the moon's surface there is, ecologically, a true space environment, and the lunar sky is the universal black space-sky with sunshine and earthshine.

The *Martian* atmosphere shows, at its ground level, the same pressure conditions as our atmosphere at about 16 kilometers (10 miles). It must, therefore, be characterized as a critical atmosphere for man. It becomes supercritical, as

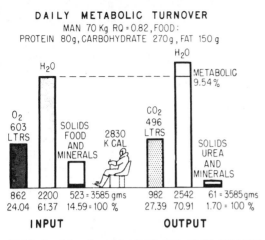

DAILY METABOLIC TURNOVER
MAN 70 Kg RQ = 0.82, FOOD:
PROTEIN 80g, CARBOHYDRATE 270g, FAT 150 g

Metabolic data of a (standard) man of 70 kilograms weight (H. G. Clamann, Aerospace Medical Division, Brooks AFB, Texas). *Official Air Force Photo.*

manifested in the occurrence of boiling of body fluids, or ebullism, at an altitude of 5 kilometers (3 miles), which corresponds to 20 kilometers (12 miles) in our atmosphere. The atmospheric environment on Mars, therefore, is space-equivalent very close to its surface. Some tests show that organic compounds—the same compounds believed to have been precursors to biological molecules on earth millions of years before man—are probably being produced by sunlight on the surface of Mars.

To sustain human life on Mars and, of course, on the moon, requires a sealed compartment of the same type as in space itself.

The development of effective *intracabin life-supporting systems* is a *conditio sine qua non* for the realization of space flight, just the same as the provision of protective capabilities of the cabin's shell against the surrounding vacuum, radiations, and meteorites, which have already been mentioned.

Space does not allow a discussion of all the vital ecological factors in the *cabin's environment,* such as pressure, composition of the air, and the control of temperature, humidity, and odor; only a few remarks can be made about the respiratory and nutritional metabolic side of the vital necessities in space flight, and their procurement.

First, for a general familiarization in this matter, the figure above shows the daily metabolic turnover of a "standard man." It can also serve as a guide for the estimation of the vital requirements for any astronautical journey.

To supply the *respiratory requirements* in space operations, the following methods are available or conceivable: First, replacement of the consumed oxygen from stored oxygen tanks

and elimination of the exhaled carbon dioxide by chemical absorbents and storage of the absorbers. This *storage method* is *the* measure of the reconstitution of the cabin's air for short-time space operations, up to perhaps two months. Beyond this duration, the logistic difficulties make this method unsuitable when we consider that for such a period an oxygen reserve of 50 kilograms per man would be required, and more than this amount for chemicals to absorb carbon dioxide and water vapor.

The solution to this problem is *recycling* of the air and of the absorbents by physicochemical means. This method might be logistically acceptable for a duration of one year. Beyond this time, especially for a permanent moon base, reconstitution of all vital necessities—air, water, and food—is necessary if we wish to stay within the payload capabilities of rockets. The method of choice, then, is *biological regeneration,* as we observe this in free nature in the biotic relationship between animals and plants: in the process of photosynthesis, found in all chlorophyl-bearing vegetation. In this process, carbon dioxide is consumed and oxygen is produced—the reverse of respiration. Algae in a nutrient solution are used as photosynthetic gas exchangers in laboratory experiments. With one and one-half pounds of algae, and even less, we can meet the respiratory requirements of one man. But in photosynthesis, carbohydrates are also produced, thus providing material for nutrition. In this manner, photosynthetic regeneration offers the possibility to include, in addition to carbon dioxide and water, all body wastes. With such total reconstruction of the vital necessities, we can achieve a true closed ecological system. But since photosynthesis requires light (and most probably solar light will be utilized) it is a sun-dependent closed ecological system. However, as already mentioned, solar illuminance drops below the effective minimum required for photosynthesis somewhere near the belt of the asteroids. The production of its own light by a nuclear power plant will, then, be necessary, and this will make the vehicle a sun-independent, or an autarch closed ecological system. Such will be the various phases in the development and utilization of the intracabin life-supporting systems.

Despite successful moon landings, all of this is still under extensive study in *space cabin simulators.* These devices also enable us to study the occupants' reaction to confinement and isolation. Experiments in a two-man space cabin simulator over a period of four or more weeks are now a matter of routine, and have given us indispensable information for life support in actual space flight. These space cabin simulators are, of course, also useful tools in the selection and training program for prospective astronauts.

An interesting topic in these space medical laboratory studies is *day-night* cycling. This sub-

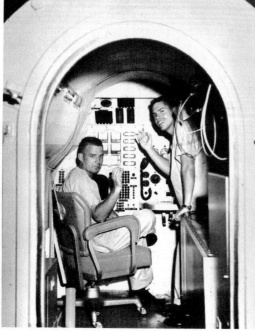

Two-man space cabin simulator, Department of Space Medicine, Aerospace Medical Division, Brooks AFB, Texas. *Official Air Force Photo.*

ject matter demands attention even in long-distance atmospheric flight, insofar as the crossing of half a dozen time zones within a quarter of a day leads to an asynchrony between the physical or geographic, and the physiological day-night cycle of the terrestrial traveler. For certain travelers—diplomats, businessmen, etc.—a fast synchronization in this respect may be sometimes important, which can be achieved by preadaptation and drugs acting as synchronizers. In space flight, there is no day and night in earthly terms. A satellite night is in the order of half an hour. In his light and shadow cycle an orbiting astronaut does not need a synchronization with his home planet any more than he would need a synchronization with the time on the moon or Mars. His physical time is the universal time. Nevertheless, he remains a terrestrial creature in his physiological nature and still needs a physiological sequence of activity, rest, and sleep; in other words, his life processes are still governed by his "physiological clock" or circadian rhythm.

In the space flight situation, however, an unfamiliar, novel factor—namely, dynamic weightlessness—enters the picture. Zero g enters the life of a basically 1-g creature, and this might lead to a modification of his sleep and activity cycle. Only actual experience *in situ,* that is, in space, by the astronauts will reveal the physiological space pattern in this respect. Exercise or space calisthenics will play an important role; and perhaps drugs—at least in the beginning of

extended space operations—may be used to facilitate the establishment of a routine earth's independent sleep and wakefulness cycle which guarantees the health and well-being of the astronauts.

With zero g another important subfield of space medicine has been considered: *biodynamics,* as manifested in the large g spectrum from some 10 g to zero g.

Increased g's are encountered during launching and atmospheric reentry, recovery operations, and landing. Experiments on large centrifuges during the past 25 years, and pertinent experiments on rocket-powered sleds have taught us the tolerable g limits of man and means of protection. We know that the transversal direction of the g forces, that is, vertical to the longitudinal body axis, is the one which makes the high accelerations and decelerations during launching and atmospheric reentry tolerable. This knowledge has been utilized in actual suborbital and orbital flights by putting the astronaut in the required position on a couch which has been specially molded for that purpose.

As for the tolerability of *zero g* or *weightlessness* which occurs during the passive phase of the space flight trajectory or during coasting, performance and well-being seem not to be disturbed during short periods of time, that is, up to several hours, as has been proved in the suborbital and orbital flights in 1961 and 1962 and in the Apollo flights of the late sixties and early seventies. Concerning longer periods of time, definite statements cannot be made at present. If it should turn out that prolonged weightlessness would lead to disturbances, similar to seasickness, which could not be handled therapeutically, then artificial gravitation will be necessary. This, of course, would have a tremendous effect upon the design of space vehicle systems. It may not be necessary to apply 1 g, rather, fractions of it may be sufficient. This—what we might call physiological gravitational minimum required for the normalization of body functions—can be found, of course, only in actual space flight of longer durations than trips to the moon and back.

If artificial gravitation should be required, then the logical g value for a Martian journey would be 37 percent of 1 g, which is the gravity on Mars.

Zero gravity has also some definite effects upon the life-supporting equipment. For instance, water and food must be consumed by means of squeeze bottles. This method was developed in parabolic flight maneuvers in jet aircraft, carried out at 10 kilometers (30,000 feet), in space medical efforts by the U.S. Air Force in 1956. This was subsequently tested and utilized by our astronauts in suborbital and orbital flights, by the Russian cosmonauts, and by U.S. astronauts during the Apollo moon flights.

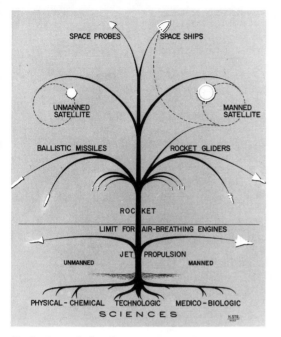

Family tree of aircraft, aerospace craft, rockets, and space vehicles. *Official Air Force Photo.*

watery environment and crawled out onto land into an unfamiliar environment—that of the atmosphere. By development of highly efficient respiratory organs they became, after an amphibian phase, exclusive air breathers. They had crossed the threshold from sea life to land life, or the border between the sea ocean and the air ocean.

Now, in the cenozoic era, man, the highest air-breathing creature, is engaged in the venture of crossing the threshold of space, or the border between the air ocean and the vacuum ocean in interplanetary space. This is not, in contrast to the sea-to-land transition of animal life, a matter of natural adaptive evolution over millions of generations; rather, it is a matter of revolutionary scientific and technological progress accomplished within a few generations. It is based on the development of artificial means such as propulsion methods and vehicles which, independent of the earth's atmosphere, carry man, after the amphibian stage of atmospheric space-equivalent flight with air-breathing engines, into the vacuum environment of space. This technological evolution is demonstrated by the genealogical family tree of various types of aircraft, aerospace craft, rockets, satellites, and space ships, as shown in the figure. And as a basic root of this technological family tree, space medicine will play a vital role.

But the activities in space medicine are not a one-way affair, serving exclusively the realization of manned space flight; rather it will pay back, and has already done so, dividends in the form of by-products valuable for the whole field of medicine. This is evidenced by the development of microinstrumentation and biotelemetry useful in hospitals, the development of novel medical concepts, and by a new terminology, which, all in all, leads to an extension of our whole earthbound medical and biological thinking into a broader cosmic spectrum.

These examples in the fields of environmental ecology and biodynamics of space flight may be sufficient to demonstrate the novelty of the problems space medicine, or bioastronautics, is faced with in this space age.

Crossing the threshold of space is, in its biological significance, comparable only with the transition of life in the oceans to life on land in geological times. This started some 300 million years ago in the paleozoicum when certain aquatic animals, such as the lungfish, left their

STATISTICAL APPENDIX

REPORTABLE DISEASES—NUMBER OF CASES REPORTED IN THE UNITED STATES: 1959 TO 1966

Disease	1959	1960	1961	1962	1963	1964	1965	1966
Typhoid fever	859	816	814	608	566	501	454	378
Brucellosis	892	751	636	409	407	411	262	262
Scarlet fever and streptococcal sore throat	334,715	315,173	338,410	315,809	342,161	402,334	395,168	427,752
Diphtheria	934	918	617	444	314	293	164	209
Whooping cough	40,005	14,809	11,468	17,749	17,135	13,005	6,799	7,717
Meningococcal infections	2,180	2,259	2,232	2,150	2,470	2,826	3,040	3,381
Tularemia	459	390	365	328	327	342	264	208
Acute poliomyelitis	8,425	3,190	1,312	910	449	122	72	113
Acute infectious encephalitis	2,437	2,341	2,248	2,094	1,993	3,587	2,703	3,085
Smallpox	—	—	—	—	—	—	—	—
Measles	406,162	441,703	423,919	481,530	385,156	458,083	261,904	204,136
Endemic typhus fever	51	68	46	32	35	30	28	33
Rocky Mountain spotted fever	199	204	219	240	216	277	281	268
Malaria	71	72	73	118	99	93	147	565
Venereal diseases:								
Gonococcal infection	240,158	258,933	264,158	263,708	278,289	300,667	324,925	351,738
Syphilis and its sequelae	120,766	122,003	124,658	126,245	124,137	114,314	112,842	126,573

Source: United States Public Health Service.

BIRTHS AND BIRTH RATES PER 1,000 POPULATION FOR BIRTH-REGISTRATION STATES: 1959 TO 1967

| Year | BIRTHS BY RACE | | | | BIRTHS BY SEX | | |
| | Number | | Rate | | | | Male births per 1,000 female births |
	White	Nonwhite	White	Nonwhite	Male	Female	
1959*	3,597,430	647,366	30.3	39.4	2,173,638	2,071,158	1,049
1960*	3,600,744	657,106	30.2	38.8	2,179,708	2,078,142	1,049
1961*	3,600,864	667,462	29.9	38.8	2,186,274	2,082,052	1,050
1962*[1]	3,394,068	641,580	28.6	37.6	2,132,466	2,034,896	1,048
1963*[1]	3,326,344	638,928	27.3	36.5	2,101,632	1,996,388	1,053
1964*	3,369,160	658,330	26.2	35.6	2,060,162	1,967,328	1,047
1965*	3,123,860	636,498	23.8	33.3	1,927,054	1,833,304	1,051
1966*	2,993,230	613,044	22.3	31.0	1,845,862	1,760,412	1,049
1967*	2,922,502	598,457	21.0	29.1	1,803,388	1,717,571	1,050

*Figures based on 50% sample.
Source: Public Health Service, National Office of Vital Statistics.
[1]Figures by color exclude data for residents of New Jersey.

HOSPITALS IN THE UNITED STATES

TYPE OF CONTROL

Year	Total Hospitals	Total Beds Number	Total Beds Rate*	Federal Hospitals	Federal Beds	State and Local Hospitals	State and Local Beds	All Other Hospitals	All Other Beds
1951	6,637	1,529,988	10.0	388	216,939	1,644	880,781	4,605	432,268
1952	6,665	1,541,615	9.9	386	211,510	1,692	888,113	4,587	441,992
1953	6,840	1,573,014	9.9	392	200,535	1,744	912,469	4,704	460,010
1954	6,970	1,577,961	9.8	430	189,233	1,800	919,870	4,740	468,858
1955	6,956	1,604,000	9.8	428	183,000	1,805	942,000	4,723	479,000
1956	6,966	1,608,000	9.6	432	184,000	1,816	930,000	4,718	494,000
1957	6,818	1,559,000	9.2	437	183,000	1,781	881,000	4,600	495,000
1958	6,818	1,578,000	9.1	440	182,000	1,819	890,000	4,559	506,000
1959	6,845	1,613,000	9.1	438	179,000	1,835	921,000	4,572	513,000
1960	6,876	1,658,000	9.2	435	177,000	1,880	953,000	4,561	528,000
1961	6,923	1,670,000	9.1	437	178,000	1,925	951,000	4,561	541,000
1962	7,028	1,689,000	9.1	447	178,000	1,968	954,000	4,613	557,000
1963	7,138	1,702,000	9.0	446	176,000	2,007	950,000	4,685	576,000
1964	7,127	1,696,000	8.9	441	175,000	2,055	935,000	4,631	586,000
1965	7,123	1,704,000	8.8	443	174,000	2,041	924,000	4,639	606,000
1966	7,160	1,679,000	8.7	425	173,000	2,104	888,000	4,631	618,000
1967	7,172	1,671,000	8.5	416	175,000	2,141	863,000	4,615	633,000
1968	7,137	1,663,000	8.4	416	175,000	2,190	839,000	4,531	649,000

TYPE OF SERVICE

Year	General Hospitals	General Beds Number	General Beds Rate*	Mental Hospitals	Mental Beds	Tuberculosis Hospitals	Tuberculosis Beds	All Other Hospitals	All Other Beds
1959	5,601	728,132	4.1	502	755,293	273	64,116	469	65,281
1960	5,659	747,779	4.2	531	789,101	251	55,693	435	65,397
1961	5,713	765,955	4.2	526	781,847	236	52,167	448	69,820
1962	5,823	784,906	4.2	535	784,240	214	47,819	456	72,449
1963	5,941	802,608	4.3	543	782,161	197	42,138	457	74,932
1964	5,949	821,981	4.3	531	758,401	194	41,385	453	74,272
1965	5,974	841,491	4.4	527	751,461	185	39,271	437	71,299
1966	6,086	891,819	4.6	513	694,261	159	31,317	402	61,261
1967	6,139	920,207	4.7	505	661,163	106	18,323	422	71,432
1968	6,069	926,756	4.7	542	646,609	118	22,431	408	67,407

*Beds per 1,000 population.
Source: American Hospital Association, Chicago, Ill., Hospitals, Guide Issue.

HOSPITAL FACILITIES, 1959 TO 1968, AND BY STATES, 1968

Year and State or Other Area	Hospitals		Beds		Bassinets		Patients Adm. (1,000)		Average Census**	
	Total	General and Special Short-term*	Total	General and Special Short-term*	Total	General and Special Short-term*	Total	General and Special Short-term*	Total	General and Special Short-term*
1959	6,845	5,364	1,612,822	619,877	101,582	96,869	23,605	21,605	1,363,217	462,010
1960	6,876	5,407	1,657,970	639,057	102,764	98,127	25,027	22,970	1,401,873	477,437
1961	6,923	5,460	1,669,789	658,521	103,393	98,720	25,474	23,375	1,392,856	489,468
1962	7,028	5,564	1,689,414	676,795	104,101	99,479	26,531	24,307	1,406,818	508,791
1963	7,138	5,684	1,701,839	698,191	104,695	100,190	27,502	25,267	1,429,586	530,318
1964	7,127	5,712	1,696,039	720,810	103,350	98,905	28,266	25,987	1,420,918	550,062
1965	7,123	5,736	1,703,522	741,292	101,287	96,782	28,812	26,463	1,402,625	563,424
1966	7,160	5,812	1,678,658	768,479	100,555	96,157	29,151	26,897	1,398,491	587,866
1967	7,172	5,850	1,671,000	788,000	99,296	95,075	29,361	26,988	1,380,000	612,000
1968, U.S.	7,137	5,820	1,663,203	805,592	97,319	93,213	29,766	27,276	1,378,398	630,368
Alabama	139	121	28,399	13,311	1,825	1,761	538	495	24,486	10,631
Alaska	26	13	1,937	578	200	92	40	19	1,285	345
Arizona	80	56	10,238	7,026	871	722	254	210	7,235	4,483
Arkansas	92	84	11,297	7,344	1,051	1,025	298	278	8,425	5,562
California	639	529	134,909	69,979	7,898	7,445	2,828	2,548	107,720	51,087
Colorado	92	73	16,337	9,178	1,129	1,033	383	336	12,451	6,931
Connecticut	65	41	24,777	9,970	1,309	1,288	384	356	21,152	8,158
Delaware	14	6	5,113	1,648	235	208	64	58	4,384	1,356
Dist. of Columbia	21	14	15,093	5,028	640	610	203	172	12,849	4,133
Florida	186	156	43,253	24,240	2,442	2,252	931	857	36,174	19,315
Georgia	162	137	34,134	14,885	2,105	1,953	703	608	28,458	11,720
Hawaii	32	21	6,290	2,091	415	316	98	73	4,940	1,523
Idaho	54	48	3,980	2,894	442	430	105	100	2,904	2,021
Illinois	314	256	102,407	49,122	5,070	4,985	1,667	1,568	85,891	39,202
Indiana	138	111	39,129	19,031	2,502	2,483	703	680	33,503	15,797
Iowa	144	130	20,568	14,562	1,718	1,710	479	458	15,626	10,985
Kansas	166	147	19,916	11,501	1,520	1,431	377	348	15,447	8,717
Kentucky	133	105	22,937	11,704	1,538	1,436	523	460	18,610	9,343
Louisiana	152	134	26,891	14,863	1,793	1,711	610	549	20,332	10,511
Maine	58	48	9,652	4,023	613	582	149	138	7,866	3,001
Maryland	84	46	33,259	11,386	1,546	1,381	441	369	28,375	9,239
Massachusetts	205	141	64,543	25,862	2,707	2,606	885	815	53,596	20,312
Michigan	251	198	71,415	32,426	3,957	3,915	1,155	1,099	60,173	26,339
Minnesota	206	183	34,115	20,412	2,548	2,533	651	623	26,919	15,514
Mississippi	104	93	16,479	7,734	1,095	1,039	326	298	13,133	5,818

HOSPITAL FACILITIES, 1959 TO 1968, AND BY STATES, 1968 (Con't.)

Year and State or Other Area	Hospitals		Beds		Bassinets		Patients Adm. (1,000)		Average Census**	
	Total	General and Special Short-term*	Total	General and Special Short-term*	Total	General and Special Short-term*	Total	General and Special Short-term*	Total	General and Special Short-term*
Missouri	146	119	39,610	20,581	2,066	2,000	720	663	33,115	16,824
Montana	65	56	4,554	3,727	522	487	132	121	3,229	2,578
Nebraska	116	102	12,943	8,064	1,129	1,074	258	234	9,364	5,890
Nevada	22	17	2,756	1,884	241	221	71	64	2,068	1,370
New Hampshire	36	32	6,668	3,033	481	481	101	98	5,479	2,242
New Jersey	141	106	52,776	23,505	2,849	2,801	870	790	44,367	19,167
New Mexico	58	40	5,918	3,242	660	517	155	123	4,272	2,229
New York	432	343	204,190	80,046	8,320	8,187	2,481	2,314	182,040	66,557
N. Carolina	164	137	35,567	18,022	2,596	2,445	759	678	29,365	14,176
N. Dakota	65	56	6,238	3,811	617	573	126	116	4,624	2,740
Ohio	247	194	81,275	39,530	4,713	4,673	1,445	1,377	69,477	32,791
Oklahoma	145	122	15,888	9,631	1,371	1,269	399	349	12,370	7,290
Oregon	87	78	15,801	8,012	856	856	302	286	11,956	5,649
Pennsylvania	321	241	116,606	52,966	5,809	5,745	1,682	1,602	99,851	43,245
Rhode Island	24	15	8,700	3,364	443	408	129	110	7,415	2,699
S. Carolina	84	70	19,002	9,202	1,626	1,493	381	325	15,477	7,169
S. Dakota	61	49	6,320	3,322	559	498	121	105	4,864	2,293
Tennessee	160	135	32,886	16,787	1,905	1,850	651	606	27,117	13,262
Texas	558	493	74,614	43,380	5,451	5,097	1,742	1,574	59,390	32,136
Utah	39	33	4,772	3,277	554	534	151	142	3,596	2,373
Vermont	25	20	4,565	1,900	274	274	69	65	3,806	1,487
Virginia	130	103	38,275	15,492	2,003	1,799	622	535	33,181	12,581
Washington	130	109	18,866	10,818	1,420	1,320	515	456	14,140	7,802
W. Virginia	89	73	15,926	8,663	966	961	329	308	13,366	6,813
Wisconsin	202	159	37,394	21,073	2,436	2,436	701	668	29,623	15,814
Wyoming	33	27	4,025	1,782	283	267	60	55	2,912	1,148
Puerto Rico	60	48	10,003	5,864	736	694	237	219	8,132	4,923

*Nonfederal hospitals.
**Average number of patients receiving hospital treatment each day.
Source: American Hospital Association, Chicago, Ill., Hospitals, Guide Issue.

DEATH RATES PER 1,000 POPULATION, IN DEATH-REGISTRATION STATES: 1951 TO 1966

Year	Total			White			Nonwhite		
	Both sexes	Male	Female	Both sexes	Male	Female	Both sexes	Male	Female
1951	9.7	11.1	8.2	9.5	11.0	8.0	11.1	12.5	9.8
1952	9.6	11.1	8.1	9.4	11.0	8.0	11.0	12.5	9.6
1953	9.6	11.1	8.1	9.4	11.0	8.0	10.8	12.3	9.4
1954	9.2	10.7	7.8	9.1	10.6	7.6	10.1	11.4	8.8
1955	9.3	10.8	7.9	9.2	10.7	7.8	10.0	11.3	8.8
1956	9.4	10.8	7.9	9.3	10.8	7.8	10.1	11.4	8.8
1957	9.6	11.1	8.1	9.5	11.0	8.0	10.5	11.9	9.1
1958	9.5	11.0	8.1	9.4	10.9	8.0	10.3	11.6	9.0
1959	9.4	10.8	8.0	9.3	10.8	7.9	9.9	11.3	8.6
1960	9.5	11.0	8.1	9.5	11.0	8.0	10.1	11.5	8.7
1961	9.3	10.7	7.9	9.3	10.7	7.8	9.6	10.9	8.4
1962	9.5	10.9	8.1	9.4	10.8	8.0	9.8	11.2	8.5
1963	9.6	11.1	8.2	9.5	11.0	8.1	10.1	11.5	8.7
1964	9.4	10.8	8.0	9.4	10.8	8.0	9.7	11.1	8.3
1965	9.4	10.9	8.0	9.4	10.8	8.0	9.6	11.1	8.2
1966	9.5	11.0	8.1	9.5	10.9	8.1	9.7	11.3	8.3

Source: Dept. of Health, Education and Welfare, Public Health Service, National Office of Vital Statistics.

INFANTS DEATHS (UNDER 1 YEAR OF AGE) PER 1,000 LIVE BIRTHS, BY AGE GROUPS, FOR BIRTH-REGISTRATION STATES: 1959 TO 1966

Age	1959	1960	1961	1962	1963	1964	1965	1966
Total under 1 year	26.4	26.0	25.3	25.3	25.2	24.8	24.7	23.7
Under 28 days	19.0	18.7	18.4	18.3	18.2	17.9	17.7	17.2
Under 1 day	10.3	10.3	10.3	10.4	10.4	10.2	10.2	9.9
1 day	2.8	2.7	2.7	2.6	2.7	2.6	2.6	2.5
2 days	1.8	1.8	1.7	1.7	1.7	1.6	1.6	1.5
3 days	0.9	0.8	0.8	0.8	0.7	0.7	0.7	0.7
4 days	0.5	0.5	0.4	0.4	0.4	0.4	0.4	0.4
5 days	0.4	0.3	0.3	0.3	0.3	0.3	0.3	0.3
6 days	0.3	0.3	0.2	0.2	0.2	0.2	0.2	0.2
7-13 days	1.1	1.0	0.9	0.9	0.9	0.9	0.8	0.8
14-20 days	0.6	0.6	0.6	0.5	0.5	0.5	0.5	0.5
21-27 days	0.5	0.5	0.4	0.4	0.4	0.4	0.4	0.4
28-59 days	1.7	1.7	1.6	1.6	1.6	1.7	1.7	1.6
2 months	1.3	1.3	1.3	1.3	1.3	1.3	1.3	1.2
3 months	1.0	1.0	1.0	1.0	1.0	1.0	1.0	0.9
4 months	0.7	0.8	0.7	0.7	0.8	0.7	0.7	0.7
5 months	0.6	0.6	0.6	0.6	0.6	0.5	0.5	0.5
6 months	0.5	0.5	0.4	0.4	0.5	0.4	0.4	0.4
7 months	0.4	0.4	0.3	0.4	0.4	0.3	0.3	0.3
8 months	0.3	0.3	0.3	0.3	0.3	0.3	0.3	0.3
9 months	0.3	0.3	0.2	0.3	0.2	0.3	0.3	0.2
10 months	0.2	0.2	0.2	0.2	0.2	0.2	0.2	0.2
11 months	0.2	0.2	0.2	0.2	0.2	0.2	0.2	0.2

Source: Dept. of Health, Education and Welfare, Public Health Service, National Office of Vital Statistics; annual report, *Vital Statistics of the United States.*

DEATHS FROM 32 SELECTED CAUSES, 1966, AND DEATH
RATES PER 100,000 POPULATION*

Cause of Death	1966 Number	1966 Rate	1966 Rate
All causes	1,863,149	951.3	954.7
Tuberculosis, all forms	7,625	3.9	6.1
Syphilis and its sequelae	2,193	1.1	1.6
Typhoid fever	15	0.0	0.0
Dysentery, all forms	172	0.1	0.2
Diphtheria	20	0.0	0.0
Whooping cough	49	0.0	0.1
Meningococcal infections	876	0.4	0.4
Acute poliomyelitis	9	0.0	0.1
Measles	261	0.1	0.2
All other infective and parasitic diseases	6,094	3.1	3.2
Malignant neoplasms, incl. neoplasms of lymphatic and hematopoietic tissues	303,736	155.1	149.2
Diabetes mellitus	34,597	17.7	16.7
Meningitis, except meningococcal and tuberculous	2,324	1.2	1.3
Major cardiovascular-renal diseases	1,021,188	521.4	521.8
Diseases of cardiovascular system	1,010,812	516.1	515.1
Vascular lesions affecting central nervous system	204,841	104.6	108.0
Rheumatic fever	15,012	7.7	10.3
Diseases of heart	727,002	371.2	369.0
Hypertension without mention of heart and general arteriosclerosis	50,287	25.7	27.1
Other diseases of circulatory system	28,682	14.6	11.0
Chronic and unspecified nephritis and other renal sclerosis	10,376	5.3	6.7
Influenza and pneumonia, except pneumonia of newborn	63,615	32.5	37.3
Ulcer of stomach and duodenum	10,321	5.3	6.7
Gastritis, duodenitis, enteritis, and colitis, except diarrhea of newborn	7,552	3.9	4.4
Cirrhosis of liver	26,692	13.6	11.3
Acute nephritis and nephritis with edema including nephrosis	1,164	0.6	0.9
Deliveries and complications of pregnancy, childbirth, and the puerperium	1,049	0.5	0.9
Congenital malformations	18,158	9.3	12.2
Symptoms, senility, and ill-defined conditions	23,960	12.2	11.4
Motor-vehicle accidents	53,041	27.1	21.3
All other accidents	60,522	30.9	31.0
Suicide	21,281	10.9	10.6
Homicide	11,606	5.9	4.7
All other causes	185,038	94.5	101.1

*Includes rheumatic fever and chronic rheumatic heart disease.

Source: Dept. of Health, Education, and Welfare, Public Health Service, National Office of Vital Statistics; annual report, *Vital Statistics of the U.S.*

EXPECTATION OF LIFE AND MORTALITY RATES AT SINGLE YEARS
OF AGE, BY RACE AND SEX: 1966

| | Expectation of Life in Years | | | | | Mortality Rate per 1,000 | | | | |
| | | White | | Nonwhite | | | White | | Nonwhite | |
Age	Total	Males	Females	Males	Females	Total	Males	Females	Males	Female
0	70.1	67.6	74.7	60.7	67.4	23.6	23.4	17.6	42.2	34.9
1	70.8	68.2	75.1	62.4	68.8	1.5	1.4	1.2	2.9	2.5
2	69.9	67.3	74.2	61.6	68.0	0.9	0.9	0.7	1.6	1.4
3	69.0	66.3	73.2	60.7	67.1	0.7	0.7	0.6	1.2	1.0
4	68.0	65.4	72.2	59.7	66.1	0.6	0.6	0.5	0.9	0.8
5	67.1	64.4	71.3	58.8	65.2	0.6	0.7	0.4	1.1	0.7
6	66.1	63.5	70.3	57.9	64.2	0.5	0.6	0.4	0.8	0.6
7	65.2	62.5	69.3	56.9	63.3	0.4	0.4	0.3	0.6	0.5
8	64.2	61.5	68.4	55.9	62.3	0.3	0.3	0.3	0.5	0.4
9	63.2	60.5	67.4	55.0	61.3	0.3	0.3	0.3	0.5	0.4
10	62.2	59.6	66.4	54.0	60.4	0.3	0.3	0.2	0.5	0.4
11	61.2	58.6	65.4	53.0	59.4	0.3	0.3	0.2	0.5	0.4
12	60.3	57.6	64.4	52.0	58.4	0.4	0.4	0.3	0.7	0.4
13	59.3	56.6	63.5	51.1	57.4	0.5	0.6	0.3	0.8	0.4
14	58.3	55.7	62.5	50.1	56.4	0.6	0.8	0.4	1.0	0.5
15	57.3	54.7	61.5	49.2	55.5	0.8	1.0	0.5	1.3	0.6
16	56.4	53.8	60.5	48.2	54.5	0.9	1.3	0.5	1.5	0.7
17	55.4	52.8	59.6	47.3	53.5	1.1	1.5	0.6	1.8	0.8
18	54.5	51.9	58.6	46.4	52.6	1.2	1.6	0.6	2.1	0.9
19	53.6	51.0	57.6	45.5	51.6	1.2	1.7	0.6	2.4	1.0
20	52.6	50.1	56.7	44.6	50.7	1.3	1.8	0.6	2.7	1.1
21	51.7	49.1	55.7	43.7	49.7	1.3	1.9	0.6	3.0	1.2
22	50.8	48.2	54.7	42.8	48.8	1.4	1.9	0.6	3.2	1.4
23	49.8	47.3	53.8	42.0	47.9	1.4	1.9	0.6	3.4	1.5
24	48.9	46.4	52.8	41.1	46.9	1.4	1.8	0.7	3.5	1.6
25	48.0	45.5	51.8	40.3	46.0	1.3	1.7	0.7	3.7	1.6
26	47.0	44.6	50.9	39.4	45.1	1.3	1.6	0.7	3.8	1.8
27	46.1	43.6	49.9	38.6	44.2	1.4	1.6	0.7	4.0	1.9
28	45.1	42.7	48.9	37.7	43.2	1.4	1.6	0.8	4.2	2.1
29	44.2	41.8	48.0	36.9	42.3	1.5	1.6	0.8	4.4	2.3
30	43.3	40.8	47.0	36.0	41.4	1.5	1.6	0.9	4.7	2.5
31	42.3	39.9	46.0	35.2	40.5	1.6	1.7	0.9	4.9	2.8
32	41.4	39.0	45.1	34.4	39.6	1.7	1.8	1.0	5.2	3.0
33	40.5	38.0	44.1	33.5	38.8	1.8	1.9	1.1	5.5	3.3
34	39.5	37.1	43.2	32.7	37.9	1.9	2.0	1.2	5.8	3.5
35	38.6	36.2	42.2	31.9	37.0	2.1	2.2	1.2	6.1	3.8
36	37.7	35.3	41.3	31.1	36.2	2.2	2.4	1.3	6.5	4.1
37	36.8	34.4	40.3	30.3	35.3	2.4	2.6	1.5	6.9	4.4
38	35.9	33.4	39.4	29.5	34.5	2.6	2.8	1.6	7.4	4.7
39	35.0	32.5	38.5	28.7	33.6	2.9	3.1	1.8	8.0	5.1
40	34.1	31.6	37.5	28.0	32.8	3.1	3.4	1.9	8.6	5.4
41	33.2	30.7	36.6	27.2	32.0	3.4	3.7	2.1	9.2	5.8
42	32.3	29.8	35.7	26.4	31.1	3.7	4.1	2.4	9.9	6.2
43	31.4	29.0	34.8	25.7	30.3	4.1	4.5	2.6	10.6	6.7
44	30.5	28.1	33.8	25.0	29.5	4.4	5.0	2.8	11.3	7.2
45	29.7	27.2	32.9	24.2	28.8	4.8	5.5	3.1	12.1	7.8
46	28.8	26.4	32.0	23.5	28.0	5.3	6.1	3.4	12.9	8.5
47	27.9	25.5	31.1	22.8	27.2	5.8	6.8	3.7	13.7	9.0
48	27.1	24.7	30.3	22.1	26.4	6.3	7.5	4.0	14.6	9.5
49	26.3	23.9	29.4	21.5	25.7	6.9	8.4	4.4	15.5	10.0
50	25.5	23.1	28.5	20.8	25.0	7.6	9.3	4.7	16.4	10.5
51	24.6	22.3	27.6	20.1	24.2	8.3	10.3	5.1	17.5	11.1
52	23.9	21.5	26.8	19.5	23.5	9.0	11.4	5.6	18.7	11.8
53	23.1	20.8	25.9	18.8	22.8	9.9	12.5	6.0	20.2	12.7
54	22.3	20.0	25.1	18.2	22.0	10.8	13.8	6.5	22.0	13.7
55	21.5	19.3	24.2	17.6	21.3	11.8	15.2	7.1	24.1	14.9
56	20.8	18.6	23.4	17.0	20.7	12.9	16.7	7.7	26.2	16.2
57	20.0	17.9	22.6	16.5	20.0	13.9	18.2	8.3	28.0	17.5
58	19.3	17.2	21.8	15.9	19.3	15.0	19.8	8.9	29.4	18.8
59	18.6	16.6	21.0	15.4	18.7	16.1	21.4	9.5	30.4	20.1
60	17.9	15.9	20.2	14.9	18.1	17.3	23.1	10.2	31.1	21.2

EXPECTATION OF LIFE AND MORTALITY RATES AT SINGLE YEARS OF AGE, BY RACE AND SEX: 1966 *(Con't.)*

| Age | | Expectation of Life in Years | | | | | Mortality Rate per 1,000 | | | |
| | | White | | Nonwhite | | | White | | Nonwhite | |
	Total	Males	Females	Males	Females	Total	Males	Females	Males	Female
61	17.2	15.3	19.4	14.3	17.4	18.6	24.9	11.1	32.1	22.5
62	16.5	14.7	18.6	13.8	16.8	20.1	26.9	12.1	34.3	24.7
63	15.9	14.1	17.8	13.3	16.3	21.9	29.2	13.3	38.3	27.9
64	15.2	13.5	17.0	12.8	15.7	24.1	31.8	14.8	43.8	32.1
65	14.6	12.9	16.3	12.4	15.2	26.4	34.5	16.5	50.4	37.0
66	13.9	12.3	15.5	12.0	14.8	28.8	37.4	18.3	57.1	41.7
67	13.3	11.8	14.8	11.7	14.4	31.4	40.5	20.3	62.7	45.3
68	12.8	11.3	14.1	11.4	14.1	33.9	43.8	22.4	66.3	46.9
69	12.2	10.8	13.4	11.2	13.7	36.5	47.3	24.8	68.0	46.7

Source: Dept. of Health, Education, and Welfare, Public Health Service, National Office of Vital Statistics; annual report, *Vital Statistics of the U.S.*

PATIENTS IN HOSPITALS FOR MENTAL DISEASE AND IN INSTITUTIONS FOR MENTAL DEFECTIVES AND EPILEPTICS, UNDER PUBLIC AND PRIVATE CONTROL: 1958 TO 1966

| | Patients in Hospitals for Mental Disease at End of Year | | | | | Mental Defectives and Epileptics in Institutions at End of Year | | | |
| | Total | | Public Hospitals | | | Total | | | |
Year	Number of Patients	Rate[1]	Veterans	Other[2]	Private Hospitals	Number of Patients	Rate[1]	Public Institutions	Private Institutions
1958	619,508	361.4	59,855	545,182	14,471	161,815	94.4	153,699	8,116
1959	618,211	352.7	62,632	541,883	13,696	165,889	95.0	157,736	8,153
1960	611,432	343.2	62,097	535,540	13,795	171,511	96.3	163,730	7,781
1961	603,044	332.9	62,569	527,456	13,019	169,664	93.7	162,456	7,208
1962	591,285	321.8	61,889	515,640	13,756	182,118	99.1	173,638	8,480
1963	578,819	310.3	61,234	504,604	12,981	183,864	98.6	176,516	7,348
1964	565,354	298.6	61,300	490,754	13,300	186,735	98.6	179,353	7,382
1965	550,721	287.0	61,760	475,761	13,200	193,766	101.0	187,305	6,461
1966	527,000	272.0	62,000	452,000	13,000	197,000	102.0	191,000	6,000

[1]Per 100,000 estimated civilian population.
[2]Comprises state, psychopathic, and county hospitals.
Source: Department of Health, Education, and Welfare, Public Health Service, National Institute of Mental Health; annual report, "Patients in Mental Institutions."

TEN LEADING CAUSES OF DEATH IN THE UNITED STATES

	1966			1960		
	Number of Deaths	Rate*	Rank Order	Number of Deaths	Rate*	Rank Order
Diseases of heart	727,002	371.2	1	661,712	369.0	1
Malignant neoplasms	303,736	155.1	2	267,627	149.2	2
Vascular lesions affecting central nervous system	204,841	104.6	3	193,588	108.0	3
Accidents	113,563	58.0	4	93,806	52.3	4
Influenza and pneumonia	63,615	32.5	5	66,806	37.3	6
Certain diseases of early infancy	51,644	26.4	6	67,094	37.4	5
General arteriosclerosis	38,907	19.9	7	35,876	20.0	7
Diabetes mellitus	34,597	17.1	8	29,971	16.7	8
Other diseases of circulatory system	28,682	14.6	9	—	—	—
Other bronchopulmonic diseases	28,371	14.5	10	—	—	—
Congenital malformations	—	—	—	21,860	12.2	9
Cirrhosis of liver	—	—	—	20,296	11.3	10

*Rate per 100,000 population.
Source: U.S. Department of Health, Education and Welfare, Public Health Service, National Office of Vital Statistics.

WEIGHT-HEIGHT-AGE TABLE FOR GIRLS BETWEEN SIX AND EIGHTEEN YEARS
(IN SCHOOLROOM CLOTHING, WITHOUT SHOES)*

Height in inches	AVERAGE WEIGHT IN POUNDS FOR EACH SPECIFIED AGE											
	6-7 years	7-8 years	8-9 years	9-10 years	10-11 years	11-12 years	12-13 years	13-14 years	14-15 years	15-16 years	16-17 years	17-18 years
38												
39												
40	36											
41	37											
42	39											
43	41	41										
44	42	42										
45	45	45	45									
46	47	48	48									
47	50	50	50	50								
48	52	52	52	53	53							
49	54	55	55	56	56							
50	56	57	58	59	61	62						
51	59	60	61	61	63	65						
52	63	64	64	64	65	67						
53	66	67	67	68	68	69	71					
54	—	69	70	70	71	71	73					
55	—	72	74	74	74	75	77	78				
56	—	—	76	78	78	79	81	83				
57	—	—	80	82	82	82	84	88	92			
58	—	—	—	84	86	86	88	93	96	101		
59	—	—	—	87	90	90	92	96	100	103	104	
60	—	—	—	91	95	95	97	101	105	108	109	111
61	—	—	—	—	99	100	101	105	108	112	113	116
62	—	—	—	—	104	105	106	109	113	115	117	118
63	—	—	—	—	—	110	110	112	116	117	119	120
64	—	—	—	—	—	114	115	117	119	120	122	123
65	—	—	—	—	—	118	120	121	122	123	125	126
66	—	—	—	—	—	—	124	124	125	128	129	130
67	—	—	—	—	—	—	128	130	131	133	133	135
68	—	—	—	—	—	—	131	133	135	136	138	138
69	—	—	—	—	—	—	—	135	137	138	140	142
70	—	—	—	—	—	—	—	136	138	140	142	144
71	—	—	—	—	—	—	—	138	140	142	144	145

*Bureau of Education, United States Department of the Interior.

WEIGHT-HEIGHT-AGE TABLE FOR BOYS BETWEEN SIX AND EIGHTEEN YEARS
(IN SCHOOLROOM CLOTHING, WITHOUT SHOES)*

Height in inches	AVERAGE WEIGHT IN POUNDS FOR EACH SPECIFIED AGE											
	6-7 years	7-8 years	8-9 years	9-10 years	10-11 years	11-12 years	12-13 years	13-14 years	14-15 years	15-16 years	16-17 years	17-18 years
41	38											
42	39	39										
43	41	41										
44	44	44										
45	46	46	46									
46	48	48	48									
47	50	50	50	50								
48	53	53	53	53								
49	55	55	55	55	55							
50	58	58	58	58	58	58						
51	61	61	61	61	61	61						
52	63	64	64	64	64	64	64					
53	66	67	67	67	67	68	68					
54	—	70	70	70	70	71	71	72				
55	—	72	72	73	73	74	74	74				
56	—	75	76	77	77	77	78	78	80			
57	—	—	79	80	81	81	82	83	83			
58	—	—	83	84	84	85	85	86	87			
59	—	—	—	87	88	89	89	90	90	90		
60	—	—	—	91	92	92	93	94	95	96		
61	—	—	—	—	95	96	97	99	100	103	106	
62	—	—	—	—	100	101	102	103	104	107	111	116
63	—	—	—	—	105	106	107	108	110	113	118	123
64	—	—	—	—	—	109	111	113	115	117	121	126
65	—	—	—	—	—	114	117	118	120	122	127	131
66	—	—	—	—	—	—	119	122	125	128	132	136
67	—	—	—	—	—	—	124	128	130	134	136	139
68	—	—	—	—	—	—	—	134	134	137	141	143
69	—	—	—	—	—	—	—	137	139	143	146	149
70	—	—	—	—	—	—	—	143	144	145	148	151
71	—	—	—	—	—	—	—	148	150	151	152	154
72	—	—	—	—	—	—	—	—	153	155	156	158
73	—	—	—	—	—	—	—	—	157	160	162	164
74	—	—	—	—	—	—	—	—	160	164	168	170

*Bureau of Education, United States Department of the Interior.

WEIGHT-HEIGHT-AGE TABLE FOR GIRLS BETWEEN ONE AND SIX YEARS OF AGE (WITHOUT CLOTHES)*

Height in inches	AVERAGE WEIGHT IN POUNDS FOR EACH SPECIFIED AGE						
	1 year but less than 1½	1½ years but less than 2	2 years but less than 2½	2½ years but less than 3	3 years but less than 4	4 years but less than 5	5 years but less than 6
25	14½						
26	16						
27	17	17½					
28	18½	18½	18½				
29	20	20	20				
30	21	21	21½	21½			
31	22½	22½	22½	22½	23		
32	23½	24	24	24	24		
33	25	25	25	25½	25½	25½	
34	26½	26½	26½	26½	26½	27	
35	27½	27½	28	28	28	28	
36	—	29	29	29	29½	29½	29½
37	—	30½	30½	30½	30½	31	31
38	—	—	31½	32	32	32	32½
39	—	—	33	33	33	33½	33½
40	—	—	—	34½	34½	34½	35
41	—	—	—	35½	36	36	36
42	—	—	—	—	37	37½	37½
43	—	—	—	—	38½	38½	39
44	—	—	—	—	40	40	40
45	—	—	—	—	—	41	41½
46	—	—	—	—	—	42½	42½
47	—	—	—	—	—	—	44
48	—	—	—	—	—	—	45½
49	—	—	—	—	—	—	46½

*From 'The Child from One to Six', Children's Bureau Publication No. 30.

WEIGHT-HEIGHT-AGE TABLE FOR BOYS BETWEEN ONE AND SIX YEARS OF AGE (WITHOUT CLOTHES)*

Height in inches	AVERAGE WEIGHT IN POUNDS FOR EACH SPECIFIED AGE						
	1 year but less than 1½	1½ years but less than 2	2 years but less than 2½	2½ years but less than 3	3 years but less than 4	4 years but less than 5	5 years but less than 6
25	15						
26	16½						
27	17½	18					
28	19	19					
29	20½	20½	20½				
30	21½	22	22	22			
31	23	23	23	23½			
32	24½	24½	24½	24½	25		
33	25	26	26	26	26		
34	27½	27	27	27½	27½	27½	
35	28½	28½	28½	28½	28½	29	
36	—	29½	30	30	30	30	30½
37	—	31	31	31½	31½	31½	32
38	—	32½	32½	32½	32½	33	33
39	—	—	34	34	34	34	34½
40	—	—	35	35	35½	35½	35½
41	—	—	—	36½	36½	37	37
42	—	—	—	38	38	38	38½
43	—	—	—	—	39½	39½	39½
44	—	—	—	—	40½	41	41
45	—	—	—	—	—	42	42½
46	—	—	—	—	—	43½	43½
47	—	—	—	—	—	45	45
48	—	—	—	—	—	—	46½
49	—	—	—	—	—	—	47½

*From 'The Child from One to Six', Children's Bureau Publication No. 30.

WEIGHT-HEIGHT-AGE TABLE FOR BOYS FROM BIRTH TO ONE YEAR
(WITHOUT CLOTHES)*

AVERAGE WEIGHT IN POUNDS FOR EACH MONTH OF AGE

Height in inches	Less than 1 month	1 month but less than 2	2 months but less than 3	3 months but less than 4	4 months but less than 5	5 months but less than 6	6 months but less than 7	7 months but less than 8	8 months but less than 9	9 months but less than 10	10 months but less than 11	11 months but less than 12
17	$5^1/_2$											
18	$6^1/_2$											
19	$7^1/_2$	$7^1/_2$										
20	8	$8^1/_2$	9									
21	9	$9^1/_2$	10	$10^1/_2$	$10^1/_2$							
22	10	$10^1/_2$	11	$11^1/_2$	$11^1/_2$	$11^1/_2$	12					
23	$10^1/_2$	$11^1/_2$	12	$12^1/_2$	13	13	13	$13^1/_2$				
24	$11^1/_2$	$12^1/_2$	13	$13^1/_2$	14	14	$14^1/_2$	$14^1/_2$	15	15	15	
25	$12^1/_2$	$13^1/_2$	14	$14^1/_2$	15	$15^1/_2$	$15^1/_2$	$15^1/_2$	16	16	16	$16^1/_2$
26	—	14	15	$15^1/_2$	16	$16^1/_2$	$16^1/_2$	17	17	17	$17^1/_2$	18
27	—	—	16	$16^1/_2$	17	$17^1/_2$	18	18	$18^1/_2$	$18^1/_2$	$18^1/_2$	19
28	—	—	—	$17^1/_2$	18	19	19	19	$19^1/_2$	$19^1/_2$	$19^1/_2$	20
29	—	—	—	—	$19^1/_2$	20	20	$20^1/_2$	$20^1/_2$	$20^1/_2$	$20^1/_2$	21
30	—	—	—	—	—	$21^1/_2$	$21^1/_2$	$21^1/_2$	$21^1/_2$	$21^1/_2$	22	22
31	—	—	—	—	—	—	$22^1/_2$	23	23	23	23	23
32	—	—	—	—	—	—	—	24	24	24	24	24
33	—	—	—	—	—	—	—	—	—	—	$25^1/_2$	25

*From 'Infant Care', Children's Bureau Publication No. 8.

WEIGHT-HEIGHT-AGE TABLE FOR GIRLS FROM BIRTH TO ONE YEAR
(WITHOUT CLOTHES)*

AVERAGE WEIGHT IN POUNDS FOR EACH MONTH OF AGE

Height in inches	Less than 1 month	1 month but less than 2	2 months but less than 3	3 months but less than 4	4 months but less than 5	5 months but less than 6	6 months but less than 7	7 months but less than 8	8 months but less than 9	9 months but less than 10	10 months but less than 11	11 months but less than 12
17	$5^1/_2$											
18	$6^1/_2$	$6^1/_2$										
19	7	$7^1/_2$	8									
20	8	$8^1/_2$	9	9								
21	$8^1/_2$	$9^1/_2$	$9^1/_2$	10	$10^1/_2$	11	11					
22	$9^1/_2$	10	$10^1/_2$	11	$11^1/_2$	12	12	12	$12^1/_2$			
23	10	11	$11^1/_2$	12	$12^1/_2$	13	13	13	$13^1/_2$	$13^1/_2$	$13^1/_2$	
24	11	12	$12^1/_2$	13	$13^1/_2$	14	14	14	$14^1/_2$	$14^1/_2$	$14^1/_2$	$14^1/_2$
25	$11^1/_2$	13	$13^1/_2$	14	$14^1/_2$	15	15	$15^1/_2$	$15^1/_2$	$15^1/_2$	16	16
26	—	14	$14^1/_2$	15	$15^1/_2$	16	16	$16^1/_2$	$16^1/_2$	$16^1/_2$	17	17
27	—	—	$15^1/_2$	16	$16^1/_2$	17	17	$17^1/_2$	$17^1/_2$	18	18	18
28	—	—	—	17	$17^1/_2$	18	$18^1/_2$	$18^1/_2$	19	19	19	19
29	—	—	—	—	19	19	$19^1/_2$	20	20	20	20	20
30	—	—	—	—	—	20	$20^1/_2$	21	21	21	21	$21^1/_2$
31	—	—	—	—	—	—	$21^1/_2$	22	22	22	$22^1/_2$	$22^1/_2$
32	—	—	—	—	—	—	—	—	23	$23^1/_2$	$23^1/_2$	$23^1/_2$
33	—	—	—	—	—	—	—	—	—	—	—	$24^1/_2$

*From 'Infant Care', Children's Bureau Publication No. 8.

DESIRABLE WEIGHTS FOR MEN OF AGE 25 AND OVER*
WEIGHT IN POUNDS ACCORDING TO FRAME (AS ORDINARILY DRESSED)

HEIGHT (with shoes on)		FRAME		
Feet	Inches	Small	Medium	Large
5	2	116-125	124-133	131-142
5	3	119-128	127-136	133-144
5	4	122-132	130-140	137-149
5	5	126-136	134-144	141-153
5	6	129-139	137-147	145-157
5	7	133-143	141-151	149-162
5	8	136-147	145-156	153-166
5	9	140-151	149-160	157-170
5	10	144-155	153-164	161-175
5	11	148-159	157-168	165-180
6	0	152-164	161-173	169-185
6	1	157-169	166-178	174-190
6	2	163-175	171-184	179-196
6	3	168-180	176-189	184-202

DESIRABLE WEIGHTS FOR WOMEN OF AGE 25 AND OVER*

HEIGHT (with shoes on)		FRAME		
Feet	Inches	Small	Medium	Large
4	11	104-111	110-118	117-127
5	0	105-113	112-120	119-129
5	1	107-115	114-122	121-131
5	2	110-118	117-125	124-135
5	3	113-121	120-128	127-138
5	4	116-125	124-132	131-142
5	5	119-128	127-135	133-145
5	6	123-132	130-140	138-150
5	7	126-136	134-144	142-154
5	8	129-139	137-147	145-158
5	9	133-143	141-151	149-162
5	10	136-147	145-155	152-166
5	11	139-150	148-158	155-169

*These tables reproduced by courtesy of Metropolitan Life Insurance Co.

INDEX AND GLOSSARY

NAME INDEX

Page numbers in *italics* refer to illustrations and charts.

SUBJECT INDEX AND GLOSSARY

This subject index and glossary have been compiled to include general definitions which are likely to prove of value for quick reference. Uncommon and rarely used terms which require lengthy definitions are indexed only. Self-evident terms with which most people are familiar usually are not defined, but are indexed. The contexts of all indexed terms are clearly shown with extensive subheads. Page numbers in *italics* refer to illustrations and charts.

mone. A secretion from the pituitary gland which acts upon the adrenal gland to cause production of cortisone. 358, 359.

adrenal gland overactivity and, 360

allergy and, 241

rheumatoid arthritis and, 305

Actinomyces. A genus of vegetable parasites; also called *ray fungus.*

Actinomyces bovis, *244*

actinomycosis. A disease caused by the fungus *Actinomyces bovis,* affecting cattle, hogs, and sometimes human beings; called "lumpy-jaw" in cattle because of the characteristic pus-producing tumors in the jaw.

chronic osteomyelitis and, 311

dermatitis and, 244

lung fungus diseases and, 170

mouth disorders and, 444

action

idea to, *99*

active immunity, 101

viruses and, 107

actuarial tables, *893*

acute (adjective). 1. Having a rapid onset, severe symptoms, and a relatively short duration; not chronic. 2. Sharp or severe.

active pulmonary tuberculosis, 163

bacterial endocarditis, 217

bronchitis, 149ff

catarrhal conjunctivitis, 561

diarrhea, 464ff

draining middle ear infection, 586

frontal sinusitis, 142

glaucoma, 567

laryngitis, 146

leukemia, 185

mastoiditis, 586

maxillary sinusitis, 142

miliary tuberculosis, 162ff

myringitis, 584

necrotizing gingivitis, 433

otitis media, 160

pharyngitis, 144

pneumococcal endocarditis, 160

prostatitis, 507

puerperal mastitis, 548

sinusitis, 142

small intestine inflammation, 459

sphenoid sinusitis, 142ff

suppurative otitis media, 586

vesiculitis, 508

Adam and Eve, *541*

Adams-Stokes attack, 226

Addison's disease. A disease caused by malfunction of the adrenal glands. It is characterized by a bronze color of the skin, prostration, anemia, disturbance of electrolyte metabolism, and diarrhea. 360

adenine, 3

adenoids, 77ff

adenoma. A benign epithelial tumor, glandlike in structure.

adenosis. Any disease of a gland, or glands.

breast, 548

adenovirus

pneumonia and, 157

adherent pericarditis, 225

adhesion. Abnormal union of tissues or organs; a sticking together.

adipocere. The waxy substance formed during decomposition of animal bodies, occurring especially in human bodies buried in moist places. 775

adipose capsule, 545

adiposogenital syndrome, 332

adolescence. The period of youth extending from the beginning of· puberty to adulthood.

breast and, 546

carbohydrates and, 670

menstrual periods and, 516

mind and, 603ff

physical development during, 529

adolescent idiopathic scoliosis, 315

adolescent peer culture, 69ff

adontia, 425

adoption

medicolegal aspects of, 789ff

adrenal cortex

hormones of, 358ff

adrenal cortical hormones, 358ff

aldosterone, 359

hydrocortisone, 359

adrenal disorders

Addison's disease, 360

adrenal gland, *suprarenal gland.* One of the paired glands of internal secretion located over each kidney; elaborates and secretes adrenalin and other hormones. *358*

Addison's disease and, 360

adrenalin and, 94

allergy and, 234

kidneys and, 482

rheumatoid arthritis and, 305

adrenal hormones, 358

adrenal overactivity, 360ff

adrenalin. The trade name for *epinephrine,* a hormone produced by the suprarenal glands. It acts to constrict blood vessels, control bleeding, and raise blood pressure. 94, 358

diarrhea and, 465

nervous system and, 329

overproduction, 360ff

adrenocorticotrophic hormone see ACTH

adrenogenital syndrome. A group of symptoms which is regarded as clinical evidence of overactivity of the adrenal cortex. 360

adult diabetes mellitus, 366

adult flies

fly control and, 758

adult myxedema, 345

adult teeth, 421

Aedes aegypti. The species of mosquito which transmits yellow fever and dengue. 112ff, 743, 749

control of, 758ff

life cycle of, 761

aerobic (adjective). Requiring atmospheric oxygen to live. See also **bacteria.** 116

aero-otitis media. Traumatic inflammation of the middle ear, caused by variation of the pressure of air in the tympanic cavity and the surrounding atmosphere. 584

first aid for, 698

aerosol. A type of spray in which liquid or powdered material is placed under gas pressure in a "bomb" apparatus, fitted with a nozzle for releasing the spray substance. 160

aerospace craft

family tree of, *883*

African sleeping sickness, 390, 748

Flagellata and, 121

trypanosomes and, 121

tsetse fly and, 121

African trypanosomiasis, 390

afterpains

postbirth uterine changes and, 34

aged

food needs and, 671

aged, homes for

nonprofit, 651

proprietary, 651

public, 651

aged, increase in

problems of, 635

aged patient

home care and, 686

aggression

adolescent and, 66

aging

alcohol and, 637ff

arteriosclerosis and, 204

cancer and, 641

changes in, 636

clubs for, 649

committees on, 649

damaged heart and, 641

degenerative arthritis and, 300ff

dying patient and, 645

exercise and, 638

eye degeneration and, 569

family and, 646

fractures and, 641

health rules for, 636ff

homes for, 651

life span and, *638*

malnutrition and, 637

medicaid and, 651

medicare and, 649ff

mental disorders and, 645ff

mental health and, 645ff

nutritional requirements of, 670ff

obesity and, 637

older worker and, 646ff

physical disorders and, 640ff

physical rehabilitation and, 645

physiology of, 636

presbyopea and, 571
rest and, 639ff
retirement and, 646ff
sex and, 640
sleep and, 638ff
social facilities and, 648
social security and, 649
social welfare for, 648ff
stroke and, 641
surgical operations and, 640
tobacco and, 637ff
work and, 646ff
aging population
problems of, 635
agitation
anxiety reaction and, 607
agranulocytosis. An acute disease marked by an increase in agranulocytes (nongranule-containing leucocytes). 191
agriculture
occupational accidents in, 732
AHF (antihemophilic factor), 184
air
combustion and, 126
composition of, 126
respiratory system and, 126
aircraft
family tree of, *883*
air embolus, 174
air-lock incubator, *40*
air pollution, 754
airsickness, 589, 697
albinism. Congenital or hereditary absence of pigment from the skin and eyes. 257ff
albino. An individual affected with albinism or absence of skin pigment. *257*
pedigree of, *257*
Albright's syndrome
sexual precocity and, 353
albumen. A protein substance soluble in water or dilute salt solution and coagulable by heat, such as egg white.
albumin. A protein substance composing the major portion of many tissues.
kidney stones and, 486
albuminuria. The presence of albumin in the urine. 488
Bright's disease and, 488
alchemistry
pharmacists and, 833
alcohol
aging and, 637ff
drug abuse and, 619
germicides and, 770
sexual intercourse and, 539
alcohol blood levels, 789
alcohol intoxication tests
criminology and, 788ff
alcoholic
personality disorders and, 619
alcoholism. 1. An acute toxic condition resulting from excessive alcohol in the system. 2. Compulsive or chronic consumption of alcohol.
beri beri and, 660
deaths from, *619*

aldosterone, 359
aldosteronism, 359
Aldobrandini Marriage, *525*
Alexandria rat, 766
alimentary canal, 439ff
mouth and, 86
stomach and, 86
alkylating agents
cancer and, 643
all clear
Civil Defense and, 856
allantois. A blind sac in the intestine of the embryo, which later forms the bladder and the umbilical cord and placenta.
allele. One of paired genes having corresponding locations in like chromosomes.
dominant, 4
gene locus and, 4
heredity and, 5
recessive, 4
allergenic (adjective). Pertaining to the production of allergy.
allergens
antigens and, 234
chemical, 238ff
allergist. A physician who specializes in the diagnosis and treatment of patients with allergies.
allergy. A reaction to a specific substance in an individual who is sensitive to that substance.
ACTH and, 333
European olive tree and, *235*
hay fever and, 132
headache and, 406
migraine headaches and, 409ff
skin, 233ff
hand, *265*
alopecia. Loss of hair, baldness. Loss may be partial or total, congenital, premature, or senile.
alopecia areata, *277*
alopecia congenitalis. A congenital form of baldness in which there is partial or complete absence of hair follicles. Also called *hypotrichosis.*
alphabet
one-hand, *593*
two-hand, *591*
alpha cells
islets of Langerhans and, 364
alpha rays, 841
alum. Alumen, which may be ammonium or potassium alum, occurring as colorless, odorless crystals, soluble in water; used as an emetic and astringent, and also as a coagulant in water purification plants.
aluminum. A metallic element of light weight (Symbol, Al).
artificial limbs and, 317
alveolar bone. Bony process of the upper and lower jaw.
teeth and, 419
alveoli
respiration and, 90ff

alveolus (plural, alveoli). 1. An air cell of the lung. 2. A cavity or depression. 3. Bony socket of a tooth.
lactiferous duct and, 545
periodontal membrane and, 419
AMA
medical organizations and, 825
amalgam. In dentistry, an alloy of mercury in combination with silver which is used for filling teeth.
amastia. Absence of breasts. 548
Amblyomma americanum, 114
amblyopia
strabismus and, 568
treatment for, 568
ambulance service
atomic warfare and, 865
ameba (plural, amebae). A single-celled animal belonging to the class Sarcodina, some of which are pathogenic.
button-hole ulcer and, 468
disease and, 120
Sarcodina and, 120
amebic dysentery, 120
food-borne infections and, 756
intestinal parasites and, 468
amelanotic nevus (plural, nevi). Nonpigmented mole. 254
amenorrhea. Absence of menstruation. 356
American Annals for the Deaf, 592
American College of Surgeons
hospital accreditation and, 828
American Public Health Association
state health departments and, 836
American Red Cross, 690
American trypanosomiasis, 748
amino acid. An organic acid; one of the main intermediary products of protein metabolism; from amino acids the body resynthesizes its proteins. 85, 655
digestion of, 443
essential, 655
milk and, 670
villi and, 443
amino acid sequencing, 8
Amish
dwarfism and, 335
amnesia
brain injury and, 415
dissociative reaction and, 609
amniocentesis, 16
amnion. A thin, transparent sac, usually filled with fluid in which the fetus is suspended until birth. 11
rupture and labor, 24
amniotic cavity, 11
amphetamines
drug abuse and, 618
ampulla
lactiferous duct and, 545
amputations, 316ff
bone cancer and, 314
complications of, 316ff
cosmetic gloves and, *322*

ment of microorganisms without necessarily destroying them. 769ff
bacteria and, 116
antiseptic surgery, *808*
antisocial psychopath, 615
antitoxin. 1. A substance made and elaborated in the body to neutralize a specific bacterial, plant, or animal toxin. 2. One of the class of specific antibodies.
bacterial, 120
tetanus and, 389
antivenom. An antitoxic serum used to counteract the action of snake bites. 721
anvil
middle ear and, 581
ANTU. Alpha-naphylthiourea, a rodenticide, used in destruction of rodents which transmit endemic typhus, Weil's disease, and bubonic plague. 768
anuria. Suppresion of urine formation by the kidneys. 496
anus. The terminal portion of the rectum, which forms an external opening.
anxiety
indigestion and, 451
anxiety reaction. A type of neurosis in which there is some degree of depression accompanied by worry, apprehension, and agitation; generalized dread often accompanied by somatic symptoms. 606, 607
aorta. The largest artery in the body. It receives all of the blood from the heart before it is circulated throughout the body.
aneurysm of, 210
arteriosclerosis and, 204
bacterial endocarditis and, 218
blood pressure and, 201
blue babies and, 223
coarctation of, 225
congenital anomalies of, 224
stenosis of, 224
valve, 197
aphasia. Loss of the ability to use words as symbols of ideas. 597
brain tumor and, 410
aphthous stomatitis
mouth disorders and, 444
aplastic anemia, 182
apocrine (adjective). Pertaining to a type of sebaceous gland or its secretion, in which part of the secreting gland is pinched off, the remaining cells losing part of their cytoplasm while functioning for the entire gland. 233
appendicitis. Inflammation of the vermiform appendix. 460
abdominal pain and, 697
deaths from, *461*
signs of, 460
appendicular support
skeleton and, 282

appendix removal, 461
appendix, vermiform. A small blind sac extending as an outpouching of the cecum. *460*
appetite. Complex reaction consisting of a craving for food, which is developed by past enjoyment of savory food.
child and, 53ff
apples
arteriosclerosis and, 205
pectin and, 205
APRL hook, *323*
aqueous humor, 559
Arachnida. A large class of arthropods which includes scorpions, spiders, mites, and ticks. The adult organism usually lacks wings and antennae, and has four pairs of legs. 765
arachnoid. Delicate, cobweb-like middle layer of the three tissues covering the brain and spinal cord. 390
meningitis and, 390
arched fingerprint, 777
area baldness, 277
areola. The darkened circular area about the nipple of the breast. 544
argasidae. A family of Ixodidae to which the hard ticks belong. 766
argonin. The trade name for silver caseinate, a compound insoluble in cold water but soluble in hot water.
disinfectants and, 770
argyrol. A silver oxide compound containing protein, used as a nonirritating antiseptic in infection of the mucous membranes. 770
arm
artificial replacements for, 319
humerus of, 285
radius of, 285
ulna of, 285
arm fracture
first aid for, 709
arrhythmia, 226
coronary thrombosis and, 217
pacemaker and, 226
arsenic. A toxic chemical element, compounds of which are sometimes used in medicine in small amounts (Symbol, As).
arsenical keratosis
precancerous skin and, 267
arsphenamine, 519
arterial circulation, *201*
arterial grafts, *228*
arterial spasm, 396ff
arteriolar nephrosclerosis
Bright's disease and, 488
arteriography. Roentgenography of the arteries after the injection of an opaque dye.
brain tumor and, 410
arteriole. One of the small arteries connecting the larger arteries with the capillaries.

arteriosclerosis, 203
aging and, 204
aneurysm and, 210
arterioles and, 203
diabetes mellitus and, 368
hardening of the arteries or, 203ff
signs of, 204
stroke and, 396
symptoms of, 204
artery. One of the blood vessels which transport the aerated blood from the heart to the various organs and tissues of the body. 199, *201*
circulatory system and, 87
contraction of, 199
transplantation of, *227ff*
arteriovenous communications
aneurysm and, 210
arthritis. Inflammation of the joints. 300ff
degenerative, 300ff
food requirements and, 670
rheumatoid, *306*
signs of, 301ff
traumatic, 301
treatment for, 302ff
arthropods
viruses and, 111
artificial atmosphere
space medicine and, 877ff
artificial corneas, 565
artificial hands
types of, 319
artificial heart, 227, 818
artificial insemination. Introduction of semen into the vagina by means of surgical instruments.
medicolegal problems of, 793
sterility and, 535
artificial joints
rheumatoid arthritis and, 306
artificial kidney, 489ff
artificial larynx, 149
laryngectomy and, 149
artificial lung
heart-lung bypass machine and, 225
artificial organs
artificial heart and, 227
artificial replacements
arms, 319
body parts, 316ff
children and, 319ff
face, 321
immediate postoperative prostheses and, 318
legs, 318
materials in, 317ff
myo-electric arms and, 319
artificial respiration, 722ff, *inside back cover*
manual methods of, 726ff
respiratory failure and, 132
nondrowning needs for, 723
Ascaris. Nematode worms belonging to the family Ascaridae; commonly infesting the intestinal tract of man. 123
life cycle of, 123
ascending colon
large intestine and, 438
ascites. An abnormal accumulation of fluid in the ab-

dominal cavity. 481
diuretics and, 481
portal cirrhosis and, 477
ascorbic acid, 662ff
aseptic (adjective). Free of infectious material.
precautions, 194
asphyxia. Suffocation; unconsciousness resulting from deprivation of oxygen.
artificial respiration and, 723
aspiration pneumonia, 158
aspirin
rheumatic fever and, 221
asthma. An affection of the upper respiratory tract characterized by dyspnea, coughing, wheezing, and pain in the chest. 139ff
allergy and, 235
diagnosis of, 139ff
long-term therapy for, 140
psychosomatic disorders and, 613
symptoms of, 139ff
therapy during an attack of, 140ff
astigmatism. A form of defective vision in which there is distortion of the visual image. The distortion may be vertical, horizontal, or compound, and is caused by a deviation in the curvature of the lens or cornea. 571
atabrine. A quinine substitute used for therapy and prophylaxis in malaria; quinacrine hydrochloride. 739
A. T. 10. Antitetanic substance 10. A synthetic preparation of dihydrotachysterol, used to counteract parathyroid tetany, by increasing the calcium content of the blood. 349
ataxia
cerebral palsy and, 395
atelectasis. A collapsed or airless state of the lungs, caused by occlusion of the small bronchial tubes or a bronchus.
pneumonia and, 159
pulmonary, 174ff
athetosis. A series of constantly recurring involuntary motions, especially of the hands, that are slow and wormlike in nature, resulting usually from a brain lesion. 394
athlete's foot. A skin disease occurring usually between the toes, caused by a variety of fungi. 264ff
dermatitis and, 244, *265*
hand allergy and, *265*
intertriginous, 264
squamous-hyperkeratotic, 264
treatment for, 265ff
types of, 264
atmosphere
space medicine and, 877
atmospheric zones, *878*
atom. The smallest unit of an element that can take part

in a chemical reaction and retain its identity, and which cannot be further divided without changing its structure. 840
atomic blast injuries
first aid for, 848
atomic bomb
lethal effects of 20 megaton, *846*
atomic bomb shelter
basement concrete block, *859*
basement lean-to, *858*
below-ground corrugated steel culvert, *861*
atomic energy
principles of, 839
Atomic Energy Commission
radioactive isotopes and, 867
atomic explosions
effects of, 729
heat effects of, *846*
injury prevention during, 730
injury treatment after, 730
atomic pile. An arrangement of highly radioactive elements in graphite blocks or other apparatus; elements placed in such apparatus are radioactivated thereby.
atomic radiation measurement
dosimeter and, *845*
atomic structure, 840ff
radioactivity and, 841ff
atomic warfare
casualties of, 847ff
civil defense for, 854
first aid in, 864
population evacuation and, 856ff
recovery from attack, 864ff
atomic warfare casualties
blast injuries and, 848
burns, 848ff
radiation injury and, 850
radiation injury in Japan, 850
radiation sickness, 852ff
atomic warfare recovery
casualty evacuation, 864ff
first aid, 864
home fire fighting, 865ff
radiological decontamination, 866ff
atomic weapons, 839
employment of, 845ff
medical aspects of, 839
atomic weight, 840
ATP
shock and, 699
atrial-septal defect, 224
atrial-ventricular defect, 224
atrophic chronic pharyngitis, 144
atrophic pyelonephritis, 487
atrophic rhinitis, 145
atrophy. Physiologic or pathologic reduction in size of a mature cell or organ; usually with some degree of degeneration.
Fröhlich's syndrome and, 336
pituitary, 336
atropine. A drug which causes paralysis of response to stimulation of nerves of the parasympathetic system. Used internally in bronchial

asthma, intestinal and biliary colic; topically it is used extensively in ophthalmology for dilating the pupil and in various eye conditions.
peptic ulcer and, 454
salivary glands and, 445
attenuated oral vaccine
poliomyelitis and, 384
atypical facial neuralgia, 403ff
atypical neuralgia, 403
atypical pneumonia
mycoplasmas and, 115
auditory (adjective). Pertaining to the sense of hearing.
auditory canal, 581
auditory nerve. A part of the eighth cranial nerve; it is a sensory nerve composed of two kinds of fibers; the cochlear nerves of hearing, and the vestibular nerves of the equilibrium. 583
auditory vesicle. One of the expansions of the neural embryonic canal from which the external ears are developed. 13.
aura. Peculiar sensations or unusual perceptions that precede an epileptic seizure.
migraine headache and, 408ff
aureomycin. An antibiotic substance derived from the mold, *Streptomyces aureofaciens.*
auricle. 1. Either of the two smaller and upper chambers of the heart. The auricles receive the blood from the veins and empty it into the ventricles. 2. The external ear. 581
heart and, 196
hematoma of, 589
auriculoventricular (adjective). Pertaining to both the auricle and ventricle, or the junction between them.
node, 197
authority
childhood behavior problems and, 62
autoantibodies, 192
autografts, 279
autoimmune diseases
blood disorders, 192
multiple sclerosis and, 412
nervous system disorders, 412
rheumatoid arthritis, 303
automatism. Automatic actions or behavior without conscious purpose or awareness.
coma and, 414
automobile accidents
broken neck and, 295
deaths from, *733*
autonomic (adjective). Pertaining to automatic or unconscious activity.
autonomic nervous system, 94
environmental influences, 94
peripheral nerves and, 380
psychosomatic disorders and, 611

autopsy. Examination of organs of the body after death; a postmortem examination. 774
  history of, 773
  legal permission for, 773ff
  medicolegal identification and, 774
autosome. Any chromosome as distinguished from the sex chromosome. 3
axial support
  skeleton and, 282
axillary line
  fractured ribs and, 171
axon. 1. The body axis. 2. A thread-like process given off of a nerve cell body. 382

baby
  childhood behavior problems and, 64
Babylonia
  medical history of, 796ff
bacillus (plural, bacilli). A group of rod-shaped bacteria. 115
Bacillus anthracis, *248*
back-pressure, arm-lift artificial respiration, *726*
backrest, 677
  how to make, *676*
bacteremia. Presence of bacteria in the blood stream. 182
bacteria (singular, bacterium). One-celled vegetable microorganisms. 115ff
  aerobic, 116
  anaerobic, 116
  bacillus, 115
  cocci, 115
  common types of, *116*
  dermatitis and, 243ff
  destruction of, 116ff
  digestion and, 87, 442
  Diplococcus, 115
  facultative anaerobes, 116
  flagella and, 115
  Micrococcus, 115
  pathogenic, 116
  rickettsial diseases and, 113ff
  Sarcina, 115
  spirochetes, 115
  Spirillum, 115
  spores and, 115
  Staphylococcus, 115
  Streptococcus, 115
  types of, 115ff, *117*
  usefulness of, 115
  Vibrio, 115
  white cells and, 177
bacterial diseases
  bacterial endocarditis, 217ff
  blepharitis, 562
  chlamydia and, 114
  diphtheria, 76ff
  laryngitis and, 146
  mycoplasmas and, 114ff
  onychia, 274
  Oroya fever, 747
  paronychia and, 274
  pneumonia, 157
  pyorrhea, 432
  rickettsial, 113ff
  symptoms of, 118
  table of, *118*
  tetanus, 388

  transmission of, 118ff
  tropical diseases and, 747ff
  Weil's disease and, 747
  whooping cough, 76
  yaws, 737
bacterial embolus
  hemorrhagic bronchopneumonia and, 218
  mycotic aneurysm and, 218
  nephritis and, 218
bacterial endoarteritis, 217
bacterial endocarditis, 217ff
  prevention of, 219
  signs of, 217ff
  symptoms of, 217ff
  treatment for, 218ff
bacterial infection
  bladder, 491ff
  endocardium, 217
  nephritis and, 487ff
bacterial pneumonia, 157
  treatment for, 160
bactericide, 769
bacteriological blood tests, 195
bacteriology. The science and study of bacteria. 823
bacteriophage. An ultramicroscopic virus which destroys bacteria.
bacteriostasis. Prevention of bacterial growth. 116
Baker Day
  aftercloud of, *840*
  plume of, *841*
balance
  semicircular canals and, 99, 583
Balantidium. A genus of ciliated, parasitic protozoans.
  dysentery and, 121, 468
baldness
  disease and, 277
  heredity and, 276ff
  pedigree of, *277*
  sex-influenced heredity and, 6
  skin disorders and, 276ff
  symptomatic, 277ff
ballistocardiography. A method of recording body movements resulting from the impact and recoil of the blood after ejection from the ventricles; it is used to estimate cardiac output.
bamboo spine, 305
bandages, *708*
  burn, *714ff*
barber's itch, 245ff
barbiturates
  drug abuse and, 618
  hypersensitivity to, *236*
bargaining
  dying and, 645
barium carbonate. A heavy odorless, tasteless compound which is poisonous to rats and, in larger doses, lethal to dogs, cats, and larger animals. 767
bars and handrails
  paralytics and, *400*
Bartholin's gland. One of a pair of major vestibular glands in the vagina. 504
Bartonella bacilliformis. The bacterium that causes Oroya fever. 747

basal cell. One of the cells forming the deepest layer of the epithelium.
  carcinoma. *270, 271*
basal ganglia. Collections of nerve cells located deep within the brain substance.
  cerebral palsy and, 394
basal metabolic rate. The amount of energy expended per unit of time under basal conditions (the basic body processes such as respiration, circulation, etc., of an individual completely at rest). The basal rate is usually expressed as large calories per square meter of body surface (or kilograms of body weight) per hour. 333, 339ff
basal metabolism test, *340*
basement concrete block shelter, *859*
basement lean-to shelter, *860*
bathing
  home care and, 678
  infants and, 48
  pregnancy and, 21
bathing trunk nevus, 254
battered children
  first aid for, 712
battered child syndrome
  medicolegal problems of, 794
Bayer 7602. A compound used in therapy of patients in the early stages of trypanosomiasis.
BCG (Bacillus Calmette Guerin), 165
beautiful indifference
  conversion reaction and, 610ff
Becker Hand, *323*
bed
  home care and, 676ff
  how to make occupied, *682ff*
bedbug. A common domestic parasite; a bloodsucking insect of genus *Cimex,* not pathogenic. *250*
  control of, 763
  dermatitis and, 250
Bedlam, *612*
bed making
  home care and, 682ff
bedpan
  bedrest equipment and, 677
bedrest equipment
  home care and, 677
bed rest
  hypertension and, 213
  preparation for, 673ff
bed wetting, 63
  urination disturbances and, 496ff
behavior problems
  brain injury and, 63
  childhood and, 60ff
  correction of, 64ff
  dominance-submission and, 61ff
  dyslexia and, 63
  emotional factors and, 60ff
  environment and, 62
  expression of, 63ff
  mental retardation and, 62ff
  physical causes of, 62
BEI test, 340

belching
speech class and, *150*
below-ground corrugated steel culvert shelter, 862
benadryl. An antihistaminic drug used in various allergic conditions such as contact dermatitis, erythema, rhinitis, drug sensitization, hay fever, serum reactions, urticaria, some forms of dysmenorrhea, and irradiation sickness.
motion sickness and, 697
bends, 734
benign (adjective). Not malignant; favorable for recovery.
benign blood disorders
agranulocytosis, 191
infectious mononucleosis, 190ff
benign breast disorders, 548ff
abnormal nipple conditions, 550
breast injuries, 550
fat necrosis, 549
hypertrophy, 549
skin eruption, 549
benign bronchial tumors, 151ff, 175ff
benign lymph disorders, 190ff
benign skin tumors, 253
precancerous skin and, 268ff
benign tertian malaria, 738
benign tumor, 641
sinus, 143
skin, 253
benzene. A clear, volatile, inflammable organic solvent.
benzene hexachloride. An isomer of hexachlorocyclohexane, used extensively as an insecticide and fumigant. The drug is important in the control of chiggers, ticks, fleas, cockroaches, lice, and *Acarus scabiei.* Also called *gammexane.* 762
benzidine test. A test used to determine the presence of blood in which benzidine and hydrogen peroxide are added to 1 cc. of the unknown material. A blue color indicates the presence of blood in the specimen being tested. 775
benzyl benzoate. A parasiticide, used topically in scabies and for eradication of head lice; also used as an antispasmodic in spasms of smooth muscles, particularly the uterine muscle. 745
beri beri. A disease resulting from the absence of adequate amounts of vitamin B_1 or thiamin in the diet. 660, 747
Berlin Medical Papyrus
medical history and, 797
bermuda grass, *136*
Bertillon system. The system of recorded physical measurements and descriptions of criminals used for future identification, originated by

Alphonse Bertillon in 1879. 778
beta cells, 364
beta rays
radioactive iodine and, 341
Bettinger Hand, *323*
bezoar. A concretion in the gastrointestinal tract caused by the ingestion of hair or other indigestible materials, such as those with high cellulose content. 458
bifocal glasses, 572
Bikini atomic test
cloud chamber effect, *843*
bilateral pneumonia, 156
bile. A bitter alkaline fluid secreted by the liver into the duodenum, which aids in the digestion of food. 441
gallstones and, 441, 478
hepatic ducts and, 441
jaundice and, 476
liver and, 441
stomach and, 438
vitamin A deficiency and, 659
bile ducts
gallbladder and, 441
bile pigments, 441
bile salts, 441
bilharziasis. Infestation with blood flukes of the genus *Schistosoma;* also called schistosomiasis. 492
biliary cirrhosis, 477
biliary colic
gallstones and, 478
binocular (adjective). Pertaining to both eyes.
binocular vision
strabismus and, 568
bioastronautics
space medicine and, 877
biochemical brain disorders, 412ff
biochemistry of thought, 634
biodynamics of space flight, 878
bioelectric currents
electrocardiograph and, 197
biological chemistry, 823
biological clock
pineal gland and, 363
biological regeneration
air requirements in space and, 881
biological warfare
first aid during, 729
biology
radioactive isotopes and, 867ff
biophysics. The science and study of the physical changes involved in life processes.
biopsy. Removal and microscopic examination of a portion of living tissue to establish a diagnosis.
breast cancer and, 553
skin cancer and, 269
birds
ornithosis and, 159
birth, 11, 24ff
cesarean section and, *33*
delivery and, *29*
episiotomy and, *28*
forceps and, *28*
head rotations and, *29*

labor and, 25ff
placenta and, *31*
preparation for, 24
progress of labor and, 25
recording of, 795
second stage of, *27*
seventeenth century Dutch, *528*
umbilical cord and, *30*
birth-cry, 44
birth control
marriage and, 535ff
sex and, 535ff
birth rates, *885*
bisexual dispositions, 538
black bile
adrenals and, 358
black eye
ecchymosis and, 569
blackheads, 258ff
black tongue
niacin deficiencies and, 661
blackwater fever. A complication of one type of malaria; characterized by chills, fever, jaundice, and dark urine. 739
black widow spider, 703ff
dermatitis and, 251
bladder, 485
hourglass, *493*
urine and, 484ff
bladder control, 53
bladder disorders, 491ff
developmental abnormalities, 491
fistulae, 491
hernia, 491
inflammations, 491ff
tumors, 493
bladder inflammation
flatworms and, *492*
bladder tumors, 493
blanket drag
short-distance transfer and, 694
blast effects
atomic bomb explosion and, 846
blast injuries
atomic warfare casualties and, 848
blastodisc. The primitive inner germ layer from which the primary germ layers develop. 11
Blastomyces, *244*
blastomycosis and, 170
blastomycosis. A disease, usually occurring in the lungs, in the skin, or systematically, caused by the fungus *Blastomyces.* 170
blast waves
atomic explosions and, 729
bleeding
do nots, 701
dos, 701ff
first aid for, 691
first aid for severe, 701
blepharitis
eyelids and, 562
blind
care for, 574ff
care for the newly, 575ff
education for, 576
legal benefits for, 577ff

multiple handicapped and,
578ff
opportunities for, 574ff
schools for, 576ff
blind education, *579ff*
blindness
causes of, 574
childhood behavior problems
and, 63
determination of, 574ff
blisters
allergy and, 236
blood. The fluid tissue which
circulates through the heart,
arteries, veins, and capillaries, carrying nourishment
and oxygen to the tissues
and taking away waste
products and carbon di-
oxide. It is composed of
plasma and cellular ele-
ments. 87ff
absorption and, 88
definition of, 177
hemoglobin and, 90ff
manufacture of, 178
storage of, 178
white cells, 177ff
blood cells, *185*
bone marrow and, *179*
leukemia and, *185*
blood changes
radiation injury and, 850
blood circulation
blue babies and, 223
pathway of, 196
blood clotting
fibrin and, 178
hemophilia and, 183
platelets and, 178
thromboplastin and, 178
blood components
blood transfusion and, 192ff
blood count
blood tests and, 195
blood disorders
agranulocytosis, 191
anemia, 179ff
autoimmune diseases, 192
benign, 190ff
benign lymph disorders and,
190ff
blood poisoning, 182ff
bone marrow deficiencies,
181ff
flukes and, 124ff
hemophilia, 183ff
hemorrhagic diseases, 184
Hodgkin's disease, 188ff
infectious mononucleosis, 190ff
Letterer-Siwe disease, 312
leukemia, 184ff
lymphosarcoma, 188ff
malignant, 188ff
multiple myeloma, 189ff
nutritional anemias, 180ff
posthemorrhagic anemias, 179
red cell overproduction, 189
reticuloendothelial system and,
191ff
schistosomes, 124ff
blood factors, 194
blood flow
nephron unit and, *484*
blood flukes, 124ff
life cycle of, 125
symptoms of, 125

blood groups
inheritance of, *194*
blood letting, *192, 194*
blood loss
menstruation and, 355
blood plasma, 178
blood poisoning, 182ff
causative agents of, 182ff
prevention of, 183
signs of, 183
symptoms of, 183
treatment for, 183
wound and, 701
blood pressure. The force exerted against the walls of
the blood vessels by the circulating blood. 199ff
high, 211ff
low, 211ff
manometer and, 199ff
normal, 212
sphygmograph and, 787
vasoconstrictors and, 201
vasodilators and, 201
blood storage
liver and, 201
blood sugar
diabetes mellitus and, 364
insulin shock and, 367
blood supply
shock and, 699
blood test. Examination made of
blood sample to determine
content and composition of
the blood as diagnostic aid.
194ff
alcohol intoxication and, 788
bacteriological, 195
chemical, 195
hematological, 195
immunological, 194ff
serological, 194ff
blood type. The classification
of blood depending upon
the agglutinogen in the red
cells and the agglutinins in
the serum. When different
bloods are mixed, as in
blood transfusion, if these
blood factors are incom-
patible, dissolution of the
cells (hemolysis)or clumping
(agglutination) will result.
Generally, the various blood
types are classified as O, A,
B, and AB. 193ff
blood identification and, 776
disputed parentage and, 776
kidney transplantation and,
490
negative identification and,
776
blood transfusion. Intravenous
administration of blood to
a patient. 192ff
animal, *194*
hemorrhage and, 179
blood vessels
bone and, 282
composition of, 198
tissue layers of, 198
bluegrass, *136*
blue babies. Babies born with
congenital cyanotic heart
disease. Surgery is the only
successful method of treatment. 223

tetralogy of Fallot and, 223
Blue Cross, 831
blue moles, 254
Blue Shield, 831
**Board of Registry of Medical
Technologists,** 831
body
cells and, 80ff
coordination of, 93
duplication of, 96ff
efficiency of, 102ff
environment and, 99ff
functioning of, 79ff
machine functioning of, 79ff
movement of, 97ff
smaller parts of, 80
body louse, *250*
body movement, *97*
boiling
water purification and, 750
boils
dermatitis and, 245
earache and, 584
bolus. A mass of masticated
food within the mouth or
alimentary canal. 438
bone. The hard, calcified tissue
which forms the major part
of the skeletal system of the
body. 280ff
blood vessels and, 282
body movement and, 97
eosinophilic granuloma and,
191
growth of, 280
infant and, 42
long, 281
nerves and, 282
periosteum and, 97
transverse cut of macerated,
82
bone calcium
parathyroids and, 348
bone cancer, 312ff
treatment for, 314
bone growth
vitamin D and, 663
bone hypertrophy
degenerative arthritis and, 301
bone inflammation
Letterer-Siwe disease, 312
rheumatoid spondylitis, 312
osteitis fibrosa, 311
osteochrondritis dissecans, 312
Paget's disease (osteitis deformans), 311ff
bone injuries
first aid for, 706ff
bone marrow, *178*
aplastic anemia and, 182
blood cells and, *179*
blood transfusion and, 193
deficiency diseases, 181ff
granulocytes and, 178
macrocytic anemia and, 181
Paget's disease and, 311
red blood cells and, 178
bone pain
chronic osteomyelitis, 311
skeletal disorders and, 310ff
bone tumor, *313*
lower femur, *313*
upper femur, *313*
bony labyrinth, *582*
internal ear and, 583
borax. *Sodium borate,* a colorless, odorless preparation,

occurring either in crystal or powder form.
housefly breeding and, 758
boric acid. A water-soluble substance used externally as a mild antiseptic. It is extremely poisonous if taken internally.
cockroach control and, 765
Borrelia recurrentis
relapsing fever and, 747
botulin
botulism and, 755
botulism. A type of food poisoning caused by eating foods contaminated with toxin produced by the bacterium *Clostridium botulinum*. 457, 755
bowel, 438ff
bowel musculature
constipation and, 466
boys
weight-height-age table and, *821*
brachydactyly. Abnormal shortness of the fingers or toes.
dominant inheritance and, 4
bradycardia, 226
Braille system. A system of printing or writing for the blind in which letters and characters are represented by raised dots or points which are discernible to the touch. Invented by Louis Braille, a French teacher of the blind, in 1829. 576
brain. The large, soft mass of nerve tissue contained within the cranium; the *encephalon*. It consists of four major parts; the *cerebrum, cerebellum, pons Varolli,* and *medulla oblongata*. The brain and spinal cord together constitute the *central nervous system*. 93, 377ff
cerebral cortex and, 94, 100
cross section of, *380*
description of, 377ff
electroencephalogram and, *393*
function of, 377ff
hypothalamus and, 336
lateral view of, *380*
organ differentiation, 13
sagittal section of, *380*
sensory perception and, 100
sleep and, 102
underside of, *380*
vocal communication and, 100
voluntary movement and, 100
brain disorders
biochemical, 412ff
brain tumors, 409ff
brain damage
whiplash and, 292
brain function
epilepsy and, 392
research on, 631ff
studies on, *631ff*
brain injury
artificial respiration and, 723
behavior problems and, 63
childhood and, 63
head injuries and, 413ff

brain lesions
encephalography and, 383
brain tumor
electroencephalogram and, *410*
headaches and, 406
nervous system disorders and, 409ff
brain tumor imaging
radionuclides and, 871
brassiere, 548
breakbone fever, 749
breast. The upper aspect of the chest; one of mammary glands. 544ff
development of, 66ff
development of female, *67ff*
estrogen and, 354
infant feeding and, 45
new mother and, 34ff
progesterone and, 354
breast cancer, 550ff
deaths from, *551*
diagnosis of, 553
male, 552
mammogram and, *553*
melphalan and, *554*
orange peel skin and advanced, *552*
Paget's disease of the nipple, 552
pregnancy and, 552
reconstruction for, 555
rehabilitation for, 555
retracted nipple and, *552*
self-examination for, *555ff*
symptoms of, 552
thermogram and, *553*
treatment for, 553ff
types of, 551ff
breast care
pregnancy and, 21
breast changes
pregnancy and, 18
breast disorders
benign, 548ff
cancer, 550ff
breastbone fracture, 171
breast hygiene
pregnancy and, 546
breast injuries, 550
breast sarcoma, *551*
breast shape
pregnancy and, *546*
breath analysis
alcohol intoxication and, 788
breathing
diaphragm and, 98
mechanism of, 127
muscles and, 98
breathing mechanism, *128*
breath stoppage
first aid for, 691
breech delivery, 31
bridge
dental restorations and, 433
Bright's disease, 488
broad ligament. A peritoneal layer of tissue which extends laterally from the uterus to the pelvic wall and contains blood vessels, lymphatics, and nerves, 502
broken bones
atomic warfare first aid and, 864

broken neck, 295
transportation and, *693*
broken ribs
x-ray appearance of, *173*
bromides
drug abuse and, 618
bronchi, 129
foreign bodies in, 705
lobar, 131
respiratory, 131
terminal, 131
bronchial disorders, 149ff
bronchial tumors
benign, 151ff
bronchiectasis. An inflammatory or degenerative condition of the bronchi and bronchioles in which the tubes are dilated; usually associated with abscess formation. 151, *152*
bronchiolitis
influenza and, 155
bronchitis
acute, 149ff
chronic, 151
bronchopneumonia. Pneumonic infection of the bronchi and bronchioles of one or both lungs; may result from many causative organisms. 157
bronchopulmonary segments, 131
bronchoscopic examination
benign bronchial growths and, 151
bronchoscopy. Internal visual examination of the bronchi by means of a tubelike instrument, the bronchoscope, which contains a light; the bronchoscope is introduced into the mouth and passed through the throat into the bronchial tree.
lung cancer and, 167
bronchus (plural bronchi). One of the two main divisions of the trachea, which penetrate the lungs and terminate in the bronchioles.
brown recluse spider, 704
bruises
first aid for, 712
purpura and, 184
bubonic plague (*black death*). An acute, infectious bacterial disease characterized by enlargement of the lymphatic glands, severe toxic symptoms, and high mortality. Caused by the bacterium *Pasteurella pestis*, transmitted to man by the rat flea. 766
budding
fungi and, 121
Buerger's disease, 204
bullet wounds
brain injury and, 414
medicolegal aspects of, 781
respiratory disorders and, 171
bulbar poliomyelitis, 384
bulbo-spinal poliomyelitis, 384
bulbo-urethral gland. One of the two mucous glands situated

anterior to the prostate gland. 499

Bullis fever
Amblyomma americanum and, 114
rickettsial diseases and, 114
bullous keratopathy, 563
bundle of His, 197
burn. The tissue reaction or injury resulting from contact with heat, caustics, or electricity.
atomic warfare casualties and, 848ff
atomic warfare first aid and, 864
do nots, 714
dos, 714
esophageal, 450
first aid for, 712ff
first degree, 712, *713*
second degree, 712, *713*
shock and, 699
third degree, 712, *713*
ulcerated, *268*
burn bandages, *714ff*
burning clothing, 729
burping
colic and, 49
infant feeding and, 45
bursa. A small sac of connective tissue, usually interposed between joints, lined by synovial membrane and filled with fluid, which reduces friction.
burweed marsh elder, *135*
button-hole ulcer, 468

caffeine
drug abuse and, 618
caisson disease, 734
calcaneoscaphoid (adjective). Pertaining to the heel bone, *calcaneous,* and the *scaphoid* bone of the foot.
calcification
arteriosclerosis and, 203ff
calcitonin
thyroid and, 338
calcium. A silver-white metallic element; an important constituent of the mineral matter of bone. (Symbol, Ca).
endocrine-producing tumors and, 329
feedback mechanism for, 348ff
nutritional need for, *656*
osteitis fibrosa and, 348
parathyroids and, 348
tetany and, 348
thyrocalcitonin and, 348
vitamin D and, 663
calcium deficiencies, 656ff
calcium disodium edetate
lead poisoning and, 169
calcium salts
dentin and, 418
calculi (singular calculus). An abnormal concretion of bone or teeth composed of mineral salts. When such concretions occur within soft tissue they are commonly called "stones."
pyorrhea and, 432
urethra and, 494

Californium-252, *873*
callus. 1. An area of thickened skin. 2. New growth of bony tissue at the site of a fracture which has been reunited. 297
dermatitis and, 243
calorie. The amount of heat necessary to raise the temperature of one gram of water one degree centigrade. In dietetics and metabolic measurement, a unit 1000 times as large is used, designated *Calorie* (capitalized). 84
underweight and, 668
weight control and, 665
calyx (plural calyces). One of the cuplike divisions of the renal pelvis.
cambium. The inner, cellular layer of the periosteum of bone. 281
cancer. 1. A malignant tumor. 2. Cytologically, hyperplasia of epithelial or glandular cells with infiltration and destruction.
aging and, 641
anal, 472
bone, 312ff
breast, 550ff
cause of, 643
cell transformation and, 113
chemotherapy for, 643
crab and, *472*
deaths from, *642*
diagnosis of, 642ff
estrogen and, 505
gallbladder, 479
head and neck, *272*
larynx, 147ff
lung, 166ff
liver, 477ff
pancreas, 480ff
prostate, 508
radiotherapy for, 643
rectal, 471ff
sinus, 143
skin, 269ff
stomach, 455ff
surgical therapy for, 643
symptoms of, 642
testes, 506
tissue growth and, 83
treatment for, 643ff
viruses and, 113
cancer diagnosis, 813
Candida. A genus of yeastlike, disease-producing microorganisms. 122
canning
botulism and, 457
capillary. A small blood vessel connecting an artery with a vein.
circulatory system and, 87
endothelium and, 198
skin color and, 231
temperature regulation and, 201
capping
dental restoration and, 433
capsule
cortex and, 483
kidney corpuscle and, 483

capture
marriage by, 523
car
paralytics and, *400*
carbohydrate. Any of the organic substances containing carbon, hydrogen, and oxygen which are the chief sources of energy used by the body. Typical substances include sugars, starches, dextrins, and cellulose. 654
adolescent diet and, 670
combustion, 334
diabetes mellitus and, 370
weight control and, 666
carbon. A nonmetallic element, the characteristic constituent of organic compounds. It is found in all living organisms in various forms and occurs naturally as coal. (Symbol, C).
universal antidote and, 718
carbon dioxide. The chemical combination of carbon and oxygen. It is one of the major constituents of exhaled air and a product of combustion. (Symbol, CO_2). 91, 127
plasma and, 91
respiration rate and, 91
respiratory center and, 127
carbon-14
age determination and, 875ff
carbon monoxide. An odorless, poisonous gas resulting from the combustion of carbon compounds in the presence of insufficient oxygen. (Symbol, CO).
carbuncle. A hard, delineated, deeply rooted, painful, suppurative inflammation of the subcutaneous tissue; larger than a boil, having a flat surface and discharging pus from multiple points. 245
carcinogen. Cancer-inducing agent. 643
precancerous skin and, 267
carcinoma. A malignant tumor originating in epithelial tissue; *cancer.* 642
basal cell, *270,* 271
gastric, *452*
skin cancer and, 271
squamous cell, 271
metatypical, 271
cardiac catheterization
heart disease and, 203
cardiac massage
artificial respiration and, 723
heart failure and, 696
cardiac muscle fibers, *82*
cardiac sphincter. The muscle at the lower end of the esophagus at the entrance to the stomach.
cardiologist. A physician who specializes in diseases of the heart.
cardiospasm. Spasmodic contraction of the sphincter muscle

between the esophagus and the stomach. 450, 451

cardiovascular disorders
angina pectoris, 225ff
carditis, 225
congenital, 223ff

carditis. Inflammation of the heart. 225

caries. Decay of a bone or tooth; a progressive decalcification and proteolysis of the enamel and dentin. See also **cavity.**
fluoride deficiencies and, 657

carotene. Any of the oily yellow to red pigments from plants that may be converted by the body to vitamin A. 658.
myxedema and, 346
skin color and, 231

carotenemia. Presence of carotene in the blood; when excessive, it may cause yellow pigmentation of the skin. 231.

carotenoid. A plant and animal substance that closely resembles carotenes. 658.

carpopedal (adjective). Pertaining to the hands and feet.
spasm, 349

cartilage
child and, 52
degenerative arthritis and, 300ff
joints and, 286
skeleton and, 280

caruncle. An abnormal small, red nodule; in women, the mass occurs in the opening of the urethra usually about the time of the menopause. 495ff

castration. Removal, destruction, or inactivation of the testicles or ovaries. 508

cataract. An opacity of the lens of the eye or its capsule. 565
operation for, 567

catarrhal (adjective). Pertaining to inflammation and flowing of exudate from mucous membranes.

catarrhal chronic pharyngitis, 144

catarrhal stomatitis, 443ff

cathartic. A drug or medicinal preparation used to produce evacuation of the bowels.

catheter. A tube for removing or injecting fluids through a natural body passage; made of plastic, rubber, glass, or metal.
cystoscope and, 487
hydronephrotic atrophy and, 487
premature infant feeding and, 42
puerperium and, 35ff

catheterization
cardiac, 203

cauda equina. The taillike lower end of the spinal cord. 379

cauliflower ear, 589

causalgia. A burning pain associated with disorder of the sensory nerves to the affected part.
skin disorders and, 278

caustic soda. *Sodium hydroxide,* used mainly as a chemical reagent.

cavity
tooth decay and, 427

cecum. The large blind sac at the beginning of the large intestine. 438

cell. The protoplasmic substance constituting the basic unit of life; a complete organism having a nucleus with or without a limiting wall. *81*
division, 2
somatic, 1

cell division
chromosomes and, 2
fertilized ovum and, *2*
process of, 2

cell poisons
cancer and, 644

cells, 1
body and, 80ff
cytoplasm and, 1
energy and, 80
food transportation and, 85ff
germ, 1
human machine and, 80
mitosis and, 80
plasma membrane and, 1
protoplasm and, 1
waste materials and, 91
white blood, 80ff

cell transformation
cancer and, 113
viruses and, 113

cellular antibodies, 191

cellulose. The complex carbohydrate material, insoluble in water, of which paper, linen, cotton, and wood are largely composed. 664ff

cementum. The layer of bony material on the root of a tooth. 417

centigrade. A scale of temperature measurement, in which the boiling point is 100° and the freezing point is 0°. (Symbol, C).

central incisors
infants and, 43

central nervous system. One of the two main divisions of the nervous system, composed of the brain and spinal cord. *381*
vascular lesions and, *214*

centrosphere, *81*

cercaria. The second, or tailed, stage of the larval life of trematode worms.
bilharziasis and, 492

cerebellum. The second largest division of the brain, consisting of a middle lobe and two lateral lobes. It occupies the back lower part of the skull. It is concerned with the coordinating of muscular movements. 377
cerebral palsy and, 394

cerebral arteriosclerosis
psychoses and, 628

cerebral cortex. The outer layer of the brain substance, composed of grey matter or nerve cells. It is concerned with abstract reasoning. 94, 100, 378

cerebral hemispheres. The two large, rounded halves of the cerebrum. 378

cerebral hemorrhage
aged and, 641

cerebral palsy. A group of disorders resulting from brain injury, usually manifested by some type of paralysis and incoordination. 394ff

cerebrospinal fluid. The watery fluid which circulates in the ventricles of the brain, the subarachnoid space, and the central canal of the spinal cord. 383
hydrocephalus and, 383

cerebrum. The largest portion of the brain. It consists of right and left halves called hemispheres, and occupies the upper part of the skull. 377
ear and, 583

cervical cancer
irregular menstruation and, 516
radiotherapy for, 514
surgical therapy for, 514

cervical vertebrae, 282

cervix. The lower part of the uterus. It is conical in shape and protrudes into the vagina, penetrated by the cervical canal through which menstrual blood and the fetus are expelled. 503
cancer of, 513

cesarean section. Surgical removal of the fetus through an incision into the uterus, usually made through the abdominal wall, *33*

cess pools, 752

cestoda. Any of the flatworms belonging to the class, *Cestoda,* which includes the tapeworms. 124

Chagas' disease. A febrile disease occurring in South America, caused by *Trypanosoma cruzi,* transmitted by the bite of a blood-sucking bug. 748
reduviids and, 763ff

chain reaction
nuclear fission and, 842

chain rescue technique, *724*

chalazion (plural chalazia). A tumor developing on the eyelid, formed by infection and distention of a sebaceous gland.
eyelids and, 562
sebaceous cysts and, 273

chancre. An ulcerating lesion, usually the first sign of syphilis.

chancroid. A lesion produced by infection with *Hemophilus ducreyi,* which involves the genitalia. 520

character inheritance
identical twins and, 7

chastity belt, *537*

chaulmoogra oil
leprosy and, 736ff

cheilosis. A lip disorder caused by vitamin deficiency.

chemical allergens, 238ff

chemical assays
circulatory disorders and, 203

chemical blood tests, 195

chemical burns
first aid for, 712ff
eye and, 569

chemical contraceptives, 535

chemical poisoning
first aid for, 718
jaundice and, 476ff
table of, *719ff*
urethra and, 494

chemical tests
alcohol intoxication and, 788

chemicals
dermatitis and, 252

chemical warfare
first aid during, 729

chemotherapy
cancer and, 643
leukemia and, 185

chest carry, *724*

chest cavity
breathing and, 127

chest cold
acute bronchitis and, 149

chest diseases
percussion and, 203

chest injuries
breastbone fracture, 171
bullet wounds, 171
mediastinal emphysema, 174
mediastinitis and, 174
pneumonia and, 173ff
pulmonary embolism and, 174
respiratory disorders and, 171ff
stab wounds, 171
traumatic pneumothorax, 172

chest pain
coronary thrombosis and, 215

chest wall
congenital abnormalities of, 176

chest wounds
open, 172ff

chicken pox. A contagious, infectious disease, characterized by eruptions on the skin and mucous membranes; caused by a virus, *Varicella.* 71ff
complications of, 72
hygiene and, 72
symptoms of, 71
transmission of, 71

chigger. A larval mite of the genus *Trombicula,* the bite of which causes inflammatory lesions. *250,* 765

chignon
childbirth and, 26
vacuum extractor and, 26

Chigoe
disease caused by, 765

chilblain
dermatitis and, 242

child
premature, 37ff
mother and, *38*

child-bearing women
children per, *531*

childbirth. Expulsion of the child with placenta and membranes at birth. 97
retrodisplacement and, 510
without fear, 26
without pain, 26

childhood, 52ff
anxiety reaction and, 607
behavior problems and, 60ff
brain injury and, 63
communicable diseases and, 56ff
development during, 52ff
discipline and, 60
dominance-submission and, 61ff
dyslexia and, 63
emotional factors and, 60ff
emotional growth and, 52ff
environment and, 62
mental growth of, 52ff
mental retardation and, 62ff
mind and, 601ff
postural defects and, *58*

childhood diseases, 71ff
adenoids and, 77ff
chicken pox, 71ff
diphtheria, 76ff
measles, 72
mumps, 75ff
rubella, 72ff
scarlet fever, 74ff
tonsils and, 77ff
whooping cough, 76
Wilms' tumor, 489

children
child-bearing women per, *531*
growth rate of, *60, 88ff*
home care and, 685

chills
malaria and, 738ff

China
medical history of, 796ff

China bedbugs
control of, 763ff

chlamydia, 114

chloasma. The appearance of light brown patches of irregular shape and size on the skin surface, sometimes associated with endocrine imbalance. 257

chlordane. A chlorinated hydrocarbon insecticide which is highly toxic to arthropods, but not as long-lasting in effects as DDT. It is used extensively in control of flies and cockroaches, but is highly toxic to man and animals. 764, 769
mosquito control and, 762

chlorination. The process of treating with chlorine, used in disinfecting water or sewage.

chlorinator, *753*

chlorine. A greenish-yellow gaseous element with a sharp odor; the active principle in germicides, bleaches, and deodorants. (Symbol, Cl). 750

chloroform. *Trichloromethane;* a colorless volatile liquid used as a solvent, an anesthetic, and an antispasmodic. It is more potent and more rapid in effect than ether.

chloromycetin. An antibiotic substance obtained from cultures of the organism, *Streptomyces venezuelae.*

chlorophyll. The green coloring matter found in plants which enables them to manufacture their own food.
fungi and, 121

chloroquine
malaria and, 740
resistant malaria, 740

chlorosis. 1. Iron-deficiency anemia characterized by greenish coloration of the skin. 2. A symptom of plant disease marked by loss of green pigmentation. 180

chlorpromazine
psychoses and, 628

choking
cyanosis and, 696
first aid for, 696ff
stridor and, 696
tracheostomy and, 696

cholera. An acute infectious disease caused by the bacterium, *Vibrio comma.* It is transmitted by drinking polluted water, is usually epidemic, and has a high mortality.
digestive tract disorders and, 470ff
disinfection chamber and, *469*
symptoms of, 470

cholera epidemic
water carrier and, *470*

cholesterol. A form of alcohol found in animal fats and oils, especially in the bile; it is also found in the brain and blood.
arteriosclerosis and, 204
circulatory disturbances and, 670
gallstones and, 478
Hand-Schuller-Christian's disease, 191
heart and circulation disorders and, 202
saturated fatty acids and, 655
triiodothyropropionic acid and, 205

choline. One of the B complex group of vitamins. Believed to be important in fat metabolism and as a raw material from which other important tissue substances are made.

chondriosomes, 81

chondroma (plural, chondromata). A tumor derived from cartilage. 176
ulna, *312*

chondrodysplasia, *292*

chorea. A nervous convulsive

disease characterized by involuntary jerking movements of the body.

chorioid. The dark brown, vascular coat of the eye, located between the sclera and the retina.

chorion. The membrane which envelops, protects, and supplies nourishment to the embryo, and later becomes the placenta. 14
  mesoderm and, 11

chorionic gonadotrophin, 329

Christianity
  marriage and, 523ff

chromatin, *81*

chromium
  trace elements and, 657
  glucose tolerance abnormalities and, 657

chromophytosis, 244

chromosomal abnormalities
  radiation injury and, 852

chromosome. One of the deeply staining bodies in the cell nucleus which carries the hereditary factors, or *genes.* 1, 3
  fetal human spleen, *542*
  fly salivary gland, *542*
  map. A schematic drawing showing location of genes along the chromosomes. 4
  cell division and, 2

chronic (adjective). Of long duration, applied to a disease that is not acute.
  atrophic laryngitis, 147
  bronchitis, 151
  constrictive pericarditis, 225
  cystic mastitis, 548
  diarrhea, 465
  frontal sinusitis, 142
  glaucoma, 567
  hypertrophic laryngitis, 147
  interstitial mastitis, 548
  laryngitis, 146ff
  leukemia, 185
  marginal gingivitis, 432
  mastitis, 548
  mastoiditis, 586
  maxillary sinusitis, 142
  middle ear infection, 585
  myelogenous leukemia, *186*
  osteomyelitis, 311
  pancreatitis, 480
  pharyngitis, 144
  prostatitis, 507
  pulmonary tuberculosis, 163
  simple pharyngitis, 144
  sinusitis, 142

chronic illness
  home care and, 686

cilia. Fine threadlike hairs located in various parts of the body which serve as filtering mechanisms to protect body areas from foreign particles, e.g. the eyelashes.
  nose and, 127
  pneumonia and, 156
  trachea and, 129ff

ciliary body. A thickened annular structure extending from the base line of the

iris to the anterior part of the choroid, consisting of secretory processes and ciliary muscle. 559
  iridocyclitis and, 565

Ciliata. A class of protozoa characterized by the possession of cilia.

Cimex lectularius
  bedbugs and, 763

cinchona. The dried bark of the *Cinchona succirubra* tree found in South America from which quinine is prepared. 739

cineplastic hand, 319

circadian rhythm
  space medicine and, 882

circulating swing
  insane treatment and, *602*

circulation. Movement in a circle or regular course, as the ciculation of the blood or lymph. 87ff, *198,* 199ff, *200*
  arterial, *201*
  heart and, 196ff
  Persian drawing of, *90*
  venous, *201*

circulation disorders
  aneurysm, 210ff
  diagnostic procedures for, 202ff
  dye injection and, 203
  high blood pressure, 211ff
  hypertension and, 212ff
  hypotension and, 214
  low blood pressure, 211ff
  prevention of, 202
  varicose veins, 205ff
  x-rays and, 203

circulatory disturbances
  food requirements and, 670

circulatory system
  food and, 85ff

circumcision. Surgical removal of the foreskin of the penis. *46ff,* 500

circumvallate papillae. The relatively large flat projections, each surrounded by a trench, which together make an inverted V-shape at the back of the tongue. 445

cirrhosis. A chronic liver disease characterized by nodular regeneration of undestroyed liver cells and associated with proliferation of the connective tissue within the liver. 477
  biliary, 477
  Laennec's, *476*
  portal, 477

cisterns
  water sources and, 752

civil defense
  atomic warfare and, 854
  food protection and, 863
  home protection and, 862ff
  home shelters, 858ff
  organization of, 854
  population evacuation and, 856
  public shelters and, 856ff
  supplies and, 855ff
  warning systems and, 856
  water protection and, 863

what to do in an attack, 863

civil defense signs, *857*

civil rights
  medicolegal aspects of, 789ff

clarifiers
  sewage and, 753

claustrophobia. Fear of being in a confined space.

clavicle. The curved bone between the scapula and the sternum; the *collar bone.* 285
  fracture of, 709

claw hand
  leprosy and, *736*

classical typhus, 744

Class I malocclusion, *422*

Class II malocclusion, *422*

Class III malocclusion, *422*

cleft
  oblique facial, 448

cleft palate. A fissure through the roof of the mouth which is present from birth. 447ff

climate
  kidney stones and, 486

climacteric. 351

clinical crown
  teeth and, 417

CLINITEST, *372*

clitoris. An organ composed of erectile tissue; the analogue, in the female, of the penis. 504
  epispadias and, 495

clonic spasm
  diaphragm and, 175

Clonorchis. The *Chinese liver fluke,* transmitted to man by ingestion of raw or improperly cooked fish. 124

closed fracture, 706

closed skull fracture, 413

Clostridium botulinum, 755
  food poisoning and, 456

Clostridium perfringens
  food-borne infections and, 755ff

Clostridium tetani. A long, motile, rod-shaped, anaerobic bacterium which causes tetanus.

clothing
  allergies and, 238
  pregnancy and, 21ff

clotting
  platelets and, 178

clubbed fingers
  bronchiectasis and, 151

clubs
  aging and, 648

coagulation. Clotting; the process of congealing of a fluid.

coarctation of the aorta, 225

cobalt-60
  radiotherapy and, 874

cocaine, *403*
  drug abuse and, 617

cocci
  bacteria and, 115

Coccidiodes immitis. A fungus which causes a lung disease in man. 122, 170

coccidioidomycosis. A disease usually occurring in the lungs, caused by inhalation

consumption
tuberculosis and, 161
contact dermatitis
nail disorders and, 274
contact lenses, 572
making of, *574*
refractory defects and, 574
contact poisons
insecticides, 768ff
contagious diseases
utensils and, *685*
chicken pox, 72
reportable diseases and, 795
contraction
muscle, 286
contusion
brain injury and, 414
convalescence. The period of recovery from a disease or injury.
rheumatic fever and, 221
convalescent patient
home care for, 686ff
convergence. The coordinated movement of the two eyes toward fixation of the same "near-point"; the eyes rotate inward to make the lines of vision meet at the object or point. 559, 570
conversion reaction. A psychiatric term denoting a repressed emotion that becomes manifest through a physical reaction; "hysterical paralysis" is an example, 610ff
emotional stress and, 606
convulsion. A violent, uncontrollable contraction, or series of contractions, of voluntary muscles. It may or may not be accompanied by loss of consciousness.
first aid for, 695
infants and, 49
convulsive capacity
epilepsy and, 392
convulsive disorders
brain tumor and, 410
electroencephalogram and, *393*
convulsive seizures
head injuries and, 415ff
coordination
cerebellum and, 378
child and, 53ff
copper. A metallic element required in the diet in minute amounts. (Symbol, Cu). 657
iron deficiencies and, 657
nutritional anemia and, 181
trace elements and, 657
copper deficiencies, 657
coral snakes, 721
cornea. The clear, transparent, portion of the fibrous outer coat of the eye which lies in front of the iris. 558
astigmatism and, 571
eye disorders and, 562ff
corneal disorders, 562ff
corneal transplantation and, 563ff
keratitis, 562ff
keratopathy, 563
ulcers, 562

corneal lens
contact lenses and, 572
corneal microscope, 572
corneal transplantation, 563ff
corneal type contact lenses, 574
corneal ulcers, 562
cornified layer, 231
corns
dermatitis and, 243
coronary (adjective). Resembling a crown; a term applied to vessels which completely encircle organs, especially those encircling the heart.
thrombosis. The formation of a blood clot in the coronary arteries resulting in obstruction of the blood supply to the heart muscle. 216ff
coronary arteries, 201
coronary thrombosis and, 214ff
coronary thrombosis
drug treatment for, 216ff
heart and, *215*
heart disorders and, 214ff
mechanism of, 214ff
surgical treatment for, 217
symptoms of, 215
what to do, 215ff
corpuscle
kidney, 483
corpus luteum. The yellow body which develops on the surface of the ovary after rupture of the Graffian follicle and which secretes the hormone, *progesterone.* 9
ovulation and, 354
pregnancy and, 22
corpus mammae. The body of the breast; the mass of breast tissue excluding the nipples. 545
corrosion
ionizing radiation and, 875
corrosive. 1. A substance that destroys tissue, either by direct chemical action, or by causing inflammation and suppuration. 2. Eating away.
poisons and, 717
cortex. The outer layers of an organ, as distinguished from its inner substance.
adrenal glands and, 332
kidneys and, 482
cortical hormones
ACTH, 332
miscellaneous, 359ff
secondary sex characteristics and, 359
cortisol
Addison's disease and, 360
cortisone. A hormone produced by the adrenal cortex; influences a number of metabolic functions; used as a therapeutic agent in various diseases, particularly in rheumatoid arthritis.
Addison's disease and, 360
allergy and, 241
rheumatoid arthritis and, 303, 305, *306*

Corynebacterium diphtheriae. A small rodlike microorganism that causes diphtheria. 76ff
cosmetic gloves, *322*
cosmetics
allergies and, 238
freckles and, 256ff
cough
infants and, 48
lung cancer and, 166
respiration and, 132
coumarin. An anticoagulant compound occurring naturally in sweet clover, derivatives of which are used as ingredients in rodenticides. Also prepared synthetically.
coronary thrombosis and, 216
red clover and, *216*
Cowper's glands. Two small glands located beneath the male urethra which produce a mucous secretion into the urethra; analogous to Bartholin's glands in the female.
cowpox. A virus disease of cows which is transmissible to man by contact and by vaccination. Cowpox vaccination bestows immunity to smallpox. 262
CPK (creatine phosphokinase)
muscular dystrophy and, 315
crab
cancer and, *472*
cracked nipples, 550
cranial arteries
migraine headaches and, 408
cranial artery dilatation
headaches and, 405
cranial inflammation
headaches and, 406
cranial nerve. One of the twelve pairs of nerves originating in the brain, which have both sensory and motor function.
cranium. That part of the skull which encloses the brain.
creatine phosphokinase
muscular dystrophy and, 315
creatinine. A waste product in the blood, excreted in the urine; it is a waste product of muscular contraction.
kidneys and, 484
creeping eruption, 251
creosols
germicides and, 770
crepitation. 1. The crackling sound heard in some diseases, as the rales heard in pneumonia. 2. The grating sound produced by fractured bones rubbing together. 171
cretinism. A congenital condition, characterized by lack of mental and physical development, resulting from abnormal thyroid function. 345
goiter and, 341
pituitary gland and, 332
teeth and, 425
thyroid and, *346*

crib deaths
    United States, 50ff
cricothyroid membrane
    choking and, 696
crime laboratory, *790, 793*
criminals
    medical studies of, 785ff
criminology
    alcohol intoxication tests and,
        788ff
    drug abuse and, 789
    lie detector tests and, 786ff
    medical studies of criminals
        and, 785ff
    medicolegal aspects of, 784ff
critical size
    nuclear fission and, 842
Crohn's disease
    small intestine and, 459
crossed ectopy
    kidneys and, 486
cross-eyes, *568*
    strabismus and, 568
crossing over. The process of
    exchange of genes between
    paired chromosomes which
    occurs before the reduction
    division of the germ cells. 3
crossmatching. Mixing of sam-
    ples of blood of donor
    and recipient to determine
    whether the bloods are
    compatible. 193
cross-sensitivity
    drug allergies and, 237
croup. A disease characterized
    by a noisy cough, inflamma-
    tion of the larynx, and dif-
    ficult breathing.
    infants and, 49
cryoextraction
    cataract removal and, 565
cryosurgery
    cataract removal and, 565
    Ménière's syndrome and, 588
    retinal detachment and, 566
cryothalamotomy
    Parkinson's disease and, 412
cryptorchism. A developmental
    defect in which the testes
    do not descend, but rather
    remain within the abdomen
    or inguinal canal. 351, 505
crystallin insulin. A form of
    purified insulin containing
    zinc, used mainly by insulin-
    allergic patients.
Culex mosquitoes
    control of, 758
Cushing's disease. A condition
    characterized by the symp-
    toms of Cushing's syn-
    drome, without adrenal
    gland involvement. 335ff
Cushing's syndrome. A group
    of symptoms consisting of
    obesity of the abdomen,
    face, and buttocks, decalci-
    fication of the bones, and
    increased blood pressure;
    caused by a tumor in the
    pituitary gland in conjunc-
    tion with excessive adrenal
    cortical hormone produc-
    tion. *336,* 360ff
    endocrine-producing   tumors
        and, 329

pituitary and, 335ff
curettage. Scraping of a cavity
    with a curette or other in-
    strument. 432
curie
    radioactivity and, 844
cuspid. One of the four teeth
    with cone-shape crowns; the
    canine tooth.
    infants and, 43
cutaneous horn, *272*
cutaneous neuroses, 278
cutaneous nodular leprosy, 736
cutaneous porphyria, 253
cutis, 229
cuts
    do nots, 702
    dos, 702
    first aid for, 702
cyanosis. A bluish tint to the
    skin caused by a lack of
    sufficient oxygen in the
    blood.
    asthma and, 139
    atelectasis and, 175
    blue babies and, 223
    choking and, 696
    congenital circulatory dis-
        orders and, 223
    laryngitis and, 146
cycloid (adjective). In psy-
    chiatry, a term denoting pe-
    riodic recurrence of extreme
    variation of mood, from
    elation and overactivity to
    depression and immobility.
    personality, 620 ff
cyclopentate
    eye dilation and, 572
cyst. A sac containing fluid or
    other substances; a bladder.
    amoebic dysentery and, 120
    kidney disorders and, 489
    lung and, 175
    mucous, 273
    sebaceous glands, *273*
    sinus, 143
cystic disease
    breast and, 548
cystic duct. Tube leading from
    the gall bladder to the com-
    mon bile duct.
    gallstones and, 478
cystic epithelioma, 273
cystine. An amino acid which is
    a component of many pro-
    teins.
    kidney stones and, 486
cystitis. Inflammation of the
    bladder. 491ff
cystocele. Protrusion of the
    bladder into the vagina. 491
cystoscope. A tubelike instru-
    ment for insertion through
    the urethra into the bladder,
    used in the diagnosis and
    treatment of diseases of the
    urinary tract. 487, 492, 507
cytoplasm. Cellular material not
    including the nucleus.
    cells and, 80
    living tissue and, 1
    protoplasm and, 1, 80
cytosine, 3

Dacron
    aneurysm and, 211

artificial arteries and, 205, 227
    arteriosclerosis and, 205
dacryocystitis
    lacrimal apparatus and, 562
daily living
    emotional stress and, 606ff
damaged heart
    aging and, 641
dandruff. Scales formed upon
    the scalp as a result of ex-
    cessive secretion of the
    sebaceous glands or ab-
    normal quality of sebum.
    260, 275ff
dapsone
    leprosy and, 737
dark adaptation
    rods and, 559
David Hook, *322*
daydreams
    mind and, 597
    schizophrenia and, 624
day-night cycling
    space medicine and, 881ff
D-cell adenoma, 365
D-cells
    islets of Langerhans and, 364
DDT. Abbreviation of *dichloro-
    di-phenyl-trichloro-ethane,* a
    powerful insecticide used in
    powdered or liquid form.
    bedbug control and, 763
    chigger control and, 765
    cockroach control and, 764
    flea control and, 765
    fly control and, 758
    insecticides and, 769
    louse control and, 763
    mosquito control and, 744,
        762
    yellow fever and, 744
dead air
    respiration and, 132
deaf
    education of, 592ff
    hearing aids and, 593ff
    opportunities for, 592ff
    problems of, 595
    schools for, 592ff
deafness
    causes of, 589ff
    childhood behavior problems
        and, 63
    conductive, 590
    ear disorders and, 589ff
    noise and, 591ff
    occupational, 591ff
    otosclerosis and, 590ff
    sensorineural, 590
    types of, 589ff
death (see also various diseases
    for rates of)
    heart transplantation and, 227
    human machine and, 79
    medicolegal identification and,
        775
    recording of, 795
    ten leading causes of, *895*
    32 selected causes of, *891*
death definition
    heart transplantation and, 227
death time
    organ transplantation and, 795
decalcification
    tooth decay and, 427
deciduous dentition, *419, 420*
    infants and, 43

tropical sprue and, 749
vitamin A deficiency and, 659
diastole. The phase of the heart beat in which the ventricles are expanded or relaxed. 198
diastolic pressure, 211
diathermy
retinal detachment and, 566
dicumarol. The trade name for *dicoumarin,* a compound which interferes with the normal clotting property of blood; it is used in treating patients with thrombosis.
vitamin K deficiencies and, 664
coronary thrombosis and, 216
diencephalon, 336
diet
acne vulgaris and, 260
aging and, 637
arteriosclerosis and, 205
asthma and, 140
constipation and, 466
diabetes mellitus and, 370
diarrhea and, 465
gallstones and, 478
gastritis and, 451
gout and, 307
hypertension and, 213
irritable bowel habits and, 464
kidney stones and, 486
liver cancer and, 477
modified, 668ff
peptic ulcer and, 454
pregnancy and, 20
puerperium and, 35ff
reducing, *669*
sterility and, 533
teeth and, 421
underweight and, 668
diet control
tooth decay and, 428ff
dietary supplements
nutrition and, 671
dietetics. The science of diet regulation for hygienic or therapeutic purposes.
dietitian. One who specializes in dietetics. 830
differential blood count. Enumeration of the relative proportions of the various types of cells in the blood. 195
differential diagnosis
ACTH and, 333
digester
sewage treatment and, 753
digestion. The complex physiological and chemical process of converting foods to forms assimilable by the body cells. 85ff
chemical process of, 442ff
food preparation and, 85ff
mouth and, 86
pancreatic juice and, 441
digestive cancer
deaths from, *473*
digestive enzymes, *86*
digestive juices, 86ff
digestive rhythm
infant feeding and, 45
digestive system. The aggregation of organs which are concerned with ingestion,

digestion, and elimination. *436,* 438ff
child and, 52
esophagus, 437
food and, 85ff
liver, 41
pancreas, 41ff
peritoneal cavity, 441
pharynx, 437
salivary glands, 437
stomach, 437
tongue, 445
digestive tract disorders
cholera and, 470ff
insecticides and, 768
parasites, 467ff
typhoid fever, 469ff
diguanides
diabetes mellitus and, 367
dilantin. A drug used in the control of epilepsy. 394
dilation. 1. Expansion of an organ or vessel. 2. Expansion of an orifice with an instrument. 3. Expansion of the pupil of the eye.
capillary, 201
eye examination and, 572
dementia praecox, 623
dimethyl phthalate, 762
typhus fever and, 745
diphtheria. An acute infectious disease characterized by formation of a false membrane on any mucous surface, accompanied by pain and fever. Caused by Klebs-Loeffler bacillus.
childhood disease and, 76ff
deaths from 76
dermatitis and, 247
mouth disorders and, 444
toxic diphtheric myocarditis and, 225
Diphyllobothrium. A genus of tapeworms parasitic in the intestinal tracts of fish, transmitted to man by the ingestion of improperly cooked fish. 124
macrocytic anemia and, 181
Diplococcus. A genus of spherical bacteria which occur in pairs. 115
Diplococcus pneumoniae, 157
diplopia. Double vision.
multiple sclerosis and, 412
strabismus and, 568
disaster
first aid in, 728ff
discharge
nipple, 550
discipline
childhood and, 60
disclosing wafers
dental hygiene and, 430
disease barriers
immunity, 101
skin, 101
white blood cells and, 101
Disease of Children
The First Treatise on, *54*
disease of the first year of life, *48*
disinfectant. An agent which destroys or inhibits pathogenic organisms. 769ff

bacteria and, 116
disinfection chamber
cholera and, *469*
displacement
mind and, 598
phobic reaction and, 607
dislocation. The displacement of a bone or an organ from its normal joint or position. 291ff
first aid for, 711
hip, *293*
mechanism of, 293
shoulder, *294*
subglenoid, *294*
disputed parentage
blood factors and, 194
medicolegal identification and, 776ff
dissociative reaction. Negation of consciousness of a phase of personality or being. 606
neuroses and, 609
distention
large intestine and, 461ff
diuretic. Any substance that increases the volume of urine.
ascites and, 481
water and, 654
diverticulitis. Inflammation of a diverticulum. 467
diverticulum (plural, diverticula). A blind sac or pouch branching off from a hollow organ.
esophagus and, 450
urethra and, 494
divorces
number of, *530*
DNA
adenine and, 3
copying of, 4
cytosine, 3
gene-protein interactions and, 4
genes and, 96
guanine, 3
nucleus and, 3ff, 80
structure of, 3ff
thymine, 3
viruses and, 105
doctor
fees, 825
medical organizations and, 825ff
medical profession and, 822ff
medical school training and, 823ff
specialization of, 824ff
dog tick, *249*
domestic mosquitoes
control of, 758
dominancy-submission
behavior problems and, 61ff
childhood and, 61ff
dominant (adjective). Pertaining to a characteristic inherited from one parent that develops to the exclusion of a contrasting character from the other parent. See **gene.**
dominant allele, 4
Huntington's chorea and, 5
dominant inheritance
brachydactyly, 4
domination
parenthood and, 604ff

Don Juanism
  satyriasis and, 538
donor (Medicine). One who gives blood, tissue, or organ for transfusion or transplantation.
Donovania granulomatosis, 521
doorbell
  sickroom and, *679*
Dorrance Hook, *322*
dosimeter
  atomic radiation measurement and, *845*
double ureter, 490
douche
  sex hygiene and, 540
  home care and, 679ff
Dramamine. The trade name for *dimenhydrinate*, a compound with antihistaminic properties, used in prevention and treatment of motion sickness. 589, 697
draw sheet
  patient's bed and, 677
dreams
  mind and, 605
  sleep and, 102
dressings
  home care and, 681
drooling
  cerebral palsy and, 395
dropsy
  heart failure and, 226
drowning
  medicolegal aspects of, 782
drug abuse, 616
  criminology and, 789
  history of, 616
  medicolegal aspects of, 789
Drug Abuse Control Amendments, 789
drug addiction. A physiological and emotional dependence on an abnormal use of habit-forming drugs.
drug allergies, 236ff
  symptoms of, 237
drug industry, 833ff
drugs
  asthma and, 139ff
  human milk and, 547
drunken drivers, 731
dry bronchiectasis, 151
dry pericarditis, 225
dry pleurisy, 160
drying beds
  sewage treatment and, 753
Duchenne types
  muscular dystrophy, 315
duct. A tubular vessel which conveys blood or other secretions of the body.
  gastrointestinal tract and, *440*
ductus
  epididymis and, 499
ductus arteriosus. A portion of the aortic arch in the fetus which connects the pulmonary artery and the aorta; normally, this is closed at birth, or shortly thereafter. *224*
duodenum. The first portion of the small intestine, about eight to ten inches in length; it contains the open-

ings of the pancreatic duct and common bile duct.
  digestion and, 86ff
  intestines and, 86ff
  peptic ulcer of, 459
  small intestine and, 438
dura mater. The tough, outermost layer of the three coverings of the brain and spinal cord. 383
duralumin. A noncorrosive alloy of aluminum and copper. Because of its light weight and relatively high tensile strength, it is used extensively in surgical splints and prosthetic appliances.
dust
  occupational disease and, 732
dust allergy, 238
dwarfism
  achondroplasia, 335
  pituitary, 334
dwarf tapeworm, 767
dye injection
  circulation disorders and, 203
  liver function tests and, 475ff
dying patient
  aging and, 645
dysentery. Inflammation of the colon characterized by diarrhea with the passage of mucus and blood.
  amoeba and, 120
  Balantidium coli and, 121
  deaths from, *465*
  diarrhea and, 465
dyslexia, 63
  behavior problems and, 63
  childhood and. 63
dysmenorrhea, 356
dyspareunia. Painful or difficult sexual intercourse in women.
  frigidity and, 537
dysphagia, 449
dyspnea
  aneurysm and, 210
  asthma and, 139
  atelectasis and, 175
  laryngitis and, 146
  lung cancer and, 166
dysuria, 496

ear. The organ of hearing, consisting of the external, middle, and internal ear. 581
  external, 581, *582, 583*
  foreign bodies in, 705
  function of, 583
  horizontal section of, *586*
  internal, 583
  middle, 581ff
  nervous system and, 100
  receptors and, 100
  vertical section of, *586*
ear disorders
  acute draining middle ear infection, 586
  aero-otitis media and, 584
  boils, 584
  cauliflower ear, 589
  congenital malformations, 589
  deafness, 589ff
  earache, 584ff
  eardrum inflammation, 584
  eardrum puncture, 587

  equilibrium disturbances, 589
  fungus infection, 584
  furuncles, 584
  mastoid, 586ff
  Ménière's syndrome, 588
  middle ear, 586ff
  middle ear nondraining infection, 584ff
  motion sickness, 589
  tinnitus, 587
earache
  acute draining middle ear infection and, 586
  aero-otitis media and, 584
  boils and, 584
  eardrum inflammation and, 584
  fungus infection and, 584
  furuncles and, 584
  middle ear nondraining infection and, 584ff
  outer ear infection and, 584
eardrum
  diagnosis of puncture of, 587
  earache and, 584
  growths following puncture of, 587
  punctures of, 587
  receptors and, 100
  treatment for punctures of, 587
ear infection
  deafness and, 590
early medical history, 796ff
early rising
  advantages of, 34
  new mother and, 32ff
eating
  cleft palate and, 448
Ebers Papyrus
  medical history and, 797
Eberthella typhosa, *756*
Ebstein's malformation of tricuspid valve, 224
ebullism
  space medicine and, 879
ecchymosis, 569
eccrine glands
  sweat glands and, 233
Echinococcus. A genus of tapeworms, commonly infesting sheep and dogs, but also parasitic to man. 124
ecology
  pollution and, 754
ectoderm. The outer layer of germinal cells of an embryo from which are developed skin structures, the nervous system, organs of special sense, the pineal, and part of the pituitary and suprarenal glands. 11
ectopic (adjective). In an abnormal position.
  kidneys and, 486
  pregnancy, 9
ecythema
  dermatitis and, 246
eczema. An acute or chronic, noncontagious, itching, inflammatory condition of the skin in which reddened, scaly, and vesicular lesions occur.
  allergy and, 235
  food allergies and, 236

Endamoeba histolytica
intestinal parasites and, 468
amoebic dysentery and, 120
food-borne infections and, 756
endarterectomy
arteriosclerosis and, 205
endemic (adjective). Occurring in a certain locality; used to designate an outbreak of a disease which occurs more or less constantly in that particular area.
endemic diseases
cholera, 470
goiter, 341
endoarteritis. Inflammation of the inner wall of an artery.
endocarditis. Inflammation of the endocardium.
endocardium. A thin layer of tissue lining the inner surfaces of the heart.
bacterial infection of, 217
endocrine (adjective). Internal secretion; refers especially to the ductless glands of the body which secrete their products directly into the blood stream.
endocrine disorders
Addison's disease, 360
adrenal overactivity, 360ff
Cushing's disease, 335ff
Cushing's syndrome, 335ff
diabetes mellitus, 365ff
Fröhlich's syndrome, 336
Graves' disease (hyperthyroidism), 343ff
growth and, 334ff
hypothyroidism, 345ff
islet cell disorders, 365
myxedema, 345ff
nodular goiter, 343
parathyroid diseases, 349
thyroid and, 341ff
thyroid tumors, 346ff
thyroiditis, 347ff
endocrine glands, 94
adrenal glands, 358ff
distribution of, *95*
gonads, 349ff
hypothalamus, 336ff
ovary, 352ff
parathyroids, 348ff
pars intermedia, 334
pituitary, 330ff
pancreas, 363ff
pineal gland, 362ff
thyroid, 337ff
thymus gland, 361ff
endocrine imbalances
sterility and, 533
endocrine system, 328
function of, 328ff
nervous system and, 329
placenta and, 329
endocrinologist. One who specializes in the science of the ductless glands and their function.
endocrinology. The science of the ductless glands. 823
endoderm. Innermost layer of germinal cells of an embryo which forms the gastrointestinal lining and its derivatives. 11

endogamy. The custom of marriage within the tribe, caste, or social group; *inbreeding.*
marriage ceremony and, 523
endolymph. The watery fluid in the labyrinth of the ear.
endometriosis. The abnormal presence of endometrial tissue outside the uterus, throughout the pelvis, or in the abdominal wall. 511
irregular menstruation and, 516
endometrium. The mucous membrane and glandular tissue which lines the inner surface of the uterus. 503
menstruation and, 354
endoscope. An instrument equipped with lighting and lens systems used for visual examination of the interior of a body organ or cavity.
endothelium. A layer of simple cells which completely lines the inner surface of blood vessels and hollow organs of the body.
capillaries and, 198
enema
apparatus, *471*
flexible tube, *679*
home care and, 679ff
energy
cells and, 80
metabolic rate and, 83
needs, 83ff
nuclear fission and, 842
nuclear reactor and, 874ff
requirements, 84
England
nineteenth century medicine in, 809ff
English plantain, *134*
Engineering Service
Civil Defense and, 855
entomologist. One who specializes in entomology.
death time and, 775
entomology. The branch of zoology which deals with the study of insects.
enuresis. Urinary incontinence, usually at night; bed-wetting. 497
urethra and, 493
environment
autonomic nervous system and, 94
behavior problems and, 62
body and, 99ff
body conflict and, 100ff
childhood and, 62
criminals and, 785
infant and, 43ff
environmental health
fly control, 756ff
food-transmitted diseases, 754
germicides, 768ff
insect control, 762ff
insecticides, 768ff
mosquito control, 758ff
pollution, 754
rat control, 766ff
sewage disposal, 750ff
water purification, 750ff
Environmental Health Service, 836

environmental medicine
space medicine and, 878
environmental poisoning, 783
Environmental Protection Agency
environmental poisoning and, 783
enzyme. A complex chemical substance found mainly in the digestive juices, which acts upon other substances to cause splitting into simpler substances.
cataract removal and, 565
digestion and, 86
digestive, *86*
gout and, 307
pepsin, 86
enzyme abnormalities
brain damage and, 412
Mongolism, 413
eosinophile. A cell, especially a white blood cell, which stains easily with eosin. Normally eosinophiles constitute from 0.5 to 2% of the normal white cells.
eosinophilic granuloma, 191
ephedrine. An alkaloid drug made from *ephrada equisetna* or produced synthetically and used in the treatment of patients with hay fever, asthma, shock, and other conditions.
epidemics
influenza, 155ff
poliomyelitis, 384
epidemic parotitis, 75ff
epidermis. The protective epithelial outer portion of the skin.
fingerprints and, 777
skin and, 231
skin growth and, 231
sunburn and, 713
Epidermophyton. A genus of fungi that causes skin infections.
inguinale, 265
epididymis. The small, oblong body resting upon the posterior surface of each testis, composed of a convoluted tube 18 to 20 feet long, covered by the tunica vaginalis and ending in the vas deferens. 498, 499
spermatazoa and, 10
epigastric (adjective). Pertaining to the upper middle portion of the abdomen.
epiglottis
pharynx and, 129
epilation
atomic explosion and, *851*
radiation injury and, 851
epilepsy. A condition giving rise to periodic disturbances of brain function, diverse in nature, abrupt in onset, usually brief in duration, and often accompanied by a disturbance in consciousness and involuntary muscular contractions. 695
first aid for, 695

development of, *67ff*

female gonads
menstrual cycle and, 354ff
ovaries, 352ff
ovulation and, 353ff

female hormones
ovaries and, 349

female reproductive system, 501ff
menopause and, 504ff

female sex hormone
prostatic cancer and, 508

femoral artery
transplantation of, *228*

femoral fracture, *296*

femoral hernia, 299

femur. The proximal bone of the leg; the thigh bone.

fenestration. The act of perforating or the condition of being perforated with a windowlike opening.

fermentation. Chemical change of an organic product by the action of the enzymes of yeast or bacteria.

fertility
pregnancy and, 23
radiation injury and, 852

fertilization. Union of the egg cell from the female with the sperm cell from the male. 10, 11, 500
corpus luteum and, 9
Fallopian tube and, 8ff

fertilized ovum, 2
chromosomes and, *10*
division of, *2*
spindles and, *10*

fermentation tanks
antibiotic production and, *834*

fetal
development, 14
head size, 17
human spleen chromosome, *542*
malformation, 75
maturation, 16

fetology, 16
amniocentesis and, 16
fiberoptic camera and, 16
illuminated endoscope and, 16

fetus. The developing child in the uterus after the third month of life. 11
4 month, *15*
protected, *15*
6 month, *15*

fever
bacterial endocarditis and, 218
blisters, 243
food requirements and, 669
infants and, 49
infectious mononucleosis and, 190
malaria and, 738ff
mumps and, 75
poliomyelitis and, 384
sinusitis and, 142ff
thermometers, 680
tonsilitis and, 78

fiberoptic camera
fetology and, 16

fiberscope
peptic ulcer and, 453

fibril. One of the fine longitudinal threads of striated muscle fibers; the con-

tractile element of the muscle. 286

fibrin. An insoluble protein which makes up the fibers of a blood clot. 178
plasma and, 178

fibrinogen
liver and, 441, 475

fibrinous pericarditis, 225

fibroadenoma
breast and, 549

fibroid (adjective). Pertaining to fibrous tissue or its formation; especially tissues that have become extensively fibrosed.
irregular menstruation and, 516
uterine tumors and, 512

fibroma
benign skin tumors and, 253ff
ovarian, 509

fibroneurosarcoma
skin cancer and, 272

fibrosarcoma
skin cancer and, 272

fibrosis
pulmonary, 175

fibrositis. Inflammation of fibrous tissue; often called muscular rheumatism.
low back pain and, 310

fibrothorax
hemothorax and, 172

fibrous tissue
cauliflower ear and, 589
cirrhosis and, 477

fibula. The outer and smaller of the two bones of the leg between the knee and the ankle. 285

fibula fracture
first aid for, 711

fifth lumbar vertebra, 1
low back pain and, 308

fight or flight
autonomic nervous system and, 381

filaria (plural, filariae). A group of parasitic nematode worms.
filariasis and, 123
life cycle of, 123

filariasis. A disease caused by the presence of filarial worms in the body, characterized by hypertrophy of body tissues caused by obstruction of lymphatic or blood vessels by the filariae.
Culex mosquitoes and, 758
diagnosis of, 746
elephantiasis and, 123, 745ff
roundworms and, 123
treatment for, 746
worms and, 745ff

filiform papillae. The small, threadlike projections which occur over the dorsal surface of the tongue. 445

fillings, 427ff

filtering
water purification and, 750

filters
viruses and, 105

fimbriae
Fallopian tubes and, 502

financial security
retirement and, 647

fingers
degenerative arthritis of, 301
amputation, *317*
sucking, *425*

fingernail
section of, *274*

fingerprint. An imprint of the skin ridges of the fleshy portion of the fingertips, used as a means of identification.
arched, 777
Bertillon system and, 778
composite, 777
identification classification, *780*
looped, 777
medicolegal identification of, 777ff
patterns, *779*
whorled, 777

fireman's carry, 694

fires
first aid in, 728ff

Fire Service
Civil Defense and, 855

fire storm
atomic bomb explosion and, 847

first aid. The immediate and temporary assistance given to a sick or injured person before the services of a physician can be secured.
abdominal pain, 697
abrasions, 702
aero-otitis media, 698
animal bites, 702ff
arm fracture, 709
artificial respiration, 722ff
asthma, 141
atomic blast injuries, 848
atomic warfare, 864
battered children, 712
biological warfare, 729
boils, 245
bone injuries, 706ff
bruises, 712
burns, 712ff
chemical burns, 712ff
chemical poisoning, 718
chemical warfare, 729
choking, 696ff
clavicle fracture, 709
cold exposure, 716
convulsions, 695
coronary thrombosis, 215ff
cuts, 702
diabetic shock, 700ff
diarrhea, 465
disaster, 728ff
dislocations, 711
electrical burns, 712ff
electric shock, 701
emergencies and, 694ff
epilepsy, 695
fainting, 694ff
febrile convulsions, 695
fibula fracture, 711
fires, 728ff
floods, 728ff
food poisoning, 718
foreign bodies, 704ff
frostbite, 716
general considerations of, 690ff

heart failure, 696
heat exhaustion, 716
hiccough, 697
hip fractures, 708
hysteria, 697
infant convulsions, 49
insect bites, 703ff
insulin shock, 701
joint injuries, 706ff
lacerations, 702
long-distance transfer and, 694
lower leg fracture, 708ff
man-of-war bites, 704
metal poisoning, 718
motion sickness, 697ff
moving major fractures and, 694
muscle injuries, 706ff
neck fracture, 707
need for, 690
nosebleed, 697
pelvic fractures, 708
poisonous plants, 718ff
poisonous snakes, 721
poisons, 716ff
puncture wounds, 702
purposes of, 690ff
rib fracture, 709
scorpions, 704
severe bleeding, 701
shock, 698ff
short-distance transfer and, 693ff
skull concussion, 706ff
skull fracture, 706ff
spider bites, 703ff
spinal column fracture, 707
sprains, 711
status asthmaticus, 141
strains, 711
sunburn, 713ff
sunstroke, 716
thigh fractures, 708
tibia fracture, 711
transportation of injured and, 692ff
unconsciousness, 415, 695
upper body fracture, 707ff
warfare, 729ff
water rescue, 724ff
woolly worm, 704
wounds, 701
first aid kits, 692
first aid stations
atomic warfare and, 864ff
first degree burns, 712
first year of life, 42ff
fission. 1. Cleavage or division. 2. In biology, asexual reproduction by division of the organism.
amoeba, and, 120
bacteria reproduction and, 115
fissure. A crack or crevice.
nipple, 550
fistula. An abnormal tube or canal leading from a body organ.
anal, 472ff
bladder, 491
fixed joints, 285
flagella
bacteria and, 115
Flagellata and, 121
Flagellata. A class of protozoa possessing flagella, the slen-

der whiplike processes that aid in movement.
diseases produced by, 121
flagellum (plural, flagella). A small whiplike structure on some microorganisms, used as a means of locomotion.
flat feet, 293
flatworms, 124ff
bladder inflammation and, 492
flea. A bloodsucking insect of the order Siphonaptera, which acts as host and transmitter for disease. 251, 764
control of, 765
dermatitis and, 251
flea control
typhus fever and, 745
flea hunting, 766
FLEX
physician licensing and, 771
flexion. The act of bending, in contrast to extending. 286
reflex activity and, 379
floods
first aid in, 728ff
floss, dental
how to use, 430
fluid absorption
large intestine and, 439
fluid infectious principle
viruses and, 104
fluke. Any of the small parasitic flatworms belonging to the class, Trematoda.
blood, 124ff
Clonorchis and, 124
flatworms, 124
life cycle of, 124
fluorescent (adjective). Pertaining to the property of certain substances to radiate light of a greater wave length than that of the incident light.
fluoridation
dental caries and, 431
fluoride deficiencies, 657
fluorine. A gaseous chemical element occurring rarely in the free state but found in the soil in combination with calcium. (Symbol, F).
fluorine compounds
insecticides and, 768
fluoroscope. The x-ray apparatus with which fluoroscopy is performed.
fluoroscopy. Examination of the movement and form of internal body organs by means of a fluorescent screen in conjunction with a roentgen tube which emits rays by which shadows of objects interposed between the tube and screen are made visible.
fly control, 756ff
adult flies and, 758
breeding places and, 757ff
life cycle and, 757
flying glass injuries
atomic explosion and, 848
fly salivary gland chromosome, 542

fly-transmitted disease
Loa loa, 123
focal seizures
Jacksonian epilepsy, 393
folic acid. One of the B complex group of vitamins, organic in nature and believed to be essential in the diet to sustain life, found in liver, yeast, and green leaves. In pure form, it is a yellow crystalline material.
essential food elements and, 662
pernicious anemia and, 181
folic acid deficiencies, 662
tropical sprue and, 749
follicle. A small excretory duct; a small sac or tubular gland.
hair and, 232
skin and, 229
thyroid and, 338
fontanel. The space in the skull of the newborn child before the cranial bones fuse; commonly known as "the soft spot." 42
food
absorption, 439
allergies, 236
building material and, 84ff
deficiencies of, 653
essential, 654ff
handling, 470
human machine and, 79ff
intoxications, 755
metabolism and, 83
poisoning, 456ff, 718
preparation, 85ff
recommended servings of, 666
-transmitted diseases, 754ff
transportation, 85ff
Food and Drug Administration, 836
foot
care, 375ff
muscles of, 289
foramina papillaria
kidneys and, 482
forceps
birth and, 28
labor and, 26ff
forearm amputation, 317
forearm muscles
major, 98
forebrain. The anterior portion of the brain of the embryo.
foreign bodies
first aid for, 704ff
foreign material
white cells and, 177
forensic psychiatry, 793
forensics
medical education and, 823
foreskin
circumcision and, 46
forge at Gretna Green, 526
formalin. Trade name for formaldehyde, a gas dissolved in water and alcohol, used as a fixative for the preservation of tissue for study and as a germicidal agent.
fossae
skull and, 383
four humours
medical history and, 799

dal material in the spleen. 191

gavage, *41*

Geiger counter. An instrument used to detect and measure radioactivity. 845

gene. The ultramicroscopic particle which is the basic unit in the transmission of hereditary characteristics. 1
DNA and, 96
germ cells and, 96
heredity and, 1ff
RNA and, 96

gene action, 3
heredity and, 3

gene behavior, 4

gene locus, 4
chromosome map and, 4

generalized acute miliary tuberculosis, 163

generalized mouth disease, 443ff

generalized osteitis fibrosa, 311

general paresis
syphilis and, 519

genetic(s). The branch of biology which deals with the phenomena of heredity and the variations between parents and offspring.
action, 4
counseling, 7
dwarfism, 335
engineering, 113
independent assortment and, 4
Klinefelter's syndrome, 351
marriage and, 525
radiation injury and, 852
sex determination by, 3

geniculate neuralgia, 403

genotype. Basic hereditary combination of genes characterizing an individual or group. 4
heterozygous and, 5
homozygous and, 4

germ. 1. Protoplasmic unit capable of developing into a new individual especially an egg or sperm cell. 2. A microorganism, particularly a disease-producing bacterium.
cells, 1, 96

German measles. Acute contagious disease resembling measles and scarlet fever; characterized by a rash of short duration.

German precisionists
nineteenth century medicine and, 809

germ cell division
crossing over and, 3
heredity and, 2ff
process of, 2ff
reduction division and, 2ff

germ theory
medical history and, 808

germicide. An agent that kills germs. 768ff

germinal epithelium. The embryonic tissue which gives rise to the epithelium and to the germ cells. 502

gestation. The period of intrauterine fetal development.

See **pregnancy.**

giant
pituitary, *332*

giant cell tumors
bone cancer and, 314

giant ragweed, *135*

giantism. Exaggerated body growth resulting from excessive pituitary function.
human growth hormone and, 335
pituitary tumors and, 335

gingival tissues, 419

gingivitis
chronic marginal, 432

girls, weight-height-age table, *820*

gland. A cell, tissue, or organ which elaborates and secretes substances which are used elsewhere in the body or are discharged.
differentiation of, 13
endocrine, 94ff

glanders. An acute febrile disease, caused by *Malleomyces mallei* and transmitted by animals. 246

glans clitoris. The area at the distal end of the clitoris.

glans penis. The conical body which forms the distal end of the penis. 495

glass eyes, *573*
eye disorders and, 573

glasses, 572ff
bifocal, 572
refractory defects and, 569ff, 572ff
trifocal, 573

glaucoma. A disease of the eye characterized by increase in pressure within the eye which causes atrophy of the optic nerve with resultant gradual loss of vision and blindness.
acute, 567
chronic, 567
corneal transplantation and, 563
eye disorders and, 567ff

globin insulin. Insulin preparation modified by the addition of beef blood, hemoglobin, and zinc; effective for longer periods of time than regular insulin. 369

globulin. A member of a group of proteins characterized by being insoluble in water, but being soluble in dilute salt solutions.

globulin metabolites
multiple myeloma and, 189

glomerulonephritis. Inflammation of the glomeruli of the kidney.
Bright's disease and, 488

glomerulus. A small knotlike grouping of capillaries in the renal corpuscle. 483

Glossina. A genus of blood-sucking flies to which the tsetse flies belong.

glossitis. An inflammation of the tongue.

croup and, 49
riboflavin deficiencies and, 661

glossopharyngeal neuralgia, 403

glucagon, 364
islets of Langerhans and, 364

glucose. A simple sugar that is present in normal blood; it is oxidized by the body as a source of heat or energy; 58% of the proteins in the body are converted to glucose, which is formed from the chemical breakdown of glycogen.
diabetes mellitus and, 365
glucagon and, 364
insulin and, 364
liver and, 364, 475

glycogen. Animal starch, the form in which carbohydrates are stored in the animal body for future conversion into sugar for energy to perform muscular work or to liberate heat.
carbohydrates and, 654
liver and, 475

goiter. Enlargement of the thyroid gland.
cretinism and, 341
food-caused, 342
iodine deficiencies and, 657
nodular, 343
simple, 342ff
thyroid and, 341

goiterous figure, *341*

gold salts
rheumatoid arthritis and, 305

Golgi bodies, *81*

gonad. A general term referring to both the male sex gland or testis and the female sex gland or ovary.
endocrine glands and, 95, 349ff
female, 352ff
male, 350ff
ovaries, 352ff
reproduction and, 96ff
testes, 350ff

gonadal dysfunction
hypothalamus and, 337

gonadal hormones
extraction of, 350
functions of, 350
secondary sex characteristics and, 350
synthesis of, 350

gonadotrophic (adjective). Gonad-stimulating, 322
reproductive hormones and, 8

gondadotrophin. Any of the hormones, produced by the anterior lobe of the pituitary gland, which directly stimulate the gonads. 19, 24

gonococcus. Name commonly used to designate the diplococcus which causes gonorrhea, *Neisseria gonorrhoeae.* *117*
ophthalmia neonatorum and, 561

gonorrhea. A contagious catarrhal inflammation of the genital mucous membrane.

It may also affect other structures such as the conjunctiva, oral mucosa, the rectum, and the joints. Caused by the diplococcus. *Neisseria gonorrhoeae.* 517ff
  complications of, 517ff
  prevention of, 518
  symptoms of, 517ff
  treatment for, 518
  types of, 517ff

Gonyaulax catenella. A species of shellfish, the eating of which causes a paralytic type of poisoning in man. 458

goose pimples
  erectores pilorum and, 232

gout. An arthritic disease caused by abnormal uric acid metabolism. *306*
  food requirements and, 670
  skeletal disorders and, 306ff
  uric acid and, 670

Graafian follicle. One of the vesicles in the ovaries which contains the ovum. It appears externally, rupturing and freeing the ripened ovum; it secretes hormones which affect the menstrual cycle. 353

grafts
  arterial, *228*
  skin, 279

grand mal seizures
  epilepsy and, 392
  status epilepticus and, 392

grandparents
  childhood behavior problems and, 62

granulocyte. A cell which contains granules, generally leucocytes.
  Bone marrow and, 178

granulocytic leukemia, 185

granuloma. A granular tumor, composed usually of lymphoid or epithelial cells.
  tooth decay and, 428

granuloma inguinale, 521ff

grasses
  hay fever and, 133

Graves' disease (hyperthyroidism)
  radioactive iodine and, 345
  thyroid and, 343ff
  treatment for, 344ff

gravid hypertrophy, 549

gravitational factors
  space time and, 882

gravitational forces
  space medicine and, 878

gray matter. Gray colored part of the nervous system which is composed of nerve cell bodies.
  central nervous system and, 382

greater curvature. The outer curved edge of the stomach. 437

Greece
  medical history of, 797ff

green nails, 274

green-stick fracture, *295*

Gretna Green
  forge at, *526*

Grievance Committee
  medical fees and, 825

griseofulvin
  athlete's foot and, 266
  ringworm and, 263

grooming
  home care and, 678

ground zero
  atomic bomb explosion and, 846

group identification
  adolescence and, 603
  teen-ager and, 69ff

group therapy
  alcoholism and, 619

growing pains
  subclinical rheumatic fever and, 220

growth
  child, 52
  children's rate of, *60, 88ff*
  disorders, 334ff
  growth hormone and, *330*
  infants and, 43
  pituitary gland and, 330
  pituitary tumors and, *353*
  premature child and, 42
  radiation injuries and, 852ff
  relative human-animal, *70*
  somatotrophic hormone and, 334
  tissue, 83

guanine
  DNA base, 3

guide dogs
  blind and, 576

guilt
  melancholic and, 621

guilt feelings
  frigidity and, 537

guinea pigs
  Wassermann test and, 521

gumma. The specific lesion of tertiary or late syphilis, which may occur in many tissues, but most often occurs in the brain, liver, and heart. 519

gums
  pyorrhea and, 432
  scurvy and, 663
  teeth and, 419
  Vincent's infection, 433

gut
  anatomy of, 439

guttate keratopathy, 563

gynecology. The medical science which deals with diseases of women, especially diseases of the female reproductive system.
  Galen and, *523*

gynecomastia. Abnormally large mammary glands in the male. 549

habits
  obsessive-compulsive reaction and, 608

hair
  falling out of, *232*
  follicles, 229
  medicolegal identification of, 778ff
  photomicrograph of, *777*
  scalp and, *233*
  skin and, 232ff

hair follicle. A small gland from which hair grows. *232*

hairy nevus, *253*

hairy raised nevus, *256*

halazone. A potent chloride disinfectant used in water purification. 750

half-life
  radioactivity and, 842

hallucinations, *615, 621*

hallucinogens
  drug abuse and, 617ff
  LSD, 618
  marijuana, 618

hammer
  middle ear and, 581

handicaps
  criminals and, 785

Hand-Schuller-Christian's disease. A disease of children marked by deposition of cholesterol in the bones and subcutaneous tissues. 191

Hansen's bacillus
  leprosy and, 735

hard chancre, 518

hardening arteries
  heart disorders and, 203ff

hard ticks, 766

harelip, *447, 448*
  mouth disorders and, 447ff
  rehabilitation of, *447*

Harrison Narcotic Act
  drug abuse and, 789

Hashimoto's struma. A type of diffuse thyroid enlargement characterized by atrophy of the thyroid parenchyma and fibrosis. 347

hay fever. An allergic disease of the upper respiratory tract and the nasal passages induced by external irritation, usually by pollen; formerly called *rose fever.* 235
  nonseasonal, 132, 138
  plants and, 133ff
  recognition of, 138
  relief from, 139
  seasonal, 132, 133
  skin tests for, 138ff
  symptoms of, 138

head
  embryo and, *21*

headache, *405*
  mechanisms of, 405ff
  meningitis and, 390
  migraine, 408ff
  nervous system disorders and, 405ff
  pain-sensitive structures and, 405
  sinusitis and, 142ff

head and neck cancer, *272*

head injuries, 413ff
  brain injuries and, 413ff
  care for, 415
  complications of, 415
  convulsive seizures and, 415ff
  skull fractures, 413

head-trunk sizes
  relative, *70*

health organizations, 835ff
  federal, 836
  local, 835
  state, 836
  voluntary, 836ff

Health Service
Civil Defense and, 855
Health Services and Mental Health Administration, 836
hearing
aids, 593ff, *594*
cochlea and, 583
infant and, 42
middle ear infections and, 585ff
noise and, 591ff
temporal lobe and, 583
tests, *590*
Hearst Medical Papyrus
medical history and, 797
heart. The muscular organ that pumps the blood.
child and, 52
coronary arteries and, 201
coronary thrombosis and, *215*
description of, 196ff
differentiation of, 13
rear view of, *197*
heart beat, 196
electrocardiogram and, *198*
mechanism of, 196ff
vagus nerve and, 196
heartburn. A burning sensation felt under the breastbone; usually caused by cardiospasm. 450
heart disease
aneurysm, 210ff
angina pectoris, 225ff
bacterial endocarditis, 217ff
coronary thrombosis, 214ff
deaths from, *217*
diagnostic procedures for, 202ff
hardening of arteries, 203ff
high blood pressure, 211ff
home care and, 686
prevention of, 202
rheumatic fever, 219ff
rheumatic heart disease, 222
thyrotoxic, 226
varicose veins and, 205ff
heart failure. Failure of the heart to pump the amount of blood required for proper circulation. 226
cardiac massage and, 696
first aid for, 695ff
heart-lung bypass machine, 225
pulmonary embolism and, 205
heart surgery
medical history and, 817
heart transplantation, 227
heat
allergy, 239
exhaustion, 716
human machine and, 79ff
insane treatment and, *606*
prostration, 733ff
heat radiation
atomic bomb explosion and, 846ff
space medicine and, 879
Heberden's nodes. Nodular enlargements located about the terminal joints of the fingers in certain arthritic patients. 301
heliophobe. A person who is morbidly sensitive to the effects of sun light. 713
helix. The rim or margin of the external ear.

hellebore
housefly breeding and, 758
hemangioma. A tumor made up of blood vessels. *256*
cavernosum, 255ff
skin disorders and, 255ff
hematocrit. The per cent of the blood volume occupied by the red cells when closely packed, the normal content being generally around 45%. 195
hematological, (adjective). Pertaining to the blood.
blood tests, 195
hematology. The science which deals with the blood and its diseases.
hematoma. A swelling or tumor filled with blood.
auricle, 589
breast, 550
headaches and, 406
hematuria
bladder cancer and, 493
kidney cancer and, 489
kidney stones and, 486
hemianopsia
brain tumor and, 410
hemicorporectomy patient, *325*
hemoglobin. A protein substance that constitutes the coloring matter of the red blood corpuscles, and has the chemical property of combining with and releasing oxygen. 90ff, 177
iron deficiencies and, 657
oxygen and, 90ff, 126
respiration and, 90ff, 126
sickle-cell anemia and, 180
skin color and, 231
hemolysis. The destruction of red blood cells and the resultant release of hemoglobin.
hemolytic anemia, 179ff
jaundice and, 179
hemolytic disease
Rh blood groups and, 193
hemolytic streptococci, *220*
hemophilia. A hereditary blood condition in which the blood fails to coagulate; an abnormal tendency to bleed. Transmitted by females, but occurs in severe form only in males. 183ff
pedigree of, *7*
sex-linked inheritance and, 6
Hemophilus. A genus of bacteria which cause hemolytic infections.
ducreyi, 520
influenzae, 155
pertussis, 76
hemorrhage. Bleeding; escape of blood from the vessels.
atomic casualties first aid, 864
blood transfusion and, 179
hemorrhagic bronchopneumonia
bacterial embolus and, 218
hemorrhagic diseases
blood disorders and, 184
hemorrhagic effusion. An outpouring of bloody fluid,

usually into the pleural space. 161
hemorrhoids, *472*
anal disorders and, 473
anal pruritus and, 473
constipation and, 466
varicose veins and, 206
hemothorax. A collection of blood in the pleural cavity.
chest injuries and, 172
decortication and, 172
empyema and, 172
fibrothorax and, 172
organized, 172
hemotoxins, 717
hemp, *134*
Henle's loop. The U-shaped portion of the uriniferous tubule of the kidney.
ascending portion of, 483
descending portion of, 483
heparin. An anticoagulant substance found normally in the liver and other tissues, commonly used in blood transfusions to inhibit clotting.
coronary thrombosis and, 216
hepatic artery, 201
hepatic ducts. Two bile ducts leading from the liver into the common bile duct. 441
hepatic vein
vena cava and, 201
hepatitis, infectious. An acute infectious disease of the liver, caused by a virus; causes jaundice, nausea, and vomiting. 110ff, 476
hepatotoxins, 717
hereditary diseases
baldness, 276ff
hereditary spastic paralysis. A rare hereditary disease manifested by a slow, progressive stiffness and paralysis of the legs. It usually begins around age 5 to 7 years.
heredity, 3
alleles and, 5
allergy and, 132
blood types and, 776
chromosomes and, 1ff
DNA and, 3ff
eye color and, 5
gene action and, 3
gene behavior and, 4
genes and, 1ff, 96
genetic counseling and, 7
genotype and, 4
germ cell division and, 2ff
mutation and, 4
pattern baldness, 276
phenotype and, 5
races and, 8
sex-influenced, 6
sex-linked, 6
single factor, 4
skin color and, 5, 7
heritable diseases
albinism, 257ff
allergy, 234
diabetes mellitus, 366
hemophilia, 183
muscular dystrophy, 315
nearsightedness, 571

nervous system and, 411
sickle-cell anemia, 180
hermaphrodite, *353*
hermaphroditism. A condition characterized by presence of both ovarian and testicular tissue.
adrenal gland and, 360
hernia. Abnormal protrusion of a part or organ through the containing wall of its cavity; applies usually to the abdominal cavity and implies a covering or sac over the protrusion.
acquired, 299
bladder disorders and, 491
congenital, 299
cryptorchism and, 506
diaphragm and, 175
diaphragmatic, 449
femoral, 299
hiatus, 449
incisional, 300
inguinal, 299
irreducible, 299
lung, 176
reducible, 299
traumatic diaphragmatic, 449
umbilical, 300
hernial ring, 299
heroin
drug abuse and, 616
hero-worship
adolescence and, 70
herpes diseases, 112
herpes simplex
dermatitis and, 243
dermatropic viruses and, 112
herpes zoster
dermatitis and, 244
dermatropic viruses and, 112
mouth disorders and, 444
heterografts
kidney transplantation and, 490
skin grafts and, 279
heterozygous (adjective). Pertaining to an individual in which the members of a given pair of genes are unlike. 5
hetrazan
elephantiasis and, 746
hexachlorophene
germicides and, 770
hiatus hernia, 449
hiccough
first aid for, 697
high blood pressure, 211ff
hypertension and, 212ff
strokes and, 396
high risk groups
breast cancer and, 551
hilus. A recess or depression in the kidney contour at the point where the renal artery and renal vein enter and leave the kidney. 482
hindbrain. The posterior portion of the brain of the embryo.
hip
congenital dislocation of, 294
degenerative arthritis of, 302
dislocation of, *293*
fractures, 297ff, 708
pelvis and, 285

hip-lift, back-pressure artificial respiration, *727*
Hippocratic Oath
medical history and, 798
physicians as witnesses and, 772
Hirschsprung's disease
colon distention and, 462
histamine. A substance occurring in the body wherever tissues are damaged. It stimulates visceral muscles, salivary, pancreatic, and gastric secretions, and dilates capillaries. Used in various allergies, as a diagnostic agent, and to contract the uterus. 234
histology. The science which deals with the study of the microscopic anatomy of tissues.
Histoplasma capsulatum, 122
histoplasmosis and, 122
hives, *235*
allergy and, 235
edema and, 235
hoarseness
laryngeal cancer and, 148
Hodgkin's disease, 188ff
radiotherapy for, *187*
x-ray appearance of, *187*
Hodson Community Center
aged and, 648
homatropine. A hydrobromide or hydrochloride of a synthetic alkaloid which has the same dilatory action as atropine. 572
home
accidents, 731
aged and, 651ff
canning, 755
fire fighting, 865ff
nurse, 674
protection, 862ff
shelters, 858ff
home care
advantages of, 673
aged patient and, 686
atmosphere and, 674
bathing and, 678
bed and, 676ff
bed making and, 682ff
bed rest equipment and, 677
chicken pox, 72
children and, 685
chronic illness and, 686
communicable diseases and, 684ff
daily routine of, 677ff
diabetic patient and, 686
douches and, 679ff
enemas and, 679ff
feeding and, 684
grooming and, 678
heart disease and, 686
measles and, 73
medication and, 678ff
mumps, 75
nursing facilities and, 688ff
occupational therapy and, 687
patient records and, 684
physical care and, 678ff
pulse and, 680ff
recreational facilities and, 687
rehabilitation and, 686ff
respiration and, 680ff

sanitary procedures and, 681ff
scarlet fever, 74
sickroom and, 675ff
steam tent and, 680ff
temperature and, 680ff
tonsilitis, 77ff
tuberculosis and, 685
whooping cough, 76
homicide
medicolegal aspects of, 781ff
homografts
skin grafts and, 279
kidney transplantation and, 490
homosexuality. A form of sexual deviation in which the sexual interest is directed toward persons of the same sex. 538ff, 615
homozygous (adjective). Pertaining to an individual in which the members of a given pair of genes are alike. 4
hookworm. Any of the nematodes belonging to the family *Strongyloides,* particularly *Ancylostoma duodenale* and *Necator americanus,* which are intestinal parasites in man. *251*
dermatitis and, 251
life cycle of, 122
roundworms and, 122
hordeolum. Inflammation of a sebaceous gland of the eyelid; stye or sty. 561.
hormone. A chemical substance which is secreted by the ductless glands into the blood and conveyed to another part of the body, upon which it exerts a regulatory effect.
adrenal cortex and, 358ff
adrenalin, 94, 358
aldosterone, 359
blood and, 177
cancer and, 644
endocrine glands and, 94ff
endocrine system and, 328ff
hydrocortisone, 359
hypothalamic, 337
lactation and, 547
manager, 328
messenger, 328
nonendocrine tumors and, 329
pituitary, 95
placenta and, 15, 22, 329
pregnancy and, 22ff
reproductive, 8
therapy for breast cancer, 554ff
hospital, *886*
administrator, 830
admission to, 831ff
atomic warfare and, 865
care, 673
components of, 829ff
costs, 830ff
facilities, *887ff*
medicaid and, 831
medical profession and, 828ff
medicare and, 831
national health insurance and, 831
professions in, 830

types of, 829
weight control and, 667
host
-virus relationship, 106ff
hourglass bladder, *493*
house fly, *756ff*
human-animal growth rates
relative, 70
human flea, *251*
human louse, *763*
human milk
composition of, 547
humerus. The bone of the upper arm from the shoulder to the elbow. 285
fracture of, *294*
humoral antibodies
reticuloendothelial system and, 191
humoral pathology, 799
humpback
chronic osteomyelitis and, 311
hunger
infant crying and, 44
stomach and, 443
Huntington's chorea. A chronic progressive, hereditary disease characterized by irregular movements, speech disturbance, and mental deterioration.
dominant allele and, 5
hyaline cartilage, *82*
hyaline membrane disease, 52
hyaluronidase. An enzyme which increases permeability of connective tissue.
hydration. The addition of water; or the property of acquiring or containing water. 654
hydrocele. A collection of serous fluid within the tunica vaginalis or other structures of the testes. *299*
cryptorchism and, 506
hydrocephalus. A condition characterized by abnormally large amounts of cerebrospinal fluid around or within the brain, usually associated with enlargement of the cerebral ventricles. 383
meningitis and, 390
hydrochloric acid. *Hydrogen chloride,* a dilute form of which is normally present in the stomach.
digestion and, 442
oxyntic cells and, 442
peptic ulcers and, 452
hydrocortisone
ACTH and, 333
adrenal cortex and, 359
disease treated by, 359
hydrogen. The lightest known gaseous element, occurring naturally in water and many organic compounds. (Symbol, H).
hydronephrosis. An abnormal collection of urine in the kidney pelvis caused by an obstruction of the ureter. 493
urine obstruction and, 487

hydrophobia
animal bites and, 703
rabies or, 391
hydrotherapy. Treatment of patients by use of external application of water. 833
hygiene
acne vulgaris and, 260
athlete's foot and, 265
breast feeding and, 35
chicken pox and, 72
communicable diseases and, 684ff
diabetes mellitus and, 369ff
food poisoning and, 457
infant feeding and, 45
measles, 73
new mother and, 35ff
pink-eye and, 561
poliomyelitis and, 386
pregnancy and, 19ff
premature baldness and, 276
puerperal sepsis and, 32
ringworm and, 263
sex and, 539ff
sickroom and, 675
spinal cord injury and, 399
tuberculosis patients and, 685
hymen. A membrane partially blocking the opening of the vagina. *502, 503*
virginity and, 503, 528
Hymenolepis. A genus of tapeworms, many of which are parasitic to man.
hyperemia
allergy and, 235
hyperfunctioning adenoma. A form of nodular goiter; characterized by production of large quantities of thyroid hormone. 343
hyperinsulinism. A condition resulting from excessive production of insulin by the pancreas, causing intermittent or continuous loss of consciousness; *insulin shock.* 365
hyperopia. A defect in refraction of light into the eye which diminishes ability to see at close range; *farsightedness, hypermetropia.*
hyperplasia
intraductal papillary, 549
hypersexuality, 537ff
hypertension. The condition of abnormally elevated blood pressure.
aged and, 641
blood pressure and, 212
circulation disorders and, 212ff
essential, 212
high blood pressure or, 212ff
renal, 213
symptoms of, 213
treatment for, 213
hyperthyroidism. A condition of overactivity of the thyroid gland. See also **osteitis fibrosa cystica.**
hypertrophy
benign breast disorders and, 549
gravid, 549
infantile, 549

virginal, 549
hypertropic chronic pharyngitis, 144
hypervitaminosis
vitamin A and, 659
hypnosis. A trancelike state resembling sleep, induced by means of verbal suggestion or intense concentration on some object. Hypnosis is characterized by the subject's extreme responsiveness to suggestions made by the hypnotist.
neuroses and, 609ff
hypocalcification. Lack of normal deposition of calcium within the tissues of the body.
teeth and, 426
hypochondria, *622*
hypochromic anemia, 179
hypogonadism
male hormone and, 351
hypomanics
cycloid personality and, 620
hypomastia. Abnormal smallness of the breasts. 548
hypoparathyroidism. Deficient functioning of the parathyroids. 349
hypophysis, *331*
pituitary gland or, 330
hypoplasia. Defective or insufficient development of any tissue.
teeth and, 427
hypoprothrombinemia. Lack of adequate amounts of prothrombin in the blood resulting in tendency to hemorrhage from impairment of the clotting mechanism.
vitamin K deficiencies and, 664
hyposexuality, 537ff
hypospadias. The condition wherein the urinary meatus opens on the undersurface of the penis posterior to the glans. *495*
hypostome. A rodlike organ arising at the base of the beak of certain mites and ticks; in some of these it is armed with teeth that serve to retain it in the skin of the host. 766
hypotension. Blood pressure below the normal range.
Bright's disease and, 488
essential, 214
low blood pressure, 214
orthostatic, 214
postural, 214
hypothalamus, 378
dystrophia adiposogenitalis, 336
endocrine glands and, 336ff
endocrine-nervous system interaction and, 329
endocrine system and, 329
Fröhlich's syndrome and, 336
hormones of, 337
nervous system and, 329
pituitary and, 334
releasing factors of, 337

hypothyroidism. A condition in which there is an insufficient amount of secretion from the thyroid glands. 345ff

hypotrichosis. A congenital form of baldness. See **alopecia congenitalis.** 276

hysterectomy. Total or partial removal of the uterus.

hysteria. A conversion reaction characterized by loss of normal control of bodily or emotional function without structural disease of the nervous system; caused by unconscious emotional conflict. 610

first aid for, 697
general, 697

ice bag, *678*
idea to action, *99*
identical twins, 23
character inheritance and, 7
fertilization and, 500

identification. The mental process by which an individual imagines himself in the role of another personality; this may be conscious or unconscious.
medicolegal aspects of, 774ff
mind and, 598

idiopathic (adjective). Of unknown cause.
epilepsy, 392
hypochromic anemia, 180
scoliosis, 315

idiot. An individual with a congenital form of feeblemindedness, in which the mental age remains less than three years.

idle thought
mind and, 597

ileocecal valve. The valve located at the junction of the ileum and cecum which prevents reflux from the cecum. 438

ileum. The lower portion of the small intestine, extending from the jejunum to the large intestine. 438

iliac crest. The upper border of ilium.

iliolumbar ligaments
low back pain and, 310

illness
infants and, 48ff

illuminated endoscope
fetology and, 16

imbecile. An individual with deficient mental development, in which the mental age remains between three and seven years and the intelligence quotient ranges between 20 and 49.

immediate postoperative prostheses
artificial replacements and, 318

immune reaction
organ transplantation and, 490
vaccination and, 262

immune system
thymus and, 361ff

immunity. The state of being resistant to attack from a specific disease organism.
active, 101
allergy and, 234
antibodies and, 101
antigen and, 101
bacterial disease resistance and, 120
disease barriers and, 101
influenza and, 154ff
natural, 101
passive, 101
placenta and, 636
tuberculosis and, 162
viral diseases and, 107ff

immunization. The process of rendering an individual resistant to a specific disease organism, by the formation of antibodies.
diphtheria, 77
infant illness and, 48
viral diseases and, 111
whooping cough, 76

immunization route
viruses and, 110

immunological blood tests, 194ff
immunological pregnancy tests, 19

imperforate (adjective). Without the normal opening.
anus, 472
hymen, 503
urethra, 493

impetigo. A contagious inflammation of the skin characterized by blisters which rupture and become encrusted. *245*
chicken pox and, 72
dermatitis and, 246
neonatorum, 246

implantation. The embedding of the human embryo into the uterine wall, usually about the tenth day of its growth. 11

impotence
emotional, 536
marriage and, 536ff
onset of, *529*
sex and, 536ff

inadequate personality, 619ff
incision
snake bite first aid and, 721

incisional hernias, 300

incisor. One of the four front teeth of either jaw having sharp or cutting edges.

inclusion body. A small particle which is formed within a body cell in the presence of viral infection. 106

inclusion conjunctivitis
chlamydia and, 114

inclusion cyst. A cyst caused by embryonal or traumatic implantation of epithelium.
vaginal tumors and, 515

incontinence. 1. Inability to control the excretion of feces or urine. 2. Lack of sexual restraint.
epispadias and, 495

hydronephrosis and, 493
prolapse and, 511
urethra and, 493
urination disturbances and, 496

incubation period. Interval between exposure to infection and the appearance of the first symptom.
chicken pox and, 71
gonorrhea and, 517

incubator. Apparatus in which the temperature can be regulated; used primarily in the care of premature babies. *39, 41*
air-lock, *40*
eighteenth century, *42*
infant feeding and, *41*
premature infant and, 37ff

incus
middle ear and, 581

independent assortment. The chance assorting of genes in chromosome transmission.
genetic action and, 4

India rubber skin
myxedema and, 253

indigestion. Imperfect or incomplete digestion. 450ff

industrial diseases
keratitis, 563
lead poisoning and, 169
primary irritant dermatitis and, 252
respiratory disorders and, 169ff
silicosis and, 169

industrial medicine
space medicine and, 878

industrial nurse, 827

industrial training
deaf and, 595

industrial wastes
water pollution and, 754

industry
childhood and, 602
radioisotopes and, 874ff

infancy
mind and, 599ff

infant
bathing, 48
cerebral palsy and, 395
circumcision and, 46ff
clothing and, 48
colds and, 49
colic and, 49ff
convulsions and, 49
croup and, 49
deaths, *44, 890*
dental development of, 43
diet, 670
feeding of, *41, 44,* 50
fever and, 49
growth, 43
hyaline membrane disease, 52
illnesses of, 48ff
impetigo neonatorum, 246
iron-deficiency anemia and, 180
learning and, 43ff
mental growth of, *51*
mortality in U.S., 50ff
secondary hair and, 232
sleep and, 45
weight gain, *44*

kidney. One of a pair of bean-shaped organs located in the lateral areas of the abdominal cavity; these organs aid in regulating the concentration of various blood constituents by removing water and certain waste products in the form of urine. *92*
artificial, 489ff
congenital abnormalities of, 485ff
cross-section of, *483*
scans, 871ff
transplantation, 490
urinary system and, 482ff
kidney disorders, 485ff
artificial kidney and, 489ff
Bright's disease, 488
cysts, 489
infection, 487ff
kidney transplantation and, 490
malfunction, 219
noninfectious diseases of, 488
obstruction, 487
physiological albuminuria, 488ff
stones, 486
tuberculosis, 488
tumors, 489
kidney failure
diabetes mellitus and, 368
kidney perforation
tympanic membrane and, *588*
kind treatment
insane and, *625*
kinesiology. The study of muscular movements, especially the therapeutic aspect of muscular movements.
muscle contraction and, 286ff
kings
healing powers of, *302*
king's touch
curative powers of, *163*
kissing bug
Chagas' disease and, 748
Klebsiella. A genus of bacteria associated with infections of the respiratory tract and other body organs.
Klebs-Loeffler bacillus. The microorganism causing diphtheria; *Corynebacterium diphtheriae*. 145
Klinefelter's syndrome
hypogonadism and, 351
sex chromosomes and, 3
knee
degenerative arthritis of, 301
joints and, 285
knee derangements
internal, 294
Koch-Weeks bacillus. The causative organism of one form of conjunctivitis or "pink-eye."
Kolmer test, 195
syphilis, 195
Koplik's spots. Eruptions occurring in measles, having the appearance of small raised white nodules surrounded by a flat area of reddened mucous membrane

and found opposite the molars in the cheek. 73
kraurosis penis
skin cancer and, 268
kraurosis vulvae
skin cancer and, 268
Kwarshiorkor
protein deficiency and, 747
kyphosis. A pronounced outward curvature of the spine; humpback or hunchback.
chronic osteomyelitis and, 311

labia majora, 503
labia minora, 504
labor. The physiological process by which the child is expelled from the uterus; *childbirth.*
amnion rupture and, 24
birth and, 24ff
complications of, 31ff
contractions, 25
ergot mold and, *23*
forceps and, 26ff
hypothalamic hormones and, 337
inducement of, 25
natural childbirth and, 25ff
oxytocin and, 25, 337
second stage of, 25
signs of, 24ff
stages of, *24*
uterus and, *23*
labyrinth. Any intricate communicating network of passages.
laceration
brain injury and, 414
breast, 550
first aid for, 702
lacrimal (adjective). Pertaining to the tears, or the secretion of tears.
apparatus, 562
lacrimal duct, 558
lactase. An enzyme found in the body which hydrolyzes lactose to dextrose and galactose.
lactation. The function of secreting milk by the mammary glands.
breast and, 547
hormones and, 547
mammary glands and, 22
postbirth breast changes and, 34
lacteal. One of the lymph vessels connected to the intestines. Most of the fat used in the body passes through these vessels. 199
lactic acid. A colorless, syrupy acid found in muscle tissue as a waste product of sugar oxidation; it causes a feeling of fatigue.
liver and, 475
muscle contraction and, 286
lactiferous duct
breast and, 545
nipple and, 545
lactiferous sinus, 545
lactose. Milk-sugar, the sugar found in the milk of mammals, and occasionally in

the urine of nursing women.
Laennec's cirrhosis, *476*
Lamaze method
natural childbirth, 26
lamellated bone, 280
lanugo. The downy covering of hair over the fetus. 231
premature infant and, 37
lap belt
traffic accidents and, 731
large intestine, 438
large intestine disorders
constipation and, 465ff
diarrhea, 464ff
distention, 461ff
irritable bowel, 462ff
parasites, 467ff
tumor, 467
larva (plural, larvae). An early stage in the life cycle of various lower animals. 758
larva migrans. A skin disorder characterized by inflamed linear eruptions, formed by burrowings of the larval form of parasitic nematodes.
laryngeal cancer
symptoms of, 148
treatment for, 148ff
laryngeal pharynx, 129
laryngectomy patients
laryngeal cancer and, 148
speech class for, *150*
laryngitis. Inflammation of the larynx. 449
chronic, 146ff
chronic hypertrophic, 147
edematous, 147
myasthenic, 147
respiratory disorders and, 146ff
laryngopharynx. That area of the pharynx located between the oropharynx and the cricoid cartilage of the larynx.
laryngoscope. An instrument for visual examination of the larynx. See also **endoscope.** *147*
nineteenth century, *148*
vocal cords and, *132*
larynx. A cartilaginous organ of the throat which contains the vocal cords and produces most of the sound in phonation; the voice-box. *128*
artificial, 149
communication and, 100
foreign bodies in, 705
lasers
retinal detachment and, 566ff
latent consciousness, 596
latent period
rheumatic fever and, 220
latent phase
diabetes mellitus and, 366
lateral (adjective). Pertaining to the side; at or belonging to the side.
lateral incisors
infants and, 43
lateral semicircular canals, 583
late summer pollens
geographic incidence of, *137*
latex. A rubberlike substance used in making prostheses

and many commercial products.

facial reconstruction and, 321

law
medicine and, 771ff
patient and, 771
physician and, 771

law of contracts
physician-patient relationship and, 772

laxatives
irritable bowel habits and, 463

lazy eye
strabismus and, 568

Leach-Nyham syndrome
gout and, 307

lead. A metallic element, compounds of which are poisonous. (Symbol, Pb).

lead poisoning
paint and, 718

learning
infants and, 43ff

leather
artificial limbs and, 317
clothing, *770*
dermatitis and, *237*

left flexure
large intestine and, 438

leg
artificial replacements for, 318
amputation, *318*
bones, 285
muscles, *98*
veins, *209*

legal contracts
physician-patient relationship and, 772

legal permission
autopsy and, 773ff
surgical treatment and, 773

legalized abortion, 784

Legg-Calve-Perthes disease
osteochondritis and, 312

Leishman-Donovan body. One of the small oval bodies found in the spleen and liver of patients with kala-azar. These bodies are the intracellular forms of the protozoan *Leishmania.*

Leishmania. A genus of protozoa, many species of which cause disease in man, transmitted by *Phlebotomus* flies.

Chagas' disease and, 748
espundia and, 749
kala-azar and, 749
oriental sore and, 749

leishmaniasis, 737

leiomyoma (plural, leiomyomata). A benign fibroid tumor of muscle tissue origin, especially of the uterus.
benign skin tumors and, 254
uterine tumors and, 512

lens. 1. The crystalline lens of the eye. 2. A transparent refracting medium of glass. 100, 559
farsightedness and, 570
nearsightedness and, 570
disorders, 565

leopard frog
pregnancy test and, *534*

lepromatous leprosy, 736

leprosy. A chronic, infectious disease characterized by lesions on the skin which cause mutilations; the disease is produced by *Mycobacterium leprae; Hansen's disease. 736*
claw hand and, *736*
cutaneous nodular, 736
diagnosis of, 736
lepromatous, 736
maculo-anesthetic, 736
microorganisms and, 735ff
treatment for, 736ff
tuberculoid, 736
types of, 736

Leptospira icterohaemorrhagiae. The species of bacteria which causes leptospiral jaundice or *Weil's disease.* 747

Leptotrichia buccalis. An organism normally found in the oral cavity.

lesser curvature. The inner curved surface of the stomach. 437

Letterer-Siwe's disease, 191, 312

leucocyte. A white blood corpuscle; a nonpigmented cell present in blood and lymph. The leucocytes act as scavengers and aid in resisting infection.
lymph and, 77
plasma and, 77

leucorrhea
pregnancy and, 21

leukemia. A malignant condition marked by increased numbers of circulating leucocytes. 184ff, *185*
chemotherapy for, 188
Philadelphia chromosome and, *186*
radiation injury and, 851
radiophosporus and, 873
radiotherapy for, 188
signs of, 185ff
symptoms of, 185ff
treatment for, 187ff
viruses and, 113

leukoderma, 258

leukonychia. White spots appearing on the nails. 275

leukopenia. A condition characterized by a decreased number of white blood cells in the peripheral blood.

leukoplakia. Irregular white patches on the mucous membranes which are considered to be precancerous lesions. *268*
mouth disorders and, 444
skin cancer and, 268
tongue cancer and, 446
vulva and, 515ff

leukorrhea. A whitish mucous discharge from the cervical canal or vagina.
irregular menstruation and, 516

levels of consciousness, 596

lever
body movement and, *97*

lice
control of, 762ff
dermatitis and, 250
pediculosis and, 250

licensing
physician, 771ff

lichen planus. An inflammatory skin disease of uncertain etiology, characterized by eruptions of skin papules; may be either acute or chronic. 254

lie detector, *786*
criminology and, 786ff
recording, *787*

life
beginning of, 1
expectancy, *650*

life fuel
nutrition and, 83ff

life insurance
medicolegal aspects of, 791ff

life island
infection and, *830*

life-saving
fires and, 728
floods and, 729

life span
aging and, *638*

life-support
space medicine and, 878
zero gravity and, 882

ligament. A fibrous band of tissue which connects bones or supports organs.
dislocations and, 711
joints and, 285
sprains and, 291, 711

ligament of Cooper. Bands of fibrous tissue which connect the external capsule of the mammary gland to the skin. 545

ligamentum flavum
low back pain and, 310

ligation
varicose veins and, *209*

ligature. 1. The thread used in surgery for tying vessels. 2. The operation of tying vessels.

light
allergy, 239
eye fatigue and, 570
sickroom and, 675
vitamin A deficiency and, *660*

light irradiation
space medicine and, 880

limb fracture
do nots, 711
dos, 711

limbs
muscles of, *288*

lime deposits
middle ear infection and, 587

linear nevus, 255

lingual tonsil. One of a pair of lymphatic tissue masses located at the base of the tongue. 77

lipases
digestion and, 87

lip cancer, 446

lipoid granulomatosis, 191

lipoid histiocytosis, 191

lipoma
benign skin tumors and, 254

liposarcoma, *644*

litholapaxy. The surgical procedure whereby a stone in the urinary bladder is crushed and then removed by irrigation. 493

lithotrite. An instrument for crushing stones in the urinary bladder. 493

liver. The largest organ in the body, consisting of four lobes and located in the upper abdominal cavity; its functions are multiple, including the secretion of bile for digestion, the breakdown of proteins into simpler compounds, the storage of blood sugar and fat, the maintenance of chemical levels within the blood, and the clearing of foreign matter from the blood. 41, *438, 440*

atrophy, 477
blood and, 201
cancer, *477*
cirrhosis, 477
Clonorchis and, 124
diabetes mellitus and, 365ff
disease, *476*
disorders, 475ff
flukes and, 124
function tests, 475ff
glucose and, 364
hepatic artery and, 201
jaundice, 476ff
location of, *439*
macrocytic anemia and, 181ff
scans, 871

living tissue, 1

Loa loa. An infection of the conjunctiva or subcutaneous tissues of the body, caused by a roundworm belonging to a subgenus of Filariae. 123.

lobar bronchi, 131

lobar pneumonia
x-ray appearance of, *158*

lobe. A round-shaped part or projection of an organ, separated from adjacent structures by fissures or constrictions.
breast, 545

local health departments, 835

localized suppuration, 165

lochia
postbirth uterine changes and, 34

locked back syndrome, 310

lockjaw, 388ff
prevention of, 388ff
puncture wounds and, 702
symptoms of, 388
treatment for, 389

Loeffler's syndrome. A condition characterized by infiltration of the lungs by an increased number of eosinophilic leucocytes; also called *Loeffler's eosinophilia.* 175

lonely personality, 620

long bones, 281

long-distance transfer, 694

looped fingerprint, 777

louse. An animal parasite which infests hairy parts of the body.
body, *250*
human, *763*

louse control
typhus fever and, 745

low back pain, 308
intervertebral disc syndrome and, 309
lumbosacral syndrome and, 308ff
sacroiliac syndrome, 309ff
sciatica, 307ff
skeletal disorders and, 307ff
slipped vertebra and, 309
treatment for, 310

low blood pressure, 221ff

lower leg fracture
first aid for, 708ff

lower lip cancer, 446

LSD
drug abuse and, 618
hallucinogens and, 618

lumbago. An aching in the lower back region.
low back pain and, 310
lumbosacral syndrome and, 309

lumbar vertebrae, 282

lump
breast cancer and, 551ff

lung. One of a pair of cone-shaped, spongy organs of respiration located in the chest cavity; concerned with the interchange of oxygen and carbon dioxide in the blood. *91, 131*
abscess of, 165ff
cancer, 166ff, *167*
carcinoma, *167*
child and, 52
differentiation of, 13
exercise function of, 131ff
foreign bodies in, 705ff
respiration and, 90ff, 126
scans, 871
transplantation, 168ff
tumor, *168, 175ff*
volatile wastes and, 92

lung fungus diseases, 170ff
actinomycosis, 170
blastomycosis, 170
coccidioidosis, 170
moniliasis, 170

lung with metal bolt
x-ray appearance of, *152*

lung with nail
x-ray appearance of, *152*

lunula, 233

lupus erythematosus. Usually a chronic, but at times an acute, disease of the skin marked by the appearance of red, scaly patches of various sizes and configuration which induce atrophy and scar formation. The acute form may be fatal. 254

luteinizing hormone
amino-acid sequencing of, 8

lymph. An alkaline fluid of the body, contained in the lymphatic vessels; it differs from blood in that it is

more diluted and contains no red blood corpuscles. 87
leucocytes and, 77
plasma and, 178
stratum mucosum and, 231
tonsils and, 77

lymphadenitis. Inflammation of the lymph glands.
elephantiasis and, 746

lymphangiography
cancer and, 643

lymphatic system, 199
plasma and, 178
tonsils and, 77
vessels, *199*

lymph channels
elephantiasis and, 746

lymph duct
tissue fluid and, 199

lymph nodes, *199*
head and neck, *199*
infection and, 199
lymphocytic leukemia and, 185
plasma and, 178
tonsils and, 77

lymphocytes. A white blood cell which originates in the reticular tissue of the lymphatic system. 178
thymosin and, 362

lymphocytic leukemia, 185

lymphogranuloma venereum, 520ff
chlamydia and, 114

lymphoma, *187*
x-ray appearance of, *186*

lymphosarcoma. A malignant neoplasm of the lymphatic system. 188ff
stomach ulcer and, *452*

lymph vessels
lacteals and, 199

lysosomes
cytoplasm and, 80

macerated bone
transverse cut of, *82*

maceration. A softening and sloughing away of tissue.

machine
body and, 79ff

macrocytic anemia, 179
bone marrow and, 181

macule. A discolored spot on the skin, nonelevated and nondepressed, of various colors, sizes and shapes.
chicken pox and, 71

maculo-anesthetic leprosy, 736

madura foot. A disease caused by a variety of parasitic molds, affecting usually the feet. Also called *mycetoma, maduromycosis.* 737, 748

maduromycosis. A tropical fungus disease common among persons who go barefooted.
fungi and, 122

magic
disease and, 796

magnesium. A white mineral element found in soft tissue, muscles, bones and, in minute amounts, in the body fluids. (Symbol, Mg).

magnesium oxide
universal antidote and, 718

major calyces, 482
major fractures
moving, 694
malaise. Discomfort, a feeling of generalized illness.
malaria. An infectious disease caused by the *Plasmodium* parasite, transmitted by the bite of the *Anopheles* mosquito. 761ff
antimalarial drugs for, 739ff
benign tertian, 738
chills, 738ff
chloroquine-resistant, 740
complications of, 739
deaths from, *740*
distribution of, *759*
falciparum, 738
fever and, 738ff
malignant tertian, 738
medical history and, 812
microorganisms and, 737ff
mosquito control and, 761ff
parasite life cycle, 738
protozoan disease and, 121
relapses of, 739
research on, 741ff
sporozoa and, 121
suppressive drugs for, 739ff
malaria research
mosquitos and, *741*
malathion
fly control, 758
male breast cancer, 552
male gonads
testes, 350ff
male reproductive system, 498ff
malignant (adjective). That which threatens life; having a tendency to become progressively worse.
malignant melanoma, *269*
eye tumors and, 569
moles and, 254
skin cancer and, 268
treatment for, 271
malignant tertian malaria, 738
malignant tumors
large bowel, 467
Malleomyces mallei, *248*
malleus
middle ear and, 581
malnutrition. A condition associated with a deficiency of the body's essential food requirements, or their improper assimilation and distribution.
aging and, 637
dermatitis and, 252
yaws and, 737
malocclusion. An abnormality of closure of the upper and lower teeth, usually associated with abnormal development of the jaws. *422, 423*
finger sucking and, *425*
jaw and, 422ff
teeth and, 422ff
maltose
ptyalin and, 437
mammalian (adjective). Pertaining to the highest order (*mammalia*) of vertebrate animals, including man, that nourish their young with milk.

mammary cancer
menopause and, *553*
mammary gland. One of the glands in the breast which secretes milk; in the male the mammary glands are normally nonfunctioning. 544
estrogen and, 22
lactation and, 22
mammitis
mumps and, 75
mammogram
breast cancer and, 642
breast carcinoma and, *553*
manager hormones, 328
mandible
facial bones and, 285
infant and, 42
malocclusion and, 422
manganese
trace elements and, 657ff
manic-depressive psychosis. A form of mental disorder characterized by alternating moods of depression and elation with characteristic changes in physical activity. *Mania* is the psychosis characterized by exhilaration and overactivity; *hypomania* is the less intense form, and *hypermania,* the more acute reaction. 625ff
manners
child and, 54ff
man-of-war
first aid for, 704
manometer. Any instrument that measures the pressure of liquids or gases.
blood pressure and, 199ff
Marie's ataxia. A disease the symptoms of which include muscular incoordination, and speech and eye disturbances. It is an hereditary disease of early adult life.
Marie-Strumpell disease
rheumatoid spondylitis and, 312
marijuana
drug abuse and, 618
Marijuana Tax Act
drug abuse and, 789
marriage
birth control and, 535ff
family forms and, 522ff
frigidity and, 537
genetic aspects of, 525
impotence and, 536ff
number of, *530*
sex and, 522ff
sexual activity and, 528ff
sexual drive and, 525
sterility and, 532ff
marriage ceremony, 523
marriage legal requirements, *524*
marrow. A vascular, soft tissue filling the cavities of most bones. *178, 281*
Mars environment
space medicine and, 880ff
Marshall Islands
radiation sickness and, 853
massage
home care and, 678

mass reflex
spinal cord injury and, 398
mastectomy
patient, *324*
simple, *554*
mastication. The process of chewing. 421
mastitis. Inflammation of the breasts, occurring most commonly during lactation; *mammitis.*
acute puerperal, 548
chronic, 548
chronic cystic, 548
chronic interstitial, 548
postbirth breast changes and, 34
traumatic, 548
mastodynia. Pain in the breasts. 548
mastoid. 1. A nipple-shaped process of the irregular bone at the side and base of the skull directly behind the ear and encasing the hearing organs. 2. Nipple-shaped. 586ff
mastoid antrum, 581
mastoidectomy, 587
mastoiditis. Inflammation of the mastoid process.
acute, 586
chronic, 586
middle ear and, 581
masturbation. Self-stimulation of the genital area.
puberty and, 65ff
matriarchal family, 522
matrix. The intercellular substance of a tissue.
bone and, 280
skeletal muscles and, 286
matter interconvertibility
atomic bomb and, 843
maturation. The process of maturing or ripening of the germ cells which includes exchange of genes and reduction of chromosomes to half their original number.
adolescent and, 70ff
fetal, 16
germ cell, 3
mature personality, 605
maxilla
facial bones and, 285
infant and, 42
malocclusion and, 422
maxillary sinus, 127
anatomy of, 141
McNaughton rules
criminally insane and, 785ff
meals
rest and, 639
measles. A contagious disease characterized by catarrhal symptoms and a red skin rash; caused by a virus.
childhood disease and, 72
complications of, 73
deaths from, *73*
dermatropic viruses and, 112
infant deaths from, *49*
symptoms of, 73
transmission of, 73
measles pneumonia, 159
meatotomy. Surgical enlargement

of the opening of the meatus.

meatus. A passage or opening.
abnormalities of, 495ff
urethra and, 485

mechanical hands
problems of, 319

mechanical obstruction
artificial respiration and, 722ff

Meckel's diverticulum
small intestine and, 459

Medex
physicians' helpers and, 824

media. 1. The middle layer of an artery. 2. A nutrient substance upon which bacteria are cultivated.
arteriosclerosis and, 203

medial (adjective). 1. Pertaining to the middle. 2. Internal.

median (adjective). Central, or middle.

mediastinitis Inflammation of the mediastinum. 174

mediastinum The partition in the middle of the chest between the two pleural cavities.
open chest wounds and, 173

medicaid
aging and, 651
hospital and, 831
schedule of benefits of, 651

medical aid
first aid and, 691

medical corps personnel
Medex and, 824

medical education
doctors and, 823
medical history and, 804

medical history
early, 796ff
eighteenth century, 804ff
Greek, 797ff
medieval, 799ff
Mohammedan, 799
nineteenth century, 807ff
primitive, 796
Renaissance, 800ff
Roman, 798ff
seventeenth century, 802ff
twentieth century, 812ff

medical organizations
doctor and, 825ff

medical profession
dentist, 837ff
doctor and, 822ff
drug industry and, 833ff
health organizations and, 835ff
hospital and, 828ff
nurse, 826ff
occupational therapists, 833
pharmacist, 833
physical therapists, 833
practical nurse, 828
technologists, 832

medical radioisotopes, 870ff
physiological function studies and, 871
radionuclide imaging procedures and, 871ff
therapy with, 872ff

medical schools
number of, *829*
doctor and, *823ff*

medical service
medical history and, 805

medical tag
first aid and, 691

medical technologists
procedures performed by, 832
schools for, 831

medical treatment
psychosomatic disorders and, 611

medical universities
medical history and, 800

medicare
aging and, 649ff
home care and, 689
hospital and, 831
schedule of benefits, 649

medication
home care and, 678ff

medicine. 1. A substance used in treating the ill. 2. The science and art of treating the ill.
law and, 771ff
pouring of, *678*
radioactive isotopes and, 870ff
space, 877ff
time of dosage, *674*

medicolegal (adjective). Relating to medical jurisprudence or forensic medicine; aspects of medicine which have legal implications.

medicolegal aspects
abortion, 784
accidental death, 781ff
civil rights, 789ff
criminology, 784ff
drug abuse and, 789
federal, 794
homicide, 781ff
legislation, 794ff
life insurance, 791ff
mental illness, 792ff
notifiable diseases, 795
organ transplantation and, 794ff
poisoning, 782ff
rape, 784
suicide, 781ff
vital statistics and, 795
workmen's compensation, 791
wounding, 781

medicolegal identification
disputed parentage and, 776ff
fingerprints and, 777ff
hair and, 778ff

medieval times
medical history of, 799ff

medulla. 1. Bone marrow. 2. Any structure resembling marrow in composition or relation to other parts. 3. The central portion of an organ.
Henle's loop and, 483
kidneys and, 482

medulla oblongata. A part of the brain which is continuous below with the spinal cord and above with other sections of the brain. 377

megacolon. Abnormally large colon caused by reduction in or absence of mesenteric nerve supply; *Hirschsprung's disease.*

megaloureter. Abnormal enlargement of the ureter. 490

melancholia. A depression of mental condition characterized by despondency and apathy.

melanin. Black or dark brown pigments produced by metabolic activity; occurring naturally in the eye, skin, hair, heart muscle, and brain.
albinism and, 257
hair and, 232
melanocytes and, 229
skin and, 229
skin pigment and, 229
sunlight and, 231

melanocytes
albinism and, 257
melanin and, 229

melanoma
malignant, *260*

Melarsen B. An arsenical compound used therapeutically in trypanosomiasis. 748

melatonin, 362

melphalan
breast cancer and, *554*

membranous labyrinth, *582*
internal ear and, 583

memory protein, 634

memory RNA, 634

Ménière's syndrome, 588

meningeal acute miliary tuberculosis, 162ff

meninges. The covering membranes of the brain and spinal cord.

meningitis
encephalitis and, 389
nervous system disorders and, 390
pneumonia and, 160

meningoencephalitis. Inflammation of the brain and its membranes.
brain injury and, 415
mumps and, 76

menopause. The period which marks the permanent cessation of menstruation; the *climacteric.*
cervical cancer and, 516
chronic mastitis and, 548
female reproductive system and, 504ff
involutional melancholia and, 626
mammary cancer and, *553*
menstrual cycle and, 356ff
symptoms of, 357ff, 504

menorrhagea. Abnormally profuse menstrual bleeding.

menorrhalgia. Difficult or painful menstruation. 356

menstrual periods
adolescence and, 516
disorders of, 356
irregular bleeding, 516ff
irregular discharge, 516ff
menopause and, 356ff
ovaries and, 354ff
pain and, 356
pituitary gland and, 352
pregnancy and, 18
temperature variation and, *532*

mucous patches
syphilis and, 519
mucus. A secretion produced by the mucous gland.
chronic bronchitis and, 151
mulatto. The first generation offspring of pure white and pure negro parents.
multiple benign cystic epithelioma, 273
multiple-factor inheritance, 6ff
race and, 8
skin color and, 7ff
multiple handicapped
blind and, 578
multiple myeloma
blood disorders and, 189ff
multiple sclerosis. A chronic disease which may have remission of symptoms that include weakness, muscular incoordination, jerking movements of the legs and arms, speech disturbance, and involuntary movement of the eyes.
autoimmunity and, 412
nervous system and, 412
mumps. An acute, contagious, febrile disease, characterized by swelling of the parotid and other salivary glands; probably caused by a filterable virus. 75ff
complications of, 75ff
pneumotropic viruses and, 112
salivary glands and, 446
symptoms of, 75
transmission of, 75
municipal sewage disposal, 753ff
municipal water supply, 752
murine typhus, 744, 767
murmur
heart disease and, 202ff
mitral stenosis and, 203
patent ductus arteriosus and, 203
rheumatic fever and, 221
stethoscope and, 202ff
Musca domestica. The species to which the common housefly belongs. The housefly carries and transmits the causal agents of a number of diseases, including typhoid, dysentery, cholera, tuberculosis, and infantile diarrhea. *757*
control of, 756
muscle. Elastic connective tissue of three types; that composed of striped or striated fibers which is connected principally with the skeleton and designated *voluntary muscles;* that composed of smooth or unstriated fibers, designated *involuntary muscles,* which is not under control of the will, found principally in walls of hollow organs; and the specialized tissue of the heart muscle. *284,* 286ff
body movement and, 97
breathing and, 98
cancer, 290ff

cells, 286
contraction of, 286, 406
control, 43ff
development, 52
foot, *289*
injuries, 706ff
major forearm, *98*
major leg, *98*
muscular dystrophy and, 315ff
peristalsis, 98
rheumatism and, 303ff
strains and, 711
striated, 98
tendons and, 98
tissue, 81
tone, 379ff
trichinosis and, 287ff
trunk and limbs, *288*
unstriated, 98
muscle training
cerebral palsy and, 396
muscular layer
alimentary canal and, 439
mushrooms
food poisoning and, 458
mutants
viruses and, 106
mutation. 1. A change or transformation. 2. A change in the germ plasm of an organism, producing a permanent alteration in the characteristics of the succeeding generations.
heredity and, 4
influenza virus and, 154ff
myasthenia. Pertaining to muscular debility, causing weakness and exhaustibility.
myasthenia gravis, 411
thymus and, 362
myasthenic laryngitis, 147
Mycobacterium leprae. Bacterium thought to be the cause of leprosy. 735
Mycobacterium tuberculosis. Rod-shaped organism which causes tuberculosis. 161
Mycoplasma hominis
respiratory disease and, 115
Mycoplasma pneumoniae, 157
mycoplasmas
bacterial diseases and, 114ff
mycosis. Any infection caused by a vegetative microorganism such as a fungus.
mycotic (adjective). Pertaining to a mycosis.
mycotic aneurysms, 210
bacterial embolus and, 218
myelofibrosis
anemia and, 182
myeloma. A malignant tumor of bone marrow. 314
myocardial anoxia
angina pectoris and, 226
myocardial infarction. Death of an area of tissue in the heart muscle, caused by decreased blood supply to the heart. 204
myocarditis. Inflammation of the heart muscle.
myocardium. The heart muscle. It causes contraction and expansion of the chambers of the heart.

rheumatic heart disease and, 222
myo-electric arms, 319
myoma
benign skin tumors and, 254
myopia. A defect in vision in which objects can be seen distinctly only when very close to the eyes; *nearsightedness.* 570ff
myositis
low back pain, 310
myringitis. Inflammation of the tympanic membrane.
acute, 584
myxedema. One of the types of hypothyroidism, *Gull's disease.*
adult, 345
anemia and, 182
dermatitis and, 253
India rubber skin and, 253
juvenile, 345
thyroid diseases and, 345ff
myxedema madness, 346

nails, 233
disorders, 273ff
injuries, 275
narcotic. 1. A drug which produces sleep or stupor, and also relieves pain. 2. (adjective) Producing sleep or stupor.
nares. The paired external openings of the nose.
narrow-leaved marsh elder, *135*
nasal
cavity, 127
conchae, 127
congestion, 142ff
pharynx, 129
septum, 127
nasopharynx. The area of the pharynx immediately above the palate.
National Board of Examiners
physician licensing and, 771
National Conference on Aging, 649
national health insurance, 831
National Institutes of Health, 836
National Safety Council, 690, 730ff
native resistance
tuberculosis and, 162
natural childbirth
labor and, 25ff
natural immunity, 101
nausea
peptic ulcer and, 453
pregnancy and, 18
radiation sickness and, 852ff
nearsightedness
refractory defects and, 570ff, *571*
Necator americanus. A species of hookworm; it infests man and is found in the Western Hemisphere.
neck fracture
first aid for, 707
necrosis. Degeneration or death of areas of tissue or bone surrounded by healthy tissue.
corneal ulcer and, 562
nephrosis and, 488

ovaries and, 501
reproduction and, 96ff
sperm and, *10*
spindles and, *10*
uterus and, *11*
oxalates
urine and, 486
oxalic acid. An acid used chiefly
as a chemical reagent.
oxidation. The process by which
a substance combines with
oxygen. The rate of oxidation in the human body depends upon cellular activity,
not the intake of oxygen or
food.
oxygen. A nonmetallic element
occurring in the atmosphere;
a colorless, odorless, tasteless gas which constitutes
65% of the elements of the
body and 20% of the at-
mosphere at sea level. (Symbol, O).
airplanes and, 698
angina pectoris and, 225
anomalous drainage of pulmonary veins and, 225
asthma and, 140ff
coronary thrombosis and, 216
emphysema and, 153
hemoglobin and, 90ff, 126
respiration and, 90ff
space medicine and, 878ff
thyroid and, 339
oxyhemoglobin. Hemoglobin
which has been saturated
with oxygen. 126
oxyntic cells
digestion and, 442
oxytocin. Trade name of a preparation obtained from the
posterior lobe of the pituitary gland; stimulates uterine contractions.
hypothalamus and, 337
labor and, 25
posterior pituitary and, 334

pacemaker
arrhythmia and, 226
heart and, 197
heart disease and, 641
sino-auricular node and, 197
Paget's disease. 1. A malignant
disease of the areola and
nipple.   2.   Osteitis   deformans.
bone inflammation and, 311ff
breast cancer and, 552
skin eruption and, 549
pain
dysuria and, 496
fractured ribs and, 171
heart failure and, 695
pancreas infection and, 480
pancreatic cancer and, 480
peptic ulcer and, 453
spinal cord tumor and, 411
tongue, 445
palate. The roof of the mouth,
which is divided into a *hard*
palate and a *soft* palate. 435
palatine tonsil. Either of a pair
of tonsils situated at the
sides of the aperture lead-

ing from the mouth into
the throat. 77
palp. A feeler, one of the pointed
sensory organs attached to
the mouth of an insect.
Anopheles mosquitoes and,
761
pancreas. An elongated glandular organ located in the
midportion of the abdom-
inal cavity; it secretes juices
which aid in digestion, and
certain of its cells produce
the endocrine hormone *insulin,* which aids in the regulation of blood sugar
levels. *364,* 441ff
amylases and, 87
cancer, 480ff
diabetes mellitus and, 365ff,
481
disorders, 480ff
duct, 441
endocrine glands and, 363ff
infection and, 480
insulin and, 95
islet cell disorders and, 365
juice, 363, 438, 441
lipases and, 87
proteases and, 87
pancreatitis. Inflammation of the
pancreas.
chronic, 480
gallstones and, 479
mumps and, 76
pandemic. An epidemic occurring throughout a wide geographic area.
influenza, 155ff
pannus
rheumatoid arthritis and, 303
pantothenic acid. One of the B
complex group of vitamins,
not presently known to be
essential in the human diet.
It is marketed as its calcium
salt, in which form it is a
white powder.
papilla, kidney. The point of any
one of the renal pyramids
which projects into the renal
pelvis.
papillae
tongue and, 437, 445
papillary ducts, 482
**papillary squamous cell carci-
noma,** 271
Pap test
cervical cancer and, 513
papular urticaria, 235
papule. A small circumscribed
solid elevation of the skin.
allergy and, 235
lymphogranuloma   venereum
and, 520
paradoxical incontinence, 496
paraffin
tooth decay and, 431
paralysis. Temporary or permanent loss of function, especially loss of sensation or
voluntary motion.
diaphragm and, 175
hysteria and, 697
nervous system disorders and,
396ff
poliomyelitis and, 384

rehabilitation for, 400ff
spinal cord injury and, 398ff
spinal cord tumor and, 411
strokes and, 396ff
ticks and, 766
paralyzed patient
rehabilitation of, *400ff*
paranasal sinuses, 127
anatomy of, 141
paranoia. A chronic psychosis
characterized by delusions
of persecution.
psychoses and, 626
paraplegia, 398
parasite. An organism that lives
in or on another organism,
known as the *host,* from
which it derives nourish-
ment during all or part of
its existance.
food-transmitted disease and,
756
fungi, 121
large intestine, 467ff
parasitic (adjective). Like, caused
by, or pertaining to a para-
site.
parasitic diseases
leishmaniasis, 737
typhus fever, 744
parasitology. The science and
study of parasites.
parathyroid gland. One of four
small bodies located at the
back and at the lower edge
of the thyroid gland. They
control the calcium-phos-
phorus balance of the body.
Tumors or hyperfunctions
result in various body disturbances. 95, 348ff
calcium deficiencies and, 657
diseases of, 349
functioning of, 348ff
osteitis fibrosa and, 311
osteodystrophy, 311
thyroid and, *339*
para-urethral glands
urethra and, 485
parentage
disputed, 776ff
parental attitudes
adolescent and, 71
childhood behavior problems
and, 60ff
mental retardation and, 62ff
paresthesia. Abnormal burning
or prickling sensation which
occurs as a result of neural
disorders.
multiple sclerosis and, 412
parietal (adjective). Pertaining to
the large flat bones which
form the sides of the skull;
also a cerebral lobe of the
brain corresponding in position to this bone.
lobe, 378
peritoneum, 439
Paris green. A salt of copper
and arsenic used mainly as
an insecticide; it is especially
effective as a larvicide.
mosquito control and, 762
stomach poisons and, 768
Parkinsonism
encephalitis and, 389ff

Parkinson's disease. A condition characterized by rigidity of the muscles, a tremor which tends to disappear on voluntary movement, loss of associated and automatic movements, and a masklike facial expression. Also known as *palsy*. 412
encephalitis and, 389ff
encephalitis lethargica and, 412
paronychia. Inflammation of the skin surrounding the finger or toe nail. *274*
parotid gland. Largest of the paired salivary glands located on each side of the face below and in front of the ear. 435, 437
mumps and, 75
parotitis
salivary glands and, 446
pars intermedia. The middle portion of the pituitary gland; connects the anterior and posterior lobes. 331, 334
particle rays
space medicine and, 879
passive immunity, 101
viruses and, 107
passive incontinence, 496
Pasteurella pestis. A species of rod-shaped bacillus which is the cause of bubonic plague. 766
Pasteurella tularensis, *248*
pasteurization. A process by which fermentation is inhibited and pathogens destroyed by heating to a temperature of 60–70° C for 40 minutes. 115ff
Pasteur treatment
rabies and, 703
pasture sage, *134*
patch test
allergy diagnosis and, 241
tuberculosis and, 165
patent ductus arteriosus. A congenital disorder of the blood vessels. A small duct connecting the aorta and pulmonary artery fails to close at birth, resulting in faulty circulation of the blood. 203, 223
pathogens. Disease-producing agents. 116
pathologic fractures, 294
pathologist, 774
pathology, 823
patient
law and, 771
-physician relationship, 772ff
records, 684
patriarchal family, 522
pattern baldness, 276
Pavlov's principles
natural childbirth and, 26
PBI test
thyroid function and, 340
pectin
arteriosclerosis and, 205
pectus carinatum. A condition characterized by the chest projecting outwardly; pigeon-breast.

pectus excavatum. A condition characterized by the chest projecting inwardly; funnel chest.
pediatrics. The branch of medical science which is concerned with the care and treatment of children. 824
pediculosis. Infestation by lice. 250, 763
Pediculus. A genus of parasitic insects; lice. 762, *763*
classical typhus and, 744
pedigree. A table or chart indicating the derivation of inherited factors; a graphic genealogical tree which depicts such derivation.
pedodontics, 838
pellagra. A disease resulting from the lack of adequate amounts of nicotinic acid and other B complex vitamins in the diet. 181
dermatitis and, 252
niacin deficiencies and, 661
pelvic examination
cervical cancer and, 513
pelvic fractures
first aid for, 708
pelvis, 285
hip joint and, 285
kidney, 484
sacroiliac joints and, 285
pemphigus. An acute or chronic disease of the skin marked by the appearance of large blisters which develop in crops or continuous succession. 254
penetrating wounds, 171
penicillin. An antibiotic drug obtained from growths of the mold.
Penicillium. A mold from which penicillin is extracted; effective in many infections. *119*
aerosol, 160
bacteria and, 117
rheumatic fever and, 219
Penicillium notatum, *119*
penis. The external sexual organ of the male. It is cylindrical and pendulous, and contains the urethra, which functions as a passage for the urine and for the discharge of semen during copulation. 498
anatomy of, 500
erection of, 10
male reproductive system and, 498, 500
Pentamidine. A derivative of diamidine used in treatment of protozoan infections. 748
pepsin. An enzyme secreted in the stomach, which aids in the digestion of proteins. 86, 442
peptic ulcer and, 452
proteins and, 86
zymogenic cells and, 442
peptic ulcer. An inflamed lesion of the gastric or duodenal mucosa caused by the action of the digestive juices on

the mucosa.
complications of, 454ff
diagnosis of, 452
Dragstedt operation for, *454*
duodenum and, 459
stomach disorders and, 452ff
surgical procedure for, 455
treatment for, 454
perception. Awareness of stimuli received by the senses. 596
percussion (Medicine). The act of tapping the body with the fingers or a small instrument to produce sounds to determine position, size, and consistency of underlying structures.
chest diseases and, 203
pneumonia and, 157
perforation
peptic ulcers and, 455
perfusion
cancer chemotherapy and, 644
periapical (adjective). About or near the apex of a tooth.
pericarditis
adherent, 225
chronic constrictive, 225
dry, 225
fibrinous, 225
pericardium and, 225
pneumonia and, 160
pericardium. A sac containing a small amount of fluid which completely envelopes the heart. 198
pericarditis and, 225
perilymph. The watery fluid contained in the space between the membranous and bony labyrinths of the internal ear.
perimysium
skeletal muscles and, 286
perineal muscles
urination and, 485
perineum. The region between the anus and the scrotum in the male; between the anus and the vulva in the female.
hypospadias and, 495
labia majora and, 504
periodontal membrane. The membrane which covers the cementum of a tooth, joining it to the alveolar bone. 418ff
periodontal pocket
pyorrhea and, 432
periodontics, 838
periodontitis, 432
periodontoclasia, 432
periodontosis, 432
periosteum. The connective tissue membrane surrounding all bone except at articular surfaces. 97, 281
bone inflammation and, 311
cambium and, 281
peripheral (adjective). Located, or pertaining to the outer surface of an organ.
nerves, 381ff
vascular disease, 226
peristalsis. A progressive muscular wave of contraction occurring in certain of the tubular organs of the body.
intestinal muscles and, 98, 438

swallowing and, 442
ureters and, 484
peritoneal cavity. That cavity enclosed by the peritoneum. 41
peritoneum. The membrane which lines the interior of the abdominal cavity, covering the intestines, stomach, and other organs.
alimentary canal and, 439
kidneys and, 482
peritonitis. Inflammation of the peritoneum.
appendicitis and, 460
peritoneal cavity and, 441
pneumonia and, 160
peritonsillar abscess, 145ff
permanent cuspids
eruption of, 426
permanent dentition, *420,* 421
pernicious anemia, 181
spinal cord and, 412
tongue coating and, 445
persecution
paranoia and, 626
persimmons
bezoars and, 458
personality disorders
alcoholic, 619
inadequate personality, 619ff
lonely personality (schizoid), 620
mind disorders and, 614ff
moody personality (cycloid), 620ff
senility and, 645ff
social problem types, 615ff
suspicious personality (paranoid), 622
pertussis. An inflammatory infectious disease characterized by catarrh of the respiratory tract and paroxysms of cough ending in a prolonged whooping inspiration; caused by *Hemophilus pertussis; whooping cough.* 76
perversion. Deviation from the average or from the accepted norm.
pessary. 1. A device inserted in the vagina to support the uterus. 2. Any vaginal suppository.
prolapse and, 511
retrodisplacement and, 510
uterine position and, *512*
pesticides
water pollution and, 754
petit mal. A mild form of epilepsy in which the period of unconsciousness is brief and in which the muscular contractions are mild or absent. 393
Peyer's patches. Aggregations of lymph tissue in the mucosa of the ileum and jejunum. 439
phagedena. A rapidly spreading ulceration; the condition occurs in warm, moist tropical areas. 737
phantom limb. An imaginary leg or arm often fantasied

by amputees, who claim to feel pain in the lost member. 317
pharmacist. One who specializes in compounding and dispensing medicines; *apothecary.* 833ff
pharmocology. The science of the nature, properties, and actions of drugs. 823
pharyngeal speech
laryngeal cancer and, 149
laryngectomy and, 149
pharyngeal tonsil. An unpaired tonsil located in back of the nasopharynx, referred to as the "adenoids." 77
pharynges. In zoology, it refers to the mouth parts of lower animals. In the insects these are often protrusible, have teeth, and are used as powerful sucking organs.
chiggers and, 765
pharyngitis. Inflammation of the pharynx; sore throat. 144ff
acute, 144
chronic, 144
infectious mononucleosis and, 190
influenza and, 155
sore throat and, 144
pharynx. A musculomembranous tube which extends from the oral cavity to the esophagus. Functions as a resonating cavity, passage for air and food. 127, 437
laryngeal, 129
nasal, 129
oral, 129
sore throat and, 144
phenobarbital. A white, colorless, material used as a sedative for nervous excitement, or to control the convulsions in epilepsy. 394
phenol. Hydroxybenzene, an organic compound derived from coal tar, used as a cauterizing agent, disinfectant germicide, and local anesthetic. Also called *carbolic acid.* 770
phenotype. The visible traits which characterize the members of a group. 5
phenylketonuria. A congenital disorder of metabolism by which *phenylpyruvic acid* appears in the urine. Usually detected in first month of life and may be associated with mental defects.
Philadelphia chromosome
chronic myelogenous leukemia and, *186*
phlebitis. Inflammation of a vein.
varicose veins and, 206
Phlebotomus. A genus of small blood-sucking sandflies which transmit several febrile diseases to man.
Oroya fever and, 747
phobic reaction. A form of neurosis in which the individual

experiences a feeling of fear related to some object or situation which symbolizes something else which he unconsciously fears. 606, 607ff
phocomelia
thalidomide and, 17
phosphates
urine and, 486
phosphatide. Fatlike material containing phosphate. 191
Niemann-Pick's disease and, 191
phosphoric acid. A colorless, odorless acid used in making phosphates and lacto-phosphates.
phosphorus. A nonmetallic element not found in a free state but present in body tissues. (Symbol, P).
insecticides and, 769
parathyroids and, 348
stomach poisons and, 768
photocoagulation
retinal detachment and, 566ff
photophobia
blepharitis and, 562
cornea and, 562
photosynthetic regeneration
space medicine and, 880
phrenic nerve. The motor nerve which innervates the diaphragm. 175
hiccough and, 697
Phthirius pubis. A species of lice which infests the pubic region of the body and is thought to transmit typhus and relapsing fever.
pubic lice and, 762
phylum (plural, phyla). A major category in biological nomenclature. The common categories in the systematic arrangement of plants and animals are, in order, *phylum, class, order, family, genus, species, variety.*
Physalia
Portuguese man-of-war and, 704
physical abilities
intellectual capacity and, *650*
physical development
adolescence and, *529*
physical examinations
aging and, 637
industrial diseases and, 169
physical maturity
adolescent and, 70ff
physical needs
infant mind and, 599
physical senility, 645
physical therapists, 833
physical therapy. The use of physical agents in treatment, such as electricity, heat, light, water, massage, etc.
degenerative arthritis and, 303
muscular dystrophy and, 315
physician
law and, 771
licensing of, 771ff
number of, *829*
-patient relationship, 772ff

witness and, 772
physiological albuminuria
  kidney disorders and, 488ff
physiological function studies
  medical radioisotopes and, 871
physiological measurements
  Bertillon system and, 778
physiology. The science of the
  function of living organisms
  and their organs. 823
PKU
  brain damage and, 412
  infant and, 42
pia mater. The innermost of
  the three membranes covering the brain.
  meningitis and, 390
  skull and, 383
pick-a-back carry, 694
piebald skin, 258
pigeon breast, 176
pigmented moles, *253*
pigmented nevus, *255*
pile
  nuclear fission and, 844
pill
  contraception and, 535ff
pimples, 258ff
pineal gland. A small gland attached to the posterior part
  of the brain, behind and
  above the third ventricle.
  95, 362ff, *363*
  pituitary gland and, *363*
pinealoma, 363
pinguecula, 561
pink-eye, 561
pinworm, 123ff
Pithecanthropus erectus. A prehistoric primate thought to
  be an ancestor of the
  human species.
pit toilet
  construction of, 752
pituitary gland. The small endocrine gland attached by a
  stalk to the floor of the
  brain. It regulates the production of other endocrine
  glands and produces at
  least six hormones con-
  cerned with growth, sex,
  metabolism, blood pressure,
  and body temperature. 95,
  330ff, *331*
  adrenocorticotrophic hormone
  and, 332ff
  atrophy of, 336
  Cushing's disease and, 335ff
  Cushing's syndrome and, 335ff
  dwarfism, 334
  feedback mechanism and,
  331ff
  Fröhlich's syndrome and, 336
  function of, 95
  giant, *332*
  gonadotrophic hormone and,
  332
  growth disorders and, 334ff
  growth hormone and, *330*
  hypothalamus and, 334
  infantilism, 334
  metabolism regulation and,
  333ff
  ovaries and, 352
  pars intermedia and, 334
  pineal gland and, *363*

posterior lobe of, 334
pregnancy and, 22
reproductive hormones and, 8
Simmonds-Sheehan disease
  and, 336
tumors, 330, *353*
pit viper
  poisonous snakes and, 721
pityriasis rosea. A skin disease
  limited to the trunk, usually
  acute, characterized by pale
  red patches with light centers. The causative agent is
  unknown. 248, *249*
pityriasis versicolor. A chronic
  skin disease marked by yellowish brown flaky spots;
  involves principally the
  trunk and is caused by the
  fungus *Malasșezia furfur.*
  244
placenta. The oval spongy structure in the uterus through
  which the fetus derives its
  nourishment. 14
  aging and, 636
  amniotic sac and, 15
  birth and, *31*
  chorion, 14
  endocrine system and, 329
  estrogen and, 22
  hormones, 15, 22
  immunity and, 636
  lactogen, 329
  mesoderm and, 11
  postbirth, 31
  premature infant and, 37
  sinuses, 14
  supportive role of, 15
  unborn and, 14
plants
  allergies and, 238
  dermatitis and, 249ff
  hay fever and, 133ff
plaque
  dental caries and, 427
  dental hygiene and, 430
  mercurochrome and, *428*
plasma
  blood, 178
  carbon dioxide and, 91
  cell myeloma, 189
  composition of, 178
  glomerulus and, 484
  leucocytes and, 77
  membrane, 1
  transfusion, 34, 192ff
plasmochin. A trade name for
  a drug used as a substitute
  for quinine.
Plasmodium. The genus of parasitic protozoa to which the
  malarial parasites belong.
  falciparum, *739*
  malariae, *739*
  vivax, *740*
plasmosome, *81*
plastics
  artificial limbs and, 317
plastic surgery. That branch of
  surgery concerned with repairing a defective area of
  the body by transferring to
  it sound tissues from other
  body areas or from other
  persons.

congenital ear malformations,
  589
facial deformities and, 321
nose and, *801*
platelets
  blood, 178
  replacement therapy, 188
Platyhelminthes. The phylum to
  which the intestinal parasites commonly called *flatworms* belong.
play
  child and, 53ff
pleura. The covering membrane
  of the lungs. 131
  pleurisy, 160
pleural cavity. The space enclosed by the pleura; the
  lung cavity. 131
pleural friction rub
  pleurisy and, 160
pleurisy
  dry, 160
  respiratory disorders and, 160ff
  wet, 160
pleuro-pneumonia-like organism,
  157
pneumograph. A part of the
  polygraph apparatus which
  is used for recording respiration. 787
pneumonia. Inflammation of the
  lung with exudation into
  the lung tissue. 158
  atelectasis, 159
  bacterial, 157
  bilateral, 156
  chemical, 158
  chest injuries and, 173ff
  chest wounds and, 173
  chicken pox and, 72
  death rates from, *159*
  Friedlander's, 157
  history of, 156
  infant deaths from, 155
  influenzal, 154
  measles and, 73, 159
  ornithosis, 159
  pneumococcal, 157
  postoperative, 157ff
  respiratory disorders and, 156ff
  secondary complications of,
  159ff
  staphylococcal, 157
  streptococcal, 157
  terminal, 159
  traumatic, 159
  viral, 157
  x-ray appearance of lobar,
  158
pneumothorax. A collection of
  air or gas in the pleural
  cavity which causes partial
  or complete collapse of the
  lungs. Results from perforation of pleura by injury,
  spontaneous rupture, or by
  surgical procedure.
pneumotropic (adjective). Having an affinity for the lungs.
  virus, 112
pneumoventriculography. X-ray
  examination of the ventricular system of the brain after
  removal of fluid content and
  injection of air or gas.

poison
dilution, 717
first aid for, 716ff
general treatment principles
for, 717
groups of, 783ff
universial antidote for, 718
poison baits
insecticides and, 768
poisoning
do nots, 717ff
dos, 717
food, 456ff
medicolegal aspects of, 782ff
poison ivy, *239,* 718
allergies and, 238ff
blisters, *239*
poisonous gases
occupational diseases and, 733
poisonous plants
first aid for, 718ff
poisonous snake bites
do nots, 722
dos, 722
first aid for, 721
poisonous vapors
occupational diseases and, 733
poison sumac, *240*
polarograph
antibiotic production and, 834
Police service
Civil Defense and, 855
poliomyelitis. Inflammation of
the gray matter in the
spinal cord, thought to be
caused by a filterable virus;
infantile paralysis.
abortive, 384
bulbar, 384
bulbo-spinal, 384
encephalitic, 384
muscle contraction and, 286
nervous system disorders and,
384ff
neurotropic viruses and, 112
nonparalytic, 384
paralytic, 384
prevention of, 386
rehabilitation for, 386ff
season of, 384
spinal, 384
symptoms of, *57,* 384ff
treatment for, 385ff
polio vaccine
administration schedule of, 385
pollen. The fertilizing or male
substance produced by
flowering plants.
allergies and, 238
counting of, 138
geographic incidence of fall,
137
hay fever and, 133
pollen extract
hay fever relief and, 139
pollution, 754
air, 754
control, 754
water, 754
polyandry. A form of marriage
in which one woman may
have more than one legal
husband. 522
polyarthritis. Inflammation of
several joints. 304
polycystic (adjective). Contain-

ing or composed of many
cysts.
disease, 489
polycythemia, 189
polycythemia vera. A disorder
of unknown etiology char-
acterized by an increase in
the number of circulating
red blood cells. 189
radiophosphorus and, 873
polygraph. The recording apparatus which is used in making tracings on the same
recording surface of the
blood pressure, respiration,
and activity of the sweat
glands of a subject during
verbal questioning. The various recording devices, the
pneumograph, the galvano-
graph, and the sphygmo-
graph, are parts of the
apparatus which measure
respiration, activity of the
sweat glands, and blood
pressure, respectively. Also
known as the *lie detector.*
786
medical criminology and, 786ff
principles of, 787
polygyny. A form of marriage
in which a man may have
more than one legal wife.
522
polymastia. The presence of
more than two breasts. *547,*
548
polyp. A tumor with a pedicle,
or slender base.
intussusception and, 467
large intestine tumors and,
467
rectal cancer and, 471
sinus, 143
stomach and, *451*
stomach tumors and, 456
urethra and, 494
uterine, *513*
polyunsaturated fats
heart and circulation disorders
and, 202
polyuria. The excretion of an
abnormally large quantity
of urine. 496
pons. 1. Any slip of tissue connecting two parts of an
organ. 2. A rounded white
mass of tissue, directly continuous with the medulla
oblongata below and the
midbrain above. 377ff
popliteal artery
arteriosclerosis and, 204
population
control, 821
pores
skin and, 229
pork
trichinosis and, 123, 290, 756
pork tapeworm, *755*
porphyria
congenital photosensitive, 253
cutaneous, 253
dermatitis and, 253
variegate, 253
porphyrins
porphyria and, 253

portal cirrhosis, 477
ascites and, 477
esophageal varices and, 477
portal vein. A large trunk vein
which conveys blood from
the abdominal viscera into
the liver. 201
port-wine hemangioma, 255
port-wine nevi, *255*
postconcussion syndrome, 416
posterior lobe. The posterior
lobe is the smaller of the
two lobes of the pituitary
gland which produces some
of the pituitary hormones.
331
posterior semicircular canals, 583
posthemorrhagic anemia, 179
postmenopausal bleeding, 357
postnatal (adjective). Occuring
after birth.
postoperative pneumonia, 157ff
posttraumatic amnesia, 415
postural defects
childhood and, *58*
scoliosis and, 315
walker and, *59*
postural hypotension, 214
posture
degenerative arthritis and, 301
postvaricella encephalitis
chicken pox and, 72
potassium. An alkaline mineral
element found in combina-
tion with other elements in
the body. Salts of potassium
and magnesium help to
maintain osmotic pressure
and the ion balance. Found
in most foods. (Symbol, K).
potency
sterility and, 532
PPLO
pneumonia and, 157
practical nurse, 828
home care and, 689
pre-adolescence
sex play and, *529*
precancer of the skin, 266ff
precipitin test
blood identification and, 775
preclinical phase
diabetes mellitus and, 366
prednisone
thyroiditis and, 347
pregnancy. The state of being
with child. The term of
pregnancy is usually about
280 days. 18ff
breast and, 546
breast cancer and, 552
breast hygiene and, 546
breast shape and, *546*
clothing and, 21ff
colostrum and, 21, 546
conception and, 18
date of confinement and, 22
death from, *533*
disorders of, 23
examination for, 18ff
fertility and, 23
frigidity and, 537
hormones and, 22ff
hygiene, 19ff
leucorrhea and, 21
menopause and, 505
menstrual period and, 18

spine. The spinal column, consisting of 33 vertebrae; 7 cervical, 12 thoracic, 5 lumbar, 5 sacral, 4 coccygeal. The bones of the sacrum and coccyx are ankylosed in the adult and are counted as one each; the *backbone*.
degenerative arthritis of, 302
spinous process. Bony projection from the summit of the neural arch, to which muscles are attached.
vertebrae and, 282
Spirillum
bacteria and, 115
spirochetal jaundice. 767
spirochete. Any of the microorganisms belonging to the order Spirochaetales. 115
spirometer. An instrument used to determine the vital capacity of the lungs.
spleen. A ductless, glandlike organ, highly vascular, located under the diaphragm. It lies back of the 9th, 10th, and 11th ribs, on the left side of the body. The spleen is the largest lymphatic organ—about 5 inches long and weighing about 6 ounces—and is dark red in color. One of its principal functions is the manufacture of red corpuscles; it also acts to resist microbic infection. Extracts of the organ have some action upon the smooth muscles.
splenectomy. Surgical removal of the spleen.
splenomegaly. Enlargement of the spleen.
splints, *297, 710*
fractures and, 706, 710ff
hip fracture and, *298*
patient moving and, 693
spondylolisthesis. Deformity of the spinal column caused by forward displacement of one vertebra over another, especially the separation of the 5th lumbar vertebra over the sacrum.
spongy bone, 280
spontaneous dislocations, 293
spontaneous fractures, 295
spore. The reproductive cell of a protozoan, bacterium, or plant, invested with a firm cell wall which enables the cell to survive in adverse environment. 115
botulism and, 755
fungi and, 121
sporotrichosis. A fungus disease characterized by ulceration of the skin and mucous membranes, caused by *Sporotrichum schenckii*.
Sporotrichum schenckii. A cigar-shaped fungus which causes skin ulceration in man. 122
Sporozoa. The class of protozoan organisms which are spore-producing, to which

the malarial parasites belong.
coccidiosis and, 121
malaria and, 121
toxoplasmosis and, 121
sporozoite. The stage in the life cycle of the malarial parasite during which it is infectious to man. 738
sports
blind and, 576
sprain. A sudden or violent wrenching of a joint, causing ligaments to stretch or rupture; the injury resulting from such violent tension. 291ff
first aid for, 711
sprue. A disorder of uncertain etiology characterized by loose stools and various other symptoms that may result secondarily from the poor absorption of various nutritional essentials. 181
sputum. Substance expectorated from the mouth, containing saliva, mucus, and sometimes pus.
sputum test
lung cancer and, 167
squamous cell cancer of lung
x-ray appearance of, *167*
squamous cell carcinoma
cross-section of lung, *167*
papillary, 271
skin cancer and, 271
ulcerating, 271
squamous-hyperkeratotic athlete's foot, 264
stab wounds
respiratory disorders and, 171
stag-horn calculi
kidney stones and, 486
standing
varicose veins and, 208
Stanford Research Institute's Radiation Engineering Laboratory, *874*
St. Anthony's fire, *247*
dermatitis and, 246
stapedectomy
conductive deafness and, 591
stapes, 581
Staphylococcus. A genus of spherical bacteria characterized by growth in irregular bunches. 115
bacteremia and, 182
bone inflammation and, 311
food intoxications and, 755
food poisoning and, 456
pneumonia and, 157
state health departments, 836
state hospitals
insane and, 792
status asthmaticus, 141
status epilepticus. A series of epileptic convulsions without periods of consciousness between them.
grand mal seizures and, 392
steam tent
home care and, 680ff
how to make, *680ff*

steapsin. An enzyme which aids in digestion of fat.
steatorrhea. Presence of excess fat in the stools. 181
stenosis. A constriction or narrowing, especially of a channel or aperture.
sterility
cryptorchism and, 506
marriage and, 532ff
mumps and, 75
orchitis and, 75
sex and, 532ff
sterilization, 875
sternum. A longitudinal plate of bone forming the anterior wall of the chest; the breast bone. 131
esophagitis and, 449
ribs and, 285
steroid. The generic name for compounds comprising the sterols, bile acids, heart poisons, and sex hormones.
gonadal hormones and, 350
oral contraceptives and, 536
stethoscope. An instrument for listening to sounds originating within the body, especially of the heart and lungs
circulatory disease and, 202
lung and, 131
murmurs and, 202ff
Réné Laennec and, *132*
sphygmomanometer and, 212
stiffness
degenerative arthritis and, 301
tetanus and, 388
stimulants
drug abuse and, 618
psychoses and, 628ff
stirrup
middle ear, 581
stomach. The relatively large, hollow organ of the digestive system which receives the food from the esophagus, and in which processes of digestion are performed. 437
alimentary canal and, 86
bezoars and, 458
cancer, 455ff
congenital abnormalities of, 458ff
disorders, 450ff
food poisoning and, 456ff
gastric juice and, 86
gastritis and, 451ff
infant deaths and, *458*
peptic ulcers and, 452ff
polyps of, *451*
stomach emptying
poison first aid and, 717
stomach poisons
insecticides and, 768
stomach ulcer, *451*
deaths from, *456*
lymphosarcoma and, *452*
stomatitis. Inflammation of the mouth.
Stomoxys calcitrans. The species to which the common stable fly belongs; this insect transmits trypanosomiasis and anthrax.

tendon. A fibrous band of connective tissue uniting a muscle with some other part and transmitting the force which the muscle exerts; a sinew. 98, 287, 711

Tenenbaum Hand, *323*

tentorium cerebelli. A horizontal fold of the dura mater which separates the cerebellum from the cerebrum. 383

tensions
dreams and, 605

terminal bronchi, 131

terminal pneumonia, 159

terramycin. An oral antibiotic derived from cultures of *Streptomyces rimosus*.

tertiary hair, 232

testis (plural, testes). The testicle; the male reproductive gland in the scrotum, which secretes the sperm cells. *501*
cancer, 506
descent, 505ff, *506*
disorders, 505ff
gonadotrophic hormones and, 332
male gonads and, 350ff
male reproductive system and, 498
reproductive organs and, 9
scrotum and, 9
seminiferous tubules and, 9
temperature control of, 499
tumors, 352

testosterone. One of the male sex hormones produced chiefly in the testicles.

tetanus. 1. An acute infectious disease manifested by more or less persistent spasm of the voluntary muscles, particularly those about the head, caused by the toxins produced by the bacillus *Clostridium tetani; lockjaw.* 2. Any continuous spasm or steady contraction of a muscle. 388
puncture wounds and, 702
vaccination, 388

tetany. A disease characterized by intermittent painful spasms of the muscles.
calcium and, 348
parathyroid and, 348

tetraiodophenolphthalein
gallstones and, 478

tetralogy of Fallot. A congenital heart disease characterized by four disorders in the heart and large blood vessels. It is the most common abnormality of "blue babies." 223

thalamus. The mass of gray tissue at the base of the brain which relays sensation and other stimuli on to the cerebral cortex. 378

thalidomide
mechanisms of, 17
phocomelia and, 17
rehabilitation for, 17
treatment for, 17

unborn enemies, 17

thallium sulfate. A metallic slat, the action of which is similar to that of arsenic. It is used as a rat poison and as a depilatory. 768

therapeutic abortions, 784
medicolegal problems of, 793

therapeutic radiopharmaceuticals, 870

therapeutics. The branch of medical science concerned with medical treatment.

Theratron unit
radiation therapy and, *872*

thermodynamics. The study of the relationship between heat and other forms of energy.

thermogram
breast cancer and, *553*

thermometer
infant fever and, 49

thermonuclear reaction, 844

thiamine
deficiencies, 660
underweight and, 668

thigh fractures
first aid for, 708

thiouracil. A drug used in treating patients with thyrotoxicosis.
Graves' disease and, 345

third degree burns, 712

third molars
eruption of, 426

thirst
pharynx and, 443

thoracic cage. The bony structure formed by the twelve pairs of ribs and the sternum. 285

thoracic cavity, 131

thoracic duct, 87

thoracic lymphatic ducts, 199

thoracic vertebrae, 282

thoracopagus. Twins which are united in the thoracic regions.
congenital chest wall abnormalities, 176
Siamese twins and, 176

thoracoplasty. The complete or partial removal of one or more ribs to cause collapse of the lung; used in treating patients with pulmonary tuberculosis. 165

thorax
mosquitoes and, 758

threadworms, 469
Stongyloidiasis and, 469

throat
cancer, 449
diseases, 449
infection, 449

thromboangiitis obliterans, 204
embolism and, 204

thrombocyte. Blood platelet; a small colorless disk in the circulating blood. It contains thromboplastin, believed to be important in the clotting of blood.

thrombocytopenia. An abnormal decrease in the number of platelets in the blood.

purpura, 188

thromboembolism, 174

thromboplastin. A substance in the tissues which is believed to function in the conversion of prothrombin to thrombin in blood clotting. Also called *thrombokinase*. 178

thrombosis
coronary, 215
stroke and, 396

thrush. A mouth infection characterized by small white spots inside the mouth, caused by a fungus. 122
dermatitis and, 244
infant illness and, 48
mouth disorders and, 444

thumb sucking
malocclusion and, 422ff

thymosin
lymphocytes and, 362
thymus and, 362

thymus gland. A lymphoid, ductless organ, located in the upper thorax which is included in the endocrine system. It attains full size at puberty, after which it atrophies. 95, 361ff

thyrocalcitonin
calcium and, 348
thyroid and, 338

thyroid. An endocrine gland located in front of the trachea, consisting of a right and left lobe and a connecting lobe called the isthmus. 95, 337ff
diseases of, 341ff
function test for, 339ff
nodular goiter and, 343
parathyroid gland and, *339*
radioactive iodine and, 340ff
thyroxin and, 95

thyroid cancer
radiation injury and, 851

thyroid cartilage. The largest cartilage of the larynx which has the appearance of a shield and forms the Adam's apple. 129

thyroid disorders
anemia and, 182
food requirements and, 670
Graves' disease, 343ff
hypothyroidism, 345ff
myxedema, 345ff
nodular goiter, 343
thyroiditis, 347ff
tumors, 346ff

thyroidectomy. Surgical removal of the thyroid gland.

thyroiditis. Inflammation of the thyroid gland. 347ff

thyroid scans
radionuclides and, 871

thyrotoxic (adjective). Pertaining to thyrotoxicosis.
heart disease, 226

thyrotoxicosis. A systemic condition caused by excessive activity of the thyroid glands.

thyrotrophic (adjective). Pertaining to a hormone of the

excretion of urine; the component organs are the kidneys, ureters, bladder, and urethra. 485
definition of, 482
kidneys and, 482ff
urethra, 485
urination. The discharge of urine from the bladder.
acute prostatitis and, 507
nephritis and, 487ff
pregnancy and, 18
process of, 485
prostatic hypertrophy, 506
stricture, 494
urination disturbances, 496ff
abnormal output, 496
bed-wetting, 496ff
difficulty, 496
incontinence, 496
pain, 496
urine. The fluid secreted from the blood by the kidneys, stored in the bladder, and discharged by the urethra. In health, it is amber colored, and contains urea, inorganic salts, pigments and other end products of protein and mineral metabolism.
composition of, 92
urea and, 92
urine analysis
diabetes mellitus and, 369
urine sugar
CLINITEST and, *372*
diabetes mellitus and, 366
uriniferous tubule. The small tube extending from Bowman's capsule to the collecting tubule in the kidney. 484
urologist. A physician who specializes in diseases of the urogenital system.
urology. The branch of medicine dealing with the diseases of the urogenital tract in the male and the urinary tract in the female.
kidney stones and, 486
urticaria. Hives or nettle rash; a skin condition characterized by the appearance of intensely itching wheals or welts; may be an allergic reaction. 235
uterine disorders, 510ff
endometriosis, 511
tuberculosis, 514
tumors, 512ff, *513*
uterus. The muscular, hollow, pear-shaped organs of gestation. The upper portion is called the fundus, the lower part, the cervix.
embryo and, *12*
endometriosis and, 511
female reproductive system and, 503
labor and, *23*
new mother and, 34
normal, *511*
ovum and, *11*
polyps, and *513*
pregnancy and, *19*

retrocession of, *512*
retroflexion of, *511*
ureters and, 484
utricule
vestibule and, 583
uvula. The soft, fleshy, pendulant mass that hangs from the soft palate above the root of the tongue.
cleft palate and, 448
mouth and, 435

vaccination. Inoculation with an organism, previously treated to render it harmless, to develop immunity to a specific infectious disease.
eczema vaccinatum and, 262
immune reaction to, 262
inactivated viruses and, 107
influenza, 154ff
mumps, 75
procedure for, 262
production of, 107
rabies and, 391
reactions to, 262
rubella, 73
smallpox, *57, 262*
tetanus, 388
viral diseases and, 111
viruses and, 107
yellow. fever, 744
vacuoles, *81*
vacuum extractor, 26
vagina. The internal sexual organ of the female; the passageway between the uterus and external orifice, functioning as a passage for sexual intercourse, discharge of the menses, and as the birth canal. 9, 503
bleeding, 23
congenital absence of, 515
disorders, 515ff
infections, 515
Pap test and, 513
tumors, 515
vaginismus
frigidity and, 537
sexual intercourse and, 515
vagus nerve. The tenth cranial nerve. It has motor and sensory functions, stimulating the heart, lungs, larynx, esophagus, stomach, and most of the intestines. 196
valves
circulation and, 198
venous, *206*
vanity
paranoid personality and, 622
vapona
fly control and, 758
varicele. Abnormal distention and varicosity of the veins of the spermatic cord inside the scrotum. 206
varicose (adjective). Pertaining to a swollen, distended, and tortuous vein with the loss of normal elasticity.
greater saphenous vein, *207*
hemorrhoids and, 473
leg, *209*

lesser saphenous vein, *207*
ligation and, *209*
pregnancy and, *208*
prevention of, 206ff
symptoms of, 206
treatment for, 208ff
ulceration and, *207*
veins, 205ff, *206*
variegate porphyria, 253
variola, 261ff
vasa deferentia, 498
vasa efferentia, 499
vascular (adjective). Pertaining to or composed of blood vessels.
lesions, *214*
vascular lesions
central nervous system and, *214*
deaths from, *214*
vascular headaches, 405
vas deferens. One of a pair of ducts which carries the sperm from the testis to the seminal vesicle. *500*
epididymis and, 499
ureters and, 484
vasectomy
medicolegal problems of, 794
vas efferens. The lymphatic vessel of a lymph node, especially the excretory ducts of the testes.
vasoconstrictor. A drug which causes narrowing of the blood vessels. 201
vasodilator. A drug which causes enlargement or dilation of the blood vessels. 201
vasopressin. A hormone produced by the posterior lobe of the pituitary gland which raises blood pressure and stimulates intestinal muscles, and acts as an antidiuretic.
hypothalamus and, 337
posterior pituitary and, 334
vein. One of the blood vessels which transports the blood from the organs and tissues and the body back to the heart to be oxygenated. 87
lymphatic vessels and, *202*
varicose, *206*
vein dilation
varicose veins and, 205ff
vena cava. Either the *inferior* or *superior* **vena cava,** the large veins which return the blood to the right auricle.
heart and, 196
hepatic vein and, 201
venereal disease, 517ff
chancroid, 520
gonorrhea, 517ff
granuloma inguinale, 521ff
lymphogranuloma venereum, 520ff
reportable diseases and, 795
sex hygiene and, 539
syphilis, 518ff
venesection.
polycythemia vera and, 189
venous (adjective). Pertaining to the veins, or blood passing through them.
circulation, *201*

x-chromosome. One of the sex-determining chromosomes; it apparently carries genes for femaleness.

xenon-133
physiological function studies and, 871

Xenopsylla cheopsis. The species of Indian rat flea which is found in tropical regions. The flea is parasitic to man and other animals and transmits bubonic plague and tapeworms.

xeroderma pigmentosum. A rare disease of the skin usually beginning in childhood and characterized by disseminated pigment spots and shrinking of the skin. Warty lesions occur that develop into malignant growths. Also called *Kaposi's disease.* 267

xerosis. Abnormal dryness of the skin.
vitamin A deficiency and, *662*

xerostomia. Insufficient flow or production of saliva, causing dry mouth. 445

x-ray. Radiation similar to light but of extremely short wave length, emitted principally as the result of a sudden change in the velocity of electrons striking a target in

a vacuum tube. Primary properties are: ionization of gases, penetration of solids, production of image on a photographic plate.
circulation disorders and, 203
defractometer, *790*
dye injection and, 203
examination, 210
gallstones and, 478
kidney stones and, 486
medicolegal aspects of, 792
radioactivity measurement and, 845
tooth decay and, 428
technology, 831

yaws. An infectious disease occurring in the tropics, caused by *Treponema pertenue,* transmitted by flies. It is characterized by open sores on the skin; *frambesia.* 737, 747, *748*

y-chromosome. The sex-determining chromosome; it apparently carries genes for maleness.

yellow fever. A viral disease transmitted by the mosquito. *Aedes aegypti,* characterized by fever, jaundice, and albuminuria. 112ff
control of, 743ff
distribution of, *759*

generalized viruses and, 112ff
jungle (sylvan), 743
medical history and, 812
microorganisms and, 740ff
mosquito control and, 758ff
prevention of, 743ff
sylvan, 743

yellow marrow, 281

yolk. The nutritive portion of the ovum.
sac, 11

young adulthood
mind and, 604ff

Your Medicare Handbook, 649

zero gravity, 882

zinc. A bluish-white, crystalline, metallic element; occurs naturally as silicate and carbonate, known as *calamine.* (symbol, Zn).
deficiencies, 657
trace elements and, 657
phosphide, 768

Zollinger-Ellison syndrome, 365

zooglea
plaque and, 427

zoology. The science of animal life.

zygote. The cell produced by the union of two germ cells. 10

zymogenic cells. Those cells of the stomach that secrete pepsin. 442